Handbook of
Experimental Pharmacology

Continuation of Handbuch der experimentellen Pharmakologie

Vol. 63

Editorial Board

G. V. R. Born, London · A. Farah, Rensselaer, New York
H. Herken, Berlin · A. D. Welch, Memphis, Tennessee

Advisory Board

S. Ebashi · E. G. Erdös · V. Erspamer · U. S. von Euler · W. S. Feldberg
G. B. Koelle · M. Rocha e Silva · J. R. Vane · P. G. Waser

Allergic Reactions to Drugs

Contributors

M. Alexander · H. E. Amos · K. E. Andersen · A. Arnaud
E. S. K. Assem · J. Aubert · H. Bundgaard · J. Charpin
M. C. Conroy · A. L. de Weck · J. Dewdney · L. Dostálová
A. A. Fisher · L. Gamba · J.-P. Girard · H. Hedin · R. Hoigné
L. Juhlin · D. Kraft · H. I. Maibach · P. Middleton · C. W. Parker
J. Pepys · W. Richter · W. Schalch · C. H. Schneider
K. H. Schulz · F. Stocker · A. Szczeklik · S. Zawodnik

Editors

A.L. de Weck and H. Bundgaard

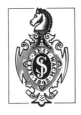

Springer-Verlag Berlin Heidelberg New York Tokyo 1983

Professor Dr. ALAIN L. DE WECK
Institut für klinische Immunologie, Inselspital,
CH-3010 Bern

Professor Dr. HANS BUNDGAARD
The Royal Danish School of Pharmacy,
Department of Pharmaceutical Chemistry AD, 2, Universitetsparken,
DK-2100 Copenhagen

LIBRARY

FEB 8 1984

UNIVERSITY OF THE PACIFIC

415169
Science

With 96 Figures

ISBN 3-540-12399-7 Springer-Verlag Berlin Heidelberg New York Tokyo
ISBN 0-387-12399-7 Springer-Verlag New York Heidelberg Berlin Tokyo

Library of Congress Cataloging in Publication Data. Main entry under title: Allergic reactions to drugs. (Handbook of experimental pharmacology; v. 63) Bibliography: p. Includes index. 1. Drug allergy–Addresses, essays, lectures. I. Alexander, M. (Meta), 1924–. II. Weck, Alain L. de. III. Bundgaard, Hans. IV. Series. [DNLM: 1. Drug hypersensitivity–Congresses. W1 HA51L v. 63/WD 320 A434] QP905.H3 vol. 63 [RC594.D7] 615′.s [616.97′5] 83-4756

This work is subject to copyright. All rights are reserved, whether the whole or part of the material is concerned, specifically those of translation, reprinting, re-use of illustrations, broadcasting, reproduction by photocopying machine or similar means, and storage in data banks. Under § 54 of the German Copyright Law where copies are made for other than private use, a fee is payable to "Verwertungsgesellschaft Wort", Munich.

© by Springer-Verlag Berlin Heidelberg 1983.
Printed in Germany.

The use of registered names, trademarks, etc. in this publication does not imply, even in the absence of a specific statement, that such names are exempt from the relevant protective laws and regulations and therefore free for general use.

Product liability: The publisher can give no guarantee for information about drug dosage and application thereof contained in this book. In every individual case the respective user must check its accuracy by consulting other pharmaceutical literature.

Typesetting, printing, and bookbinding: Brühlsche Universitätsdruckerei, Giessen
2122/3130-543210

Preface

According to most studies, allergic reactions represent 35%–50% of all untoward reactions to drugs, yet the pharmacological literature concerning the clinical aspects, diagnosis, and pathophysiological mechanisms of drug allergy is markedly less extensive than reports dealing with the toxicological or pharmacological effects of drugs. The main reasons for this state of affairs may be on the one hand that until a few years ago the pathophysiological mechanisms of the various types of allergic reactions were not well understood, and on the other hand that objective diagnosis of a drug allergy is still fraught with serious difficulties. Drug allergy is still an unpopular topic for most allergologists and pharmacologists; this is reflected by the fact that despite their frequency, allergic reactions to drugs still occupy a relatively small proportion of space in most pharmacology handbooks and in classical books devoted to the side effects of drugs.

There has recently been considerable progress in research into the immunological and pathophysiological events occurring in allergic reactions, and on that basis investigations of various drug allergies have also yielded new objective findings. Consequently, it was natural to attempt a review of the most frequent and important drug allergies in the form of a handbook. We originally intended to present a comprehensive review of all drug allergies, but the realization of this goal soon became more difficult than we had at first imagined. Whereas for some frequent allergies to drugs that have been in clinical use for over 20 years, such as the beta-lactam antibiotics, the clinical forms as well as the pathophysiological and immunological features have been thoroughly studied by numerous investigators, the reports concerning other drugs are often limited to clinical descriptions and to hypothetical considerations without objective elements that permit a secure diagnosis and an understanding of the mechanisms.

Accordingly, the level and extent of information contained in this volume have become somewhat unbalanced, since for many drugs causing allergic reactions, little can be said about the pathogenic and immunological or para-immunological mechanisms involved. An additional complicating factor is the recent finding that many "allergic" reactions to drugs are in fact "pseudoallergic," i.e., they may be due to the same inflammatory mediators but are not initially triggered by an immunological reaction and are not dependent on specific sensitization to the drug implicated.

For the compilation of this book, which reflects the still fragmentary state of our knowledge, we owe particular gratitude to the authors, who have continued their collaboration despite a fairly long gestation period. Special thanks also go to the publisher and his competent staff.

Bern   A. L. DE WECK
Copenhagen   H. BUNDGAARD

List of Contributors

M. ALEXANDER, Abteilung für Innere Medizin mit Schwerpunkt Infektions-krankheiten, Freie Universität Berlin, Klinikum Charlottenburg, Spandauer Damm 130, D-1000 Berlin 19

H. E. AMOS, Pharmaceuticals Division, Imperial Chemical Industries, PLC, Mereside Alderley Park, GB-Macclesfield, Cheshire SK10 4TG

K. E. ANDERSEN, Københavns Amts Sygehus i Gentofte, Dermatology, Afdeling, Niels Andersens vej 65, DK-2900 Hellerup

A. ARNAUD, Hôpital Sainte-Marguerite, B.P. 29, F-13274 Marseille Cedex 2

E. S. K. ASSEM, Department of Pharmacology, University College London, Gower Street, GB-London WC1E 6BT

J. AUBERT, Service de Pneumologie, Hôpital Saint-Joseph, 26, Bd. de Louvain, B.P. 265, F-13285 Marseille Cedex 8

H. BUNDGAARD, The Royal Danish School of Pharmacy, Department of Pharmaceutical Chemistry AD, 2, Universitetsparken, DK-2100 Copenhagen

J. CHARPIN, Université Aix-Marseille, Faculté de Medecine, Clinique de Pneumo-Phtisiologie, Allergologie, Hôpital Sainte-Marguerite, B.P. 29, F-13277 Marseille Cedex 9

M. C. CONROY, Institut für klinische Immunologie, Inselspital, CH-3010 Bern

A. L. DE WECK, Institut für klinische Immunologie, Inselspital, CH-3010 Bern

J. DEWDNEY, Research Division, Beecham Pharmaceuticals, Biosciences Research Centre, Great Burgh, Yew Tree Bottom Road, GB-Epsom, Surrey KT18 5XQ

L. DOSTÁLOVÁ, Abteilung VF (Department of Vitamin and Nutrition Research), Hoffmann-La Roche & Co., Ltd., Grenzacher Strasse 124, CH-4002 Basel

A. A. FISHER, 45–14 48th Street, Woodside, Long Island, NY 11377/USA

L. GAMBA, Division of Immunology and Allergology, Department of Medicine, Hôpital Cantonal Universitaire, CH-1211 Geneva 4

J.-P. GIRARD, Division of Immunology and Allergology, Department of Medicine, Hôpital Cantonal Universitaire, CH-1211 Geneva 4

H. HEDIN, Department of Biomedical Research, Pharmacia AB, Box 181, S-751 04 Uppsala 1

R. HOIGNÉ, Medizinische Abteilung, Zieglerspital, Postfach 2600, CH-3001 Bern

L. JUHLIN, Centre International de Recherches Dermatologiques, Sophia Antipolis, F-06565 Valbonne Cedex

D. KRAFT, Institut für Allgemeine und Experimentelle Pathologie der Universität Wien, Währinger Strasse 13, A-1090 Wien

H. I. MAIBACH, Department of Dermatology, School of Medicine, University of California, San Francisco, CA 94143/USA

P. MIDDLETON, 11 St. Anne's Court, Northenden Road, GB-Sale/Cheshire M33 3HB

C. W. PARKER, Department of Medicine, Washington University School of Medicine, 650 South Euclid, St. Louis, MO 63110/USA

J. PEPYS, Clinical Immunology, University of London (Cardiothoracic Institute), 34 Ferncroft Avenue, GB-Hampstead, London NW3 7PE

W. RICHTER, Department of Biomedical Research, Pharmacia AB, Box 181, S-751 04 Uppsala 1

W. SCHALCH, Abteilung VF (Department of Vitamin and Nutrition Research), Hoffmann-La Roche & Co., Ltd., Grenzacher Strasse 124, CH-4002 Basel

C. H. SCHNEIDER, Institut für klinische Immunologie, Inselspital, CH-3010 Bern

K. H. SCHULZ, Universitäts-Hautklinik, Martinistrasse 52, D-2000 Hamburg 20

F. STOCKER, Comprehensive Hospital Drug Monitoring, Zieglerspital, CH-3007 Bern

A. SZCZEKLIK, Instytut Medycyny Wewnetrznei, Klinika Alergii i Immunologii, ul. Skawinska 8, PL-31-066 Krakow

S. ZAWODNIK, Division of Immunology and Allergology, Department of Medicine, Hôpital Cantonal Universitaire, CH-1211 Geneva 4

Contents

Section I: General Aspects of Drug Allergies

CHAPTER 3

**Immunopathological Mechanisms and Clinical Aspects
of Allergic Reactions to Drugs**
A. L. DE WECK. With 4 Figures

CHAPTER 4

Cutaneous Manifestations of Drug Allergy
K. H. SCHULZ

CHAPTER 5

Allergy of the Respiratory Tract to Low Molecular Weight Chemical Agents
J. PEPYS

CHAPTER 6

Epidemiology of Drug Allergy: Drug Monitoring
R. HOIGNÉ, F. STOCKER, and P. MIDDLETON. With 3 Figures

CHAPTER 7

Diagnostic Procedures in Drug Allergy
J.-P. GIRARD and S. ZAWODNIK

CHAPTER 8

Prevention and Treatment of Drug Allergies
A. L. DE WECK

Section II: Allergic Reactions to Specific Drugs

CHAPTER 9

Major Drugs Acting on the Central Nervous System
C. W. PARKER

CHAPTER 10

General and Local Anaesthetics
E. S. K. ASSEM. With 6 Figures

CHAPTER 11

Analgesics and Nonsteroidal Anti-Inflammatory Drugs
A. SZCZEKLIK. With 2 Figures

CHAPTER 12

Neuromuscular Blocking Drugs
E. S. K. ASSEM. With 8 Figures

CHAPTER 13

Drugs Used Topically
K. E. ANDERSEN and H. I. MAIBACH

CHAPTER 14

Antihistamines

A. A. FISHER

CHAPTER 15

Drugs Acting on the Cardiovascular System
H. E. Amos. With 9 Figures

CHAPTER 16

Penicillins and Cephalosporins
A. L. DE WECK. With 10 Figures

CHAPTER 17

Other Antibiotics
D. KRAFT. With 8 Figures

CHAPTER 18

Other Antibacterial Drugs

M. ALEXANDER

CHAPTER 19

Antifungal, Anthelmintic, and Antiprotozoal Drugs
J. DEWDNEY. With 9 Figures

CHAPTER 20

Solutions and Emulsions Used for Intravenous Infusions
W. RICHTER and H. HEDIN. With 7 Figures

CHAPTER 21

Gastrointestinal Drugs
L. JUHLIN

CHAPTER 24

Corticotrophins and Corticosteroids
J. CHARPIN, A. ARNAUD, and J. AUBERT. With 6 Figures

CHAPTER 25

Hypersensitivity Reactions to Hormones
M. C. CONROY and A. L. DE WECK

CHAPTER 26

Allergy to Insulin
J. AUBERT and J. CHARPIN

CHAPTER 27

Radiologic Contrast Media
J.-P. GIRARD and L. GAMBA

Section I:
General Aspects of Drug Allergies

CHAPTER 1

Immunochemical Basis
of Allergic Reactions to Drugs

C. H. SCHNEIDER

A. Introduction

It is well established that almost any chemical entity, from macromolecule to metallic ion, can be brought to function as an antigen under appropriate conditions. Drugs are no exception to this and a general although brief introductory discussion of antigenicity seems in order. Most of the present knowledge about antigenicity has been obtained from experiments in laboratory animals and more rarely from careful and enlightened observation of naturally occurring immunologic reactions in animals or humans. It is assumed that as far as the more general phenomena are concerned, an extrapolation from one species to another is possible, particularly when the same observations can be made in a variety of species. This aspect will not be further discussed but the understanding is that mechanisms established from animal data may, with due caution, be regarded as relevant to the human organism.

I. Definitions

An antigen can in principle exert several types of immunologic functions and it is consistent therefore to regard "antigenicity" as a broad term comprising all the specialized function. The main antigenic functions may be defined, taking into account earlier published proposals (SELA 1969; SCHNEIDER and DE WECK 1970; DE WECK 1974), as follows:
1. Immunogenicity – capacity to induce an immune response manifested by formation of specific immunoglobulins and/or specifically committed lymphocytes
2. Antigenicity sensu stricto – capacity to react with and bind to specific immunoglobulins and cellular receptors; this function could also be called "haptenicity" but the term is rarely used in the literature
3. Allergenicity – capacity to elicit various types of allergic reactions and tissue lesions in already sensitized individuals possessing specific immunoglobulins and/or specifically committed lymphocytes
4. Tolerogenicity – capacity to induce specific immunologic unresponsiveness
   Further differentiations are useful within all of the above categories. For instance most immunogens need assistance from T-lymphocytes in order to be fully effective whereas certain (usually polymeric and undegradable) immunogens do not show this requirement. The terms T-dependent and T-independent immunogens are thus well established in the newer literature (see Sect. B.I). In allergy, the term "sensitizing capacity" is frequently used instead of immunogenicity. This

seems appropriate although not obligatory whenever the immune response involves manifestations of immediate or delayed hypersensitivity.

Receptor binding is clearly the specialized capacity of a hapten. Originally, the term "hapten" was used by LANDSTEINER (1921) in a description of the immunogenicity of tissue extracts containing the Forssmann antigen. It defined a substance with the capacity to react with an antibody but not to immunize and was – in this particular instance – a polysaccharide representing a segment of a larger immunogenic molecule. The size of the haptenic compound was not implied. In the more recent literature the name "hapten" is also used to describe reactive chemicals, usually of low molecular weight, capable of binding covalently (conjugating) to larger carrier molecules such as proteins. Since the classical series of experiments on antigenic specificity by LANDSTEINER (1945), hapten–protein conjugates have become established tools in immunologic research. The haptenic group on such conjugates represents the known portion of the entire, usually more extended antigenic determinant, which is newly created by the attachment of the chemical (see Sect. B.II). The term "haptenic determinant," as opposed to "carrier determinant," has quite recently been used to distinguish determinants of hapten–protein conjugates that react with B-lymphocytes and which may be called B-cell determinants from those that react with T-lymphocytes and thus are T-cell determinants (ISHIZAKA 1976).

The term "allergenicity" is sometimes used to describe sensitizing capacity, i.e., immunogenicity, which is not included in the definition proposed above. On the other hand, a more detailed classification of allergenicity according to molecular parameters essential for elicitation of allergic reactions of immediate types I and II, immune complex type III, and delayed type IV (GELL and COOMBS 1964) seems desirable since different molecular properties of the antigen may be required for elicitation of these various reactions (see Sect. C.IV). Finally, in describing tolerogenicity one may at least wish to indicate whether the effect is on B-lymphocytes or T-cells.

II. Miscellaneous Parameters in Sensitization

A variety of factors affect the immunogenicity of any antigen and the description of a molecule as "immunogenic" or "nonimmunogenic" can only be given in operational terms. In particular, the claim of "nonimmunogenicity" of a compound, which rests solely on its demonstrated incapacity to induce an antibody response, is not acceptable, since T-cell activation is necessary for an antibody response to most antigens. It would appear that manifestations of cellular immunity, e.g., delayed hypersensitivity are a better criterion of immunogenicity (PAUL et al. 1971). Among the factors which affect immunogenicity, chemical and biochemical characteristics of the antigen have been considered as well as circumstantial effects such as route of administration, dose and eventual adjuvants used, and finally genetic characteristics of the organism to be immunized. It should be realized that some of these parameters cannot be discussed in very general terms since their influence on the immunization process may be markedly dependent on the antigen under consideration. Detailed reviews, e.g., by GILL (1972), BOREK (1972), MITCHISON

(1972), CRUMPTON (1973), DE WECK (1974), and ARNON and GEIGER (1977) are available.

1. Chemical Characteristics of the Antigen

In many instances, high molecular weight of antigen correlates with strong immunogenicity whereas low molecular weight compounds are usually weak immunogens or nonimmunogenic under a variety of conditions. It also seems that particulate antigens such as bacteria, viruses, or tissue cells may be highly immunogenic and by the same token immunogenicity can be enhanced by insolubilization of antigens, e.g., by heat aggregation (PARKHOUSE and DUTTON 1967) or cross-linking (ANDERER and SCHLUMBERGER 1969). On the other hand, there are macromolecules such as fully succinylated polylysines as well as other amino acid polymers, various polysaccharides (RICHTER et al. 1979), and even proteins such as gelatin (SELA and ARNON 1960) which are poorly immunogenic or even nonimmunogenic under various conditions. It appears that large molecules normally possess a number of antigenic determinants, which may be selected by competent lymphocytes, whereas small or highly ordered polymeric molecules offer only a restricted and eventually insufficient number of these sites (see Sects. B.II, III).

The question of the minimal molecular size necessary for immunogenicity has attracted considerable interest. The most definitive study (SCHLOSSMAN et al. 1965; SCHLOSSMAN and LEVINE 1967) used a series of oligo-L-lysines of increasing size, substituted on the α-amino terminus by a single 2,4-dinitrophenyl (DNP) group. It showed that the heptalysine derivative was the smallest molecule inducing anti-DNP antibody formation as well as cell-mediated reactions in the guinea pig. A similar series of DNP-oligolysines, in the hands of STUPP et al. (1971 a, b), confirmed the heptamer as the smallest molecule which could induce delayed hypersensitivity. However, anti-DNP antibody formation could also be induced with smaller DNP-oligolysines, provided high doses of mycobacterial adjuvant were employed. Very small immunogens which produce cellular immunity in guinea pigs are p-azobenzene arsonate derivatives of tyrosine and histidine (BOREK et al. 1965; LESKOWITZ et al. 1966; ALKAN et al. 1972 a, b). It appears that the minimal size required for immunogenicity varies with the chemical composition of the antigen and is related to the ability of a molecule to induce T-cell/B-cell cooperation. Indeed, evidence is available showing that at least two determinants are required on an immunogen capable of inducing an antibody response (RAJEWSKY et al. 1969). On the other hand, a single T-cell-activating determinant appears sufficient for induction of cellular immunity, as in the azobenzene arsonate derivatives.

Electrical charge as such is not required for immunogenicity. SELA and FUCHS (1963) clearly showed that a synthetic polypeptide containing tyrosine which was nonionizable in neutral aqueous solution induced an antibody response in rabbits. Analogous evidence was also presented by MAURER et al. (1966) and MAURER (1970). Furthermore uncharged hapten–polysaccharide conjugates, namely benzylated or nitrobenzylated dextrans of molecular weight 20,000 daltons were found to induce delayed skin reactions in guinea pigs (SCHNEIDER et al. 1971 a). The effect of charge on the immune response was systematically studied with a series of (Lys, Glu, Tyr) copolymers in which the proportion of the two charged amino acids Glu and Lys were varied (Gill et al. 1967). It was concluded that charge variation over a wide range does not influence the amount of antibody induced but extremely high charge density appears to depress it. On the other hand, evidence is available to show that basic peptides or proteins containing clusters of positive charge are particularly good immunogens (Gill et al. 1964 b; Maurer 1970). Furthermore, nucleic acids and oligonucleotides, which are acidic polymers, can be made into effective immunogens by complexing them with basic protein carriers such as methylated bovine serum albumin (Plescia et al. 1964, 1965 a, b).

An interesting case is constituted by poly-L-lysine conjugates, which carry one or a small number of haptenic groups such as DNP or BPO (benzylpenicilloyl) and retain their polybasic character. Such conjugates are immunogenic but lose this capacity after succinylation, which transforms them into polyacidic compounds (Parker et al. 1962 a, b; Levine 1964, de Weck and Schneider 1968). One may speculate that the polybasic conjugates are able to associate with an immunogenic carrier, perhaps within the adjuvant mixture used, whereas the polyacidic molecules are unable to do so. On the other hand, by changing the charge of these molecules by succinylation, one may also affect other characteristics such as their rate of degradation or distribution within the organism.

2. Antigen Metabolism

It is well established that antigenic determinants are surface structures (Sela et al. 1962) and in various instances, antibody responses against conformational determinants have been described, e.g., in lysozyme (Arnon and Sela 1969; Atassi and Habeeb 1977), hemoglobin (discussed by Goodman 1969) and bovine serum albumin (Wright and Rothberg 1971). Even the haptenic structure p-azo-β-benzoyl propionate is to be included here, since it was found that antibodies against it were directed against a resonance-stabilized, coiled conformation. Haptens of similar structure but unable to coil, such as p-azo-β-benzoyl acrylate, showed very poor cross-reaction (Pressman and Siegel 1953). This evidence suggests that processing and digestion of antigen is not an obligatory step in the induction of antibody formation and certainly not in antigen recognition. Reports concerning the detection of "hidden determinants" (Ishizaka et al. 1960), which are exposed after discrete in vivo degradation, are not at variance with this, since they simply illustrate the fact that during biochemical degradation of the antigen–protein, antigen fragments, with distinct determinants and of sufficient half-life to be immunogenic, are created.

Macrophage ingestion of some antigens may considerably enhance their immunogenicity (Unanue 1970; Shortman and Palmer 1971; Feldman and Palmer 1971), but again this effect is not primarily related to the digestion of the antigen within the macrophage but seems mainly due to suitable presentation of the antigen within the macrophage membrane to immunocompetent lymphocytes (Unanue and Cerottini 1970). A more direct effect of degradability on immunogenicity has been observed with pairs of linear copolymers, which comprise an all-D-amino acid and a similar all-L-amino acid chain. With a $(Glu^{55} - Lys^{38} - Tyr^6)$ sequence pair, Gill et al. (1964 a) found that both enantiomers were immunogenic but the D-polymer induced considerably less antibody than the L-polymer. Similarly, JANEWAY and SELA (1967) found that the primary response in mice to a D-Tyr-D-Glu-D-Ala copolymer in adjuvant was highly dose dependent, in contrast to the response inducible with a polymer of the opposite L configuration, which was largely dose independent. At low doses, the D-polymer was as immunogenic as the L-polymer. The D-polymer was highly potent in inducing specific tolerance whereas the L-polymer was at least fifty times less efficient. In modern terms, one would state that where degradation of an antigen is slow or absent its tolerogenic function, in particular involving B-cell tolerance, may become prominent at higher dosage (SELA et al. 1972; see also COUTINHO and MÖLLER 1975).

3. Genetic Aspects

In addition to the Ig genes which control antibody structure, immune response or Ir genes, which control certain T-cell functions, have been detected during the past decade. An important finding has been the genetic linkage of these Ir genes to the major histocompatibility complex (MHC) in mice, guinea pigs, rats, monkeys, and humans, i.e., in every species thus far studied. In more detail, this means that Ir genes are on the same chromosome and closely linked to those genes that code for molecules bearing various alloantigens and provoking rejection of tissue grafts. A number of recent reviews on several aspects of the genetic control of the immune response are available (BENACERRAF and McDEVITT 1972; BENACERRAF and KATZ 1975; GECZY and DE WECK 1974; MOZES 1975) and a lucid introductory chapter is provided by KABAT (1976).

The first Ir gene to be described was the so-called poly-L-lysine (PLL) gene which controls the carrier-specific response to haptenic conjugates with a number of polybasic polymers including poly-L-lysine, poly-L-ornithine, and poly-L-arginine (LEVINE et al. 1963; BEN-EPHRAIM et al. 1966). The GA gene controls responses to copolymers of glutamic acid and alanine whereas the GT gene regulates the responses to glutamic acid–tyrosine copolymers. Strain 2 guinea pigs possess the PLL and GA genes but do not respond to GT polymers; strain 13 guinea pigs possess the GT gene but are unresponsive to PLL and GA polymers. Unresponsive guinea pigs exhibit neither delayed hypersensitivity nor T-cell-dependent humoral responses (BLUESTEIN et al. 1971). In addition, no anti-hapten response is obtained in unresponsive animals which have been exposed to these polypeptide carriers after chemical attachment of haptenic groups (GREEN and BENACERRAF 1971). Thus, cellular immunity as well as carrier function, which are both T-cell dependent, are not operative in the unresponsive animals.

The significance of the close genetic linkage between Ir genes and MHC genes is not definitively established, but it is likely that the responsive defect in unresponsive animals has a cellular basis since such animals can be converted to responsive individuals with lymphoid cells from responsive donors (FOERSTER et al. 1969; TYAN et al. 1969). The failure of carrier recognition and the T-cell defect can be overcome by means of high doses of mycobacterial adjuvants or complexes involving methylated bovine serum albumin, at least in experiments with polylysine (GREEN et al. 1966, 1968). It should also be noted that in some cases genetic control was only apparent when low doses of antigens were used (VAZ and LEVINE 1970; VAZ et al. 1971; GREEN and Benacerraf 1971). Furthermore, when the immunization process is continued over a period of several months, unresponsive guinea pigs in an outbred stock may convert to apparent responsive status, although usually of lower intensity than immediately responding animals (DE WECK 1972; SCHNEIDER et al. 1972).

A rather different kind of genetic control, that of the IgE antibody response in mice, was reported by LEVINE (1971). Strains were found that showed a poor IgE antibody response to six different antigens but at least moderate titers of IgG antibody to some of these antigens. There seemed to be no dose effect. Breeding experiments showed that the genetic control is not linked to the MHC of the mouse and is influenced by more than one locus.

Evidence for human Ir loci is beginning to accumulate as well. Family studies revealed that members of a family having the HL-A1, HL-A8 haplotype had pronounced immediate skin reactivity to antigen E whereas none of the individuals exhibiting other HL-A haplotypes had any such reactivity (LEVINE et al. 1972). The authors also showed that sensitivity to other allergens had no relationship to the haplotype associated with ragweed hay fever and suggested that the HL-A-linked control of responsiveness towards antigen E has antigenic specificity.

MARSH et al. (1973) found a relationship between HL-A haplotypes and the response to a minor, and relatively simple structured ragweed allergen, the Ra5 component. In another human study (MARSH et al. 1974; GLEICH et al. 1971), it was suggested that IgE synthesis is genetically controlled and that the inheritance of high levels of serum IgE is a simple mendelian recessive trait. There appeared to be no linkage between HL-A haplotype and IgE level. Rather it seemed that in most allergic families a gene controlling IgE levels in the serum was able to mask the possible role of Ir genes linked to a HL-A haplotype, which would control the expression of specific IgE antibody responses to different allergens.

B. Cellular and Immunochemical Elements in Antigenicity

I. Cellular Aspects

In allergy, a dichotomy of the immune response recognized by the terms "immediate" and "delayed" reaction has been of long standing. The recognition of a requirement for the thymus in the immune response and for at least two different lymphoid cell populations for an antibody response to specific antigens (CLAMAN et al. 1966; MILLER and MITCHELL 1968) laid the foundation for an appreciation of this dichotomy in more general terms at the cellular level.

Immunologically reactive or immunocompetent cells are lymphocytes which, together with granulocytes and erythrocytes, originate from common hemopoietic stem cells (WU et al. 1967). The sites of primary lymphopoiesis are the bursa of Fabricius (in birds) and the thymus; in mammals no bursa has been found but an equivalent organ is inferred (MITCHELL and MILLER 1968; PEREY et al. 1968; OWEN and RITTER 1969). Lymphocytes which differentiate within the thymus independent of antigenic influence become thymus-derived or thymus-processed lymphocytes, so-called T-cells. It is now generally accepted that a cooperation between T-cells and bursa-equivalent lymphocytes (B-cells) is necessary for induction of IgM and IgG antibody responses and considerable evidence shows that an equivalent collaborative interaction is also required for IgE antibody responses (TADA 1975; ISHIZAKA 1976). Obviously, the bulk of the evidence comes from animal experimentation but a recent review points to applications of the T-cell/B-cell concept in human studies (DWYER 1976).

B-lymphocytes eventually differentiate to become antibody-synthesizing and antibody-secreting plasma cells and there is convincing evidence that the B-cell receptor is ordinary antibody identical to the product secreted by the plasma cells. On the other hand, T-cells regulate the magnitude and duration of the antibody response. Under antigenic stimulation, they give rise to helper cells, suppressor cells, and also specific effector cytotoxic cells (LOOR and ROELANTS 1977). In contrast to the recognition function of B-cells, which is well understood in molecular terms, that of T-cells has remained controversial. What complicates their recognition function is the fact, established under a variety of conditions, that association with the appropriate syngeneic MHC is required. Furthermore, a role of macrophages as antigen-presenting cells may be inferred (NEVEU 1977; SPRENT 1978; YAMASHITA and SHEVACH 1978). Some of the characteristics of B- and T-lymphocytes are summarized in Table 1.

The cellular collaborative process seems to require a close proximity of B-cells and helper T-cells. This is usually achieved by presenting B-cell and T-cell determinants on the same antigen molecule. The antigen is thought to bridge the cells involved, thus establishing the required contact (GOODMAN 1975; WOODS et al. 1975; FONG et al. 1978). In addition, bacterial endotoxin or lipopolysaccharide and also allogeneic T-cells which recognize and react with the (mouse) H-2 determinants on B-cells (allogeneic effect) may provide the necessary T-cell activation. The effect of T-cells is mediated by soluble factors, since such factors are able to replace helper T-cells in their function, as shown for the IgM response (SCHIMPL and WECKER 1972; DUTTON 1975; WALDMANN 1975) and less regularly also for the IgG response (NORTH et al. 1977).

The T-cell dependence of the IgE antibody response was shown in a number of instances with different antigens containing efficient T-cell determinants, such as protein from *Ascaris suum* (HAMAOKA et al. 1972; KATZ et al. 1974), antigen from *Nippostrongylus brasiliensis* (KOJIMA and OVARY 1975) or ragweed antigen (KISHIMOTO and ISHIZAKA 1973). In these and other experiments, evidence for an enhancing soluble factor was obtained, which mediates the helper function of T-cells in the IgE response. In a preliminary study, KISHIMOTO and ISHIZAKA (1975) showed that the IgE-enhancing factor may be distinct from the IgG-enhancing factor.

II. Antigenic Determinants Reacting with Antibody

B-cell determinants or haptenic determinants, as they are frequently called, are comparatively well defined with regard to dimensions and specificity relationships. The problem of their size has attracted considerable interest during the last two decades and seems now satisfactorily elucidated. A recent careful review of these aspects has been provided by GOODMAN (1975). It has been known for some time that haptenic groups such as DNP and BPO do not comprise the entire deter-

Table 1. Characterization of B- and T-lymphocytes[a]

Parameters	B-lymphocytes (from bursa of Fabricius in birds or "bursal equivalent")	T-lymphocytes (from thymus)
Receptors on surface specific for antigen	Immunoglobulins IgG, IgM, IgD, or IgA may occur alone or combined	IgT or non-immunoglobulin (heavy chain?)
Antigenic markers on cell membrane	MBLA (mouse) Fc-receptor C_3-receptor H-2/HL-A Ia	θ, TL (mouse) H-2/HL-A Ia
Inactivation by X-irradiation	Sensitive	Primed cells for helper effect, cytotoxic effect and cell-mediated immunity: resistant; unprimed cells: sensitive
Corticosteroid	Sensitive	95% of thymocytes: sensitive; population of residual 5%: resistant
Antilymphocyte serum plus complement	Slightly sensitive	Senitive
Tolerogens	Sensitive	Sensitive (tolerance induction easier than in B-cells)
Involved in		
Helper function		Active
Cellular immunity		Active
Secretion of antibody	Active	
Immunologic memory	Active	Active
Proportion (%) in		
Blood	10–15	85–90
Thoracic duct lymph	10–15	85–90
Lymph node	25	75
Spleen	60–65	35–40

[a] Mainly from KATZ and BENACERRAF (1972)

minant, since the free haptens, i.e., dinitrophenol and benzylpenicilloic acid respectively, are always weaker inhibitors of the interaction of the haptenic conjugates with their antibody than the haptens combined with lysine derivatives, lysine being the amino acid to which most of these haptenic groups are attached in a protein (EISEN and SISKIND 1964; LEVINE 1963; LOCHER et al. 1969). It was even found that N^{ε}-BPO-N^{α}-formyl lysine was a slightly better inhibitor of BPO–BGG-specific antibody precipitation (where BGG is bovine gamma-globulin) than N^{ε}-BPO-aminocaproic acid (LOCHER et al. 1969). This suggests that the formyl side chain which stands for a (very short) portion of the protein chain is recognized by the antibody and thus is part of the determinant.

More precise information became available through a series of conceptually simple experiments which used polysaccharides, in particular dextran, or homopolymers of amino acids as immunogens. By studying the binding of graded oligo-mers of these antigens to their antibodies, one finds that the binding becomes stronger with increasing size of the oligomer up to a rather well-defined limit. This size limit may, with due consideration for conformational effects, be interpreted as the maximal dimension of the determinant. In most cases, binding was simply stud-ied by observing the inhibition of antigen–antibody precipitation by the oligomers. It was similarly found that dextran determinants comprise hexasaccharide units in rabbits (MAGE and KABAT 1963) and humans (KABAT 1966). Polylysine which was attached to protein carriers for immunization exhibited a penta- or hexalysine de-terminant in the rabbit (VAN VUNAKIS et al. 1966; ARNON et al. 1965), whereas N^α-DNP-polylysine in the guinea pig showed a N^α-DNP-trilysine determinant (SCHLOSSMAN et al. 1968). The most straightforward evaluation, with a minimum of conformational complications, was possible with oligo-D-alanylglycyl proteins. Antigens of this type, with one to four alanyl residues in their peptidyl moieties, were used for obtaining peptide-specific antibodies in rabbits. Mono-, di-, tri-, and tetra-D-alanine, as well as mono-, di-, and tri-D-alanylglycyl-ε-aminocaproic acid, were used as inhibitors of precipitation. It was found that the determinant was a tetrapeptide and that the lysine residue of the protein carrier was a part of this de-terminant only when the peptidyl moiety on the protein was smaller than a tetra-peptide (SCHECHTER et al. 1970). There seems to be little difference in the dimen-sions of the combining sites of IgG and IgM antibody classes, since IgG as well as IgM antibodies to poly-D-alanine gave quite similar precipitin inhibition data with tri-, tetra-, and penta-D-alanine (HAIMOVICH et al. 1969).

Another major approach to the study of antigenic determinants uses direct im-munochemical analysis of proteins and includes fragmentation to obtain deter-minant-containing peptides, synthesis and immunologic evaluation of a large num-ber of peptides with a variety of overlaps, as well as immunochemical study of spe-cific chemical derivatives of determinant-bearing peptides. The most advanced studies in this field are those by ATASSI on sperm whale myoglobin (ATASSI 1975, 1977). In brief, the work on myoglobin which is a globular protein revealed that there are five regions consisting of hexa- or heptapeptide sequences which consti-tute antigenic determinants. These determinants are located mainly in the non-heli-cal corners, at the outer surface of the protein, and are separated from each other by immunosilent areas. It appears likely that, assuming other requirements are sat-isfied, antibodies are preferentially formed against the most exposed moieties of the protein surface.

All determinants discussed in this section so far may be characterized as so-called sequential determinants, which are composed of chemically linked units. One may expect that both the native determinant in a macromolecule and the iso-lated determinant-bearing fragment will specifically and efficiently react with anti-body raised against the native antigen. If the determinant has a fixed conformation within the macromolecule, which is only partially or not at all retained by the frag-ment, then fragment binding to antibody will become poor and eventually un-measurable. In such cases, one deals with so-called conformational determinants. It is most important that the work on lysozyme (ATASSI and HABEEB 1977) has now clearly established quite a different type of B-cell determinant which is non-sequen-tial and radically dependent on native conformation. There are three antigenic reactive sites in lysozyme. Site 1 comprises the side chains of Arg-14, Lys-13, Glu-7, Cys-6, Gly-126, and Arg-128. Site 2 also contains six residues namely Trp-62, Lys-97, Lys-96, Asn-93, Thr-89, and Asp-87. Site 3 is made up of the seven residues Tyr-20, Arg-21, Lys-116, Asn-113, Arg-114, Phe-34, and Lys-33. These residues are spatially adjacent in the native protein but many are, as revealed by the numbering, quite distantly positioned from each other within the primary sequence. It is interesting to note that this type of determinant was found not to exist in myoglobin, contrary to some earlier speculation (ATASSI and KOKETSU 1975).

The antibody response to all defined determinants ever studied has been characterized by its high degree of specificity. Antibody specificity is a classical theme (LANDSTEINER 1945) which has hardly lost its attractiveness and a more recent and very detailed review has been made by PRESSMAN and GROSSBERG (1968). Much of the information comes from work using chemically prepared hapten–protein conjugates and shows that very small differences in haptenic structure may be distinguished. Such differences include presence or absence of a methyl group, lengthening or shortening of an aliphatic chain by one methylene unit, ortho, meta, and para positions of aromatic substituents, and optical isomerism.

It appears that in certain genetically controlled instances, antibody raised against an immunogen may have a higher binding affinity for a closely related antigen which was not used for immunization. Such so-called heteroclitic antibodies are for instance produced in C57BL/6-mice towards 4-hydroxy-5-nitrophenylacetyl residues. They react more strongly with derivatives in which carbon-3 of the benzene ring is additionally substituted by an iodo or a nitro group. CBA-mice did not show this effect in their antibody response (IMANISHI and MÄKELÄ 1974).

Structural heterogeneity of the antibody response even towards rigid haptenic groups is a common feature. It is related to structural parameters of the immunogen, in contrast to heterogeneity controlled by genetic factors (SINGER 1964). Indeed, haptenic groups attached to a protein should not be regarded as structurally homogeneous entities, since some might lie embedded in the protein surface in close contact with discrete constellations of amino acid residues, while others at the other extreme would protrude outwards from the protein matrix. Thus, depending on the attachment positions of the haptenic group, structural varieties for the entire determinant can be envisaged.

Experimental evidence from various studies confirms a considerable heterogeneity of the antibody response to haptenic determinants. Thus, ATSUMI et al. (1967) showed that antibody populations raised in a single rabbit against benzylpenicilloylated rabbit serum albumin were directed towards different parts of the BPO residue. Similar observations were mady by using passive cutaneous anaphylaxis (PCA) techniques and inhibition studies with various penicillin derivatives (DE WECK and SCHNEIDER 1978 unpublished). On the other hand, LEVINE (1963) found no antibodies in a pooled rabbit anti-BPO serum globulin fraction which were directed towards the benzyl side chain or the thiazolidine moiety and concluded that the bulk of the antibody reacted with the entire BPO haptenic group. DANDLIKER et al. (1967) studied anti-penicillin antibodies in human sera by means of fluorescence polarization of fluorescent penicilloyl hapten and found rather high affinities $(2.2 \times 10^6 M^{-1} - 3.8 \times 10^8 M^{-1})$ and relatively low heterogeneity (0.78–0.92 for the index values) in a variety of cases.

Heterogeneity of antibody is most readily appreciated from haptenic binding studies, using either classical equilibrium dialysis and even simple hapten binding at high dilution (OTZ et al. 1976), or quantum-sensitive techniques that use differences in quantum levels of atoms related to energy changes effected by binding interactions (see, for example, STRYER and GRIFFITH 1965; where a spin-labeled hapten was used, or HAUGLUND et al. 1967; where a nuclear magnetic resonance technique was applied). The most important of these techniques has been fluorescence quenching, as pioneered by EISEN (VELICK et al. 1960). This method elegantly allowed one to confirm for a DNP-hapten the then uncertain notion, that high binding affinities of the order of $10^8\ M^{-1}$ may be common. It was also established that the average binding constant progressively increases with time after immunization, whereas the heterogeneity index of the binding remains largely unchanged (EISEN and SISKIND 1964). The phenomenon has later been called "maturation of the immune response." It is not the result of selective removal of high affinity antibody by excess antigen early after immunization, but rather reflects changes in the cell population producing the antibodies (STEINER and EISEN 1967).

III. Antigenic Determinants in Cellular Reactions

Precise information on antigenic determinants reactive in T-cell activation, delayed hypersensitivity, and other manifestations of cellular immunity is quite limited. What has clearly emerged, however, is the notion that B- and T-cells react normally or at least frequently to different determinants on the same molecule. The classical example is that of GELL and BENACERRAF (1959), where heat-denatured proteins lost their capacity to react with antibody against the native protein, whereas delayed reactions could be provoked with either native or denatured antigen. This finding was open to at least two possible interpretations namely that cellular immunity has a broader specificity than antibody responses, or that the structural entities serving as determinants in humoral and cellular immunity are not the same.

Present evidence strongly favors the second possibility. GOODMAN and associates (SENYK et al. 1971 a, b), studying the immune response to the nonacosapeptide, glucagon in guinea pigs, found that animals developed antibodies predominantly against the NH_2 terminal heptadecapeptide and showed virtually no reactivity with the COOH terminal undecapeptide. On the other hand, cellular reactions could be elicited by the COOH terminal peptide as well as by the entire glucagon molecule. These findings demonstrated a functional dissection of the antigen into a haptenic B-cell-reactive determinant and a distinct determinant for cellular immunity.

Similar evidence was obtained with an entirely artificial antigen. Relying on previous information (LESKOWITZ et al. 1966) that azobenzene-p-arsonate tyrosine (RAT) was able to evoke delayed hypersensitivity without concomitant antibody production in guinea pigs, ALKAN et al. (1972a) prepared a series of conjugates involving RAT and DNP moieties. They found that RAT–DNP induced an anti-DNP antibody response in guinea pigs, which was improved when an 6-aminocaproic acid (EACA) residue was inserted to give RAT–EACA–DNP. Preimmunization with RAT clearly enhanced the anti-DNP antibody response to RAT–EA-

CA–DNP. On the other hand, conjugates such as RAT–EACA–RAT induced delayed hypersensitivity or helper activity but no anti-RAT antibody. Thus RAT and DNP in this system are distinctive T-cell and B-cell determinants.

What about the size of T-determinants? The RAT moiety is obviously rather small, but it should be kept in mind that this is a rather special T-cell activator and no data are available to show that this residue would entirely fill the T-cell receptor. More detailed information comes again from peptide studies with glucagon, which show that stimulation of lymph node cell cultures from glucagon-sensitized guinea pigs was best achieved by the COOH terminal undecapeptide, whereas the dodecapeptide and smaller peptides of the glucagon COOH terminus were markedly less active in most experiments (GOODMAN 1975). It may also be taken into account that cellular immunity in guinea pigs can be induced with DNP–poly-L-lysines larger than the hexamer (SCHLOSSMAN and LEVINE 1967; STUPP et al. 1971 a, b). Thus it could appear that T-cell determinants are of comparable size and certainly not much larger than B-cell determinants.

Can T-cell determinants function as B-cell determinants? This is to be expected, because in contrast to the much more restricted selection of T-cell determinants, B-cell responses seem possible to almost any imaginable structure. In fact, with a glucagon–protein conjugate in which the peptide hormone was protein linked via the tyrosines at positions 10 and 13, an antibody response specific for one or more determinants of the COOH terminus previously involved in T-cell activation of unconjugated glucagon was obtained (SENYK et al. 1972). Similarly, when the flexible EACA spacer chain in RAT–EACA$_n$–RAT was replaced by rigid oligoproline chains, antibody responses to RAT could also be evoked (BUSH et al. 1972). It appears that only in such rigid molecules are both RAT determinants sufficiently effective in intercellular bridging required for T-cell/B-cell cooperation (FONG et al. 1978; see also Sect. B.I).

In certain instances, the opposite situation, namely that "ordinary" haptenic groups can serve as T-cell determinants, is also implied. Thus, good delayed skin reactions can be induced in guinea pigs by means of BPO-polysaccharides and benzyl- or nitrobenzylpolysaccharides of modest molecular weight. No immediate reactions develop and no antibody can be found by precipitation or hemagglutination; only in a small proportion of the animals is anaphylactic antibody detectable. The delayed reactions show both haptenic and polysaccharide specificity (SCHNEIDER and DE WECK 1967; SCHNEIDER et al. 1971 a).

C. Antigenicity and Drugs

I. Agents of Intrinsic Immunogenicity

In modern terms, any compound possessing T-cell activating determinants may be expected to induce an immune response and possibly allergic manifestations. Heterologous proteins and other complex macromolecules usually satisfy this condition and, less regularly, this may also be said of peptides and other derivatives of medium size. The azobenzenearsonate tyrosine derivatives described in Sect. B.III no doubt constitute the lowest end of the scale in this respect. Many of the medium-sized compounds may not be intrinsically immunogenic but may recruit T-cell help by association with a carrier within the body, as discussed in more detail in Sect. C.III. There are in addition the thymus-independent antigens, which apparently do not require T-cells in order to activate B-cells optimally (KATZ and BENACERRAF 1972). These antigens are large polymers with many repetitions of the same determinants, e.g., pneumococcal polysaccharides, polyfructose, polyvinylpyrrolidone, polymerized flagellin, and some viruses. They are commonly highly resistant to degradation by host enzymes. Their antibody responses differ in various ways from those induced by the T-cell-dependent antigens and are in the first place characterized by being primarily or exclusively of the IgM class (KATZ and BENACERRAF 1972; BARTHOLD et al. 1974). It is also noteworthy that their repeated injection does not induce IgG memory (BRALEY-MULLEN 1978).

Potent protein antigens produce hypersensitivity reactions in a high proportion of patients, particularly if repeated doses have to be administered. In experimental animals, three dosage ranges producing different effects have been defined, namely a very low dosage which leads to partial tolerance (low-zone tolerance), an intermediate range resulting in immunization, and a very high dosage range which results in an early, limited response followed by a state of so-called high-zone tolerance (DRESSER and MITCHISON 1968).

It is probable that these observations are applicable to immune responses in humans, but this is not established on a sufficient scale. Unfortunately it appears that many therapeutic applications of proteins are within the intermediate, immunogenic dose range. A survey, taken from the world literature, of 146 patients with anaphylactic shock from heterologous sera, shows that the incidence of this complication has considerably declined owing to less widespread use of such sera (BIANCHI et al. 1967).

Very low doses of complex protein antigens are used in long-term hyposensitization therapy of hay fever patients which classically consists of a series of injections of the specific allergens in the native or in modified form. The major effects of this treatment are a considerable increase of IgG antibody and a gradual decline of IgE antibody, as measured in ragweed-sensitive patients. In addition, secondary IgE antibody responses appear suppressed (ISHIZAKA 1976). Additional studies in mice showed that the primary effect of the repeated antigen injections resulting in abrogation of the secondary IgE response was on T-cell function (TAKATSU and ISHIZAKA 1975; BACH and BRASHLER 1975); it appears now that suppressor T-cells are formed thereby in effective numbers.

Allogeneic material requires special consideration. Antigens of this type were thought for many years to be exclusively cellular, yet several proteins such as haptoglobins, transferrins, or some β-lipoproteins have now been characterized as alloantigens. Furthermore, the allogeneic forms of immunoglobulins, the so-called allotypes were very important tools in studying the genetics and structure of antibody molecules. Alloantigens are defined as constituents from certain individuals that are immunogenic in some other individuals of the same species but not in the donor. The term isoantigen is an older synonym still widely used. Examples of isoantigens extensively applied in humans are commercial preparations of human gamma-globulin. ELLIS and HENNEY (1969) discuss reactions due to denatured, in particular aggregated, components which in part involve newly created determinants and consider native protein containing allogeneic determinants. Earlier, human plasma protein preparations containing ethylene oxide as a preservative were shown to become permanently altered and inducers of delayed hypersensitivity in humans (MAURER 1961).

Proteins and other more or less potent intrinsic immunogens have to be considered not only as essential constituents of vaccines, allergen extracts for hyposensitization, plasma protein preparations, enzyme preparations, and hormone preparations, but also as possible contaminants of certain low molecular weight compounds and even as additives in pharmaceutical formulations. Widely discussed are protein and macromolecular polymeric impurities in penicillins and cephalosporins (DE WECK et al. 1968; DEWDNEY 1977; AHLSTEDT et al. 1979) and an example of an antigenically active additive in certain formulations, namely carboxymethyl cellulose, comes from the penicillin field. Penicilloylated carboxymethyl cellulose is readily formed by reaction of penicillin with the polysaccharide during remarkably short storage in cold solutions. Although potentially immunogenic under certain conditions, it was primarily studied as an elicitor of immediate hypersensitivity (SCHNEIDER et al. 1971 b).

II. Low Molecular Weight Drugs as Immunogens

1. The Formation of Antigenic Determinants

The notion that low molecular weight compounds (less than about 600 daltons) are not immunogenic unless covalently attached to proteins or other macromolecular carriers, is based on classical evidence. In modern terms, it is quite clear that such compounds may be recognized as B-cell determinants or parts of such determinants, but only after conjugation to a carrier containing effective T-cell determinants are these structures ready to evoke specific antibody responses. On the other hand, low molecular weight compounds may give rise to T-cell determinants after conjugation and much of the information about low molecular weight sensitizers is in fact based on manifestations of T-cell activity such as delayed and contact hypersensitivity.

One of the questions which still requires clarification is whether covalent linkage is indeed necessary, although it is evident that it is sufficient for the establishment of antigenic determinants. This in turn raises the question why ionic and van der Waals bonds do not seem to suffice, although they are adequate for somewhat larger haptens, as discussed in Sect. C.III.

The first piece of evidence that covalent linkage, or by the same token reactive chemicals, are necessary for the sensitization process was obtained by LANDSTEINER and JACOBS (1935), who used a large number of chloro- and nitrobenzenes. They found a marked parallelism between the capacity of these derivatives to induce contact sensitivity in guinea pigs and their chemical reactivity with aniline. These observations were confirmed by parallel studies in humans (SULZBERGER and BAER 1938). It was inferred that effective sensitizers are capable of forming protein conjugates in vivo. Later, GELL et al. (1946) found that intraperitoneal injection of rabbits with a variety of protein-reactive chemicals induced chemical-specific antibodies, which could be quantitated in the sera by precipitation with gelatin conjugates of the chemicals. With 2-phenyl-4-ethoxymethylene oxazolone, antibody concentrations as high as 3 mg/ml were obtained.

EISEN et al. (1952) demonstrated that four protein-reactive DNP derivatives were able to sensitize humans, whereas four structurally similar but unreactive compounds were found to be non-sensitizers. In particular, 2,4-dinitrophenol does not form covalent 2,4-dinitrophenyl–protein conjugates but strongly associates with serum albumin. This compound is unable to induce DNP-specific sensitization or to elicit allergic skin reactions. On the other hand, 2,4-dinitrobromobenzene, a good inducer of DNP-specific skin hypersensitivity, readily reacts with protein to yield dinitrophenylated conjugates but it binds reversibly to serum albumin only to a slight extent. It is also noteworthy that, among the 2,4-dinitrobenzene sensitizers, there is a parallelism between rate of reaction with protein and potency for inducing DNP-specific anaphylactic antibody, the order for both activities being 2,4-dinitrofluorobenzene »2,4,-dinitrochlorobenzene > 2,4,-dinitrobenzenesulfonate (EISEN 1959).

There is very little evidence to show that low molecular weight drugs and chemicals may, as an exception to the rule, not need chemical conjugation to a carrier in order to be immunogenic. In two instances detailed data have been provided. One is azobenzene arsonate tyrosine, already described as an inducer of cellular immunity in Sect. B.III (see also GOODMAN 1975). The other involves picric acid, a compound well known in preparative organic chemistry for its associative power, which is used to isolate various derivatives in the form of "picrates". Good contact skin reactions are evoked in guinea pigs with picric acid by a special "split-adjuvant" technique. The sensitized animals react positively to contact tests with picryl chloride, which presumably binds to skin proteins very rapidly; they do not respond to intradermal tests with picryl chloride or picrylated protein (MAGUIRE and CHASE 1972; CHASE and MAGUIRE 1973). It was originally considered that picric acid would be reduced in vivo to picramic acid, which could then conjugate covalently to protein carriers. However, in the light of recent evidence that picramic acid is only occasionally able to sensitize, this is now thought to be unlikely (CHASE and MAGUIRE 1974). It is also to be noted that guinea pigs treated by daily intradermal injections of a mixture of picric acid and horse serum, developed anaphylactic antibody detectable with picrylated casein (CHASE and MAGUIRE 1973).

Why is covalent attachment of a drug or low molecular weight chemical to suitable carriers not only a sufficient but, except for special cases, also a necessary condition for determinant formation? Earlier thinking emphasized that antigen degradation was an important and obligatory step during immunization. It was believed that only covalently linked haptenic groups would survive as functional entities during the fragmentation. However, with the demonstration of conformational determinants as described in Sect. B.II this notion became definitively obsolete, although not all of its elements should be so readily discarded. If speculation is permitted, it would seem that the covalent bond possesses one important property which ionic as well as van der Waals bonds lack, namely the high degree of stability and irreplacibility by other moieties under physiologic conditions. Indeed, the hapten on a hapten–protein conjugate stays on its carrier in vivo, presumably until the entire molecule is enzymatically processed. There are, in exceptional cases, some implications that transconjugation of a hapten to another carrier may take place, for instance with aminoazo derivatives (FIERZ et al. 1939) or certain DNP derivatives (FREY et al. 1969). There also are unstable immunogens such as penicilloylated polysaccharides which lose their penicilloyl-haptens by chemical hydrolysis, i.e., the hapten is replaced by a proton on the hydroxyl groups (SCHNEIDER and DE WECK 1967; SCHNEIDER et al. 1978). But in this case, as well as with the aminoazo conjugates, the replacement reactions are sufficiently slow or restricted and do not abolish the immunogenicity of the conjugates.

In contrast single ionic bonds are reversible and a haptenic group bound ionically to a carrier is expected to dissociate in vivo very rapidly. Direct evidence for this was obtained with a solution of polylysine containing one molar equivalent of benzylpenicilloic acid for each ε-amino residue. Penicilloic acid forms a salt with the lysines by either of its two carboxyls or by both if sterically possible. In any case, this solution contains sufficient penicilloyl residues ionically bound to polylysine, which should be functionally equivalent to penicilloyl residues of a penicilloyl polylysine obtained by chemical reaction. Whereas penicilloylated polylysine, even when containing considerably less than one penicilloyl group for each lysine in the chain, is an efficient elicitor of BPO-specific passive cutaneous anaphylaxis in the guinea pig, the penicilloic acid–polylysine mixture was virtually ineffective (SCHNEIDER et al. 1976, unpublished). By the same token, the reversibility of van der Waals binding may lead to a rapid redistribution of a small hapten associated with a carrier upon injection into an organism. The hapten will then become associated with autologous carriers, which do not recruit T-cell assistance for immunization as such, i.e., without modification leading to T-cell determinants. The hapten may also become buried within protein or other body constituents, be conjugated by detoxification processes, metabolized in other ways and rapidly excreted. In short, the non-covalently bound small hapten may be consumed by a variety of processes, which compete most sucessfully with the immunogenic one. It may be noteworthy that direct infusion of dinitrophenol into an afferent lymphatic vessel of Large White pigs proved to be contact sensitizing but much less efficiently so than similar infusion of 1-fluoro-2,4,-dinitrobenzene (SOEBERG et al. 1978 b).

What are the conjugation reactions available to low molecular weight sensitizers or (to use a different term) chemical immunogens? In addition to the classical examples of EISEN, GELL, or LANDSTEINER already cited, many more reactive chemicals have been shown to be sensitizers and more recent cases include drugs such as β-lactam antibiotics, which are chemical acylators of amino and other nucleophilic groups (SCHNEIDER and DE WECK 1968), and cyclophosphamide, which is an alkylating agent (LAKIN and CAHILL 1976). Toluenediisocyanate and phenylglycine acid chloride, both highly reactive toward amino groups in the first place, are occupational hazards to industrial workers (BUTCHER et al. 1976; KAMMERMEYER and MATHEWS 1973). Benzoyl peroxide, a strong oxidant, is a contact sensitizer in guinea pigs and in humans (POOLE et al. 1970); it is not clear, however, whether the antigenic determinant involves the benzoyl group. Since reactive functional groups on proteins and other constituents available as carriers are of the nucleophilic type, it seems straightforward to conclude that most chemical immunogens have to be electrophilic reagents. This would be true even for oxidizing agents converting hydroxyls into carboxyls or thiols into disulfides and sulfonates. On the other hand, reducing agents, which could also react with disulfides, would not fit into this general statement.

It is common knowledge that most of the sensitizing drugs and many low molecular weight sensitizers do not exhibit any relevant chemical reactivity in vitro. For these cases, the concept has been developed that metabolic transformation or chemical degradation in vivo will yield chemically reactive immunogens. This concept has been quite fruitful in explaining hypersensitivity reactions induced by sulfonamides and a variety of aromatic amines, nitro derivatives, catechols, and azo compounds, the common denominator being the ability of these sensitizers to be transformed into protein-reactive *ortho-* or *para-*quinones, quinoneimine or quinonediimine derivatives. The subject has been extensively treated in a review by MAYER (1954), which is still worth consulting. The reaction of benzoquinone with amine and proteins has been more recently studied in some detail (MORRISON et al. 1969) and an interesting assay for the study of quinone–protein coupling related to sensitizing catechols of poison ivy has been developed (BYCK and DAWSON 1968).

A variety of biochemical pathways are known which may lead to reactive quinoid derivatives. They include dihydroxylation of aromatic or heterocyclic compounds and epoxide formation and hydrolysis to *o*-diphenolic compounds (BOOTH and BOYLAND 1957); *o*- and *p*-hydroxylations of phenols or arylamines (INSCOE et al. 1965; MILLER et al. 1960; BOOTH and BOYLAND 1957) and rearrangement of *n*-hydroxyarylamines to *o*-aminophenols (MILLER and MILLER 1960). It now appears that "aromatic hydroxylations" proceed via highly reactive arene oxides, i.e., compounds in which a formal aromatic double bond has undergone epoxidation. Depending on the compound, arene oxides may give rise to other electrophilic reactive species, including quinoid structures, but react as such readily with nucleophiles and thus provide a basis for understanding covalent attachment of aromatic hydrocarbon derivatives to protein and nucleic acids (JERINA and DALY 1974).

Most, if not all of this more recent evidence has come from the field of chemical carcinogenesis. This specialty requires detailed information about how, inter alia, low molecular weight carcinogenic compounds may become covalently linked to the informational macromolecules of target cells (MILLER 1970; MILLER and MILLER 1974; MAGEE et al. 1975). This is of course directly related to the interests of the immunochemist who wishes to know how low molecular weight sensitizers may become attached to macromolecular carriers of the organism. This basic relationship between the two fields has been taken into account by MAYER in his review on group sensitization to quinoid compounds already cited. Very recently, delayed hypersensitivity to the powerful carcinogen benzo[a]pyrene was studied in some detail in the guinea pig (LEWIS et al. 1978).

In a variety of instances, the metabolic concept has encountered difficulties in explaining the sensitizing capacity of low molecular weight compounds. Thus, in the early 1960s, penicillenic acid was held to be a major sensitizing intermediate in penicillin allergy. This is not a true metabolite, in the sense that it does not require metabolic processes for its formation, but it was thought to form spontaneously from penicillin. The notion met a number of problems, one being that penicillenic acid forms only at acid pH and hardly at all at blood pH levels. A distinct situation, of course, is constituted by the prior formation of penicillenic acid disulfide or other oxazolone derivatives in vitro. By ultraviolet (UV) spectroscopy, their generation in unbuffered penicillin solutions is readily demonstrable after auto-acidification (DE WECK et al. 1968).

2. The Formation of Complete Immunogens

Complete immunogens capable of inducing an immune response as such possess one or several T-cell determinants for evoking manifestations of cellular immunity; they also induce antibody responses if distinctive B-cell determinants are present, or if at least one of the T-cell determinants may also be recognized by B-cells. Autologous carriers in steady contact with the immunocompetent cells possess determinants for which no cells of the host are ready to become activated. Formation of complete immunogens therefore requires transformation of parts of the autologous carrier into distinctly different moieties, which may then be recognized as T-cell determinants and eventually as B-cell determinants. This is what appears to be sucessfully accomplished by the chemical immunogens discussed in Sect. C.II.1.

However, there is evidence that not every autologous carrier becomes readily immunogenic after haptenic conjugation. Furthermore, adjuvants are used in most animal experiments with ill-defined effects in many instances, lacking of course in human sensitization to drugs. Thus, in order to understand human sensitization to drugs, one should not only know how antigenic determinants may be formed but where, with what carriers, and in what numbers. Unfortunately, such complete information is hardly available in any single case, but indirect evidence pertinent to the issue is accumulating at an encouraging rate. In any case, it is clear that the pathway from reactive drug or metabolite to complete and effective immunogen is complex and many factors may influence the process. Some of these have been briefly mentioned in Sect. A.II.

In one clinical situation, the nature of the autologous carrier may be rather clearly defined: this is in drug-induced hemolytic anemia based on immunologic mechanisms. It has been shown that destruction of erythrocytes is due to interaction of IgG antibodies with the red cell membrane after its appreciable penicilloylation during therapy with high doeses of penicillin (LEVINE and REDMOND 1967). The antibodies involved were penicilloyl specific but it appeared possible that modified structures of the red cell surface are also contributing to the specificity. If this can be substantiated, the erythrocyte will be definitively implicated as the actual immunogenic carrier.

In the guinea pig, in which contact sensitivity to 1-fluoro-2,4-dinitrobenzene can be readily induced after application to the skin, suggestive evidence for a role in immunization of dinitrophenylated leukocytes was obtained (GECZY and BAUMGARTEN 1972). There is also evidence, however, that DNP–epidermal protein conjugates are involved in the development and elicitation of contact reactions (PARKER et al. 1970; LEWIS and HEISE 1977). It also appeared that multiple hapten carriers may play a role and that in particular circulating serum proteins could serve as carriers. Very informative studies on Large White pigs using intralymphatic infusion of various DNP-conjugated materials have recently shown that contact sensitivity is efficiently induced by in vivo conjugated afferent lymph cells and by lightly conjugated autologous peripheral white cells. Comparatively weak sensitizers were DNP-conjugated serum albumin or lymph node cell membranes (SOEBERG et al. 1978 a, b). Similarly, in vivo penicilloylated serum proteins of mice induced very weak antibody responses when injected together with Freund's adjuvant (AHLSTEDT et al. 1979).

The establishment of effective immunogens may require the formation of new antigenic determinants (NAD), distinct from those formed around the hapten after conjugation to the autologous carrier. Such determinants may be generated by conformational changes of the carrier induced by the conjugation reaction, e.g., via altered electrical charge distribution. These NAD may be T-cell determinants and as such would be important in those instances where the haptenic determinants are not T-cell activating.

Evidence for NAD generation after haptenic conjugation has been obtained in a number of experiments. Thus, rabbit serum albumin conjugated with sulfanilic acid by diazotization induced antibodies in rabbits which were directed against the sulfanilic hapten but also against a NAD which was created by the coupling procedure (RUBIN 1972). NAD created by different conjugation reactions may be different. Thus, rabbits immunized with DNP+-rabbit serum albumin obtained by diazotization produced NAD antibodies which exhibited almost no serologic cross-reaction with a directly dinitrophenylated rabbit serum albumin (RUBIN and AASTED 1973). At the cellular level, spleen cells from B-10 mice incubated with trinitrophenylated syngeneic spleen cells produced a cytotoxic lytic response. There was no significant lysis of native syngeneic cells or trinitrophenylated allogeneic cells. It was concluded that the cell-mediated cytotoxicity was against a NAD generated by the trinitrophenylation (SHEARER 1974; SHEARER et al. 1975).

III. Immunogenic Complexes not Involving Covalent Linkage Between Hapten and Carrier

The immunogens discussed in this section are a heterogeneous group of chemical substances and include molecules of medium size (molecular weight above 600–800 daltons), but also some large compounds and, on the other hand, several metal salts. These compounds do not possess T-cell determinants and need combination with a carrier to acquire such sites. They thereby form complete immunogens capable of inducing cellular immunity and/or antibody responses. Why is non-covalent linkage between larger haptens and carrier sufficient for establishing immunogenic function? In the first place, one should consider that with increasing size of the hapten, multiple associative and ionic bonds may form. This polyvalent attachment, although still reversible, is much less easy to break than single bonds. In the second place, a larger molecule may become closely associated with and enclosed within a carrier matrix but still possess moieties sticking out from the surface to serve as determinants.

This group of immunogens is theoretically quite well defined and it seems straightforward to include large haptens which become immunogenic after complexing with heterologous carriers. On the other hand, evidence for association of large haptens with autologous carriers as a basis for immunogenicity is not readily found in the literature, although it is conceivable that multiple associative binding to protein may create NAD similar to chemical modification. In any case, large and medium-sized molecules may be expected to provoke T-cell activation in their own right.

A different classification problem is raised by immunogens produced by metal salts. In these cases, autologous carriers are thought to become modified by metal ion interaction, and NAD which contain the metal and others which may not contain it can be envisaged. The question here is rather whether the coordinate bonds which are inferred for the transition metals should not be simply considered as covalent.

Various immunogenic substances requiring association with carriers are listed in Table 2. Picric acid, discussed as an exceptional low molecular weight sensitizer in Sect. C.II.1, may be cited with some confidence as a compound which associates with autologous carriers, giving rise to an immunogenic complex. This may be inferred from the cross-reactivity data already mentioned, namely that reactions in contact-sensitized animals may only be evoked by contact application of picryl chloride, not by intradermal application or by means of picrylated protein.

Many small peptides require prior complexing with a carrier to be immunogenic and/or adjuvant mixtures, which also might provide carriers. For instance the charcoal used for immunization to vasopressin could mediate association with and denaturation of autologous protein. However, other peptides could be intrinsically immunogenic. Thus, in the case of BPO-bacitracin, almost half the guinea pigs of a group of 21 animals showed BPO-specific, antibody-mediated skin responses and/or strong BPO-specific delayed skin reactions. It may be inferred therefore that the BPO moiety of the peptide was also T-cell activating and may have done this in its own right. With regard to the DNP-polylysines of SCHLOSSMAN, it has to be taken into account that DNP-poly-D-lysine was not immunogenic under the conditions used. If the DNP-polylysines were simply haptens associated with an immunogenic carrier, the D-chains should be as immunogenic as the L-chains. Therefore the DNP-poly-L-lysines are probably intrinsically immunogenic.

The lipids are classical substances to be complexed for immunization with heterologous proteins, formerly called Schlepper proteins. On the other hand, nucleic acids and nucleotides have only recently been found to be immunogenic, provided these polyacidic derivatives are combined with polybasic carriers like methylated serum albumin.

A number of metal salts have been found to induce delayed hypersensitivity, mainly of the contact type, in humans or in laboratory animals. Sensitivity to ions of chromium, mercury, platinum, nickel, beryllium, and others seem well established and Table 2 shows some recent findings. The best studied metal sensitizers are the chromium salts, since chromium eczema due to cement is the most important occupational dermatosis (POLAK et al. 1973). Hexavalent chromium, in the form of potassium dichromate, is a better sensitizer than trivalent chromium. This seems related to the much better skin penetrating capacity of the dichromate, since numerous studies have shown that trivalent chromium compounds as opposed to hexavalent salt are the actual sensitizers (POLAK et al. 1973). The same authors conclude that chromium is probably a component of the determinants formed with autologous carriers and does not produce autoantigens without further participation of the metal ion. In particular, oxidation reactions as generators of determinants seem inoperative in chromium hypersensitivity, since other strong oxidizers like

Table 2. Some immunogens effective after non-covalent association with carriers[a]

Immunogen	Carrier	Adjuvant	Response	Species	Reference
Low molecular weight chemicals					
Picric acid	Autologous	"split-adjuvant"	DH	GP	CHASE and MAGUIRE (1973)
Peptides					
Oxytocin	Carboxymethylcellulose	IFA	Ab	RB	SCHÄCKER et al. (1967)
Vasopressin	Charcoal	CFA	Ab	RB	CZERNICHOV et al. (1974)
Fibrinopeptide B	Polymethylmethacrylate	Incomplete	Ab	RB	BERGLUND (1965)
BPO_1-bacitracin F	None	CFA	Ab, DH	GP	de WECK and SCHNEIDER (1968)
N^α-DNP-hepta-L-lysine-butylamide	None	CFA	Ab, DH	GP	SCHLOSSMAN et al. (1965)
Lipids					
Glucosylceramide	Cholesterol + HSA	None	Ab	RB	ZALC et al. (1979)
Sulfatide	Lecithin + cholesterol + MBSA	None	Ab	RB	ZALC et al. (1977)
Triphosphoinositide	Lecithin + cholesterol + MBSA	None	Ab	RB	GREENBERG et al. (1979)
Nucleic acids					
sRNA	MBSA	CFA	Ab	RB	PLESCIA et al. (1965a)
DNA	MBSA	CFA	Ab	RB	PLESCIA et al. (1964)
Oligonucleotides	MBSA	CFA	Ab	RB	PLESCIA et al. (1965b)
Metal salts					
Beryllium sulfate	Autologous	None	DH	RB	KANG et al. (1977)
Ferric chloride	Autologous	None	DH	H	BAER (1973)
Chloroplatinates	Autologous	None	Ab	H	FREEDMAN and KRUPEY (1968)
Potassium dichromate	Autologous		DH	GP	POLAK and FREY (1973)

[a] MBSA = methylated bovine serum albumin; CFA = complete Freund's adjuvant; DH = delayed hypersensitivity; Ab = antibody response; RB = rabbits; GP = guinea pigs; H = humans; IFA = incomplete Freund's adjuvant.

potassium permanganate or hydrogen peroxide did not produce eczematous reactions.

On the other hand, few leads pointing to the actual antigenic chromium conjugate formed in vivo have been obtained, since attempts to sensitize animals with conjugates between chromium salts and albumins, globulins, and skin extracts prepared in vitro were unsuccessful. These preparations were also unsuccessful in eliciting skin reactions in already sensitized animals or in patients (Gross et al. 1968; Samitz et al. 1969). Chromium chloride conjugates with heparin, human serum albumin, and gamma-globulin were however able, in another study, to evoke positive skin reactions in patients who reacted positively to potassium dichromate (Cohen 1966a, b).

IV. Molecular Parameters in Elicitation and Inhibition of Allergic Reactions

Natural macromolecular antigens are usually capable of exhibiting the full range of antigenic functions (except inhibition), and a detailed differentiation of the molecular characteristics required for one or the other function seemed unnecessary. With the introduction of synthetically prepared antigens, in particular of low molecular weight antigens, such distinctions became important and indeed readily apparent in a number of instances. However, the different molecular requirements for induction of immune responses and elicitation of allergic reactions are not fully appreciated in parts of the more recent literature. A section concentrating on these aspects seems therefore in order.

Since antigens with a restricted number of functions, or even with a single functional capacity are not only theoretically interesting but may eventually be applied in human medicine, it is not surprising that the most complete understanding of these aspects has been achieved by using penicillin allergy as a model. Rather detailed summaries are available (de Weck 1974; de Weck and Schneider 1969) and only a general outline is presented here. Table 3 shows a series of BPO-antigens which represent different categories and are characterized in the first place by the number of BPO-ligands. BPO-protein represents a "complete antigen" which is immunogenic, i.e., able to evoke delayed hypersensitivity as well as antibody formation. It precipitates antibody and elicits the various reactions of immediate and delayed hypersensitivity. The highly or fully penicilloylated poly-L-lysine, on the other hand, is an "incomplete antigen" since it lacks immunogenicity; it is however a fully competent multivalent hapten and elicits the various types of allergic responses. The low molecular weight bivalent BPO-conjugate BPO_2-HEX is nonimmunogenic and does not precipitate antibody nor elicit Arthus reactions; it elicits, however, anaphylactic reactions. BPO-bacitracin is a counterpart to BPO_H-PLL; it is a "pure immunogen" which evokes antibody formation as well as delayed hypersensitivity but does not generally elicit any of the reactions listed. On the contrary, it is an inhibitor of, for example, BPO-specific antibody precipitation in sufficient excess. BPO-EACA is neither immunogenic nor eliciting and may be used in high doses as an inhibitor of anaphylactic reactions. It is a true monovalent inhibitor. In modern terms, the difference between the two monovalent antigens

Table 3. Some antigenic functions of BPO-conjugates

Antigens[a]	Immunogenicity		Precipitation of anti-BPO antibody	Elicitation of hypersensitivity[b]					Delayed local intradermal reactions
	Induction of anti-BPO antibody	Induction of delayed hypersensitivity		Anaphylactic reactions			Arthus reactions		
				PCA	SA	WE	RB	GP	
Multivalent									
BPO-protein (BPO [box] BPO / BPO BPO BPO)	+	+	+	+	+	+	+	+	+
BPO$_H$-PLL (BPO BPO BPO / BPO BPO BPO)	−	−	+	+	+	+	+	+	−
Bivalent									
BPO$_2$-HEX (BPO—BPO)	−	−	−	+	+	+	−	−	−
Monovalent									
BPO-BAC (BPO—[box])	+	+	− Inh	−	−	−	−	−	−
BPO-EACA (BPO—)	− Inh	−	− Inh	− Inh	− Inh	− Inh	−	−	−
Pseudomonovalent									
BPO$_1$-PLL (BPO +++)	+	+	− Inh	+	+	+	+[c]	+[c]	+

[a] BPO-protein = highly penicilloylated bovine, gamma-globulin and human serum albumin were mainly studied; BPO$_H$-PLL = highly or fully penicilloylated poly-L-lysine (chain length 12 or 20 lysines) were studied; BPO$_2$-HEX = N^1-N^6-bis-benzylpenicilloyl diaminohexane; BPO-BAC = Bacitracin F; monopenicilloylated at the ε-amino function of lysine; BPO-EACA = N^ε-benzylpenicilloylaminocaproic acid; BPO$_1$-PLL = Poly-L-lysine (12 lysines) carrying on the average one BPO-group

[b] PCA = passive cutaneous anaphylaxis in the guinea pig; SA = systemic anaphylactic shock in the guinea pig; WE = wheal and erythema reactions in human penicillin allergics; RB = rabbits; GP = guinea pigs; Inh = specific inhibition

[c] In part nonspecific reactions, reaction elicitable at higher dosage also in non-sensitized animals

+ = occurs; − = does not occur

seems clear – both are monovalent with respect to BPO but BPO-bacitracin possesses in addition T-cell-activating capacity as discussed in Sect. C.III.

The so-called pseudomonovalent BPO_1-PLL apparently functions as an almost complete antigen. It is immunogenic and elicits most hypersensitivity responses, including Arthus reactions, although it does not precipitate antibody in vitro. The example shows the limits of the classification based on haptenic structure as illustrated in Table 3. Indeed, one would expect that only tri- or multivalent haptenic conjugates will be able to mediate immune-complex-mediated manifestations, such as the Arthus reactions. Similarly, anaphylactic reactions mediated by IgE antibody require bridging of antibody molecules on the membrane of histamine-releasing cells. Accordingly, such triggering may normally only be accomplished by divalent or multivalent antigens (OVARY 1965; DE WECK and SCHNEIDER 1968; ISHIZAKA et al. 1978).

The mechanism by which BPO_1-PLL exerts its eliciting functions is not established. The case is exceptional but there is evidence that several different monovalent compounds may be effective elicitors of anaphylaxis. Thus monohaptenic carbohydrates such as penicilloylated carboxymethylcellulose mentioned in Sect. C.I and BPO_1-dextrans are elicitors of BPO-specific passive cutaneous anaphylaxis in the guinea pig (MOLINARI et al. 1973). Even monopenicilloylated raffinose, a trisaccharide but not glucose, is an anaphylactogen under these conditions. In another series of experiments, it was found that 1,6-diaminohexane carrying two different groups, namely dinitrocarboxyphenyl (DNCP) on one NH_2 terminus and BPO on the other (DNCP-BPO-HEX), was an elicitor of passive cutaneous anaphylaxis in guinea pigs sensitized by anti-DNCP antiserum (but not in anti-BPO-sensitized animals). This "monovalent elicitation" required intravenous application of the elicitor whereas intradermal administration was always ineffective (SCHNEIDER et al. 1979). These findings are related to earlier studies with similar compounds (AMKRAUT et al. 1963; FRICK et al. 1968; LEVINE 1965). It appears that certain hydrocarbon residues may act as helper groups and enable a monovalent hapten to become an elicitor of anaphylaxis under certain conditions. In the DNCP-BPO-HEX elicitation, the benzyl side chain of the penicilloyl group, possibly in conjunction with other structural elements of the BPO moiety, acts as an efficient helper group. More recent experiments make it likely that this type of elicitation requires hetero- or homocytotropic IgG antibodies whereas IgE-mediated reactions do not occur (SCHNEIDER and TOFFLER 1979, unpublished). A direct relationship of these experiments to clinical problems is thus not readily envisaged since the bulk of immediate hypersensitivity reactions appears to be IgE mediated. However, a recent report of anaphylaxis to protamine sulfate as well as earlier observations show that complement-dependent IgG antibody reactions may also be involved in human reaginic hypersensitivity (LAKIN et al. 1978; PARISH 1970, 1971).

Since elicitation of antibody-mediated hypersensitivity reactions requires as a rule at least divalent or trivalent antigens, and is usually best achieved with multivalent conjugates, the specific inhibition of such reactions by monovalent haptens seems theoretically possible and depends primarily on the concentrations of inhibiting and eliciting haptens and on antibody affinity and concentration. It has been shown that anaphylactic reactions in vivo assessed by the PCA technique, or by observation of systemic shock or urticarial skin reactions, can be completely inhibited by a sufficiently high concentration of haptenic inhibitor (OVARY and KARUSH 1960; PARKER et al. 1962b; LOCHER et al. 1969; DE WECK and SCHNEIDER 1972). More recently, successful haptenic inhibitions with N^ε-BPO-N^α-formyl-L-lysine in clinical cases has been reported (DE WECK and GIRARD 1972; DE WECK and JEUNET 1975). With regard to inhibition of clinical manifestations, it should be kept in mind that in cases where high therapeutic doses of drug are administered, the drug itself may act as a monovalent inhibitor and mitigate or abolish allergic reactions elicited by conjugates. This effect has been considered for explaining low incidences of immediate reactions to the BPO major antigenic determinant in penicillin allergy, in the presence of presumably anaphylactic anti-BPO antibody and may be called "inbuilt inhibition".

Inhibition of cellular hypersensitivity, such as contact sensitivity, is not readily achieved with simple haptens. DNP-lysine, for instance, did not markedly depress contact reactions to 1-chloro-2,4-dinitrobenzene in guinea pigs whereas 2,4-dinitrobenzene sulfonate, which is able to conjugate in vivo, temporarily abolished contact reactions after parenteral injection (DE WECK et al. 1964).

With regard to the inhibition of primary antibody responses, it may prove difficult to maintain sufficiently high concentrations of low molecular weight hapten in vivo. Thus, N^ε-BPO-N^α-formyl-L-lysine did not inhibit the primary anti-BPO response to a BPO–BGG conjugate injected intravenously into rabbits, whereas with in vitro induction systems, specific inhibition of anti-hapten antibody responses can be observed in a number of instances. Secondary anti-hapten responses are easier to inhibit and N^ε-BPO-N^α-formyl-L-lysine strikingly abolished anti-BPO antibody synthesis in primed rabbits secondarily injected with BPO–BGG (for review see DE WECK 1974).

More recently, inhibitions of anti-BPO antibody responses in mice have also been achieved with a variety of multivalent BPO-conjugates including BPO-oligolysines of modest molecular weight ($< 10{,}000$ daltons) and penicilloylated high molecular weight polymers and copolymers of D-lysine, D-glutamic acid, D-alanine, and D-tyrosine (OTZ et al. 1978). The anti-BPO response could be specifically abolished by a single injection of conjugate, either before or after priming, and during anamnestic responses. The refractory state persisted for many weeks and could be reestablished by additional injection of conjugate in those cases where anti-BPO responses began to reappear following booster injections. Since the dose in these cases is in the milligram range and the effect of long duration, the mechanism involved is not simple haptenic inhibition and is probably better described as B-cell tolerance. Similar results have also been obtained by CHIORAZZI et al. (1976) with a multivalent BPO-D-glutamic-D-lysine copolymer, by KATZ et al. (1972) with a polymeric DNP conjugate and by ESHHAR et al. (1975) with a nucleoside conjugate.

References

Ahlstedt S, Kristofferson A, Pettersson E (1979) Antigens in penicillin allergy. III. Antigen and antibody levels in mice treated with pure and contaminated penicillins. Int Arch Allergy Appl Immunol 58:20–29

Alkan SS, Williams EB, Nitecki DE, Goodman JW (1972a) Antigen recognition and the immune response. Humoral and cellular immune responses to small mono and bifunctional antigen molecules. J Exp Med 135:1228–1246

Alkan SS, Bush ME, Nitecki DE, Goodman JW (1972 b) Antigen recognition and the immune response. Structural requirements in the side chain of tyrosine for immunogenicity of L-tyrosine-azobenzenearsonate. J Exp Med 136:387–391

Amkraut AA, Rosenberg LT, Raffel S (1963) Elicitation of PCA by univalent and divalent haptens. J Immunol 91:644–650

Anderer FA, Schlumberger HD (1969) Antigenic properties of proteins cross-linked by multidiazonium compounds. Immunochemistry 6:1–10

Arnon M, Sela M (1969) Antibodies to a unique region in lysozyme provoked by a synthetic antigen conjugate. Proc Natl Acad Sci USA 62:163–170

Arnon R, Geiger B (1977) Molecular basis of immunogenicitiy and antigenicity. In: Glynn LE, Steward MW (eds) Immunochemistry: an advanced textbook. Wiley-Interscience, New York Chichester

Arnon R, Sela M, Yaron A, Sober HA (1965) Polylysine-specific antibodies and their reaction with oligolysines. Biochemistry 4:948–953

Atassi MZ (1975) Antigenic structure of myoglobin: the complete immunochemical anatomy of a protein and conclusions relating to antigenic structures of proteins. Immunochemistry 12:423–438

Atassi MZ (1977) The complete antigenic structure of myoglobin. In: Atassi MZ (ed) Immunochemistry of proteins, vol II. Plenum, New York

Atassi MZ, Habeeb AFSA (1977) The antigenic structure of hen eggwhite lysozyme: A model for disulfide-containing proteins. In: Atassi MZ (ed) Immunochemistry of proteins, vol II. Plenum, New York

Atassi MZ, Koketsu J (1975) Immunochemistry of sperm-whale myoglobin. XXIII. Investigation of the independence of the five antigenic reactive regions by immunoabsorbent studies. Immunochemistry 12:741–744

Atsumi T, Nishida K, Kinoshita Y, Shibata K, Horiuchi Y (1967) The heterogeneity of combining sites of anti-benzylpenicilloyl antibodies obtained from individual rabbits. Fractionation of antibodies with specific immunoadsorbent. J Immunol 99:1286–1293

Bach MK, Brashler JR (1975) IgE antibody-specific abrogation of an established immune response in mice by modified antigens. J Immunol 114:1799–1807

Baer RL (1973) Allergic contact sensitization to iron. J Allergy Clin Immunol 51:35–38

Barthold DR, Prescott B, Stashak PW, Amsbaugh DF, Baker PJ (1974) Regulation of the antibody response to type III pneumococcal polysaccharide. III. Role of regulatory T cells in the development of an IgG and IgA antibody response. J Immunol 112:1042–1050

Benacerraf B, Katz DH (1975) The histocompatibility immune response genes. Adv Cancer Res 21:121–174

Benacerraf B, McDevitt HO (1972) Histocompatibility-linked immune response genes. Science 175:273–279

Ben-Ephraim S, Arnon R, Sela M (1966) The immune response of inbred strains of guinea pigs to polylysyl rabbit serum albumin. Immunochemistry 3:491–494

Berglund G (1965) Preparation of antiserum to an antigen of low molecular weight. Nature 206:523–524

Bianchi, Däppen U, Hoigné R (1967) Der anaphylaktische Schock des Menschen auf artfremdes Serum. Helv Chir Acta 34:257–272

Bluestein H, Green I, Benacerraf B (1971) Specific immune response genes of the guinea pig I. Dominant genetic control of immuno responsiveness to copolymers of L-glutamic acid and L-alanine and L-glutamic acid and L-tyrosine. J Exp Med 134:458–470

Booth J, Boyland E (1957) The biochemistry of aromatic amines. III. Enzymatic hydroxylation by rat liver microsomes. Biochem J 66:73–78

Borek F (1972) Molecular size and shape of antigens. In: Borek F (ed) Immunogenicity. North-Holland, Amsterdam Oxford New York

Borek F, Stupp Y, Sela M (1965) Immunogenicity and role of size: response of guinea pigs to oligotyrosine and tyrosine derivatives. Science 150:1177–1178

Braley-Mullen H (1978) Antigen requirements for induction of B-memory cells. Studies with dinitrophenyl coupled T-dependent and T-independet carriers. J Exp Med 147:1824–1831

Bush ME, Alkan SS, Nitecki DE, Goodman JW (1972) Antigen recognition and the immune response. "Self help" with symmetrical bifunctional antigen molecules. J Exp Med 136:1478–1483

Butcher BT, Salvaggio JE, Weill H, Ziskind MM (1976) Toluene diisocyanate (TDI) pulmonary disease: immunologic and inhalation challenge studies. J Allergy Clin Immunol 58:89–100

Byck JS, Dawson CR (1968) Assay of protein-quinone coupling involving compounds structurally related to the active principle of poison ivy. Anal Biochem 25:123–125

Chase MW, Maguire HC (1973) Studies on the sensitization of animals with simple chemical compounds. XIV. Further studies on sensitization of guinea pigs with picric acid. Int Arch Allergy Appl Immunol 45:513–542

Chase MW, Maguire HC (1974) Further studies on sensitization to picric acid. Monogr Allergy 8:1–12

Chiorazzi N, Eshhar Z, Katz DH (1976) Induction of immunological tolerance to the major antigenic determinant of penicillin: a therapeutic approach to penicillin allergy. Proc Natl Acad Sci USA 73:2091–2095

Claman HN, Chaperon EA, Triplett RF (1966) Thymus-marrow cell combinations. Synergism in antibody production. Proc Soc Exp Biol Med 122:1167–1171

Cohen HA (1966a) Carrier specificity of tuberculin-type reaction to trivalent chromium. Arch Dermatol 93:34–40

Cohen HA (1966b) Tuberculin-type reaction to heparin-chromium complex. Arch Dermatol 94:409–412

Coutinho A, Möller G (1975) Thymus-independent B-cell induction and paralysis. Adv Immunol 21:113–236

Crumpton MJ (1973) Antigenicity and immunogenicity. In: Porter RR (ed) Defence and recognition. Butterworths, London

Czernikov P, Reinharz A, Valloton MB (1974) Immunochemical analysis of rabbit antibodies against vasopressin. Immunochemistry 11:47–53

Dandliker WB, Alonso R, Meyers CY (1967) The synthesis of fluorescent penicilloyl haptens and their use in investigating penicillin antibodies by fluorescence polarization. Immunochemistry 4:295–302

Dewdney JM (1977) Immunology of the antibiotics. In: Sela M (ed) The antigens, vol IV. Academic Press, New York

de Weck AL (1972) Molecular models for induction of the immune response and their relationship to the genetic control of histocompatibility antigens. Transplant Rev 10:3–35

de Weck AL (1974) Low molecular weight antigens. In: Sela M (ed) The antigens, vol II. Academic Press, New York

de Weck AL, Girard JP (1972) Specific inhibition of allergic reactions to penicillin in man by a monovalent hapten. II. Clinical studies. Int Arch Allergy Appl Immunol 42:798–815

de Weck AL, Jeunet F (1975) Clinical trial of Ro 6-0787 a monovalent specific hapten inhibitor of penicillin allergy. Z Immunitaetsforsch Immunbiol 150:138–160

de Weck AL, Schneider CH (1968) Immune and non-immune responses to monovalent low molecular weight penicilloyl-polylysines and penicilloyl-bacitracin in rabbits and guinea pigs. Immunolog 14:457–473

de Weck AL, Schneider CH (1969) Molecular and stereochemical properties required of antigens for the elicitation of allergic reactions. In: Westphal O, Bock HE, Grundmann E (eds) Current problems in immunology. Springer, Berlin Heidelberg New York

de Weck AL, Schneider CH (1972) Specific inhibition of allergic reactions to penicillin in man by a monovalent hapten. I. Experimental immunological and toxicological studies. Int Arch Allergy Appl Immunol 42:782–797

de Weck AL, Frey JR, Geleick H (1964) Specific inhibition of contact dermatitis to dinitrochlorobenzene in guinea pigs by injection of haptens and protein conjugates. Int Arch Allergy Appl Immunol 24:63–87

de Weck AL, Schneider CH, Gutersohn J (1968) The role of penicilloylated protein impurities penicillin polymers and dimers in penicillin allergy. Int Arch Allergy Appl Immunol 33:535–567

Dresser DN, Mitchison NA (1968) The mechanism of immunological paralysis. Adv Immunol 9:129–174

Dutton RW (1975) Separate signals for the initiation of proliferation and differentiation in the B cell response to antigen. Transplant Rev 23:66–77

Dwyer JM (1976) Identifying and enumerating human T and B lymphocytes. Prog Allergy 21:178–260

Eisen HN (1959) Hypersensitivity to simple chemicals. In: Lawrence HS (ed) Cellular and humoral aspects of hypersensitivity states. Hoeber, New York

Eisen HN, Siskind GW (1964) Variations in affinities of antibodies during the immune response. Biochemistry 3:996–1008

Eisen HN, Orris L, Belman S (1952) Elicitation of delayed skin reactions with haptens: the dependence of elicitation on hapten combination with protein. J Exp Med 95:473–487

Ellis FE, Henney CS (1969) Adverse reactions following administration of human gamma globulin. J Allergy 43:45–54

Eshar Z, Benacerraf B, Katz DH (1975) Induction of tolerance to nucleic acid determinants by administration of a complex of nucleoside D-glutamic acid and D-lysine (D-GL). J Immunol 114:872–876

Feldman M, Palmer J (1971) The requirement for macrophages in the secondary immune response to antigens of small and large size in vitro. Immunology 21:685–699

Fierz HE, Jadassohn W, Kleemann A (1939) Zum Problem der Anaphylaxie mit chemisch bekannten Substanzen. Helv Chim Acta 22:3–18

Foerster G, Green I, Lamelin JP, Benacerraf B (1969) Transfer of responsiveness to hapten conjugates of poly-L-lysine and a copolymer of L-glutamic acid and L-lysine to lethally irradiated non-responder guinea pigs by bone marrow or lymph node and spleen cells from responder guinea pigs. J Exp Med 130:1107–1122

Fong S, Nitecki DE, Cook RM, Goodman JW (1978) Spatial requirements between haptenic and carrier determinants for T-dependent antibody responses. J Exp Med 148:817–822

Freedman SO, Krupey J (1968) Respiratory allergy caused by platinum salts. J Allergy 42:233–237

Frey JR, de Weck AL, Geleick H, Lergier W (1969) The immunogenicity of dinitrophenyl amino acids. J Exp Med 130:1123–1143

Frick OL, Nye W, Raffel S (1968) Anaphylactic reactions to univalent haptens. Immunology 14:563–568

Geczy AF, Baumgarten A (1972) Distribution of a contact sensitizer, 1-fluoro-2,4-dinitrobenzene, in the tissues of the guinea pig. Immunology 22:381–392

Geczy A, de Weck AL (1974) Genetic control of sensitization to chemically defined antigens and its relationship to histocompatibility antigens in guinea pigs. Monogr Allergy 8:83–88

Gell PGH, Benacerraf B (1959) Studies on hypersensitivity. II. Delayed hypersensitivity to denatured proteins in guinea pigs. Immunology 2:64–72

Gell PHG, Coombs RRA (1964) Clinical aspects of immunology. Blackwell, Oxford

Gell PGH, Harington CR, Rivers RP (1946) The antigenic function of simple chemical compounds: production of precipitins in rabbits. Br J Exp Pathol 27:267–286

Gill TJ (1972) The chemistry of antigens and its influence on immunogenicity. In: Borek F (ed) Immunogenicity. North-Holland, Amsterdam Oxford New York

Gill TJ, Kunz HW, Gould HJ, Doty P (1964a) Studies on synthetic polypeptide antigens. XI. The antigenicity of optically isomeric synthetic polypeptides. J Biol Chem 239:1107–1113

Gill TJ, Gould HJ, Kunz HW (1964b) Studies on synthetic polypeptide antigens. XIII. The effects of systematic variation in composition and chemical modifications of synthetic polypeptides on the antibodysynthetic polypeptide antigen interaction. J Biol Chem 239:3083–3092

Gill TJ, Kunz HW, Papermaster DS (1967) Studies on synthetic polypeptide antigens. XVIII. The role of composition, charge and optical isomerism in the immunogenicity of synthetic polypeptides. J Biol Chem 242:3308–3318

Gleich GJ, Averbeck AK, Swedlund HA (1971) Measurement of IgE in normal and allergic serum by radioimmunoassay. J Lab Clin Med 77:690–698

Goodman JW (1969) Immunochemical specificity: recent conceptual advances. Immunochemistry 6:139 149

Goodman JW (1975) Antigenic determinants and antibody combining sites. In: Sela M (ed) The antigens, vol III. Academic Press, New York

Green I, Benacerraf B (1971) Genetic control of immune responsiveness to limiting doses of proteins and hapten-protein conjugates in guinea pigs. J Immunol 107:374–381

Green I, Paul WE, Benacerraf B (1966) The behavior of hapten-poly-L-lysine conjugates as complete antigens in genetic responder and as haptens in nonresponder guinea pigs. J Exp Med 123:859–879

Green I, Paul WE, Benacerraf B (1968) Hapten carrier relationships in the DNP-PLL foreign albumin complex system: induction of tolerance and stimulation of cells in vitro. J Exp Med 127:43–53

Greenberg AJ, Trevor AJ, Johnson DA, Loh HH (1979) Immunochemical studies of phospholipids: production of antibodies to triphosphoinositide. Mol Immunol 16:193–196

Gross PR, Katz SA, Samitz MH (1968) Sensitization of guinea pigs to chromium salts. J Invest Dermatol 50:424–427

Haimovich J, Schechter I, Sela M (1969) Combining sites of IgG and IgM antibodies of poly-D-alanyl specificity. Eur J Biochem 7:537–543

Hamaoka T, Katz DH, Benacerraf B (1972) Radioresistance of carrierspecific helper thymus-derived lymphocytes in mice. Proc Natl Acad Sci USA 69:3453–3458

Hauglund RP, Stryer L, Stengle TR, Baldeschweiler JD (1967) Nuclear magnetic resonance studies of antibody-hapten interactions using a chloride ion probe. Biochemistry 6:498–502

Imanishi T, Mäkelä O (1974) Inheritance of antibody specificity. I. Anti(4-hydroxy-3-nitrophenyl)-acetyl of the mouse primary response. J Exp Med 140:1498–1510

Inscoe JK, Daly J, Axelrod J (1965) Factors affecting the enzymatic formation of o-methylated dihydroxy derivatives. Biochem Pharmacol 14:1257–1263

Ishizaka K (1976) Cellular events in the IgE antibody response. Adv Immunol 23:1–75

Ishizaka T, Campbell DH, Ishizaka K (1960) Internal antigenic determinants in protein molecules. Proc Soc Exp Biol Med 103:5–9

Ishizaka T, Ishizaka K, Conrad DH, Froese A (1978) A new concept of triggering mechanisms of IgE-mediated histamine release. J Allergy Clin Immunol 61:320–330

Janeway CA, Sela M (1967) Synthetic antigens composed exclusively of L- or D-amino acids. I. Effect of optical configuration on the immunogenicity of synthetic polypeptides in mice. Immunology 13:29–38

Jerina DM, Daly JW (1974) Arene oxides: a new aspect of drug metabolism. Science 185:573–582

Kabat EA (1976) The nature of an antigenic determinant. J Immunol 97:1–11

Kabat EA (1976) Structural concepts in immunology and immunochemistry, 2nd edn. Holt, Rinehart & Winston, New York

Kammermeyer JK, Mathews KP (1973) Hypersensitivity to phenylglycine acid chloride. J Allergy Clin Immunol 52:73–84

Kang K, Bice D, Hoffmann E, D'Amato R, Salvaggio J (1977) Experimental studies of sensitization to beryllium, zirconium and aluminium compounds in the rabbit. J Allergy Clin Immunol 59:425–436

Katz DH, Benacerraf B (1972) The regulatory influence of activated T cells on B cell responses to antigen. Adv Immunol 15:1–94

Katz DH, Hamaoka T, Benacerraf B (1972) Immunological tolerance in bone marrow derived lymphocytes. I. Evidence for an intracellular mechanism of inactivation of haptenspecific precursors of antibodyforming cells. J Exp Med 136:1404–1429

Katz DH, Hamaoka T, Newburger PE, Benacerraf B (1974) Hapten-specific IgE antibody responses in mice. IV. Evidence for distinctive sensitivities of IgE and IgG B lymphocytes to the regulatory influences of T cells. J Immunol 113:974–983

Kishimoto T, Ishizaka K (1973) Regulation of antibody response in vitro. VII. Enhancing soluble factors for IgG and IgE antibody response. J Immunol 111:1194–1205

Kishimoto T, Ishizaka K (1975) Immunologic and physicochemical properties of enhancing soluble factors for IgG and IgE antibody responses. J Immunol 114:1177–1184

Kojima S, Ovary Z (1975) Effect of Nippostrongylus brasiliensis infection on anti-hapten IgE antibody response in the mouse. II. Mechanism of potentiation of the IgE antibody response to a heterologous hapten-carrier conjugate. Cell Immunol 17:383–391

Lakin JD, Cahill RA (1976) Generalized urticaria to cyclophosphamide: type I hypernsensitivity to an immunosupressive agent. J Allergy Clin Immunol 58:160–171

Lakin JD, Blocker TJ, Strong DM, Yocum MW (1978) Anaphylaxis to protamine sulfate mediated by a complement-dependent IgG antibody. J Allergy Clin Immunol 61:102–107

Landsteiner K (1921) Über heterogenetisches Antigen und Hapten. XV. Mitteilungen über Antigene. Biochem Z 119:294–306

Landsteiner K (1945) The specificity of serological reactions. Harvard University Press, Cambridge

Landsteiner K, Jacobs J (1935) Studies on the sensitization of animals with simple chemical compounds. J Exp Med 61:643–657

Leskowitz S, Jones VE, Zak SJ (1966) Immunological study of antigenic specificity in delayed hypersensitivity. V. Immunization with monovalent low molecular weight conjugates. J Exp Med 123:229–237

Levine BB (1963) Studies on the dimensions of the rabbit anti-benzyl-penicilloyl antibody combining sites. J Exp Med 117:161–183

Levine BB (1964) Studies on antigenicity. The effect of succinylation of ε-amino groups on antigenicity of benzylpenicilloyl-poly-L-lysine conjugates in random-bred and in strain 2 guinea pigs. Proc Soc Exp Biol Med 116:1127–1131

Levine BB (1965) The nature of the antigen-antibody complexes which initiate anaphylactic reactions. J Immunol 94:111–120

Levine BB (1971) Genetic factors in reagin production in mice. In: Austen KF, Becker EL (eds) Biochemistry of the acute allergic reactions. Blackwell, Oxford

Levine BB, Redmond AP (1967) Immunochemical mechanisms of penicillin-induced Coombs positivity and hemolytic anemia in man. Int Arch Allergy Appl Immunol 31:594–606

Levine BB, Ojeda A, Benacerraf B (1963) Studies of artificial antigens. III. The genetic control of the immune response to hapten-poly-L-lysine conjugates in guinea pigs. J Exp Med 118:953–957

Levine BB, Stember RH, Fotino M (1972) Ragweed hay fever: genetic control and linkage to HL-A haplotypes. Science 178:1201–1203

Lewis FA, Heise ER (1977) Isolation of dinitrophenyl-skin protein conjugates by immunoadsorbent chromatography. Int Arch Allergy Appl Immunol 53:123–131

Lewis FA, Heise ER, Tulis JJ (1978) Delayed hypersensitivity to hapten-skin protein conjugates in guinea pigs sensitized to benzo(a) pyrene. Int Arch Allergy Appl Immunol 57:535–541

Locher GW, Schneider CH, de Weck AL (1969) Hemmung allergischer Reaktionen auf Penicillin durch Penicilloyl-Amide und chemisch verwandte Substanzen. Z Immunitaetsforsch Immunobiol 138:299–323

Loor F, Roelants GE (1977) B and T cells in immune recognition. Wiley, New York

Mage RG, Kabat EA (1963) Immunochemical studies on dextran. III. The specificities of rabbit antidextrans. Further findings on antidextrans with 1,2- and 1,6-specificities. J Immunol 91:633–640

Magee PN, Pegg AE, Swann PF (1975) Molecular mechanisms of chemical carcinogenesis. In: Grundmann E (ed) Handbuch der allgemeinen Pathologie, vol VI. Springer, Berlin Heidelberg New York

Maguire HC, Chase MW (1972) Studies on the sensitization of animals with simple chemical compounds. XIII. Sensitization of guinea pigs with picric acid. J Exp Med 135:357–375

Marsh DG, Bias WB, Hsu SH, Goodfriend L (1973) Associations between major histocompatibility (HL-A) antigens and specific reaginic antibody responses in allergic man. In: Goodfriend L, Sehon AH, Orange RP (eds) Mechanisms in allergy. Dekker, New York

Marsh DG, Bias WB, Ishizaka K (1974) Genetic control of basal serum immunoglobulin E level and its effect on specific reaginic sensitivity. Proc Natl Acad Sci USA 71:3588–3592

Maurer PH (1970) Antigenicity of polypeptides (poly-α-amino acids): immunogenicity of chemically modified polymers II. Proc Soc Exp Biol Med 134:663–666

Maurer PH, Gerulat BF, Pinchuck P (1966) Antigenicity of polypeptides (poly-α-amino acids). XIX. Studies with chemically modified polymers. J Immunol 97:306–312

Mayer RL (1954) Group-sensitization to compounds of quinone structure and its biochemical basis: role of these substances in cancer. Prog Allergy 4:79–172

Miller EC, Miller JA (1960) A mechanism of o-hydroxylation of aromatic amines in vivo. Biochim Biophys Acta 40:380–382

Miller EC, Miller JA (1974) Biochemical mechanisms of chemical carcinogensis. In: Busch H (ed) Molecular biology of cancer. Academic Press, New York

Miller JA (1970) Carcinogenesis by chemicals: an overview. GGA Clowes memorial lecture. Cancer Res 30:559–576

Miller JA, Cramer JW, Miller EC (1960) The N- and ring-hydroxylation of 2-acetylaminofluorene during carcinogenesis in the rat. Cancer Res 20:950–962

Miller JFAP, Mitchell GF (1968) Cell to cell interaction in the immune response. I. Hemolysin-forming cells in neonatally thymectomized mice reconstituted with thymus or thoracic duct lymphocytes. J Exp Med 128:801–820

Mitchell GF, Miller JFAP (1968) Cell to cell interaction in the immune response. II. The source of hemolysin-forming cells in irradiated mice given bone marrow and thymus or thoracic duct lymphocytes. J Exp Med 128:821–837

Mitchison NA (1972) Dose, frequency and route of administration of antigen. In: Borek F (ed) Immunogenicity. North-Holland, Amsterdam Oxford New York

Molinari M, Schneider CH, de Weck AL (1973) Über pseudo-monovalente Penicilloyl-Kohlehydrate. Z Immunitaetsforsch Immunobiol 146:225–238

Morrison M, Steele W, Danner DJ (1969) The reaction of benzoquinone with amines and proteins. Arch Biochem Biophys 134:515–523

Mozes E (1975) Expression of immune response (Ir) genes in T- and B-cells. Immunogenetics 2:397–410

Neveu PJ (1977) Stimulation and inhibition of macrophages prior to immunization with a hapten-carrier conjugate. Immunology 33:269–273

North JR, Kemshead JT, Askonas BA (1977) Non-specific factor replaces T cells in an IgG response to soluble antigens. Immunology 33:321–329

Otz U, Schneider CH, de Weck AL (1976) Charakterisierung von Immunseren durch Bindung von monovalentem Penicilloylhapten. Chimia 30:89–91

Otz U, Schneider CH, de Weck AL, Gruden E, Gill TJ (1978) Induction of immunological tolerance to the penicilloyl antigenic determinant. I. Evaluation of penicilloylated amino acid polymers and copolymers in mice. Eur J Immunol 8:410–414

Ovary Z (1965) PCA reaction and its elicitation by specific immunoglobulin species and fragments. Fed Proc Fed Am Soc Exp Biol 24:94–97

Ovary Z, Karush F (1960) Studies on the immunologic mechanism of anaphylaxis. I. Antibody-hapten interactions studied by passive cutaneous anaphylaxis in the guinea pig. J Immunol 84:409–415

Owen JJT, Ritter MA (1969) Tissue interaction in the development of thymus lymphocytes. J Exp Med 129:431–442

Parish WE (1970) Short-term anaphylactic IgG antibodies in human sera. Lancet 2:591–592

Parish WE (1971) Detection of reagin and short-term sensitizing anaphylactic or anaphylactoid antibodies to milk in sera of allergic and normal persons. Clin Allergy 1:369–380

Parker CW, de Weck AL, Kern M, Eisen HN (1962a) The preparation and some properties of penicillenic acid derivatives relevant to penicillin hypersensitivity. J Exp Med 115:803–819

Parker CW, Kern M, Eisen HN (1962b) Hypersensitivity to penicillenic acid derivatives in humans with penicillin allergy. J Exp Med 115:821

Parker D, Aoki T, Turk JL (1970) Studies on the ability of the soluble proteins from skin, painted in vivo with DNFB, to cause contact sensitivity in the guinea pig. Int Arch Allergy Appl Immunol 38:42–56

Parkhouse RME, Dutton RW (1967) The effect of physical and chemical modifications on antigen in the secondary response in vitro. Immunochemistry 4:431–439

Paul WE, Stupp Y, Siskind GW, Benacerraf B (1971) Structural control of immunogenicity. IV. Relative specificity of elicitation of cellular immune responses and of ligand binding to anti-hapten antibody after immunization with mono-ε-DNP-nona-L-lysine. Immunology 21:605–616

Perey DYE, Cooper MD, Good RA (1968) Lymphoepithelial tissues of the intestine and differentiation of antibody production. Science 161:265–266

Plescia OJ, Braun W, Palczuk NC (1964) Production of antibodies to denatured deoxyribonucleic acid (DNA). Proc Natl Acad Sci USA 54:1281–1285

Plescia OJ, Palczuk NC, Cora-Figueroa E, Mukherjee A, Braun W (1965 a) Production of antibodies to soluble RNA. Proc Natl Acad Sci USA 54:1281–1285

Plescia OJ, Palczuk NC, Braun W, Cora-Figueroa E (1965 b) Antibodies to DNA and a synthetic polydecaribonucleotide produced by oligodeoxyribonucleotides. Science 148:1102–1103

Polak L, Frey JR (1973) Studies on contact hypersensitivity to chromium in the guinea pig. Int Arch Allergy Appl Immunol 44:51–61

Polak L, Turk JL, Frey JR (1973) Studies on contact hypersensitivity to chromium compounds. Prog Allergy 17:145–226

Poole RJ, Griffith JF, MacMillan FSK (1970) Experimental contact sensitization with benzoyl peroxide. Arch Dermatol 102:635–639

Pressman D, Grossberg AL (1968) The structural basis of antibody specificity. Benjamin, New York

Pressman D, Siegel M (1953) The steric configuration of β-benzoylpropionate ion in aqueous solution as determined by immunochemical means. J Am Chem Soc 75:1376–1379

Rajewsky K, Schirrmacher V, Nase S, Jerne NK (1969) The requirement of more than one antigenic determinant for immunogenicity. J Exp Med 129:1131–1143

Richter AW, Ryde EM, Zetterström EO (1979) Non-immunogenicity of a purified sodium hyaluronidate preparation in man. Int Arch Allergy Appl Immunol 59:45–48

Rubin B (1972) Studies on the induction of antibody synthesis against sulfanilic acid in rabbits. I. Effect of the number of hapten molecules introduced in homologous protein on antibody synthesis against the hapten and the new antigenic determinants. Eur J Immunol 2:5–11

Rubin B, Aasted B (1973) Characterization of new antigenic determinants introduced into homologous serum albumin by dinitrophenylation and sulphanylation. Immunology 25:399–408

Samitz MH, Katz S, Scheiner DM, Gross PR (1969) Chromium-protein interactions. Acta Derm Venereol (Stockh) 49:142–146

Schäker W, Sterba G, Ambrosius H (1967) Der immunologische Nachweis von Isoleucin[3]-Leucin[8]-Oxytocin nach Immunisierung mit einem Oxytocin-Carboxymethyldextran-Komplex. Pfluegers Arch 297:166–173

Schechter B, Schechter I, Sela M (1970) Antibody combining sites to a series of peptide determinants of increasing size and defined structure. J Biol Chem 245:1438–1447

Schimpl A, Wecker E (1972) Replacement of T cell function by a T cell product. Nature New Biol 273:15–17

Schlossman SF, Levine H (1967) Immunochemical studies on delayed and arthus-type hypersensitivity reactions. I. The relationship between antigenic determinant size and antibody combining site size. J Immunol 98:211–219

Schlossman SF, Yaron A, Ben-Efraim S, Sober HA (1965) Immunogenicity of a series of ,N-DNP-L-lysines. Biochemistry 4:1638–1645

Schlossmann SF, Levine H, Yarou A (1968) Studies on the specificity of antibody to 2,4-dinitrophenyl-poly-L-lysines. Biochemistry 7:1–7

Schneider CH, de Weck AL (1967) The reaction of benzylpenicillin with carbohydrates at neutral pH with a note on the immunogenicity of hapten polysaccharide conjugates. Immunochemistry 4:331–343

Schneider CH, de Weck AL (1968) Studies on the direct neutral penicilloylation of functional groups occurring on proteins. Biochim Biophys Acta 168:27–35

Schneider CH, de Weck AL (1970) Antigenfunktion und Molekularstruktur. Chimia 24:10–12

Schneider CH, Michl J, de Weck AL (1971a) Zur Antigenität von Hapten-Polysaccharid-Konjugaten. Eur J Immunol 1:98–106

Schneider CH, de Weck AL, Stäuble E (1971b) Carboxymethyl cellulose additives in penicillins and the elicitation of anaphylactic reactions. Experientia 27:167–168

Schneider CH, de Weck AL, Schenkel E, Wirz W, Lazary S (1972) Immunogenicity of fully defined lysine LAG dodecapeptides in guinea pigs with a note on an antigenic cooperation effect in the delayed immune response. Immunology 23:911–920

Schneider CH, Otz U, Gruden E (1978) Induction of immunological tolerance to the penicilloyl antigenic determinant. II. Evaluation of stable and unstable penicilloyl dextrans. Eur J Immunol 8:410–414

Schneider CH, Gruden E, Wälti M, Toffler O, de Weck AL, Jost R (1979) Monovalent elicitation of passive cutaneous anaphylaxis by N^1-DNCP-N^6BPO-diaminohexane. Mol Immunol 16:269–279

Sela M (1969) Antigenicity: some molecular aspects. Science 166:1365–1374

Sela M, Arnon R (1960) Studies on the chemical basis of the antigenicity of proteins. 1. Antigenicity of polypeptidyl gelatins. Biochem J 75:91–102

Sela M, Fuchs S (1963) A synthetic polypeptide antigen devoid of charge. Biochim Biophys Acta 74:796–798

Sela M, Fuchs S, Arnon R (1962) Studies on the chemical basis of the antigenicity of proteins 5. Synthesis, characterization and immunogenicity of some multichain and linear polypeptides containing lysine. Biochem J 85:223–235

Sela M, Mozes E, Shearer GM (1972) Thymus-independence of slowly metabolized immunogens. Proc Natl Acad Sci USA 69:2696–2700

Senyk G, Nitecki DE, Goodman JW (1971a) Immunogenicity of glucagon. Determinants responsible for antibody binding and lymphocyte stimulation. Science 171:407–408

Senyk G, Williams EB, Nitecki DE, Goodman JW (1971b) The functional dissection of an antigen molecule. Specificity of humoral and cellular responses to glucagon. J Exp Med 133:1294–1308

Senyk G, Nitecki DE, Spitler L, Goodman JW (1972) The immune response to glucagon in conjugated form. Immunochemistry 9:97–110

Shearer GM (1974) Cell mediated cytotoxicity to trinitrophenyl modified syngeneic lymphocytes. Eur J Immunol 4:527–533

Shearer GM, Rhen TG, Garbarino CA (1975) Cell mediated lympholysis of trinitrophenyl modified autologous lymphocytes. Effector cell specificity to modified cell surface components controlled by the H-2K and H-2D serological regions of the murine major histocompatibility complex. J Exp Med 141:1348–1364

Shortman K, Palmer J (1971) The requirement for macrophages in the in vitro immune response. Cell Immunol 2:399–410

Singer SJ (1964) On the heterogeneity of anti-hapten antibodies. Immunochemistry 1:15–20

Soeberg B, Sumerska T, Binns RM, Balfour BM (1978a) Contact sensitivity in the pig. II. Induction by intralymphatic infusion of DNP-conjugated cells. Int Arch Allergy Appl Immunol 57:114–125

Soeberg B, Sumerska T, Binns RM, Balfour BM (1978b) Contact sensitivity in the pig. III. Induction by intralymphatic infusion of DNP-conjugated cell membranes and soluble proteins, free DNFB and some small molecular weight derivatives. Int Arch Allergy Appl Immunol 57:481–487

Sprent J (1978) Role of the H-2 complex in induction of T helper cells in vivo. J Exp Med 148:478–489

Steiner LA, Eisen HN (1967) Sequential changes in the relative affinity of antibodies synthesized during the immune response. J Exp Med 126:1161–1183

Stryer L, Griffith OH (1965) Aspin-labeled hapten. Proc Natl Acad Sci USA 54:1785–1791

Stupp Y, Paul WE, Benacerraf B (1971a) Structural control of immunogenicity. II. Antibody synthesis and cellular immunity in response to immunization with mono-ε-oligo-L-lysines. Immunology 21:583–594

Stupp Y, Paul WE, Benacerraf B (1971 b) Structural control of immunogenicity III. Preparation for and elicitation of anamnestic antibody responses by oligo- and poly-lysines and their DNP derivatives. Immunology 21:595–603

Sulzberger MB, Baer RL (1938) Sensitization to simple chemicals. III. Relationship between chemical structure and properties, and sensitizing capacities in the production of eczematous sensitivity in man. J Invest Dermatol 1:45–58

Tada T (1975) Regulation of reaginic antibody formation in animals. Prog Allergy 19:122–194

Takatsu K, Ishizaka K (1975) Regulation of anti-ovalbumin (OA) IgE and IgG antibody responses in the mouse by administration of urea-denatured OH. Fed Proc Fed Am Soc Exp Biol 34:1000

Tyan ML, McDevitt HO, Herzenberg LA (1969) Genetic control of the antibody response to a synthetic polypeptide. Transfer of response with spleen cells or lymphoid precursors. Transplant Proc 1:548–560

Unanue ER (1970) Thymus dependency of the immune response to hemocyanin: an evaluation of the role of macrophages in thymectomized mice. J Immunol 105:1339–1343

Unanue ER, Cerottini JC (1970) The immunogenicity of antigen bound to the plasma membrane of macrophages. J Exp Med 131:711–725

van Vunakis H, Kaplan J, Lehrer H, Levine L (1966) Immunogenicity of polylysine and polyornithine when complexed to phosphorylated bovine serum albumin. Immunochemistry 3:393–402

Vaz NM, Levine BB (1970) Immune responses of inbred mice to repeated low doeses of antigen: relationship of histocompatibility (H-2) type. Science 168:852–856

Vaz NM, Phillips-Quagliata JM, Levine BB, Baz EM (1971) H-2-linked genetic control of immune responsiveness to ovalbumin and ovomucoid. J Exp Med 134:1335–1348

Velick SF, Parker CW, Eisen HN (1960) Excitation energy transfer and the quantitative study of the antibody hapten reaction. Proc Natl Acad Sci USA 46:1470–1482

Waldmann H (1975) T cell dependent mediator in the immune response III. The role of nonspecific factor (NSF) in the in vitro immune response. Immunology 28:497–507

Woods V, Nitecki DE, Goodman JW (1975) The capacity of bifunctional antigens to bridge antibody molecules and to mediate cell cooperation. Immunochemistry 12:379–382

Wright RN, Rothberg RM (1971) The reactions of pepsin-trypsin digestion products of bovine serum albumin with antisera from rabbits ingesting this protein. J Immunol 107:1410–1418

Wu AM, Till JE, Siminovitch L, McCulloch EA (1967) A cytological study of the capacity for differentiation of normal hemopoietic colony-forming cells. J Cell Physiol 69:177–184

Yamashita U, Shevach EM (1978) The histocompatibility restrictions on macrophage T-helper cell interaction determine the histocompatibility restrictions on T-helper cell B-cell interaction. J Exp Med 148:1171–1185

Zalc B, Jacque C, Radin NS, Duponey P (1977) Immunogenicity of sulfatide. Immunochemistry 14:775–779

Zalc B, Duponey P, Coulon-Morelec MJ, Baumann NA (1979) Immunogenic properties of glucosylceramide. Mol Immunol 16:297–300

CHAPTER 2

Chemical and Pharmaceutical Aspects of Drug Allergy

H. Bundgaard

A. Introduction: Routes of Formation of Drug Antigens

Generally, a low molecular weight compound is incapable of constituting per se a sensitizing antigen. In order to induce an immune response, a low molecular weight chemical must first bind irreversibly, i.e., covalently, to a large carrier molecule, e.g., tissue proteins such as serum proteins or cell membrane proteins (Eisen 1959; Levine 1968; de Weck 1971 a). Most drugs are of low molecular weight (< 500–1,000 daltons), and an explanation of the immunochemical mechanisms underlying the allergic reactions produced by several of such drugs must accordingly be based on the "irreversible binding theory." The arguments which have been advanced during the last few years to establish this concept are summarized in Chap. 1.

However, most allergenic drugs do not react, or cannot be demonstrated in vitro to react covalently with proteins, and in such cases it seems reasonable to postulate that metabolites, in vitro degradation products, or synthesis impurities present in the clinical drug preparations may be the chemically reactive agents (proantigens) responsible for immunogenicity. These various possibilities of formation of the complete immunogens are depicted in Fig. 1.

The only drugs which in fact have been shown to be capable of reacting covalently with proteins in vitro and for which such conjugation reactions in vivo appear to be of marked immunologic significance are the β-lactam antibiotics, penicillins and cephalosporins (for a recent review, see Dewdney 1977).

In recent years, a number of drugs have been shown to undergo biotransformation with the production of chemically highly reactive metabolites which are capable of combining covalently with proteins or other tissue macromolecules in the body. For example, chemically reactive metabolites can be formed from aromatic amines by N-hydroxylation and subsequent formation of glucuronate, sulfate, or phosphate esters (Weisburger and Weisburger 1973). The metabolic conversion of aromatic compounds into phenols and the hydroxylation of carbon–carbon double bonds in other compounds have in several cases been shown to proceed through an intermediate formation of epoxides (e.g., Daly et al. 1972; Jerina and Daly 1974; Mitchell et al. 1975). In particular, aromatic epoxides (arene oxides) are extremely reactive agents, being capable of alkylating various nucleophiles including functional nucleophilic groups in proteins (Fig. 2; Jerina et al. 1973; Bruice and Bruice 1976). The metabolic hydroxylation of several drugs has been shown to involve an intermediate formation of epoxides, for example diethylstilbestrol (Metzler 1975), glutethimide (Stillwell et al. 1973), imipramine (Kap-

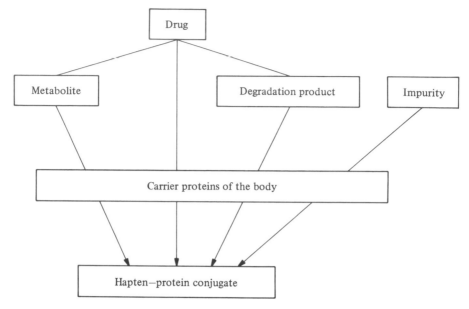

Fig. 1. Various possibilities of formation of hapten–protein conjugates in vivo

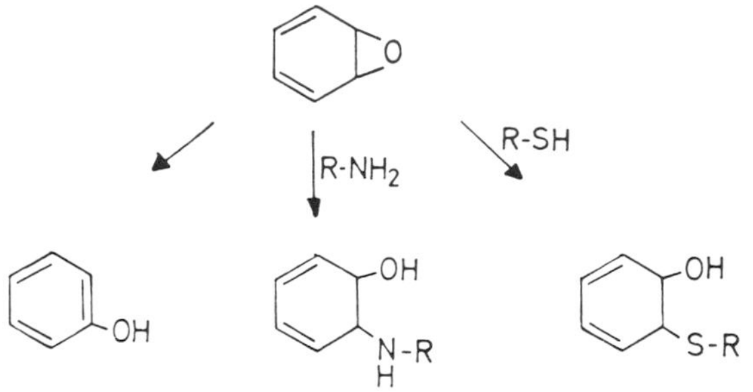

Fig. 2. Reactions of arene oxides. Spontaneous aromatization into phenols and nucleophilic addition reactions by amines and thiols

PUS and REMMER 1975), acetanilide (GRANTHAM et al. 1974), and furosemide (MITCHELL et al. 1976). Therefore, it is tempting to speculate that such metabolites or other protein-reactive metabolites formed by oxidative metabolism as, for example, quinones (e.g., from rifampicin, BOLT and REMMER 1976), methyldopa (SAS-SETTI and FUDENBERG 1971; GOTTLIEB and WURZEL 1974), or quinone imines (e.g., from paracetamol, MITCHELL et al. 1975) constitute the pro-antigens involved in several drug-induced allergic reactions. Immunochemical studies along this line are largely absent, but are certainly warranted.

In the last few years, the problem of impurities in drug preparations and their role in drug allergy has received increasing attention. Since microgram quantities of antigen often suffice to induce an immunologic response, and since many drugs are given therapeutically in gram amounts, it is apparent that the hapten–protein conjugate presumably involved in an allergic reaction may well be formed from a chemically reactive contaminant present in only trace amounts in the drug formulations. Among immunologically active substances, which may be present as contaminants of drug preparations, the following three types are distinguishable (BUNDGAARD 1977c):

1. Low molecular weight chemicals which are chemically reactive with proteins (pro-antigens);
2. Antigenic divalent and multivalent conjugates per se, formed by polymerization of the drug or by chemical reactions between the drug and a pharmaceutical adjuvant or an additive;
3. High molecular weight substances which are immunogenic and antigenic per se.

Whereas the sensitization of an organism nearly always requires an antigen of a certain macromolecular character, the elicitation of reactions in an already sensitized organism requires no macromolecular antigen. Instead, an eliciting antigen should be at least divalent, i.e., carry at least two antigenic determinants or haptenic groups on each molecule (DE WECK 1974). The second type of contaminants refers to substances fulfilling this requirement.

In the following, specific examples of contaminants of these three types are described along with aspects of the formulation, manufacture, and storage of drug preparations, which may be of importance for the formation of antigenic products. The main part of the presentation is devoted to penicillins, owing to the fact that penicillin allergy, an important therapeutic problem, has been the subject of extensive immunochemical and immunologi studies by several investigators.

B. Immunologically Active Macromolecular Contaminants of Penicillins

About a decade ago, British investigators observed the presence of small amounts of immunologically active high molecular weight materials in commercial benzylpenicillin and 6-aminopenicillanic acid (6-APA) (BATCHELOR et al. 1967; STEWART 1967; KNUDSEN et al. 1967; WESTON 1968). The contaminant was isolated by gel filtration and dialysis and was shown to be of proteinaceous nature, to carry benzylpenicilloyl groups, and to be a potent penicilloyl-specific immunogen and antigen. Such impurities were consequently suggested by these investigators to be the cause of, or at least contribute to, allergic reactions of benzylpenicillin. Since they occur in very minute amounts, their importance for the development of reactions has been questioned by some investigators (DE WECK et al. 1968; OTTENS et al. 1971; WALSH et al. 1971) and their role in penicillin allergy has been a controversial topic for a long time.

The protein contaminants in benzylpenicillin derive from the fermentation manufacturing processes used in production of the antibiotic. During the course of fermentation, proteins of the medium become penicilloylated and may be extracted in minute amounts into the final preparations. The semisynthetic penicillins are prepared from 6-APA, which in turn is obtained through either enzymatic or chemical removal of the side chain in benzylpenicillin (CARRINGTON 1971). Penicilloylated proteins originating from the enzymes or from the original benzylpenicillin may then appear in the final semisynthetic penicillin preparations.

The amounts of penicilloylated proteins in commercial benzylpenicillin and semisynthetic penicillins seem to vary considerably. Whereas up to 200–300 parts/10^6 of penicilloyl-protein in benzylpenicillin preparations were reported by BATCHELOR et al. (1967) and also by BUTCHER and STEWART (1970), other groups have only detected less than 10 parts/10^6 of proteinaceous impurities in commercial benzylpenicillin (DÜRSCH 1968; PREUD'HOMME and LUNEL 1969; WEIDENMÜLLER and ZIEGLER 1970; WALSH et al. 1971; OTTENS et al. 1971; VILIM et al. 1976). As described by OTTENS et al. (1971), the methods used for the determinations, i.e., dialysis, membrane filtration, and gel filtration followed by penicilloyl and protein analysis, have several drawbacks. Penicillin degradation products and polymers were found to influence the determinations, making these somewhat unreliable.

SCHNEIDER and DE WECK (1970) have reported a different approach to evaluate the immunologic significance of penicilloyl-protein contaminants in penicillin preparations. By subjecting the preparations to mild hydrolysis, the penicillin molecule looses its penicilloylating capacity and thus its ability to conjugate with proteins in vivo, whereas the contaminants remain unchanged. Measuring the immunogenicity of the sample before and after such treatment would then give an estimate of the overall immunogenicity of the sample and of the contaminants. By applying the method to some commercial benzylpenicillin and phenoxymethylpenicillin preparations, it was found that the penicilloyl-specific immunogenicity of the preparations was largely due to the intact penicillin molecules, since the selective hydrolytic treatment reduced the immunogenicity of the preparations considerably, although the effect was not completely abolished.

The presence of protein in ampicillin has been shown to have a significant effect upon the immunogenicity of the antibiotic (KNUDSEN et al. 1970). Removal of protein markedly reduced the immunogenicity as well as the antigenicity. Immunogenicity was, however, not completely abolished and low levels of antibody were detected in the rabbits used in the immunization experiments. A similar reduction in immunogenicity and antigenicity of ampicillin preparations (and 6-APA preparations) by reduction of protein levels was shown by SHALTIEL et al. (1970, 1971).

Results recently obtained by AHLSTEDT, KRISTOFFERSON, and co-workers at Astra Pharmaceuticals in Sweden are of considerable interest. These investigators have developed a sensitive and reproducible radioimmunoassay for the determination of high molecular weight penicilloylated protein impurities in penicillin preparations (KRISTOFFERSON et al. 1977a; KRISTOFFERSON 1979). The method requires prior isolation by gel filtration of the impurities and enables the determination of penicilloylated protein in various penicillins in concentrations less than 1 part/10^6. Since the radioimmunoassay, in contrast to methods previously used, takes into account the antigenic activity of penicilloylated impurities, it may directly reveal the immunogenic potency of the high molecular weight impurities present in penicillin preparations (KRISTOFFERSON et al. 1977b). On applying the method to 60 commercially available ampicillin preparations, the presence in all of them of penicilloylated protein impurities was demonstrated (AHLSTEDT et al. 1979). The quality of the preparations differed markedly, some batches being of high purity and others very contaminated. In contrast to the findings of OTTENS et al. (1971), the results did not reveal that ampicillin prepared from 6-APA obtained by chemical side chain cleavage of benzylpenicillin was less contaminated than ampicillin preparations made from 6-APA obtained via enzymatic cleavage of the benzylpenicillin. The levels of impurities in most of the contaminated preparations corresponded to 1–3 parts/10^6.

Although these amounts of impurities recorded are low, they were shown to influence the immunogenicity of the ampicillin preparations to a significant degree (AHLSTEDT et al. 1979). The immunogenic potency of a pure and a representative contaminated ampicillin preparation was investigated by treating mice subcutaneously with the preparations according to a schedule simulating the therapeutic use of penicillin. Whereas considerable antibody formation was observed in animals injected with the impure ampicillin preparation, only a very weak antibody response was recorded after treatment with ampicillin of high purity. It has further been found (KRISTOFFERSON 1979) that pure ampicillin preparations experimentally contaminated with 3–15 µg of a penicilloyl bovine gamma-globulin conjugate per g ampicillin, but not the pure preparation itself, induced the formation of penicilloyl-specific IgE, IgG, and IgM antibodies in mice treated repeatedly for 10-day periods.

Further support to the concept that the penicilloylated protein impurities in the penicillin preparations are the main causates of penicillin allergy is that the administration of a penicilloylated foreign protein would be expected to stimulate a greater immunologic response than a penicilloylated autologous protein. The protein impurities are heavily penicilloyl substituted owing to the large excess of penicillin during manufacturing, whereas penicilloylated autologous proteins formed in vivo may be assumed to be only lightly substituted and therefore less immunogenic (KRISTOFFERSON et al. 1977 b).

The conclusion reached by these investigators, that pure penicillin alone does not induce any penicilloyl-specific antibody formation when administered to mice in a schedule simulating clinical use of penicillins, contrasts with the results of other groups, indicating that the bulk of the penicilloyl-specific immunogenicity is due to penicilloylation of proteins or other macromolecular carriers in vivo (DE WECK et al. 1968; SCHNEIDER and DE WECK 1970; SCHNEIDER 1970). Obviously, further studies are needed to clarify this important question. In any case, it seems obvious that minute amounts of penicilloyl-protein impurities can be present in clinically used penicillin preparations and that they are of significant immunogenic potency. These impurities should therefore preferably be removed from clinically used penicillins. With the development of the sensitive and specific radioimmunoassay for penicilloylated high molecular weight impurities, it has become possible to control and establish the purity of the preparations.

C. Polymerization of β-Lactam Antibiotics

I. Penicillin Polymers

In 1967 BATCHELOR et al. (1967) described the formation of a higher molecular weight substance in concentrated aqueous solutions of benzylpenicillin when they were left to stand for a short time at room temperature. The substance was shown to derive from the penicillin molecule and found to be antigenic in the guinea pig passive cutaneous anaphylaxis test, using rabbit antiserum raised to benzylpenicil-loylated proteins. Antigenic polymerization products were also shown to be formed upon leaving aqueous solutions of 6-APA to stand, and the structures of these products were thought to be similar to that of a linear polymer comprising 7–8 units of 6-APA isolated by GRANT et al. (1962) some years ago from an aged neutral aqueous solution of 6-APA.

Since these observations of BATCHELOR and co-workers, a large amount of work has been concerned with polymerization of penicillins and 6-APA and con-siderable knowledge of the chemical structure, rate and mechanism of formation, and the immunologic properties of penicillin polymers has been obtained.

1. Formation and Structure of Polymers

It has been demonstrated by various groups that storage at room temperature of concentrated aqueous solutions of benzylpenicillin, phenoxymethylpenicillin, 6-APA, and a number of semisynthetic penicillins (ampicillin, methicillin, pheneticil-lin, and carbenicillin) leads to the formation of higher molecular weight (1,000–5,000 daltons) substances, socalled penicillin polymers (BATCHELOR et al. 1967; DE WECK et al. 1968; STEWART 1968, 1969; BUTCHER and STEWART 1969, 1970; GRANT 1970; SMITH and MARSHALL 1971; DEWDNEY et al. 1971; SMITH et al. 1971; SHAL-TIEL et al. 1971; KUCHINSKAS and LEVY 1982; BUNDGAARD 1974b; BUNDGAARD and LARSEN 1977; LARSEN and BUNDGAARD 1977; 1978a). The generally used methods for detection and isolation of these polymerization products have been dialysis, ul-trafiltration, or gel chromatography of the penicillin solutions, followed by chemi-cal and physicochemical characterization of dialysis retentate, ultrafiltrate, or chromatographic fractions, respectively. With respect to the mechanism of forma-tion of polymers and hence with respect to the structure of the polymers, it is ap-propriate to divide the penicillins into two classes, those containing an amino group in the side chain (e.g., ampicillin) and those penicillins without such a side chain group.

a) Benzylpenicillin

For benzylpenicillin and other penicillins without an amino group in the side chain, the polymerization is thought to be initiated by a reaction between the primary degradation products, penicillenic acid and penicilloic acid (STEWART et al. 1970). By spontaneous hydrolysis of the β-lactam bond in the penicillin, the correspond-ing penicilloic acid is formed. This results in a decrease of the pH of the penicillin solution (provided the solution is not effectively buffered) and hence an accelerated formation of penicillenic acid (SCHWARTZ and WU 1966; DE WECK et al. 1968; BUNDGAARD 1971, 1980a; BUTLER et al. 1972; DUDLEY et al. 1974). Penicillenic acid is a strong acylating agent and may certainly be capable of penicilloylating the sec-ondary amino group in penicilloic acid, with the formation of a penicillin dimer (Fig. 3). This amino group possesses a pK_a value of 5.2 (FAZAKERLEY et al. 1976) and therefore, it will to a large extent occur in the reactive unprotonated form in the partially degraded penicillin solutions. Direct penicilloylation of the

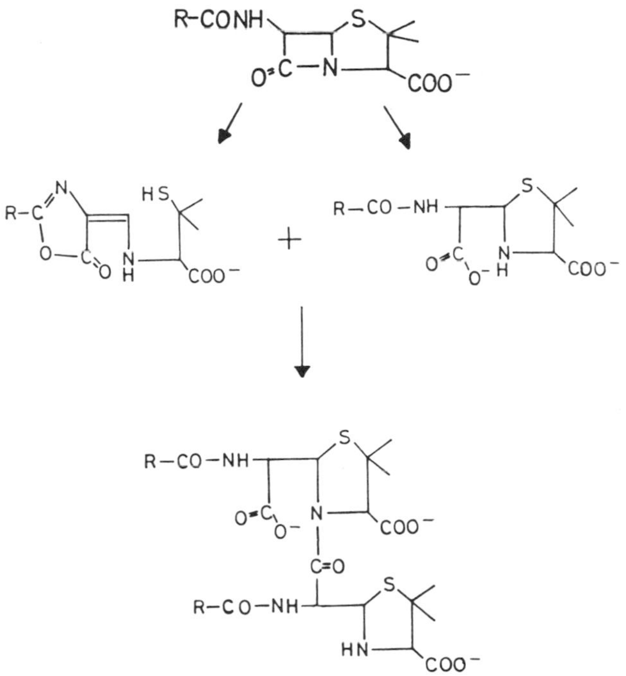

Fig. 3. Dimerization of benzylpenicillin ($R=$benzyl) via reactions between the degradation products benzylpenicillenic acid and benzylpenicilloic acid

thiazolidine nitrogen in penicilloic acid by penicillin itself would also result in the formation of dimer shown in Fig. 3, but this is a less effective process than penicilloylation by the more reactive penicillenic acid. Similar penicilloylation of the thiazolidine nitrogen atom in the dimer by another molecule of penicillenic acid results in the formation of a trimer which can undergo further N-penicilloylation. Such a series of reactions would lead to the formation of products of the general structure shown in Fig. 4. Experimental support for this structure has been provided by SMITH and MARSHALL (1971). By gel chromatography of 14-day-old aqueous solutions of benzylpenicillin sodium (25% W/V), polymeric substances with analytic data agreeing with the given structure ($n=1.5$) were isolated. The isolated polymers amounted to 0.8% and the pH of the penicillin solution had dropped from 7 to 5. In a similar way, AHLSTEDT et al. (1976) and MUNRO et al. (1976) have isolated polymers with a mean chain length of 5–11 units.

SMITH et al. (1971) have determined the amount of polymers (i.e., substances which elute in the higher molecular weight range on Sephadex G-25 gel chromatography) formed in aqueous solutions (25% W/V) of a number of penicillins stored at room temperature. The solutions were not buffered. The results obtained are shown in Table 1. In another study, these investigators (DEWDNEY et al. 1971) have demonstrated that the amounts of polymers formed in a 25% W/V solution of benzylpenicillin sodium are greatly reduced if a phosphate buffer (pH 7.5) is included in the solution. A similar observation has also been made by DE WECK et al. (1968) in the case of a 10% W/V penicillin solution. This reduction in polymerization

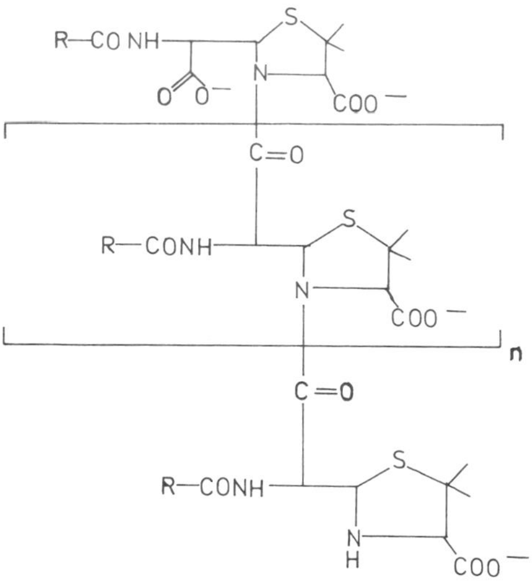

Fig. 4. Chemical structure of benzylpenicillin polymers (R = benzyl)

Table 1. Penicilloyl-specific antigenicity and amounts of penicillin polymers formed in aqueous solutions of some penicillins after standing for 14 days at room temperature. (SMITH et al. 1971)

Penicillin (sodium salts; 25% W/V)	Polymers (%)	Antigenicity (μg)[a]
Benzylpenicillin	4	10
Carbenicillin	8	1
6-APA	9	0.001
Ampicillin	12.4	0.03
Hetacillin	8	0.1

[a] Minimum amount of polymer required to elicit a passive cutaneous anaphylaxis reaction

through keeping the pH in the range 7–7.5 is in accordance with the postulated mechanism for the polymerization, since penicillenic acid is formed only very slowly at neutral pH.

More detailed investigations of the rate and factors affecting the rate of dimerization and polymerization of benzylpenicillin and similar penicillins remain to be carried out.

b) Aminopenicillins

SMITH and MARSHALL (1971) have also investigated the structure of polymers formed in aqueous solutions of 6-APA and ampicillin. From 14-day-old 25% W/V solutions of the sodium salts of these compounds 1.6% (ampicillin) and 3.4% (6-APA) of polymeric substances were isolated. The analytic data for the ampicillin polymer ($n = 4.1$) were reported to be consistent with the structure suggested by

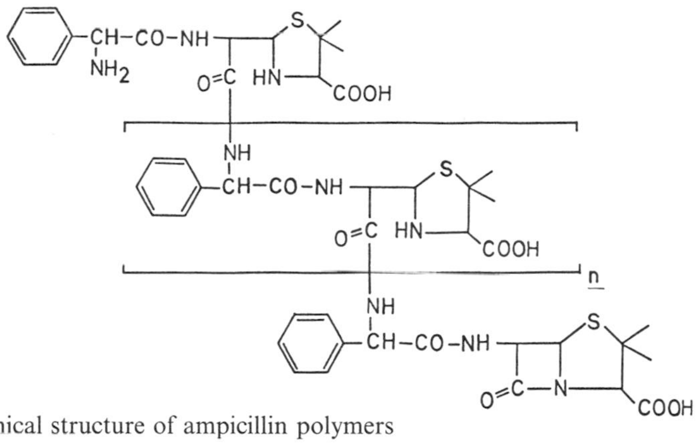

Fig. 5. Chemical structure of ampicillin polymers

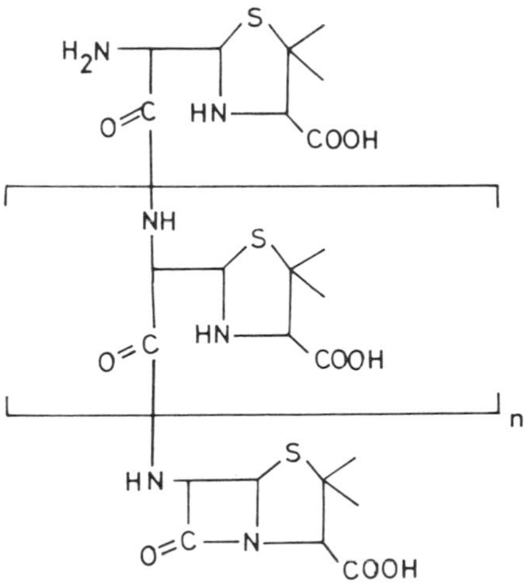

Fig. 6. Chemical structure of 6-APA polymers

GRANT (1970) shown in Fig. 5 and those for the 6-APA polymer ($n=2.7$) with the structure previously proposed by GRANT et al. (1962) shown in Fig. 6. The isolated polymers were mixtures which contained products both with an intact β-lactam ring and a hydrolyzed ring in the terminal non-amino units. The depicted structure has been supported by other workers (BUTCHER et al. 1971; KUCHINSKAS and LEVY 1972; BUNDGAARD 1967 a) and was conclusively confirmed by recent investigations in this laboratory (BUNDGAARD and LARSEN 1977). In this study, polymeric substances formed from ampicillin sodium in aqueous solution were separated according to charge by anion exchange chromatography using a linear salt gradient at a constant pH of 7.4. Homogeneous well-defined ampicillin dimer, tetramer, and hexamer were isolated from the effluent in high yields and were characterized by various functional group analyses. Figure 7 shows the elution patterns of a 20% W/V aqueous ampicillin sodium solution kept at room temperature for various times. Why polymers with an even degree of polymerization, e.g., dimer, tetramer,

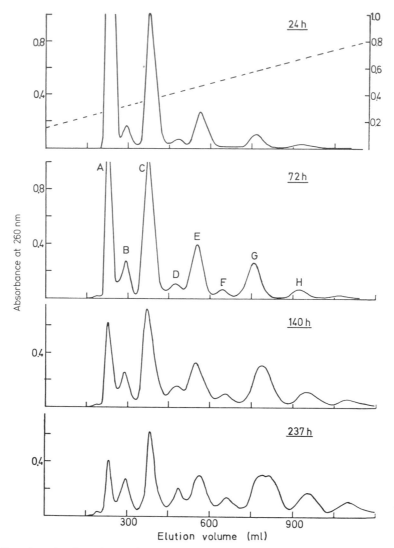

Fig. 7. Fractionation by anion exchange chromatography of 1 ml portions of a 20% aqueous solution of ampicillin sodium (initial pH 8.5) kept at 22 °C for the specified periods. The DEAE-Sephadex A-25 column was eluted with 0.05 M phosphate (pH 7.4), with a linear sodium chloride gradient. Peak identities: A, ampicillin; B, α-aminobenzylpenicilloic acid; C, dimer; D, mixture of a trimer having a closed β-lactam ring and a dimer having an open β-lactam ring; E, tetramer; F, mixture of a tetramer having an open β-lactam ring and a pentamer with an intact β-lactam ring; G, hexamer; H, octamer. (BUNDGAARD and LARSEN 1977)

appear to be formed to a much larger extent than polymers composed of an uneven number of monomeric units remains unexplained.

On the basis of the established structure of ampicillin polymers and from kinetic investigations of the decomposition of ampicillin in aqueous solution, including an examination of the influence of pH and ampicillin concentration on the

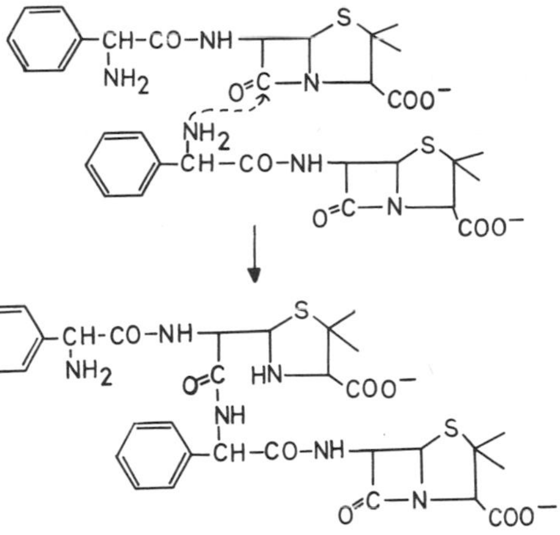

Fig. 8. Dimerization of ampicillin by auto-aminolysis

degradation rate (BUNDGAARD 1976a), it can be stated that the polymerization of ampicillin starts with a reaction involving nucleophilic attack of the amino group of the side chain in one ampicillin molecule on the reactive β-lactam moiety of a second molecule (auto-aminolysis; Fig. 8). A similar aminolysis may also be considered to initiative the polymerization of 6-APA. The dimeric substance formed, which in the case of ampicillin has been isolated by BUNDGAARD and LARSEN (1977) and in the case of 6-APA by DENNEN (1967), can then react with another penicillin molecule or with a second dimer in various ways with the formation of a trimer or tetramer:

$$A–NH_2 + Di–lactam \rightarrow Tri$$
$$A–lactam + Di–NH_2 \rightarrow Tri$$
$$Di–lactam + Di–NH_2 \rightarrow Tet$$

where A is aminopenicillin, Di is dimer, Tri is trimer, and Tet is tetramer. Through similar aminolysis reactions higher polymers may be formed.

In order to obtain a knowledge of factors influencing the rate of formation of dimeric and polymeric substances, a study of the kinetics and mechanism of dimerization of ampicillin in aqueous solutions has been made (BUNDGAARD 1976a). The rate of ampicillin dimer formation in the pH range 7–9 was found to follow the equation:

$$\frac{d[Di]}{dt} = k_1[A^-][A]_T + k_2[A^-]^2[A]_T + k_3[A^-][AH^\pm][A]_T \qquad (1)$$

where [Di] is the concentration of dimer, $[A]_T$ is the total molar ampicillin concentration, $[A^-]$ is the concentration of anionic ampicillin, and $[AH^\pm]$ is the concentration of zwitterionic ampicillin (i.e., $[A]_T = [A^-] + [AH^\pm]$). The individual rate constants in Eq. (1) have the following designations: k_1, unassisted or water-assisted nucleophilic attack of the unprotonated side chain amino group in one ampicillin molecule on the β-lactam carbonyl moiety of another molecule (Fig. 8); k_2,

Table 2. Rate constants for the dimerization of aminopenicillins in aqueous solution at 35 °C and ionic strength 1.0. (BUNDGAARD 1977b)

Penicillin	k_1 $(M^{-1}h^{-1})$	k_2 $(M^{-2}h^{-1})$	k_3 $(M^{-2}h^{-1})$
Ampicillin	0.039	0.16	0.81
Epicillin	0.066	0.29	0.65
Cyclacillin	≤ 0.002	≤ 0.008	≤ 0.04
Amoxycillin[a]	0.09	0.4	
	0.5	2.0	
		1.6	

[a] The various rate constants refer to reactions of the different ionic species of amoxycillin

aminolysis assisted by neutral side chain amino groups in molecules other than the attacked one and the attacking ones (general base catalysis of aminolysis); and k_3, aminolysis assisted by protonated side chain amino groups (general acid catalysis of aminolysis). The values obtained for k_1, k_2, and k_3 at 35 °C and ionic strength 1.0 are listed in Table 2.

As can be seen from Eq. (1), the rate of dimerization shows both a second-order and a third-order dependence upon ampicillin concentration. This means that the rate increases very strongly with increasing initial ampicillin concentration. On the basis of Eq. (1) and the values of the rate constants, the dependence of the rate of dimerization upon pH has been calculated. The results, given in Fig. 9, show that the rate is almost independent of pH at values greater than 7, but decreases strongly with decreasing pH at pH < 7.

Using a sensitive high performance liquid chromatographic (HPLC) procedure, which enables separation and simultaneous quantitation of ampicillin and the individual polymers from the dimer to the octamer (LARSEN and BUNDGAARD 1978 a) an investigation of the time courses of formation of dimers and polymers in aqueous solutions of ampicillin sodium over a broad range of initial ampicillin concentration has been carried out (LARSEN and BUNDGAARD 1977). The solutions studied correspond to those used clinically for parenteral therapy. It was found that in 10%–20% solutions and at room temperature dimers, tetramers, and hexamers account for more than 90% of the products formed up to a total degradation of ampicillin of 20% (Table 3). It can further be seen from Table 3 that, as discussed previously, the rate of ampicillin degradation (as expressed in terms of $t_{20\%}$) and consequently the rate of dimerization, increases very strongly with increasing initial ampicillin sodium concentration, but is almost invariant with pH in the range 8.5–10.

In the studies reporting on the immunologic and especially the eliciting properties of ampicillin polymers, which are described subsequently, a mixture of polymeric materials has apparently been used and no individual dimers and polymers have yet been tested. A priori the dimer molecule should be expected to be a poor elicitor of penicilloyl-specific reactions because it contains only one penicilloyl group. In contrast, the tetramer with its three penicilloyl groups might be expected

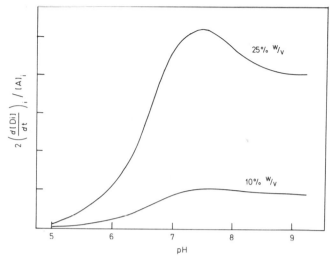

Fig. 9. Calculated effect of pH on initial rate of dimerization of ampicillin in aqueous solution at two different ampicillin concentrations. Subscript i indicates initial rates and concentrations. (BUNDGAARD 1976 a)

Table 3. Amounts of dimers and polymers formed in 20% degraded aqueous solutions of ampicillin sodium of various initial concentrations and pH values. (LARSEN and BUNDGAARD 1977)

Ampicillin sodium (% W/V)	pH initial	$t_{20\%}$[a] (h)	Dimer (% W/W)	Tetramer (% W/W)	Hexamer (% W/W)
20	10.0	4	17	2	0.5
10	9.6	13	17	3	0.2
5	9.5	20	13	1	0.1
1	9.3	41	1		
20	8.5	5	14	4	0.5
10	8.5	15	14	4	0.3
5	8.5	24	15	3	0.2
1	8.5	45	2	0.1	

[a] At 22 °C

to be quite efficient. Assuming the finding of AHLSTEDT et al. (1976), that the eliciting effect of polymers in admixture with monomeric ampicillin can be observed at a concentration of 0.1%, to be valid for the tetramer, it is possible on the basis of the results obtained by LARSEN and BUNDGAARD (1977) to calculate the time needed for the production of eliciting activity in ampicillin solutions of various concentrations. Figure 10 shows the rate of formation of tetramer in 10% and 20% W/V aqueous solutions of ampicillin sodium at room temperature. From Fig. 10 the time required to produce 0.1% W/W tetramer is found to be 0.5 h (20% W/V solution) and 1.2 h (10% W/V solution). These values are seen to be considerably

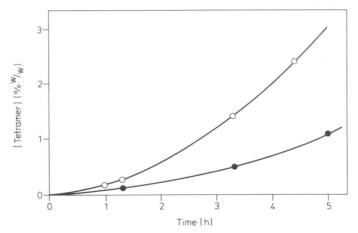

Fig. 10. Time course of formation of ampicillin tetramer in 10% (*solid circles*) and 20% W/V (*open circles*) aqueous solutions of ampicillin sodium kept at 22 °C. (LARSEN and BUNDGAARD 1977)

lower than the generally accepted utilization times, i.e., periods during which there will be less than 10% or 20% (if a 10% excess is used) loss in biologic activity, as shown in Table 3 ($t_{10\%}$ is approximately the half of $t_{20\%}$). As already pointed out by us (LARSEN and BUNDGAARD 1977), however, testing of the individual polymers in admixture with ampicillin and subsequent comparison of the data with the rate data might be a more fruitful means of obtaining more exact information about the influence of storage time on the eliciting activity of ampicillin sodium solutions. Another and more direct approach may be determination of the eliciting activity of ampicillin sodium as a function of storage time.

In an attempt to get information about structural effects influencing the tendency of aminopenicillins to polymerize, the kinetic ampicillin study by the present author has been extended to include three other clinically used aminopenicillins: epicillin, amoxycillin, and cyclacillin. These penicillins all contain a primary side chain amino group. The investigations (BUNDGAARD 1977 a, b) have shown that the dimerization of the amino-penicillins proceeds by similar mechanisms, but with rates that differ widely. For amoxycillin, however, the mechanism is somewhat more complicated as the ionized phenol group, in addition to the amino group, may exhibit general base catalysis of the aminolysis. The values of the various rate constants in the expression (Eq. 1) for the dimerization of these penicillins at 35 °C are listed in Table 2. Table 4 shows the relative order of dimerizing tendency at pH 9 and at equal penicillin concentrations. Whereas both amoxycillin and epicillin dimerize more readily than ampicillin, cyclacillin shows a strikingly low and almost undetectable tendency to dimerize and polymerize. It should be noted that several independent techniques have been used to confirm this order of rate of dimerization (BUNDGAARD 1977 b, e).

In considering structural factors influencing the rate of dimerization of amino-penicillins and possibly accounting for the observed differences in the rates, account must be taken of: (1) the susceptibility of the β-lactam moieties to attack by

Table 4. Relative rates of dimerization of some aminopenicillins in aqueous solution, pH 9.0; 35 °C; concentration range 0.05–0.6 M. (BUNDGAARD 1977b)

Side chain R	Penicillin	pK_a ($-NH_3^+$)	Relative rate of dimerization
	Ampicillin	7.04	1.0
	Epicillin	7.38	1.7
	Amoxycillin	7.33; 8.24[a]	4.2
	Cyclacillin	7.28	≤ 0.05

[a] The value 8.24 is for the protonated amino group in the amoxycillin ionic species in which the phenolic group is ionized

amines nucleophiles; (2) the basicity of the side chain amino groups; and (3) the steric location of the amino group in the side chains. With respect to the first of these factors, the four aminopenicillins were found to possess almost equal β-lactam reactivities. For the penicillins in which the α-amino groups are in similar steric positions, i.e., ampicillin, epicillin, and amoxycillin, the difference in rate of dimerization has been found to be fully accounted for by the difference in amino group basicity (given in Table 4). Finally, the greatly reduced predisposition of cyclacillin to dimerize and polymerize could most likely be ascribed to a considerable steric hindrance of the cyclohexyl amino group, making nucleophilic attack on the β-lactam bond of another molecule difficult. The amino group is bound to a tertiary carbon atom and an examination of molecular models of the aminopenicillins shows clearly that the amino group in cyclacillin is sterically much more hindered than the amino groups in the other penicillins.

In addition to being formed upon standing of ampicillin solutions, ampicillin polymers may arise during the production of the drug and its pharmaceutical prep-

Table 5. Contents of dimeric and polymeric impurities in different clinically used ampicillin formulations as determined by high performance liquid chromatography. (BUNDGAARD 1978a)

Formulation and form of ampicillin	Supplier	Dimers and polymers (% W/W)[a]						
		Dimer		Tetramer		Hexamer		Sum of dimer and polymer
		A[b]	B	A	B	A	B	
Injectable, sodium salt	I	1.6	0.6	0.9	1.8	0.2	<0.05	5.1
Injectable, sodium salt	I	1.4	0.3	0.4	2.3	0.4	<0.05	4.8
Injectable, sodium salt	II	1.0	1.3	1.7	0.3	0.1	<0.05	4.4
Injectable, sodium salt	III	1.7	1.0	1.7	3.3	0.2	0.1	5.0
Capsule, potassium salt	IV	1.0	0.3	5.4	0.7	0.1	1.0	8.5
Capsule, trihydrate	III	1.2	0.3	2.4	2.6	0.1	0.5	7.1
Tablet, trihydrate	I	1.2	0.4	0.3	0.2	0.4	0.1	2.6

[a] Expressed relative to concentration of ampicillin determined by the same HPLC procedure
[b] The designations A and B for dimers and polymers refer to molecules with an intact terminal β-lactam ring and with an open β-lactam ring, respectively

arations and hence be present as contaminants of the clinically used preparations. The previously mentioned HPLC method for analysis of ampicillin dimers and polymers (LARSEN and BUNDGAARD 1978 a) has recently been used for determining the content of polymerization products in various clinically used ampicillin formulations commercially available in Denmark (BUNDGAARD 1978 a). Table 5 shows the data obtained for various injectables, tablets, and capsules. All of the preparations contained substantial amounts of ampicillin dimers and tetramers and smaller amounts of hexamers. The content of octamers, if any, was in all preparations below the detection limit of about 0.1%.

2. Immunologic Effects of Polymers

Several immunologic studies have been carried out on isolated polymers derived from 6-APA and various penicillins. The substances have been shown to be strongly antigenic in various animal experiments. SMITH et al. (1971) have made a comparative estimation of the antigenicity of the higher molecular weight substances obtained by gel chromatographic fractionation of aged aqueous penicillin solutions. The antigenicity was assessed by measuring the ability of the materials to react with antibodies of benzylpenicilloyl specificity raised in rabbits and tested in guinea pigs by passive cutaneous anaphylaxis. As seen from the results given in Table 1, the polymers formed by 6-APA, ampicillin, and the ampicillin pro-drug, hetacillin were found to be markedly more antigenic than those formed by the non-amino penicillins. In a later study, the same group (MUNRO et al. 1976) has studied the antigenicity of more well-defined polymers. It was found that, when tested in the guinea pig passive cutaneous anaphylaxis test, the 6-APA and ampicillin polymers with the largest degree of polymerization were substantially more antigenic than lower polymers. In a similar study, AHLSTEDT et al. (1976) have found that ampicillin polymers are potent elicitors, the eliciting capacity being about 1,000-fold higher than polymers of benzylpenicillin. This difference may certainly be explained on a structural basis since the ampicillin (and 6-APA) polymers have a greater similarity to the penicilloyl group bound to a protein amino group than the polymers of benzylpenicillin. In both these studies the specificity of the reactions observed was demonstrated to be predominantly penicilloyl, as verified by hapten inhibition experiments or immunosorbent experiments. Other investigators (BATCHELOR et al. 1967; DE WECK et al. 1968; BUTCHER and STEWART 1969; MURANAKA et al. 1974, 1978; IGARASHI et al. 1978) have similarly demonstrated the antigenicity of polymeric substances derived from various penicillins.

The polymers isolated from ampicillin and benzylpenicillin solutions have further been shown to give wheal and flare reactions in a number of penicillin allergic patients, all of whom have given skin reactions also to a penicilloyl–polylysine conjugate (JUHLIN et al. 1977). Finally, a limited clinical study by PARKER and RICHMOND (1976) has indicated that the use of so-called polymer-free ampicillin may reduce the incidence of certain exanthematic adverse reactions to ampicillin preparations.

Whereas several investigators (BATCHELOR et al. 1967; BUTCHER and STEWART 1969; MUNRO et al. 1976; LIAKOPOULOU and VILIM 1976) have been unable to demonstrate any induction of antibody formation by penicillin polymers in guinea pigs, rabbits, rats, or baboons, AHLSTEDT et al. (1977) have recently shown higher ampicillin polymers as well as unfractionated polymers to be capable of inducing antibody formation in mice, when tested by a hemolytic plaque assay. Under the same test conditions, monomeric ampicillin was found to be without any significant immunogenicity. Immunization of baboons with ampicillin polymer by injection in Freund's complete adjuvant has been found to lead to the development of lymphocyte-mediated hypersensitivity reactions (MUNRO et al. 1976). No information has been given as to whether the ampicillin polymers tested for immunogenicity in these studies contained an intact β-lactam ring in one of the terminal units. If so, the observed immunogenicity may be ascribed to reaction of the β-lactam group with amino groups of proteins in vivo and not to the polymer per se. Since a method of preparing homogeneous, well-defined ampicillin polymers both with and without an intact terminal β-lactam ring has recently become available (BUNDGAARD and LARSEN 1977), it seems relevant to investigate further the immunogenic effects of the individual polymers, including the dimer. It would also be of interest to examine whether ampicillin polymers (and other penicillin polymers) might be capable of inducing a polymer-specific immune response besides the penicilloyl-specific reactions.

In summary, it seems firmly established that penicillin polymers, and especially polymers formed from aminopenicillins, exhibit a strong penicilloyl-specific antigenicity and it is likely that they may play a part in the elicitation of some clinical allergic reactions to penicillin preparations. The question of immunogenicity of penicillin polymers is still to be fully resolved.

3. Prevention of Penicillin Polymerization

Because of the immunologic effects of penicillin polymers which are strongly supposed to be of clinical importance, their presence in clinically used penicillin preparations should be controlled and kept at the lowest possible level.

For penicillins without an amino group in the side chain, the polymerization is thought to depend strongly on the presence of the reactive penicillenic acid. Thus attempts to depress the polymerization of these penicillins should primarily be concerned with preventation of formation of penicillenic acid. Since the compound is formed by an acid-catalyzed isomerization, its formation can be depressed by keeping the pH of penicillin solutions to at least pH 6, e.g., by using a citrate buffer.

For ampicillin and other aminopenicillins, the polymerization proceeds through a number of consecutive intermolecular aminolysis reactions initiated by a reaction between two penicillin molecules. As regards formulation, only limited possibilities seem to exist by which the formation of polymers in aqueous solutions can be depressed. Since the rate of dimerization and polymerization increases very strongly with increasing penicillin concentration, it is important to prepare and use solutions at the lowest possible concentrations. The rate of dimerization is only slightly dependent on pH in neutral and basic solution but falls sharply with pH lower than 7. Aqueous solutions of ampicillin salts have a pH between 9 and 10, and a lowering of pH to 7.5–8 would accordingly not result in any depression of dimerization and polymerization. Adjusting the pH to 5–6 would be effective, but the low solubility of ampicillin and other aminopenicillins in the pH range 4–6 (Hou and Poole 1969; Tsuji et al. 1978), however, prevents the preparation of solutions of such acidity at concentrations required for intramuscular administration (10%–25% W/V). Thus, it is only for more dilute penicillin solutions ($\leqq 2\%$ W/V) that an adjustment of pH to about 5 would be a useful means of depressing polymerization.

The results of the study referred to, on structural factors influencing rate of dimerization of aminopenicillins (Bundgaard 1977b), may provide a rational basis for the design of aminopenicillins with a reduced tendency to undergo dimerization and polymerization. The basicity and the structural location of the side chain α-amino groups greatly influence the polymerization tendency and by placing the amino group in a sterically hindered position, polymerization can be almost completely avoided as in the case of cyclacillin. Although the newer aminopenicillins such as epicillin and cyclacillin may offer neither bacteriologic nor pharmacologic superiority to ampicillin (Neu 1975a, b; Freiesleben and Sack 1976), it seems clear that cyclacillin preparations to be given parenterally would have considerable advantages to similar ampicillin preparations with respect to chemical stability and formation of undesirable polymerization products. In fact, some extensive clinical studies (Hertz 1973; Stüttgen and Masuch 1973; Rüefli 1976; Gold et al. 1979) have shown that cutaneous rashes are approximately twice as frequent in patients treated with ampicillin as in those treated with cyclacillin. Whether this difference is in any way related to the difference in polymerization behavior of the two penicillins is, however, not known.

Since the introduction of ampicillin in 1961, a great number of broad-spectrum aminopenicillins have been developed and certainly will continue to be developed.

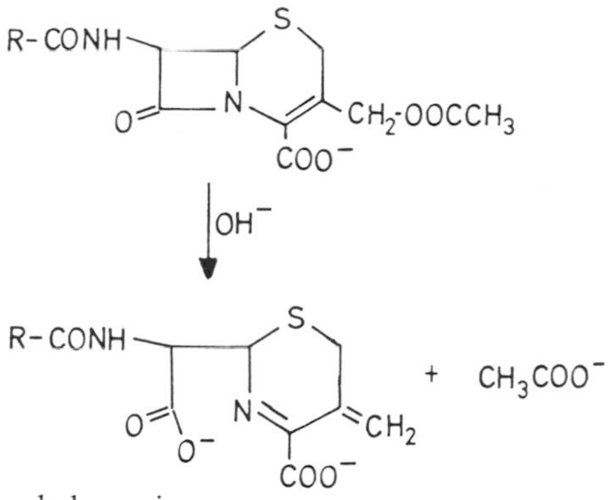

Fig. 11. Hydrolysis of cephalosporins

It seems relevant to stress that when assessing the clinical usefulness of such antibiotics, account should be taken of the polymerizing propensity of the penicillins in addition to other factors normally considered.

II. Cephalosporin Polymers

The structural analogs of penicillins, cephalosporins, may also show the formation of higher molecular weight polymerization products in aqueous solution. Using gel filtration and membrane filtration, STEWART and co-workers (STEWART 1968, 1969; STEWART et al. 1970; BUTCHER and STEWART 1979; BOYD et al. 1973) have detected the presence of polymers with a molecular weight of 1,000–5,000 daltons in solutions of cephalothin and cephaloridine and using dialysis, WALSH et al. (1971) have isolated similar products from cephalothin. Using gel filtration, DEWDNEY and co-workers (DEWDNEY et al. 1971; MUNRO et al. 1976) have isolated polymers from 14-day-old concentrated aqueous solutions of cephaloridine and cephalothin and further shown that the polymers are capable of evoking reactions in guinea pigs passively sensitized with antiserum raised in rabbits to cephalosporin–protein conjugates and also, although more weakly, to penicilloyl-specific antisera.

In contrast to penicillin polymers, the chemical structures of the polymers formed from cephalosporins remain unknown. Furthermore, the mechanism and rate of cephalosporin polymerization have not been studied. Cephalosporins cannot, apparently, undergo an intramolecular rearrangement into a reactive oxazolone structure. By hydrolysis of the β-lactam bond products are formed which are unstable (NEWTON et al. 1968; HAMILTON-MILLER et al. 1970; BUNDGAARD 1975 a) and which by reactions with each other may possibly form higher molecular weight products. It may be suggested that the primary product of hydrolysis of cephalothin and cephaloridine, 3,3^1-dehydrodeacetoxy-Δ^4-cephalosporoate (Fig. 11), is implicated in the polymerization since the stability of this product in neutral and basic solution has been observed to be concentration dependent (NEWTON et al. 1968). The stability decreases with increasing concentration, indicating that the disappearance of the compound is due to intermolecular reactions, possibly a dimerization.

For cephalosporins containing an amino group in the C_7 side chain such as cephalexin, cephaloglycin, and cephradine, a polymerization can be imagined to occur by intermolecular aminolysis in the same way as the polymerization of ampicillin and other aminopenicillins. Such as reaction can, however, be expected to be much less effective for the cephalosporins since an autocatalyzed intramolecular aminolysis with the formation of piperazine-2,5-dione derivatives may occur to a much larger extent than an intermolecular aminolysis (BUNDGAARD 1976c, d).

D. Reactions Between Penicillins and Pharmaceutical Adjuvants

An additional source of preformed antigenic penicilloyl-specific substances in penicillin preparations may be penicilloyl–carbohydrate conjugates.

In 1962 SIEGEL (1962) observed that benzylpenicillin incubated with the additive carboxymethylcellulose was capable of producing a wheal and flare reaction in sensitive patients. Later, SCHNEIDER et al. (1971 a) have shown that the antigenic product produced in the reaction between penicillin and the additive is a penicilloylated carboxymethylcellulose conjugate.

In an earlier work, SCHNEIDER and DE WECK (1967) showed that a number of other carbohydrates such as glucose, lactose, sucrose, raffinose, inulin, and various dextrans can also be penicilloylated by benzylpenicillin in neutral aqueous solutions. The products from reaction with raffinose, inulin, and the dextrans have been isolated by gel filtration and found to be capable of eliciting penicilloyl-specific passive cutaneous anaphylaxis reactions in guinea pigs (SCHNEIDER and DE WECK 1969; SCHNEIDER et al. 1971 b; MOLINARI et al. 1973). From a practical and clinical point of view, it is worth noting that even very lightly substituted penicilloyl–carbohydrate conjugates; e.g., conjugates containing less than one penicilloyl group in each molecule, could be shown to possess antigenic properties. The antigenicity is apparently not dependent on a transconjugation with protein amino groups in vivo (SCHNEIDER and DE WECK 1967). The observed eliciting capacity of monovalent carbohydrate conjugates may possibly be ascribed to adsorption of the conjugates on tissue macromolecules or cell membranes, resulting in formation of pseudomultivalent conjugates capable of bridging antibodies.

Whereas the antigenic effect of penicilloylated carbohydrates is considerable, the immunogenicity seems to be low but possibly significant. Penicilloyl–carbohydrate conjugates have been found to be capable of producing delayed hypersensitivity (but not antibody formation) in guinea pigs (SCHNEIDER and DE WECK 1967, 1969; SCHNEIDER et al. 1971 b).

Several therapeutically used penicillin preparations contain carbohydrates. Thus, penicillins are commonly infused in glucose or fructose solutions, sucrose is a common ingredient of penicillin syrups and benzylpenicillin procaine suspensions may contain carboxymethylcellulose as an additive. Because of the antigenic and potentially allergenic effect of penicilloyl–carbohydrate conjugates, their presence in penicillin preparations must be avoided. Information about the kinetics of reaction of penicillins with carbohydrate and factors affecting the reaction rate have recently been reported.

BUNDGAARD and LARSEN (1978 a) have studied the kinetics and mechanism of the sucrose-accelerated degradation of benzylpenicillin and a number of semisyn-

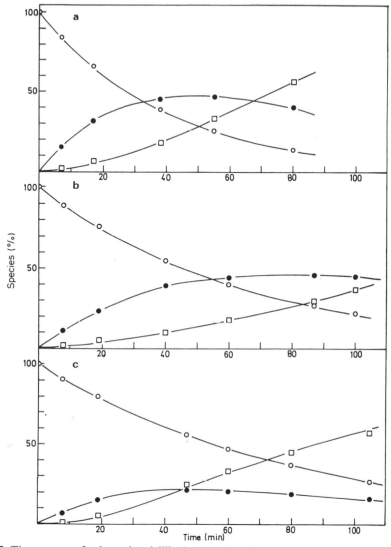

Fig. 12. Time courses for benzylpenicillin (*open circles*), benzylpenicilloyl ester (*solid cirles*), and benzylpenicilloic acid (*squares*) in the reaction between benzylpenicillin ($1.4 \times 10^{-3}M$) and sorbitol (**a**), glycerol (**b**), or dextran 40 (**c**) (all 10% W/V) at pH 9.25 (0.2 M carbonate) and 35 °C. (BUNDGAARD and LARSEN 1978 b)

thetic penicillins in aqueous sucrose solutions of pH 6–10. A linear relationship between the degradation rate and the sucrose concentration up to 10% W/V was observed and the accelerating effect of sucrose was found to be directly proportional to the hydroxide ion concentration in the pH range investigated. It was further demonstrated that the effect of sucrose on the reaction rate was entirely due to a nucleophilic reaction mechanism, involving formation of penicilloyl sucrose esters which subsequently undergo a slow hydrolysis to yield penicilloic acid. An efficient

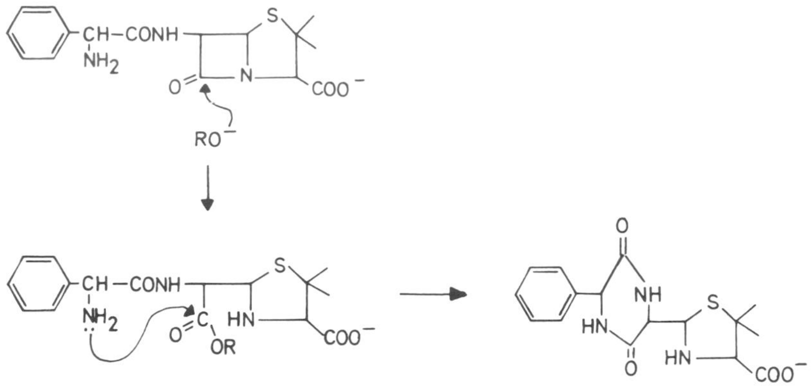

Fig. 13. Alcoholysis of ampicillin and intramolecular aminolysis of the intermediate penicilloyl ester

means of preventing the formation of penicilloylated sucrose was reported to consist in keeping the pH of the solutions at 6–6.5.

In further investigations (Bundgaard and Larsen 1978 b; Larsen and Bundgaard 1978 b) the reaction of penicillins with a number of other carbohydrates (glucose, fructose, and dextrans) as well as with polyhydric alcohols (sorbitol, mannitol, and glycerol) was studied. Like sucrose, these carbohydrates and alcohols were shown to exhibit a strong accelerating effect on the degradation of penicillins in neutral and alkaline aqueous solution. The reactions proceed entirely through a nucleophilic pathway with the intermediate formation of penicilloyl esters. Figure 12 shows the time courses for benzylpenicillin, benzylpenicilloyl ester, and benzylpenicilloic acid in the reaction with some hydroxy compounds at pH 9.25 and 35 °C.

Like that of benzylpenicillin, the reaction of ampicillin with the various hydroxy compounds also involves a nucleophilic displacement reaction at the β-lactam carbonyl moiety by the corresponding oxygen anions at produce penicilloyl esters, but instead of undergoing simple hydrolysis into penicilloic acid, these esters of ampicillin undergo an intramolecular aminolysis by the side chain amino group to produce a stable piperazine-2,5-dione derivative (Fig. 13) (Bundgaard and Larsen 1979). Figure 14 shows the time courses for the various species in the reaction of ampicillin with glucose at pH 9.4 and room temperature. Ampicillin is often administered by infusion of carbohydrate-containing intravenous fluids and the addition of ampicillin salts to such fluids usually gives them an alkaline pH (Stjernström et al. 1978), corresponding to the conditions used in the experiment described in Fig. 14. It is seen that although the piperazinedione derivative constitutes the predominant degradation product, the penicilloyl carbohydrate ester is present in significant amounts in the reaction pathway and – what is important from a practical and immunologic point of view – the relative concentrations of the ester is greatest in the early phase of ampicillin decomposition. Besides glucose, this was also found to be the case for sorbitol and various commercial dextran-containing infusion fluids (Bundgaard and Larsen 1979).

The formation of penicilloyl esters can, for all penicillins, be greatly depressed or avoided by adjusting the pH of penicillin solutions containing the hydroxy com-

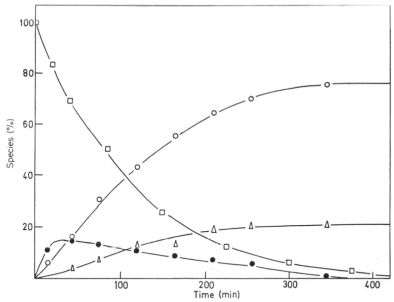

Fig. 14. Time courses for ampicillin (*squares*), α-aminobenzylpenicilloyl glucose (*solid circles*), piperazine-2,5-dione derivative (*open cirles*), and α-aminobenzylpenicilloic acid (*triangles*) in the reaction between ampicillin ($1.55 \times 10^{-3}M$) and glucose (10% W/V) at pH 9.40 (0.2 *M* carbonate) and 22 °C. (BUNDGAARD and LARSEN 1979)

pounds to 6–6.5 (BUNDGAARD and LARSEN 1978 b). This is apparent by inspection of Fig. 15 in which the pH–rate profile for degradation of benzylpenicillin in aqueous solution is shown along with the pH–rate profiles for the degradation due to hydroxy compounds at a concentration of 10% W/V. Figure 15 shows that at pH > 7 the carbohydrate or alcohol reactions are the dominant degradation reactions, while at pH 6–6.5 these reactions make the same contribution to the overall degradation as the spontaneous hydrolysis. Below these pH values the latter degradation predominates and to an increasing extent with falling pH. Thus, a pH of about 6 would be optimal as regards both depression of penicilloyl ester formation and overall stability of benzylpenicillin (and other penicillins, BUNDGAARD and LARSEN 1978 b). It should finally be noted that trace amounts of iron(II) ions have been found to exhibit a marked catalysis of the fructose-accelerated degradation of benzylpenicillin and ampicillin (LANDERSJÖ et al. 1977; STJERNSTRÖM et al. 1978). This catalytic effect, which is a catalysis of penicilloyl ester formation rather than a catalysis of hydrolysis (LARSEN and BUNDGAARD 1978 b), can be eliminated by addition of a metal-complexing agent such as edetate or citrate (STJERNSTRÖM et al. 1978).

E. Chemically Reactive Impurities and Degradation Products

Several drug substances and clinically used drug formulations have been found to contain small amounts of impurities or degradation products which are chemically

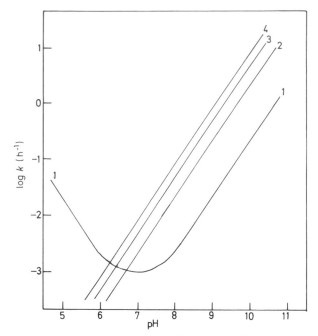

Fig. 15. pH–rate profiles for the degradation of benzylpenicillin in aqueous solution (*1*) and for the degradation due to glycerol (*2*), sorbitol (*3*), and sucrose (*4*) all at a concentration of 10% W/V, at 35 °C; k denotes a pseudo-first-order rate constant for penicillin degradation. (Bundgaard and Larsen 1978 b)

highly reactive with proteins or "protein-model" compounds (amino acids and small peptides) and therefore are to be considered as potentially immunogenic substances. For some of the contaminants, the chemically predicted immunogenicity has been confirmed in immunologic animal experiments. Specific examples are described in this section.

I. Acetylsalicylic Acid

It is generally agreed that the majority of clinical hypersensitivity reactions to acetylsalicylic acid, such as bronchial asthma are not due to any immunologic mechanism and thus are of a nonallergic nature (e.g., Schlumberger et al. 1974; Abrishami and Thomas 1977; Weltman et al. 1978). On the other hand, several authors have detected the presence of salicyloyl-specific antibodies or sensitized lymphocytes of salicyloyl specificity in a number of persons intolerant to acetylsalicylic acid and indicated that some of the occurring hypersensitivity reactions in humans appear to be associated with an immunologic pathogenesis and to be mediated by antibodies of salicyloyl specificity (Weiner et al. 1963; Giraldo et al. 1969; Girard et al. 1969; Amos et al. 1971; de Weck 1971 b; Lazary et al. 1972; Phills and Perelmutter 1974; Patriarca et al. 1976). Such reactions, certainly accounting for only a minor part of all hypersensitivity reactions, may include reactions of the anaphylactic type (Phills and Perelmutter 1974).

The formation of salicyloyl-specific antibodies implies a formation of salicyloyl–protein conjugates in the organism upon ingestion of acetylsalicylic acid. It has

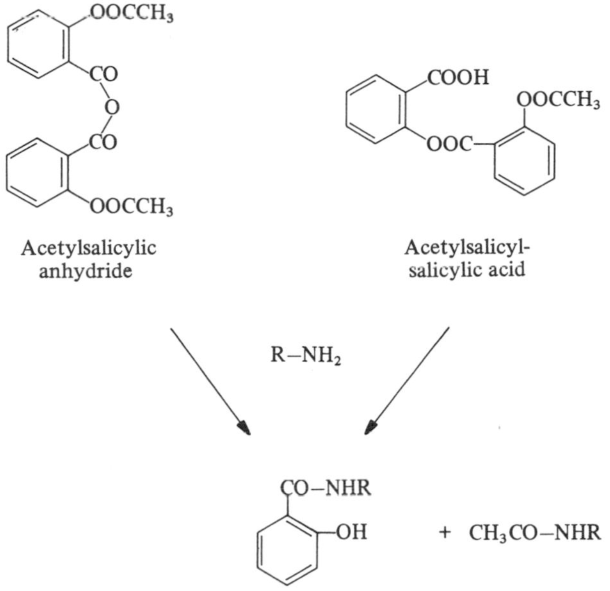

Fig. 16. Formation of *N*-salicyloyl amines by aminolysis of acetylsalicylic anhydride and acetylsalicylsalicylic acid

been suggested (SCHWARTZ and AMIDON 1966) that these postulated conjugates may arise directly from acetylsalicylic acid through an intermediate mixed acetic virqule salicylic anhydride. These authors observed that upon incubation of acetylsalicylic acid with amino acids, such as glycine and ε-aminocaproic acid, in alkaline aqueous solution, very small amounts (0.01%–0.1%) of *N*-salicyloyl derivaties were formed. Later investigations (BUNDGAARD 1974a, 1976b; BUNDGAARD and DE WECK 1975) have shown, however, that the observed formation of the salicyloyl derivatives is due to reaction of the amino acids with impurities in commercial acetylsalicylic acid, acetylsalicylic anhydride, and acetylsalicylsalicylic acid, and not to reaction with acetylsalicylic acid itself (Fig. 16). The presence of these impurities in commercial acetylsalicylic acid was first described by DE WECK (1971 b) and by PATEL et al. (1972) and has subsequently been confirmed with the use of various analytic techniques (BUNDGAARD and BUNDGAARD 1973; BUNDGAARD 1976b, e; ALI 1976a, b; JANSSON and ANDERSSON 1977; SPITZ 1977). The amounts of acetylsalicylic anhydride found are in the range 0.001%–0.03% and those of acetylsalicylsalicylic acid in the range 0.01%–0.8%.

By producing acetylsalicylic acid according to several different patents it has been proved that the impurities arise as by products during the synthesis of the acid (BUNDGAARD 1976e). However, the contaminants may also be considered as degradation products of acetylsalicylic acid. Thus it has been found (BUNDGAARD and LARSEN 1976; BUNDGAARD 1976e) that by heating acetylsalicylic acid in the solid state, or dissolved in non-hydroxylic organic solvents such as benzene, chloroform, or acetone, a partial transformation into anhydride and acetylsalicylsalicylic acid readily takes place.

Being a carboxylic anhydride and a phenolic ester respectively, the acetylsalicylic acid contaminants are highly reactive. They have been shown to react readily

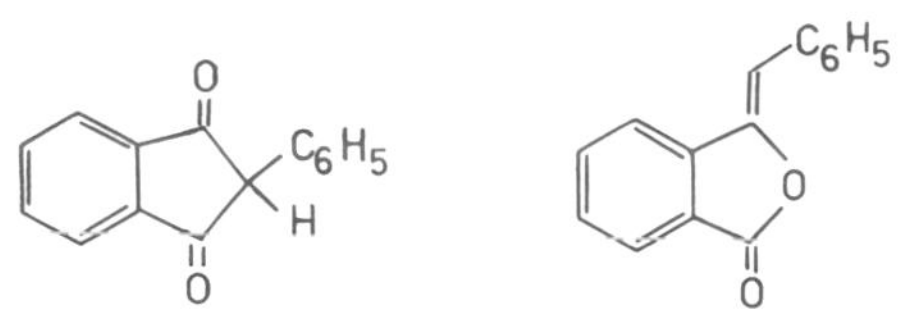

Fig. 17. Chemical structures of phenindione (*I*) and a contaminant of phenindione tablet preparations, 3-benzyl-idenephthalide (*II*)

with amino acids, polypeptides, and with various proteins under physiologic conditions of pH and temperature to give *N*-salicyloyl derivatives (DE WECK 1971b; BUNDGAARD 1974a).

In accordance with their high chemical reactivity, the contaminants were found to be highly immunogenic in experimental animals, being capable of inducing salicyloyl-specific contact hypersensitivity as well as formation of anti-salicyloyl antibodies (DE WECK 1971b; BUNDGAARD and DE WECK 1975; SCHLUMBERGER 1975). Under standardized conditions, different commercial acetylsalicylic acid preparations were found to sensitize animals to varying extents (DE WECK 1971b). However, preparations purified by repeated recrystallization until no impurities were detectable completely failed to induce any antibody formation or contact hypersensitivity (BUNDGAARD and DE WECK 1975).

These results strongly suggest that the immunogenic effect of acetylsalicylic acid preparations as observed in experimental animals is due to acetylsalicylic anhydride and/or acetylsalicylsalicylic acid present as impurities in the preparations and not to the acetylsalicylic acid itself. By extrapolation of these findings to clinical acetylsalicylic acid allergy, it may appear that the impurities rather than the drug substance itself are responsible for the appearance of anti-salicyloyl antibodies in patients treated with acetylsalicylic acid.

A formal direct proof that these impurities are responsible for or implicated in clinical allergic reactions to acetylsalicylic acid does not exist and has even been questioned by some authors (JUHLIN et al. 1972; SCHLUMBERGER 1975), but owing to the definite immunologic effects of the products, it appears justifiable to suggest that steps be taken to reduce the content of the impurities in clinically used acetylsalicylic acid preparations.

II. Phenindione

The anticoagulant phenindione (2-phenylindane-1,3-dione, compound I in Fig. 17) has been reported (PERKINS 1962; BAKER and LEVENE 1969, and references cited therein) to be a frequent cause of presumably allergic hypersensitivity reactions in humans. An attempt has been made to identify a mechanism by which antigenic hapten–protein conjugates may be formed in vivo. This investigation (BUNDGAARD 1975b) has demonstrated that whereas phenindione itself cannot be shown to form stable conjugates with proteins in vitro, e.g., through formation of a Schiff base with amino groups, a contaminant of clinically used phenindione tablets, 3-benzyl-idenephthalide (compound II in Fig. 17), is highly reactive with simple amines and

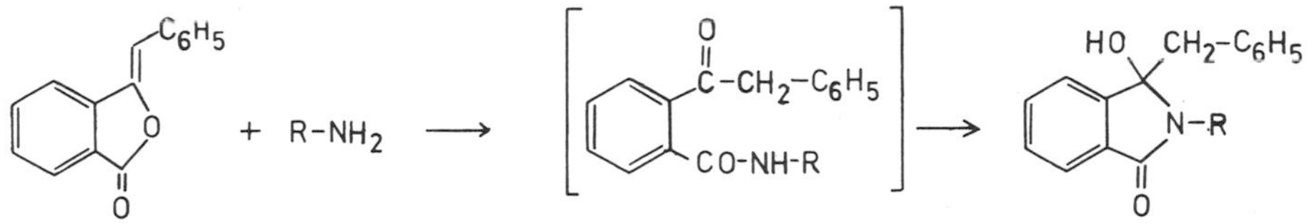

Fig. 18. Formation of 3-benzyl-3-hydroxyphthalimidine derivatives by aminolysis of 3-benzylidenephthalide

with proteins. 3-Benzylidenephthalide is an intermediate or a starting material in most of the commercially used processes for the preparation of phenindione and it was found to be present in various tablet formulations in amounts ranging from 0.006% to 0.016%. The compound was shown to react readily with the ε-amino groups of lysine residues of proteins in aqueous solutions under physiologic conditions of pH and temperature with the formation of stable N-substituted 3-benzyl-3-hydroxy-phthalimidine conjugates (Fig. 18).

Immunologic investigations of the 3-benzylidenephthalide contaminant have not yet been performed. The phthalimidine group is, however, most certainly immunologically powerful, and since the capacity of the compound to react covalently with proteins and protein-model compounds as measured in vitro is very high, it was characterized as a potentially immunogenic substance. In order to evaluate the possible involvement of this contaminant in clinical hypersensitivity reactions to phenindione preparations, it is suggested that a conjugate with, for example, polylysine be prepared and used as a skin testing reagent for the detection of antibodies.

III. Phenylbutazone

Another example of the possible implication of a chemically reactive contaminant in drug allergy is phenylbutazone. Although this drug and its structural analog oxyphenbutazone have been implicated frequently in a variety of allergic reactions including generalized urticaria, angioedema, contact dermatitis and various erythematous rashes (e.g., LITTLEJOHNS et al. 1973; VAN JOOST et al. 1974; VOOYS and VAN KETEL 1977), apparently no studies of the immunochemical mechanism involved had been carried out until recently (BUNDGAARD 1977d).

An examination of the reactivity of phenylbutazone with various protein-model compounds, such as primary amines and amino acids, did not reveal the occurrence of any aminolysis in neutral and basic aqueous solutions. The resistance of the amide bonds in phenylbutazone to opening by hydrolysis or aminolysis may be ascribed to the tautomeric character of the structure (Fig. 19). On the other hand, the great mobility of the proton at C-4 in conjunction with the two neighboring carbonyl groups makes phenylbutazone highly susceptible to oxidation at this carbon atom. Thus, simple air oxidation in aqueous solutions or in the solid state gives rise to the formation of 4-hydroxyphenylbutazone (Fig. 19). This oxidation product is a frequently occurring (in percentage amounts) contaminant of various phenylbutazone preparations (BECKSTEAD et al. 1968; PAWELCZYK and WACHOWIAK 1969; SLINGSBY and ZUCK 1972; AWANG et al. 1973; BUNDGAARD 1978c; MATSUI et al. 1978).

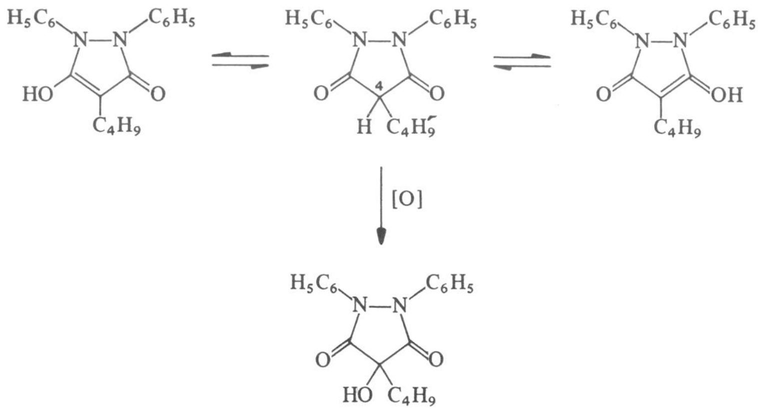

Fig. 19. Tautomeric forms of phenylbutazone and its oxidation to 4-hydroxyphenylbutazone

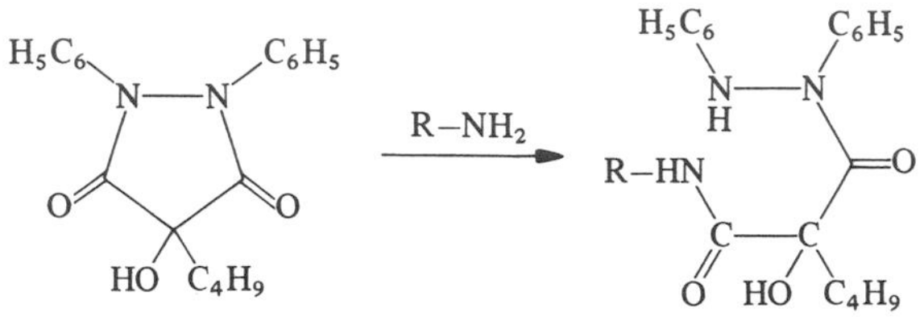

Fig. 20. Reaction scheme for aminolysis of 4-hydroxyphenylbutazone

In 4-hydroxyphenylbutazone, keto–enol tautomerism is no longer possible, and this product may therefore be expected to be much more labile than the parent drug. The investigation carried out by the present author (BUNDGAARD 1977 d) has shown that the compound is, in fact, highly reactive. It reacts readily with various amines and simple peptides as well as with free amino groups in serum albumin in aqueous solutions to yield amides of butyltartronic acid mono- (N,N-diphenyl)-hydrazide (Fig. 20). A kinetic study of the reactions showed that 4-hydroxyphenyl-butazone is about 20 times more reactive than benzylpenicillin with the dipeptide glycylglycine in aqueous solution at 37 °C.

On basis of the high chemical reactivity of 4-hydroxyphenylbutazone along with its frequent occurrence in phenylbutazone formulations it was suggested that the substance may be immunogenic and possibly involved in clinical allergic reactions to phenylbutazone. Preliminary experiments in guinea pigs have indicated that the compound does possess a fairly strong sensitizing effect (DE WECK personal communication).

IV. Corticosteroids

Several cases of allergic hypersensitivity reactions including anaphylactic reactions, urticaria, and contact dermatitis to various corticosteroid preparations have been reported (ALANI and ALANI 1972; GUTZWILLER 1974; KOUNIS 1976; TEGNER 1976; and references cited therein), but the immunochemical mechanisms involved have apparently not been studied as yet.

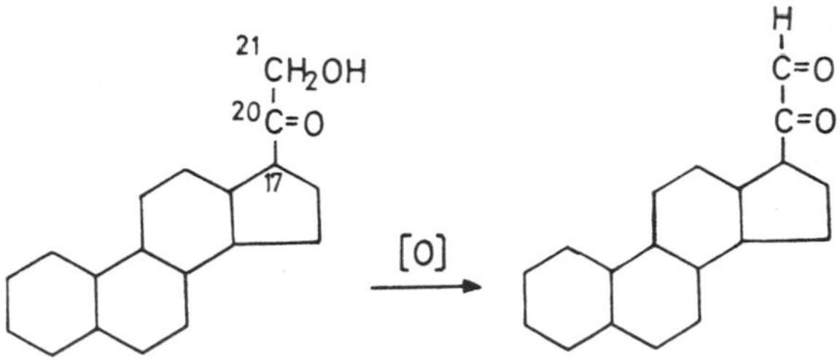

Fig. 21. Oxidation of 21-hydroxycorticosteroids to 21-dehydro corticosteroids

The hypothesis has been advanced (BUNDGARD 1977c, 1980b) that the allergic reactions may be due to reaction of proteins in the body with degradation products of corticosteroids, 21-dehydrocorticosteroids. In the following, this hypothesis is outlined in some detail.

21-Dehydrocorticosteroids are readily formed by autoxidation of the parent drugs (e.g., cortisone, hydrocortisone, prednisone) in aqueous solution (Fig. 21; SUNAGA and KOIDE 1968; MONDER 1968b; BUNDGAARD and HANSEN 1979) and they may certainly be present in substantial amounts in some corticosteroid formulations. Furthermore, the products can occur as impurities in the drug substances, as demonstrated by MONDER and WALTER (1970a) for some tritium-labeled hydrocortisone preparations and by BUNDGAARD (1978b) for some ordinary clinically used hydrocortisone, prednisone, and prednisolone samples. For these samples the content of the corresponding 21-dehydro derivatives was found to be in the range 0.04%–0.25%.

21-Dehydrocorticosteroids are substituted glyoxals and, like glyoxal itself and other glyoxal derivatives (TAKAHASHI 1968), highly reactive with arginine residues of proteins with formation of stable conjugates (SUNAGA and KOIDE 1968; MONDER 1968a; MONDER and WALKER 1970b; DUNCAN and DUNCAN 1973). These studies have also shown that, while the 21-dehydro derivatives react rapidly with proteins in neutral aqueous solutions, no reaction occurs with the parent drugs.

Glyoxal itself has been reported to be a strong contact sensitizer in humans (KLIGMAN 1966). This effect may be supposed to be due to its reaction with arginine residues of proteins in the organism. Since monosubstituted glyoxals such as phenylglyoxal and methylglyoxal are more reactive with arginine than unsubstituted glyoxal (TAKAHASHI 1968), and 21-dehydrocorticosteroids are, in fact, monosubstituted glyoxals, it may be expected that these steroid glyoxals are at least as reactive with protein as glyoxal and thus, for this reason alone, may be considered as potentially immunogenic substances.

V. Penicillins

Degradation of penicillins in aqueous solutions leads to a number of different products, some of which are chemically reactive with proteins or protein-model compounds and have been implicated in penicillin allergy. Such reactive degradation products include penicillenic acid, penicillenic acid disulfide, penicilloic acid,

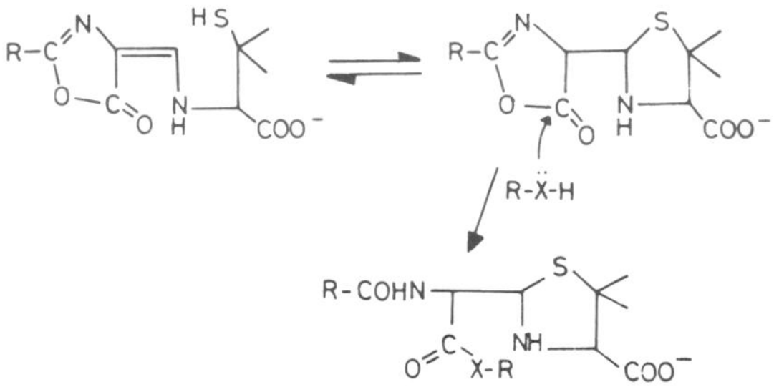

Fig. 22. Penicilloylation of nucleophiles by penicillenic acid

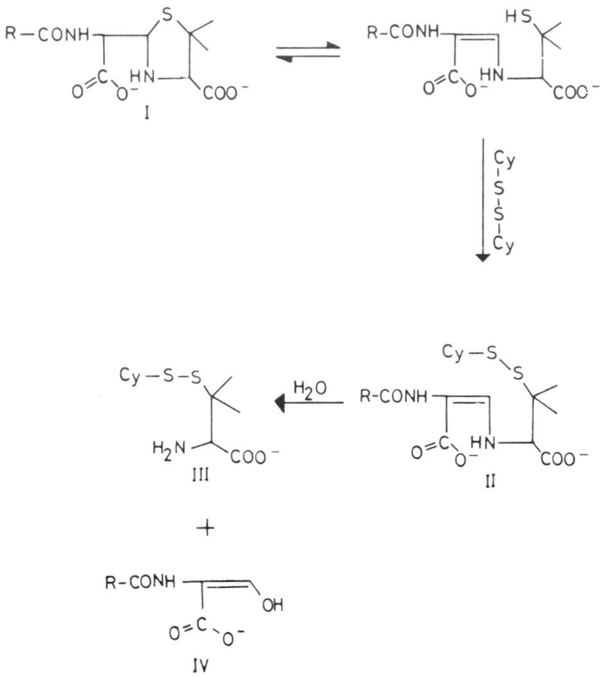

Fig. 23. Reaction of penicilloic acid (*I*) with cystine to yield penamaldic acid–cysteine mixed disulfide (*II*). Subsequent hydrolysis of II yields penicillamine–cysteine mixed disulfide (*III*) and penaldic acid (*IV*)

penilloic acid, and penicillamine (for detailed reviews, see SCHWARTZ 1969; DEWD-NEY 1977).

Penicillenic acids are readily formed in aqueous solutions of penicillins by an intramolecular rearrangement, as described in Sect. C.I.1.a, and they are present in small amounts in almost all penicillin preparations (e.g., MEULENHOFF 1965; SEITZINGER 1973; BRANDT et al. 1974). The rate of formation of penicillenic acid increases strongly with decreasing pH of the penicillin solutions and it shows a high dependence on the inductive effect of the side chain structure of the penicillins (SCHWARTZ and WU 1966). The compounds are highly reactive with proteins and various protein-model compounds, with the formation of penicilloyl derivatives (Fig. 22; LEVINE and OVARY 1961; LEVINE 1961; PARKER et al. 1962; WAGNER et al. 1969). They are, as expected from their high chemical reactivity, potent sensitizers (LEVINE 1960; CARON 1963; BATCHELOR and DEWDNEY 1968), and may play a role in penicillin allergy. As discussed in Sect. C.I, the most useful means of avoiding the formation of penicillenic acid in penicillin solutions is to maintain pH not lower than 6–6.5.

In addition to the penicilloyl determinant several other antigenic determinants are involved in penicillin allergy, the so-called minor antigenic determinants. Although much work has been carried out to establish the chemical structure of these determinants and the pathways to their formation (as reviewed by SCHWARTZ 1969; DEWDNEY 1977) no firm conclusions have been reached as yet.

Penicilloic acid, which is the major degradation product of the penicillins derived by hydrolysis of the β-lactam ring, has been shown to elicit wheal and flare reactions in a certain group of penicillin allergic patients and is thought to be implicated in immunologic responsiveness to penicillins (e.g., LEVINE and REDMOND 1969; SCHNEIDER 1974; JUHLIN et al. 1977). Similar eliciting effects were observed with penicilloic acids, which are formed by decarboxylation of the penicilloic acids. It has been suggested (LEVINE and REDMOND 1969; SCHNEIDER et al. 1973) that the formation of antigenic determinants from penicilloic acid and penilloic acid in vivo proceeds through reaction with cystine disulfide linkages in tissue proteins yielding a penamaldic acid–cysteine mixed disulfide conjugate and a penicillamine conjugate (Fig. 23). By intradermal skin testing ASSEM and VICKERS (1974) have found that a high proportion of the penicillin allergic patients tested gave a positive response to a penicillamine–protein conjugate and accordingly, the penicillamine grouping may be an important antigenic determinant in penicillin allergy.

Recently, penicillamine has been detected in neutral benzylpenicillin solutions and shown to be a degradation product of penicillenic acid at neutral pH (JEMAL et al. 1978).

References

Ahlstedt S, Kristofferson A, Svärd PO, Thor L, Örtengren B (1976) Ampicillin polymers as elicitors of passive cutaneous anaphylaxis. Int Arch Allergy Appl Immunol 51:131–139

Ahlstedt S, Kristofferson A, Svärd PO, Strannegaard Ö (1977) Immunological properties of ampicillin polymers. Int Arch Allergy Appl Immunol 53:247–253

Ahlstedt S, Kristofferson A, Pettersson E (1979) Antigens in penicillin allergy. III. Antigen and antibody levels in mice treated with pure and contaminated penicillins. Int Arch Allergy Appl Immunol 58:20–29

Abrishami MA, Thomas J (1977) Aspirin intolerance – a review. Ann Allergy 39:28–37

Alani MD, Alani SD (1972) Allergic contact dermatitis to corticosteroids. Ann Allergy 30:181–185

Ali SL (1976a) Gas-chromatographic determination of traces of acetylsalicylic anhydride and acetylsalicylsalicylic acid in acetylsalicylic acid. Z Analyt Chem 278:365–366

Ali SL (1976b) Application of gas-liquid chromatography and high-performance liquid chromatography to the analysis of trace amounts of salicylic acid, acetylsalicylic anhydride and acetylsalicylsalicylic acid in aspirin samples and aspirin formulations. J Chromatogr 126:651–663

Amos HE, Wilson DV, Taussig MJ, Carlton SJ (1971) Hypersensitivity reactions to acetyl-
    salicylic acid. I. Detection of antibodies in human sera using acetylsalicylic acid attached
    to proteins through the carboxyl group. Clin Exp Immunol 8:563–572
Assem ESK, Vickers MR (1974) Immunological response to penicillamine in penicillin-al-
    lergic patients and in normal subjects. Postgrad Med J [Suppl] 50:65–70
Awang DVC, Vincent A, Matsui F (1973) Pattern of phenylbutazone degradation. J Pharm
    Sci 62:1673–1676
Baker H, Levene GM (1969) Cutaneous reactions to anticoagulants. Br J Dermatol 81:236–
    238
Batchelor FR, Dewdney JM (1968) Some aspects of penicillin allergy. Proc R Soc Med
    61:897–899
Batchelor FR, Dewdney JM, Feinberg JG, Weston RD (1967) A penicilloylated protein im-
    purity as a source of allergy to benzylpenicillin and 6-aminopenicillanic acid. Lancet
    1:1175–1177
Beckstead HD, Kaistha KK, Smith SJ (1968) Determination and thin-layer chromatogra-
    phy of phenylbutazone in the presence of decomposition products. J Pharm Sci 57:1952–
    1957
Bolt HM, Remmer H (1976) Implication of rifampicin-quinone in the irreversible binding
    of rifampicin to macromolecules. Xenobiotica 6:21–32
Boyd JF, Butcher BT, Stewart GT (1973) The nephrotoxic effect of cephaloridine and its
    polymers. Int J Clin Pharmacol Ther Toxicol 7:307–315
Brandt E, Gapp F, Knauseder F, Kuntscher H, Riedl K (1974) Untersuchungen über die
    Reinheit und Haltbarkeit von Natrium-Penicillin-G. Sci Pharm 42:209–221
Bruice TC, Bruice PY (1976) Solution chemistry of arene oxides. Accounts Chem Res 9:378–
    384
Bundgaard H (1971) Kinetic demonstration of a metastable intermediate in isomerization
    of penicillin to penicillenic acid in aqueous solution. J Pharm Sci 60:1273–1275
Bundgaard H (1974a) Acetylsalicylsalicylic acid: A potentially immunogenic impurity in
    acetylsalicylic acid. J Pharm Pharmacol 26:18–22
Bundgaard H (1974b) Spectrophotometric determination of ampicillin sodium in the pres-
    ence of its degradation and polymerization products. J Pharm Pharmacol 26:385–392
Bundgaard H (1975a) Chemical studies related to cephalosporin allergy. I. Kinetics of
    aminolysis of cephalosporins and effect of C-3 substituents on β-lactam reactivity. Arch
    Pharm Chem Sci 3:94–123
Bundgaard H (1975b) Identification and quantitation of a 3-benzylidenephthalide contam-
    inant of phenindione tablets and its characterization as a potentially immunogenic sub-
    stance. Acta Pharm Suec 12:333–348
Bundgaard H (1976a) Polymerization of penicillins: kinetics and mechanism of di- and
    polymerization of ampicillin in aqueous solution. Acta Pharm Suec 13:9–26
Bundgaard H (1976b) Colorimetric analysis of immunogenic impurities in acetylsalicylic
    acid. J Pharm Pharmacol 28:544–547
Bundgaard H (1976c) Hydrolysis and intramolecular aminolysis of cephalexin and ce-
    phaloglycin in aqueous solution. Arch Pharm Chem Sci 4:25–43
Bundgaard H (1976d) Chemical studies related to cephalosporin allergy. II. Competitive
    amine-catalyzed intra- and intermolecular aminolysis of cephalexin and cephaloglycin
    in aqueous solution. Acta Pharm Suec 13:299–312
Bundgaard H (1976e) High-pressure liquid chromatographic determination of immuno-
    genic contaminants of acetylsalicylic acid preparations. Arch Pharm Chem Sci 4:103–
    113
Bundgaard H (1977a) Polymerization of penicillins. II. Kinetics and mechanism of dimer-
    ization and self-catalyzed hydrolysis of amoxycillin in aqueous solution. Acta Pharm
    Suec 14:47–66
Bundgaard H (1977b) Polymerization of penicillins. III. Structural effects influencing rate
    of dimerization of aminopenicillins in aqueous solution. Acta Pharm Suec 14:67–80
Bundgaard H (1977c) Allergic reactions to drugs mediated by chemically reactive impurities
    or degradation products. In: Bundgaard H, Juul P, Kofod H (eds) Drug design and ad-
    verse reactions. Alfred Benzon Symposium X, Copenhagen 1976. Munksgaard, Copen-
    hagen, pp 165–183

Bundgaard H (1977 d) 4-Hydroxyphenylbutazone: a potentially immunogenic contaminant of phenylbutazone preparations. Arch Pharm Chem Sci 5:87–96

Bundgaard H (1977 e) Quantitative determination of amino-penicillins in the presence of their degradation and polymerization products. Arch Pharm Chem Sci 5:141–148

Bundgaard H (1978 a) Impurities as a factor in therapeutic equivalence of drugs: analysis of ampicillin formulations for antigenic polymerization products. Arch Pharm Chem Sci 6:63–68

Bundgaard H (1978 b) A new stability-indicating spectrophotometric assay for 21-hydroxy corticosteroids and a kinetic assay for 21-dehydro corticosteroid impurities. Arch Pharm Chem Sci 6:127–140

Bundgaard H (1978 c) High-performance liquid chromatographic determination of phenyl-butazone and its major degradation products in pharmaceuticals. Arch Pharm Chem Sci 6:223–230

Bundgaard H (1980 a) Kinetics and mechanism of the rearrangement of penicillin to penicil-lenic acid in acidic aqueous solution. Arch Pharm Chem Sci 8:161–180

Bundgaard H (1980 b) The possible implication of steroid-glyoxal degradation products in allergic reactions to corticosteroids. Arch Pharm Chemi Sci 8:83–90

Bundgaard H, Bundgaard C (1973) Spectrophotometric determination of microgram quan-tities of acetylsalicylic anhydride in acetylsalicylic acid. J Pharm Pharmacol 25:593–598

Bundgaard H, de Weck AL (1975) The role of amino-reactive impurities in acetylsalicylic acid allergy. Int Arch Allergy Appl Immunol 49:119–124

Bundgaard H, Hansen J (1979) A new stability-indicating spectrophotometric method for the determination of corticosteroids in aqueous media. Arch Pharm Chem Sci 7:19–32

Bundgaard H, Larsen C (1976) Intramolecular and intermolecular transformations of as-pirin in nonhydroxylic solvents. J Pharm Sci 65:776–778

Bundgaard H, Larsen C (1977) Polymerization of penicillins. IV. Separation, isolation and characterization of ampicillin polymers formed in aqueous solution. J Chromatogr 132:51–59

Bundgaard H, Larsen C (1978 a) Kinetics and mechanism of the sucrose-accelerated degra-dation of penicillins in aqueous solution. Int J Pharm (Amst) 1:95–104

Bundgaard H, Larsen C (1978 b) Kinetics and mechanism of reaction of benzylpenicillin and ampicillin with carbohydrates and polyhydric alcohols in aqueous solution. Arch Pharm Chem Sci 6:184–200

Bundgaard H, Larsen C (1979) Piperazinedione formation from reaction of ampicillin with carbohydrates and alcohols in aqueous solution. Int J Pharm (Amst) 3:1–11

Butcher BT, Stewart GT (1969) Immunochemical properties of macromolecular residues in β-lactam antibiotics. Antimicrob Agents Chemother 1968:515–518

Butcher BT, Stewart GT (1970) Experimental studies on macromolecules from β-lactam antibiotics. In: Stewart GT, McGovern JP (eds) Penicillin allergy, clinical and immuno-logical aspects. Thomas, Springfield, pp 111–134

Butcher BT, Stanfield MK, Stewart GT, Zemelman R (1971) Antibiotic polymers: α-Aminobenzylpenicillin (ampicillin). Mol Cryst Liq Cryst 12:321–333

Butler TC, Dudley KH, Johnson D (1972) Chemical studies of potential relevance to penicil-lin hypersensitivity: kinetics of formation and disappearance of benzylpenicillenic acid and its derivatives in solutions of benzylpenicillin. J Pharmacol Exp Ther 181:201–211

Caron GA (1963) The role of penicillenic acid and penicillamine in contact-type sensitivity to penicillin. Immunology 6:81–93

Carrington TR (1971) The development of commercial processes for the production of 6-aminopenicillanic acid. Proc R Soc Lond [Biol] 179:321–333

Daly JW, Jerina DM, Witkop B (1972) Arene oxides and the NIH shift: The metabolism, toxicity and carcinogenicity of aromatic compounds. Experientia 28:1129–1264

Dennen DW (1967) Degradation kinetics of 6-aminopenicillanic acid. J Pharm Sci 56:1273–1276

Dewdney JM (1977) Immunology of the antibiotics. In: Sela M (eds) The antigens, vol IV. Academic Press, New York, pp 73–245

Dewdney JM, Smith H, Wheeler AW (1971) The formation of antigenic polymers in aqueous solutions of β-lactam antibiotics. Immunology 21:517–525 de Weck AL (1971 a) Drug reactions. In: Samter M (eds) Immunological diseases, 2nd edn, vol I. Little, Brown, Boston, pp 415–440

de Weck AL (1971 b) Immunological effects of aspirin anhydride, a contaminant of commercial acetylsalicylic acid preparations. Int Arch Allergy Appl Immunol 41:393–418

de Weck AL (1974) Low molecular weight antigens. In: Sela M (ed) The antigens, vol 2. Academic Press, New York, pp 141–249

de Weck AL, Schneider CH, Gutersohn J (1968) The role of penicilloylated protein impurities, penicillin polymers and dimers in penicillin allergy. Int Arch Allergy Appl Immunol 33:535–567

Dudley KH, Butler TC, Johnson D (1974) Chemical studies of potential relevance to penicillin hypersensitivity: kinetic studies of methicillin, phenoxymethylpenicillin and their penicillenic acids. J Pharmacol Exp Ther 188:491–503

Duncan MR, Duncan GR (1973) Binding studies with calf thymus histones and ^{3}H-cortisol. Can J Pharm Sci 8:115–119

Dürsch F (1968) Search for protein contaminants in benzylpenicillin. Lancet 1:1005–1007

Eisen HN (1959) Hypersensitivity to simple chemicals. In: Lawrence HS (ed) Cellular and humoral aspects of the hypersensitivity states. Hoeber, New York, pp 89–122

Fazakerley GV, Jackson GE, Linder PW (1976) Equilibrium studies of benzylpenicillinate-thiaprolinate-hippurate- and benzylpenicilloate-proton and transition metal (II) ion systems. J Inorg Nucl Chem 38:1397–1400

Freiesleben H, Sack H (1976) Comparative assessment of cyclacillin and ampicillin by experimental therapy and by serum level determinations in rats and mice. Chemotherapy 22:75–83

Giraldo B, Blumenthal MN, Spink WW (1969) Aspirin intolerance and asthma. A clinical and immunological study. Ann Intern Med 71:479–496

Girard JP, Hildebrandt F, Favre H (1969) Hypersensitivity to aspirin: clinical and immunological studies. Helv Med Acta 35:86–95

Gold JA, Hegarty CP, Deitch MW, Walker BR (1979) Double-blind clinical trials of oral cyclacillin and ampicillin. Antimicrob Agents Chemother 15:55–58

Gottlieb AJ, Wurzel HA (1974) Protein-quinone interaction: In vitro induction of indirect antiglobulin reactions with methyldopa. Blood 43:85–97

Grant NH (1970) Penicillin polypeptides and their relevance to allergenicity. In: Weinstein B, Lande S (eds) Peptides: chemistry and biochemistry. Dekker, New York, pp 487–498

Grant NH, Clark DE, Alburn HE (1962) Poly-6-aminopenicillanic acid. J Am Chem Soc 84:876–877

Grantham PE, Mohan LC, Weisburger EK, Fales HM, Sokoloski EA, Weisburger JH (1974) Identification of new water-soluble metabolites of acetanilide. Xenobiotica 4:69–76

Gutzwiller P (1974) Zum Problem der Kortikosteroid-Allergie. Dermatologica 148:253–256

Hamilton-Miller JMT, Newton GGF, Abraham EP (1970) Products of aminolysis and enzymic hydrolysis of the cephalosporins. Biochem J 116:371–384

Hertz CG (1973) The low incidence of side effects with cyclacillin. Arzneim Forsch [Suppl] 25:151–156

Hou JP, Poole JW (1969) The amino acid nature of ampicillin and related penicillins. J Pharm Sci 58:1510–1515

Igarashi H, Koizumi K, Muranaka M (1978) Eliciting antigenicities of benzylpenicillin, ampicillin and carbenicillin preparations examined with the reagin-mediated passive cutaneous anaphylaxis system. Int Arch Allergy Appl Immunol 57:341–348

Jansson S-O, Andersson I (1977) Determination of salicylic acid, acetylsalicylic anhydride and acetylsalicylsalicylic acid in acetylsalicylic acid by high-performance liquid chromatography. Acta Pharm Suec 14:161–170

Jemal M, Hem SL, Knevel AM (1978) Demonstration of penicillamine as a product in benzylpenicillenic acid degradation in neutral media using differential pulse polarography. J Pharm Sci 67:302–305

Jerina DM, Daly JW (1974) Arene oxides: a new aspect of drug metabolism. Science 185:573–582

Jerina DM, Yagi H, Daly JW (1973) Arene oxides-oxepines. Heterocycles 1:267–326

Juhlin L, Ahlstedt S, Andal L, Ekström B, Svärd PO, Wide L (1977) Antibody reactivity in penicillin sensitive patients determined with different penicillin derivatives. Int Arch Allergy Appl Immunol 54:19–28

Juhlin L, Michaëlsson G, Zetterström O (1972) Urticaria and asthma induced by food – and drug – additives in patients with aspirin hypersensitivity. J Allergy Clin Immunol 50:92–98

Kappus H, Remmer H (1975) Irreversible protein binding of ^{14}C-imipramine with rat and human liver microsomes. Biochem Pharmacol 24:1079–1084

Kligman AM (1966) The identification of contact allergens by human assay. III. The maximization test: a procedure for screening and rating contact sensitizers. J Invest Dermatol 47:393–409

Knudsen ET, Robinson OPW, Croydon EAP, Tees EC (1967) Cutaneous sensitivity to purified benzylpenicillin. Lancet 1:1184–1188

Knudsen ET, Dewdney JM, Trafford AP (1970) Reduction in incidence of ampicillin rash by purification of ampicillin. Br Med J 1:469–471

Kounis NG (1976) Untoward reactions to corticosteroids: intolerance to hydrocortisone. Ann Allergy 36:203–206

Kirstofferson A (1979) On the antigens in penicillin allergy. Thesis, University of Göteborg

Kristofferson A, Ahlstedt S, Pettersson E, Svärd PO (1977a) Antigens in penicillin allergy. I. A radioimmunoassay for detection of penicilloylated protein contaminants in penicillin preparations. Int Arch Allergy Appl Immunol 55:13–22

Kristofferson A, Ahlstedt S, Svärd PO (1977b) Antigens in penicillin allergy. II. The influence of the number of penicilloyl residues on the antigenicity of macromolecules as determined by radioimmunoassay (RIA), passive cutaneous anaphylaxis (PCA) and antibody induction. Int Arch Allergy Appl Immunol 55:23–28

Kuchinskas EJ, Levy GN (1972) Comparative stabilities of ampicillin and hetacillin in aqueous solution. J Pharm Sci 61:727–729

Landersjö L, Stjernström G, Lundgren P (1977) Studies on the stability and compatibility of drugs in infusion fluids. IV. Factors affecting the stability of benzylpenicillin in carbohydrate solutions. Acta Pharm Suec 14:293–308

Larsen C, Bundgaard H (1977) Polymerization of penicillins. VI. Time-course of formation of antigenic di- and polymerization products in aqueous ampicillin sodium solutions. Arch Pharm Chem Sci 5:201–209

Larsen C, Bundgaard H (1978a) Polymerization of penicillins. V. Separation, identification and quantitative determination of antigenic polymerization products in ampicillin sodium preparations by high-performance liquid chromatography. J Chromatogr 147:143–150

Larsen C, Bundgaard H (1978b) Penicilloyl ester intermediates in glucose- and fructose-accelerated degradation of benzylpenicillin in aqueous solution. Arch Pharm Chem Sci 6:33–40

Lazary S, Toffler O, de Weck AL (1972) Detection of hypersensitivity to aspirin by serological and skin test techniques. In: Dash CH, Jones HH (eds) Mechanisms in drug allergy. A Glaxo symposium. Churchill Livingstone, Edinburgh London, pp 65–71

Levine BB (1960) Formation of D-penicillamine-cystein mixed disulphide by reaction of D-benzylpenicilloic acid with cystine. Nature 187:940–941

Levine BB (1961) Studies on the formation of the penicillin antigen. II. Some reactions of D-benzylpenicillenic acid in aqueous solution at pH 7.5. Arch Biochem Biophys 93:50–55

Levine BB (1968) Immunochemical mechanism of drug allergy. In: Cain CK (ed) Annual reports in medicinal chemistry, 1967. Academic Press, New York, pp 240–251

Levine BB, Ovary Z (1961) Studies on the mechanism of the formation of the penicillin antigen. III. The N-(D-α-benzylpenicilloyl) group as an antigenic determinant responsible for hypersensitivity to penicillin G. J Exp Med 114:875–904

Levine BB, Redmond AP (1969) Minor haptenic determinant-specific reagins of penicillin hypersensitivity in man. Int Arch Allergy Appl Immunol 35:445–455

Liakopoulou A, Vilim AB (1976) Immunological properties of dialysis retentates from penicillin. Acta Allergol 31:255–264

Littlejohns DW, Assem ESK, Kennedy CTC (1973) Immunological evidence of two forms of allergy to pyrozolone drugs. Rheumatol Rehabil 12:57–61

Matsui F, Robertson DL, Lafontaine P, Kolasinski H, Lovering EG (1978) Stability studies of phenylbutazone and phenylbutazone-antacid oral formulations. J Pharm Sci 67:646–650

Metzler M (1975) Metabolic activation of diethylstilbestrol: indirect evidence for the formation of a stilbene oxide intermediate in hamster and rat. Biochem Pharmacol 24:1449–1453

Meulenhoff JS (1965) The presence and formation of penicillenic acid in penicillin solutions. Pharm Weekbl 100:1325–1337

Mitchell JR, Potter WZ, Hinson JA, Snodgrass WR, Timbrell JA, Gillette JR (1975) Toxic drug reactions. In: Gillette JR, Mitchell JR (eds) Concepts in biochemical pharmacology, part 3. Springer, Berlin Heidelberg New York Handbook of experimental pharmacology, vol 28/3, pp 383–419

Mitchell JR, Nelson WL, Potter WZ, Sasame HA, Jollow DJ (1976) Metabolic activation of furosemide to a chemically reactive hepatotoxic metabolite. J Pharmacol Exp Ther 199:41–52

Molinari M, Schneider CH, de Weck AL, Gouden E, Pfeuti C (1973) Über pseudomonovalente penicilloyl-Kohlenhydrate. Z Immunitaetsforsch Immunobiol 146:225–238

Monder C (1968a) Studies on the reaction of cytochrome C with corticosteroids. Biochim Biophys Acta 164:369–380

Monder C (1968b) Stability of corticosteroids in aqueous solutions. Endocrinology 82:318–326

Monder C, Walker MC, (1970a) Identification of 11 β, 17 α-dihydroxy-3,20-dioxo-4-pregnene-21-al-1,2-^{3}H(21-dehydrocortisol-1,2-^{3}H) and 11 β-hydroxy-4-androstene-3,17-dione-1,2-^{3}H as contaminants in preparations of cortisol-1,2-^{3}H. Steroids 15:1–10

Monder C, Walker MC (1970b) Interactions between corticosteroids and histones. Biochemistry 12:2489–2497

Munro AC, Dewdney JM, Smith H, Wheeler AW (1976) Antigenic properties of polymers formed by β-lactam antibiotics. Int Arch Allergy Appl Immunol 50:192–205

Muranaka M, Igarashi H, Koizumi K, Okumura H, Takeda K, Suzuki S (1974) Elicitation of homologous passive cutaneous anaphylactic reactions by a penicillin preparation. J Allergy Clin Immunol 54:329–338

Muranaka M, Suzuki S, Koizumi K et al. (1978) Benzylpenicillin preparations can evoke a systemic anaphylactic reaction in guinea pigs. J Allergy Clin Immunol 62:276–282

Neu HC (1975a) Aminopenicillins-clinical pharmacology and use in disease states. Int J Clin Pharmacol 11:132–144

Neu HC (1975b) New broad-spectrum penicillins. Drugs 9:81–87

Newton GGF, Abraham EP, Kuwabara S (1968) Preliminary observations on the formation and breakdown of "cepholosporoic acids". Antimicrob Agents Chemother 1967:449–455

Ottens H, Haan E de, Sengers CHJ (1971) A search for high molecular impurities in penicillin G. Int Arch Allergy Appl Immunol 41:575–591

Parker AC, Richmond J (1976) Reduction in incidence of rash using polymer-free ampicillin. Br Med J 1:998

Parker CW, de Weck AL, Kern M, Eisen HN (1962) The preparation and some properties of penicillenic acid derivatives relevant to penicillin hypersensitivity. J Exp Med 115:803–819

Patel S, Perrin JH, Windheuser JJ (1972) GLC analysis of aspirin from solid dosage forms. J Pharm Sci 61:1794–1796

Patriarca G, Venuti A, Schlavino D, Fais G (1976) Intolerance to aspirin: clinical and immunological studies. Z Immunitaetsforsch Immunobiol 151:295–304

Pawelczyk E, Wachowiak R (1969) Chemical characteristics of decay products of drugs. IV. Chemical mechanisms of the decay of phenylbutazone in pharmaceutical preparations. Acta Pol Pharm 26:433–438

Perkins J (1962) Phenindione sensitivity. Lancet 1:127–130

Phills JA, Perelmutter L (1974) IgE mediated and non-IgE mediated allergic-type reactions to aspirin. Acta Allergol 29:474–490

Preud'homme J, Lunel J (1969) Penicillin G. Recherche des impuretés allergisantes. Therapie 24:531–541

Rüefli P (1976) Ciclacillin versus Ampicillin im Doppelblindversuch. Praxis 65:1130–1134

Sassetti RJ, Fudenberg HH (1971) Alpha-methyldopa melanin. Synthesis and stabilization in vitro. Biochem Pharmacol 20:57–66

Schlumberger HD (1975) Immunogenicity of aryl esters of salicylic or acetylsalicylic acid in guinea pigs. Int Arch Allergy Appl Immunol 48:467–474

Schlumberger HD, Löbbecke E-A, Kallos P (1974) Acetylsalicylic acid intolerance. Acta Med Scand 196:451 458

Schneider CH (1970) Immunochemistry of penicillin. In: Stewart GT, McGovern JP (eds) Penicillin allergy, clinical and immunological aspects. Thomas, Springfield, pp 23–58

Schneider CH (1974) Specific reactions to specific drugs: penicillin. In: Yamamura Y, Frick OL, Horiuchi Y, Kishimoto S, Miyamoto T, Naranjo P, de Weck AL (eds) Allergology. Proceedings of the VIIIth International Congress on Allergology, Tokyo 1973. Excerpta Medica, Amsterdam, pp 438–444

Schneider CH, de Weck AL (1967) The reaction of benzylpenicillin with carbohydrates at neutral pH with a note on the immunogenicity of hapten polysaccharide conjugates. Immunochemistry 4:331–343

Schneider CH, de Weck AL (1969) Immunochemical aspects of penicillin chemistry. Int Arch Allergy Appl Immunol 36:129–139

Schneider CH, de Weck AL (1970) Evaluation of intrinsic and extrinsic penicilloyl-specific immunogenicity of penicillins. The use of penicillin hydrolysis catalyzed by 3,6-bis-(dimethylaminomethyl)catechol. Immunochemistry 7:157–166

Schneider CH, de Weck AL, Stäuble E (1971 a) Carboxymethyl cellulose additives in penicillins and the elicitation of anaphylactic. Experientia 27:167–168

Schneider CH, Michl J, de Weck AL (1971 b) Zur Antigenität von Hapten-Polysaccharid-Konjugaten. Eur J Immunol 1:98–106

Schneider CH, Pfeuti C, de Weck AL (1973) Aspects of formation of the D-penicillamine-antigenic determinant from penicilloyl compounds. Helv Chim Acta 56:1235–1243

Schwartz MA (1969) Chemical aspects of penicillin allergy. J Pharm Sci 58:643–661

Schwartz MA, Amidon GL (1966) Reaction of aspirin with amines. Potential mechanism for aspirin allergy. J Pharm Sci 55:1464–1465

Schwartz MA, Wu G-M (1966) Kinetics of reactions involved in penicillin allergy. I. Mechanism of reaction of penicillins and 6-aminophenicillanic acid with glycine in alkaline solutions. J Pharm Sci 55:550–555

Seitzinger IRWT (1973) De bepaling van ontledingsprodukten van penicillenen. Pharm Weekbl 108:961–968

Shaltiel S, Mizrahi R, Stupp Y, Sela M (1970) Reduction in immunological manifestations of 6-aminopenicillanic acid by treatment with water-insoluble pronase. Eur J Biochem 14:509–515

Shaltiel S, Mizrahi R, Sela M (1971) On the immunological properties of penicillins. Proc R Soc Lond [Biol] 179:411–432

Siegel BB (1962) Studies on penicillin hypersensitivity. V. Further studies on the antigenic properties of altered penicillin. J Allergy 33:349–355

Slingsby J, Zuck DA (1972) The kinetic behaviour of phenylbutazone in four solvent systems. Can J Pharm Sci 7:115–116

Smith H, Marshall AC (1971) Polymers formed by some β-lactam antibiotics. Nature 232:45–46

Smith H, Dewdney JM, Wheeler AW (1971) A comparison of the amounts and the antigenicity of polymeric materials formed in aqueous solutions by some β-lactam antibiotics. Immunology 21:527–533

Spitz HD (1977) Analysis of trace amounts of acetylsalicylic anhydride in acetylsalicylic acid. J Chromatogr 140:131–133

Stewart GT (1967) Allergic residues in penicillins. Lancet 1:1177–1183

Stewart GT (1968) Macromolecular residues contributing to the allergenicity of penicillins and cephalosporins. Antimicrob Agents Chemother 1967:543–549

Stewart GT (1969) Proteinaceous and polymeric residues in β-lactam antibiotics and bacitracin. Antimicrob Agents Chemother 1968:128–135

Stewart GT, Butcher BT, Wagle SS, Stanfield MK (1970) Biopolymerization of peptide antibiotics. In: Johnson JF, Porter RS (eds) Liquid crystals and ordered fluids. Plenum, New York, pp 33–51

Stillwell WG, Stafford M, Horning MG (1973) Metabolism of glutethimide (doriden) by the epoxide-diol pathway in the rat and guinea pig. Res Commun Chem Pathol Pharmacol 6:579–590

Stjernström G, Olson OT, Nyqvist H, Lundgren P (1978) Studies on the stability and compatibility of drugs in infusion fluids. VI. Factors affecting the stability of ampicillin. Acta Pharm Suec 15:33–50

Stüttgen G, Masuch E (1973) Exantheme und Hauttestreaktionen auf die Derivate der Penicillansäure Ampicillin und Ciclacillin. Med Klin 68:123–126

Sunaga K, Koide SS (1968) Identification of a prednisolone derivative interacting with calf thymus histones. J Pharm Sci 57:2116–2119

Takahashi K (1968) The reaction of phenylglyoxal with arginine residues in proteins. J Biol Chem 243:6171–6179

Tegner E (1976) Contact allergy to corticosteroids. Int J Dermatol 15:520–523

Tsuji A, Nakashima E, Hamano S, Yamana T (1978) Physicochemical properties of amphoteric β-lactam antibiotics. I. Stability, solubility, and dissolution behaviour of amino-penicillins as a function of pH. J Pharm Sci 67:1059–1066

Van Joost T, Asghar SS, Cormane RH (1974) Skin reactions caused by phenylbutazone. Immunological studies. Arch Dermatol 110:929–933

Vilim AB, Wilson WL, Hughes DW (1976) High molecular weight impurities in benzylpenicillin. Can J Pharm Sci 11:78–81

Vooys RC, Van Ketel WG (1977) Allergic drug eruption from pyrazolone compounds. Contact Dermatitis 3:57–58

Wagner ES, Davis WW, Gorman M (1969) The reaction of benzylpenicillenic acid with thiol-containing compounds. The formation of a possible penicillin antigenic determinant. J Med Chem 12:438–487

Walsh WE, Markowitz H, Jones JD, Gleich GJ (1971) Macromolecular contaminants in penicillin and cephalosporin antibiotics. J Allergy 47:159–169

Weidenmüller HL, Ziegler W (1970) On the proteinaceous impurity of penicillin. Arzneim Forsch 20:585–586

Weiner LM, Rosenblatt M, Howes HA (1963) The detection of humoral antibodies directed against salicylates in hypersensitivity states. J Immunol 90:788–792

Weisburger JH, Weisburger EK (1973) Biochemical formation and pharmacological, toxicological, and pathological properties of hydroxylamines and hydroxamic acids. Pharmacol Rev 25:1–66

Weltman JK, Szaro RP, Settipane GA (1978) An analysis of the role of IgE in intolerance to aspirin and tartrazine. Allergy 34:273–281

Weston RD (1968) Penicilloylated protein contaminating 6-aminopenicillanic acid and benzylpenicillin. Antimicrob Agents Chemother 1967:553–559

CHAPTER 3

Immunopathological Mechanisms and Clinical Aspects of Allergic Reactions to Drugs

A. L. DE WECK

A. Introduction

Untoward reactions to drugs may be due to many different mechanisms. The terms used for the classification of such drug reactions have varied widely. It may therefore be useful to define the most commonly used terms:

Overdosage. The untoward effects are directly related to the administered amount of drug (e.g., absolute overdosage, as in barbiturate suicide) or to its unexpected accumulation due to some excretory or metabolic abnormality in the patient (e.g., kidney or liver failure).

Intolerance. The untoward reaction represents a qualitatively normal pharmacological effect of the drug which, however, is quantitatively increased (e.g., cinchonism after low doses of quinine).

Idiosyncrasy. The reaction to the drug is qualitatively abnormal and does not correspond to the drug's usual pharmacological action. Such reactions do not, however, depend on an immunological mechanism (e.g., hemolytic anemia after primaquine in 6 GPD-deficient individuals).

Side effects. This term should be restricted to the undesirable but unavoidable pharmacological actions of the drug (e.g., sedative effects of antihistaminic drugs).

Secondary effects. These are indirect but not inevitable consequences of the primary action of the drug (e.g., disturbance of the normal bacteriological flora in patients receiving long-term antibiotic therapy).

Allergic reactions. Hypersensitivity or allergic reaction is the result of an immune response of the organism leading to the formation of specific antibodies, sensitized lymphocytes, or both.

This chapter will deal exclusively with adverse reactions due to immunological mechanisms. Ideally, an objective diagnosis of drug allergy should always rest on the demonstration of specific antibodies and/or sensitized lymphocytes to the offending drug. Unfortunately, this is still difficult to achieve in most drug allergies.

In a number of cases, the drug may also trigger the inflammatory cells also responsible for true allergic reactions by different mechanisms than those involving antibodies or sensitized cells. This is the case, for example, of the direct nonimmunological activation of mast cells (STANWORTH 1980) or of the activation of the alternate pathway of complement (HAENSCH et al. 1980; VOIGTLAENDER et al.

1980). In such cases, the mediators released and the sequence of events may be identical or very similar to those occurring during the course of true immunologically mediated allergic reactions. The clinical aspects may also closely mimic immunologically mediated reactions, even if the initial triggering event is of nonimmunological nature. Such reactions have frequently been denominated pseudoallergic reactions (DUKOR et al. 1980).

The first well-documented human allergic reactions to therapeutic agents were recognized early in the twentieth century after the introduction of heterologous antitoxic antisera. Serum sickness from foreign protein injections was for a long time the primary cause of therapeutically mediated allergic reactions. However, with the introduction of new synthetic chemotherapeutic drugs, the phenomenon of drug allergy became more concrete. Only a few years after the introduction of aspirin by Hoffmann in 1897, untoward reactions started to appear (HIRSCHBERG 1902). Phenobarbital was introduced in therapy in 1912, and by 1928 the type of reactions occurring in about 3% of patients treated had become recognized (MENNINGER 1928). One of the earliest papers on drug allergy was published in 1919 and also included aspirin reactions (COOKE 1919). The introduction of the highly sensitizing sulfonamides in the late 1930s contributed to making drug allergy a better-recognized problem, but it is probably the introduction of penicillins at the end of World War II, with their high incidence of sometimes dramatic reactions, which played the biggest part in bringing drug-allergic reactions to the forefront of medical attention. The concept that low-molecular-weight chemicals as well as foreign proteins can cause allergic reactions was considerably fostered by the work of Landsteiner in the early 1930s on the sensitizing potential of simple chemical compounds (LANDSTEINER 1945). This work has indeed remained the basis on which our current thinking on the sensitizing potential of drugs is still based.

The true incidence of allergic reactions to drugs is still a matter of debate (HURWITZ 1969; HURWITZ and WADE 1969). According to a number of reports, about 5% of medical admissions to hospitals are due to some kind of drug reactions, and at least 10%–15% of hospitalized patients experience at least one untoward reaction to drugs (KLEIN et al. 1972). However, probably only 30%–40% of such reactions may be qualified as allergic, although some figures are as low as 6% (BORDA et al. 1968). A recent analysis of the incidence of skin reactions, which constitute the great majority of allergic reactions to drugs, gives a lower figure than has been usually thought, substantially less than 2% for most drugs (ARNDT and JICK 1976). Among the present most commonly used drugs, only ampicillin, other semisynthetic penicillins, trimethoprim-sulfoxazole combinations, corticotrophin, and erythromycin were associated with reaction rates over 2%, as were blood transfusions. The macropapular or morbilliform exanthematous rash appears to be the most common reaction to drugs. In a recent survey (KUOKKANEN 1972), it accounted for 46% of 464 drug reactions. Urticaria occurred in another 23%, fixed drug eruptions in 10%, erythema multiforme in 5.4%, exfoliative dermatitis in 3.7%, and photosensitivity in 2.8%. Steven-Johnson syndrome (erythema multiforme bullosum) and Lyell's syndrome (toxic epidermal necrolysis) accounted for another 5.4% of reactions between them.

Life-threatening reactions to drugs, such as fluid overload or potassium toxicity, are more than three times as frequent as anaphylaxis (JICK et al. 1970). Death from an allergic reaction to a drug is sufficiently rare for few physicians to have seen more than one case. A rough estimate of risk based on hospital surveys is 1:10,000 (Boston collaborative drug surveillance program 1973). For penicillin, the most common cause of anaphylactic drug reactions, the risk has been estimated to be 1:50,000 or less (IDSOE et al. 1968). Even though this is a small risk, it is certainly not acceptable if treatment was inappropriate or not given for a serious therapeutic indication.

As indicated in greater detail in Chap. 6, the diagnosis of allergic reaction to a drug cannot always been made on the basis of an objective demonstration of specific antibodies and/or sensitized lymphocytes (GIRARD et al. 1976). In fact, the diagnosis of drug allergy is more frequently established at the bedside than in the laboratory. Among the clinical criteria which may indicate an allergic drug reaction are the following:

1. The reaction occurs only after repeated exposure to the drug: if reactions occurred during the first administration of a drug, the free interval is usually 8–9 days.
2. The reaction may occur at doses which are far below the usual therapeutic ranges.
3. Clinical manifestations are unrelated to the pharmacological effect of the drugs and are restricted to a limited number of syndromes (see below).
4. Blood and tissue eosinophilia may be present
5. Renewed drug challenge causes the same syndrome
6. Antibodies or sensitized T-lymphocytes reacting to the drug or to its metabolites may be demonstrated.

In addition, the symptoms usually subside promptly when treatment is stopped, but this feature is common to most untoward reactions to drugs regardless of their mechanisms.

B. Chemical Properties Involved in the Allergenic Potential of Drugs

Foreign proteins such as horse serum antitoxin or hormones or enzymes from foreign species (e.g., insulin, ACTH) used in the treatment of human disease are complete antigens and may stimulate IgE and/or IgG antibody formation in most individuals, provided a sufficient dose is administered over a given period of time. When isotypic variations in a protein exist or when the protein is congenitally absent (as in some immunoglobulin deficiencies) immunization may occur even to human proteins (e.g. formation of anti-IgA antibodies in selective IgA deficiency). However, the immune system can also respond to a wide range of low-molecular-weight organic chemicals of pharmacologic or industrial importance, although in this case the occurrence of allergic hypersensitivity is usually rare. Compounds of molecular weight less than 5,000 daltons are usually considered to be poorly or nonimmunogenic (DE WECK 1974). In the case of synthetic polypeptides, molecules with fewer than seven amino acids (1,080 daltons for DNP-polylysine) were shown to be non immunogenic whereas those with seven or more amino acids could induce an immune response (SCHLOSSMANN et al. 1965).

Most drugs are simple chemicals with molecular weights under 1,000 daltons. Our understanding of the immunochemical mechanisms involved in drug allergy is largely based on experimental studies with such low-molecular-weight simple chemical compounds (or haptens). The use of haptens as antigenic determinants in experimental animals has provided an efficient method of investigating the structural basis of immunological specificity (reviewed in LANDSTEINER 1945; PRESSMANN and GROSSBERG 1968). From these studies, a certain number of rules have emerged which appear to be valid also in allergy to low molecular weight chemotherapeutic agents.

I. Formation of Immunogenic Conjugates

The formation of immunogenic conjugates between a simple chemical (or hapten) and a carrier molecule appears to be an absolute requirement for the induction of an immune response to the hapten. It has for a long time been considered that the formation of an immunogenic conjugate required covalent binding between the hapten and some protein or other macromolecular carrier (GELL et al. 1946). The importance of the formation of stable bonds with proteins in the induction of antibody response to organic molecules was suggested originally by Landsteiner, based on the apparent correlation between sensitizing capacity in vivo and the chemical reactivity determined in vitro by conjugation to the amino group of aniline. Eisen and his colleagues (EISEN 1959) confirmed and extended this observation using a homologous series of halopolynitrobenzenes or polynitrobenzene sulfonates, which differ in their protein reactivity but form identical haptenic determinants on proteins. A good correlation between sensitizing capacity and protein reactivity was established. Furthermore, it was shown that substituted nitrobenzenes reacting with proteins in vitro also form stable bonds with skin proteins in vivo. The applicability of the principle of covalent binding to drug allergy in man has been demonstrated also in the case of penicillin allergy (PARKER 1970 a, 1980).

As a rule, simple chemicals which are potent sensitizers are also highly reactive and can readily be shown to form conjugates with proteins in vivo. Those chemicals unable to form covalent bonds with proteins in vitro show no or only a very low incidence of sensitization. The extent to which a simple chemical is reversibly bound to serum proteins such as albumin has no apparent influence on its ability to sensitize. In several instances, the antibodies formed on sensitization with a simple chemical in vivo are specific not for the original compound injected, but for the modified haptenic structure formed on covalent binding to a protein carrier.

In experimental studies on the formation of antibodies to a hapten-protein conjugate, it appears that the more immunogenic the protein, the better the response. Although proteins are usually the most efficient carriers, polypeptides, polysaccharides, lipid membranes, or even polynucleotides may be sufficient to impart immunogenicity. In recent years, direct conjugation of simple chemicals to structural elements of cell membranes (especially of monocytes and macrophages) has been thought to play an important role in the induction of sensitization (DE WECK 1975; SHEARER 1975). The protein carrier or cell membrane structure of the host may contribute to the specificity of the response (partial autoimmunity).

On the basis of numerous experimental studies, it has been assumed that only conjugates formed by covalent binding are immunogenic. Experiments using methylated albumins or electrostatically charged polypeptides as carriers indicate, however, that molecules strongly attached to such carriers by noncovalent bonds may also behave as immunogens (PLESCIA et al. 1968). However, the reversible ionic and hydrophobic interactions most drugs undergo with albumin and other serum proteins are apparently ineffective in promoting immunization. When covalent interactions take place, the hapten usually binds with functional amino acid residues of the proteins, that is amino acids capable of assuming a charge on their side chains, such as lysine, tyrosine, cysteine, and histidine. Obviously, a minimal stability in binding strength is required.

II. Reactive Derivatives and Metabolites

Organic compounds that are known to form covalent bonds with carrier proteins are acid anhydrides, acyl chlorides, reactive aromatic halides, isocyanates, isothiocyanates, mercaptans, quinones, oxazolones, and diazonium salts. While some compounds of this nature are frequently encountered in the chemical and manufacturing industries and may be responsible for cases of industrial allergy, they will seldom if ever be present in drugs, precisely because of their sensitizing potential. However, when an in vivo immune response has occurred following injection of chemicals which appeared by themselves to be nonreactive with proteins in vitro, further investigations invariably show that the immunological activity is due to some antigenic contaminants or to metabolic degradation of the administered compound to some reactive intermediate. The transformation into reactive derivatives may also occur for some unstable drugs without the influence of metabolism. This is the case for penicillins, which in solution spontaneously form penicillenic acids with a highly reactive oxazolone group.

Most drugs do not possess protein reactivity, and it is therefore necessary to assume that reactive metabolites are formed in vivo. Many drugs are converted to chemically reactive metabolites in the liver (REMMER and SCHUPPEL 1972), and this conversion may also mediate different types of direct toxicity in addition to allergy. Direct verification in man that metabolites of drugs are responsible for human allergy has up to now been limited. In a single case of thrombocytopenia produced by acetaminophen, an antibody to a sulfate conjugate of the drug could be demonstrated (EISNER and SHAHIDI 1972). Tentative identification of possible metabolites has also been made in allergic reactions to mesantoin, phenylbutazone, phenacetin, phenindione, amidopyrine and p-amino salicylic acid (PARKER 1980; BUNDGAARD this volume Chap. 2). The concept that quinones are the reactive intermediates responsible for sensitization by arylamines such as paraphenylenediamine, azodyes, p-aminobenzoic acid and its derivatives, including some local anesthetics, sulfonamides, and nitro compounds was thoroughly reviewed 25 years ago by MAYER (1955). However, this concept has not been conclusively verified in human drug allergy.

An exception to the rule that immunogenic conjugates may only be formed by covalent binding appears to be the strong absorption of some low-molecular-weight compounds to cell membranes, as is the case with some metal salts, e.g., nickel, beryllium and chromium salts. These form coordinating complexes with proteins, and the specificity of the reactions induced probably involves the modified autologous protein carriers as well (HUTCHINSON et al. 1975).

III. Requirements for Allergens Eliciting Antibody-Mediated Reactions

Elicitation of allergic reactions of the immediate type due to antibodies requires multivalent antigens acting as a passive link between antibody-combining sites. In the case of anaphylactic reactions due to the interaction of antigen with homocytotropic antibodies (reagins, IgE) bound to the mast cell membrane, bridging of adjacent immunoglobulin molecules by antigens which must be at least bivalent (i.e. two antigenic determinants per molecule) appears to be required (DE WECK et al. 1973; LEVINE 1965; PARKER et al. 1962a). It has been shown convincingly in the penicillin system that antigens carrying three to six penicilloyl determinants per molecule at some suitable distance from each other are optimal elicitors (DE WECK and SCHNEIDER 1969; LEVINE and REDMOND 1968). Elicitation of anaphylactic reactions by univalent haptens, on the other hand, has remained an exception (FRICK et al. 1968; DE WECK et al. 1973). Reactions to univalent haptens are probably the result of nonspecific aggregation of the hapten in vivo or of binding to cell membranes yielding multivalent antigens.

Drugs which elicit clinical anaphylactic reactions in vivo in sensitized individuals may do so only if they possess a relatively high degree of protein reactivity and form multivalent hapten-carrier conjugates within a short time. A higher degree of chemical reactivity is required to elicit an anaphylactic reaction than to sensitize, since anaphylaxis requires significant amounts of multivalent conjugates. Even if this requirement is met, which is rarely the case, some unconjugated drug will often still be present in large excess and will compete for available antibody-combining sites ("built-in inhibition"), provided that the sensitizing antigenic determinant formed on conjugation and the unconjugated drugs have sufficient structural similarities to permit cross-reactivity. Therefore, immediate-type skin tests with unconjugated chemicals or drugs are frequently negative even in sensitized animals or individuals who react readily to preformed multivalent conjugates. In some cases, eliciting antigens may be formed directly without conjugation to protein carriers if the drug is able to dimerize or polymerize, thereby yielding multivalent antigenic determinants. Such polymers may be nonimmunogenic, since their potential conjugating capacity has been exhausted by the formation of the polymer. Accumulation of dimers and polymers in penicillin solutions is probably responsible for the bulk of anaphylactic reactions to penicillin (DE WECK et al. 1968; DEWDNEY 1977). Of significance may also be the presence of macromolecular contaminants, e.g., protein impurities or macromolecular additives capable of functioning as carriers (BATCHELOR et al. 1967; STEWART 1967; KRISTOFFERSON et al. 1977; DE WECK et al. 1969; KNUDSEN et al. 1970).

While bivalent antigens may suffice to induce anaphylactic reactions, the induction of Arthus reactions and activation of complement require the formation of a tridimensional multimolecular antigen-antibody lattice. Accordingly, Arthus reactions may be elicited only by trivalent antigens and are rarely observed in drug allergy.

IV. Requirements for Allergens Eliciting Cell-Mediated (Delayed-Type) Allergic Reactions

Delayed-type allergic reactions occur when T-lymphocytes have been sensitized to simple chemicals, forming conjugates in vivo. Conjugates eliciting delayed-type reactions must have a chemical structure (hapten and carrier) very similar if not identical to that responsible for sensitization (GELL and BENACERRAF 1961). Experimental evidence suggests that the mononuclear infiltration characteristic of delayed-type reactions is due to synthesis and release of inflammatory mediators (lymphokines) from specific T-lymphocytes following renewed contact with the sensitizing simple chemical. Although the molecular mechanism which triggers these events is not yet elucidated, indirect evidence suggests that it is basically different from the mere bridging of adjacent immunoglobulin receptors by multivalent antigens, as observed for mast cells in anaphylaxis. Experiments on the stimulation of penicillin-sensitive T-lymphocytes in vitro suggest that their activity may be triggered only by antigenic determinants actively presented on the membrane of other living cells, preferentially monocytes (DE WECK 1975). Whether B-lymphocytes may, like mast cells, also be activated by passive bridging of immunoglobulin receptors through multivalent antigens has not been conclusively established. In vitro at least, the presence of monocytes or macrophages (acting as antigen-presenting cells) appears to be necessary to stimulate sensitized T- and/or B-lymphocytes with soluble hapten-protein conjugates. Nonconjugates haptens or monovalent hapten-amino acid conjugates are definitely unable to stimulate sensitized lymphocytes to proliferate or to produce lymphokines (SPENGLER et al. 1974). In delayed-type reactions initiated by lymphokines, secondary antibody response in situ by infiltrating B-lymphocytes, as well as antibody-dependent reactions involving cytophilic antibodies on monocytes and infiltrating mast cells, probably contributes to the inflammatory events in later stages of the reaction (ASKENAZE 1977).

V. Impurities and Galenic Factors Involved in Sensitization

As already discussed above, the presence of reactive contaminating chemicals may sometimes be responsible for sensitization, rather than the drug itself. This was shown to be the case for aspirin anhydride and acetylsalicylsalicylic acid, two contaminants present in aspirin which appear to be responsible for the induction of antiaspiryl and antisalicyloyl antibodies in a number of patients (DE WECK 1971; BUDGAARD and DE WECK 1975; AMOS et al. 1971). It has not been demonstrated, however, that these contaminants are responsible for symptoms of intolerance to aspirin. In some cases of drug allergy, the presence of macromolecular contaminants, e.g., protein impurities, has been considered to play a major role. In the initial years following the introduction of penicillins, which were extracted from a fermentation medium containing numerous macromolecular components, protein impurities were considered to play an important role in the allergic reactions which had been observed since the beginning of therapy with penicillins. Improvements in the techniques of purification and extraction decreased the incidence of such reactions considerably. However, as recently as 1967 the demonstration of penicilloylated protein impurities in commercial penicillins (BATCHELOR et al. 1967) renewed interest in this possible cause of penicillin allergy. A controversy developed at that time over the effective role of such protein traces in the induction of sensitization and the elicitation of allergic reactions in sensitized patients, since further purification measures did not appear to abolish penicillin hypersensitivity (DE WECK et al. 1968). The possible role of protein impurities in penicillin hypersensitivity has been reviewed recently by AHLSTEDT et al. (1980), and a more thorough discussion of this problem is presented in Chap. 10.

Various types of additives introduced in the galenic presentation of drugs such as dyes (e.g., tartrazine) preservatives (e.g., parabens) or filling material (e.g., carboxymethylcellulose, starch) may function themselves as sensitizers or as inert macromolecular carriers facilitating the formation in vitro of eliciting hapten conjugates. Indeed, it has been shown that carboxymethylcellulose, for example, is an efficient carrier for penicilloyl groups, (SCHNEIDER et al. 1971) and may by itself act as sensitizer in cattle (DE WECK et al. 1969).

C. Induction of Immune Responses to Drugs: Main Factors Involved

The induction of the immune response to drugs appears to be governed by the same rules and factors that play a role in experimental sensitization to simple chemical compounds. Some factors are inherent to the sensitizing drug, whereas others involve the host.

I. Factors Involving the Sensitizing Drug

1. Chemical Structure and Reactivity

Most drugs in clinical use are not such highly reactive chemicals as to form stable conjugates readily when incubated with proteins in vitro. Furthermore, the incidence of clinical allergic reactions to drugs is generally low, and correlation between chemical reactivity and sensitization index is usually difficult to establish. However, highly reactive chemicals such as dinitrochlorobenzene and chloramine-T have a high sensitization index in man. Furthermore, when the incidence of the immune response is evaluated not from the incidence of overt clinical reactions but by objective immunological procedures, good correlations may be demonstrated between chemical reactivity and sensitizing capacity (e.g., penicillins). The involvment of enzymatic and metabolic processes in the coupling of drugs to proteins in vivo is increasingly recognized (REMMER and SCHUEPPEL 1972), even though in many instances the reactive derivatives responsible for drug allergy have not been identified.

The fact that antibodies detected in drug-allergic patients may be specific for modified structures derived from the original structure of the drug, such as the penicilloyl group in penicillin allergy (DE WECK 1979; PARKER 1980) or a sulfate conjugate in the case of thrombocytopenia induced by acetaminophen (EISNER and SHAHIDI 1972), attests that metabolic degradation and in vivo conjugation effectively play a role in the induction of drug hypersensitivity.

2. Cross-Sensitization

Cross-sensitization occurs when allergic reactions induced by one compound are subsequently elicited by one or more related compounds. The range of cross-sensitization to drugs is extremely variable. Among the clinically frequent causes of cross-reactions, substances of the so-called para group (i.e., possessing a free amino group in the para position of a benzene ring) such as benzocaine, p-aminobenzoic acid, paraphenylenediamine, procaine, and sulfonamides, compounds with the phenothiazine structure, and those possessing the penicilin nucleus (penicillins and cephalosporins) should be emphasized. The range of cross-sensitization may vary with time and repeated exposure, as observed also in experimental sensitization to haptens (STEINER and EISEN 1966). Immunochemical studies have shown wide individual variations in range of cross-sensitization to penicillins with various side chains and have also demonstrated heterogeneity in the affinity of antibodies formed in individual patients.

3. Dose, Duration, and Number of Courses of Therapy

There is a general feeling that the higher the dose and the longer the period of administration, the greater the probability of sensitization, but it is very difficult to collect reliable data in this regard. With penicillin or insulin, courses of therapy with moderate doses repeated at various intervals seem to lead more frequently to sensitization than prolonged treatment without free intervals. On the other hand, minute doses are certainly capable of inducing sensitization in some genetically predisposed individuals.

   With most drugs, the risk of allergy probably increases with the daily dose or when there is interference with the drug excretion (hepatic or renal insufficiency, congenital enzyme defects). For the induction of hemolytic anemia by penicillin, adequate penicilloylation of the erythrocytes require high and sustained penicillin blood levels. Under these conditions, however, other manifestations of penicillin allergy, such as anaphylaxis and serum sickness, appear to be rare. It is well known that IgE synthesis requires rather small doses of antigen; accordingly, high doses of penicillin may cause high-dose tolerance as far as IgE antibodies are concerned.

4. Mode of Administration

Except for contact dermatitis, the route of administration appears to be of little importance in determining the type of hypersensitivity and clinical symptoms produced. Application of allergenic drugs to the skin is usually associated with a high incidence of sensitization (favorable conditions for the formation of conjugates?), whereas the oral route appears to be less likely to foster sensitization. Allergic reactions occur in about 2.5% of patients given penicillin G parenterally, in 5%

of those receiving procaine penicillin intramuscularly, and in approximately 0.3% of those receiving benzathine penicillin intramuscularly or phenoxymethyl- or ben- zylpenicillin orally (WEINSTEIN and WEINSTEIN 1974). The initial route of exposure may influence the site of reactions, as shown by the fact that workers repeatedly exposed to penicillin dust frequently develop asthma when later exposed to the drug by the oral route (DAVIES et al. 1974). Some drugs, such as chlorprothixene, which on topical application frequently cause contact dermatitis, have an extreme- ly low sensitization index when given orally. To what extent this phenomenon may be related to the fact that feeding with haptens may induce immunological toler- ance (CHASE 1946) is not clear. Oral administration of drugs such as penicillin and sulfonamides to sensitive patients can also induce severe allergic reactions such as anaphylactic shock (KRAPIN 1962; SPARK 1971). The oral route therefore is by no means entirely "safe." Additives and solvents, of which oils, carboxymethylcel- lulose, and emulsifiers may be examples, may have an adjuvant effect by favoring retention of antigen and by causing local inflammation. The depot forms of insulin, for example, induce an immune response more readily than rapidly resorbed prep- arations (FANKHAUSER 1969).

II. Factors Involving the Patient

In general, it can be said that the patient rather than the drug determines the in- cidence of sensitization. Allergic reactions occur in a comparatively small number of patients who take drugs, since drugs with an unusually high allergic potential (e.g., phenylethylhydantoin) are either kept from distribution or soon withdrawn.

1. The Immune System and the Regulation of Immune Responses to Drugs

The immune system is composed of lymphoid cell populations of various origins and functions (monocytes/macrophages, T- and B-lymphocytes), distributed in various lymphoid organs (spleen, lymph nodes, thymus, Peyer's patches, tonsils, etc.) and which differentiate from the bone marrow under the influence of various factors and hormones (Fig. 1). Upon interaction with antigen, various subsets of T-lymphocytes may arise with helper, suppressor, and/or cytotoxic functions, while B-lymphocytes may differentiate into antibody-producing plasma cells, re- sponsible for the large scale synthesis of immunoglobulin of various classes.

Aside from the presence of appropriately differentiated subsets of lymphoid cells ready to cooperate, the induction of an immune response requires suitable presentation of the antigen to T- and/or B-lymphocytes carrying the corresponding antigen-specific T-receptors or immunoglobulins respectively and ready to under- go clonal expansion. It is generally considered that the macrophages play a decisive role in antigen presentation. The regulation of the immune response is currently understood as the interplay of several immunoregulatory circuits involving various subpopulations of suppressor and helper T cells, macrophages, and B cells (GER- MAIN et al. 1981). Antigen-specific T cell helper and suppressor factors, as well as nonspecific amplifying factors produced by the macrophages (interleukin 1) or subsets of T-lymphocytes (interleukin 2), are also required for a full-fledged re-

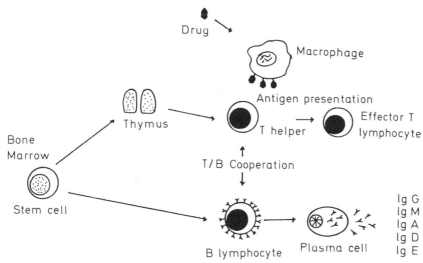

Fig. 1. Schematic representation of the possible reactions of the immune system to drugs. A drug is probably presented as antigen most efficiently after binding to macrophage membranes and interacting with T-helper lymphocytes, which may either generate effector-sensitized T-lymphocytes or cooperate with B-lymphocytes in the production of antidrug antibodies. This scheme of T/B cooperation is extremely oversimplified, since the various circuits of T-helper and suppressor cells are not represented (GERMAIN et al. 1981)

sponse. As such, the immune response to a drug should not be regulated differently than the response to other antigens, with the exception that the formation of antigenic conjugates may obey special rules. Furthermore, some drugs may influence the immune response itself and/or some of the lymphoid cell subsets involved through their own pharmacological effects.

2. Age and Sex

Allergic reactions to drugs appear to be less frequent in children than in adults (BERKOWITZ et al. 1953; BIERMAN and VAN ARSDEL 1969). This may represent the effect of accumulated exposure rather than an intrinsic difference between children and adults in the capacity to respond. Severe allergic reactions may also be observed in very small infants; death from anaphylactic shock after penicillin may occur even in babies (passive sensitization from maternal blood or milk). Indeed, the capacity to synthesize antipenicilloyl antibodies arises as early as the 6th month of gestation. Aged people seem somewhat less prone to become sensitized. There is no definite evidence, with some exceptions (BOLTON and DAMESHEK 1956; KUOKANNEN 1972), that the incidence of drug reactions on similar exposure would be higher in females than in males.

3. Genetic Factors

Genetic factors play an important role in the development of hypersensitivity to drugs. It has been claimed that patients with an atopic constitution are predisposed to develop immediate-type hypersensitivity to drugs, especially penicillin (Miller 1967; Rajka and Skog 1965), but this statement does not appear to hold true (Green and Rosenblum 1971). Immediate-type allergy to injected allergens such as penicillin, insect venoms, and insulin (in contrast to inhaled or ingested allergens) does not appear to be more common in atopic than in nonatopic patients (Parker 1980; Horowitz and Parker 1975). Anaphylactic sensitivity to penicillin frequently develops in nonatopic individuals, and many patients with allergy to drugs have no allergic background. Genetic factors probably also condition an individual specifically for sensitization to a given drug or chemical. In experimental sensitization to various chemicals, it has become evident that the immune response is specifically under the influence of genetic factors, among which the so-called immune response (Ir) genes, which are linked to major histocompatibility complex genes, have attracted the most attention (Benacerraf and Germain 1978). Genetic differences in the sensitivity of guinea pigs to various drugs such as phenetidin, aspirin, hydralazine, and penicillin have been established (Ellmann et al. 1971; Geczy and de Weck 1974). The rapidly evolving field of pharmacogenetics also provides evidence that a number of individual variations in the metabolism of drugs are genetically determined. Genetic factors could therefore intervene at several levels in the biochemical pathways leading to sensitization, such as the formation of reactive metabolites or the selectively inherited ability to form antibodies specific for a given chemical structure. However, typing for histocompatibility antigens of the HLA system in patients allergic to penicillins has not yet revealed any clear-cut association with any allele of the HLA-A or HLA-B locus (Spengler and de Weck 1977).

The rate of drug metabolism, which is in part under genetic control, may be of importance. The population with low levels of hepatic acetyltransferase activity seems at greater risk of developing the hydralazine-induced lupus syndrome (Perry et al. 1970), but this does not hold for procainamide-induced lupus. Genetic factors have also been implied in pseudoallergic reactions, such as aspirin intolerance (Lockey et al. 1963).

4. Underlying Diseases

The incidence of drug allergy may be influenced by diseases affecting the metabolism and excretion of the drug, such as chronic hepatic or renal disease, although these probably have a more direct influence on toxic effects. Theoretically, drug reactions should occur less frequently in patients whose immunological responsiveness is impaired. However, hypogammaglobulinemic patients are still capable of developing exanthematous eruptions to drugs (Good et al. 1962). Patients with sarcoidosis and viral diseases with impaired cellular hypersensitivity seem less prone to develop contact dermatitis and drug exanthemas, but they still manifest urticarial and anaphylactic reactions (Chase 1966).

On the other hand, some diseases are associated with a very high incidence of drug-induced reactions. This seems to be the case for systemic lupus erythematosus (SLE) (Brown and Kanwar 1967) although penicillin allergy does not seem to be more frequent in such patients (Von Maur et al. 1975). Individuals with hyperuricemia on allopurinol treatment, infectious mononucleosis, or lymphatic leukemia have a very high incidence of maculopapular skin rashes when treated with ampicillin (BROWN and KANWAR 1967; PULLEN et al. 1967), but it is not certain that such reactions occur through immunological mechanisms (McKENZIE et al. 1976). Immunosuppression may paradoxically enhance the sensitization potential of drugs by depressing suppressor T cells, which regulate IgE antibody synthesis. In a patient immunosuppressed following a bone marrow transplant, an IgE-mediated reaction to polymyxin B has been documented (LAKIN et al. 1975).

Another factor possibly predisposing to allergic reactions is therapy with several drugs activating enzymatic liver systems such as cytochrome P-450. The rate of reactions seems to increase in patients treated with 12 or more drugs (SMITH et al. 1966). The clinical observation of multiple drug "sensitivities" is quite common and has sometimes been documented (GIRARD et al. 1971). Inductive effects on enzymes responsible for drug metabolism, interference of drugs with their respective metabolisms (GOLDMAN and BRAMAN 1972), or enhancing effects on the immune responsiveness may play a role. Although simultaneous allergies to several drugs can sometimes be documented, it is likely that untoward reactions to a large number of chemically unrelated drugs are usually of toxic rather than immunological nature.

5. Variable Relationship Between the Immune Response to a Drug and the Incidence of Clinical Allergic Symptoms

Studies of the immune response to penicillins have shown that the incidence of an immune response after administration of a drug may be considerably higher than would be expected from the mere incidence of overt clinical allergic reactions. For example, a large percentage of patients receiving penicillin develop IgM antibodies. According to the sensitivity of the hemagglutination technique used, the percentage reported has varied between 20% and 100% (LEVINE et al. 1966 b; DE WECK 1964). It is now certain that an immune response to a drug may not be evident clinically. Caution should therefore be exercised in the interpretation of clinical data not based on immunochemical investigations and the use of suitable techniques for antibody detection. The clinical manifestations of the hypersensitivity state may be governed not only by the types of antibodies formed, but also by the relative proportion of the various immunoglobulins present at various times. For example, in most cases, the presence of IgM antibodies to penicillin does not lead to clinical symptoms and the presence of IgG antibodies sometimes appears to be protective. In patients developing IgE antibodies and anaphylactic reactivity, high titers of IgG antibody may be sufficient to compete for antigens and prevent anaphylactic reactions. In penicillin urticaria and in the serum sickness syndrome, the disappearance of skin lesions often coincides with a marked rise of the antipenicilloyl IgG level in the serum. A summary of the immunoglobulins formed on administration of penicillin and of their biological and pathological properties is given in Table 1.

There is an increasing awareness of the role of delayed-type hypersensitivity in clinical drug reactions (REDMOND and LEVINE 1968). Drug fever and especially the typical maculopapular exanthemas common to several drug reactions might be the expression of delayed-type hypersensitivity. The development of suitable test reagents and methods of investigation for sensitized lymphocytes in vitro has re-

Table 1. Clinical forms of allergic reactions to penicillins: immunological parameters

Clinical reaction	Interval between penicillin administration and symptoms	Main symptoms	Antibodies involved	Specificity[a]
No reaction	Undetermined	None	IgM or IgG	BPO
Anaphylactoid reaction	1–5 min after IV injection	Neurological and sensorial	None	None
Anaphylactic shock	5–120 min	Cardiovascular collapse	IgE	BPO and minor determinants
Immediate urticaria	2–14 h	Urticaria	IgE	BPO
Serum-sickness-like disease	1–3 weeks	Urticaria, fever arthralgias, adenopathies	IgG and IgE	BPO and minor determinants
Chronic urticaria	Variable	Urticaria and pressure urticaria	IgE	Minor determinants and BPO
Exanthema	5–10 days	Morbilliform exanthema, rash	Sensitized lymphocytes or IgG immune complexes	BPO and minor determinants
Hemolytic anemia	Variable	Anemia with positive Coombs test	IgG and IgM	BPO

[a] BPO, benzylpenicilloyl; major determinant

vealed that specific sensitized T-lymphocytes are frequently present in the peripheral blood of patients allergic to drugs. However, the mere presence of lymphocytes reacting to the drug in lymphocyte culture is not sufficient to predict the outcome of therapy. In numerous patients treated with high doses of penicillin without untoward symptoms, lymphocyte tests may be positive, at least for a while (SAURAT et al. 1976; NEFTEL et al. 1981).

In allergic patients, drug-sensitive lymphocytes usually persist in the circulation for several years (SPENGLER et al. 1974). Drug-specific IgE antibodies, on the other hand, may decrease within a few months of last exposure to the drug, as well documented with penicillin (KRAFT et al. 1977; DE WECK 1978). Skin reactivity also appears to decrease with time, although at a slower pace than IgE antibodies, probably due to a differences in half-life between free or cell bound IgE antibodies (2.4 vs 14–21 days).

D. Immunopathological Mechanisms of Allergic Reactions to Drugs

I. Antibody-Mediated Reactions

It is classical to divide allergic reactions into four types according to the classification of GELLS and COOMBS (1962). Whereas this classification may still appear valid as far as some of the initial triggering events of allergic or immunologically mediated reactions are concerned, it has become obvious that it represents a rather simplistic approach to the complex reality of immunologically mediated reactions in tissues.

1. Anaphylactic Reactions

It is generally agreed upon that the initial event in anaphylactic reactions is the interaction of allergen with IgE antibodies bound to special receptors on the membrane of tissue mast cells and blood basophils (ISHIZAKA and ISHIZAKA 1978). The capacity of IgE antibodies (previously denominated reagins) to bind firmly to such cellular receptors is the main feature of this type of antibodies, also called homocytotropic. In most animal species, however, a second type of homocytotropic antibody, usually a subclass of IgG, has been shown to bind to similar receptors on the same cells, although with lesser avidity. These antibodies are also able to elicit anaphylactic reactions (PARISH 1970). It is still disputed at the present time whether IgG4 or some subclass of immunoglobulins carrying IgG4 determinants represent the long sought second class of homocytotropic antibodies in men (STANWORTH and SMITH 1973; VAN TOORENENBERGEN and AALSBERSE 1981). In any case, bridging of IgE molecules by antigen on the surface of tissue mast cells and blood basophils appears to provide a triggering event required to induce these cells to produce and/or release their mediators. Recent studies (ISHIZAKA and ISHIZAKA 1978) have demonstrated that it is in fact the bridging of the IgE receptors which is the required triggering event. This can be brought about by bifunctional reagents acting on the IgE receptors themselves (e.g., by anti-IgE receptor antibody), in which case the presence of IgE is not even required for triggering the reaction. Experimentally, the bridging of IgE molecules and/or their cellular receptors can be achieved by a variety of bi- or plurifunctional agents (Fig. 2). The bridging of IgE receptors appears to trigger on the one hand the activation of adenyl cyclase and on the other hand the transmethylation of enzymes affecting the production of arachidonic acid metabolites such as prostaglandins and related inflammatory mediators, e.g., slow-reacting substance of anaphylaxis (Marone et al. 1981). Activation of the mast cells and blood basophils by IgE-mediated interactions also leads to an influx of intracellular calcium, which appears instrumental in causing the expulsion of intracellular granules, in which a number of preformed mediators such as histamine and heparin are being stored. Although it is no longer certain that all mediators, either preformed or formed by the mast cell only after triggering, are being released simultaneously, it appears that mast cell and blood basophil degranulation occurs in most instances of anaphylactic reactions.

Several of the mediators stored or synthesized and released by the mast cells have an effect on capillary permeability. An increase in capillary permeability permits the influx of several blood proteins into the adjacent tissues, thereby causing disturbances in osmotic equilibrium and tissular edema. In the skin, this is manifested by the formation of an urticarial wheal and by erythema. In addition, contraction of the nonstriated muscle fibers wherever they occur and increase in the secretion from exocrine glands are common features. Since the major mediators present in tissue mast cells and blood basophils are either preformed (e.g., histamine) or arise within seconds following the triggering event, it is understandable that anaphylactic reactions develop very rapidly following contact with antigen; they also have a relatively limited duration.

However, a number of secondary reactions are the consequence of anaphylactic triggering, since several mast cell mediators interact with other cell types. For example, release of eosinophil chemotactic factors (ECF-A) is probably the main reason for the secondary involvement of eosinophils in most anaphylactic reactions. Although the full role of eosinophils in allergic reactions is not yet definitely established, it appears certain that they represent "cleaning-up" cells, capable on the one hand of phagocytosing excess antigen and on the other hand of destroying some of the inflammatory mediators produced by tissue mast cells (histaminase, arylsulfatase) (Ottesen and Cohen 1978). Another type of cell which probably also plays an important role in some immediate-type allergic reactions is the platelet (Benveniste 1974). A drop in circulating blood platelet counts is frequently observed in systemic allergic reactions and appears to be due to platelet aggregation in lung capillaries. Release of platelet activating factor (PAF) during immediate-type allergic reactions has been demonstrated. Since platelets contain large amounts of serotonin, this may also be the reason why serotonin can be detected in man in some immediate-type skin reactions. (Kaplan et al. 1975) even if no or very little serotonin is present in human mast cells and blood basophils, in contrast to other species. Chemotactic factors for neutrophils (NCF) have also been described; since neutrophils are also able when stimulated to produce various inflammatory mediators, e.g., slow-reacting substance of anaphylaxis (SRS-A) their potential role in the late phases of IgE-mediated reactions should not be overlooked (Askenaze 1980).

In recent years, it has been shown that IgE antibodies may be bound not only to the mast cells and basophils mediating anaphylactic reactions, but also to mac-

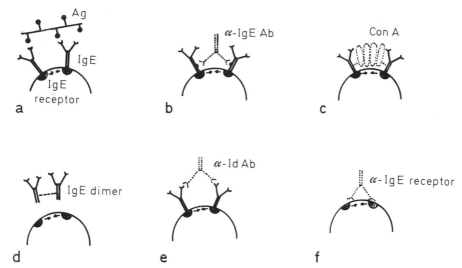

Fig. 2a–f. Triggering of mast cells and blood basophils by bridging of IgE receptors. The bridging of IgE receptors, which is the triggering event leading to mediator release from mast cells and basophils, may be caused by several mechanisms. **a** Bridging of adjacent IgE molecules by a plurivalent antigen (*Ag*). **b** Bivalent anti-IgE antibody (*α-IgE Ab*) directed against the Fc portion. **c** Leucoagglutinin (e.g., *con A*) interacting with IgE. **d** Soluble IgE dimer or polymer. **e** Bivalent anti-idiotypic antibody (*α-Id Ab*) reacting with IgE idiotypes. **f** Bivalent anti-IgE receptor antibody

rophages (CAPRON et al. 1975) and to subsets of T-lymphocytes (SPIEGELBERG 1981). Indeed, IgE bound to macrophages has been shown to play a role in the cytotoxic elimination of parasites. The possible interaction of allergen with IgE on lymphocytes also raises the still theoretical possibility that lymphokines produced by such activated T-lymphocytes could be responsible for the delayed reactions which have been described in IgE-possessing individuals and which had been attributed to IgE, through mechanisms which are not yet elucidated (SOLLEY et al. 1976). Recently, it has been shown that human monocytes passively sensitized by incubation with sera from allergic individuals and triggered by anti-IgE antibodies or allergen release lysosomal enzymes (JOSEPH et al. 1977) and become cytotoxic (SPIEGELBERG 1981).

The fact that IgE-mediated reactions require the bridging of IgE receptors brings some special constraints to the elicitation of such reactions by drugs. As clearly shown by several authors (LEVINE 1965, 1976; DE WECK and SCHNEIDER 1969), only compounds possessing at least two antigenic determinants per molecule are capable of producing such a bridging (Fig. 2). The chance that bi- or plurivalent conjugates of a drug, i.e., conjugates possessing two or more haptenic groups on the same carrier, would be formed in vivo is rather remote, unless the drug is highly reactive chemically and present at high concentration. This may be the reason why anaphylactic reactions immediately following administration of drugs are relatively seldom, with the exception of highly reactive chemicals (such as chloramine-T or phthalic anhydride), of drugs capable of polymerizing, and of compounds of biological origin which may contain high-molecular-weight impurities. These three criteria apply to penicillins, and this may be the reason why penicillins are by far the most frequent cause of anaphylactic reactions to drugs.

It must be remembered, however, that in experimental allergy anaphylactic reactions may also in some cases be elicited by molecules which appear, on paper at least, to be monovalent and to be able to combine with a single antibody combining site (AMKRAUT et al. 1963; CAMPBELL and McCASLAND 1944; SCHNEIDER et al. 1979; DE WECK et al. 1973). The mere impact of one antigenic determinant in a single antibody combining site does not appear to be sufficient to trigger the reaction, but on the contrary usually inhibits it (GARDNER and OVARY 1960; FARAH et al. 1960). Our current working hypothesis to explain anaphylaxis by monovalent antigens is that a part of the molecule acts as antigenic determinant and interacts with an IgE molecule of high affinity, while some other portion of the monovalent elicitor interacts either with a membrane protein or nonspecifically with another IgE molecule. This might suffice to achieve the required bridging of IgE receptors within the mast cell membrane.

2. Cytotoxic Reactions

According to the Gell/Coombs classification, in type II or cytotoxic reactions, specific antibodies interact with antigen present on the surface of target cells. Activation of complement following this interaction is then responsible for the cytotoxic damage to the target cell. In recent years, however, there has been increasing realization that immunologically mediated cytotoxic damage to target cells by drugs can come about by different mechanisms. These include:

1. Interaction of antibodies, especially of the IgM and IgG type, with antigenic determinants present on the membrane of target cells, followed by classical activation of complement (Gell/Coombs type II).

2. Complexing of antigen with antibody in free solution, followed by the attachment of immune complexes to a target cell and activation of complement. In this case, the damaged cell plays the role of an "innocent bystander."

3. Modification by the drug of membrane proteins on the target cell, leading to an alteration in the process of self-recognition and to an autoimmune response against the modified target cell. It is conceivable that drugs might also cause autoimmune reactions by acting on elements of the immune response at other levels than the target cell, for example by interfering with suppressor cells.

4. Covering of antigenic determinants by specific antibodies on target cells, followed by deleterious effects brought about by cytotoxic T-lymphocytes (antibody-dependent cell cytotoxicity).

5. Interactions of macrophages bearing cytophilic antibodies (armed macrophages) with target cells bearing antigenic determinants.

6. Interaction of antigenic determinants on target cells with sensitized T-lymphocytes leading to the activation of such lymphocytes and to the destruction of target cells, possibly through the formation of lymphotoxins and/or of toxic peroxides.

These various cytotoxic mechanisms are represented schematically in Fig. 3. Immunologically mediated cytotoxic reactions to drugs may affect target cells in

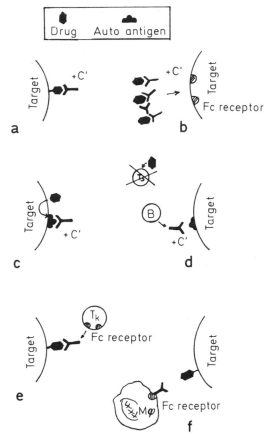

Fig. 3 a–f. Various mechanisms of immune cytotoxic target cell destruction by drugs and antibodies. **a** Direct interaction of antidrug antibody and complement with drug bound to the target cell membrane (e.g., hemolytic anemia to penicillin). **b** Formation of drug-antibody complexes, bound to a target cell possessing Fc receptors and leading to activation of complement (e.g., some thrombocytopenias). **c** Transformation of membrane structures into autoantigens by drugs, generation and binding of autoantibodies with interaction of complement (e.g., hemolytic anemia to α-methyldopa?). **d** Suppression of T suppressor cells *(Ts)* by drugs, polyclonal activation of B cells leading to the formation of autoantibodies. **e** Same mechanism as **a** (generation of antidrug antibodies), but killing by a cytotoxic cell *(Tk)* ("antibody-dependent cell cytotoxicity"). **f** Same mechanism as **e**, but killing by an activated macrophage

various organs such as the liver or the kidney, but most frequently such reactions appear to affect circulating blood cells.

3. Immune Complex Reactions

While in the original conceptions of immune complex diseases, interaction of antigen with antibody in free solution frequently led to tissue damage, it has become clear that the large majority of immune complexes arising in vivo are probably not pathogenic at all. First, the size and composition of the complex seems to play a role in tissue damage: small soluble complexes are more likely to be phagocytosed and digested by macrophages than to be deposited in tissue with corresponding lesions. Since the formation of large multimolecular complexes requires multideterminant antigens, it is unlikely that drugs will often produce in vivo the required conjugates (see Sect. B.IV). Second, complement components in serum appear in most instances to favour solubilization of the complexes. Third, deposition of complexes does not appear to occur at random; it seems that part of the complex (usually the antigen) must have some peculiar affinity for the tissue in which the complex will be deposited. Fourth, the deposition of complexes usually requires an increase in capillary permeability, which may be brought about by a concomitant sensitization of the IgE type or by complement fragments (C3a, C5a) generated upon complement activation.

For all these reasons, immune complex reactions to drugs, such as Arthus reactions in the skin, appear to be extremely rare. The most striking allergic reaction to drugs in which an immune complex mechanism is certainly involved is the serum-sickness-like disease. Other forms include hematological disorders such as hemolytic anemia, thrombocytopenia, and agranulocytosis. An immune complex mechanism is also suspected in several instances of drug fever, exanthematous skin rashes, and possibly drug-induced nephritis (see Sect. E.VI).

The pathophysiology of immune complex reactions occurs in several stages: formation of immune complexes in antigen excess, deposition of complexes in tissue, activation of complement followed by attraction at the site of plynuclear neutrophils, and liberation in tissue of proteolytic lysosomal enzymes and inflammatory cationic proteins. The importance of concomitant increase in vascular permeability for the deposition of immune complexes has been shown in vivo by the preventive effect of antihistaminic and antiserotonin drugs on the development of serum sickness to horse antidiphteric serum (KNIKER et al. 1971).

The liberation of lysosomal enzymes from neutrophils may occur through different mechanisms: ingestion of immune complexes with formation and expulsion of a vacuole filled with hydrolases (phagosome), exocytosis of lysosomes, or secretion of enzymes under the influence of C5a on the neutrophil's membrane. Macrophages stimulated by immune complexes are also able to liberate lysosomal enzymes. These enzymes damage tissues in hydrolyzing collagen, elastin, and cartilage. Other enzymes liberated by neutrophils (e.g., cationic protein) contribute to the inflammatory process by causing degranulation of mast cells.

II. Cell-Mediated (Delayed-Type) Reactions

Contact dermatitis to drugs applied topically on the skin in the form of ointments, creams, etc. is a classical example of localized cell-mediated allergic reaction. Similar reactions may occur in people professionally handling drugs with high allergenic potential. Further details on the clinical aspects of such reactions and on the large number of drugs capable of inducing them are given in Chap. 13.

The pathophysiologic mechanism of localized cell-mediated allergic reactions is to some extent at least clarified. Penetration or injection of antigen into the tissues (e.g., skin) of a sensitized individual leads to an uptake of antigen by macrophages, a role played in the skin by the Langerhans cells. Presentation of antigen to sensitized effector T-lymphocytes leads to activation of such lymphocytes, which synthesize and excrete a whole array of mediators denominated lymphokines. Whether the encounter between antigen-loaded macrophages and sensitized T-lymphocytes takes place in the tissue itself, in the pericapillary spaces, or in the draining lymphatics is not yet ascertained. It appears that several of the lymphokines produced by the activated T-lymphocytes play a key role in the sequence of pathological events occuring in the tissue within 24–48 h of encountering antigen. An increase in capillary permeability is observed early in the reaction, but follows an oscillating pattern, with new peaks of capillary permeability increase occurring at various times (VOISIN and TOULLET 1960; MORLEY 1972). Triggering of mast cells by allergen interacting with allergen-specific IgE or IgG concomitantly present in sensitized individuals and/or the production of a lymphokine increasing capillary permeability (permeability increasing factor: PIF) (SOBEL et al. 1977) may be the explanation. Lymphokines have also recently been shown to increase mast cell reactivity (IDA et al. 1980). Finally, the frequently observed late influx of basophils into the lesions may be responsible for the delayed increase in capillary permeability (ASKENASE 1980).

Mononuclear cell infiltration, composed essentially of monocytes and lymphocytes, is one of the main features of such reactions. Chemotactic factors released by activated effector T-lymphocytes are likely to be responsible for this, as well as for the influx of neutrophils, eosinophils, and basophils which appear in the reaction site at various times. The natural ultimate fate of cells constantly migrating from blood to tissues is to return to the blood through lymphatic pathways. However, the presence at the reaction site of agents impairing cell migration would have the effect of facilitating local accumulation of infiltrating cells. This is the role presently attributed to the macrophage migration inhibiting factor (MIF), one of the first lymphokines identified, which also impairs macrophage locomotion in vitro. As demonstrated by the injection of labeled ^{3}H-thymidine in animals undergoing such a contact reaction, both the local infiltrating cells and the lymphoid cells present in the draining lymph nodes undergo intense proliferation during the reaction. This is thought to be the effect in vivo of mitogenic factors released by the activated effector T-lymphocytes. Finally, damage to the tissues involved occurs in such reactions, and may be brought about by various mechanisms: cytotoxic T-lymphocytes reacting with haptens bound to cell membranes, lymphotoxins released by activated effector T-lymphocytes, or enzymatic digestion by activated macrophages. In addition, the tissular infiltration characteristic of such lesions seems to be due largely not to the infiltrating cells themselves, but to fibrin deposits, implying an activation of the clotting process. Indeed, macrophages activated by lymphokines (macrophage activating factor) have been shown to produce plasminogen activator and a procoagulant. Accordingly, the concept of cell-mediated inflammatory lesions triggered in tissues by the interaction between antigen and effector T-lymphocytes integrates the interplay of several lymphokines and inflammatory cells (Fig. 4). It is most likely, however, that this already complex picture is in fact a gross oversimplification.

When antigen is distributed systemically, and not only locally, for example following ingestion or intravenous injection, a generalized cell-mediated allergic reac-

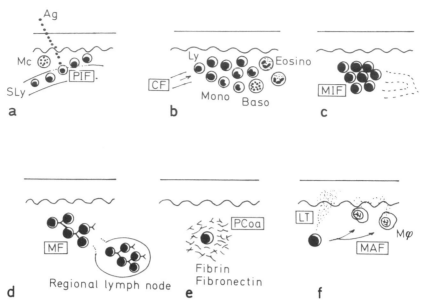

Fig. 4 a–f. Role of various lymphokines in the development of a delayed-type reaction (in the example of the tuberculin or contact skin reaction). **a** Antigen penetrates through the skin and meets either sensitized mast cells (*Mc*), releasing histamine, and/or sensitized lymphocytes (*SLy*), releasing a capillary permeability increasing factor (*PIF*). **b** The production of various chemotactic factors (*CF*) attracts to the reaction site nonspecific lymphocytes (*Ly*), monocytes (*Mono*), basophils (*Baso*), and eosinophils (*Eosino*), forming a mixed infiltrate developing dynamically with time. **c** The production of migration inhibitory factors (*MIF*) prevents the infiltrated cells leaving the tissue rapidly via lymphatic vessels. **d** Active proliferation takes place in the infiltrate and in the regional lymph node, under the influence of mitogenic factors (*MF*). **e** Activation of the coagulation system by procoagulants (*PCoa*) leads to the local deposition of fibrin and fibronection, responsible for the bulk of the induration characteristic of tuberculin-type lesions. **f** Damage to tissue may occur directly by the production and release of lymphotoxins (*LT*) or by activated lymphocytes, or indirectly through macrophages (*Ma*) activated by macrophage activating factor (*MAF*)

tion may ensue. Reactions of this type may manifest themselves clinically by fever, a state of shock (tuberculin shock?), generalized lymphadenopathies, an exanthematous skin rash, or generalized exfoliative dermatitis (PETROZZI and SHORE 1976). In such instances, the presence of lymphokines in the blood stream has been described (COHEN 1977), and it is therefore presumed that the same kind of interactions between antigen and effector T-lymphocytes with ensuing synthesis of lymphokines also occur (DE WECK 1977 a). The timing and sequence of events, as well as the distribution and effects of lymphokines throughout the organism, however, have not been precisely determined.

III. Reactions by Photosensitivity

There are two types of drug reactions by photosensitivity (HARBER and BAER 1972). In *phototoxicity*, the reaction is characterized by epidermal lesions provoked by a narrow spectrum of sun rays (285–310 nm) and is limited to the exposed areas; the reaction looks like sunburn and is followed by secondary pigmentation. This type of reaction requires a heavy exposure to light; the photosensitizing drug (e.g., psoralens, chlorothiazide, sulfonamides, or phenothiazines) will absorb photons and provoke an electron excitation leading to the appearance of free radicals or peroxides and heat, which affect cellular nuclei, lysosomes, and cytoplasmic membranes.

Reactions due to *photoallergy*, on the other hand, require less intense light, with a larger spectrum at higher wavelengths (320–450 nm). In this case, the light rays appear to transform the drug in such a way that a reactive hapten combines with skin proteins and forms a new antigen. Sensitization may ensue, as demonstrated by the formation of specific IgE antibodies or of effector T-lymphocytes. Upon renewed administration of the drug together with exposure to light, epidermal skin lesions occur, which can take the form of erythema, urticaria, or eczematous, papulovesicular, or exudative eruptions. The lesions are usually less sharply limited than in phototoxic reactions. Some of the sensitizing drugs act upon contact with the skin (e.g., promethazine or ointments containing para-aminobenzoic acid or sulfamides), while others, especially sulfamides, act preferentially after parenteral administration (SCHWARZ and SCHWARZ-PECK 1960). Further details about phototoxic and photoallergic reactions are given in Chap. 10.

IV. Pseudoallergic Reactions

This term has been given by some authors (DUKOR et al. 1980) to characterize allergic reactions which are apparently of the immediate type (anaphylactic shock, urticaria, asthma, rhinitis), but which are not mediated by IgE antibodies. However, many of these reactions seem to involve the same cells, such as mast cells and blood basophils, and the same mediators as classical anaphylactic reactions. In these cases, only the initial triggering event may be different. Accordingly, and since such reactions do not appear to occur in everyone at the therapeutic dose of the drug usually employed, they should still fit into the general frame-work of allergy, as defined originally by von Pirquet. Several mechanisms by which tissue mast cells and in some instances blood basophils can be triggered without the presence of drug-specific IgE have been identified.

1. Mast Cell and Basophil Degranulation by Complement Components (Anaphylatoxins)

Whereas complement and its role in immune complex diseases have been described above (Sect. D.I.2), there appears to be a number of instances of untoward reactions to drugs in which complement activation may play a major role. Anaphylactic reactions have been described following the development of drug-specific antibodies of the IgG type capable of activating complement. In some cases, such as an immediate-type reaction following the intravenous injection of protamine sulfate (LAKIN et al. 1978), homocytotropic antibodies of IgG type capable of passively transferring the reaction have been demonstrated. Such antibodies have a short sensitization period, are stable to heating at 56 °C and seem to require complement to induce the anaphylactic reaction.

The shocks observed after intravenous administration of plasma expanders such as dextran (Furhoff 1977) also appear to rest upon the presence of IgG-specific antibodies (see Chap. 20). Whether the effect of anaphylatoxins such as C3a or C5a on the blood basophils and tissue mast cells occur following interaction of the drug with specific IgGs in solution or only after such IgGs have fixed to the mast cell membrane is not yet certain.

It appears also in some instances that drugs may activate complement directly by the alternate pathway. The immediate-type reactions observed after the injection of radiologic contrast media (Brasch et al. 1970) has been attributed to complement activation (Arroyave et al. 1976; Lang et al. 1976; Ring et al. 1978) but may in some cases be due to IgE (Wakkers-Garritsen et al. 1976). Activation of complement in vitro (Haensch et al. 1980) and in vivo (Voigtlaender et al. 1980) following ingestion of aspirin has been implicated as a possible mechanism of aspirin intolerance. However, in neither case has it yet been demonstrated unequivocally that patients presenting allergic reactions to these drugs differ quantitatively or qualitatively in the reactivity of their complement system from those patients who tolerate the drugs without problems.

2. Liberation of Histamine Through Nonimmunologic Mechanisms

It has long been known that a number of basic peptides, as well as various drugs (e.g., opiates), are able to release histamine from tissue mast cells through triggering mechanisms which seem to be independent from those acted upon by IgE receptors or by receptors for the anaphylatoxins (Stanworth 1980). Among the drugs capable of triggering mast cells in this way, polymyxin, colistin, the ACTH tetracosapeptide, iodinated radiologic contrast media, morphine, codeine, and myorelaxants have been especially considered (Rockhoff et al. 1970; Shehadi 1975; Brashear et al. 1974; Vervloet et al. 1979). Some local anesthetics (e.g., Pantocaine) also appear to induce nonspecifically histamine liberation from skin mast cells (Conroy and de Weck 1981). A number of these agents are acting only on tissue mast cells but appear to be ineffective on blood basophils, a feature which distinguishes them from agents working through the IgE or anaphylatoxin receptors (Conroy and de Weck 1981). Experiments demonstrating in vitro the liberation of histamine in the presence of various drugs may be difficult to interpret, since release may also be due to a toxic effect of the drug on the cell membrane. However, a number of patients will release mediators at drug concentrations which do not appear to be harmful to other people. When no drug-specific antibodies of the IgE or IgG type are detected, the possibility of a nonimmunologic liberation of mediators should always be kept in mind.

The precise molecular mechanisms triggering, in the mast cell membrane and in their cytoplasm, the chain of events leading to the liberation of mediators via nonimmunological pathways is not yet precisely understood. Various aspects of this type of mediator release have been reviewed recently by Stanworth (1980). Several arguments speak for a different mechanism, at least at the initial triggering stage, from that involved in the IgE- or anaphylatoxin-mediated release. The facts that such drug-induced mechanisms appear to function preferentially on mast cells and that the addition of calcium seems to have a paradoxical inhibiting effect (Conroy and de Weck 1980) support this point of view.

3. Pseudoallergic Reactions to Drugs Interfering
with Prostaglandin Synthesis

One of the major pseudoallergic syndromes is that caused by aspirin and other nonsteroidal anti-inflammatory drugs which interfere with prostaglandin synthesis. As described in detail in Chap. 11 such drugs may cause either the well-known "aspirin triad" (asthma, rhinitis, and nasal polyposis) or a cutaneous syndrome characterized by urticaria and angioneurotic edema. Most authors have failed to detect IgE antibodies in such cases (WELTMAN et al. 1978; SCHLUMBERGER 1980). Recently, the possibility that complement activation would play a role in such situations (YURCHAK et al. 1970) has been revived by experiments demonstrating activation of complement shortly after ingestion of aspirin (VOIGTLAENDER et al. 1980). Whether this is due to a nonspecific effect of aspirin or possibly to the interaction of such compounds with IgG antibodies of aspiryl specificity has not yet been established clearly. However, the fact that the great majority of patients developing allergic reactions to aspirin also react to a whole array of chemically unrelated prostaglandin synthesis inhibitors points to the involvement of the prostaglandin system in the pathogenesis of such reactions (SAMTER and BEERS 1967, 1968). It is still rather controversial whether aspirin-sensitive patients indeed react to all other agents having similar actions on prostaglandin synthesis. While exposition experiments by SZCZEKLIK et al. (1975) indicate that indeed patients with this syndrome will react to all compounds interfering with prostaglandin synthesis, provided the dose administered is sufficiently high, other authors (MICHAELSSON and JUHLIN 1973; DOEGLAS 1975) have observed very variable patterns of reactivity: some patients react to a large variety of prostaglandin synthesis inhibitors, while others show a more selective pattern. Aspirin and other anti-inflammatory drugs such as indomethacin or mefenamic acid interfere very early in the cyclooxygenase pathway of arachidonic acid metabolism. At a time when the metabolism of arachidonic acid derivatives was not yet known in full detail, it was postulated that the allergic symptoms could be due to an imbalance between the various prostaglandins themselves, for example between bronchodilatating E and bronchoconstricting $F_{2\alpha}$ prostaglandins (HARNETT et al. 1978). However, this seems rather illogical, since the blockade of the cyclooxygenase pathway appears to affect all prostaglandins more or less equally. Indeed, it was not possible to show a difference in this respect between patients who are intolerant to aspirin and patients who are not (PATRONO et al. 1978). Since the recent discovery that the very potent mediator of allergic reactions, SRS-A, is also a product of the arachidonic acid metabolism through the lipooxygenase pathway (PARKER 1979 b; SAMUELSSON 1981), it is in this direction that most current hypotheses on the pathophysiology of aspirin intolerance reactions have developed. It may be assumed that patients intolerant to aspirin and aspirin-like drugs undergo untoward reactions because of an increased production of SRS-A, since these drugs do not interfere with the lipooxygenase pathway. Up to now, however, a direct demonstration that aspirin-intolerant patients indeed differ from normal individuals in their production of SRS-A in the presence of aspirin has not been presented.

Activation of complement might also be envisaged as playing a triggering role in such reactions YURCHAK et al. 1970), but since activation of complement after ingestion of aspirin apparently occurs in everyone (VOIGTLAENDER et al. 1980), an additional possibility to explain the hyperreactivity of aspirin-intolerant people would be to postulate a modified response to anaphylatoxins in the presence of aspirin or aspirin-like drugs. While the presence of indomethacin and other prostaglandin synthesis inhibitors usually increases histamine release triggered in blood basophils by anti-IgE antibodies and IgE-dependent mechanisms, the reverse appears to be true for mediator release induced by anaphylatoxins (CONROY and DE WECK 1981). However, it could not consistently be demonstrated that blood basophils from patients intolerant to aspirin react to anaphylatoxins in the presence of indomethacin in a different way than normal controls, although in some intolerant patients a marked increase in mediator release was observed (CONROY and DE WECK 1981).

E. Clinical Forms of Allergic Reactions to Drugs

I. Anaphylactic Shock

Systemic anaphylaxis is an acute life-threatening allergic reaction characterized by the appearance of a generalized flush, weakness, anxiety, dizziness, palpitations, tingling of the extremities or of the tongue, urticaria and angioedema, nausea and vomiting, and uterine and intestinal cramps within a few minutes of administration of a drug. If not treated, the reaction may progress to respiratory distress, hyperperistalsis, cardiac arrhythmias, cardiovascular collapse, seizures, coma, and death. Anaphylactic symptoms are most frequently produced by parenteral injections, but in highly sensitive persons oral, percutaneous, vaginal, or even respiratory exposure may produce a similar response. Anaphylaxis can in most instances be distinguished from vasovagal syncope, since the patients develop a flush and tachycardia in contrast to the blanching, diaphoresis, and bradycardia associated with vasovagal reactions (ORANGE and DONSKY 1978).

Symptoms usually develop within seconds to minutes, reaching a maximum within 5–20 min. Occasionally, especially if a depot preparation has been given, symptoms may not appear until 60–90 min or even longer has elapsed. In 35 subjects dying from anaphylactic shock to insect stings (BARNARD 1967), death occurred in 23 cases within 1 h, in 8 cases between 1 and 6 h, and only in 4 cases over 6 h after the sting. In drug allergy, the reaction is most likely to occur at the start of a new course of treatment with a previously used drug, which may or may not have caused allergic symptoms at earlier times. In view of the frequently transient character of the IgE response following drug therapy, it has been considered that the greatest risk is in the 2–8 weeks following a preceding course of therapy. However, anaphylactic hypersensitivity can also persist for many years in the absence of any known exposure to the drug. Approximately 10% of overt anaphylactic reactions are fatal. Death is usually due to hypotension, laryngeal edema, cardiac arrest, or bronchospasm.

Only a few studies (HANASHIRO and WEIL 1967; BERNREITER 1959; BOOTH and PATTERSON 1970; WEGMANN and RENKER 1976) have described the pathophysiological changes occurring during anaphylactic shock in man, obviously because during such an emergency the primary attention of the physician is concentrated on the required therapeutic measures. However, a number of case studies in patients undergoing anaphylactic reactions while monitored during the course of a surgical intervention have shown the following phenomena: hemoconcentration, leucopenia and thrombocytopenia, hypoxemia, and hypocapnia, which may be followed by hypercapnia and acidosis (WEIL and SHUBIN 1974). Alterations of blood coagulation have also been observed. In recent years, electrocardiographic changes have been repeatedly described (PAVEK and WEGMANN 1981) such as flattening or inversion of the T wave, changes in ST segment, and rhythm modifications by auricular fibrillation. Such changes may be reproduced experimentally in monkeys (PAVEK 1977). The drop in blood pressure and in cardiac output are also well known.

From an anatomopathological point of view, early authors quoted by AUSTEN (1965) only described acute lesions of pulmonary emphysema, sometimes accompanied by a massive laryngeal and tracheobronchic edema. In 50 necropsies on patients who died of anaphylactic shock, lesions were restricted in 70% of the cases to the upper respiratory tract, which was obstructed by intense edema and secretions. In some cases, diffuse vascular lesions were associated with congestion of liver and kidneys, thrombosis of the coronary arteries and hemolysis. In three cases only the central nervous system showed cerebral and meningeal edema, while in six cases no organic alterations whatsoever could be described (BARNARD 1967). The paper by DELAGE and IREY (1972) on necropsies of 40 cases of anapyhlactic shock to drugs presents similar data.

Early recognition of anaphylactic shock and the immediate use of epinephrine and other supportive measures (see Chap. 8) may be life-saving. The critical time is usually the first 30–60 min; after this initial phase, symptoms often subside completely, even in the absence of continuing therapy. However, patients with severe reactions may require treatment and medical observation for at least 24 h; delayed fatality can occur due to severe hypotension or hypoxemia leading to infarction of parenchymatous organs such as the brain, heart, kidney, or liver. Symptoms of urticaria or serum sickness may occur in the aftermath of anaphylactic reactions and last for several days.

Aside from the severe cardiovascular collapse observed in major anaphylactic shock, all symptoms may occur in a milder form such as generalized urticaria, angioneurotic edema, and asthmatic attacks. In general, the faster the symptoms appear after injection or ingestion of the drug, the more severe the reaction.

The list of drugs in current use and reported to cause anaphylactic shock is given in Table 2, which is not exhaustive. Penicillin still appears to be by far the most frequent cause: it was still implicated in 32 of 43 anaphylactic deaths reported in the American armed forces (DELAGE and IREY 1972). However, considering the large number of patients treated with penicillins, it may be stated that even penicillin does not produce anaphylaxis very often. In this respect, other macromolecular substances such as enzymes (e.g., asparaginase) or xenogenic sera are certainly much more dangerous (VAN ARSDEL 1978). Serious reactions to penicillin appeared to occur in no more than one to four cases per 10,000 injections and fatal reactions in no more than one to two cases per 100,000 injections (IDSOE et al. 1968). While in the early 1960s it was estimated that penicillin-induced anaphylaxis caused up

Table 2. Drugs and compounds most frequently involved in anaphylactic and anaphylactoid reactions. (Adapted from van Arsdel 1978)

Macromolecules

Xenogenic sera
Human gamma globulin
Allergenic extracts
Dextrans (including iron dextran)
Organ extracts
Vaccines
Venoms

Enzymes
  Asparaginase
  Chymotrypsin
  Trypsin
  Papain
  Penicillinase
  Streptokinase
  Hormones (ACTH, insulin, calcitonin)
  Heparin

Diagnostic agents

Iodinated contrast media[a]
Dyes
  Fluorescein
    Alphazurine
  Sodium dehydrocholate
    (Decholin)

Dyes
  Bromsulphalein (BSP)[a]
  Congo red
  Triphenylmethane

Antibiotics

p-Aminosalicylic acid
Amphotericin B
Bacitracin
Cephalosporins
Clindamycin
Ethambutol
Kanamycin
Linomycin

Penicillins
Penicillin-procaine[a]
Polymyxin B[a]
Streptomycin
Sulfonamides
Tetracyclines
Vancomycin

Other drugs

Alfaxolone
Aminopyrine
Aspirin[a]
Bleomycin[a]
Chlorpropamide
Colchicine
Cromolyn
Dantrolene
Ethylene oxide
Gallamine
Glafenine
Indomethacin[a]

Local anesthetics[a]
Meprobamate
Mercurial diuretics
Opiates (heroin)[a]
Procaine[a]
Probenecid
Succinylcholine
d-Tubocurarine
Vitamin B_1, B_{12}
Thiopental

[a] Most frequently anaphylactoid reactions

to 500 deaths per year in the United States, it is likely that the current mortality has considerably decreased (Parker 1980).

In classical immunologically mediated anaphylactic reactions, drug-specific IgE antibodies appear to play the main role. Such antibodies have been detected in a number of patients with histories of anaphylactic shock, including some anaphylactic deaths where blood was collected post mortem (STOFER et al. 1973). Such patients also frequently possess exquisite skin hypersensitivity of the immediate type to penicilloyl-polylysine and/or minor determinants of penicillin allergy (LEVINE 1976; DE WECK 1979; PARKER 1980). In such patients, even a scratch test with penicillin may cause a fatal anaphylactic reaction (DOGLIOTTI 1968). A number of anaphylactic shocks following skin tests with penicillins have been reported (IDSOE et al. 1968).

However, as already indicated (see Sect. D.IV), a number of substances appear to induce systemic reactions which may closely resemble in symptomatology an IgE-mediated anaphylactic shock, but which are due to different pathophysiological mechanisms. Such reactions are generally denominated *anaphylactoid*. Iodinated contrast media (LIEBERMAN et al. 1978), dyes such as fluorescein and bromsulphalein, aspirin and aspirin-like drugs, opiates (ABELSON 1970), and local anesthetics are the most frequent drugs involved in anaphylactoid reactions. Some of them may represent IgG-mediated and complement-dependent anaphylaxis (LAKIN et al. 1978); other may be due to direct activation of clomplement. A special case is represented by the Hoigné syndrome (HOIGNÉ and SCHOCH 1959) observed after injection of procaine penicillin G and sometimes of other drugs in microcrystalline form. In this case, microemboli appear to be responsible for the symptoms, which affect mostly the central nervous system. Although some of the anaphylactoid reactions may also be fatal, they are generally as a whole less severe, the cardiovascular collapse less profound, and the symptomatology less complete than in IgE-mediated "true" anaphylactic reactions.

II. Serum Sickness

Serum sickness is a systemic allergic reaction produced by circulating antigen-antibody complexes. The serum sickness syndrome usually develops 5–14 days after the first administration of the drug, and is characterized by a generalized urticarial skin rash, fever, joint swelling, and lymphadenopathy. Brief episodes of glomerulonephritis, neuropathy, and vasculitis are not rare. Clinical manifestations usually develop 6–20 days after the initiation of therapy, reflecting the time required for primary sensitization (MORRISON-SMITH and GELL 1975). However, after previous sensitizing exposure, an accelerated serum sickness syndrome can occur with development of symptoms within 12–36 h. Symptoms usually last for only a few days to a week after the drug is withdrawn, but they may persist for several weeks. Skin rashes nd lymphoadenopathy are frequent manifestations of the serum sickness syndrome, but fever is not always present, especially in children. Occasionally, an individual clinical manifestation such as fever or neuritis almost completely dominates the clinical picture. After penicillin has been withdrawn, a syndrome of chronic recurrent urticaria and arthritic symptoms persisting for several months has been described (LEVINE et al. 1966a).

The serum sickness syndrome was originally described by VON PIRQUET and SCHICK at the beginning of this century, following the injection of antidiphteric and antitetanic horse sera. In recent years, the injection of horse antilymphocyte sera in transplanted patients has given a new topicality to this cause of serum sickness (KASHIWAGI et al. 1968). Among the low-molecular-weight drugs which can pro-

Table 3. Drugs frequently involved in serum-sickness-like reactions. (Adapted from van Arsdel 1978)

Macromolecules	
Xenogenic sera[a]	Dextrans
Hormones (insulin, ACTH)	Vaccines (?)
Antibiotics	
p-Aminosalicylic acid	Penicillins[a]
Cephalosporins	Streptomycin
Griseofulvin	Sulfonamides[a]
Lincomycin	Tetracyclines (?)
Nitrofurantoin (?)	
Other drugs	
Nomifensin (Alival)	Phenylbutazone[a]
Barbiturates	Phenylhydantoin (Nirvanol)[b]
Hydantoins	Procainamide (?)
Hydralazine[a]	Procarbazine
Isoniazid	Salicylates
Mercurial diuretics	Thiouracils[a]

[a] Frequent offenders
[b] No longer in use

duce serum sickness, penicillins are probably the most frequent (Table 3). Some drugs such as Nirvanol (5-ethyl 5-phenylhydantoin), a metabolite of phenytoin used in the treatment of Sydenham's chorea, produced manifestations of serum sickness with such frequency that they had to be withdrawn (Braverman and Levin 1963).

Many of the low-molecular-weight antigens that produce serum sickness also produce anaphylaxis, suggesting the existence of direct protein reactivity or rapid metabolism to antigenic products. In this case, hapten-serum protein conjugates are formed which should remain in the circulation for prolonged periods, When antidrug antibodies first appear, intravascular or tissue-bound antigen is still present, and circulating antigen-antibody complexes capable of producing serum sickness and vasculitis can then be formed. The antibodies involved in serum sickness are probably to a large extent of the IgG class, but definite proof in this respect is not available at present. In penicillin-induced serum sickness high, agglutinating antibody titers of both the IgG and IgM classes are usually present (Levine et al. 1966a). However, drug-specific IgE may also be involved, since patients with serum sickness syndrome frequently possess and IgE-mediated skin reactivity to penicillin antigens (de Weck and Blum 1965). The skin hypersensitivity, however, frequently develops only a few weeks after the serum sickness syndrome has receded; its pathogenic role in the occurrence of the syndrome is therefore doubtful. The deposition of immune complexes in the skin lesions of serum sickness due to penicillin has been demonstrated, as well as the deposition of complement components (Fellner and Harris 1972). Altered levels of serum complement components have also been demonstrated directly at the time of active clinical symptoms in a serum-sickness-like reaction to procarbazine (Glovsky et al. 1976).

Table 4. Drugs frequently involved in allergic fever. (Adapted from VAN ARSDEL 1978; PARKER 1980)

Antibiotics	Other drugs
p-Aminosalicylic acid	Allopurinol
Cephalosporins	Barbiturates
Chloramphenicol	Hydralazine
Erythromycin	Iodides
Isoniazid	Mercurial diuretics
Kaomycin	Methyldopa
Nitrofurantoin	Penicillamine
Penicillins	Phenobarbital
Pyrazinamide	Procainamide
Streptomycin	Propylthiouracil
Sulfonamides	Quinidine
Tetracyclines	Quinine
	Salicylates

III. Fever

Fever may appear as an isolated manifestation of drug hypersensitivity, although more frequently allergic manifestations in other organs, especially the skin, are observed concomitantly. Fever is usually moderate but bouts in the 39.5–41 °C range can also occur. Leucocytosis is commonly present, increasing the possibility that fever may be erroneously attributed to infection. Ordinarily, the fever subsides within the first few days after the drug is discontinued. However, drug fever may also persist, especially when associated with widespread small-vessel vasculitis. Fever may sometimes be an early sign of drug-induced serum sickness, hepatitis, vasculitis, nephritis, pneumonitis, agranulocytosis, or thrombocytopenia.

Among the drugs frequently causing fever by immunological mechanisms, penicillins and cephalosporins as well as aminosalicylic acid, phenobarbital, and quinidine are the most frequently quoted (PARKER 1980, DE SWARTE 1972). Drugs presumed to cause fever by immunological mechanisms are listed in Table 4. The precise immunological mechanisms by which drug fever may arise are not entirely established (VAN ARSDEL 1978). On the one hand, the fact that fever frequently accompanies the serum sickness syndrome and may be experimentally induced by antigen-antibody complexes pleads in a number of cases for an antibody-mediated mechanism (CLUFF and JOHNSON 1964). On the other hand, fever may also be considered as a manifestation of generalized cell-mediated hypersensitivity (SNELL 1972); in such cases, the only immunological abnormality observed may be a positive lymphocyte culture to the drug.

Fever may be caused by many other mechanisms than an allergic one. Some effects appear to be toxic, such as a fever observed after treatment with amphotericin B, iron dextran, calcium disodium edetate, and dimercaprol, which causes fever in almost 30% of patients treated (VAN ARSDEL 1978). The endogenous release of bacterial pyrogens (e.g., Jarisch-Herxheimer reaction), the administration of exogenous pyrogenic substances contained in contaminated fluids or drugs, the release of endogenous pyrogen such as may occur after sterile inflammation fol-

Table 5. Drugs frequently involved in aplastic anemia. (Adapted from van Arsdel 1978)

Analgesics	
Acetaminophen	Oxyphenbutazone
Indomethacin	Phenylbutazone[a]
Anticonvulsants	
Carbamazepine	Phenytoin
Mephenytoin[a]	Trimethadione[a]
Antimicrobials	
Chloramphenicol[a]	Streptomycin
Methicillin	Sulfonamides
Antineoplastics	
Busulfan	Nitrogen mustards
Cytosine arabinoside	6-Mercaptopurine
5-Fluorouracil	Vinca alkaloids
Methotrexate	
Oral hypoglycemics	
Chlorpropamide	Tolbutamide
Tranquilizers	
Meprobamate	Phenothiazines
Other drugs	
Chlorothiazide	Penicillamine
Colchicine	Perchlorate
Gold salts[a]	

[a] More than 20 cases described

lowing intramuscular drug injection, and the febrile reactions accompanying various metabolic or hormonal changes due to drugs (e.g., general anesthetics, amphetamine, intoxication, etiocholanolone fever) are all examples of drug fever not caused by allergic hypersensitively.

IV. Hematologic Reactions

The peripheral destruction of erythrocytes, leucocytes, and/or platelets by immunological mechanisms must be distinguished from central cytotoxic damage to the bone marrow resulting in diminished cell formation. Many of these reactions involve toxic or idiosyncratic effects on the bone marrow, although toxic effects on the blood cells themselves resulting in shortened life span and accelerated destruction may also occur. Numerous drugs can produce toxic or idiosyncratic bone marrow depression (aplastic anemia) and a list of the drugs most frequently involved is given in Table 5. In individuals with enzymatic defects of intracellular oxidative processes in the red cell, oxidant drugs may produce a toxic hemolytic anemia. One example is the congenital glucose-6-phosphate dehydrogenase defi-

Table 6. Drugs frequently involved in hemolytic anemia. (Adapted from VAN ARSDEL 1978; PARKER 1980)

Hapten-cell type	
Penicillin	Dipyrone
Cephalosporins	
Innocent-bystander type	
p-Aminosalicylic acid	Quinidine
Carbromal	Quinine
Chlorpromazine	Rifampin
Insulin	Stibophen
Isoniazid	Sulfonamides
Melphalan	Sulfonylureas
Phenacetin	Tetracyclines
Autoimmune type	
Catergens	Mefenamic acid
Chlorpromazine (?)	Methyldopa
Hydantoins (?)	Methysergide (?)
Levodopa	Pyramidon

ciency, which is seen in more than 10% of colored people in the United States. Such individuals develop acute hemolytic anemia following administration of analgesics, antimalarials, sulfonamides, and several other drugs. In general, drug-induced granulocytopenia, anemia, or thrombocytopenia is more frequently due to direct cytotoxicity than to immunologically mediated mechanisms (PARKER 1980).

1. Hemolytic Anemia

As already discussed in Sect. D.I.2, immunologically mediated hemolytic anemia may be due to three different mechanisms, defined as the hapten-cell binding type, the innocent bystander type, and the autoimmune type. The drugs most frequently responsible are given in Table 6.

a) Hapten-Cell Binding Type

A classical example is the penicillin-induced variety, resulting from high-dose penicillin therapy over a period of several weeks (VAN ARSDEL and GILLILAND 1965; PETZ and FUDENBERG 1976). As a consequence of sustained high penicillin blood levels, the red cells become substituted with penicillin haptens through the formation of stable linkages, primarily of the penicilloyl type, on the red cell surface (THIEL et al. 1964; DE WECK 1964; LEVINE and REDMOND 1967). In patients who develop high-titer antipenicilloyl IgG antibodies, accelerated red cell destruction then occurs, leading to anemia. There is in such cases no evidence of intravascular destruction, suggesting that the cells are destroyed by the reticuloendothelial system rather than by the direct hemolytic activity of complement. The presence of an antibody on the surface of the red cells can be demonstrated with anti-immunoglobulin (COOMBS) reagents. Accordingly, individuals under high-dose penicillin treatment who are menaced by hemolytic anemia are identified by a rapid drop in hematocrit values, associated with reticulocytosis and a positive direct Coombs reaction. An indirect Coombs reactivity can also be demonstrated with the patient's serum and normal red blood cells, provided these have been sensitized by incubation with penicillin in vitro. The etiologic role of penicillin in the hemolytic process has been demonstrated in several cases by the fact that readministration of the drug caused recurrent hemolysis (PARKER 1980). Penicillin-induced hemolytic anemia is frequently an isolated manifestation of penicillin allergy. The nature of the antibody involved is not completely clear, since hemagglutinating antibodies, which are consistently demonstrated in patients with penicillin-induced hemolytic anemia, may also be present in individuals receiving high-dose penicillin who do not develop the disease. Hemagglutinating antibodies are frequently present, but in lower titers, in normal subjects (LEVINE et al. 1966 b; THIEL et al. 1964). A positive direct Coombs reaction occurs in the majority of patients receiving cephalothin, but this appears to be due to a nonspecific effect of the drug, which causes protein absorption onto the red cell surface. In this case, the clinical significance of the positive Coombs reaction is very doubtful, since few patients treated with cephalothin developed hemolytic anemia. Other pharmacologic agents which seem to attach in a stable manner to red cells and to induce hemolytic anemia are dipyrone, phenacetin (DAUSSET and CONTU 1964), and catergens (NEFTEL et al. 1981). In a number of other drug-induced hemolytic anemias, for example after stibophen and quinidine, one observes a positive antiglobulin reaction, which is readily reversible by washing, suggesting the existence of labile complexes similar to those observed with platelets in quinidine-induced thrombocytopenia (FREEDMAN et al. 1956). Accordingly, a second group of hemolytic anemias might be due to an innocent bystander mechanism.

b) Innocent Bystander Type

In that case, it appears that the drug binds only loosely, if at all, to red cells. If, however, the drug complexes first with antibody in solution, the whole complex can then bind to red cells together with complement components. Intravascular hemolysis may follow, and the more severe reactions cause hemoglobinemia, hemoglobinuria, and even renal failure. The direct Coombs antiglobulin reaction may be positive, but sometimes only if an anticomplement serum is used, since the drug-antibody complex may not remain bound to the cell. When reactions using anti-immunoglobulin sera are positive, the responsible antibody may be IgM (stibophen, rifampin) or IgG (melphalan, sulfonylurea, insulin). In such cases, prompt recovery usually occurs when drug treatment is terminated (VAN ARSDEL 1978).

c) Autoimmune Type

Some other drugs produce an autoimmune hemolytic anemia in which the antibodies are directed towards native antigens on the red cell surface, while the drug does not seem to function as a hapten in the reaction. This type of autoimmune hemolytic anemia has been described following treatment with levodopa, methyldopa, and mefenamic acid (WORRLEDGE et al. 1966; WORRLEDGE 1973). With α-methyldopa, clinically significant hemolysis develops in less than 1% of individuals receiving the drug over a period of at least several months. However, direct Coombs antiglobulin reactivity is demonstrable in as many as 10%–15% of treated individuals. Evidence of immunoglobulin binding to red cells is demonstrable only after several months of treatment, and this delay is not shortened when a patient with a previous positive reaction is started again on the drug. Other drugs possibly but not yet definitely associated with autoimmune hemolytic anemia are chlorpromazine, hydantoins, and methysergide.

The antibodies involved in α-methyldopa-induced autoimmune hemolytic anemia are of the IgG type (LOBUGLIO and JANDL 1967) and are specific for Rh determinants. α-Methyldopa needs to be present in order for the reaction to occur, and direct Coombs reactivity is demonstrable for immunoglobulins, but most of the time not for complement. After cessation of therapy, clinical improvement may take several weeks, and the antiglobulin tests may remain positive for 1–2 years. The mechanism by which autoimmune antibodies arise following α-methyldopa treatment is not clear. It has not been shown that α-methyldopa interacts directly with the red cell surface as a hapten or denatures this surface, making the Rh antigens more immunogenic (TERRITO et al. 1973). A pharmacologic effect on the immune system itself, affecting suppressor cells and the normal mechanisms of self-recognition, should possibly be considered. Occasionally, antinuclear antibodies and rheumatoid factor activity have been demonstrated in patients with a positive Coombs test while treated with α-methyldopa (PARKER 1980).

2. Agranulocytosis

The reactions due to immune destruction of granulocytes usually develop between the 2nd and 12th weeks of drug therapy, but they may also occur only after a year or more of continuous therapy (MOESCHLIN 1958; HUBULEY 1964; HARTL 1965, 1973). The symptoms develop suddenly in the form of chills, fever, and collapse as the leukocyte count drops precipitously. This may be contrasted with toxic or idiosyncratic bone marrow depression (PISCIOTTA 1973), which develops insidiously and where symptoms are usually lacking until an infection such as stomatitis, pharyngitis, or anogenital ulceration occurs. Pharyngitis with severe edema and ulcerations due to loss of host resistance and uncontrolled infection usually develop when the granulocyte count in peripheral blood drops below $1,000/mm^3$. Peripheral manifestations such as skin rash or lymphodenopathy are usually absent, with the exception of gold-induced agranulocytosis (HARTL 1965). The few remaining leukocytes show frequently toxic granulations. In severe cases, they may be a reduction in the number of monocytes and lymphocytes as well, while the change in eosinophils is erratic (e.g., eosinophilia in gold-induced agranulocytosis). Bone marrow studies reveal a diminution in mature granulocytes with a shift to the left. The granulocyte stem cells are also involved in severe cases. Withdrawal of the drug is usually associated with recovery within 1–2 weeks, although recovery may sometimes take several months. It is considered that the disease still has 5%–10% mortality.

The first drug documented as causing immunologically mediated agranulocytosis was aminopyrine. Leukoagglutinins to aminopyrine were demonstrated and granulocytopenia could be transferred passively by serum to normal volun-

Table 7. Drugs frequently involved in agranulocytosis by peripheral leukocyte destruction. (Adapted from van Arsdel 1978; Parker 1980)

Aminopyrine[a]	Methyldopa
Chloral hydrate	Phenylbutazone
Chlordiazepoxide	Phenylindanedione
Chlorpromazine	Propranolol
Chlorpropamide	Salicylazosulfapyridine
Dipyrone[a]	Sulfamethoxypyridazine[a]
Mercurial diuretics	Sulfapyridine[a]

[a] No longer in use in several countries

teers if the serum donor had received the drug immediately prior to transfer (Moeschlin and Wagner 1952). Leukoagglutinins to several other drugs have since been identified (Thierfelder et al. 1967), but may be present only transiently. Further evidence for an immunological mechanism is the fact that leukopenia occurs again within a few minutes after a renewed challenge with the drug, suggesting peripheral destruction of leukocytes (Petz and Fudenberg 1976). This has been most frequently observed with aminopyrine- or phenylbutazone-induced agranulocytosis (Barrett et al. 1976). In such cases, fever, chills, arthralgia, and even shock may accompany the reaction. These acute symptoms are probably due to leukocyte lysis and the release of leukocytic pyrogens and lysosomal enzymes in the circulation. In summary, the evidence that leukopenia may be due to immunological mechanisms, at least in some cases, involves the following: (a) presence of leukoagglutinins, especially when the patient's serum has been taken a few hours after administration of the drug; (b) passive transfer of leukopenia to normal volunteers with such sera; (c) agglutination of normal leukocytes in presence of the drug in vitro by sera from patients with agranulocytosis; (d) deleterious effects of such sera on leukocyte metabolism (Bilezikian et al. 1976), and (e) lymphocyte proliferation in vitro in presence of the drug (Wall et al. 1977). Such immunological reactivities have been demonstrated in cases of agranulocytosis to aminopyrine and sulfonamides and antithyroid agents such as propylthiouracil and methimazole (Wall et al. 1977). The drugs reported to cause peripheral leukocyte destruction are listed in Table 7.

In contrast to this, however, drugs such as phenothiazine and sulfonamides often fail to produce acute manifestations when the drug is readministered in sensitive patients; the agranulocytosis may develop only somewhat later in the course of therapy. Similar cases of isolated leukopenia without hemolytic anemia during the course of high-dose penicillin therapy have also been described (Neftel et al. 1981), and appear to rest on an immunological mechanism possibly involving both IgG antibodies and cellular immunity to the BPO determinant but a toxic effect on bone marrow stem cells is also possible. Frequently, anemia and thrombocytopenia are also present, and the prognosis for recovery becomes markedly poor. This suggest a different mechanism than peripheral leukocyte destruction, such as decreased formation and release of leukocytes from the bone marrow. Leukocyte precursors in the bone marrow appear affected in such cases.

Table 8. Drugs frequently involved in thrombocytopenia. (Adapted from VAN ARSDEL 1978; PARKER 1980)

Acetaminophen	Meprobamate
Acetazolamide	Methyldopa
Acetylsalicylic acid	Narcodorm
Allymid	Novobiocin
p-Aminosalicylic acid	Penicillamine
Antazoine	Phenacetin
Atabrine	Phenobarbital
Carbamazepine	Phenytoin
Cephalothin	Phenylbutazone
Chloramphenicol	Quinine
Chlorothiazide	Quinidine
Dicoumarol	Rauwolfia alkaloids
Digitoxin	Rifampin
Ethchlor	Sedormid[a]
Gold salts	Spironolactone
Heparin	Stilbophen
Hydantoins	Sulfonamides
Hydrochlorothiazide	Sulfonylureas
Imipramine	Thiazide diuretics
Isoniazid	Thioguanine

[a] No longer in use

3. Thrombocytopenia

Bleeding similar to that seen in other forms of thrombocytopenia is the most important symptom. Sensitized patients, on reexposure to even minute amounts of a drug, develop an acute hemorrhagic syndrome with petechiae and mucous membrane bleeding. The platelet counts can drop precipitously within 30 min of administration of the drug. These symptoms can be associated with fever, cutaneous rashes, arthralgia, and other manifestations of allergy. The thrombocytopenia usually develops during drug treatment, but may be delayed for several weeks or even months after the drug has been discontinued in the case of gold therapy (PARKER 1980). The rapidity of the fall of platelet counts following drug readministration suggests accelerated destruction of platelets in the peripheral blood rather than decreased synthesis and release of platelets from the bone marrow. The megakaryocytes in the bone marrow are usually normal or elevated. However, in prolonged reactions, decreased platelet synthesis and release may also occur. Discontinuation of the drug usually results in full recovery within 2 weeks.

A large variety of drugs (Table 8) have been shown to induce immune thrombocytopenia (MIESCHER 1973). While at one time allylisopropylacetylcarbamide (Sedormid/apronalide) was a leading cause (ACKROYD 1962), quinidine and quinine (including quinine-containing drinks) are probably at present the most frequent causes of thrombocytopenia (ASTER 1977; LIBMAN and GOLDSMITZ 1972). Levodopa has also been implicated (WANAMAKER et al. 1976). The innocent bystander mechanism appears to be responsible for most cases of drug-induced thrombocytopenia, and the antibodies involved are almost always of the IgG class (PARKER 1980; KUNICKI et al. 1978). The sera of affected patients contain anti-

Table 9. Drugs frequently involved in eosinophilia. (Van Arsdel 1978; Parker 1980)

Antibiotics

Aminosalicylic acid	Nitrofurantoin
Cephalosporins	Penicillins
Erythromycin	Rifampin
Isoniazid	Streptomycin
Kanamycin	Sulfonamides
Nalidixic acid	Tetracyclines

Other drugs

Allopurinol	Ethosuximide
Chloral hydrate	Penicillamine
Digitalis	Phenothiazines

bodies that in presence of the drug produce platelet lysis or agglutination, depending on whether or not complement is present (Ackroyd 1975; Shulman 1958). Release of serotonin by platelets and complement fixation assays seem to be the most sensitive and reproducible assays to demonstrate the effect of antibodies and drug on platelets. Mixtures of specific antibody and quinine (or Quinidine) apparently react with one or more receptor sites on the surface of normal platelets. However, the exact sequence of binding is not yet ascertained. Participation of the drug itself or its metabolites in the binding by antibody seems certain, because of the marked specificity of the response. It is not yet established whether the antibodies are specific for the drug alone or for the drug and the platelets in combination. In the case of acetaminophen and of p-aminosalicylic acid, metabolites of the drugs have been implicated in the sensitization leading to thrombocytopenia (Eisner and Shahidi 1972; Eisner and Kasper 1972). It has also been suggested in some patients that, in addition to thrombocytopenia, capillary lesions may be present, resulting in bleeding even when the platelet count is normal. A similar reaction involving antigen-antibody complexes could occur in capillary endothelial cells (Ackroyd 1975).

4. Eosinophilia

Occasionally, blood eosinophilia may be the only evidence for allergy to a drug. It might also be the first sign of an impending clinical allergic reaction. The drugs indicated in Table 9 are frequently associated with eosinophilia. However, the interpretation of an isolated eosinophilia is frequently difficult. The incidence of eosinophilia without other signs of allergy may be high during treatment with drugs such as kanamycin (up to 10% of treated patients) or during prolonged treatment with streptomycin (up to 50% of patients treated) (van Arsdel 1978). Even drugs such as digoxin or digitoxin, which very rarely cause allergic symptoms, have been associated with eosinophilia. Eosinophilia in the absence of allergic symptoms has frequently been observed in patients allergic to penicillin and nevertheless treated with the drug in the presence of a protective inhibiting monovalent penicilloyl hapten (de Weck and Jeunet 1975).

Table 10. Drugs frequently involved in hepatic damage. (Adapted from VAN ARSDEL 1978; PARKER 1980)

Primarily cholestatic

Chlordiazepoxide	Nalidixic acid
Chlorpromazine	Nitrofurantoin
Chlorzoxazone	Phenothiazines
Erythromycin estolate	Sulfamethoxazole
Ethchlorvynol	Sulfonylureas
Imipramine	Troleandomycin

Primarily hepatocellular

p-Aminosalicylic acid	Monoamine oxidase inhibitors
Amphotericin B	Nitrofurantoin
Ethacrynic acid	Oxyphenisation
Furosemide	Phenylbutazone
Gold salts	Propylthiouracil
Griseofulvin	Pyrazinamide
Halothane	Quinidine
Hydantoins	Rifampin
Indomethacin	Sulfonamides
Isoniazid	Trimethadione
Methoxyflurane	Zoxazolamine
Methyldopa	

V. Hepatic Disorders

Drug-induced hepatic damage may consist in primarily hepatocellular or primarily cholestatic alterations in hepatic functions, although some combination of the two may occur. In cholestasis, jaundice is usually the first symptom, but may be preceded by blood eosinophilia. Phenothiazines (ZELMAN 1959) and erythromycin estolate are most frequently responsible for cholestatic jaundice (Table 10). When the reaction involves hepatocellular damage, fever may be the first manifestation, or obstructive jaundice may come first followed by pain and the development of a large tender liver. The clinical picture is similar to that of viral hepatitis and the reaction may be preceded by skin rash and eosinophilia. Infiltration of the liver by eosinophils, lymphocytes, and plasmocytes is common. This type of hepatocellular damage has been reported to be rather common with pyrazinamide and rifampin (VAN ARSDEL 1978). Other drugs which have been implied in primarily hepatocellular damage are shown in Table 10.

It is frequently difficult to ascribe an immunological pathogenesis to liver reactions following the administration of drugs. Arguments for such a mechanism are: (a) the fact that such reactions occurs only in a small proportion of patients taking the drug; (b) that the onset of hepatitis is typically delayed (consistent with a primary immune response); (c) that the reaction may be associated with other signs of sensitivity such as skin rash, fever, and eosinophilia. Furthermore, in some cases, repeated episodes of hepatitis have been observed upon repeated exposure to even small doses of the drug (DUJOVNE et al. 1967; SIMPSON and WALKER 1960; ZIMMERMANN 1972). This has been the case for halothane, which only rarely causes hepatitis, but which has been responsible for repeated episodes following halothane exposure in anesthesiologists or in operated patients (KLATSKIN and KIMBERG 1969). There is little direct experimental evidence for an immunological reaction in drug-induced liver disease, although a number of reports suggest that lymphocytes from patients with hepatic reactions to isoniazid and para-aminosalicylate may indeed possess cell-mediated hypersensitivity to these drugs (HALPERN 1972; PARONETTO and POPPER 1970). The investigations of in vitro lymphocyte responsiveness to halothane have been inconsistent (DAVIES and HOLMES 1972; BRUCE and RAYMON 1972). However, the use of liver homogenates from halothane-anestesized animals as antigen in the lymphocyte culture, rather than halothane itself, may give more conclusive results (EDDLESTON 1980).

Since most drugs are actively metabolized in the liver, for example through the hepatic cytochrome P-450 system (REMMER and SCHUPPEL 1972), it is in the liver that the concentration of potentially immunogenic metabolites should be the highest. Accordingly, the incidence of hepatic damage in drug allergy should be expected to be even higher than observed. It is likely that in most forms of drug-induced hepatic damage, some direct toxic effects are present. It has been shown that drugs such as acetaminophen are converted to toxic reactive intermediates within the liver. By reacting with enzymes and other essential cellular elements, these metabolites alter the function of the liver cell, leading to acute necrosis (GILLETTE et al. 1974). Few drugs that are known to be hepatotoxic remain in use. Hepatotoxicity resulting in necrosis and cirrhosis is a calculated risk with methotrexate and mercaptopurine treatment (SCHEIN and WINOKUR 1965). High-dose intravenous tetracyclines are also hepatotoxic.

VI. Renal Diseases

Most instance of drug-induced renal disease are probably due to direct toxicity. Even cephalosporins such as cephalothin or cephaloridin, which can produce immunological reactions, more frequently damage the kidney directly (PARKER 1979 a).

Since antigen-antibody complexes localize nonspecifically in the glomeruli, serum sickness may be the most common allergic drug reaction in the kidney. While proteinuria and microscopic hematuria may occur in serum sickness, they are usually mild and are not accompanied by clinically significant changes in renal function. The *glomerulonephritis* is transient, and almost always subsides completely after treatment with the drug has been stopped. Some more severe forms of nephritis have been observed in association with drug-induced generalized vasculitis. A *nephrotic syndrome* has been produced by a variety of drugs, in particular penicillin, penicillamines, organic mercurials, Tridione, paramethadione and gold (BACON et al. 1976; PARKER 1975; RAIJ and MICHAEL 1980). The glomerular lesions produced by penicillin and penicillamine during the nephrotic syndrome contain IgG and complement deposits, as shown by immunofluorescence. Immune complexes have also been observed in the glomeruli in the course of gold-induced nephropathy (LEE et al. 1965). However, in that case, gold appeared to be localized in the proximal tubules, not in the same areas within the glomeruli where immune complexes are deposited. Accordingly, it is possible that some drugs initiate an in-

Table 11. Drugs frequently involved in kidney damage. (VAN ARSDEL 1978; PARKER 1980)

Nephrotic syndrome	
Gold salts	Penicillamine
Organic mercurials	Phenindione
Paramethadione	Tridione
Penicillin	
Interstitial nephritis	
Allopurinol	Penicillin
Azathioprine	Phenindione
Cephalothin	Phenylbutazone
Furosemide	Polymyxin B
Glafenin	Sulfonamides
Hydantoins	Thiazide
Methicillin	Tridione
Oxacillin	

jury to tubular cells, resulting in the solubilization of tubular antigens, the development of an autoimmune response, and secondary glomerular localization of immune complexes directed against such tubular antigens (SILVERBERG et al. 1970). In the case of phenindione-induced nephrotic syndrome the antigen may be 3-benzylidenephtalide, a highly reactive contaminant discovered in pharmaceutical preparations of the drug (BUNDGAARD 1975).

The most common immunologically mediated lesion of the kidney due to drugs appears to be *interstitial nephritis*. Fever, skin rash and/or eosinophilia frequently accompany the renal symptoms. These are characterized by hematuria associated with proteinuria and rapidly progressive renal failure (LYONS et al. 1973; BAKER and WILLIAMS 1963). Microscopically, degenerative changes and necrosis are observed in the tubules, as well as edema and interstitial infiltration with mononuclear cells, plasma cells, and eosinophils. Penicillins, especially methicillin, appear to be one of the most frequent causes (BALWIN et al. 1968; BORDER et al. 1974), although interstitial nephritis is a rare complication of high-dose penicillin therapy. The mechanism of the lesions may be cell-mediated, as suggested by the extensive infiltration with mononuclear cells. However, penicillin antigens, immunoglobulins, and complement have also been demonstrated by immunofluorescence on the surface of tubular cells and in the glomeruli. In some patients, the serum contained antibodies reactive with tubular basement membranes, suggesting a drug-induced autoimmune reaction. In such cases, the autoimmune process could continue even after discontinuation of the drug. Drug-induced interstitial nephritis has also been observed with a number of other drugs (Table 11). Interstitial nephritis leading to renal failure is frequently observed in patients taking large doses of analgesics for a prolonged time, in particular phenacetin. It is estimated that more than 20% of patients with a clinical diagnosis of chronic interstitial nephritis are chronic analgesic abusers (MURRAY and GOLDBERG 1975; ERNE et al. 1977; BENNETT et al. 1977). Since lymphocytic infiltration is frequently a prominent feature in the renal lesions of such people, the hypothesis that an immunological mechanism is at hand must be considered. Phenacetin produces two metabolites which are immunogenic in guinea pigs and man, paraphenetidin and 2-hydroxyphenetidine (UEHLEKE 1962; RUEGGER et al. 1973; ERNE et al. 1977; MACKLON et al. 1974). However, it has not been conclusively demonstrated upon skin testing patients with phenacetin abuse and kidney disease that hypersensitivity to such metabolites is really responsible for the disease. Indeed, such patients most of the time showed negative skin tests, suggesting either immunological tolerance brought about by the large doses of phenacetin absorbed or sequestration of phenacetin-reactive lymphocytes within the renal lesions, leading to paradoxically negative skin tests (RUEGGER et al. 1973).

VII. Reactions Affecting the Respiratory Tract

1. Asthma

Any drug that can cause IgE-mediated allergy and anaphylactic reactions can also be responsible for bronchospasm (CHARPIN et al. 1972). However, this is seldom the only manifestation of allergy, unless the drug is delivered to the lungs by aerosol of by inhalation as a powder. Enzymes and macromolecular components such as pituitary snuff are well known to produce sensitization of that type. Sensitization to simple chemicals such as penicillin (DAVIES et al. 1974), spiramycin (DAVIES and PEPYS 1975), or phenylmercuric propionate (MATHEWS and PAN 1968) can lead to asthmatic reactions through IgE-mediated mechanisms. The same has been described for the inhalation of other low-molecular-weight chemicals such as diisothiocyanate and platinum salts encountered in industrial applications (PEPYS and DAVIES 1978).

In other cases, such as inhalation of cromolyn (SHEFFER et al. 1975), quinine, and quinidine, asthma may be produced without other signs of allergy, and it may be questioned whether the reaction is due to allergic sensitization or to a nonallergic mechanism (idiosyncrasy or toxicity). The asthmatic reaction induced by drugs inhibiting prostaglandin synthesis is discussed elsewhere (see Chap. 11).

2. Infiltrative and Fibrotic Pulmonary Reactions

Acute pulmonary reactions have been described, resembling bouts of extrinsic allergic alveolitis. This is particularly the case in patients with diabetes insipidus inhaling pituitary snuff (BUETTIKOFER et al. 1970). Another form of pulmonary acute reaction, most frequently induced by nitrofurantoin, is a syndrome of fever, cough, diffuse pulmonary infiltration of an edematous nature, pleural effusion, and hilar adenopathy (ROSENOW 1972; PEARSALL et al. 1974). This syndrome appears to develop in about 1 of 400 patients treated (KOCH-WESER et al. 1971). Drugs are also responsible for a number of instances of eosinophilic pneumonitis (pulmonary infiltrates with eosinophilia) in which nodular or diffuse migratory infiltrates develop in the lungs. With some other drugs, such as gold salts, metothrexate, or hydrochlorothiazide, more chronic, progressive, and diffuse interstitial infiltrates, sometimes associated with moderate eosinophilia, are observed. In these cases, infiltrates with numerous lymphocytes and plasma cells and sometimes giant cells and noncaseating granulomas have been described (AUTRAN et a. 1977; SHARMA 1973; WINTERBAUER et al. 1976; SCHEIN and WINOKUR 1965; AKOUN and DU-VALDESTIN 1972).

Table 12. Drugs frequently involved in pulmonary reactions. (VAN ARSDEL 1978; PARKER 1980)

Probably allergic	
1. Asthma	
Anaphylactogens in anaphylactic shock	Sulfamide
Penicillins (aerosol)	Aspirin
Spiramycin	Indomethacin
2. Extrinsic alveolitis (acute onset: infiltrative)	
Pituitary snuff	
Cromolyn	
3. Eosinophilic pneumonitis	
Methotrexate	Ethiodol
p-Aminosalicylic acid	Mephenesin
Aurothioglucose	Penicillin
Carbamazepine	Penicillamine
Chlorpropamide	Sulfonamides
Cromolyn	
4. Other	
Gold sodium thiomalate	Methotrexate
Hydrochlorothiazide	Nitrofurantoin
Probably toxic (slow onset: fibrotic)	
Bleomycin	Gold salts
Busulfan	Methysergide
Cyclophosphamide	Nitrofurantoin
Ganglionic blocking drugs	

The allergic etiology is suggested by the frequent presence of eosinophilia and skin rashes, the rapid recurrence of symptoms after renewed challenge with the drug, and the usual healing after withdrawal. Drugs of the nitrofurantoin group also produce other types of allergic reactions, such as urticaria and contact hypersensitivity (SHELDON et al. 1967). There are several reports of lymphocyte positive responses to the drug in vitro (BAECK et al.. 1976), which appear to be more frequent in patients with clinical sensitivity. However, negative studies have also been published (GELLER et al. 1977). IgG antibodies to nitrofurantoin have been observed both in the presence and absence of clinical symptoms. Cases of Goodpasture's syndrome or alveolitis have also been reported with penicillamine (EASTMOND 1967). Gold therapy leading to pulmonary fibrosis has been ascribed to an immunological pathogenesis on the basis of a positive lymphocyte transformation test (GEDDES and BROSTOFF 1976). On the other hand, a number of chronic progressive fibrotic reactions of the lung's interstitium appear to be due to drugs such as methysergide, nitrofurantoin, and antineoplastic agents such as bleomycin, busulfan, and cyclophosphamide (Table 12). Bleomycin reactions are dose-related and can be reproduced in dogs; the clinical syndrome is characterized by the insidious development of cough and dyspnea after several weeks or months of treatment, and encompasses a progressive pulmonary fibrosis which may increase even after drug treatment is stopped.

Table 13. Drugs frequently involved in autoimmune reactions. (Van Arsdel 1978; Parker 1980)

SLE syndrome

Chlorpromazine	Phenytoin
Hydralazine	Practolol
Isoniazid	Procainamide
Penicillamine	Venocuran (phenopyrazone + digitoxosides)

SLE-like or other less clear-cut autoimmune reactions

p-Aminosalicylic acid	Phenylbutazone
Barbiturates	Primidone
Carbamazepine	Quinidine
Ethosuximide	Streptomycin
Griseofulvin	Sulfisoxazole
Mephenytoin	Tetracycline
Penicillins	Thiouracils
D-Penicillamine	Trimethadione
Phenolphthalein	Vinyl chloride

VIII. Drug-Induced Autoimmunity

A clinical syndrome resembling systemic lupus erythematosus (SLE) was first described in 1954 following treatment with hydralazine (Perry and Schroeder 1954). Since then, many other drugs have been implicated in similar syndromes (Lee et al. 1966) (Table 13), but the most frequent cases still appear to be due to hydralazine or procainamide (Tan 1974). The syndrome is characterized by malaise, fever, arthralgias, arthritis, polyserositis, lymphadenopathy, hepato- and splenomegaly, dermatitis, and leukopenia. A common feature of drug-induced lupus is that the drug involved has been used for at least 6–8 weeks before symptoms appear. Generally, the symptoms subside slowly after the drug is withdrawn. About 10% of patients receiving hydralazine in moderate to large doses over a period of several months develop clinical symptoms of a lupus-like syndrome. The common laboratory manifestations include an elevated erythrocyte sedimentation rate, leukopenia, mild anemia, positive SLE cell reaction, and positive tests for antinuclear antibodies. Serum complement levels are normal in contrast to those observed in spontaneously occurring clinically active SLE. Furthermore, the antibodies do not appear to react with native (double stranded) DNA. Procainamide induces the lupus-like syndrome more frequently than any other drug. Up to 68% of patients taking procainamide over a period of several months develop antinuclear antibodies (Blomgren et al. 1969; Davis et al. 1975). Antinuclear antibodies have also been demonstrated in up to 20% of patients receiving isoniazid therapy for active tuberculosis, but clinical manifestations of lupus are uncommon (Parker 1980; Alarcon-Segovia et al. 1969).

The mechanisms by which antinuclear antibodies are produced are not completely elucidated. It seems that the responsible drugs produce a lupus-like syndrome de novo rather than activating latent SLE. Hydralazine and procainamide produce immunologic and immunopathological changes resembling SLE in laboratory animals (CANNAT and SELIGMAN 1968). The clinical patterns also differ in drug-induced lupus from ordinary SLE, in that males are frequently involved and that leukopenia, anemia, and nervous system, cutaneous, and renal involvement are less frequent (HAHN et al. 1972, HOLLEY 1964). Patients with hydralazine-induced lupus possess serum antibodies which react with red cells sensitized to diazotized hydralazine. Some lymphocyte transformation tests to hydralazine have also been observed, suggesting that the drug may participate in the reaction as a hapten (HAHN et al. 1972). It has been suggested that hydralazine (TAN 1974) and procainamide (BLOMGREN et al. 1969) may affect DNA structures. These drugs may therefore produce an antigenically modified DNA. Following sensitization to the drug itself, the drug-DNA conjugates formed may act as new antigens in which the drug's haptenic determinants function as carrier presenting DNA bases as immunogens, and promote the formation of antinuclear antibodies (PARKER 1980). A second possibility is that antihapten antibodies formed in response to procainamide and hydralazine might cross-react with some bases in DNA (YAMAUCHI et al. 1975). Enzymatic abnormalities may be related to the development of that syndrome (PERRY et al. 1970).

A similar clinical syndrome has been described following treatment with Venocuran, a composed drug used for the treatment of venous diseases that contains phenopyrazone, a horse chestnut extract, and several glycosides (MULLER et al. 1975; GROB et al. 1975). The clinical manifestations include recurrent fever, myalgia, arthralgia, pleuritis, pulmonary infiltrates, pericarditis, and myocarditis. In that case, the serum contains not antinuclear but antimitochondrial antibodies. Up to 90% of patients using Venocuran for a long time were shown to possess antimitochondrial antibodies in the serum, with 30% showing minor symptoms and at least 10% developing the full clinical syndrome. The clinical manifestations developed only after a minimum of several months on the drug, and could continue for many months after the drug had been discontinued.

Several other autoimmune syndromes have been described in which drugs may be responsible. As discussed elsewhere in this chapter, tubular and interstitial nephritis, hemolytic anemia, glomerulonephritis, and pulmonary alveolitis induced by drugs may rest, at least in part, on an autoimmune mechanism. Practolol, a selective β_1-blocking agent, may induce keratoconjunctivitis simulating Sjögren's syndrome as well as other clinical symptoms such as exfoliative dermatitis, a lupus-like syndrome, a nephrotic syndrome, and fibrinous peritonitis (BEHAN et al. 1976). The clinical and immunological features of this reaction are described in detail in Chap. 15. Chronic exposure to vinyl chloride, a chemical used in the plastics industry, can cause a clinical syndrome resembling scleroderma and Raynaud's phenomenon together with impaired pulmonary functions. Hyperglobulinemia, cryoglobulinemia and abnormalities of the complement system are frequently present, together with antinuclear antibodies. It has been speculated that vinyl chloride may be metabolized to highly reactive oxides, causing immunological alterations of autologous proteins and resulting in autoimmune disease (WARD et al. 1976). Occasionally, polymyositis has also been related to drug-induced allergy, for example following treatment with D-penicillamine. A similar association has been observed with penicillin therapy (PARKER 1980).

IX. Vasculitis

Several terms have been used to describe reactions in this category, including allergic angiitis, allergic vasculitis, hypersensitivity angiitis, and allergic purpura (VAN ARSDEL 1978). Since the reactions frequently also involve the skin and other organs, the term systemic cutaneous vasculitis appears appropriate. Cutaneous lesions generally appear first on the lower legs and appear erythematous, macropapular, and purpuric. In case of systemic involvement, additional symptoms may include fever, malaise, myalgias, edema, arthritis, dyspnea, headache, and peripheral neuropathy (ZEEK 1953; McCOMBS et al. 1956; SYMMERS 1962). Abdominal pain and enteric bleeding sometimes occur. The urinary sediment may suggest glomerulonephritis. Biopsies show fibrinoid necrosis in the walls of small blood vessels associated with endothelial swelling, hemorrhage, platelet thrombi, and leukocyte infiltration. The observed disintegration of leukocyte nuclei has led to the term leukocytoclastic vasculitis (ZEEK 1953; SAMS et al. 1976). Immunoglobulins and early and late components of complement have been found in the vessel walls of early lesions, suggesting that vasculitis may be in origin an immune complex disease (SAMS et al. 1976).

Some special forms of vasculitis such as Henoch-Schönlein purpura, temporal arteritis or periarteritis nodosa are defined clinical entities (RICH 1942; BRAVERMANN 1970) which may be mimicked by drug-induced reactions (GRIEBLE and JACKSON 1958). However, it is frequently quite difficult to assess objectively the possible involvement of drug allergy in such cases. A history consistent with drug allergy has been obtained in 20%–30% of patients with pathologic changes of allergic vasculitis (MC COMBS et al. 1956). The drugs most frequently suspected of causing vasculitis are shown in Table 14. While it is important to consider drug allergy as a possible cause in any form of acute or chronic vasculitis, objective elements to implicate a drug are frequently absent. There is also no ready explanation for the observation that in these chronic vasculitis syndromes possibly induced by drug allergy, fresh lesions continue to appear long after the drug has been discontinued, unless autoimmune mechanisms, as discussed above, are postulated.

X. Digestive Tract and Other Manifestations

The majority of digestive tract symptoms following injections of drug are due to nonspecific toxicity, changes in bacterial flora, or direct effects on mucous cell secretions or smooth muscle tone. However, following the development of hypersensitivity to a drug, oral use may lead to symptoms primarily affecting the gastrointestinal tract. Such manifestations include diarrhea, edema, hemorrhage, eosinophilic infiltration, and steatorrhea (GLEICH et al. 1980). "Allergy" to a drug may be entertained by food additives presenting the same reactivity (e.g., tartrazine or prostaglandin synthesis inhibitors) even if the reactions are due to a nonimmunological mechanism.

Following oxyphenbutazone therapy, a febrile syndrome with salivary gland enlargement has been described (GROSS 1969). A generalized syndrome with hepato- and splenomegaly, generalized enlargement of lymph nodes, and fever, accompanied by a polyclonal elevation of IgGs, has been described following pro-

Table 14. Drugs frequently involved in allergic vasculitis. (VAN ARSDEL 1978; PARKER 1980)

Allopurinol	Penicillins
Busulfan	Phenothiazines
Colchicine	Phenylbutazone
Diphenhydramine	Propranolol
Ethionamide	Propylthiouracil
Indomethacin	Quinidine
Iodides	Sulfonamides
Isoniazid	Tetracyclines
Meprobamate	Thiazide diuretics
Metamphetamine	Vaccines
Hydantoins	

longed treatment with phenytoins and *p*-aminosalicylic acid, dapsone, or procainamide (SALTZEIN and ACKERMANN 1959; GAMS et al. 1968; GROB and HEROLD 1972). The evolution of the phenytoin-induced immunoblastic lymphadenopathy may be quite severe (FRIZZERA et al. 1974; KREISLER et al. 1977; PRUZANSKI et al. 1976; HYMAN and SOMMERS 1966; LUKES and TINDLY 1975; OLMER et al. 1952; VESIN et al. 1976).

XI. Skin Manifestations

The most frequent manifestations of drug allergy involve the skin. Urticaria, angioedema, exanthematous skin rashes, allergic eczematous contact dermatitis, photodermatitis, fixed drug eruptions, erythema multiforme, and the Stevens-Johnson and Lyell syndromes are the best characterized clinical manifestations. Their clinical aspects, evolution, and pathophysiological mechanisms are described in detail in the following chapter.

References

Abelson PH (1970) Death from heroin. Science 168:1289

Ackroyd JF (1962) The immunological basis of purpura due to drug hypersensitivity. Proc R Soc Med 55:30

Ackroyd JF (1975) Immunological mechanisms in drug hypersensitivity. In: Gell PGH, Coombs RRA, Lachmann PJ (eds) Clinical aspects of immunology, 3rd ed., Blackwell, Oxford

Ahlstedt S, Ekström B, Svärd PO, Sjöberg B, Kristofferson A, Oertengren B (1980) New aspects on antigens in penicillin allergy. CRC Rev Toxicol 7:219

Akoun G, Duvaldestin P (1972) Les granulomatoses pulmonaires d'origine medicamenteuse. Rev Tuberc 36:785

Alarcon-Segovia D, Fishbein E, Betancourt VM (1969) Antibodies to nucleoprotein and to hydraide-altered soluble nucleoprotein in tuberculous patients receiving isoniazid. Clin Exp Immunol 5:429

Amkraut AA, Rosenberg LT, Raffel S (1963) Elicitation of PCA by univalent and divalent haptens. J Immunol 91:644

Amos HE (1976) Allergic drug reactions. Arnold, London

Amos HE, Wilson DV, Taussig MJ, Carlton SJ (1971) Hypersensitivity reactions ro acetylsalicylic acid. I. Detection of antibodies in human sera using acetylsalicylic acid attached to proteins through the carboxyl group. Clin Exp Immunol 8:563

Arnaud A, Vervloet B (1980) Allergies medicamenteuses. In: Charpin J (ed) Traite d'Allergie. Flammarion, Paris, p 559

Arndt KA, Jick H (1976) Rates of cutaneous reactions to drugs: a report from the Boston collaborative Drug Surveillance Programm. JAMA 235:913

Arroyave CM, Bhat KN, Crown R (1976) Activation of the alternative pathway of the complement system by radiographic contrast media. J Immunol 117:1866

Askenaze PW (1977) Role of basophils, mast cells and vasoamines in hypersensitivity reactions with a delayed time course. Prog Allergy 23:199

Askenaze PW (1980) Effector cells in late and delayed hypersensitivity reactions that are dependent on antibodies or T cells. In: Fougereau M, Dausset J (eds) Immunology 80. Academic Press, London New York, p 829

Aster RH (1977) Thrombocytopenia due to platelet loss. In: Williams WJ, Beutler E, Erslev AJ, Rundles RW (eds) Hematology. Mc Graw-Hill, New York

Autran P, Garbe L, Pommier de Santi P, Baralis G, Charpin J (1977) Un cas d'accident rare de la chrysotherapie: une miliaire pulmonaire allergique. Rev Fr Mal Respir 5:713

Austen KF (1965) Histamine and other mediators of allergic reactions. In: Samter M (ed) Immunological diseases, 1st ed., Little, Brown & Co., Boston, p 211

Bäck O, Liden S, Ahlstedt S (1976) Adverse reactions to nitrofurantoin in relation to cellular and humoral immune responses. Clin Exp Immunol 28:400

Bacon PA, Tribe CR, Mackenzie JC, Jones JV, Cumming RH, Amer B (1976) Penicillamine nephropathy in rheumatoid arthritis. A clinical, pathological and immunological study. Q J Med 45:661

Baker SB, Williams RT (1963) Acute interstitial nephritis due to drug sensitivity. Br Med J 1:1655

Baldwin PS, Levine BB, McCluskey RT, Gallo GR (1968) Renal failure and interstitial nephritis due to penicillin and methicillin. N Engl J Med 279:1254

Barnard JH (1967) Allergic and pathologic findings in fifty insect sting fatalities. J Allergy 40:107

Barrett AJ, Weller E, Rozengurst N, Loggurst P, Humble JD (1976) Amidopyrine agranulocytosis: drug inhibition of granulocyte colonies in the presence of patient's serum. Br Med J 2:850

Batchelor FR, Dewdney JM, Feinerg JG, Weston RD (1967) A penicilloylated protein impurity as a source of allergy to benzylpenicillin and 6-aminopenicillanic acid. Lancet 1:1175

Behan PO, Behan WM, Zacharias FJ, Nicholls JT (1976) Immunological abnormalities in patients who had the oculomucocutaneous syndrome associated with practolol therapy. Lancet 2:984

Benacerraf B, Germain RN (1978) The immune response genes of the major histocompatibility complex. Immunol Rev 38:70

Benacerraf B, Levine BB (1962) Immunological specificity of delayed and immediate hypersensitivity reactions. J Exp Med 115:1023

Bennett WM, Plamp C, Porter GA (1977) Drug-related syndromes in clinical nephrology. Ann Intern Med 87:582

Benveniste J (1974) Platelet-activating factor, a new mediator of anaphylaxis and immune complex deposition from rabbit and human basophils. Nature 249:581

Berkowitz M, Glaser J, Johnstone DE (1953) The incidence of allergy to drugs in pediatric practice. Ann Allergy 11:561

Bernreiter M (1959) Electrocardiogram of a patient in anaphylactic shock. JAMA 170:1628

Bierman CW, Van Arsdel PP Jr (1969) Penicillin allergy in children. J Allergy 43:267

Bilezikian SB, Lalei YR, Tsan MF (1976) Immunological reactions involving leukocytes. III. Agranulocytosis induced by antithyroid drugs. Johns Hopkinks Med J 138:124

Blaser K, De Weck AL (to be published) Regulation of the IgE antibody response by idiotype-antiidiotype network. Prog Allergy 30

Blomgren SE (1973) Drug induced lupus erythematosus. Semin Hematol 10:345

Blomgren SE, Condemi JJ, Biganll MC, Vaughan JH (1969) Antinuclear antibody induced by procainamide. A prospective study. N Engl J Med 281:64

Bolton FG, Dameshek W (1956) Thrombocytopenic purpura due to quinidine. I. Clinical studies. Blood 11:527

Booth BH, Patterson R (1970) Electrocardiographic changes during human anaphylaxis. JAMA 211:627

Borda IT, Slone D, Jick H (1968) Assessment of adverse reactions within a drug surveillance program. JAMA 205:645

Border WA, Lehmann DH, Egan JD, Sass HJ, Glode JE, Wilson CB (1974) Antitubular basement-membrane antibodies in methicillin-associated interstitial nephritis. N Engl J Med 291:381

Boston collaborative drug surveillance programm (1973) Drug-induced anaphylaxis: a comparative study. JAMA 224:613

Brasch RC, Rockoff SD, Kuhn C, Chaplyvy M (1970) Contrast media as histamine liberators. II. Histamine release into venous plasma during intravenous urography in man. Invest Radiol 5:510

Brashear RE, Kelly MT, White AC (1974) Elevated plasma histamine after heroin and morphine. J Lab Clin Med 83:451

Braverman IM (1970) Skin signs of systemic disease. Saunders, Philadelphia

Braverman IM, Levin J (1963) Dilutin-induced serum sickness. Am J Med 35:418

Brown GL, Kanwar BS (1967) Drug rashes in glandular fever. Lancet 2:1418

Bruce DL, Raymon F (1972) Test for halothane sensitivity. N Engl J Med 286:1218

Bundgaard H (1975) Identification and quantitation of an 3-benzylidenephtalid contaminant of phenindione tablets and its characterization as a potentially immunogenic substance. Acta Pharm Suec 12:33

Bundgaard H (1980) Drug allergy: chemical and pharmaceutical aspects. Pharm Int 1:100

Bundgaard H, de Weck AL (1975) The role of aminoreactive impurities in acetylsalicylic acid allergy. Int Arch Allergy A PPL Immunol 49:119

Bundgaard H, Larsen C (1977) Polymerization of penicillins. J Chromatogr 132:51

Bundgaard H, Juul P, Kofod H (eds) (1977) Drug design and adverse reactions. Alfred Benzon symposium X. Academic Press, New York

Büttikofer E, De Weck AL, Scherrer M (1970) Pituitary snuff taker's lung. Schweiz Med Wochenschr 100:97

Campbell DH, Mc Casland GE (1944) In vitro anaphylactic response to polyhaptenic and monohaptenic simple antigens. J Immunol 49:315

Cannat A, Seligmann M (1968) Induction by isoniazid and hydralazine of antinuclear factors in mice. Clin Exp Immunol 3:99

Capron A, Dessaint JP, Capron M, Bazin H (1975) Specific IgE antibodies in immune adherence of normal macrophages to Schistosoma mansoni schistosomules. Nature 253:474

Charpin J, Boutin C, Gratecos LA (1972) Place actuelle de l'asthme medicamenteux. Rev Tuberc 36:841

Chase MW (1946) Inhibition of experimental drug allergy by prior feeding of the sensitizing agent. Proc Soc Biol Med 61:257

Chase MW (1953) The inheritance of susceptibility to drug allergy in guinea pigs. Trans NY Acad Sci 15:78

Chase MW (1958) Antibodies to Drugs. In: Sensitivity reactions to drugs. CIOMS Symposium. Blackwell, Oxford, p 125

Chase MW (1966) Delayed type hypersensitivity and the immunology of Hodgkin's disease, with a parallel examination of sarcoidosis. Cancer Res 26:1097

Cluff LE, Johnson JE (1964) Drug fever. Prog Allergy 8:149

Cluff LE, Carnasos GJ, Stewart RB (1975) Clinical problems with drugs. Saunders, Philadelphia

Cohen S (1977) The role of cell-mediated immunity in the induction of inflammatory responses. Am J Pathol 88:502

Conroy MC, de Weck AL (1981) The effect of aspirin and indomethacin on histamine release from leukocytes of petients with suspected intolerance to aspirin. Int Arch Allergy Appl Immunol [Suppl I) 66:152

Conroy MC, de Weck AL (1982) New aspects of pathophysiological reactions in allergic diseases. New developments in allergy. Davos (in press)

Cooke RA (1919) Allergy in drug idiosyncrasy. JAMA 73:759

Cream JJ, Turk JL (1971) A review of the evidence for immune complex deposition as a cause of skin disease in man. Clin Allergy 1:235

Dausset J, Contu LA (1964) A case of haemolytic anemia due to phenacetin allergy. Vox Sang 9:599

Davies GE, Holmes JE (1972) Drug-induced immunological effects on the liver. Br J Anaesth 44:941

Davies RJ, Pepys J (1975) Asthma due to inhaled chemical agents: the macrolide antibiotic spiramycin. Clin Allergy 5:99

Davies RJ, Hendrick DJ, Pepys J (1974) Asthma due to inhaled chemical agents: Ampicillin, benzylpenicillin, 6-amino penicillanic acid related substances. Clin Allergy 4:227

Davis DM, Beedle MA, Rawlins MD (1975) Antinuclear antibodies during procainamide treatment and drug acetylation. Br Med J 3:682

Delage C, Irey MS (1972) Anaphylactic deaths: a clinicopathologic study of 43 cases. J Forensic Sci 17:525

Dembo M, Goldstein B, Sobotka AK, Lichtenstein LM (1978) Histamine release due to bivalent penicilloyl haptens: Control by the number of cross-linked IgE antibodies on basophil plasma membrane. J Immunol 121:354

De Swarte RD (1972) Drug allergy. In: Patterson R (ed) Allergic diseases. Diagnosis and management, Lippincott, Philadelphia

Dewdney J (1977) Immunology of the antibiotics. In: Sela M (ed) The antigens, vol 4. Academic Press, New York, p 74

Dewdney J (1980) Pseudo-allergic reactions to antibiotics. In: Dukor P et al. (eds) PAR: Pseudo-allergic reactions, vol 1. Karger, Basel, p 273

De Weck AL (1964) Penicillin allergy, its detection by an improved hemagglutination technique. Nature 202:975

De Weck AL (1968) Comparison of the antigen's molecular properties required for elicitation of various types of allergic tissue damage. In: Grabar P, Miescher PA (eds) Immunopathology. Schwabe, Basel, p 295

De Weck AL (1971) Immunological effects of aspirin anhydride, a contaminant of commercial acetylsalicylic acid preparations. Int Arch Allergy Appl Immunol 41:393

De Weck AL (1974) Low molecular weight antigens. In: Sela M (ed) The antigens, vol II. Academic Press, New York, p 141

De Weck AL (1975) Molecular mechanisms of T and B lymphocyte triggering. Int Arch Allergy Appl Immunol 49:247

De Weck AL (1977a) Immune responses to environmental antigens that act on the skin: the role of lymphokines in contact dermatitis. Fed Proc 36:1742

De Weck AL (1977b) Immunologic aspects of allergic reactions to drugs. In: Bundgaard H (ed) Drug design and adverse reactions. X Alfred Benzon Symposium. Munksgaard, Copenhagen, p 141

De Weck AL (1978) Drug reactions. In: Samter M (ed) Immunological diseases, 3rd edn. Little, Brown & Co, Boston, p 413

De Weck AL (1979) Drug allergy. In: Gupta S, Good RA (eds) Cellular, molecular and clinical aspects of allergic disorders. Plenum, New York London, p 355

De Weck AL, Blum G (1965) Recent clinical and immunological aspects of penicillin allergy. Int Arch Allergy Appl Immunol 27:221

De Weck AL, Jeunet F (1975) Clinical trial of Ro 6-0787: A monovalent specific hapten inhibitor of penicillin allergy. Z Immunforsch 150:138

De Weck AL, Schneider CH (1969) Molecular and stereochemical properties required of antigens for the elicitation of allergic reactions. In: Westphal O, Bock HE, Grundmann E (eds) Problems of immunological diseases. Springer, Heidelberg, p 32

De Weck AL, Schneider CH, Gutersohn J (1968) The role of penicilloylated protein impurities, penicillin polymers and dimers in penicillin allergy. Int Arch Allergy Appl Immunol 33:535

De Weck AL, Schneider CH, Leemann W (1969) Hypersensitivity to carboxmethylcellulose as cause of anaphylactic reactions in cattle. Nature 223:621

De Weck AL, Schneider CH, Spengler H, Toffler O, Lazary S (1973) Inhibition of allergic reactions by monovalent haptens. In: Sehoin A (ed) Mechanisms of reagnic allergy. Dekker, New York, p 323

Doeglas HMG (1975) Chronic urticaria. Thesis, Groningen

Dogliotti M (1968) An instance of fatal reaction to the penicillin scratch-test. Dermatologica 136:489

Dujovne CZ, Chan CH, Zimmermann HJ (1967) Sulfonamide hepatic injury. Review of the literature and report of a case due to sulfamethoxazole. N Engl J Med 277:785

Dukor P, Kallos P, Schlumberger HD, West GB (eds) (1980) PAR: Pseudo-Allergic Reactions, vol I. Karger, Basel

Eastmond CJ (1976) Diffuse alveolitis complication of penicillamine treatment for rheumatoid arthritis. Br Med J 1:1506

Eddleston ALWF (1980) Immunology and the liver. In: Parker CW (ed) Clinical immunology. Saunders, Philadelphia, p 1009

Eisen HN (1959) Hypersensitivity to simple chemicals. In: Lawrence HS (ed) Cellular and humoral aspects of the hypersensitivity state. Hoeber, New York, p 89

Eisner EV, Kasper K (1972) Immune thrombocytopenia due to a metabolite of para-aminosalicylic acid. Am J Med 53:790

Eisner EV, Shahidi NT (1972) Immune thrombocytopenia due to a drug metabolite. N Engl J Med 287:376

Ellman L, Inman J, Green I (1971) Strain difference in the immune response to hydralazine in inbred guinea pigs. Clin Exp Immunol 9:927

Erne PE, Geczy AF, Spengler H, De Weck AL, Dubach UC (1977) Immunogenicity of p-phenetidine, 2-hydroxy-p-phenetidine and their protein conjugates in guinea pigs, rabbits and man. Int Arch Allergy Appl Immunol 53:319

Fankhauser S (1969) Neuere Aspekte der Insulintherapie. Schweiz Med Wochenschr 99:414

Farah FS, Kern M, Eisen HN (1960) Specific inhibition of wheal and erythema responses with univalent haptens and univalent antibody fragments. J Exp Med 112:1211

Fellner MJ, Harris H (1972) Adverse cutaneous reactions to drugs. In: Meyer L, Peck HM (eds) Drug induced diseases, vol 4. Excerpta Medica North-Holland, Amsterdam, p 382

Fellner MJ, Redmond AP, Levine BB, Baer RL (1967) Immediate penicillin reactions associated with penicilloyl specific skin sensitizing antibodies and low titers of blocking (IgG) antibodies. J Allergy 38:106

Freedman PL, Barr PS, Brody EA (1956) Hemolytic anemia due to quinidine: observations on its mechanism. Am J Med 20:806

Frick OL, Nye W, Raffel S (1968) Anaphylactic reactions to univalent haptens. Immunology 14:563

Frizzera G, Moran EM, Rappaport H (1974) Angioimmunoblastic lymphadenopathy with dysproteinemia. Lancet I:1070

Furhoff AK (1977) Anaphylactoid reaction to dextran. A report of 133 cases. Acta Anaesthesiol Scand 21:161

Furuya K, Urasawa S (1978) Demonstration of antibodies to chlorophenothiazine derivates. Int Arch Allergy 57:22

Gams RA, Neal JA, Conrad FG (1968) Hydantoin-induced pseudo-pseudolymphoma. Ann Intern Med 69:557

Gardner RC, Ovary Z (1960) Immunologic mechanism of anaphylaxis. III. Inhibition phenomenon in passive cutaneous anaphylaxis in the mouse. Proc Soc Exp Biol Med 105:342

Geczy AF, de Weck AL (1974) Genetic control of sensitization to chemically defined antigens and its relationship to histocompatibility antigens in guinea pigs. Monogr Allergy 8:83

Gell PGH, Benacerraf B (1961) Delayed hypersensitivity to simple protein antigens. Adv Immunol 1:319

Gell PGH, Harington CR, Rivers RP (1946) The antigenic function of simple chemical compounds: production of precipitins in rabbits. Bri J Exp Pathol 27:267

Geller M, Flaherty DK, Dickie HA, Reed CE (1977) Lymphopenia in acute nitrofurantoin pleuropulmonary reactions. J Allergy Clin Immunol 59:445

Germain RN, Sy SN, Roch K, Dietz MH, Greene MI, Nisonoff A, Weinberger JZ, Ju ST, Dorf ME, Benacerraf B (1981) The role of idiotype and the MLC in suppressor T cell pathways. In: Idiotypes and their expression, ICN-UCLA symposium, 1981

Gillette JR, Mitchell JR, Brodie BB (1974) Biochemical mechanisms of drug toxicity. Annu Rev Pharmacol 14:271

Girard JP, Vidmar B, Laugier P (1971) Diagnostic des allergies medicamenteuses. Rev Fr Aller 11:397

Girard JP, Cattin S, Cuevas M (1976) Immunological mechanisms and diagnosis tests in allergic drug reactions. Ann Clin Res 8:74

Gleich GJ, Sachs MI, O'Connel EJ (1980) Hypersensitivity reactions induced by foods. In: Parker CW (ed) Clinical immunology. Saunders, Philadelphia, p 1261

Glovsky MM, Braunwald J, Opelz G, Alenty A (1976) Hypersensitivity to procarbazine associated with angioedema, urticaria and low serum complement activity. J Allergy Clin Immunol 57:134

Goldman AL, Braman SS (1972) Isoniazid: A review with emphasis on adverse reactions. Chest 62:71

Good RA, Kelley WD, Rötstein J, Varco RL (1962) Immunological deficiency diseases. Prog Allergy 6:187

Green GR, Rosenblum A (1971) Report of the penicillin study group. American academy of allergy. J Allergy Clin Immunol 48:331

Grieble HG, Jackson GG (1958) Prolonged treatment of urinary tract infections with sulfamethoxypyridazine. N Engl J Med 258:1

Grob PJ, Herold GE (1972) Immunological abnormalities and hydantoins. Br Med J 2:561

Grob PJ, Muller-Schoop JW, Hacki MA, Joller-Jemelka HI (1975) Drug-induced pseudolupus. Lancet 2:144

Gross L (1969) Oxyphenbutazone-induced parotitis. Ann Intern Med 70:1229

Hahn BH, Sharp GC, Irwin WS, Kantor OS, Garoner CA, Bagby MK, Perry HM, Osterland CK (1972) Immune responses to hydralazine and nuclear antigens in hydralazine-induced lupus erythematosus. Ann Intern Med 76:365

Halpern BN (1972) Antibodies produced by drugs and methods for their detection. In: Samter M, Parker CW (eds) International encyclopedia of pharmacology and therapeutics, Sect 75: Hypersensitivity to drugs, vol 1. Pergamon, Oxford

Hanashiro PK, Weil MH (1967) Anaphylactic shock in man. Report of two cases with detailed hemodynamic and metabolic studies. Arch Intern Med 119:129

Hänsch GM, Voigtländer V, Rother U (1980) Effect of aspirin on the complement system in vitro. Int Arch Allergy Appl Immunol 61:150

Harber LC, Baer RL (1972) Pathogenic mechanisms of drug-induced photosensitivity. J Invest Dermatol 58:327

Harnett JC, Spector SL, Farr RS (1978) Aspirin idiosyncrasy. In: Middleton E (ed) Allergy, principles and practice. Mosby, St. Louis, p 1002

Hartl W (1965) Drug allergic agranulocytosis (Schultz disease) Semin Hematol 2:313

Hartl W (1966) On the serological diagnosis of drug-induce allergic agranulocytosis. Arch Klin Med 212:191

Hartl W (1973) Drug-indcued agranulocytosis. In: Girdwood RH (ed) Blood disorders due to drugs and other agents. Excerpta Medica, Amsterdam

Hirschberg (1902) Mitteilung über einen Fall von Nebenwirkung des Aspirin. Dtsch Med Wochenschr 1:416

Hoigné R, Schoch K (1959) Anaphylaktischer Shock und akute nicht allergische Reaktionen nach Procain-Penicillin. Schweiz Med Wochenschr 89:1350

Holley HL (1964) Drugs and the lupus diathesis (editorial). J Chronic Dis 17:1

Horowitz L, Parker CW (1975) Correspondence. N Engl J Med 292:1243

Huguley CM (1964) Drug-induced blood dyscrasias. II. Agranulocytosis. JAMA 188:817

Hurwitz N (1969) Admissions to hospital due to drugs. Br Med J 1:539

Hurwitz N, Wade OL (1969) Intensive hospital monitoring of adverse reactions to drugs. Br Med J 1:531

Hutchinson F, Mc Leod TM, Raffle EJ (1975) Nickel hypersensitivity. Br J Dermatol 93:557

Hyman G, Sommers SC (1966) The development of Hodgkin's disease and lymphoma during anticonvulsant therapy. Blood 28:416

Ida S, Hooks JJ, Siraganian RP, Notkins AL (1980) Enhancement of IgE-mediated histamine release from human basophils by immunespecific lymphokines. Clin Exp Immunol 41:380

Idsoe O, Guthe YT, Willcox RR, de Weck AL (1968) Nature and extent of penicillin side-reactions with particular reference to fatalities from anaphylactic shock. Bull WHO 38:159

Ishizaka T, Ishizaka K (1978) Triggering of histamine release from rat mast cells by divalent antibodies against IgE receptors. J Immunol 120:800

Jick H, Miettinen OS, Shapiro S (1970) Comprehensive drug surveillance. JAMA 213:1455

Joseph M, Dessaint JP, Capron A (1977) Characteristics of macrophage cytotoxicity induced by IgE immune complexes. Cell Immunol 34:247

Kaplan AP, Gray L, Shaff RE, Horakowa Z, Beaven MA (1975) In vivo studies of mediator release in cold urticaria and cholinergic urticaria. J Allergy Clin Immunol 56:491

Kashiwagi N, Brantignan CO, Brettschneider L, Groth CG, Starzl TE (1968) Clinical reactions and serologic changes after the administration of heterologous antilymphocyte globulin to human recipients of renal allografts. Ann Intern Med 68:275

Klatskin G, Kimberg DV (1969) Recurrent hepatitis attributable to halothane sensitization in an anesthesist. N Engl J Med 280:515

Klein U, Gikalov I, Keller M, Hoigné R (1972) Drug monitoring in der medizinischen Abteilung eines Regionalspitals. Schweiz Med Wochenschr 102:1083

Kniker WT, Guerra FA, Richards SEM (1971) Prevention of immune complex disease (serum sickness) by antagonists of vasoactive amines (Abstr). Pediatr Res 5:381

Knudsen ET, Dewdney JM, Trafford JAP (1970) Reduction of incidence of ampicillin rash by purification of ampicillin. Br Med J 1:469

Koch-Weser J, Sifel VW, Dexter M (1971) Adverse reactions to sulfioxazole and nitrofurantoin: manifestations and specific reaction rates during 2118 courses of therapy. Arch Intern Med 128:399

Kraft D, Roth A, Mischer P, Pichler H, Ebner H (1977) Specific and total serum IgE measurements in the diagnosis of penicillin allergy. A long term follow-up study. Clin Allergy 7:21

Krapin D (1962) Anaphylaxis with orally administered penicillin. N Engl J Med 267:820

Kreisler JM, Moreno E, Moneo I, Bootello A, Bouza A, Martinez de Letona J (1977) Immunological findings in immunoblastic lymphadenopathy. Clin Exp Immunol 27:497

Kristofferson A, Ahlstedt S, Pettersson E, Svärd PO (1977) Antigens in penicillin allergy. I. A radioimmunoassay for detection of penicilloylated protein contaminants in penicillin preparations. Int Arch Allergy Appl Immunol 55:13

Kunicki TJ, Johnson MM, Aster RH (1978) Absence of the platelet receptor for drug dependent antibodies and the Bernard-Soulier syndrome. J Clin Invest 62:716

Kuokkanen L (1972) Drug eruptions: a series of 464 cases in the Department of dermatology, University of Turku, Finnland, during 1966–1970. Acta Allergol 27:407

Lakin JD, Grace WR, Sell KW (1975) IgE anti-polymyxin B antibody formation in a T cell-depleted bone marrow transplant patient. J Allergy Clin Immunol 56:94

Lakin JD, Blockert J, Strong DM, Yocum MW (1978) Anaphylaxis to protamine sulfate mediated by a complement-dependent IgG antibody. J Allergy Clin Immunol 61:102

Landsteiner K (1945) The specificity of serological reactions. Harvard University Press, Cambridge, MA

Lang JH, Lasser EC, Kolb WP (1976) Activation of serum complement by contrast media. Invest Radiol 11:303

Lee JC, Dushkin M, Eyring EJ, Engleman EP, Hopper J Jr (1965) Renal lesions associated with gold therapy. Light and electron microscopy studies. Arthritis Rheum 8:1

Lee SL, Rivers I, Siegel M (1966) Activation of systemic lupus by drugs. Arch Intern Med 117:120

Leverre G, Baker H (1968) Ampicillin and infectious mononucleosis. Br J Dermatol 80:417

Levine BB (1965) The nature of the antigen-antibody complexes which initiate anaphylactic reactions. J Immunol 94:11

Levine BB (1966) Immunochemical mechanisms of drug allergy. Annu Rev Med 17:23

Levine BB (1976) Immunochemical mechanisms of drug allergy. In: Miescher PA, Müller-Eberhard HJ (eds) Textbook of immunopathology, 2nd edn, Grune & Stratton, New York, vol 1, 403

Levine BB (1972) Skin rashes with penicillin therapy: current management. N Engl J Med 286:42

Levine BB, Price VH (1964) Studies on the immunological mechanisms of penicillin allergy. II. Antigenic specificities of allergic wheal-and-flare skin responses in patients with histories of penicillin allergy. Immunology 7:542

Levine BB, Redmond AP (1967) Immunochemical mechanisms of penicillin induced Coombs positivity and hemolytic anemia in man. Int Arch Allergy 21:594

Levine BB, Redmond AP (1968) The nature of the antigen-antibody complexes initiating the specific wheal-and-flare reactions in sensitized man. J Clin Invest 47:566

Levine BB, Redmond AP, Fellner MJ, Voss HE, Levytska V (1966a) Penicillin allergy and the heterogeneous immune response of man to benzylpenicillin. J Clin Invest 45:1895

Levine BB, Fellner MJ, Levytska V, Franklin EC, Alisberg N (1966b) Benzylpenicilloyl-specific antibodies in man. II. Sensitivity of the hemagglutination assay method, molecular classes of the antibodies detected and antibody titers of randomly selected patients. J Immunol 96:719

Lewis JP, Austen KF (1964) Fatal systemic anaphylaxis in man. N Engl J Med 270:597

Libman LJ, Goldsmith KLG (1972) Quinidine-induced thrombocytopenia. Proc R Soc Med 65:590

Lieberman P, Siegle RL, Taylor WW (1978) Anaphylactoid reactions to iodinated contrast material. J Allergy Clin Immunol 62:174

Littner MR, Rosenfield AT, Putman CE, Ulreich S, Meadows G (1978) Evidence against histamine release as a cause of bronchospasm during intravenous urography. Am Rev Respir Dis 117:71

Lo Buglio AF, Jandl JH (1967) The nature of the alpha-methyl-dopa red-cell antibody. N Engl J Med 276:658

Lockey RF, Rucknagel DL, Vanselow NA (1963) Familial occurence of asthma, nasal polyps and aspirin intolerance. Ann Intern Med 78:57

Lukes RJ, Tindle BH (1975) Immunoblastic lymphadenopathy. N Engl J Med 292:1

Lyons H, Pinn VW, Cortell S (1973) Allergic interstitial nephritis causing reversible renal failure in four patients with idiopathic nephrotic syndrome. N Engl J Med 288:124

Macklon AF, Craft AW, Thompson M, Kerr DNS (1974) Aspisin and analgesic nephropathy. Br Med J I:597

Marone G, Kagey-Sobotka A, Lichtenstein LM (1981) Control mechanisms of histamine release from human basophils in vitro: The role of phospholipase A 2 and of lipoxygenase metabolites. Int Arch Allergy Appl Immunol [Suppl 1] 66:144

Mathews KP, Pan PM (1968) Immediate type hypersensitivity to phenylmercuric compounds. Am J Med 44:310

Mayer RL (1955) Group sensitization to compounds of quinone structure and its biological basis; role of these substances in cancer. Prog Allergy 4:79

Mc Combs RP (1965) Systemic allergic vasculitis. JAMA 194:1059

Mc Combs RP, Patterson JF, Mac Mahon HE (1956) Syndromes associated with "allergic vasculitis." N Engl J Med 255:251

McKenzie H, Parratt D, White RG (1976) IgM and IgG antibody levels to ampicillin in patients with infectious mononucleosis. Clin Exp Immunol 26:214

Menninger WC (1928) Skin eruptions from phenobarbital. JAMA 91:14

Metzger H (1978) The IgE-mast cell system as a paradigm for the study of antibody mechanisms. Immunol Rev 41:186

Michaelson G, Juhlin L (1973) Urticaria induced by preservatives and dye additives in food and drugs. Br J Dermatol 88:525

Miescher PA (1973) Drug-induced thrombocytopenia. Semin Hematol 10:311

Miller FF (1967) History of drug sensitivity in atopic persons. J Allergy Clin Immunol 40:46

Moeschlin S (1958) Agranulocytosis due to sensitivity to drugs. In: Rosenheim ML, Moulton R (eds) Sensitivity reactions to drugs. Blackwell, Oxford

Moeschlin S, Wagner K (1952) Agranulocytosis due to the occurrence of leukocyte-ag-glutinins (pyramidon and cold agglutinins). Acta Haematol 8:29

Morley J (1972) Production of increased vascular permeability by leukocytes: The role of kinin-releasing enzymes. In: Dash CH, Jones HEH (eds) Mechanism in drug allergy. Churchill-Livingstone, London, p 121

Morrison-Smith J, Gell PGH (1975) Serum sickness and acute anaphylaxis in man. In: Gell PGH, Coombs RRA, Lachmnann PJ (eds) Clinical aspects of immunology, 3rd edn. Blackwell, Oxford, p 903

Müller JW, Grob PJ, Joller HI, Guggisberg HE (1975) Pseudolupus: Eine schwere Neben-wirkung eines Venenpräparates. Schweiz Med Wochenschr 105:665

Murray G, Goldberg M (1975) Chronic interstitial nephritis: etiologic factors. Ann Intern Med 82:453

Neftel KA, Diem P, Gerber H, de Weck AL, Stucki P (1980) Durch (+)-Cyanidanol-3 (Ca-tergen) induzierte immunhämolytische Anämie. Schweiz Med Wochenschr 110:380

Neftel KA, Wälti M, Spengler H, Von Felten A, Weitzman SA, Bürgi H, de Weck AL (1981) Neutropenia after penicillins: Toxic or immune-mediated? Klin Wochenschr 59:877

Olmer J, Paillas D, Roger J, Muratore R, Badier M (1952) Manifestations ganglionnaires au cours des traitements par la methyl-3-phenyl-ethyl 5-5 hydantoine. Presse Med 60:1748

Orange RP, Donsky GJ (1978) Anaphylaxis. In: Middleton E Jr, Reed CE, Ellis EF (eds) Allergy: principles and practice. Mosby, St. Louis, p 563

Ottesen EA, Cohen SG (1978) The eosinophil, eosinophilia and eosinophil related disorders. In: Middleton E Jr, Reed CE, Ellis EF (eds) Allergy: principles and practice. Mosby, St. Louis, p 584

Parish WE (1970) Short-term anaphylactic IgG antibodies in human sera. Lancet 2:591

Parker CW (1975) Drug allergy (three parts). N Engl J Med 292:511, 732, 957

Parker CW (1977) Problems in identification of responsible antigenic determinants in drug allergy. In: Bundgaard H, Juul P, Kofod H (eds) Drug design and adverse reactions, Al-fred Benzon Symposium X. Munksgaard, Copenhagen

Parker CW (1979a) Drug allergy. In: Wolff ME (ed) Burger's medicinal chemistry, 4th edn. J Wiley & Sons, New York

Parker CW (1979b) Prostaglandins and slow-reacting substance. J Allergy Clin Immunol 63:1

Parker CW (1980) Drug allergy. In: Parker CW (ed) Clinical immunology. Saunders, Phil-adelphia, p 1219

Parker CW, de Weck AL, Kern M, Eisen HN (1962a) The preparation and some properties of penicillenic acid derivatives relevant to penicillin hypersensitivity. J Exp Med 115:803

Parker CW, Kern M, Eisen HN (1962b) Polyfunctional dinitrophenyl haptens as reagents for elicitation of immediate type allergic skin responses. J Exp Med 115:789

Paronetto F, Popper H (1970) Lymphocyte stimulation induced by halothane in patients with hepatitis following exposure to halothane. N Engl J Med 283:277

Patrono C, Ciabattoni G, Venutti A, Pugliese F, Schiavino D, Patriarca G (1978) Aspirin intolerance: unaltered susceptibility of platelet cyclo-oxygenase to inhibition by aspirin in vitro. J Allergy Clin Immunol 62:271

Pavek K (1977) Anaphylactic shock in the monkey: its hemodynamics and mediators. Acta Anesthesiol Scand 21:293

Pavek K, Wegmann A (1981) Pathophysiologie des anaphylaktischen und anaphylaktoiden Schocks. Fortschr Med 99:1994

Pearsall HR, Ewalt J, Tsoi MS, Sumida S, Backus D, Winterbauer RH, Webb DR, Jones H (1974) Nitrofurantoin lung sensitivity: report of a case with prolonged nitrofurantoin lymphocyte sensitivity and interaction of nitrofurantoinstimulated lymphocytes with al-veolar cells. J Lab Clin Med 83:728

Pepys J, Davies RJ (1978) Occupational asthma. In: Middleton E Jr, Reed CE, Ellis EF (eds) Allergy: principles and practice. Mosby, St. Louis, p 812

Perry HM (1973) Late toxicity to hydralazine resembling systemic lupus erythematosus or rheumatoid arthritis. Am J Med 54:58

Perry HM, Schroeder HS (1954) Syndrome simulating collagen disease caused by hydralazine (apresoline) JAMA 154:670

Perry HM, Tan EM, Carmody S (1970) Relationship of acetyltransferase activity to antinuclear antibodies and toxic symptoms in hypersensitive patients treated with hydralazine. J Lab Clin Med 76:114

Petrozzi JW, Shore RN (1976) Generalized exfoliative dermatitis from ethylenediamine. Arch Dermatol 112:525

Petz LD, Fudenberg HH (1966) Coombs positive hemolytic anemia caused by penicillin administration. N Engl J Med 274:171

Petz LD, Fudenberg H (1976) Immunologic mechanisms in drug-induced cytopenias. In: Brown EB (ed) Progress in hematology, vol 9. Grune & Stratton, New York

Pisciotta AV (1973) Immune and toxic mechanisms in drug-induced agarnulocytosis. Semin Hematol 10:279

Plescia OJ, Braun W, Imperato S, Cora-Block E, Jaroskova L, Schimbor C (1968) Methylated serum albumin as a carrier for oligo- and polynucleotides. In: Plescia OJ, Braun W (eds) Nuclei acids in immunology. Springer, New York

Pressmann D, Goldberg AL (1968) The structural basis of antibody specificity. Benjamin, New York

Pruzanski W, Sutton DM, Pantalony D (1976) Angioimmunoblastic lymphadenopathy: An immunochemical study. Clin Immunol Immunopathol 6:62

Pullen H, Wright N, Murdoch JM (1967) Hypersensitivity reactions to antibacterial drugs in infectious mononucleosis. Lancet 2:1176

Raij L, Michael AF (1980) Immunologic aspects of kidney disease. In: Parker CW (ed) Clinical immunology. Saunders, Philadelphia, p 1051

Rajka G, Skog E (1965) On the relation between drug allergy and atopy. Acta Allergol 20:387

Redmond AP, Levine BB (1968) Delayed skin reactions to benzylepenicillin in man. Int Arch Allergy 23:193

Remmer H, Schuppel R (1972) The formation of antigenic determinants. In: Samter M, Parker CW (eds) International encyclopedia of pharmacology and therapeutics. Section 75: Hypersensitivity to drugs, vol 1. Pergamon, Oxford

Rich A (1942) The role of hypersensitivity in periarteritis nodosa, as indicated by seven cases developing during serum sickness and sulfonamide therapy. Johns Hopkins Hosp Bull 71:123

Ring J, Arroyave CM, Fritzler MJ, Tan EM (1978) In vitro histamine release by radiographic contrast media in man. J Allergy Clin Immunol 61:145

Rockoff JD, Brash R, Kuhn C, Chaplyvy M (1970) Contrast media as histamine liberators. Invest Radiol 5:503

Rosenow EC (1972) The spectrum of drug-induced pulmonary diseases. Ann Intern Med 77:977

Rudolph AH, Price EV (1973) Penicillin reactions among patients in venereal disease clinics: a national survey. JAMA 223:499

Ruegger R, Spengler H, de Weck AL, Dubach UC (1973) Immunologische Aspekte der Sensibilisierung auf Phenacetin. Dtsch Med Wochenschr 98:762

Saltzstein SL, Ackerman LV (1959) Lymphadenopathy induced by anticonvulsant drugs and mimicking clinically and pathologically malignant lymphomas. Cancer 12:164

Sams WM Jr, Thorne EG, Small P (1976) Leukocytoclastic vasculitis. Arch Dermatol 112:219

Samter M, Beers RF (1967) Concerning the nature of intolerance to aspirin. J Allergy Clin Immunol 40:281

Samter M, Beers RF Jr (1968) Intolerance to aspirin: Clinical studies and consideration of its pathogenesis. Ann Intern Med 68:975

Samuelsson B (1981) Leukotrienes: Mediators of allergic reactions and inflammation. Int Arch Allergy Appl Immunol [Suppl 1] 66:98

Saurat JH, Ponvert C, Burtin C, Soubrane C, Lebel B, Bencher F, Paupe J (1976) Lymphocyte transformation, leucocyte migration, specific IgE, IgG, and IgM before, during and after penicillin treatment without adverse reaction. Acta Allergol 31:1

Schein PS, Winokur SH (1965) Immunosuppressive and cytotoxic chemotherapy: long term complications. Ann Intern Med 82:84

Schlossmann SF, Yaron A, Ben-Efraim S, Sober HA (1965) Immunogenicity of a series of a-N, DNP-L-lysines. Biochemistry 4:1638

Schneider CH, de Weck AL (1965) A new chemical aspect of penicillin allergy: The direct reaction of penicillin with e-amino groups. Nature 208:57

Schneider CH, de Weck AL, Stauble E (1971) Carboxymethyl-cellulose. Additives in penicillins and the elicitation of anaphylactic reactions. Experientia 27:167

Schneider CH, Gruden E, Wälti M, Toffler O, de Weck AL, Jost R (1979) Monovalent elicitation of passive cutaneous anaphylaxis by N-1-DNCP-6-diaminohexane. Mol Immunol 16:269

Schlumberger HD (1980) Drug-induced pseudo-allergic syndrome as exemplified by acetylsalicylic acid intolerance. In: Dukor P et al. (eds) PAR: Pseudo-allergic reactions, vol 1, Karger, Basel, p 125

Schwarz K, Schwarz-Speck M (1960) Experimentally induced photoallergy to sulfonilamide. Acta Allergol 7:224

Seidl LG, Thornton GF, Smith JW, Cluff LE (1966) Studies on the epidemiology of adverse drug reactions. III. Reactions in patients on a general medical service. Bull Johns Hopkins Hosp 119:299

Sharma OP (1973) Drug-induced pulmonary disease. Ann Intern Med 78:616

Shearer GM (1975) Recognition of chemically modified autologous cells. Importance of the murine major histocompatibility complex. In: Rosenthal A (ed)Immune recognition. Academic Press, New York, p 21

Sheffer AL, Rocklin RE, Goetzl EJ (1975) Immunologic components of hypersensitivity reactions to cromolyn sodium. N Engl J Med 293:1220

Shehadi WH (1975) Adverse rections to intravascularly administered contrast media: a comprehensive study based on a prospective survey. Annu J Roentgenol 124:145

Sheldon JM, Lovell RG, Mathews KP (1967) Drug allergy. In: Sheldon JM, Lvell RG, Mathews KP (eds) A manual of clinically allergy, 2nd edn. Saunders, Philadelphia

Shulman NR (1958) Immunoreactions involving platelets. I. A steric-kinetic model for formation of a complex from a human antibody, quinidine as a hapten, and platelets; and for fixation of complement by the complex. J Exp Med 107:665

Silverberg DS, Kidd EG, Shnilka TK (1970) Gold nephropathy. A clinical and pathological study. Arthritis Rheum 13:812

Simpson DG, Walker JH (1960) Hypersensitivity to para-aminosalicylic acid. AM J Med 29:297

Smith JW, Seidl LG, Cluff LE (1966) Studies on the epidemiology of adverse drug reactions. V. Clinical factors influencing susceptibility. Ann Intern Med 65:629

Snell ES (1972) Hypersensitivity fever. In: Dash CH, Jones HEH (eds) Mechanisms of drug allergy. Williams & Wilkins, Baltimore, p 93

Sobel AT, Branellec AL, Blanc CJ, Lagrue GA (1977) Physicochemical characterization of a vascular permeability factor produced by Con A-stimulated human lymphocytes. J Immunol 119:1230

Solley O, Gleich J, Jordan RE, Schroeter AL (1976) The late phase of the immediate wheal-and-flare skin reaction. Its dependence upon IgE antibodies. J Clin Invest 58:408

Spark RP (1971) Fatal anaphylaxis due to oral penicillin. Clin Pathol 56:407

Spengler H, de Weck AL (1977) Evaluation of genetic control of the immune response to penicillin in man. Monogr Allergy 11:116

Spengler H, de Weck AL, Geczy AF (1974) Studies on the molecular mechanisms of lymphocyte stimulation by penicillin and penicillin derivatives. In: Kissling R (ed) Proceedings 8th leukocyte culture conference. Academic Press, New York, p 501

Spiegelberg HL (1981) Lymphocytes bearing Fc receptor for IgE. Immunol Rev 56:199

Stanworth DR (1980) Oligopeptide-induced release of histamine. In: Dukor P et al. (eds) Pseudo-allergic reactions, vol 1. Karger, Basel, p 56

Stanworth DR, Smith AK (1973) Inhibition of reagin-mediated PCA reactions in baboons by the human IgG4 subclass. Clin Allergy 3:37

Steiner LA, Eisen HN (1966) Variations in the immune response to a simple determinant. Bacteriol Rev 30:383

Stewart GT (1967) Allergenic residues in penicillins. Lancet 1:1177

Stofer AR, Lazary S, de Weck AL (1973) Zur Diagnostik des tödlichen anaphylaktischen Shocks auf Penicillin an der Leiche. Beitr Gerichtl Med 31:270

Symmers WSC (1962) The occurrence of angiitis and of other generalized diseases of connective tissues as a consequence of the administration in drugs. Proc R Soc Med 55:20

Szczeklik A (1977) Prostaglandines et aspirine. Rev Fr Allergol 17:2

Szczeklik A, Gryglewski RJ, Czerniawska-Mysik G (1975) Relationship of inhibition of prostaglandin biosynthesis by analgesics to asthma attacks in aspirin-sensitive patients. Br Med J 1:67

Tan EM (1974) Drug-induced autoimmune disease. Fed Proc 33:1894

Territo MC, Peters RW, Tanaka KR (1973) Autoimmune hemolytic anemia due to levodopa therapy. JAMA 226:1347

Thiel JA, Mitchell S, Parker CW (1964) The specificity of hemagglutination reactions in human and experimental penicillin hypersensitivity. J Allergy Clin Immunol 35:399

Thierfelder S, Eulitz M, Karl ML (1967) Immunologische Studien an einem Pyramidon-Leukozytenantikörper. Klin Wochenschr 45:78

Uehleke H (1962) Biochemische Reaktionen als Ursache erworbener Überempfindlichkeit gegen Fremdstoffe. Z Immunforsch 123:447

Van Arsdel PP Jr (1978) Adverse drug reactions. In: Middleton E Jr, Reed CE, Ellis EF (eds) Allergy: principles and practice, vol 2. Mosby, St. Louis, p 1133

Van Arsdel PP Jr, Franz KB (1963) Nature of antibody in penicillin-induced hemolytic anemia. J Clin Invest 42:988

Van Arsdel PP Jr, Gilliland BC (1965) Anemia secondary to penicillin treatment: Studies on two patients with non allergic serum hemagglutinins. J Lab Clin Med 65:277

Van Toorenenbergen AW, Aalberse RC (1981) IgG4 and passive sensitization of basophil leukocytes. Int Arch Allergy Appl Immunol 65:432

Vervloet D, Arnaud A, Vellieux P, Kaplansky S, Charpin J (1979) Anaphylactic reactions to muscle relaxants under general anesthesia. J Allergy Clin Immunol 63:348

Vesin P, Periac P, Kalifat R, Intrator L, Tulliez M, Cattan D (1976) Lympadenopathie et anomalies protidiques apres traitement par la phenylhydantoine. Nouv Presse Med 5:1125

Voigtländer V, Hänsch GM, Rother U (1980) Effect of aspirin on complement in vivo. Int Arch Allergy Appl Immunol 61:145

Voisin GA, Toullet F (1960) Modifications of capillary permeability in immunological reactions mediated through cells. In: Wolstencroft GEW (ed) Cellular aspects of immunity. Churchill, London, p 373

Von Maur K, Turk A, Stevens MB, Adkinson NF, Lichtenstein LM (1975) Penicillin hypersensitivity in systemic lupus. Int Arch Allergy Appl Immunol 49:428

Wakkers-Garritsen BG, Howerzni J, Nater JP, Wakkers PJM (1976) IgE mediated adverse reactivity to a radiographic contrast medium. Ann Allergy 38:122

Wall J, Fang S, Ingbar S, Braverman L (1977) Studies of lymphocyte transformation to propylthiouracil and methimazole in patients with antithyroid drug-induced agranulocytosis. Clin Res 25:516

Wanamaker WM, Wanamaker SJ, Celesia GG (1976) Thrombocytopenia associated with long term levo-dopa therapy. JAMA 235:2217

Ward AM, Udnoon S, Watkins J (1976) Immunological mechanisms in the pathogenesis of vinyl chloride disease. Br Med J 1:936

Wegmann A, Renker H (1976) Das Elektrokardiogramm im anaphylaktischen Schock des Menschen. Klin Wochenschr 54:453

Weil MH, Shubin H (1974) Anaphylactic shock in man. In: Kolen JN (ed) Critical care medicine handbook. New York, p 396

Weinstein L, Weinstein AJ (1974) The pathophysiology and pathoanatomy of reactions to antimicrobial agents. Adv Intern Med 19:109

Weltman JK, Szaro RP, Settipane GA (1978) An analysis of the role of IgE in intolerance to aspirin and tartrazine. Allergy 34:273

Winterbauer RH, Wilske KR, Wheelis RF (1976) Diffuse pulmonary injury associated with gold treatment. N Engl J Med 294:919

Worlledge SM (1973) Immune hemolytic anemias. Semin Hematol 10:327

Worlledge SM, Carstairs KC, Dacie JV (1966) Autoimmune hemolytic anemia associated with alpha-methyldopa. Lancet 2:135

Yamauchi Y, Litwin A, Adams L, Zimmer H, Hess EV (1975) Induction of antibodies to nuclear antigens in rabbits by immunization with hydralazine-human serum albumin conjugates. J Clin Invest 56:958

Yurchak WM, Wicher K, Arbesman CE (1970) Immunologic studies on aspirin. J Allergy 46:245

Zeek PM (1953) Periarteritis nodosa and other forms of necrotizing angiitis. N Engl J Med 248:764

Zelman S (1959) Liver cell necrosis in chlorpromazine jaundice (allergic cholangiolitis): A serialstudy of twenty six beedle biopsy specimens in nine patients. Am J Med 27:708

Zimmermann HJ (1972) Drug-induced hepatic injury. In: Samter M, Parker CW (eds) International encyclopedia of pharmacology and therapeutics. Section 75: Hypersensitivity to drugs, vol 1. Pergamon Press, Oxford

CHAPTER 4

Cutaneous Manifestations of Drug Allergy

K. H. SCHULZ

Allergic and pseudoallergic reactions can occur in many organs and systems. The skin and adjacent mucosae are commonly the sites of such reactions, and may be the only tissues affected or may be involved as part of a wider systemic reaction. According to BRUINSMA (1972), who evaluated more than 50,000 notifications of adverse drug reactions of every conceivable kind, roughly one quarter of all side effects are associated with skin changes. Most of these were allergic manifestations such as urticarial and maculopapular eruptions.

Clinically and morphologically, drug-induced allergic skin reactions are of enormous diversity. Many of the manifestations and features of other skin diseases can be evoked or mimicked by drugs. Drug eruptions cover a wide range from simple pruritus to generalized exfoliative erythroderma, from erythematous macules to the gravest skin eruptions associated with bulla formation and sometimes ending fatally. The question of whether a given clinical condition could have arisen as a result of drug allergy, and if so which drug is responsible, is one which not infrequently presents the physician with great difficulties.

The principal criteria of drug allergy were summarized by BAER and WITTEN (1961). The following list of characteristic features is based on their work:

1. The manifestations of drug allergy are independent of the chemical and pharmacological properties of the drug.
2. Even small doses can evoke severe reactions, even if they have been well tolerated for a long time previously.
3. The same drug can produce different reactions in the same person at different times; conversely, different drugs can have similar or identical clinical manifestations.
4. There are numerous drugs which can cause allergic skin reactions, although the relative frequency (incidence) varies widely from drug to drug.
5. The opinion that renewed administration of the same or a similar drug will lead to a recurrence does not apply to all clinical forms. A specific drug allergy seldom persists for decades.

The entire range of cutaneous drug reactions can be produced by numerous therapeutic substances. However, it has become evident that certain skin manifestations are most commonly caused by narrowly defined groups of drugs. For example, allergy to penicillin G and related oral penicillins (propicillin, penicillin V, phenethicillin) generally takes the form of urticaria, while ampicillin nearly always produces maculopapular rashes. Drug-induced purpura pigmentosa progressiva is usually due to a bromine-containing hypnotic of the carbamide series, while allergic reactions to phenolphthalein or Diphesatin predominantly take the form of fixed eruptions.

Time relationships are of great importance in the analysis and interpretation of allergic reactions due to drugs (HOIGNÉ et al. 1974; HOIGNÉ 1966; LINDEMAYR 1954, 1959; MAYER 1933). The interval, elapsing from first exposure to the onset of the first symptoms and signs, designated as the incubation period, is extremely variable, but it amounts to at least 1 week, though it may be as long as several years. Sensitization of the body takes place during this time. Of more importance for diagnosis is the interval between the last dose of the drug and the onset of the first signs, an interval known as the reaction time. Its length is largely determined by immunological mechanisms, and is hence related to the clinical manifestations. In the anaphylactic syndrome it is quite short, ranging from a few minutes up to 1 h. The vast majority of cutaneous drug reactions develops within the first 24 h, but considerably longer reaction times, amounting to days or weeks, may be seen in various forms of vasculitis and in the phenomena summarized under the heading of serum sickness.

A. Pathogenesis and Classification

Several workers have attempted to classify allergic drug reactions in terms of their underlying immunological mechanisms. Such a classification presupposes knowledge of their immunopathogenesis, and there are at present very few cutaneous drug reactions for which this is understood (SCHULZ 1972, 1974):

1. Antibody-mediated:
   a) IgE: erythema, urticaria, angioedema, conjunctivitis, mucosal edema asthma
   b) IgG: serum sickness, Arthus reaction, vasculitis, thrombocytopenic purpura.
2. Cell-mediated: contact dermatitis, photoallergy, maculopapular rashes, circumscribed infiltrates following injections.

There are some other phenomena which could possibly be of immunological origin:

1. Fixed eruptions
2. Erythema multiforme; Stevens-Johnson syndrome
3. Erythema nodosum
4. Lyell's syndrome
5. Bullous eruptions
6. Lichenoid eruptions.

There are various conditions which are commonly regarded as allergic, but in fact are not, although they may conform to or resemble genuine allergic manifestations:

1. Anaphylactoid (pseudoallergic) reactions
2. Jarisch-Herxheimer reaction
3. Phototoxic reactions
3. Hemorrhagic necrosis following anticoagulants
5. Acne
6. Hyperpigmentation and depigmentation.

There are certain factors which have been claimed to exert an influence on the development of skin reactions due to drug allergy.

The possibility of hereditary factors has been raised on many occasions. Although animal experiments suggest that such factors do exist, recent research on this subject in man is scanty. All that can be gleaned from the older literature is that the existence of any such influence remains uncertain. It is nevertheless claimed that patients with an atopic predisposition or with the lupus erythematosus diathesis are more prone to drug reactions than normal people.

Some workers have concluded from statistical evidence that the underlying disease affects the incidence of sensitization. In infectious mononucleosis the incidence of eruptions following ampicillin treatment is particularly high, and in salmonellosis ampicillin seems to cause rashes more often than it does in other infections.

The sensitization rate is known to depend on the route of administration of the drug. These correlations have been most closely investigated in the case of penicillin allergy. The highest sensitization rates are produced by local application or by aerosol inhalation: oral administration gives the lowest figures, while the parenteral route – intramuscular or intravenous injection – occupies a place in the middle. There seem also to be differences between long-term continuous dosage and intermittent dosage. It seems probable that similar correlations apply to other drugs, but they are not so well documented.

Dosage appears to have some bearing on the induction of allergy, in that higher doses produce higher rates of skin rahes (BELINSON 1948; COHEN and GLINSKY 1949; LINDEMAYR 1954, 1959).

The chemical properties of the drug molecule are of crucial importance. Although there are many drugs which can produce allergic reactions, clear differences in sensitizing power have become apparent. However, the frequency of skin reactions observed in clinical practice is not necessarily proportional to the sensitizing power of the drug.

I. Anaphylaxis, Urticaria, Angioedema

The anaphylactic syndrome is characterized by the acute onset of skin and mucosal lesions, in severe cases associated with nausea, vomiting, diarrhea, asthma, peripheral vascular collapse, and shock. It nearly always begins in the skin and the adjacent mucosae. The first signs – erythema, urticaria, and angiodema – often make their appearance within a few minutes or usually at most 1 h of administration of the allergen. Signs of conjunctivities, rhinitis, asthma, and gastrointestinal involvement may develop more or less simultaneously. The initial symptoms commonly consist of itching in the palms and soles, the genital area, or the external auditory meatus; tingling in the soft palate; and a sense of oppression in the chest.

The reaction time is short and depends to some extent on the nature of the allergen and the route of administration:

Urticarial reactions are among the commonest cutaneous manifestations of drug allergy. The individual lesions vary in number and size from a single urticarial focus developing at the site of a subcutaneous or intracutaneous injection to a generalized eruption with numerous lesions involving large areas. There is every possible variation between these two extremes. The urticaria is occasionally accompanied by vesicle formation.

Urticarial lesions are caused by the liberation of histamine and other mediators as the result of an IgE-mediated immune reaction which takes place in mast cells. Histamine liberation can also occur without the intervention of an immunological mechanism. Various drugs and other foreign substances are capable, either by the pathway of complement activation or by a direct attack on the mast cells, of liberating histamine and hence producing urticarial lesions. These anaphylactoid manifestations of drug intolerance are clinically indistinguishable from IgE-mediated allergic phenomena. The differential diagnosis can be made only by immunological investigations (demonstration of antibodies), differential skin testing, and oral provocation tests (Schulz 1979).

The course of drug-induced urticaria is acute. In the vast majority of cases the lesions heal within 1–3 days without leaving any residual changes. However, the condition can assume a chronic form and the lesions can recur repeatedly over many weeks. Such events are most commonly observed in penicillin allergy. Small amounts of penicillins can be detected in foodstuffs, especially dairy products, in vaccines, secretions (saliva, semen), and furthermore they are produced by various molds (Hyphomycetes) which are found everywhere in our environment and hence gain entry to our bodies every day (Cole and Robinson 1961; McGovern et al. 1970; Jillson and Porter 1965; Stewart 1965; Un and Valu 1963). However, it is only in a small proportion of patients that the manifestations persist and it may be doubted whether the widespread occurrence of traces of penicillin is enough to explain why some cases of acute penicillin urticaria become chronic.

The causes of anaphylactic reactions include not only drugs of high molecular weight (over 5,000) but also those consisting of small molecules. Drugs known to cause urticaria and anaphylaxis are:
1. High molecular weight:
    Foreign sera
    Insulin
    ACTH and other peptide hormones
    Enzyme preparations
    Allergen extracts used for desensitization.
2. Low molecular weight:
    Penicillins
    Pyrazolone derivatives (propylphenazone, phenazone, metamizol, etc.)
    Sulfonamides
    Salicylic acid derivatives etc.

II. Late Urticarial Reactions

This form of drug-induced urticaria is most commonly due to penicillin. The manifestations do not arise until at least 3–48 h after the dose of penicillin, and in some circumstances not until 3–4 days afterwards. Transitional forms between this condition and serum sickness are not uncommon; clinically, the relationship is attested by the development of joint swellings.

III. Serum Sickness

Allergic reactions due to drugs may present under the guise of serum sickness. Skin eruptions, lymphadenopathy, and joint swellings are the essential symptoms, present in nearly every case, while other manifestations such as high fever, nephritis, vasculitis, gastrointestinal symptoms, pericarditis and myocarditis, polyneuritis, and myelitis are much less frequent. The skin manifestations take the form of urticaria or an urticarial eruption and often begin in the vicinity of the injection, though soon extending and becoming generalized. Besides the urticarial manifestations, morbilliform and scarlatiniform eruptions are also seen. The skin changes can be the only manifestation of serum sickness.

One characteristic feature is the late onset of the symptoms and signs – approximately 8–21 days after administration of the therapeutic substance. If a subsequent dose of the allergen is given the reaction time will be much shorter. In such instances the clinical features tend to resemble those of the anaphylactic syndrome (immune complex anaphylaxis).

The condition is seldom fatal, and as a rule the symptoms and signs regress within 1–3 weeks.

Apart from foreign sera, the commonest cause is penicillin, in particular depot injection preparations. Sulfonamides, insulin, and barbiturates have also been reported (HOIGNÉ 1966; HOIGNÉ and DÖPPEN 1963; HOIGNÉ and KREBS 1964; SCHULZ 1972).

IV. Maculopapular Rashes

Generalized macular or in some cases maculopapular eruptions are among the commonest cutaneous manifestations of drug allergy. In our series of nearly 1,200 patients referred because of suspected drug allergy, such eruptions (285 cases) formed the second largest category, exceeded only by urticarial-anaphylactic reactions. Similar findings have been reported by LINDEMAYR (1954, 1959) from Vienna.

The clinical appearances are often reminiscent of measles, scarlet fever, or rubella and are hence known as morbilliform, scarlatiniform, or rubelliform eruptions. However, the skin manifestations do not always mimic the rashes of virus infections. Usually they are nonspecific, and the terms maculopapular or maculovesicular are more appropriate. The individual lesions range from the size of a lentil to that of a fingernail; they are reddened and slightly raised and may merge into large confluent areas. Vesicles are not uncommon and on the dependent parts of the leg there may be a hemorrhagic component.

Rashes which evolve from contact dermatitis or which arise when patients already sensitized by exogenous contact ingest the allergen or receive it parenterally (hematogenous contact eczema) display special features. There is a dense eruption of papulovesicular lesions side by side with superficial eczematous changes.

Immunologically, maculopapular eruptions are probably due to cell-mediated allergy (MARGHESCU 1978; DE WECK 1974). This hypothesis is based on clinical observations, on the results of skin tests (patch and intracutaneous), and on in vitro investigations carried out by means of the lymphocyte transformation test and the macrophage migration inhibition test (GIRARD 1974; DE WECK 1974, 1979). It must, however, be emphasized that only in a relatively small proportion of patients do these tests give positive results. In the majority of drug eruptions, endeavors to demonstrate an allergic mechanism are unsuccessful. There is some evidence that immune complex reactions may possibly be involved in the pathogenesis.

At present, the ampicillins must be regarded as the commonest cause of drug-induced maculopapular eruptions. Rashes develop in an average of 10% of patients treated with ampicillin. As already mentioned, the underlying disease, and possibly the dose as well, has an unmistakable influence on the frequency of rashes. KENNEDY et al. (1963) found higher incidences in salmonellosis than in other bacterial infections. In infectious mononucleosis the incidence of rashes is said to be 90%–100%.

In more than half the cases the ampicillin eruption appears 8–12 days after starting treatment, though not uncommonly the lesions may arise in the first few days. This observation, together with the fact that the manifestations regress despite continuation of treatment and that in such cases allergological and immunological tests give negative results, has caused doubt to be cast on the allergic origin of the eruptions (PEVNY and RÖCKL 1975; SCHÖPF 1979; WEUTA 1972). Although the arguments advanced against the allergic hypothesis are unconvincing, most workers believe that both nonallergic and allergic ampicillin eruptions may occur. In our experience the allergic forms are more serious and more frequently assume the characteristics of erythema multiforme.

WEBSTER and THOMPSON (1974) have shown that lymphocytes can be stimulated in vitro by polymers of ampicillin and MCKENZIE et al. (1976) have found that patients with infectious mononucleosis have raised levels of IgM and IgG antibodies against ampicillin. These interesting observations may contribute to our understanding of the pathogenesis. The fact that ampicillin possesses sensitizing properties is evident from clinical observations in patients with occupational contact dermatitis. The amino group present in the side chain has been shown to play an essential part in determining specificity (SCHULZ et al. 1970).

Besides ampicillin there are numerous other drugs which cause maculopapular eruptions. The drugs most frequently mentioned are other penicillins, streptomycin, rifampicin, sulfonamides, pyrazolidine derivatives (phenylbutazone), pyrazolones, barbiturates, tricyclic antidepressants, hydantoin derivatives, indomethacin, quinine, and meprobamate (KAUPPINEN 1972; KORTING 1972; LOUIS and SCHULZ 1973; SCHUPPLI 1972; THIERS et al. 1964).

As a rule, the rash clears up within a few days after discontinuation of the drug which provoked it. However, should there be any recurrence, the condition may evolve into a more serious type of cutaneous drug reaction, such as exfoliative dermatitis or even Lyell's syndrome. Maculopapular eruptions seldom persist for long periods, though DUPONT and LACHAPELLE (1964) observed a papular eruption caused by polyvinylpyrrolidone which lasted for 4 years.

V. Erythema Multiforme and Stevens-Johnson Syndrome

Erythema multiforme is clinically a circumscribed and well-defined condition. Its salient and diagnostically most important feature are the iris-like lesions, ranging roughly from the size of a pea to that of a fingernail (elevated patches of erythema with central livid discoloration and vesicle formation). The lesions vary in size, location, and intensity of inflammation, the result being a multiform eruption located mainly on the hands, forearms, feet, and legs. Lesions may also be found on the face, and the mucosae of the mouth and the eyes are not infrequently involved. If the inflammation is very intense, vesicles may appear and vesiculation may be so severe as to dominate the picture. Bullous drug eruptions frequently assume the picture of erythema multiforme. The severest form is the Stevens-Johnson syndrome, in which the patient is febrile and gravely ill. In addition to extensive skin changes spreading outside the areas usually affected, there are widespread erosive lesions on the mucous membranes, including the conjunctivae.

The pathogenesis of erythema multiforme has not been satisfactorily elucidated. Its course and evolution seem to suggest an allergic origin, but the immunological mechanisms are disputed. Some workers regard the condition as the outcome of a cell-mediated immune reaction, but an immune coomplex mechanism seems more probable. It is conceivable that both processes – type III and type IV – may be involved. The immunological investigations so far published are incomplete and do not provide enough evidence for final assessment.

Drug-induced erythema multiforme is histologically and even clinically related to fixed drug eruptions. There also seems to be some relationship to Lyell's syndrome, as transitional cases have been observed (SCHUPPLI 1972).

The etiology is by no means the same in all cases. Erythema multiforme can be caused by various totally unconnected factors. The eruption most commonly arises after infections with herpesviruses or streptococci. In comparison with these, drugs are relatively seldom the cause. However, if drug-induced rashes of erythema multiforme type are included, much larger numbers will be recorded (e.g., ampicillin rashes).

In our own series the drugs most frequently responsible were pyrazolone analgesics and pyrazolidine derivatives (CONE et al. 1954; GELBER 1954; STEEL and MAFFAT 1954). In the 1960s there were reports, first from Australia and subsequently from other countries, claiming an increased incidence of erythema multiforme and Stevens-Johnson syndrome in patients receiving long-term sulfonamides (CLAXTON 1963; COHLAN 1960; PELZ 1962; YAFFEE 1960).

According to WEREIDE (1967) the incidence of sulfonamide-induced Stevens-Johnson syndrome in Norway is one case from two million single doses, i.e., one case from one ton of sulfonamide (HJORTH 1968).

Among other drugs which have been blamed are penicillins, streptomycin, barbiturates, oral antidiabetics, hydantoins, diuretics, quinine, and smallpox vaccine (BETSON and ALFORDT 1961; DUGOIS et al. 1957; LUTZ 1951; SAXL 1972; SCHUPPLI 1972; STREMPEL 1959; TULLETT 1966, VAYRE and COMBEY 1955; WATTS 1962; WORINGER and LEVY 1949; YAFFEE 1959, 1960).

VI. Allergic Vasculitis

Synonyms for allergic vasculitis are vasculitis hyperergica cutis, leukocytoclastic vasculitis, arteriolitis allergica cutis, and necrotizing angiitis.

The various clinical forms of allergic vasculitis are based on immunopathological reactions of type III. This hypothesis is supported by evidence of various kinds.
The Arthus phenomenon, which has been thoroughly studied in experimental animals, displays clinical, histological, immunohistological, and electro-microscopic
analogies. Circulating immune complexes have been detected in experimental animals and in the spontaneous disease in human beings. Furthermore – a point of
greater clinical relevance – they have been demonstrated as deposits in vessel walls
by direct immunofluorescence and by immunoelectron-microscopy (BRAUERMANN
and YEN 1975; GOWER et al. 1976; HOLUBAR et al. 1975; SCHERER 1979; WOLFF et
al. 1978).

In the present state of our knowledge the most plausible view of the pathogenesis of allergic vasculitis is derived from the fact that free antigen is present in the
circulating blood as well as antigen-antibody complexes. This free antigen reacts
with specific IgE antibodies on the cell membrane of basophil leucocytes. This results in liberation of histamine together with a platelet-agglutinating agent and
other factors. The histamine-induced increase in vascular permeability facilitates
the passage of immune complexes from the blood into the vessel wall, where activation of the complement system by various pathways ultimately leads to the picture of granulocytic-leucocytoclastic vasculitis associated with necrosis of the tissues (SCHERER and WOLFF 1979). Clinically, three principal types can be distinguished, though various combined forms occur.

The hemorrhagic type is the commonest and conforms to the classical picture
of Schönlein-Henoch purpura. The main feature of the condition are petechial
haemorrhages, ranging from pinhead- to coin-size and appearing preferentially
on dependent parts of the body. Urticarial lesions may accompany the purpura.
In severe cases there are also vesicular, bullous, and ulcerating lesions.

In the rarer papulonecrotic type the predominant feature are inflammatory
nodules which have central necrosis and leave depressed scars when they finally
heal.

The third variant is characterized by urticarial, papulohemorrhagic, and nodular lesions in conjunction.

The manifestations of allergic vasculitis are not confined to the skin. The kidneys, lungs, gastrointestinal tract, joints, and even the central nervous system may
be involved. The prognosis depends entirely on the extent of the changes affecting
the internal organs. McCOOMBS (1965) found arthralgia, hematuria, or gastrointestinal or central nervous manifestations in 30 of 72 patients.

Allergic vasculitis is one of those diseases in which drugs, though playing a certain part in the etiology, are of relatively small importance among the numerous
other etiological factors. In our own series of 78 patients, evaluated by SCHWIEBERT
(1967), a drug was found to be the allergen responsible in only three cases: 38 cases
were due to various infections or neoplasms, while in the other 37 cases the etiology
remained unknown.

In their review, SCHERER and WOLFF (1979) list various groups of drugs which
have been recognized as causes. The list includes insulin, penicillins, hydantoins,
phenothiazines, sulfonamides, phenobutazone, and quinine (PASCHOUD 1966).

Conventional diagnostic methods such as skin tests and in vitro testing seldom
reveal the cause. The history often fails to advance matters any further and the only

convincing proof can be obtained by a provocative test with the drugs under suspicion. However, for ethical reasons this is not always justifiable. Attempts to ascertain the cause are often unsuccessful.

VII. Erythema Nodosum

Erythema nodosum presents a typical clinical picture. There are multiple tender subcutaneous nodules of inflammatory nature mainly on the lower parts of the legs and occasionally in other sites such as the arms, the trunk, or the external ear. Fever, leukocytosis, and a rise in ESR accompany the acute skin lesions, which usually subside within 2–3 weeks, although they may recur and may become chronic.

The histological picture is characterized by inflammation localized in the connective tissue of the subcutis. Initially there is infiltration by granulocytes together with fibrin deposition and erythrocyte diapedesis; later there are granulomatous lesions (MIESCHER 1947).

It is generally accepted that erythema nodosum is of allergic origin, but the immunological mechanism is not understood. Among the possibilites suggested are reactions of the Arthus type, the cellular type (type IV), or mixed forms of the two (HAUSTEIN and KLUG 1977).

Etiologically, infections of various kinds are undoubtedly the major factors. Drugs are only occasionally responsible, but among them there are certain sulfonamides which play a part in the etiology. LOVEMAN and SIMON, as long ago as 1940, described the occurrence of erythema nodosum after administration of sulfanilamide, and after the introduction of sulfathiazole similar cases were seen in larger numbers. When this sulfonamide was withdrawn from the market the number of cases of drug-induced erythema nodosum decreased. The drugs most commonly responsible today are oral contraceptives, penicillins, aspirin, trimethoprim-sulfamethoxazole, and iodide (MARGHESCU 1978; PEVNY and RÖCKL 1975; RÖCKL et al. 1979; RÖCKL and METZ 1973).

The incidence of sulfathiazole-induced erythema nodosum varies and depends on the underlying disease which is being treated (SIMPSON 1950). Such cases were most commonly seen in association with tuberculosis (105 of 231 cases) (ROLLOF 1950) and lymphogranuloma inguinale (37 of 504 cases), and least commonly in association with gonorrhoea (1 of 1,500 cases). The allergen is difficult to identify. As a rule, skin tests are not sufficiently reliable, so that the only remaining method is the provocation test, which does not always give clear-cut results.

VIII. Purpura

In general, there are three different forms of purpura which may be seen in connexion with drug allergy:
1. Allergic vasculitis presenting as purpura
2. Thrombocytopenic purpura
3. Purpura pigmentosa progressiva (chronic pigment purpura).

The form of purpura noted under the first heading is dealt with in the section on allergic vasculitis. Drug-induced thrombocytopenic purpure is of allergic nature: antibodies can be demonstrated, the specificity of the reaction is undoubted, and the manifestations are independent of the nature and pharmacological effect of the drug which causes them.

The manifestations vary in severity and almost any organ may be affected by the hemorrhages. There is an ever-present danger of cerebral involvement. The skin is nearly always affected. The lesions appear suddenly in crops of punctate to lentil-sized petechiae, sometimes merging into larger confluent hemorrhagic patches. In contrast to Schönlein-Henoch purpura, they are not elevated above the level of the skin. Histologically, there is merely extravasation of erythrocytes without inflammatory changes.

The immunology of allergic thrombocytopenia will not be discussed in detail here, as it is dealt with elsewhere in the book (see also P. MIESCHER 1961).

Many drugs have been listed as causing allergic thrombocytopenia. The most notorious was Sedormid, withdrawn from the market long ago. Other drugs on the list include quinine, quinidine, phenylbutazone, hydantoins, and sulfonamides (for further details see DISCOMBE 1972; KARPATKIN 1971; MIESCHER 1961b; McVIE 1973).

Attempts to establish the cause should as far as possible be carried out in vitro. Trial exposure to drugs on which the patient's history casts suspicion may lead to serious hemorrhages. If a provocation test is essential, the amount of drug administered should be very small, far below the normal dose.

IX. Purpura Pigmentosa Progressiva

This term denotes a clinically and histologically well-defined form of purpura, the manifestations of which are almost entirely confined to the skin. Drugs play by far the major role in its etiology. Cases of this kind were first described by LOEB (1921) and subsequently in greater detail by MULZER and HABERMANN (1930). Even in those early days they were linked with bromine-containing carbamide hypnotics (carbromal, bromural). However, it is only in the last two decades that cases have been seen in larger numbers and the etiological correlations have become more widely known.

Clinically, the condition is characterized by a combination of minute punctate hemorrhages, resembling fleabites, with diffuse, yellow to brown hemosiderin pigmentation and dermatitis of variable intensity. Lichenoid changes may ensue. Itching is nearly always present. The lesions usually begin on the legs and dorsa of the feet and spread upwards over the thighs, buttocks, and large areas of the trunk; the arms and hands are less frequently involved and the face nearly always remains unaffected.

The histological changes extend to the outer layers of the dermis and the epidermis. In addition to extravasation of erythrocytes and deposition of hemosiderin, there is perivascular infiltration by lymphocytes and histiocytes, among which eosinophils and granulocytes are very scanty. The main feature of the epidermal changes is focal spongiosis with some tendency to immigration by mononuclear cells. ILLIG and KALKOFF (1970) described characteristic appearances on capillary microscopy.

The hypothesis that an immune mechanism is concerned in the pathogenesis of the disease did not gain general acceptance for some time. The revival of interest in carbromal (Adalin) purpura, first described some decades earlier, investigation of "textile purpura" (BATSCHUAROV and MINKOW 1968; CALNAN 1971), and the observation that the manifestations could be induced by inhalation of house dust mite antigen (HEPPLE and MACMILLAN 1973) furnished a variety of evidence which supported this view.

Between 1950 and 1970 there was a sharp increase in the consumption of carbromal and similar brominated urea derivatives in the German Federal Republic and presumably in other European countries also. The drugs were used chiefly as hypnotics and sedatives but were also included in remedies for pain, cough, and influenza. Before long they became available without prescription. The rise in consumption was followed by an increase in carbromal purpura (KRUIZINGA 1950; VELTMAN 1959). By means of the patch test (not the intracutaneous test), and more successfully with the aid of oral provocation tests, SCHULZ (1964, 1967, 1974) and VAN KETEL (1967) showed that allergic and immunological mechanisms are important in the genesis of this form of purpura. The macroscopic and microscopic appearances of the patch test reactions point to a reaction of cellular type (ILLIG and KALKOFF 1970; ILLIG 1976; SCHULZ 1964, 1974).

It was at one time believed that the platelet system was not involved and that the lesions were due to vascular damage alone, but in the light of more recent investigations this view can no longer be maintained. TRONNIER (1967) and PETTER and PERLICK (1969) found abnormalities of the coagulation system in some cases. In collaboration with TILSNER (personal communication) we carried out investigations in several patients. These showed some decrease in platelet aggregation and spreading, together with antiplatelet antibodies with specificities directed against carbromal, bromural, and related substances.

To which part of the molecular structure is the reactivity linked? This question has not yet been solved. Though we were unsuccessful in provoking purpura by giving 200 mg sodium bromide to 20 patients, GOERZ et al. (1974) saw fresh petechiae in six patients after oral administration of 20 ml of a 1% solution.

Of the drugs which cause this form of purpura, the brominated carbamides are undoubtedly the most important. When they were put on the "prescription only" list their consumption in the German Federal Republic declined and with it the incidence of carbromal rashes. However, the fact that other drugs can cause the eruption has been proved by a number of well documented cases (ILLIG 1976). In our experience, the drugs most frequently involved, other than carbromal, are benzodiazepines, other tranquillizers, and hypnotics.

Up to the present time in vitro testing has proved unsuccessful. It is therefore necessary to employ in vivo methods such as patch testing or oral provocation doses. The results which can be achieved by these methods are shown in Tables 1 and 2.

X. Fixed Eruptions

Although described more than 90 years ago, fixed drug eruptions are little known outside the world of dermatology. Whereas other allergic drug rashes exhibit a

Table 1. Results of patch tests in carbromal purpura. (From SCHULZ 1974)

Substance	Concentration in ethanol (%)	No. of cases	Results	
			Positive	Negative
Carbromal (Adalin)	2.5	93	19 (20%)	74
Bromvalurea (Bromural)	2.5	88	26 (29%)	62
Meprobamate	5	73	0	73
Sodium bromide	5	50	0	50

Table 2. Results of oral provocation tests in carbromal purpura. (From SCHULZ 1974)

Substance	Dose (mg)	No. of cases	Result	
			Positive	Negative
Carbromal (Adalin)	50–200	76	73	3
Bromvalurea (Bromural)	50–200	52	50	2
Acetylcarbromal (Abasin)	100–200	15	13	2
Meprobamate	100–200	20	2	18
Sodium bromide	200	20	0	20

huge variety of forms, this is not true of fixed eruptions. In the average case the picture is uniform almost to the point of monotony, and the diagnosis is easily made provided that the possibility of fixed eruptions is not forgotten. The picture consists of erythematous lesions – either a single patch or a small number of adjacent patches – in shape round or oval and in size from that of a coin to that of the palm of a child's hand. At first pale red, later they assume a more livid tone. Vesicle formation and hemorrhage within the lesions are relatively frequent. A gray-brown pigmented spot remains after healing, and may often persist for months or years (BURCKHARDT 1962; KLEINE-NATROP 1966). As regards location, there seems to be some preference for the hands, feet, and genital area, though any part of the skin and the adjacent mucosae (in particular the mouth) can be affected. There are less typical variants forming morphological transitions between this and other rashes such as generalized superficial eruption or drug-induced erythema multiforme. A painful burning sensation is often experienced, and can be very distressing when the lesions involve mucous membranes, the lips, or the genital area.

The essential characteristic of the disease is that on renewed exposure to the allergen the rash reappears at the same sites as before, though usually the number of lesions increases with each recurrence.

The pathogenesis is still in many respects obscure. In view of the specificity of the factors which induce the reaction, the very small doses required, and the results of skin testing, an allergic mechanism has been postulated. In the 1930s attempts were made to throw light on the pathogenesis of the condition by means of autologous and isologous transplantation experiments. NAEGELI et al. (1930) and URBACH et al. (1930) found that a piece of skin which was transplanted from a lesion to a healthy area retained its reactive capacity, while conversely a healthy piece of skin transplanted into a lesion remained nonreactive. However, these findings were not confirmed by other workers. They are refuted by the results obtained by WISE and SULZBERGER (1933), LOVEMAN (1934) and KNOWLES et al. (1936), who showed that the possibility of inducing the reaction in the transplanted skin is dependent on the lapse of time. When skin was transplanted from an affected into an unaffected area it remained at first capable of reacting, but lost its reactivity within a few weeks or months. Conversely, a piece of normal skin transplanted into a previously affected area acquired within a few weeks the capacity of reacting to a renewed dose of the allergen in the same way as the skin surrounding it. These findings, together with the fact that a positive patch test which is sometimes obtainable only within the lesion and not in normal areas of skin, underline the special peculiarities of this condition. Even if we postulate that there are fixed antibodies in the affected area, the question how they were directed to that area remains unanswered. The unique feature of fixed eruptions is that the state of sensitization is restricted to clearly demarcated areas while the major proportion of the skin remains uninvolved.

The causes of fixed eruptions are manifold. Drugs come first, but foodstuffs, spices and alcoholic drinks have also been mentioned. Compilations by ENGELHARDT (1960), WELSH (1961 a, b) and KLEINE-NATROP (1966), who reviewed the older literature, list more than 60 different drugs. In terms of frequency the following head the list:

Pyrazolones   Tetracyclines
Barbiturates   Benzodiazepines
Sulfonamides   Phenolphthalein (purgative)

SCHUPPLI (1972) added the following drugs:
Meprobamate   Ethchlorvynol
Digitalis   Triaziquone (Trenimon)
Dimenhydrinate (Dramamine)

In our own series of patients, which has been reviewed by LOUIS (1972), the drugs responsible were pyrazolone analgesics in 22 cases, barbiturates in 19, sulfonamides in five, phenolphthalein in three, tetracyclines in two, benzodiazepines in two, and a hydantoin derivative in one case. Other causes of fixed eruptions have been observed by LOVEMAN (1943), BREHM and BREHM (1963), and POST and DOUGHERTY (1964).

In fixed eruptions the specificity of the reaction is extremely pronounced. Allergic cross-reactions to chemically related compounds are less common than in other forms of drug allergy such as contact dermatitis. KENNEDY et al. (1957) found that five of their patients reacted solely to aminophenazone and not to closely related pyrazolones. In a case of barbiturate allergy we showed that reactions could be induced only by barbiturates with an aromatic side chain, namely phenobarbital and methylphenobarbital, not by barbiturates with an aliphatic side chain, such as barbital, diallylbarbituric acid, allylisobutyl barbituric acid, methylcyclohexenyl barbituric acid, and allylmethylpropyl thiobarbituric acid. In many instances the degree of hypersensitivity is remarkably high and minute amounts are sufficient to provoke recurrences, as in the following example:

A 52-year-old doctor developed a fixed eruption after taking an analgesic. There were typical lesions on the back, buttocks, arms, and legs. After recovery, wishing to ascertain the cause, he himself applied patch tests in the neighborhood of the healed lesions. Tests were carried out with caffeine, phenobarbital, and aminophenazone in sequence. Within 8–24 h after applying 0.1 ml 1% aminophenazone solution there was a severe relapse. The old lesions flared up again and new lesions appeared on the back and limbs. The small amount absorbed through the skin from a 1% solution was sufficient to induce an extensive recurrence.

A special feature of the fixed eruption is shown by certain observations of double or triple sensitization at separate sites of the skin. In a large series comprising 484 cases, Furuya et al. (1966) found double sensitization to barbital and amidopyrine in two patients, and in another sulfadiazine and phenobarbital were the causes. In a female patient investigated in collaboration with P. Schmidt (Schulz and Schmidt 1967) fixed eruptions appeared consecutively at different sites. Some of the lesions were induced by barbiturates (right hand), while a second group was due to aminophenazone (left forearm) and another lesion (on the back) was provoked by phenolphthalein. Similar phenomena have been described by Sulz-berger (1940).

Identification of the cause depends entirely on in vivo methods. All the in vitro techniques tried in this condition have given disappointing and unreliable results. The most useful methods are epicutaneous and provocation tests by oral adminis-tration. A patch test with the drug responsible can sometimes provoke the skin lesions, but only when the patch is applied at the site of the healed lesion (in-trafocal patch test) (Apolant 1898; Engelhardt 1960, Kennedy et al. 1957; Louis 1972; Schulz 1979; Welsh 1961 a, b). As Louis has shown, the results of these tests differ between one drug and another. For example, barbituric acid de-rivatives more frequently yield positive tests than pyrazolones. On healthy skin the test invariably gives negative results. Administration of an oral test dose is the most reliable method. The risk involved is minimal, especially as the manifestations are confined to the skin and the mucosae.

XI. Lyell's Syndrome (Toxic Epidermal Necrolysis)

Among the serious drug reactions involving the skin is the syndrome of toxic epidermal necrolysis described by Lyell (1956) and nowadays often known as Lyell's syndrome. The syndrome is now divided into two forms: one due to drugs and one caused by staphylococci. It is doubtful whether this covers all the possible etiological factors, as a considerable proportion of the published cases have been of unknown cause.

The illness begins with nonspecific prodromal symptoms such as prostration, pyrexia, headache, pains in the limbs, and sore throat, the picture resembling that of influenza. Skin manifestations develop after a few hours or days, the first sign being an eruption accompanied by a burning sensation. The eruption quickly spreads over large areas of the skin. It usually presents a macular appearance, the macules tending to coalesce into larger areas, but not infrequently it displays features resembling those of erythema multiforme. This is very soon followed by detachment of the epidermis and formation of large bullae in areas already in-volved by the eruption – the pathognomonic feature of the disease. Nikolsky's sign

Table 3. Internal manifestations in Lyell's syndrome. (From GOERZ and RUZICKA 1978)

Site	Manifestations
Systemic	Hyperthermia, electrolyte and fluid depletion, secondary infection leading to septicemia
Cardiovascular system	Low blood pressure, tachycardia, collapse, shock, toxic myocardial damage
Lungs	Bronchitis, pneumonia, pulmonary edema
Gastrointestinal tract	Ulceration, hemorrhage
Liver	Hepatocellular damage, cholestasis, jaundice, rises in LDH and transaminases
Kidneys	Nephritis, pyelonephritis, possibly renal failure
Central nervous system	Clouding of consciousness, agitation, confusion, convulsions, meningism
Blood	Hemorrhagic tendency, anemia

is easily demonstrated at this stage. The outer coverings of the bullae soon rupture and are left clinging to the underlying tissues like wet rags. The resulting picture resembles that of a second-degree burn or scald. High fever, burning pain, and grave deterioration of general condition accompany the skin lesions.

In serious cases, especially those due to drugs, the mucosae of the mouth, nose, or more rarely the vagina may be involved. At these sites there are erosions, and encrusted lesions. Even the eyes are not spared: conjunctivitis and subsequently corneal ulceration and clouding, pannus formation, and scarring with consequent restriction of the movements of the balls are the commonest features.

In such a severe disease it is not surprising that certain internal organs should be involved. The cardiovascular and respiratory system, gastrointestinal tract, liver, and kidneys are frequently affected. The internal manifestations most commonly observed are listed in Table 3.

Laboratory investigation fails to reveal any specific changes. In the peripheral blood there is commonly leukocytosis with a shift to the left, though there may occasionally be leukopenia. Anemia not infrequently develops during the course of the disease. There may be coagulation abnormalities with a hemorrhagic tendency, disturbances of electrolyte and water balance, and a decrease in serum albumin with elevation of alpha globulins; a fall in gamma globulin is less frequent.

The histological and electron-microscopic findings of Lyell's syndrome are highly characteristic and serve to differentiate it from other bullous skin reactions such as Stevens-Johnson syndrome and erythema multiforme (BRAUN-FALCO and BANDMANN 1970).

The hypothesis that drugs are of etiological significance in a proportion of cases of Lyell's syndrome was at first based solely on statements made by numerous patients to the effect that they had taken drugs before the first manifestation appeared. GOERZ and RUZICKA (1978) give a long list of various drugs and chemicals compiled from patient's histories. The most common, in order of frequency, were as follows:

Sulfonamides	Barbiturates
Pyrazolones and Pyrazolidines (phenylbutazone)	Salicylic acid derivatives
Penicillins	Hydantoins.

Analgesics – pyrazolones, pyrazolidines, salicylates, and derivatives – form the largest group. One remarkable feature is the large contribution made by sulfonamides, among which sulfamethoxypyridazine appears with exceptional frequency. The drugs listed under this heading are also among the most frequent causes of other forms of allergic drug reactions, as are penicillins and the analgesics of the pyrazolone and pyrazolidine groups.

The mere fact that a drug has been administered before the onset of the illness is not enough to prove that it is the cause. To obtain adequate evidence against a given drug it is necessary to show that the eruption will recur after administration of the same compound or one closely related to it.

Allergological provocation tests on patients are seldom undertaken, with good reason. However, it has become apparent that of all test procedures the patch test is the one which carries the lowest risk. In our experience, complications can be largely avoided if this test is performed sequentially with graded concentrations of the drug. Working this way, we obtained positive results in four patients (one to phenytoin, one to phenylbutazone, one to pyrazolone, and one to neomycin). The reaction to testing was similar to that seen in acute contact dermatitis. Other workers (STÜTTGEN 1973; TRITSCH et al. 1969) have employed scratch tests, intracutaneous tests, and ophthalmic tests in individual patients, but these appear to give less satisfactory results.

The in vitro methods recommended for the diagnosis of drug allergy have as yet seldom been applied in Lyell's syndrome. Specific stimulation has been demonstrated in the lymphocyte transformation test in a few cases, but only when the test was carried out within a few weeks of recovery (SCHÖPF et al. 1975).

The pathogenesis of drug-induced Lyell's syndrome has not yet been satisfactorily explained. There are various hypotheses, not all of which can be cited here. The view that immunological mechanisms are involved is supported by the results of the allergological studies described above. Immunological studies have given contradictory results. Whereas some workers have found deposits of immunoglobulins and complement in the basal cell layer of the epidermis (STEIN et al. 1972), others have been unable to confirm this finding (MISGELD 1974; STÜTTGEN 1973). We still do not understand how the immunological phenomena evolve, and we do not know whether other, nonimmunological factors are also involved. It has been postulated that there are several mechanisms operating simultaneously or consecutively, or that virus infections are combined with the sensitization process to drugs. Other workers take the view that an immunological mechanism has not been proved and regard the liberation of lysosomal enzymes as being the crucial event in the pathogenesis of the syndrome (MISGELD 1974; SCHUPPLI 1967).

The distinction between drug-induced and staphylococcal Lyell's syndrome is important for prognosis and therapy. The following criteria are helpful in distinguishing the two forms:

1. Isolation of staphylococci of phage group 2 from material from the nose, throat, ears, conjunctivae, vagina, and infected skin lesions

2. Credible evidence of drug allergy from the patient's history, together with escalation of the symptoms after further administration of the allergen
3. The patient's age
4. The histological findings, including the Tzanck test
5. The clinical picture and ultimate outcome.

Lyell's syndrome due to staphylococci occurs mainly in childhood, this form
being very seldom encountered in adults. Nevertheless, drug-induced cases may occur in children.

The prognosis depends on several factors, among them the patient's age, the
extent of the skin lesions, the existence of concurrent diseases, and the occurrence
of complications, all of which influence the course of the disease and hence the
prognosis. Localized lesions have a more favorable prognosis than the generalized
condition. The mortality of the generalized, drug-induced form is high; in adults
approximately 30%.

XII. Drug-Induced Lupus Erythematosus

The main features of systemic lupus erythematosus (LE) are arthritis, fever, skin
lesions, lymphadenopathy, pleuritis, pericarditis, myalgia, hepatosplenomegaly,
leukopenia, thrombocytopenia, raised ESR, and antibodies against DNA and
other nuclear material. All these can be evoked by drugs. The skin manifestations,
in the form of livid red inflammatory infiltrates with a tendency to hemorrhages,
usually appear first on areas of the face exposed to light, but may extent to parts
covered by clothing.

There are certain differences between drug-induced and spontaneously occurring LE. According to ALARCÓN-SEGOVIA (1969) the drug-induced form runs a milder course than spontaneous systemic LE; in most cases the changes prove reversible when the drug is discontinued, and renal involvement is relatively uncommon.

The first sporadic reports of drug-induced lupus syndrome (GOLD 1951; MIES-
CHER and DELACRÉTAZ 1953; WALSH and ZIMMERMAN 1953) appeared not long after the discovery of the LE cell phenomenon by HARGRAVES et al. (1948). Hydralazine was the first drug to be linked with an increased incidence of LE syndrome (ALARCÓN-SEGOVIA 1969; ALARCÓN-SEGOVIA et al. 1965, 1967; MORROW et
al. 1953), but it soon became apparent that other drugs produced the same effect.
The principal drugs liable to induce LE are isoniazid, procainamide, and certain
anticonvulsants such as mephenytoin, phenytoin, trimethadione, and primidone
(ALARCÓN-SEGOVIA 1969; LEE et al. 1966). In a relatively high percentage of
patients these drugs evoke anti-DNA antibodies without demonstrable clinical
signs of LE: hydralazine in 15%–20%, isoniazid in 20%, and procainamide in
50%–60% (LADD 1962; SIEGEL et al. 1967). ALARCÓN-SEGOVIA (1969) mentions in
his review article various other drugs which have been linked with the LE syndrome:

Penicillin	Phenylbutazone	Oral contraceptives
Sulfonamides	Methylthiouracil	Penicillamine (HARPEY et al. 1972)
Tetracyclines	Propylmethylthiouracil	Practolol (ALARĆON-SEGOVIA et
p-Aminosalicylic acid	Reserpine	al. 1969; RAFTERY and DERN-
Griseofulvin	Methyldopa	MAN 1973)

A few years ago MAAS and SCHUBOTHE (1973) and MAAS et al. (1974, 1975) described a syndrome clinically resembling LE in which antimitochondrial antibodies were present, but not antinuclear antibodies. Skin manifestations were, however, absent. Not long afterwards it was pointed out that in many of these cases of "pseudo-LE syndrome" there was probably a link with the substance Venopyronum (intended for diseases of veins and containing 1,4-diphenyl-3,5-dioxo-pyrazolidine together with certain plant extracts). The reported data show that the patients involved had been taking this product for several months or years (MAAS and SCHUBOTHE 1973; MAAS et al. 1974, 1975; MÜLLER-SCHOOP et al. 1975; SCHWARZ and JOST 1975).

Antibodies directed against the drug appear to play no part in the pathogenesis of drug-induced LE. Though it is true that drug-specific antibodies have been found in the serum in occasional cases of hydralazine-induced LE (HEINE and FRIEDMAN 1962), the existence of an antibody does not necessarily mean that it is responsible for the symptoms and signs. The drug which induces the syndrome does not act through a direct antigen-antibody mechanism, and the LE syndrome cannot be regarded as a phenomenon of drug allergy. From the results of various in vitro and in vivo experiments (ALARCÓN-SEGOVIA 1969; BLOMGREN and VAUGHAN 1968; CANNAT and SELIGMANN 1966, 1968) it seems reasonable to assume that the drugs stimulate the formation of antibodies directed against nuclear proteins, DNA, and other antigens present in the cell nucleus. Hydralazine, isoniazid, and other drugs are capable of reacting with nucleoproteins and modifying their molecular structure in ways still unknown, with the result that these nucleoproteins can assume the function of antigens (ACKROYD 1975). However, this hypothesis does not explain why only a proportion of patients exposed to the drug produce antinuclear antibodies. The cooperation of certain genetic factors is probably necessary ("lupus diathesis", "pharmacogenetic constellation"). Correlations have been found between the formation of antinuclear factors and the acetylation rate, while some workers have postulated a genetic polymorphism (LAPPAT and CAWEIN 1968; PERRY 1967, 1973).

As drug-induced LE is not a genuine allergic condition, it will be apparent that conventional methods of identifying the cause, such as skin tests and detection of antibodies, are of no value. The cause of the condition can be ascertained only by analyzing the patient's history and the course of the disease.

XIII. Allergic and Photoallergic Contact Dermatitis

Allergic contact dermatitis is one of the commonest allergic skin diseases caused by drugs. The main causes are attributed to the group of antibiotics, chemotherapeutics, local analgetics, antirheumatics, antimycotics, disinfectants, antihistaminics, as well as ingredients of the vehicles (preservatives, antioxidants, and others). Further details will be found elsewhere in this book (Chap. 13).

Photoallergic reactions are far less common. They occur after external application or internal administration of photosensitizing drugs, combined with exposure to sunlight. In such circumstances internal administration tends to produce a more exanthematous type of eruption, while external application leads to eczematous manifestations. Transitional cases between the two forms may be encountered.

Table 4. Drugs with photosensitizing effects: reports in the literature

Drugs	Authors
Sulfonamides	BRAUN-FALCO and GEISLER (1962), BURCKHARDT (1962), IPPEN (1967, 1976), ROTHENSTEIN et al. (1966)
Oral antidiabetics	BURCKHARDT (1962), JUNG (1972)
Diuretics (hydrochlorothiazide, furosemide)	BURCKHARDT and SUTTER (1963)
Phenothiazines	BARSA and SAUNDERS (1966), GOODMAN and CAHN (1969), IPPEN (1967, 1976), SCHULZ et al. (1956), STEVANOVIĆ (1961)
Antihistamines (diphenhydramine, carbinoxamine)	SCHREIBER and NAYLOR (1962)
Halogenated salicylanilides	HARBER et al. (1966)
Buclosamide (Jadit)	JUNG (1972)
Isatin derivatives	JUNG (1972)
Cyclamate, Saccharin	JUNG (1972)
Griseofulvin	
Some antirheumatics (Benoxaprafen, Carprofen)	
Sunscreens (p-aminobenzoic acid and derivatives; benzophenones)	HÖLZLE and PLEWIG (1982)
Nalidixic acid	FITZPATRICK et al. (1979)
Stilbenes; optical brighteners	

As regards pathogenesis, there is a close relationship with allergic contact dermatitis. The special characteristics of photoallergy depend on the formation of the antigen. A prohapten can be converted into a hapten capable of conjugation only when light energy is put into the system (oxidation, formation of reactive radicals). As soon as the antigen has been formed further events follow the same pathogenesis as in allergic contact dermatitis or other exanthematous type IV reactions. Investigations by various workers have shown that photoallergy in experimental animals can be transferred passively by means of lymphoid cells. Photochemically produced hapten-protein complexes are capable of specific stimulation of lymphocytes in vitro (see Chap. 7).

Some 40 years have passed since BURCKHARDT (1941) and EPSTEIN (1939) independently reported cases of light-dependent sensitization of the skin to sulfonamides. Since that time there has been a considerable increase in the number of substances known to cause light sensitization. However, the spectrum of photosensitizers varies from time to time; many drugs are swiftly withdrawn from the market as soon as this drawback is discovered.

The most important drugs with sensitizing effects are listed in Table 4. Tetracyclines, in particular demethylchlortetracycline, are commonly responsible for photodermatitis. However, this action does not have any immunological basis, but depends on a phototoxic effect (HARBER et al. 1961; MAIBACH et al. 1967), similar to that produced by psoralens, certain dyes, cadmium sulphide, etc.

The best method for demonstrating photoallergy is the photopatch test, which must be carried out with special care and the use of a light source rich in ultraviolet rays. As a rule, photoallergy subsides once the provoking substance has been eliminated. However, in 10%–20% of patients light sensitivity may persist for long periods after the substances which originally provoked it has been withdrawn. We do not fully understand the mechanism behind this so-called persistent light reaction. If photoallergic dermatitis persists for a long time it may evolve into actinic reticuloid, the clinical features of which are massive lichenification and infiltration of the skin mainly in areas exposed to light.

B. Diagnosis of Allergic Drug Reactions Involving the Skin

A range of tests, some long established, others developed only in the last 10–15 years, is available for the diagnosis of drug allergy. However, a universally applicable, reliable, adequately sensitive method, capable of detecting all allergic reactions, has yet to be discovered. In view of the complexity of the potential reactions and the large number of antigens, it is indeed very doubtful whether any such method will be developed in the foreseeable future.

Techniques available for the diagnosis of drug eruptions are unsatisfactory, but it would be unduly pessimistic to dismiss all such attempts as being necessarily fruitless. Deployed in isolation the various methods may indeed be of little value, but by using several tests in conjunction allergy can often be demonstrated.

Current methods can be classified into those performed in vivo and those carried out in vitro with material from the patient:

In vivo:
    Patch test
    Cutaneous tests (prick, scratch,
      intracutaneous)
    Provocation tests (exposure)

In vitro:
    RAST (radioallergosorbent test) or
      enzyme assay (IgE, IgG)
    Histamine liberation from
      granulocytes
    Basophil degranulation test
    Passive hemagglutination
    Lymphocyte transformation test
    Macrophage inhibition test
    Rosette test

Patch testing calls for certain comments. Its main sphere lies in contact dermatitis, a matter which need not be dealt with here. However, this easily managed test has wider indications and can be useful in the elucidation of many eruptions, in particular type IV reactions. In approximately one-third of his cases of maculopapular eruptions, GIRARD (1972, 1974) found positive tests for antibiotics, local anesthetics, sulfonamides, phenylbutazone, phenothiazines, and even aspirin. In our own experience, which is roughly in accordance with GIRARD's, the results depend largely on the nature of the drug and that of the predominant skin reaction. Positive results will be obtained in a certain percentage of cases of carbromal-induced pigment purpura, Lyell's syndrome, and fixed eruptions.

Intracutaneous tests, scratch tests, and prick tests can be performed with the drugs as such or with their conjugates, for example penicilloyl-polylysine. Type I reactions are the main field of usefulness, but the tests are also suitable for demonstrating late reactions (type IV). The tests seldom give positive results in immune complex reactions, e.g., allergic vasculitis.

The cutaneous tests are most reliable in cases of allergy to high-molecular-weight allergens, such as insulin and other proteohormones, and to products consisting of proteins or polysaccharides. When dealing with reactions to low-molecular-weight drugs, the results are not so convincing. Experience gained in the investigation of penicillin allergy shows that the yield of positive tests can be enhanced by using conjugates. It is regrettable that conjugates such as penicilloyl-polylysine are not yet available for the diagnosis of other drug allergies, but even the use of the unmodified drug may be valuable. The planning of the investigation is of great importance. The yield of positive tests is highest when the investigation is undertaken not less than 1 week and not more than 2–3 months after the acute episode.

Deliberate provocation of the pathological manifestations by exposure to a small dose of the drug must still be regarded as the most reliable evidence of a drug allergy. However, it must always be remembered that each fresh exposure carries a by no means negligible risk. The decision to carry out a provocation test must never be taken without careful consideration. If such a test is performed, the patient must be kept under close observation, preferably in hospital, for an adequate time. In the first instance, the dose should not exceed one-tenth of the normal single dose.

Regarding in vitro tests, the RAST and ELISA deserve first mention. They are used mainly to detect IgE antibodies, though other types of antibodies can also be detected. The main usefulness of the tests lies in the field of allergy to inhalants but they can be used to detect drug allergies of typeticular penicillin allergies (WIDE and JUHLIN 1971).

Histamine liberation from basophil leukocytes from the peripheral blood has as yet seldom been applied for the detection of allergies of type I.

The modified Coombs test (KRAFT et al. 1977) and the bacteriophage inhibition test (DE WECK 1971) have the advantage of high sensitivity and can be used for determining IgG and IgE antibodies, and in some instances also for IgM antibodies, as has been demonstrated in cases of penicillin allergy. However, their performance requires elaborate laboratory resources.

Of the various methods in which lymphocytes or macrophages from the peripheral blood are employed, the lymphocyte transformation test deserves special mention. It is regarded as the most reliable in vitro test for the diagnosis of drug eruptions (GIRARD 1972, 1974; HALPERN et al. 1967; DE WECK 1971, 1979). Specific stimulation of lymphocytes has been reported not only in late but also in immediate reactions. The results appear to depend on the nature of the drug. The highest yields have been obtained in cases of penicillin and phenylbutazone allergy. Positive results were less frequent in patients with allergic reactions to local anesthetics, pyrazolones, or sulfonamides. The nature of the disease may also exert some influence. In some manifestations, for example vasculitides, erythema multiforme, purpura, and fixed eruptions, attempts to demonstrate specific stimulation of lymphocytes in vitro have very seldom been successful.

Cell-mediated reactions can also be demonstrated in vitro by the macrophage inhibition test. With the exception of penicillin sensitivity, this test has seldom been employed in the investigation of drug allergies. The possibilities and limitations of this test in this field have not yet been adequately explored and it is too early to assess its value. The rosette test has also been used for identifying allergens in drug allergy of type IV.

The vast majority of allergic drug reactions which affect the skin are relatively harmless and respond well to treatment. However, every effort should be made to ascertain the cause so that the patient can be safeguarded against a renewed episode which might have more serious consequences.

References

Ackroyd JF (1975) Immunological mechanisms in drug hypersensitivity. In: Gell PGH, Coomb RRA, Lachmann PJ (eds) Clinical aspects of immunology, 3rd edn. Blackwell Scientific, Oxford, p 913

Alarcón-Segovia D (1969) Drug-induced lupus syndromes. Mayo Clin Proc 44:664

Alarcón-Segovia D, Worthington JW, Ward LE, Wakim KG (1965) Lupus diathesis and the hydralazine syndrome. N Engl J Med 272:462

Alarcón-Segovia D, Wakim KG, Worthington JW, Ward LE (1967) Clinical and experimental studies on the hydralazine syndrome and its relationship to systemic lupus erythematosus. Medicine (Baltimore) 46:1

Alarcón-Segovia D, Fishbein E, Betancourt VM (1969) Antibodies to nucleoprotein and to hydrazide-altered soluble nucleoprotein in tuberculous patients receiving isoniazid. Clin Exp Immunol 5:429

Apolant H (1898) Die Antipyrinexantheme. Arch Dermatol Syph 46:345

Assem ESK, Banks RA (1973) Practolol induced drug eruption. Proc R Soc Lond 66:179

Baer RL, Witten VH (1961) Drug eruptions. In: Year Book of Dermatology, 1960–1961 Series. Year Book Medical Publishers, Chicago

Barsa JA, Saunders JC (1966) A peculiar photo-sensitivity reaction with chlorpromazine. Int Arch Allergy Appl Immunol 20:488

Batschuarov B, Minkow DM (1968) Dermatitis and purpura from rubber in clothing. Trans St. John's Hosp Derm Soc 54:178

Belinson L (1948) Dis Nerv Syst 9:8

Betson JR Jr, Alford CD (1961) Stevens-Johnson syndrome secondary to phenobarbital administration in the treatment of toxemia of pregnancy. Obstet Gynecol 18:195

Blomgren SE, Vaughan HJ (1968) The immunogenicity of photo-oxidized DNA and procainamide hydrochloride. Arthritis Rheum 11:470

Braun-Falco O, Bandmann HJ (1970) Das Lyell-Syndrom – Syndrom der verbrühten Haut. Huber, Bern

Braun-Falco O, Geisler H (1962) Zur Epidermolysis acuta combustiformis (Syndrom der verbrühten Haut). Med Welt 34:1737

Braverman JM, Yen A (1975) Demonstration of immune complexes in spontaneous and histamine-induced lesions and in normal skin of patients with leukocytoclastic angiitis. J Invest Dermatol 64:105

Brehm G, Brehm J (1963) Fixe Arzneiexantheme unter Anwendung des Zytostatimus TRE-NIMON. Dermatol Monatsschr 147:134

Bruinsma W (1972) Adverse reaction of drug eruptions. Dermatologica 145:377

Burckhardt W (1941) Untersuchungen über die Photoaktivität einiger Sulfonilamide. Dermatologica 83:64

Burckhardt W (1962) Arzneiexantheme. In: Marchionini A (ed) Handbuch der Haut- und Geschlechtskrankheiten, vol II/1. Springer, Berlin Göttingen Heidelberg, pp 545–596

Burckhardt W, Sutter T (1963) Photoallergische Arzneiexantheme durch Hydrochlorothiazid. Z Hautkr 17:105

Calnan CD (1971) Purpura allergique de contact. Bull Soc Franc Dermat Syphil 78:226

Cannat A, Seligmann M (1966) Possible induction of antinuclear antibodies by isoniazid. Lancet I:185

Cannat A, Seligmann M (1968) Induction by isoniazid and hydralazine of antinuclear factors in mice. Clin Exp Immunol 3:99

Claxton RC (1963) A review of 31 cases of Stevens-Johnson syndrome. Med J Aust 50 I:963–967

Cohen AC, Glinsky GL (1949) Cutaneous lesions occurring in the course of streptomycin therapy. Arch Dermatol 60:373

Cohlan SQ (1960) Erythema multiforme exsudativum associated with the use of sulfamethoxypyridazine. JAMA 173:799

Cole M, Robinson GN (1954) 6-Aminopenicillanic acid – II. Formation of 6-aminopenicillanic acid by *Emericellopsis minima* (Stolk) and related fungi. Proc R Soc (Lond) 154:490

Cone RB, Hannigan CA, Teicher R (1954) Erythema multiforme bullosum following phenylbutazone for arthritis. Arch Dermatol 69:674

de Weck AL (1971) Critical evaluation of diagnostic methods in drug allergy. In: Allergology, 8th European Congr. of Allergology, Int. Congress Series 251. Excerpta Medica, Amsterdam

de Weck AL (1974) Neue Aspekte der Arzneimittelallergie. In: Werner H, Gronemeyer W (eds) Arzneimittelallergie. Immunitätsforsch Suppl 1:37

de Weck AL (1979) Approaches to prevention and treatment of drug allergy. In: Turk JL, Parker D (eds) Drugs and immuneresponsiveness. McMillan, London, p 211

Discombe G (1972) The formed elements of the blood. In: Samter M, Parker CW (eds) Hypersensitivity to drugs, vol I. Pergamon Oxford, p 173

Doerr R (1951) Allergie. Springer, Vienna

Dugois P, Colomb L, Fayelle G (1957) Erythème polymorphe par un hypoglycémiant per os. Bull Soc Franc Dermat 64:301

Dupont A, Lachapelle JM (1964) Dermatitis due to a drug deposit during diabetes insipidus therapy. Bull Soc Franc Dermat Syph 71:508

Engelhardt AW (1960) Die Diagnostik fixer Exantheme und deren auslösende Ursachen. Hautarzt 11:49

Epstein S (1939) Photoallergy and primary photosensitivity to sulfanilamide. J Invest Dermatol 2:43

Fitzpatrick TB, Eisen A, Wolff K, Freedberg IM, Austen KF (1979) Dermatology in general medicine. McGraw-Hill, New York, p 965 ff

Furuya T, Sekido N, Ishikawa F (1966) Beitrag zum fixen Arzneimittelexanthem. Arch Dermatol Res 225:375

Gelber A (1954) Erythema multiforme nach Phenylbutazonbehandlung. Verh Dtsch Ges Inn Med 729

Girard JP (1972) Allergic reactions to antibiotics. Helv Med Acta 36:3

Girard JP (1974) Diagnostic tests in drug allergy. In: Allergology. 8th Int. Congress of Allergology, Congress series no 23. Excerpta Medica, Amsterdam

Goerz G, Ruzicka T (1978) Lyell-Syndrom, Grosse scripta 2. Grosse, Berlin

Goerz G, Jacobi E, Lissner R (1974) Bemerkungen zur sog. Adalin-Purpura. Südwestdtsch. Dermatologen-Tag. Freiburg

Gold S (1951) Role of sulphonamides and penicillin in the pathogenesis of systemic lupus erythematosus. Lancet I:268

Goodman D, Cahn MM (1959) Contact dermatitis due to phenothiazine drugs. J Invest Dermatol 33:27

Gower RG, Sams WM, Thorne G, Claman HN (1976) Immune complex deposition in leukocytoclastic vasculitis. J Invest Dermatol 66:271

Halpern B, Ky NT, Amache N (1967) Diagnosis of drug allergy with the lymphocyte transformation test. J Allergy Clin Immunol 40:168

Harber LC, Tromovitch TA, Baer RL (1961) Studies in photosensitivity due to demethylchlortetracycline. J Invest Dermatol 37:189

Harber LC, Harris H, Baer RL (1966) Photo-allergic contact dermatitis due to halogenated salicylanilides and related compounds. Arch Dermatol 94:255

Hargraves MM, Richmond H, Morton R (1948) Presentation of two bone marrow elements: the "tart" cell and the "L.E." cell. Proc Staff Meet Mayo Clinic 23:25

Harpey JP, Caille B, Moulias R, Goust JM (1972) Drug allergy and lupus-like syndrome (with special reference to D-penicillamine). In: Dash CH, Jones HEH (eds) Mechanisms in drug allergy, Glaxo-symposium series. Churchill-Livingstone, Edinburgh, p 51

Haustein UF, Klug H (1977) Ultrastrukturelle Untersuchungen der Blutgefäße beim Erythema nodosum. Dermatol Monatsschr 103:13

Heine WI, Friedman H (1962) Hydralazine lupus syndrome associated with a possible anti-hydralazine antibody. JAMA 182:726

Hepple S, Macmillan AL (1973) Purpuric dermatosis due to house-dust mite (*Dermatophagoides* spp.) allergy: a case report. Clin Allergy 3:23

Hjorth N (1968) Drug reactions. In: Allergology, Proc. 6th congr. of the int. assoc. of allergology. Excerpta Medica, Amsterdam, p 360

Hoigné R (1965) Arzneimittelallergien. Klinische und serologisch-experimentelle Untersuchungen. Huber, Bern

Hoigné R (1966) Anaphylaktischer Schock und Serumkrankheit. Schweiz Med Wochenschr 96:1119

Hoigné R, Döppen U (1963) Das Syndrom der Serumkrankheit bei Sensibilisierungen auf Medikamente. Schweiz Med Wochenschr 93:1724

Hoigné R, Krebs A (1964) Kombinierte anaphylaktische und embolisch-toxische Reaktionen durch akzidentelle intravasculäre Injektion von Procain-Penicillin. Schweiz Med Wochenschr 94:610

Hoigné R, Sturm H, Klein U (1974) Arzneimittelallergische Manifestationen in der inneren Medizin. In: Werner M, Gronemeyer W (eds) Arzneimittelallergie, Z Immunitätsforsch Immunobiol, vol 1. Fischer, Stuttgart, p 134

Holubar K, Wolff K, Konrad K, Beutner E (1975) Ultrastructural localization of immunoglobulins in bullous pemphigoid skin. Employment of a new peroxidase-antiperoxidase multistep method. J Invest Dermatol 64:220

Hölzle E, Plewig G (1982) Photoallergische Kontaktdermatitis durch benzophenonhaltige Sonnenschutzpräparate. Hautarzt 33:391

Illig L (1976) Purpura, Folge 3: Dermatologisch relevante Purpura-Formen, Teil 2. Fortschr Med 94:1379

Illig L, Kalkoff KW (1970) Zum Formenkreis der Purpura pigmentosa progressiva (unter besonderer Berücksichtigung der Adalin-Purpura). Hautarzt 21:497

Ippen H (1967) Arzneimittelausschläge durch Malariamittel, Phenothiazine, Sulfonamide, Tetracycline und andere Medikamente, die zu Photodermatosen führen können. Z Hautkr 42:47

Ippen H (1976) Photoallergien: Pathogenese und Therapie. In: Braun-Falco O, Marghescu S (eds) Fortschritte der praktischen Dermatologie und Venerologie, vol 8. Springer, Berlin Heidelberg New York, p 177

Jillson OF, Porter PS (1965) Recent advances in the understanding of the penicillin urticarias. Arch Dermatol 92:200–204

Jung EG (1972) Photoallergie. Z Hautkr 47:329

Karpatkin S (1971) Drug-induced thrombocytopenia. Am J Med Sci 262:68

Kauppinen K (1972) Cutaneous reactions to drugs with special reference to severe bullous mucocutaneous eruptions and sulphonamides. Acta Derm Venereol (Stockh) Suppl 68:1

Kennedy CB, Davis FH, Henington VM, Sternberg MJ (1957) Dermatitis medicamentosa due to antipyrine. A study of twenty-eight cases in negroes following the use of a proprietary medication (666 cold preparations). Arch Dermatol 75:286

Kennedy WPU, Wallace AT, Murdoch J (1963) Ampicillin in treatment of certain gramnegative bacterial infections. Br Med J II:962

Kleine-Natrop HE (1966) Fixe Arzneimittelexantheme und ihre aktuellen Ursachen. Allerg Asthmaforsch 12:139

Knowles FC, Decker HB, Kandle RP (1936) Phenolphthalein dermatitis. An experimental study including reproduction of the eruption in skin transplants. Arch Dermatol 33:227

Korting GW (1972) Dermatologische Nebenwirkungen von Arzneimitteln. Med Welt 23:937

Kraft D, Roth A, Miescher P, Pichler H, Ebner H (1977) Specific and total serum IgE measurements in the diagnosis of penicillin allergy. Clin Allergy 7:21

Kruizinga EE (1950) Adaline-toxicodermie onder het beeld van dermatite lichenoide purpurique et pigmentaire (Gougerot-Blum). Ned Tijdsch Geneeskd 94:1258

Ladd AT (1962) Procainamide-induced lupus erythematosus. N Engl J Med 267:1357

Lappat EJ, Cawein MJ (1968) A familial study of procainamide-induced systemic lupus erythematosus. A question of pharmacogenetic polymorphism. Am J Med 45:846

Lee SL, Rivero I, Siegel M (1966) Activation of systemic lupus erythematosus by drugs. Arch Intern Med 117:620

Lindemayr W (1954) Arzneimittelexantheme. Wiener Beiträge zur Dermatologie, vol 6. Maudrich, Wien

Lindemayr W (1959) Arzneimittelexantheme. In: Gottron HA, Schönfeld W (eds) Dermatologie und Venerologie, vol III/1. Thieme, Stuttgart, p 327

Loeb H (1921) Über Adalinexantheme. Arch Dermatol Syph 131:128

Louis Ph (1972) Zur ätiologischen Diagnostik von fixen Arzneimittelexanthemen. Z Hautkr 47:387

Louis Ph, Schulz KH (1973) Arzneimittelallergie. Urologe 13:10

Loveman AB (1943) Experimental aspect of fixed eruption due to Alurate, a compound of Allonal. JAMA 102:97

Loveman AB, Simon F (1940) Erythema nodosum due to sulfanilamide. J Allergy Clin Immunol 12:28

Lutz W (1951) Sehr ausgedehntes fixes Arzneiexanthem nach Optalidon. Dermatologica 102:317

Lyell A (1956) Toxic epidermal necrolysis: an eruption resembling scalding of the skin. Br J Dermatol 68:355

Maas D, Schubothe H (1973) Ein Lupus-erythematodes-ähnliches Syndrom mit antimitochondrialen Antikörpern. Dtsch Med Wochenschr 98:131

Maas D, Schubothe H, Droese M (1974) Das LE-ähnliche Syndrom mit antimitochondrialen Antikörpern (Pseudo-LE-Syndrom). Z Immunitätsforsch Immunobiol 147:333

Maas D, Schubothe H, Sennekamp J, Genth E, Maerker-Alzer G, Droese M, Hartl PW, Schumacher K (1975) Zur Frage der Induzierbarkeit des Pseudo-LE-Syndroms durch Arzneimittel. Vorläufige Ergebnisse von Erhebungen bei 58 Fällen. Dtsch Med Wochenschr 100:1555

Maibach HJ, Sams WM Jr, Epstein JH (1967) Screening for drug toxicity by wavelengths greater than 3,100 Å. Arch Dermatol 95:12

Marghescu S (1978) Allergische Arzneiexantheme. Perimed-Verlag D. Straube, Erlangen

Mayer RL (1933) Toxicodermien. In: Jadassohn J (ed) Handbuch der Haut- und Geschlechtskrankheiten, vol 4/2. Springer, Berlin, pp 1–252

McCoombs RP (1965) Systematic "allergic" vasculitis. JAMA 194:1059

McGovern JP, Roberson CE, Stewart GT (1970) Incidence and manifestations of penicillin allergy. In: Stewart GT, McGovern JP (eds) Penicillin allergy – clinical and immunologic aspects. Thomas, Springfield

McKenzie H, Parratt D, White RG (1976) IgM and IgG antibody levels to ampicillin in patients with infectious mononucleosis. Clin Exp Immunol 26:214

McVie JG (1973) Drug-induced thrombocytopenia. In: Girdwood RG (ed) Blood disorders due to drugs and other agents. Excerpta Medica, Amsterdam, p 187

Miescher G (1947) Zur Histologie des Erythema nodosum. Acta Derm Venerol 27:448

Miescher G (1961) Abgrenzung des allergischen und toxischen Geschehens in morphologischer und funktioneller Hinsicht. Arch Dermatol Res 213:297

Miescher P (1961) Die Immunhämatologie der Leukocyten und Thrombocyten. In: Miescher P, Vorlaender KO (eds) Immunopathologie in Klinik und Forschung. Thieme, Stuttgart, p 160

Miescher P, Delacrétaz J (1953) Démonstration d'un phénomène „L.E." positif dans deux cas d'hypersensibilité médicamenteuse. Schweiz Med Wochenschr 83:536

Misgeld V (1974) Zur Frage der Immunpathogenese des Lyell-Syndroms. Z Hautkr 49:239

Müller-Schoop JW, Grob PJ, Joller-Jemelka HJ, Guggisberg HE (1975) Pseudolupus: eine schwere Nebenwirkung eines Venenpräparates? Schweiz Med Wochenschr 105:665

Mulzer P, Habermann R (1930) Adalinexantheme unter dem Bilde der Purpura Majocchi. Z Gesamte Neurol Psychiatr 128:374

Naegeli O, de Quervain F, Stalder W (1930) Nachweis des zellulären Sitzes der Allergie beim fixen Antipyrinexanthem (Autotransplantationen, Versuch in vitro). Klin Wochenschr 9:924

Paschoud J-M (1966) Vasculitis allergica cutis durch Phenylbutazon. Dermatologica 133:76

Pelz HH (1962) Stevens-Johnson: A hypersensitivity reaction in the spectrum of lupus erythematosus. NY State J Med 62:3982

Perry HM Jr, Sakamoto A, Tan EM (1967) Relationship of acetylating enzyme to hydralazine toxicity. J Lab Clin Med 70:1020

Perry HM Jr (1973) Late toxicity to hydralazine resembling systemic lupus erythematosus or rheumatoid arthritis. Am J Med 54:58

Petter O, Perlick E (1969) Betrachtungen zur Purpura pigmentosa progressiva – unter dem besonderen Aspekt gerinnungsanalytischer Befunde. Dermatol Monatsschr 155:213

Pevny I, Röckl H (1975) Arzneimittelbedingte allergische Hautreaktionen vom kutanvaskulären Typ. MMW 117:9

Post CF, Dougherty J (1964) Fixed drug eruption caused by tetracycline hydrochloride. JAMA 188:35

Raftery AV, Dernman AM (1973) Systemic lupus erythematosus syndrome induced by practolol. Br Med J II:452

Röckl H, Metz J (1973) Nodöse Erytheme. In: Braun-Falco O, Petzoldt D (eds) Vorträge des 7. Fortbildungskurses der Dermatologischen Klinik und Poliklinik der Universität München. Springer, Berlin Heidelberg New York, p 196 (Fortschritte der praktischen Dermatologie und Venerologie, vol 7)

Röckl H, Metz J, Amschler A (1979) Erythema nodosum. Allergologie 2:72

Rollof SJ (1950) Erythema nodosum in association with sulfathiazole in thylodone. A clinical investigation with special reference to primary tuberculosis. Acta Tuberc Scand 24:Suppl

Rothenstein J, Schwarz K, Schwarz-Speck M, Storck H (1966) Role of in vivo and in vitro formed decomposition products of sulfanilamides and phenothiazine in photoallergy: relationship of spectrophotometric findings to in vivo reactions. Int Arch Allergy Appl Immunol 29:1

Saxl O (1972) Nebenwirkungen von Barbituraten. Fortschr Med 90:50

Scherer E (1979) Immunfluoreszenzuntersuchungen in der Dermatologie. Med Klin 74:132

Scherer R, Wolff HH (1979) Vasculitis allergica. Allergologie 2:62

Schöpf E (1979) Morbilliforme, scarlatiniforme und rubeoliforme Exantheme. Allergologie 2:78

Schöpf E, Schulz KH, Kessler R, Taugner M, Braun W (1975) Allergologische Untersuchungen beim Lyell-Syndrom. Z Haut Geschlkrh 50:865

Schreiber MM, Naylor LZ (1962) Antihistamine photosensitivity. Arch Dermatol 86:58

Schulz KH (1964) Allergische Hautreaktionen und Arzneimittelgruppen. Arch Klin Exp 219:288

Schulz KH (1967) Allergic eruptions due to carbromal and related drugs. 6th Int Congr of Allergology, Montreal

Schulz KH (1972) Syndrome der Arzneimittelallergie. Z Haut Geschlkrh 47:319

Schulz KH (1974) Arzneimittelallergische Reaktionen der Haut. In: Werner M, Gronemeyer W (eds) Arzneimittelallergie Z Immunitätsforsch Suppl I:177

Schulz KH (1979) Stellenwert und Aussagekraft von Testmethoden bei allergischen Arzneiexanthemen. In: Braun-Falco O, Wolff HH (eds) Vorträge der 9. Fortbildungswoche der Dermatologischen Klinik und Poliklinik der Universität München. Springer, Berlin Heidelberg New York, p 71 (Fortschritte der praktischen Dermatologie und Venerologie, vol 9)

Schulz KH, Glowania H-J (1979) Lyell-Syndrom. Allergologie 2:49

Schulz KH, Schmidt P (1967) Fixe Exantheme durch drei verschiedene Arzneimittel mit getrennter Lokalisation. Beitrag zur Frage der Barbituratallergie. Z Hautkr 14:561

Schulz KH, Wiskemann A, Wulf K (1956) Klinische und experimentelle Untersuchungen über die photodynamische Wirksamkeit von Phenothiazinderivaten, insbesondere von Megaphen. Arch Klin Exp Dermatol 202:285

Schulz KH, Schöpf E, Wex O (1970) Allergische Berufsekzeme durch Ampicillin. Berufsder-matosen 18:132

Schuppli R (1967) Zur Frage der Abgrenzung des Lyell-Syndroms. Hautarzt 18:518

Schuppli R (1972) Drug-induced skin reactions. In: Samter M, Parker CW (eds) Hypersensitivity to drugs, vol 1. Pergamon, Oxford, p 205

Schwarz JA, Jost H (1975) Pseudo-LE-Syndrom nach Einnahme eines Venenpräparates (Venopyronum-Dragees). Dtsch Med Wochenschr 100:1590

Schwiebert E (1967) Katamnestische Erhebungen zur Vasculitis allergica. PhD Dissertation, University of Hamburg

Siegel M, Lee SL, Peress NS (1967) The epidemiology of drug-induced systemic lupus erythematosus. Arthritis Rheum 10:407

Simpson RG (1950) Erythema nodosum. Dermatologica 101:94

Steel SJ, Moffatt JL (1954) Stevens-Johnson syndrome and granulocytopenia after phenylbutazone. Br Med J 795

Stein KM, Schlappner OLA, Heaton CL, Decherd JW (1972) Demonstration of basal cell immuno-fluorescence in drug induced toxic epidermal necrolysis. Br J Dermatol 86:246

Stevanović DV (1961) Photosensitivity due to certain drugs. Br J Dermatol 73:233

Stewart GT (1965) The penicillin group of drugs. Elsevier, Amsterdam

Strempel R (1959) Betrachtungen zur Symptomatologie und Pathogenese des Erythema exsudativum multiforme. Hautarzt 10:501

Stüttgen G (1973) Toxic epidermal necrolysis provoked by barbiturates. Br J Dermatol 88:291

Sulzberger MB (1940) Dermatologic allergy. Thomas, Springfield

Tan EM (1968) The influence of hydralazine on nuclear antigen-antibody reactions. Arthritis Rheum 11:515

Thiers H, Fayolle J, Colomb D, Descos L (1964) Erythème scarlatiniforme récidivant avec hématurie microscopique contemporaine chez une tuberculeuse pulmonaire diabétique traitée par le glucidoral. Responsabilité étiologique du glucidoral. Bull Soc Franc Derm Syph 72:149

Tritsch H, Orfanos C, Lückerath J (1969) Nekrolytische Arzneiexantheme. Hautarzt 19:24

Tronnier H, Streichel DF, Ksinsik R (1967) Kasuistischer Beitrag zur Dermatitis lichenoides purpurica et pigmentosa (Gougerot-Blum) mit Störungen im Blutgerinnungssystem. Dermatol Wochenschr 153:447

Tullett GL (1966) Fatal case of toxic erythema after chlorpromazide (Diabinese). Br Med J I:148

Urbach E, Sidaravicius B (1930) Zur Kritik der Methoden der passiven Übertragung der Überempfindlichkeit. Klin Wochenschr 9:2095

Uri J, Valu G (1963) Production of 6-aminopenicillanic acid by dermatophytes. Nature 200:896–897

van Ketel WG (1967) Purpura door gebruik van carbromal. Ned Tijdschr Geneeskd 111:252

Vayre J, Combey P (1955) Toxicodermie géante à type d'erythéme polymorphe. Bull Soc Franç Dermat 62:349

Veltman G (1959) Zur Kenntnis des Adalinexanthems. Z Haut Geschlkrh 27:11

Walsh JR, Zimmerman HJ (1953) The demonstration of the "L.E."-phenomenon in patients with penicillin hypersensitivity. Blood 8:65

Watts JC (1962) A fatal case of erythema multiforme exsudativum (Stevens-Johnson syndrome) following therapy with Dilantin. Pediatrics 30:592

Webster AW, Thompson RA (1974) The ampicillin rash: lymphocyte transformation by ampicillin polymer. Clin Exp Immunol 18:553

Weirich EG (1957) Das Pyrazolonexanthem. Dtsch Med Wochenschr 1011

Welsh AL (1961) The fixed eruption. Thomas, Springfield

Welsh AL, Ede M (1961) The fixed eruption: a possible hazard of modern drug therapy. Arch Dermatol 84:1004

Wereide K (1967) Stevens-Johnson syndrome in Norway, with particular reference to its relation to sulphonamides. In: International Congress Chemotherapy, Vienna

Weuta H (1972) Das Ampicillinexanthem. Bericht über eine klinische Erfahrungsaktion. Arzneim Forsch 22:1300

Wide L, Juhlin L (1971) Detection of penicillin allergy of the immediate type by radioim-
    munoassay of reagins (IgE) to penicilloyl conjugates. Clin Allergy 1:171
Wise F, Sulzberger MB (1933) Drug eruptions. I. Fixed phenolphthalein eruptions. Arch
    Dermatol 27:549
Wolff HH, Maciejewski M, Scherer R, Braun-Falco O (1978) Immunoelectromicroscope
    examination of early lesions in histamine induced immune complex vasculitis in man.
    Br J Dermatol 99:13
Woringer F, Levy JG (1949) A propos de deux cas d'erythème polymorphe associé à de le-
    rythème noueux. Bull Soc Franç Dermat 56:536
Yaffee HS (1959) Stevens-Johnson syndrome following sulfamethoxypyridazine (Kynex)
    treated successfully with triamcinolone. US Armed Forces Med J 10:1468
Yaffee HS (1960) Stevens-Johnson syndrome caused by chlorpropamide. Arch Dermatol
    82:636

CHAPTER 5

Allergy of the Respiratory Tract to Low Molecular Weight Chemical Agents

J. PEPYS

A. Introduction

Allergy to small chemical molecules is exemplified by the respiratory allergic disorders they cause, mainly in relation to occupation. Such haptenic agents present many problems familiar in allergy to drugs, such as the nature and role of the carrier molecules, the difficulties in demonstrating antibodies, and the highly reactive nature of some of these substances. The latter may lead to non-specific combination with immunoglobulins or may combine with protein in such a way as to render the specific antigenic determinants inaccessible in test procedures.

There may be doubts as to whether a particular reaction is allergic, particularly where antibodies have not yet been shown, "Allergy" defined by VON PIRQUET can be summarised as the acquired, specific altered capacity to react, starting with the induction of an antibody response and then elicitation of reactions by minute amounts of antigen, far less than the amounts needed to sensitise. It is possible however to assume an allergic mechanism, based upon a history of previous exposure without symptoms, the subsequent appearance of sensitisation, which is often of increasing degree, and the fact that only a proportion, often small, of exposed subjects are affected. Many chemical allergens can also be irritants, but irritant effects would be expected to affect the majority of exposed subjects from the initial exposure and to require larger amounts to elicit reactions than the small amounts (of a molecular order) which elicit allergic reactions.

The study of occupational allergy to small chemical molecules has much to offer to the clarification of these problems. Certain examples will therefore be discussed in detail because they are models for other as yet unresolved questions, and others will be discussed only briefly, serving to illustrate the wide range of chemical agents identified as causes of occupational respiratory allergy and meriting much further study (POPA et al. 1969; KOBAYASHI 1974, PEPYS and HUTCHCROFT 1975; PEPYS 1977b; DAVIES et al. 1977; PEPYS and DAVIES 1978). A number of these are therapeutic agents themselves or their precursors, encountered in the pharmaceutical industry.

Investigations of occupational respiratory allergy have other advantages too. The circumstances of exposure are usually well defined so that the sequence of clinical and immunological events leading first to "sensitisation" and subsequently to "elicitation" of reactions can be assessed with confidence. Confirmation of the aetiological diagnosis in highly specific immunochemical terms is possible by provocation tests made under carefully controlled conditions with exposures often of a minute order, far less than ordinarily encountered. The reactions can be objectively measured by changes in pulmonary function. These reactions, for example of an asthmatic nature, present a variety of patterns which may be present individually or in varying combinations. There may be (1) immediate reactions maximal in about 10 min and lasting for 1.5–2 h; for these there are at least two possible immunological mechanisms, IgE- or STS-IgG-mediated reactions [1] and perhaps combinations of both; (2) non-immediate reactions, with (a) a reaction starting more than 1 h after exposure, maximal at about 1.5 h and resolving within about 5 h; (b) a reaction starting after 3–4 h, maximal at 5–8 h and resolving as a rule within 24 h; and (c) a reaction coming on in the early hours of the morning after the test and recurring with gradually decreasing intensity at about the same time each night for one or many nights thereafter. Non-immediate asthmatic reactions may be accompanied by systemic reactions, such as fever, malaise and peripheral blood leucocytosis and eosinophilia. Examples of these various reactions to chemical agents will be provided. It is probable that reactions of a non-respiratory nature to chemical agents follow similar patterns which have yet to be clearly discerned and which, when understood, may explain some of the puzzling features of reaction to chemical agents in terms of their speed of appearance, duration and recurrence of the clinical manifestations.

These observations have the further advantage of dealing, in clinical and laboratory situations, with chemical agents, inorganic or organic, of a precise chemical constitution, providing valuable models for immunochemical studies. For example, sensitisation to chemical agents requires conjugation of the agent with carrier molecules and similar conjugates are usually regarded as necessary for the demonstration of antibodies. This, however, is not always the case, as shown by the demonstration of IgE antibodies to azo and anthracene cotton dyes (ALANKO et al. 1978).

B. Inorganic Chemicals

Examples of these, providing models for such chemicals, are: (a) the complex salts of platinum encountered in the refining of the metal and ranking at the top of the list of allergenic sensitising capacity, (b) nickel sulphate, (c) potassium and ammonium persulphate used as hair bleach.

I. Halide Complex Salts of Platinum

The halide complex salts of platinum, chloroplatinites and chloroplatinates, are highly reactive with proteins, with particular affinity for sulphydryl bonds. They can also be histamine liberators (PARROT et al. 1967, 1969). These salts thus represent a polar example of a chemical molecule with most of the features which complicate study as allergens. Many of the problems have been resolved and the findings will be given "in extenso". Examples of the relevant platinum salts (molecular weight 444 daltons) are ammonium hexachloroplatinate $(NH_4)_2$ [Pt Cl$_6$] and tetrachloroplatinate $(NH_4)_2$ [PtCl$_4$].

---

1 STS stands for short-term sensitising (heat-stable mercaptoethanol-resistant) antibody (PARISH 1970)

1. Allergy to Complex Platinum Salts

These salts were recognised as potent allergens from 1911 when KARASEK and KARASEK reported on their sensitising capacity in photographic use; this was followed by further reports of sensitised refinery workers and chemists suffering from rhinitis, conjunctivitis, asthma and contact urticaria, on handling the chloride salts of platinum encountered in the extraction of this precious metal (VALLERY-RADOT and BLAMOUTIER 1929; HUNTER et al. 1945; ROBERTS 1951; BIJL 1963; FREEDMAN and KRUPEY 1968; LEVENE and CALNAN 1971; PEPYS 1977). All of these reported severe anaphylactic reactions to tests with very small amounts. ROBERTS (1951) found that the highest concentration acceptable for skin tests without bringing into play histamine-liberating effects and non-specific whealing was 10^{-3} g/ml.

Safe procedure for skin prick testing and for nasal and bronchial provocation tests with the complex platinum salts have been devised, starting with very high dilutions for skin tests and with minute amounts for other tests (PEPYS et al. 1972 b; PICKERING 1972). Thus for skin prick tests fresh solutions in Coca's fluid of $[Pt(IV)Cl_6]^{2-}$ the hexachloroplatinate, and $[Pt(II)Cl_4]^{2-}$ the tetrachloroplatinate, at 10^{-9} g/ml. The prick test introduces 3×10^{-6} ml according to (SQUIRE 1952). The absolute skin test dose of platinum salt is therefore in the region of 10^{-15} g. There are appreciable numbers of subjects who give unequivocal type I immediate whealing reaction to this amount and who would probably react to even smaller amounts. Negative tests at this concentration are followed by tests with 10^{-8}, 10^{-7} etc. up to 10^{-3} g/ml.

2. Immunochemical Analysis of Allergenicity of Platinum Salts

Little is known about the actual hapten–carrier linkages of the halide platinum salts except for their affinity for proteins in general and for sulphydryl bonds in particular. There is some limited evidence of sensitisation of rats by injection of platinum–protein conjugates (KHAN et al. 1975). Such conjugates are not effective for skin prick tests and studies of platinum–human albumin conjugates have shown the presence of 26 platinum molecules for every 10^{-6} molecules of albumin. Under these conditions steric hindrance and paucity of available platinum-specific determinants are probably responsible for the poor eliciting capacity of such conjugates.

We therefore had recourse to skin prick tests of sensitised platinum refinery workers under carefully controlled conditions with a range of platinum complexes (CLEARE et al. 1976). The aim was to correlate the structure of the complexes with their capacity to elicit type I reactions. A range of halide, nitro and amine complexes was tested. The allergic response was elicited whenever there was at least one chloro ligand in a charged complex. The number of chloro groups helped to determine this with the following sequence of potency:

$$(NH_4)_2[PtCl_6] \simeq (NH_4)_2[PtCl_4]$$
$$> CS_2[Pt(NO_2)Cl_3] > CS_2[Pt(NO_2)Cl_2]$$
$$> CS_2[Pt(NO_2)_3Cl] > K_2[Pt(NO_2)_4]$$

the latter being inactive. The use of bromo instead of chloro ligands gave similar findings, though at a reduced level.

In view of the very high degrees of sensitivity of the subjects, the occasional reaction to high concentrations of the neutral compound *cis*-[Pt(OHC$_2$H$_4$NH$_2$)Cl$_2$] may be due to slight contamination and 0.001% [PtCl$_4$]$^{2-}$ would suffice. Impurities of this order could explain the anaphylactic reactions to *cis*-[Pt(NH$_3$)$_2$Cl$_2$] used for the treatment of certain cancers, reported by Khan et al. (1975).

The allergenicity as shown by skin tests of the platinum complexes was found to be directly related to both their charge and their overall reactivity. Analysis of their structure and consideration of known chemistry throws some light on the factors underlying this.

Platinum (II) complexes, like other square planar metal systems, react via an associative mechanism with a five-coordinate transition state in which both the entering and leaving groups are partially bound to the metal. They obey a general rate law which includes a solvent-assisted path. For example,

$$PtX_3Z + Y \rightarrow PtX_3Y + Z \quad \text{direct path}$$

$$\left. \begin{array}{l} PtX_3Z + S \rightarrow PtX_3S + Z \\ \\ PtX_3S + Y \rightarrow PtX_3Y + S \end{array} \right\} \text{solvent-assisted path (S = solvent)}$$

$$\text{Rate} = k_1[PtX_3Z] + k_2[PtX_3Z][Y]$$

where K_1 is a first-order constant for the solvent-controlled path and k_2 is a second-order rate constant for the direct reaction with Y. In a good coordinating solvent such as water $k_1 \gg k_2$ and the reactivity of the complex largely depends on the leaving ability of the ligand which is being replaced (Z).

For reactions with proteins in vivo we are not in a position to say anything about the incoming group except that it is likely to be the same protein (or proteins) and site (or sites) which are involved in each case. Thus we must concentrate on the leaving groups in each platinum complex. The kinetic effect of these ligands is not completely clear as yet, but certain general conclusions can be drawn. Three important sets of data are presented in Table 1.

Equations (1) and (2) are probably most relevant as the other coordination positions (apart from the leaving group under study) are occupied by an inert trichelating N-donor ligand. Some leaving groups, such as the halogens, are consistently found to be fairly labile and can be classed as reactive, whereas others such as nitro ($-NO_2^-$) and thiocyanate ($-SCN$) are more inert and much less reactive. Similarly the platinum–amine linkage is very stable and inert to nucleophilic attack while amines are very poor leaving groups.

The allergy test results can all be explained on the previous kinetic basis. Thus complexes containing strongly bound ligands with poor leaving abilities are not allergenic, presumably owing to little or no reaction with proteins (e.g. [Pt(NH$_3$)$_4$]Cl$_2$, K$_2$[Pt(NO$_2$)$_4$] [Pt(thiourea)$_4$]Cl$_2$). When reactive halogen groups are present, the complex often elicits some degree of allergic response, with chloro complexes more effective than bromide as would be forecast from Eq. (1) (the relative reactivities of chloro, bromo, and iodo complexes are not consistent for different reasons, depending on such factors as the nature of the incoming group). The only exceptions are the neutral diamine species. For most of the others, the activity appears to increase with an increasing number of halide ligands. Table 2 shows that the acid hydrolysis rate constants do not vary greatly for any member of the chloroammine series although the equilibria for the removal of one chloride

Table 1. Relative lability $k_2[X]/k_2[N_3]$ of ligands displaced from Pt(II) complexes

Ligand displacement reaction	Reference
$[Pt(dien)X]^+ + py \rightarrow [Pt(dien)(py)]^{2+} + X^-$ (water, 25 °C) $Cl > Br > I > N_3 > SCN > NO_2 > CN$ 40 27 12 1.0 0.36 0.056 0.02	BASOLO et al. (1960)
$[Pt(dien)X]^+ + \rightarrow [Pt(dien)Y]^+ + X^-$ (water, 30 °C) $I > Br > Cl > N_3 > (NO_2)$ 73 70 33 1.0 ?	BELLUCO et al. (1966)
$[Pt(bipy)(NO_2)X] + Y^- \rightarrow [Pt(bipy)(NO_2)Y] + X^-$ (methanol, 25 °C) $I > Br > Cl > NO_2 > N_3$ 900 240 140 7 1.0	CATTALINI and MARTELLI (1967)

Ligands are as follows: dien = diethylenetriamine, $H_2N \cdot CH_2 \cdot CH_2 \cdot NH \cdot CH_2 \cdot CH_2 \cdot NH_2$;

py = pyridine, ; bipy = 2,2′-bipyridyl, .

Table 2. Acid hydrolysis of Pt (II) chloroamine species

Complex		Equilibrium constants $(M \times 10^5)$		Rate constants $(s^{-1} \times 10^5)$	
		1st	2nd	1st	2nd
$[PtCl_4]^{2-}$		1,500	50	3.9	3.3
$[Pt(NH_3)Cl_3]^-$	cis	1,300		0.62	
	trans	130	4	5.6	
cis-$[Pt(NH_3)_2Cl_2]$		330	40	2.5	3.3
trans-$[Pt(NH_3)_2Cl_2]$		32	< 2	9.8	<5
$[Pt(NH_3)_3Cl]^+$		27		2.6	

vary by up to 50-fold. Generally the rates of substitution in Pt(II) complexes are independent of charge and this makes the inactivity of the neutral species somewhat puzzling as the chloro groups should be sufficiently reactive to cause an effect. Neutral compounds are more lipophilic than charged ones and can penetrate cell membranes more readily. We can hypothesise about the following aspects of the platinum–protein interaction.

a) As some compounds containing only one reactive group appear to elicit an allergic response, this tends to eliminate protein reactions in which more than one platinum coordination position is involved, e.g. protein bridging.

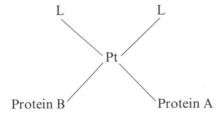

This assumes that several different types of protein interaction are not involved. However [Pt(dien)Cl]Cl, which is likely to have low $[PtCl_4]^{2-}$ contamination, was inactive. The reactions elicited by these compounds were always at the higher concentrations and contamination cannot be eliminated with absolute certainty.

b) The fact that a number of different platinum compounds can cause allergic effects in people orginally sensitised to either $[PtCl_6]^{2-}$ or $[PtCl_4]^{2-}$ salts, indicates that the antibodies formed due to the $[PtCl_6]^{2-}$ / $[PtCl_4]^{2-}$ – carrier conjugate can accommodate different structures within the approximately planar coordination around the Pt(II) centre which is presumably bound to a protein or other macromolecule. However, we have not introduced any ligands of large bulk which might be expected to cause steric hindrance in the antigen–antibody compounds. This latter point could be a reason for the inactivity of the $[Pt(dien)X]^+$ series, as diethylenetriamine is the bulkiest ligand employed in our tests.

c) The Pt(IV) and Pt(II) chloro species appear to be equally effective against the same sensitised persons. As has been postulated in the anti-cancer research, it may be that in vivo reduction of Pt(IV) to Pt(II) occurs. Pt(IV) species are usually rather inert kinetically unless a reaction occurs through a Pt(II) intermediate. However, in a biological area which is sensitive to such small quantities, it is possible (though unlikely) that Pt(IV) reacts in its own right. If this is so, it is surprising that Pt(II), the more kinetically labile species, is not a lot more allergenic than $[PtCl_6]^2$ unless this is due to the fact that the persons tested have become initially sensitised to $[PtCl_6]^{2-}$ under refinery conditions.

The observations on the nature of the sensitising material on the one hand and the eliciting agents on the other suggest the following hypotheses.

If chlorine ligands are still attached in the conjugate formed from $[PtCl_4]^{2-}$ or $[PtCl_6]^{2-}$, which are known to be sensitising agents for refinery workers, then the antibodies may have a specific preference for Pt complexes containing Pt–Cl bonds or those containing such bonds after conjugate formation. This may account for the observations that complexes containing several halide ligands are the most successful in eliciting responses in sensitive refinery personnel. Thus both kinetic and antibody specificity factors may be at play in the elicitation of reactions.

The charge on the antibodies could also be of considerable importance. Highly chlorinated species such as $[PtCl_4]^{2-}$ carry a negative charge and are more likely to give rise to positively charged antibodies, depending on the exact nature of the conjugate, than species containing fewer or no halide ligands. The latter might well give rise to negatively charged antibodies, being positively charged species. As the workers have been sensitised by inhalation to fully chlorinated species, this might explain their lack of reaction to compounds such as the neutral cis-$[Pt(NH_3)_2Cl_2]$ compound. However, it does not eliminate the possibility that the less chlorinated and differently charged compounds which are reasonably reactive may not be sensitisers in their own right and this might be an explanation for the different results reported by KHAN et al. (1975, 1977) for cis-$[Pt(NH_3)_2]$ given intravenously.

Thus, in sum, the platinum compounds eliciting reactions are confined to a small group of charged compounds containing reactive ligand systems such as chloride and, to a lesser extent, bromide. The allergenicity of the complexes is directly related to both their charge and overall reactivity. New compounds could be assessed on this basis.

Table 3. Comparison of inhalation tests with complex platinum salts

Patient	Platinum salt	Exposure time (min)	Decrease in FEV_1 (%)[a]
1	$(NH_4)_2PtCl_6$	15	38
	$(NH_4)_2PtCl_4$	10	49
	Na_2PtCl_6	10	35
2	$(NH_4)_2PtCl_6$	4	28
	$(NH_4)_2PtCl_4$	5	45
	Na_2PtCl_6	30	16
3	$(NH_4)_2PtCl_6$	6	31
	$(NH_4)_2PtCl_4$	10	38
	Na_2PtCl_6	15	23
4	$(NH_4)_2PtCl_6$	10	32
	$(NH_4)_2PtCl_4$	10	34
	Na_2PtCl_6	30	0
5	$(NH_4)_2PtCl_6$	30	0
	$(NH_4)_2PtCl_4$	30	18 (L_1)[a]
	Na_2PtCl_6	30	0
6	$(NH_4)_2PtCl_6$	30	0
	$(NH_4)_2PtCl_4$	30	15.5 (L_1)[b]
7	$(NH_4)_2PtCl_6$	30	26
	$(NH_4)_2PtCl_4$	15	30
	Na_2PtCl_6	30	0
8	$(NH_4)_2PtCl_6$	15	29
	$(NH_4)_2PtCl_4$	20	29
	Na_2PtCl_6	20	19
9	$(NH_4)_2PtCl_6$	30	17
	$(NH_4)_2PtCl_4$	30	17
	Na_2PtCl_6	30	0

[a] FEV_1 = forced expiratory volume in 1 s
[b] L_1 = late asthmatic reaction

In addition to the basic immunochemical interest of these findings emphasis is laid upon the value of a simple, though precise, clinical research investigation in obtaining revealing information of this nature. There are almost certainly other examples where studies of a similar nature could be made.

3. Inhalation Tests with Platinum Salts

Simulated occupational exposure tests to the dust from mixtures of low concentrations of platinum salts in lactose (PEPYS et al. 1972 b), decanted repeatedly from one receptacle to another, show the degree of reactivity to different salts with $(NH_4)_2[PtCl_6]$ and $(NH_4)_2[PtCl_4]$ being of similar potency and both more potent than $Na_2[PtCl_6]$ (Table 3) and the reproducibility of reactions to the test procedure

Table 4. Effect of disodium cromoglycate on and reproducibility of inhalation tests – ammonium hexachlorplatinate

Patient	Percentage decrease in FEV_1			Exposure time (min)
	Initial test	Pretreatment with Intal (disodium cromoglycate)	Pretreatment with lactose	
1	38	7.5	41	15
2	28	19	38	4
3	31	7	28.5	6
4	32	0	20.3	10
5	17	0	36	30

(Table 4). The latter also shows that sodium cromoglycate can block this reaction in the same way as it blocks IgE-mediated bronchial reactions to common allergens. This, together with the nature of the skin, nasal, and bronchial reactions suggest that IgE antibodies are present against the platinum salts and this will be discussed later.

Most subjects give immediate asthmatic reactions; some give non-immediate reactions and some give both. There is suggestive evidence of the presence of antibodies in other immunoglobulin classes which might be responsible for type III reactions such as the serum-sickness-like reactions induced by repeated injections of platinum salts (LEVENE and CALNAN 1971).

4. Serological Findings

Reaginic antibodies against platinum complex salts were first shown by passive transfer (Prausnitz–Küstner) of the immediate reactivity to intracutaneous tests in humans by FREEDMAN and KRUPEY (1968). Although suggestive results were obtained in radioallergosorbent tests (RAST) in our laboratories for specific IgE antibodies made with a wide range of platinum conjugates these were regarded as negative (CLEARE et al. 1976). There was difficulty in distinguishing between exposed sensitive subjects and non-exposed subjects.

a) Passive Transfer Tests in Humans and Monkeys

Passive transfer tests with the sera of six sensitive refinery workers were made with unheated serum for IgE, long-term sensitising antibody and with heated serum for short-term sensitising, presumably IgG antibody to prick tests (PEPYS et al. 1979). Table 5 shows positive reactions with all of the unheated sera in one or more of the three human Prausnitz–Küstner recipients and with two and probably three of the sera in Prausnitz–Küstner tests in the monkey. These findings support the possibility of specific IgE antibodies to the platinum salts.

In addition STS-IgG antibodies were shown by the reactions elicited by prick tests at sites passively sensitised with heated serum and tested within 2 h, in one of three human recipients and in the monkey. Thus the sensitised donors had both

Table 5. Passive transfer tests. Human and monkey unheated serum $(NH_4)_2PtCl_4$

Subject	Prick test minimum concentration in sensitive donors (g/ml)	Prausnitz–Küstner human prick test 24–48 h (10^{-3} g/ml); wheal diameter (mm)[a]			Prausnitz–Küstner monkey intra-cutaneous test 24 h ($50\,\mu g/10^{-5}$ g/ml) blue diameter (mm)
		A	B	C	
1	10^{-9}	15.0	8.0	8.0	13.0
2	10^{-8}	0	0	7.5[b]	0
3	10^{-6}	0	3.0	0	6
4	10^{-5}	8.0	10.5	9.0	0
5	10^{-5}	2.5	6.0	5.0	$\pm$
6	10^{-3}	2.0	2.0	0	0

[a] Serum IgE concentrations: A 640; B normal range; C 45 IU/ml
[b] Slow reaction – maximum 25 min

Table 6. RAST values–platinum salt conjugates: total IgE. A, B Sepharose/HSAPt; C Sepharose HSA/Pt

Compound	RAST quotient (test serum versus cord blood)		
$(NH_4)_2PtCl_4$:HSA (mg:mg)	0.133	0.027	0.036
Pt content of solid phase ($\mu g/mg$)	3.29	0.64	0.55
Mean RAST count for eight cord sera $\pm$ standard deviation (ct/min) (total IgE all 8 IU/ml)	$2,505\pm18.9$	$1,594\pm91.3$	$2,114\pm94.8$
IgE (IU/ml)	A	B	C
9,000	1.54	1.72	1.52
6,400	1.39	1.25	1.01
5,000	1.71	1.45	1.31
4,600	1.53	1.44	1.05
4,111	1.27	1.42	0.96
2,320	1.16	1.17	1.02
1,000	1.31	1.20	0.98
603	1.36	1.36	1.02
377	1.15	1.21	0.80
235	1.08	1.13	0.80

specific IgG and STS-IgG against the platinum salts. Challenge with platinum salts of whole blood and washed leucocytes resulted in significant release of histamine in most cases.

b) RAST for IgE Antibodies

The previous problems with the RAST against platinum conjugates were found to be due largely to non-specific reactivity of the conjugates with immunoglobulins (CROMWELL et al. 1979). This was particularly evident with the sera from patients with allergic aspergillosis, which contain high levels of total IgE.

Two main forms of conjugate were compared. The first was made by conjugating the platinum salt with human serum albumin and then linking this to the solid phase, i.e. Sepharose/HSAPt. The second consisted of linking the HSA to the solid phase and then conjugating the platinum salt with this, i.e. Sepharose HSA/Pt. Table 6 shows that, in a comparison of the RAST on cord blood sera and on control sera from subjects with high levels of total IgE and not exposed to platinum salts, two preparations of Sepharose/HSAPt conjugates gave ratios greater than unity, indicating non-specific uptake of IgE. The Sepharose HSA/Pt conjugate gave values around unity, except for sera with the highest total IgE levels.

RAST with the Sepharose HSA/Pt conjugate gave positive results in most exposed subjects with positive skin tests. Negative results in some of this group are attributable to cessation of exposure some time before the serum was taken for testing, and evidence was obtained of falls in total and specific IgE when exposure ceased (Pepys et al. 1979).

These findings confirm the suggestion that immediate reactions to appropriate concentrations of platinum complex salts are mediated by specific IgE antibody, possibly with a contribution by STS-IgG antibody in some cases. They also illustrate some of the problems of serological tests with highly reactive small molecular chemical compounds.

II. Nickel Sulphate

Nickel sensitivity is a common cause of contact dermatitis mediated by type IV allergy. Respiratory allergy with pulmonary infiltrations has been reported by Arvidsson and Bogg (1959) and Sunderman and Sunderman (1961). Asthma caused by inhalation of nickel sulphate, $NiSO_4 \cdot 6H_2O$ (molecular weight 262.85 daltons) has been reported by McConnell et al. (1973). There was indirect evidence of circulating antibodies and immediate type I skin test reactions were elicited by a scratch test with the $NiSO_4$ solution and delayed type IV reactions were given to a patch test. A bronchial provocation test with a solution of nickel sulphate provoked an immediate and prolonged asthmatic reaction.

III. Allergy to Potassium and Sodium Persulphate

Hairdressers exposed to hair bleaches containing potassium persulphate to which H_2O_2 was added can develop allergic respiratory disease (Pepys et al. 1976). In one of two such patients, an atopic subject, the application of the persulphates in 0.1%–5% solutions to unbroken skin gave an immediate whealing reaction which took 60–90 s to develop, in contrast to the 10–20 s taken for the onset of immediate reactions to extracts of common allergens. An exposure with mixing of the bleach to a paste with hydrogen peroxide in a pestle and mortar, simulating the exposure at work, was followed by an acute immediate asthmatic reaction. The skin and bronchial reactions are very suggestive of type I IgE-mediated reactions; antibodies have not as yet been sought.

In the second patient, a non-atopic subject, there were no skin reactions. The simulated occupational exposure elicited a non-immediate reaction which was inhibited by pretreatment with inhaled beclomethasone dipropionate. This corresponds to the inhibitory effect of corticosteroids on non-immediate asthmatic reactions to common allergens (PEPYS and HUTCHCROFT 1975).

In some of these, for example, in allergic bronchopulmonary aspergillosis there is evidence to support a type III reaction (PEPYS 1977 b). No skin reactions were elicited in either of the two subjects with other oxidizing agents such as potassium permanganate, potassium chlorate, sodium perchlorate, and potassium sulphate. Ammonium persulphate has also been reported to cause urticaria and dermatitis, giving both immediate and non-immediate skin test reactions (CALNAN and SHUSTER 1963).

C. Chemical Organic Dusts

A wide range of chemical organic dusts encountered at work and in the pharmaceutical industry can cause allergic respiratory disease. There is at present no discernible well-connected chemical similarity between these and they will therefore be discussed separately.

I. Amprolium Hydrochloride

Amprolium Hydrochloride, $C_{14}H_{19}ClNH_4HCl$ is of low molecular weight, 315.25 daltons. It is a white, odourless substance, readily soluble in water. It is a thiamine antagonist and is used in poultry feeds to prevent coccidioidomycosis.

Occupational exposure to dusty atmospheres containing amprolium hydrochloride has been reported as a cause of asthma and confirmed by simulated occupational provocation tests by GREENE and FREEDMAN (1976). The asthmatic reaction was immediate and suggestive of type I allergy. It dissociates to give positively charged "amprolium" and chloride ions, the latter possibly acting as leaving ligands, and in this sense perhaps comparable to the role of chloride ligands in the allergenicity of the platinum halide complex salts.

II. Chloramine-T

Chloramine-T, $CH_3 \cdot C_6H_4 \cdot SO_2 \cdot NClNa$, benzene sulphonamide N-chloro-4-methyl sodium salt (molecular weight 281.7 daltons), has many commercial names. It can react with amino acids in the gut with the probable formation of toxic cyanogen compounds (SERIN 1949). It is highly reactive, being widely used for the radiolabelling of proteins. It exerts its effects as an oxidising agent, releasing chlorine which is the leaving ligand.

Allergic sensitivity to it was first reported by FEINBERG and WATROUS (1945), who elicited positive reactions to scratch tests in sensitised pharmaceutical workers. Rhinitis and asthma in subjects exposed to it as a sterilising agent is reported by BOURNE et al. (1979). They elicited positive type I reactions to skin prick tests with unconjugated materials.

The possible role, in allergenic potency for eliciting reactions, of the leaving chlorine ligands needs to be examined here, as has been done with the halide complex platinum salts (see Sect. B.I) and as also seems indicated for amprolium hydrochloride (see Sect. C.I).

III. Piperazine Hydrochloride

Piperazine hydrochloride is produced by conversion of piperazine hydrate with hydrochloric acid. The dry solid product is broken up, then milled and sieved. Piperazine products may be present in the air as vapours or as dust.

Two industrial chemists suffering from non-immediate rhinitis and asthma on exposure gave similar reactions to a simulated occupational provocation test (PEPYS et al. 1972c). These reactions were inhibited by inhalation of sodium cromoglycate. The slow development of reactions in these cases may make it difficult to identify the causal exposure and the provocation tests are therefore of great value. Cutaneous and respiratory sensitivity to piperazine products was reported from many factories by McCULLAGH (1968).

IV. Antibiotic Dusts: Ampicillin, Benzylpenicillin, 6-Aminopenicillanic Acid and Related Substances

Sensitisation of workers engaged in the manufacture of antibiotics by the preparations which may be present in the air is not uncommon.

In the investigation of asthma in workers making antibiotics it is necessary to identify the causal allergen or allergens amongst the complex mixture of substances to which they are exposed. Simulated occupational tests with dust-containing atmospheres of the different agents show a high degree of specific identification of the aetiological cause, though much time may be needed for careful clinical studies under controlled conditions. The findings in individual patients will be described in response to tests with: two commercial ampicillin preparations used for treatment, one prepared with the use of *Escherichia coli* amidase enzyme and the other without; *E. coli* amidase itself; commercial 6-aminopenicillanic acid (6-APA); purified 6-APA and ampicillin prepared by an absorption process to remove high molecular weight impurities; commercial benzylpencillin; benzylpenicilloylpolylysine.

6-Aminopenicillanic acid, 6-amino-3,3-dimethyl-7-oxo-4-thia-1-azabicyclo [3.2.0]heptane-2-carboxylic acid, $C_8H_2N_2O_3S$, (molecular weight 216 daltons), is the nucleus of penicillin to which side chains are added for the manufacture of benzylpencillin and ampicillin. Ampicillin, D-(2-aminophenylacetomido)-3,3-dimethyl-7-oxo-4-thia-1-azabicyclo[3.2.0]heptane-2-carboxylic acid, $C_{16}H_{19}N_3O_4S$, (molecular weight 349.42 daltons), prepared by linking phenylglycine to the 6-APA nucleus. Phenylglycine acid chloride is itself a recognised inhalant allergen and affected subjects have given immediate skin and asthmatic reactions and their sera also gave positive Prausnitz-Küstner reactions (KAMMERMEYER and MATTHEWS 1973).

Individual patients will be discussed to illustrate the specificity of their sensitivities, for which they provide valuable models for other such studies (DAVIES et al. 1974). The test method consisted of simulated occupational exposure to atmospheric dusts of the particular agents.

Patient 1. Tests with commercial ampicillin in its purified form and its *E. coli* amidase prepared form, elicited identical strong non-immediate asthmatic reactions coming on after 3–4 h, maximal at 7–11 h, resolving in 24 h and blocked by corticosteroid in the form of inhaled beclomethasone dipropionate. The commercial and purified 6-APA preparations also elicited identical asthmatic reactions, which were however less vigorous than the ampicillin reactions, coming on after about 10 h, maximal at 16 h and resolving within 24 h.

The 6-APA nucleus is converted into ampicillin by the linking of phenylglycine acid chloride, and the latter appears in this case to be of major, though not exclusive, allergenic importance. No reactions were given to benzylpenicilloylpolylysine.

Patient 2. This subject gave non-immediate asthmatic reactions, coming on after 2–3 h, maximal at about 4 h and resolving within 10 h, to the two commercial preparations of ampicillin but unlike Patient 1 gave no reaction to the purified ampicillin. Tests with commercial 6-APA gave a very similar non-immediate reaction to the commercial ampicillin and once again, as with the ampicillin, no reaction was given to the purified form. A positive reaction was also elicited with commercial benzylpencillin, but not with purified material which was tested to see if this would also show evidence for a role of an impurity present in both 6-APA and ampicillin. Thus in this patient the allergenic determinants were not in the 6-APA or ampicillin (as in Patient 1), but in an impurity. Tests with the 6-APA protein impurities and with *E. coli* amidase extract gave no reactions. The identity of the reacting impurity is not known, and without the use of precise exposure tests, this information on its presence would not have been available. There were no reactions to benzylpenicilloyl-polylysine.

Patient 3. Positive asthmatic reactions were given by both purified and commercial ampicillin, and to purified and commercial benzylpencillin. No reaction was given to the 6-APA preparations. This would suggest that the subject was sensitive to both benzylpencillin and to ampicillin or that antigenic determinants common to both were present but not demonstrable in the 6-APA.

Patient 4. This patient was working in another antibiotic factory, making the macrolide antibiotic, spiramycin (Davies and Pepys 1975). There are three different components in this, spiramycin I, $C_{43}H_{74}N_2O_{14}$ (R = H); spiramycin II, $C_{45}H_{67}N_2O_{15}$ (R = COCH$_3$); and spiramycin III, $C_{46}H_{78}N_2O_{15}$ (R = COCH$_2$CH$_3$). Non-immediate asthmatic reactions were elicited, coming on after about 3 h, maximal at 5 h and resolving in about 24 h. The symptoms improved when he left the factory, but only cleared completely when his wife, a clerk there, also left.

Tests with individual components of such materials, if available in pure form, might add to the specificity of aetiological identification.

Oral Challenge of Sensitised Workers. In view of the possible future importance of antibiotics should these subjects need them for treatment, tests were made with the usual treatment preparations given by mouth. Patient 1 gave no reaction to two capsules of 500 mg ampicillin; patient 2 gave a non-immediate asthmatic reaction to two capsules of 500 mg ampicillin identical to that elicited by the inhalation test. This was accompanied by diarrhoea and colic within 1 h of administration lasting for 10 h. The gastrointestinal reaction is presumably allergic as well. Patient 3 gave a non-immediate asthmatic reaction, identical to the inhalation test, on taking two capsules of 500 mg benzylpenicillin. This started after 1 h and was accompanied by extensive urticaria, the latter presumably allergic as well. Patient 4 reported back after some months with recurrences of symptoms on visiting a friend who worked in the same factory and also on eating eggs. Spiramycin is used for egg-laying poultry and is present in minute amounts in the egg white (1 Part/10^6) (Yoshida et al. 1971), and presumably this was responsible.

The inhalation tests must be accompanied by swallowing of some of the material and this could contribute to reactions. Among the many points illustrated by these findings and particularly relevant to drug allergy, is the differences in the causal agents affecting different subjects and otherwise inlikely to be identified without provocation tests. Antibodies were not sought in these cases and it would clearly be desirable to have serological test to replace the time-consuming and costly inhalation test procedure, which, however, would still be required for confirmation where there is doubt and because of its high precision.

V. Salbutamol

Salbutamol is a selective β_2-adrenoceptor stimulant and whilst there are no reports of allergic reactions to it, a worker engaged in its manufacture has been found to be sensitive to an intermediate product and not to the precursors or final product (FAWCETT et al. 1976).

The stages in the production of salbutamol are as follows: the starting material is "diacetate", 4'-hydroxy-3'-hydroxymethylacetophenone diacetate which is a waxy powder and a series of reactions produces in turn "glycyl compound", 2-(N-benzyl-N-tert-butylamino)-4'-hydroxy-3'-hydroxymethylacetophenone diacetate, then "benzyl compound", 2-(N-benzyl-tert-butylamine)-4'-hydroxy-3'-hydroxy-methylacetophenone hydrochloride and finally salbutamol, α-tert-butyla-minomethyl-4-hydroxy-m-xylene-α,α'-diol.

High precision of the simulated occupational exposure test is shown in this case, where no reactions were given to the "diacetate" or the salbutamol, and a vigorous non-immediate reaction was given to the "glycyl compound", with a weak reaction to its successor, the "benzyl compound". The reaction to the latter could be due to some structural antigenic similarly or to carry-over of some "glycyl compound" from the previous stage.

VI. Azo and Anthraquinone Dyes

The low molecular weight dye molecules contain a chromophoric system, usually of the azo or anthroquinone, hydrophilic groups for water solubility and reactive groups, such as a heterocyclic halogen or an alphatic chain with reactive sites. The reactive groups can form covalent bonds with hydroxy and amino groups.

Respiratory allergy has been reported in workers exposed to such dyes, e.g. Levafix brilliant yellow E-36; Drimaren brilliant yellow K3GL; Drimaren brilliant blue K-BL; Civacrom Pront scarlet 3R (ALANKO et al. 1978). Scratch and inhalation tests with unconjugated dyes gave immediate, type I reactions and specific IgE antibodies were demonstrable using paper discs which had been dyed with the praticular dyes, without other conjugation, as the solid phase immunosorbent.

D. Organic Chemical Fumes and Vapours

Attempts are made to establish acceptable atmospheric concentrations, so-called threshold limit values (TVL) of chemical fumes and vapours in industry in order to prevent or reduce sensitisation. Such sensitisation may be induced by small amounts. In sensitised subjects, however, minute and often extremely minute amounts can elicit reactions. Examples of a number of these will be discussed.

I. Aminoethylethanolamine

Asthma can be caused by the fumes of aminoethylethanolamine (1-[(2-amino-ethyl)amino]-2-propanol-N-(2-hydroxypropyl)ethylenediamine, $CH_3CH(OH)CH_2NHCH_2CH_2NH_2$, molecular weight 118.18 daltons). It is used in aluminium soldering flux and such reactions were first reported by STERLING (1967). A ban has been placed on its use in the United Kingdom. In the investigation of three cases (PEPYS and PICKERING 1972) simulated occupational exposure to as few as one to six inhalations of the fumes gave dual, immediate followed by non-immediate, asthmatic reactions in two subjects and a non-immediate reaction in the third. The immediate reactions were blocked by sodium cromoglycate.

The reactions elicited were of the same nature as those elicited by common allergens in sensitive subjects, suggesting that similar antibody mechanisms, yet to be sought, are probably involved.

II. Diisocyanates

This group of reactive chemicals of low molecular weight and in particular toluene diisocyanate (TDI), $C_9H_6N_2O_2$, molecular weight 174.15 daltons), is widely used in the manufacture of plastics, foams and paints. Like so many of the reactive chemicals so far discussed, TDI is an irritant, in this case at atmospheric concentrations greater than 0.05 parts/10^6 (HENSCHLER et al. 1962). Like them too it is also a potent sensitiser and, in sensitised subjects suffering mainly from asthma, minute smounts suffice to elicit the different patterns of astmatic reaction. The first report of asthma due to TDI was made by FUCHS and VALADE in 1951, and this problem is now widely recognised (BRUGHSCH and ELKINS 1963; GLASS and THOM 1964; MARKHAM and FISHBURN 1967; PAISLEY 1969; PETERS and MURPHY 1971; US DEPARTMENT of HEALTH, EDUCATION, and WELFARE 1973; VAN ERT and BATIGELLI 1975; BUTCHER et al. 1977; DAVIES et al. 1977; O'BRIEN et al. 1979 a, b).

Tests for the aetiological diagnosis of TDI sensitivity were made possible by the introduction of a simulated occupational exposure to gaseous emanations from the use of the appropriate TDI preparations such as paints or varnishes, from the fumes of heated polyurethane materials containing TDI or of the other diisocyanates themselves where heat is required to cause volatilisation (PEPYS et al. 1972 a; CARROLL et al. 1976; FAWCETT et al. 1977; O'BRIEN et al. 1979 a, b). In these tests atmospheric concentrations of 0.001 parts/10^6 or less are created and inhalation in most cases for 30 min is sufficient, except where clinical findings or ventilatory tests show that a reaction has begun before this time. Measurement of the atmospheric concentration of TDI is made with a model 700 UEI monitor (Universal Environmental Instrument, Ltd., Polde, Dorset) and has been compared with readings from a personal monitor sampling air 10–15 cm from the subject's mouth. A high correlation (0.9539) was obtained. The asthmatic reactions elicited can be immediate, starting within about 10 min and blocked by sodium cromoglycate, or may start after about 1 h and resolve within 5 h, start after 3–4 h and last about 24 h, or may occur in the early hours of the morning after the test and may recur for many nights thereafter at the same time following a single test exposure. Nocturnal recurrent reactions of this type have been observed with a variety of other agents (NEWMAN-TAYLOR et al. 1979). Non-immediate reactions may also be blocked by sodium cromoglycate, but may require repeated 3-hourly administration. Combination of these patterns of reaction occur and their recognition may help to explain the patterns of responses to chemical agents in other organs.

Sensitisation may be produced by non-occupational environmental exposure. For example, three subjects were shown to be TDI sensitive by the simulated occupational test, where the causal exposure was from the exhaust fumes from an adjoining factory which had been sucked into the ventilating system of their warehouse. TDI was found in the air filters (CARROLL et al. 1976). Sensitisation at home by two-can "do it yourself" polyurethane–TDI foam aerosol cans (PETERS and MURPHY 1971) and other forms of domestic exposure have been reported. Patients of this sort would, in the absence of histories of sensitivity or reactions to the common allergens, and the adult (late) onset of their asthma, be classified as having cryptogenic (intrinsic) asthma. The extent to which sensitivity of this sort to chemical environmental pollutants may be responsible for some cases of cryptogenic asthma will obviously need to be determined.

1. Reactions to Diisocyanates Other than TDI

It can be difficult to know whether workers are exposed to one or more of the diisocyanates, thus creating problems in terms of possible cross-reactivity. In a study of such workers with respiratory diseases, of those reacting to TDI one-half also reacted to diphenylmethane diisocyanate (MDI), molecular weight 250.13 daltons. One-third of the subjects also reacted to hexamethylene diisocyanate (HDI), molecular weight 168 daltons. Less volatile diisocyanates such as MDI, which requires heating for the test, are being tried as substitutes for TDI, but respiratory disease has been reported with MDI (LONGLEY 1964; MUNN 1965; TANSER et al. 1973), and although it is considered safer this may not apply in terms of eliciting reactions in subjects already sensitive to TDI. We have, however, found three workers exposed and reacting only to naphthalene diisocyanate (molecular weight 210 daltons). Precise knowledge of the purity of the diisocyanates used and of the actual exposures of workers is needed for better assessment of possible cross-reactivity.

2. Modes of Action of TDI

It has been found that TDI acts as a β-adrenoceptor blocking agent, inhibiting the isoprenaline-induced increase of 3,5-cyclic AMP (DAVIES et al. 1977).

Tolyl-specific IgE antibodies have now however also been demonstrated in exposed sensitive workers by KAROL et al. (1978a; KAROL and ALARIE 1980). p-Tolyl(mono)isocyanate was coupled with human serum albumin for the paper (disc) radioimmunosorbent test (PRIST). There was no correlation between high titres of tolyl-specific IgE antibodies and levels of total serum IgE, in contrast to the findings with the platinum salts described earlier in which non-specific uptake of IgE could occur. The level of tolyl-specific antibodies decreased with cessation of exposure, as was the case with the platinum salts. The use of the monofunctional isocyanate prevented cross-linking of the carrier proteins which usually occurs with TDI, and ensured that the tolyl group was sterically exposed. The tolyl specificity of the IgE antibodies was confirmed by hapten inhibition and by the use of two antigens, both containing tolyl groups in tests on TDI-sensitive workers (KAROL and ALARIE 1980). One of the antigens, formed by reaction of p-tolylisocyanate with human serum albumin, to give p-tolylureido–human serum albumin, gave positive results and the majority of the sera gave positive results to the second antigen, a p-tolylchloro–human serum albumin complex to give p-tolylamino–human serum albumin which lacked isocyanate linkages. It is suggested that tolyl isocyanate coupled to a synthetic polypeptide might given even better results. The TDI-sensitive subjects also had small amounts of IgE antibody to human serum albumin, suggesting that the denatured TDI–human serum albumin conjugates formed in vivo were also antigenic in vivo.

These demonstrations of specific IgE antibodies will in all probability be matched by demonstration of specific IgG antibodies. Together with earlier immunological evidence suggestive of the presence of reaginic and complement-fixing antibodies in exposed workers (TAYLOR 1970), of lymphocyte transformation to a TDI-conjugated protein (AVERY et al. 1969) and of TDI antibodies in rabbits after prolonged inhalation (SCHEEL et al. 1964) all point towards allergic mechanisms in TDI sensitivity. The patterns of reaction to provocation tests and their responses to sodium cromoglycate are comparable to those elicited by common allergens, where there are long-standing immunological findings, and these findings also justify the assumption in the absence, at that time, of reproducible immunological findings, that the clinical reactions could have an immunological pathogenesis (PEPYS et al. 1972a). Participation together of immunological and non-immunological mechanisms is also very likely.

3. Antibodies to Other Diisocyanates

In two sensitised workers exposed to diphenylmethane diisocyanate (MDI), used for coating pipes with a polyurethane foam, tests with an MDI–human serum albumin conjugate showed the presence of specific IgE antibodies as measured by polystyrene tube radioimmunoassay (PTRIA) procedures (ZEISS et al. 1979). High levels of specific IgG antibody were found, with some cross-reactivity with a TDI–human serum albumin conjugate. The serum of one of the workers gave a positive precipitin reaction in the double diffusion test in gel. The authors suggest that these antibodies may be related to the respiratory reactions to the inhaled chemical.

III. Epoxy Resin System Activating Agents

A large number of small molecular reactive chemicals are used in epoxy resin systems and a number have already been found to be sensitising agents. Provocation testing of the occupational type has identified specific agents, such as phthalic anhydride, o-benzenedicarboxylic acid anhydride ($C_8H_4O_3$, molecular weight 148.11 daltons); trimellitic anhydride (1,2,4-benzenetricarboxylic acid 1,2,4-tricarboxybenzene, $C_9H_6O_6$, molecular weight 210.14 daltons); and triethylenetetramine ($C_5H_{16}N_4$ molecular weight 146.24 daltons; FAWCETT et al. 1977) and antibodies have also already been demonstrated against phthalic anhydride (MACCIA et al. 1976) and against trimellitic anhydride (ZEISS et al. 1977).

The basic components of the epoxy resin systems are the uncured resin and a curing agent or hardener. The resins vary in composition, but all are long chain polymers commonly produced as condensation products of epichlorohydrin and bisphenol A. They vary from low viscosity liquids to solids, depending on molecular weight. The resins, relatively stable in themselves, contain terminal reactive epoxy groups and side chain hydroxyl groups. The resins are converted to hard solids by the addition of a curing agent or hardener. External heat is needed in some, commonly those using acid anhydrides, or cold curing is used, notably with amine compounds. During the curing process fumes of resins and curing agents are emitted (MALTEN and ZIELHUIS 1964; LEE and NEVILLE 1967). The epoxy resin systems are among the most important causes of industrial contact dermatitis. The uncured resin is the commonest cause but curing agents or even the cured resin may cause dermatitis (BOURNE et al. 1959; FISHER 1973; GRANDJEAN 1957; MALTEN and ZIELHUIS 1964; RYCROFT and CALNAN 1976).

Asthma due to exposure to ethylene amines in manufacture has been reported by DERNEHL (1951), and after exposure to aliphatic polyamine or epoxy resin curing agents (DERNEHL 1963). Phthalic anhydride, often used in hot curing systems, is a recognised irritant of the respiratory tract and asthma has been reported (AMERICAN INDUSTRIAL HYGIENE ASSOCIATION JOURNAL 1967; MALTEN and ZIELHUIS 1964; PETIT et al. 1961).

In six patients exposed to epoxy resin curing agents (FAWCETT et al. 1977) reactions were elicited in one subject to triethylene tetramine fumes arising from painting with it, which elicited a non-immediate asthmatic reaction. This required a 2-h test exposure, much longer than for other simulated occupational exposure tests; four subjects reacted to phthalic anhydride, giving immediate or dual reactions in three cases to the fumes and, in one case, to as little as one breath of the fumes from heating epoxy resin prepared with phthalic anhydride. Another less sensitive subject reacted to the fumes from heated phthalic anhydride crystals and, in the third and least sensitive of the three, to inhalation of a dust "cloud" of phthalic anhydride; another subject working with epoxy resins prepared with trimellitic acid gave a dual reaction to one breath of fumes from heated resin. The patterns of asthmatic reaction elicited were once again comparable to those elicited by common allergens and the minute doses required to elicit them suggest that they are of an immunological nature.

1. Phthalic Anhydride-Specific IgE Antibodies

In a subject with rhinitis, conjunctivitis and asthma due to phthalic anhydride and giving immediate skin and bronchial reactions to appropriate solutions, MACCIA et al. (1976) have obtained a positive RAST for specific IgE antibodies to a conjugate of phthalic anhydride and bovine serum albumin. Passive transfer of skin test sensitivity to phthalic anhydride has been reported (KERN 1939), and lymphocyte transformation has also been reported (GERVAIS et al. 1972).

The reactions to phthalic anhydride are attributed to its possession, as with other chemical agents causing allergic reactions, of highly reactive sites capable of conjugating with proteins. MACCIA et al. (1976) claim that phthalic anhydride has a chemical structure which has this property, because the anhydride forms an in-side linkage with amino groups of the protein to give stable conjugates, whereas unconjugated material was necessary for the RAST.

2. Trimellitic Acid-Specific IgE and IgG Antibodies

In workers exposed to trimellitic acid and suffering from rhinitis and immediate and non-immediate asthma, the latter together with systemic symptoms, ZEISS et al. (1977) have demonstrated the presence of specific IgE and IgG antibodies to a hapten–human serum albumin conjugate. The late asthmatic and systemic symptoms, consisting of malaise, chills, fever, and myalgia (TMA-'flu) were associated with specific IgG antibody. Other positive immunological findings, such as skin tests, lymphocyte transformation, leucocyte histamine release, the presence of rheumatoid factor and passive cutaneous anaphylaxis (PCA) tests in the monkey were also obtained. Trimellitic acid anhydride like phthalic anhydride, is a simple, but biologically reactive chemical.

IV. Miscellaneous Agents

As can be seen from the foregoing discussion, the list of chemical agents capable of sensitisation of the respiratory tract at work and also in the ordinary environment is extensive and certain to be extended even further. Several causes will be cited only briefly to bring attention to them and not because they are of less importance or of less basic immunochemical interest. Amongst these are: sensitisation to the fumes of formaldehyde causing asthma, in contrast to the well-known contact dermatitis (POPA et al. 1969; HENDRICK and LANE 1975), sensitisation to fumes from pyrolysis products of polyvinyl chloride encountered in the wrapping and sealing of meat with the production of immediate asthmatic reactions (SOKOL et al. 1973; ANDRASCH et al. 1975), sensitisation has been reported to ethylenediamine, used as an accelerator in the rubber industry and a solvent in the laquer industry, with type I skin test and Prausnitz–Küstner reactions and immediate asthmatic reactions, and also to monoethanolamine (GELFAND 1963); sensitisation to paraphenylenediamine with immediate and non-immediate asthmatic reactions has been reported (SHILKRET and SWARTZ 1942; SILBERMAN and SORRELL 1959). Asthma in nurses and factory workers handling sulphathiazole as a powder has been described (ROSBERG 1946; SEEBERG 1944).

Finally, small molecular organic acids from vegetable materials have been found, or are thought to be responsible for respiratory sensitisation. Amongst these are; chlorogenic acid from green coffee beans (BARIANA et al. 1965), plicatic acid from Western Red Cedar (CHANG-YEUNG et al. 1973) abietic acid in colophony, pine resin, widely used in soldering processes in the electronics industry, the fumes of which are a potent cause of respiratory sensitisation (FAWCETT et al. 1976; BURGE et al. 1978).

E. General Comments

The direct clinical interest in specific aetiological diagnosis in respiratory allergy of small chemical molecules is supplemented by the better understanding of asthma from the patterns of reaction elicited in testing. The basic immunochemical interest in chemical well-defined haptens is facilitated by the known exposures and the ethical acceptability and indeed desirability of re-exposure to suspected agents under controlled conditions. The possibilities of chemical modifications of the particular agents for further clinical and laboratory study can yield information otherwise difficult to obtain, thus providing invaluable opportunities for clinical research in this field.

References

Alanko K, Keskinen H, Bjorksten F, Oganen S (1978) Immediate type hypersensitivity to reactive dyes. Clin Allergy 8:25–31

American Industrial Hygiene Association Journal (1967) Phthalic anhydride. Hygiene Guide Series July/August, 295

Andrasch RH, Koster F, Lawson WH, Bardana EJ (1975) Meatwrapper's asthma – an appraisal of a new occupational syndrome. J Allergy Clin Immunol 55:130

Arvidsson J, Bogg A (1959) Transitory pulmonary infiltrations Loefflers syndrome – in acute generalized dermatitis. Acta Derm Venereol (Stockh) 39:30–34

Avery SB, Stetson DM, Pan PM, Matthews KP (1969) Immunological investigation of individuals with toluene di-isocyanate asthma. Clin Exp Immunol 4:585–596

Bariana DS, Krupey J, Scarpati LM, Freedman SO, Sehon AH (1965) Chlorogenic acid: further evidence for its antigenic and allergic activity. Nature 207:1155–1157

Basolo F, Gray HB, Pearson RG (1960) Mechanism of substitution reactions of complex ions. XVII. Rates of react on some platinums (II) complexes with pyridoxine. J Am Chem Soc 82:4200–4203

Belluco U, Ettorre R, Basolo F, Pearson RG, Turco A (1966) Activation parameters for some substitution reactions of acidodiethylenetriamineplatinum (II) complexes. Inorg Chem 5:591–593

Bijl WJF (1963) Asthma als Berufskrankheit Allergie gegen Platinammoniumchlorid. Allergy Asthma 9:155–157

Bourne LB, Milner FJM, Alberman KB (1959) Health problems of epoxy resins and amine curing agents. Br J Ind Med 16:81–97

Bourne MS, Flindt MIH, Miles Walker J (1979) Asthma due to industrial use of chloramine. Br Med J 3:10–12

Brugsch HG, Elkins HB (1963) Toluene di-isocyanate (TDI) toxicity. N Engl J Med 268:353–357

Burge PS, Harries MG, O'Brien IM, Pepys J (1978) Respiratory disease in workers exposed to solder flux fumes containing colophony (pine resin). Clin Allergy 8:1–14

Butcher BT, Salvaggio JE, O'Neill CE, Weill H, Garg O (1977) Toluene di-isocyanate pulmonary disease: immunopharmacologic and mecholyl challenge studies. J Allergy Clin Immunol 59:223–227

Calnan CD, Shuster S (1963) Reactions to ammonium persulphate. Arch Dermatol 88:812–815

Carroll KB, Secombe CJP, Pepys J (1976) Asthma due to non-occupational exposure to toluene (tolylene) di-isocyanate. Clin Allergy 6:99–104

Cattalini L, Martelli M (1967) Relazione tra reattivita di complessi planari del platino e natura del grouppo uscente, in reazioni di sostituzione nucleofila. Gazz Chim Ital 97:498–508

Chan-Yeung M (1973) Maximum expiratory flow and airways resistance during induced bronchoconstriction in patients with asthma due to Western Red Cedar (Thuja plicata) Am Rev Respir Dis 108:1103

Chan-Yeung M, Barton GM, Maclean L, Graybowski S (1971) Bronchial reactions to western red cedar (Thuja Plicata). Can Med Assoc J 105:56–58

Cleare MJ, Hughes EG, Jacoby B, Pepys J (1976) Immediate (type 1) allergic response to platinum compounds. Clin Allergy 6:183–195

Cromwell O, Pepys J, Parish WE, Hughes EG (1979) Specific IgE antibodies to platinum salts in sensitized workers. Clin Allergy 9:109–117

Davies RJ, Pepys J (1975) Asthma due to inhaled chemical agents – the macrolide antibiotic spiramycin. Clin Allergy 5:99–108

Davies RJ, Hendrick DJ, Pepys J (1974) Asthma due to inhaled chemical agents: ampicillin, benzyl penicillin, 6 amino-penicillanic acid and related substances. Clin Allergy 4:227–248

Davies RJ, Butcher BT, O'Neill CE, Salvaggio JE (1977) The in vitro effect of toluene di-isocyanate on lymphocyte cyclic adenosine monophosphate production by isoproterenol, prostaglandin and histamine – a possible mode of action. J Allergy Clin Immunol 60:223–229

Dernehl CU (1951) Clinical experiences with exposures to ethylene amines. Ind Med Surg 20:541

Dernehl CU (1963) Hazards to health associated with the use of eopxy resins. J Occup Med 5:17–21

Fawcett IW, Pepys J, Eroaga MA (1976) Asthma due to "glycyl compound" powder – an intermediate in production of salbutamol. Clin Allergy 6:405–409

Fawcett IW, Newman-Taylor ALJ, Pepys J (1977) Asthma due to inhaled chemical agents – epoxy resin systems containing phthalic acid anhydride, trimellitic acid anhydride and triethylene tetramine. Clin Allergy 7:1–14

Feinberg SM, Watrous RM (1945) Atopy to simple chemical compounds, sulfonechloramides. J Allergy 16:209–220

Fisher AA (1980) Contact dermatitis, 2nd edn. Lea & Febiger, Philadelphia, p 180

Freedman SO, Krupey J (1968) Respiratory allergy caused by platinum salts. J Allergy 42:233–237

Fuchs S, Valade P (1951) Etude clinique et experimentale sur quelques cas d'intoxication par le desmodur T (di-isocyanate de toluylene 1-2-4 et 1-2-6). Arch Mal Prof 12:191–196

Gelfand HH (1963) Respiratory allergy due to chemical compounds encountered in the rubber, lacquer, shellac and beauty culture industries. J Allergy 34:374–381

Gervais P, Efthymious ML, Hebert S, Diamant-Berger O (1972) Diagnostic et physiopathologie de l'asthma du a l'anhydride phthalique: interet – du test de transformation lymphoblostique. Eur J Toxicol 2:106–109

Glass WI, Thom NG (1964) Respiratory hazards associated with toluene di-isocyanate in polyurethane foam production. NZ Med J 63:642–647

Grandjean E (1957) The danger of dermatoses due to cold setting ethoyline resins, epoxide resins. Br J Med 14:1–4

Greene SA, Freedman S (1976) Asthma due to inhaled chemical agents – amprolium hydrochloride. Clin Allergy 6:105–108

Hendrick DJ, Lane DJ (1975) Formalin asthma in hospital staff. Br Med J 1:607–608

Henschler D, Assman W, Meyer KO (1962) The toxicology of the toluene di-isocyanates. Arch Toxicol 19:364–387

Hunter D, Milton R Perry KMA (1945) Asthma caused by the complex salts of platinum. Br J Ind Med 2:92–101

Kammermeyer JK, Mathews KP (1973) Hypersensitivity to phenylglycine acid chloride. J Allergy Clin Immunol 52:73–84

Karasek SR, Karasek M (1911) Preliminary report of the injurious effect of metal, platinum, chromates, cyanides, hydrofluoric acid, and of materials used in silvering mirrors. Report the Illinois State Commission on Occupational Disease

Karol MH, Alarie YC (1980) Antigens which detect IgE antibodies in workers sensitive to toluene di-isocyanate. Clin Allergy 10:101

Karol MH, Ioset HH, Alarie YC (1978) Tolyl-specific IgE antibodies in workers with hypersensitivity to toluene di-isocyanate. Am Ind Hyg Assoc J 39:454–458

Kern RA (1939) Asthma and allergic rhinitis due to sensitization to phthalic anhydride – report on a case. J Allergy 10:164

Khan A, Hill JW, Grater W, Loeb E, Machallan A, Hill N (1975) Atopic hypersensitivity to cis-dichloro-diamineplatinum (II) and other platinum complexes. Cancer Res 35:2766–2770

Khan A, Wakasugi K, Hill B, Richardson D, Disabato J, Hill JM (1977) Platinum complexes: immunology and allergy. J Clin Hematol Oncol 7:797–813

Kobayashi S (1974) Occupational asthma due to inhalation of pharmacological dusts and other chemical agents with some reference to other occupational asthma in Japan. In: Yamamura Y, Fick OL, Hariuchi Y, Kishimoto S, Miyamoto T, Naranjo P, De Weck AL (eds) Allergology. Excerpta Medica, Amsterdam

Lee H, Neville K (1967) Handbook of epoxy resins. McGraw-Hill, New York London

Levene GM, Calnan CD (1971) Platinum sensitivity and treatment by specific hyposensitization. Clin Allergy 1:75–82

Longley EO (1964) Methane di-isocyanate: a respiratory hazard. Arch Environ Health 8:898

Maccia CA, Bernstein IL, Emmett EA, Brooks SM (1976) In vitro demonstration of specific IgE in phthalic anhydride hypersensitivity. Am Rev Respir Dis 113:701–704

Malten EKE, Ziehuis RL (1964) Industrial toxicology and dermatology in the production and processing of plastics. Elsevier, Amsterdam Oxford New York

Markham TN, Fishburn CW (1967) Sensitivity to toluene di-isocyanate in an adhesive. J Occup Med 9:471–473

McConnell LH, Fink JN, Schlueter DP, Schmidt MG (1973) Asthma caused by nickel sensitivity. Ann Intern Med 78:888–890

McCullagh SF (1968) Allergenicity of piperazine: a study in environmental allergy. Br J Med 25:319–325

Munn A (1965) Hazards of isocyanates. Ann Occup Hyg 8:163–169

Newman-Taylor AJ, Davies RJ, Hendrick DJ, Pepys J (1979) Recurrent nocturnal asthmatic reactions to bronchial provocation tests. Clin Allergy 9:213–220

O'Brien IM, Harries MG, Burge PS, Pepys J (1979a) Toluene di-isocyanate-induced asthma. 1: Reactions to TDI, MDI, HDI, and histamine. Clin Allergy 9:1–6

O'Brien IM, Newman-Taylor AJ, Burge PS, Harries MG, Fawcett IW, Pepys J (1979b) Toluene di-isocyanate-induced asthma. 2: Inhalation challenge tests and bronchial reactivity studies. Clin Allergy 9:7–15

Paisley DPG (1969) Isocyanate hazard from wire insulation: an old hazard in a new guise. Br J Ind Med 26:79–81

Parish WE (1970) Short-term anaphylactic IgG antibodies in human sera. Lancet 2:591–592

Parrot JL, Saindelle A, Ruff F (1967) Platine et platinose. Liberation – d⁺ histamine par certain sels de platine et allergie au platine. Nouv Presse Med 75:2817–2820

Parrot JL, Hebert R, Saindelle A, Ruff F (1969) Platinum and platinosis: allergy and histamine release due to some platinum salts. Arch Environ Health 19:685–691

Pepys J (1977a) Allergy to platinum compounds. In: Medical and biologic effects of environmental pollutants – platinum group metals. National Research Council. National Academy of Sciences, Medicine and Engineering. Washington, DC, p 105–124

Pepys J (1977b) Clinical and therapeutic significance of patterns of allergic reactions of the lungs to extrinsic agents. Am Rev Respir Dis 116:573–588

Pepys J, Davies RJ (1978) Occupational asthma. In: Allergy, principles and practice, 1st edn. Mosby, St. Louis, Mo

Pepys J, Hutchcroft BJ (1975) Bronchial provocation tests in etiological diagnosis and analysis of asthma. Am Rev Respir Dis 112:829–859

Pepys J, Pickering CAC (1972) Asthma due to inhaled chemical fumes – amino-ethyl ethanolamine aluminium soldering flux. Clin Allergy 2:197–204

Pepys J, Pickering CAC, Breslin ABX, Terry DJ (1972a) Asthma due to inhaled chemical agents – tolylene di-isocyanate. Clin Allergy 2:225–236

Pepys J, Pickering CAC, Hughes EG (1972b) Asthma due to inhaled chemical agents – complex salts of platinum. Clin Allergy 2:391–396

Pepys J, Pickering CAC, London HWG (1972c) Asthma due to inhaled chemical agents – piperazine hydrochloride. Clin Allergy 2:189

Pepys J, Hutchcroft BJ, Breslin ABX (1976) Asthma due to inhaled chemical agents – persulphate salts and henna in hairdressers. Clin Allergy 6:399

Pepys J, Parish WE, Cromwell O, Hughes EG (1979) Passive transfer in man and the monkey of Type I allergy to heat labile and heat stable antibody to complex salts of platinum. Clin Allergy 9:99–108

Peters JM, Murphy RLM (1971) Hazards to health: do it yourself polyurethane foam. Am Rev Respir Dis 104:432–433

Petit JM, Troquet J, Melon J (1961) Influence des resines ethoxylines sur les voies respiratoires. Arch Mal Prof 22:718–725

Pickering CAC (1972) Inhalation tests with chemical allergens: complex salts of platinum. Proc R Soc Med 65:272

Popa V, Teculescu D, Stanescu D, Gavrilescu N (1969) Bronchial asthma and asthmatic bronchitis determined by simple chemicals. Dis Chest 56:395–403

Roberts A (1951) Platinosis – a five year study of the effects of soluble platinum salts on employees in a platinum laboratory and refinery. Arch Ind Health Occup Hyg 4:549–559

Rosberg M (1946) Asthma bronchiale caused by sulfathiazole. Acta Med Scand 126:185–190

Rycroft RJ, Calnan CD (1976) Industrial skin diseases. Br J Hosp Med 15:457–464

Scheel LD, Killens R, Josephson A (1964) Immunochemical aspects of toluene di-isocyanate (TDI) toxicity. Am Ind Hyg Assoc J 25:179–184

Seeberg G (1944) Gewerbekrankheit der Haut bei Sulfathiazolarbeitern. Acta Derm Venereol (Stockh) 24:317

Serin F (1949) Formation of cyanogen compounds from amino-acids as factor in chloramine T poisoning. Acta Pharmacol Toxicol (Copenh) [Suppl] 5:1-12

Shilkret HH, Swartz HF (1942) Studies on hypersensitivity due to substances employed in fur industry significance of cutaneous reactions to fur dye dust extracts. J Allergy 14:538–543

Silberman DE, Sorrell AH (1959) Allergy in fur workers with special reference to paraphyenylenediamine. J Allergy 30:11–18

Sokol WN, Aelong Y, Beall GN (1973) Meatwrapper's asthma: new syndrome? JAMA 226:639–641

Squire JR (1952) Tissue reactions to protein sensitisation. Br Med J 1:1–7

Sterling CM (1967) Asthma due to aluminium soldering flux. Thorax 22:533–537

Sunderman FW, Sunderman FW Jr (1961) Loffler's syndrome associated with nickel sensitivity. Arch Intern Med 107:405–408

Tanser AR, Bourke MP, Blandford AG (1973) Isocyanate asthma: respiratory symptoms caused by diphenyl-methane di-isocyanate. Thorax 28:596–600

Taylor GL (1970) Immuno responses to tolylene di-isocyanate (TDI) exposure in man. Proc R Soc Med 63:379–380

U.S. Department of Health, Education, and Welfare (1973) Occupational exposure to toluene di-isocyanate. U.S. Government Printing Office, Washington, DC

Vallery-Radot L, Blamoutier R (1929) Sensibilisation au chloroplatinite de potassium: accidents graves de choc survenus a la suite d'une cutireaction avec ce sel. Bull Soc Med Hop Paris 45:222–230

Van Ert M, Battigelli MC (1975) Mechanisms of respiratory injury by TDI (Toluene di-isocyanate). Ann Allergy 35:142–147

Yoshida M, Kubota D, Yonezawa S, Nakamura H, Azechi H, Terakado N (1971) Transfer of dietary spiramycin into the eggs and its residue in the liver of laying hens. Jpn Polutry Sci 8:103

Zeiss CR, Patterson R, Pruzansky JJ, Miller MM, Rosenberg M, Levitz D (1977) Trimellitic anhydride-induced airways syndromes: clinical and immunological studies. J Allergy Clin Immunol 60:96–103

Zeiss CLR, Kanellakes T, Bellone J, Levitz D, Pruzansky JJ, Patterson R (1979) IgG and IgE antibody in two workers with diphenylmethane di-isocyanate induced respiratory reactions (Abstr). J Allergy Clin Immunol 63:150

CHAPTER 6

Epidemiology of Drug Allergy: Drug Monitoring

R. Hoigné, F. Stocker, and P. Middleton

A. Introduction

The interval between the initial observation of symptoms and syndromes and the final recognition of a disease entity, with known pathogenesis or aetiology, may be a long one and much careful investigation may be necessary. At one end of the whole procedure is clinical observation and at the other, medical science and epidemiology. This principle also holds true for adverse drug effects and drug-induced illnesses. In any system designed to detect adverse reactions to drugs it is of fundamental importance to observe each syndrome or symptom and to record it, independently of its interpretation (Hoigné 1978). Evaluation can follow two distinct routes: a review of interpreted, individual data, or a statistical analysis of non- or not extensively interpreted events.

A first provisional interpretation involves five important points:

1. The probability of an adverse drug reaction compared with the probabilities of the occurrence of the same reactions from non-drug causes
2. The specific drug involved
3. The severity of the reaction with regard to permanent damage or contribution to a life-threatening reaction
4. The frequency of the reaction compared with the number of patients treated, the number of treatment courses, the duration of treatment, the dosages given and the method of administration
5. The factors related to the patient or to the environment which favour the reaction.

For both the conventional practising physician, with direct patient responsibility, and the pharmacist, a knowledge of clearly established adverse drug reactions and accepted contra-indications is important. With the unprecedented increase in drug information, the risks of many drugs have to be obtained from books, scientific journals and packaging inserts. However, for the drug research orientated physician, clinical pharmacologist, pharmacologist, pharmacist and epidemiologist, not only established and probable adverse reactions, but those which are possible or questionable have to be carefully followed. This group may contain a lot of unimportant reactions, but it may also contain some not yet fully recognised damaging and life-threatening effects. Some currently accepted adverse drug reactions were scarcely recognised for years, or even decades, after the drug had been marketed (e. g. agranulocytosis to amidopyrine; embolic-toxic reactions to penicillin depot preparations; malformations of the newborn due to thalidomide).

A further group of adverse reactions to drugs are those only recognisable by statistical methods, the so-called hidden risks. To establish the relationship, e. g. an increase of the occurrence of a disease or laboratory finding during administration of a specific drug, systematic epidemiological research is necessary.

Whether an adverse drug reaction is of the allergic, the toxic, the idiosyncratic or any other type, may be at first unclear and debatable. The first step is observation, recognition and study of the reaction. Interpretation may take years of research or, it may not be possible at all with the methods currently available.

B. Methods of Epidemiology and Drug Monitoring

Epidemiological methods and drug monitoring of adverse reactions to drugs pursue four different goals (Bruppacher 1979, personal communication):

1. A signal function, if an event (disease, syndrome, mortality rate) increases or shows up under special conditions (Finney 1974; Koch-Weser 1968)
2. A search function, offering the possibility of finding other comparable situations previously observed in the same or in another system of epidemiology or drug monitoring (Finney 1974; Koch-Weser 1968)
3. A review of adverse drug reactions or drug risks by case documentation, scanning lists, tables etc.
4. Statistical monitoring with the possibility of indicating so-called hidden risks.

Usually the methods applied to a drug in the post-marketing phase of a drug are different from those in the pre-marketing period, or the clinical trial. This chapter is concerned with adverse reactions or illnesses induced by drugs which are already on the market.

Experience of drug development, which has taken place principally during the last thirty years, has shown that the number of patients in clinical trials, normally several thousands, will give a fairly good appraisal of the effect of a new drug. However, many adverse reactions and drug-induced illnesses have been observed only after tens, or hundreds, of thousands of patients have been treated with the drug after it has been marketed. Special dispositions in groups of patients, some underlying diseases, drug combinations or a drug in combination with other environmental factors are responsible for this situation. The time lag between the introduction of a new drug and the detection of an adverse effect may be reduced by a variety of epidemiological methods, including drug monitoring.

The methodology employed to study an effect of a drug is normally clearly established, as one knows what has to be looked for throughout the study. In direct contrast, difficulties are encountered with adverse reactions to drugs as it is not known which organ or system will be affected. Also the time from the exposure of the patient to the drug to the appearance of the symptoms may vary from a few seconds to months or years, or the symptoms may not occur until the second generation.

The methods for detecting adverse reactions include a continued clinical trial with a reduced number of clinical and laboratory controls, a kind of post-marketing surveillance (Slone et al. 1979); case-referent studies in which patients with an illness of interest are compared with a group of people without that illness; and a planned cohort study, mostly in the form of a follow-up, in which the choice of drug regimen is dictated by ordinary clinical practice rather than by the criterion of scientific comparison (FRIEDMAN 1974; JICK 1977). These methods are applied mainly to drug-induced diseases or illnesses with the same symptoms as a non-drug counterpart.

Systematic research is also used to study characteristic acute or sometimes chronic side effects and includes inpatient and outpatient monitoring of adverse drug reactions and spontaneous reporting to a collecting centre (FINNEY 1974; WHO 1969). Also the procedure of "record linkage" may be used for drug surveillance. The choice of the method in relation to the problem is of great importance. The system of research should be well designed so as to permit satisfactory retrospective analysis of the data recorded. This involves a considerable amount of forward planning to avoid the situation where either insufficient data have been recorded or certain data have not been recorded at all (FRIEDMANN et al. 1971).

As adverse reactions to drugs with an allergic mechanism are usually observed after relatively short exposure times of a few days to several weeks, inpatient monitoring with close observation of the patient is an especially appropriate method for frequent adverse reactions (HOIGNÉ et al. 1978; MILLER 1973). For rare adverse reactions, methods of spontaneous reporting which involve a much higher number of patients exposed to the drug are necessary (BÖTTIGER and WESTERHOLM 1973; DUNNE 1978; KÖHLER and KIMBEL 1978).

I. Comprehensive Inpatient (Intensive) Drug Monitoring

In comprehensive drug monitoring, all patients are monitored to all drugs which are received during a given time (e. g. the duration of the hospital stay) (ARNDT and JICK 1976; BAUMGARTNER et al. 1982; HURWITZ 1969 a, b; JICK et al. 1970; KLEIN et al. 1976; LAWSON and JICK 1976; MILLER 1973; PORTER and JICK 1977; SHAPIRO et al. 1969; SMITH et al. 1966 b; STREIT 1979; TÖRÖK et al. 1982). The frequency of an adverse reaction to one drug, or a combination of two or more drugs is related to the total number of patients exposed. If the number of drugs administered to each patient is small, ideally only one drug, the frequency of a characteristic adverse reaction can easily be calculated as a percentage of the number of patients treated. If, however, as with inpatients, the number of drugs is about 3–10, and the kind of reaction is not typical of one drug, the frequency of an adverse reaction has to be calculated in accordance with the probabilities given by an Euler–Venn diagram (Sect. B.I.1) or by weighted attributions (ARNDT and JICK 1976) (Sect. B.I.2).

1. Euler-Venn Diagram[1]

An example of the application of Euler–Venn diagrams is the occurrence of maculopapular rashes in patients of the Comprehensive Hospital Drug Monitoring, Bern (CHDMB) (1974–1976 Zieglerspital, Bern, 1976 Anna-Seiler-Haus, Inselspital, Bern). Only inpatients and the drugs given during the whole of their stay

---

[1] Prof. H. RIEDWYL, Director of the Institute for Mathematical Statistics, University of Bern and Dr. phil. nat. M. DOZZI were kind enough to be consultants for this section

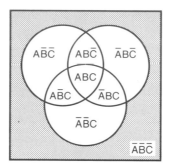

Fig. 1. Euler–Venn diagram of the occurrence of patients with maculopapular rashes. Explanation of symbols: A = ampicillin, B = other penicillins, C = cotrimoxazole or sulphonamides alone. Patients treated with drug A but not with drugs B and C are represented by $A\bar{B}\bar{C}$. Patients treated with drugs excluding drug groups A, B and C are represented by the dotted area. Each patient is represented only in one area of the diagram, even if more than one maculopapular rash occurred

at the hospital or the last seven days before the appearance of the exanthema were considered.

Table 1 gives the frequencies of rash in relation to the drug groups given to these patients. In Fig. 1, the patients are classified according to the three groups of drugs most often found in relation to the appearance of a maculopapular rash: ampicillin, other penicillins, and cotrimoxazole or sulphonamides alone.

In patients exposed to drugs outside of these three drug groups, maculopapular exanthema was observed in only 1.21% (35/2891). In the combination of cotrimoxazole with other penicillins and of all three drug groups, the small number of observations does not permit any conclusion.

That the frequencies of occurrence of a rash (Table 1) are too high is caused by two different errors. The first error is due to the fact that each drug given during the whole hospital stay is considered. This can be corrected by different approaches. The principle followed here is to reduce the exposures to the drugs to the time before the maculopapular rash occurred and to limit the time after exposure to 7 days (FLEISS 1973; SHAPIRO et al. 1969). For this calculation all patients receiving the drug A, B, or C were considered (the area of each whole circle in the Euler–Venn diagram; Fig. 1). In the case of ampicillin-treated patients (A), for example, the total number exposed ($A\bar{B}\bar{C} + AB\bar{C} + A\bar{B}C + ABC$) is 724, and the number with adverse reactions is 101.

Table 1. Frequency of rash in adult patients in relation to the number of drug-exposed patients

Medication	$\bar{A}\bar{B}\bar{C}$	$A\bar{B}\bar{C}$	$\bar{A}\bar{B}\bar{C}$	$\bar{A}\bar{B}C$	$AB\bar{C}$	$A\bar{B}C$	$\bar{A}BC$	ABC
Number of patients with adverse reaction	35	56	5	40	19	23	3	3
Number of patients exposed	2891	469	104	592	121	113	23	21
Frequencies (%)	1.21	11.94	4.81	6.76	15.70	20.35	13.04	14.29

Table 2. Number of patients with adverse reaction in relation to exposure periods

Patients treated with drug group	Full exposure period	Corrected exposure period
Ampicillin (A)	101	93
Other penicillins (B)	30	23
Cotrimoxazole or sulphonamides alone (C)	69	35

For the corrections of the numbers of patients with the adverse reaction in relation to exposure periods see Table 2. Of the 101 patients with ampicillin treatment, only 93 received the drug before the appearance of the maculopapular rash under the above-mentioned condition; the incidence therefore is 12.8% (93/724). Similar calculations for patients treated with other penicillins (B) show an incidence of this adverse reaction of 8.6% (23/269); and with cotrimoxazole or sulphonamides alone (C) of 4.7% (35/749). These frequencies, however, still contain an error, as the whole areas of the circles do not take into account that a rash occurring after exposure to more than one of the three groups of antibiotics is usually caused only by a single drug. Therefore, the above calculations should rather rely on the frequencies of the fields $A\bar{B}\bar{C}$, $\bar{A}B\bar{C}$ and $\bar{A}\bar{B}C$ instead of the whole areas of the circles. Thus in the example of ampicillin-treated patients, only the area $A\bar{B}\bar{C}$ is considered and the incidence of adverse reaction 11.94% (Table 1) is reduced by the factor 93/101 (Table 2): $11.94\% \cdot 93/101 = 11.0\%$. For other penicillins ($\bar{A}B\bar{C}$) the corrected incidence is $4.81\% \cdot 23/30 = 3.7\%$, and for cotrimoxazole or sulphonamides alone ($\bar{A}\bar{B}C$) the corrected incidence is $6.76\% \cdot 35/69 = 3.4\%$. This procedure is possible because an approximately equal distribution of the frequencies of the adverse reaction in the overlapping fields (Table 1) can be shown; furthermore, we assumed that the proportion of patients receiving, for example, drug A before and after the onset of the adverse drug reaction is not significantly different between the groups $A\bar{B}\bar{C}$, $AB\bar{C}$, $A\bar{B}C$, and ABC.

Our results agree approximately with those obtained by weighted attributions by SHAPIRO et al. (1969), who obtained percentages for drug rash with ampicillin of 7.7%, with other penicillins of 2.7%, and in patients not given these drugs of 1.8%. They used the above-mentioned corrections of time of exposure. The 1.8% basic frequency in their paper was discounted. Cotrimoxazole had not been introduced at that time.

2. Weighted Attributions

The frequencies of the reaction by weighted attributions, in the overlapping fields are distributed to the non-overlapping fields according to their proportions (ARNDT and JICK 1976). This can be done as long as no drug interactions occur.

The methods of Euler–Venn diagrams or weighted attributions can be used only with a large number of observations. For both methods the result can be expressed either as a frequency in terms of the percentage of patients exposed or, as a coefficient by which the natural occurrence of a clinical syndrome has to be multiplied to give the frequency with a defined exposure to a given drug or drug combination.

If a number of drugs is given, the drug exposure, which should be compared in patients with and without a given adverse reaction, poses a difficult problem. For patients with an adverse reaction, the exposure time can be clearly related to an event. It is logical that a drug administered after this event, e. g. during a hospital stay, will not be responsible for the reaction. Also drugs given a long time before this event, at least if the adverse reaction is of an acute nature, will scarcely be the probable cause. In contrast, for patients without adverse reactions, the only possible criterion for drug exposure is the number of drugs given during a defined time, e.g. during the hospital stay (Hurwitz 1969a, b; Jick 1977; Miller 1973; Smith et al. 1966b) or the last week before the event (Sect. B.I.1; Arndt and Jick 1976).

II. Outpatient Drug Monitoring

The distinction between inpatient and outpatient monitoring is only a procedural one. For many adverse reactions to drugs, a comprehensive study requires both inpatient and outpatient data even though either setting alone may provide sufficient information to incriminate the drug (Friedman et al. 1971; Kurland et al. 1978; Maronde et al. 1978; Skegg 1978).

III. Spontaneous Reporting of Adverse Reactions to Drugs

In spontaneous reporting, as a rule, suspected unusual and severe adverse effects of newly marketed drugs are given priority. In this situation, the number of patients exposed to the suspected drug is usually unknown or can only be estimated (Dunne 1978; Finney 1974; Köhler and Kimbel 1978; Maronde et al. 1978; WHO 1969).

Studies of drug utilisation may be interesting for comparisons of various centres on a national and even international level (Dukes 1978; James et al. 1978; Lawson and Jick 1976). Computer studies should help to compare changing drug utilisation with changing patterns of complications and causes (Böttiger and Westerholm 1973).

IV. Use of Record Linkage for Drug Surveillance

Disease occurrence and mortality statistics in special groups of diseases or age may be an important source of epidemiological information (Dukes 1978; Dunne 1978; Finney 1974; Inmann and Adelstein 1969; Skegg 1978; Speizer et al. 1968). As an example, the mortality of children with asthma in England and Wales increased seven-fold from 1960 to 1966. A close correlation to the use of pressurised aerosols containing sympathomimetics was obtained (Speizer et al. 1968). The subsequent decline in mortality has resulted from a greater awareness by doctors and patients of the dangers of over-use (Inman and Adelstein 1969).

Table 3. Frequency of adverse drug reactions in atopic patients compared with non-atopic controls

Patient characteristic	Number of patients		Patients (%)
Atopy	A	B	C
Present	240	49 (17)	17.0 (5.9)
Not known	1,271	247 (82)	16.3 (5.4)
Not present	3,116	645 (220)	17.1 (5.8)
	4,627	941 (319)	
	5,568		

A = patients without adverse reaction (AR) or with AR to drug as questionable or possible cause; B = patients with AR (causal relationship certain or probable); the number in parentheses shows those patients with at least one allergic AR; C − percentage of patients with one or more AR considered to be certain or probable; the number in parentheses shows the percentage of patients with at least one allergic AR

C. The Patient

I. Disposition

1. Allergy to Small Molecular Drugs

A few patients sensitise easily to a number of small molecular drugs. Often, the time of exposure to the particular allergenic drug in these patients is relatively short, less than 5–7 days (HOIGNÉ et al. 1978). A biochemical difference from other patients has not yet been found. Sometimes, in the same family, other members show the same tendency to develop drug allergies. Probably two types of reaction should be distinguished: patients with generalised systemic reactions or organ disease, and patients with allergic contact eczema. From personal experience, the second group may also show reactions to non-drug chemicals.

2. Atopy and Adverse Drug Reactions: Drug Allergies

The epidemiological study in our medical division on inpatients from 1974 to 1978 shows no increased frequency of adverse drug reactions in subjects with personal atopy (hay fever, allergic rhinitis to other common allergens, reaginic asthma or neurodermatitis) (Table 3; ETTLIN et al. 1981; HOIGNÉ et al. 1981). Our results resemble those obtained by SMITH et al. (1966 b) in Baltimore, but not those of SMITH et al. (1966 a). In this last paper, two different groups of patients (inpatients and outpatients) were mixed and the conclusion drawn that atopic individuals may develop adverse reactions to drugs more frequently than other individuals, especially penicillin allergies. Our results on adverse drug reactions in general and in drug allergies on 5568 patients (HOIGNÉ et al. 1978, 1981) agree with the Study Group of the American Academy of Allergy (GREEN and ROSENBLUM 1971), which did not find any correlation between atopy and the frequency of allergic reactions to penicillin. In spite of this fact, many packaging inserts for penicillins still contain a warning against the use of penicillin in atopic patients. (Our study, devoted to penicillin allergies however, does not include a sufficient number of patients with type I reactions to penicillin preparations to allow one to draw any definite conclusion about immediate reactions.)

The patients considered to have allergic reactions to drugs ranged over the whole spectrum of clinical syndromes from systemic reactions, generalised exanthemas, haematological diseases, to allergic contact dermatitis.

3. Idiosyncrasy

Idiosyncratic reactions are most often due to an inborn error of metabolism caused by an enzyme deficiency, which may be unmasked by drugs and show similar clinical symptoms and syndromes to drug allergies. Examples are:

a) The haemolytic reaction after administration of a number of drugs (e. g. sulphonamides) in individuals with 6-phosphate dehydrogenase or diaphorase deficiency of the erythrocytes (Meyer 1978).

b) The haemolytic reactions in situations of a pathological haemoglobin such as Hb H, Hb Zürich etc., again sulphonamides may elicit the reaction (Meyer 1978). Both groups a) and b) show clear-cut biological differences from an immunological haemolytic reaction, such as the classical example of penicillin-induced haemolysis. Some drugs may induce haemolysis by all three mechanisms!

c) Systemic lupus erythematosus (SLE) or lupus-like syndrome and drugs. Drugs may induce three different clinical and biological situations similar to, or the same as SLE (Hoigné et al. 1975; Lee et al. 1966): (i) An exacerbation of pre-existing SLE; (ii) The elicitation of SLE in a patient with SLE disposition or diathesis; (iii) An allergic reaction of the serum-sickness syndrome type resembling SLE, not only clinically, but also serologically.

In situations (i) and (ii), two main mechanisms seem to exist, depending on:
A) The pharmacological properties of the drug (hydralazine, diphenylhydantoin, procainamide, isonicotinic acid hydrazine and possibly sulphonamides)
B) A hypersensitivity to the drug as in other drug allergic reactions (sulphonamides, penicillins, tetracyclines and a number of other drugs).
In type A reactions, exposure and often re-exposure time is usually longer than 1–2 months; in type B reactions, it is hours, days or up to 1–2 months (Lee et al. 1966).

Even in the drug-induced forms of systemic lupus erythematosus, the reaction may last weeks, months and even years, with the necessity of continuing a maintenance dose of corticosteroids during this long period, e. g. 5.0–12.5 mg/day prednisone (Hoigné et al. 1975).

4. Intolerance

Two different forms of intolerance to a drug have to be distinguished.

a) A pharmacological adverse effect, usually associated with overdosage, is observed with a low dosage, e. g., to quinidine, morphine or digitalis preparations.

b) An adverse effect with symptoms quite specific to a special group of patients which seems not to be due to allergy and for which a precise mechanism of idiosyncrasy is not yet known, e. g. aspirin intolerance.

Asthmatic attacks due to non-narcotic analgesics, mostly occur in patients with so-called intrinsic or idiosyncratic asthma (often associated with nasal polyposis, sinusitis and eosinophilia of the blood) (McFADDEN and AUSTEN 1977). About 10% of patients with this kind of asthma show severe reactions to aspirin, methylsalicylate, pyrazolone derivatives, indomethacin, ibuprofen, diclofenac and sometimes even phenacetin and paracetamol. (Sodium salicylate is often tolerated.) The special reactivity may appear only in later life and concerns a number of chemically unrelated drugs. In some of these patients analgesic therapy with a morphine derivative such as pentazocine (Fortalgesic) or hyoscine butylbromide (Buscopan) may be necessary. However, in other patients, those with aspirin urticaria rather than asthma, the reaction may also rely on a drug-specific allergic mechanism (DE WECK 1971).

II. Basic Diseases

Adverse reactions of toxic origin are mainly influenced by the function of the kidney. If, however, creatinine values of the patients are considered with respect to dosage or dosage interval, or both, adverse effects do not seem unduly influenced by this important organ of elimination. For aminoglycosides, cephalosporins, other antibiotic drugs, digoxin and also a number of other drug groups, dosage adaptation is necessary in the case of reduced kidney function.

Some allergic or allergy-like reactions are markedly influenced by basic diseases:
1. The increase of maculopapular exanthemas by aminopenicillins in infectious mononucleosis and in lymphatic leukosis
2. Erythema nodosum, encountered in 5% of children with tuberculosis. This rate increased to 45% if a sulphonamide preparation (sulphathiazole) was administered (ROLLOF 1950).

In both examples, the pathogenesis is not clear and an allergic origin has not been proved.

D. Criteria Important to Epidemiology and Drug Monitoring

I. The Patient and the Adverse Reaction

1. Characteristics of Clinical and Laboratory Adverse Reactions: Distinction from Non-Drug Reactions

As already mentioned in Sect. B, the systematic research applied may differ according to the situation (type a, b or c, Table 4).

a) The adverse reaction is characteristic and can also be distinguished from non-drug reactions by a time relationship. In this type of situation, usually one or more of the following criteria can be applied to prove the connection with the drug:

Table 4. Epidemiological data and the individual patient

Type of situation	Relationship to drug in all patients with the disease		
	a	b	c
Drug and non-drug origin in individual patients	Established	Not known	Partially known
Method of research	Usual statistical methods	Formal epidemiological research	Combined methods
Identification of drug cause in individual patients	Possible	Impossible (except if drug is the most important or unimportant cause)	Variable

I) The disappearance of symptoms after the withdrawal of the drug. This is of extremely variable significance, because a number of allergic reactions seem to be transient, even if the drug is continued, especially maculopapular eruptions (Hoigné et al. 1978)

II) The reappearance of symptoms on re-exposure to the same, or a chemically related drug. These re-exposures are often not intended. We do not think that a patient should be re-exposed to a drug, which has probably elicited an allergic reaction

III) The symptoms correspond to a well-known allergic reaction to the specific drug, e. g., maculopapular rash, allergic contact eczema

IV) The results of specific tests in the field of allergy and immunology (mainly skin and in vitro reactions); or in the field of clinical pharmacology (drug levels, drug metabolites, drug distribution etc.) help to identify the drug causing the reaction.

Systems for combining criteria to evaluate a reaction have been proposed (Karch and Lasagna 1977). However, in reports of adverse drug reactions one should not demand a high degree of certainty about the cause and effect relationship. Most reactions which eventually become firmly established and generally recognised begin as vague suspicions in an alert and prepared mind (Koch-Weser 1968). Selective research on each single patient may be helpful. However, in many instances of drug-induced syndromes or diseases, tests are either not available, or they will not help one to understand the pathogenesis of the reaction. This is especially true for pharmacological side effects in the restricted sense (i.e. excluding relative overdosage) and for drug intolerance (i.e. when the usual adverse effect of the drug is caused by a low dosage).

b) The use of a drug increases the risk of an already occurring defect or disease, e. g. malformation of the newborn, endometrial cancer, thromboembolism. Usually in this situation, clinical observation has to be supplemented by case-referent studies, cohort studies or even formal research (Jick 1977), including record linkage. The type of investigation depends largely upon the absolute frequency of the illness when the drug is used and the absolute frequency in the non-drug situation. At the present time, only the epidemiological methods can be applied.

c) Situations between type a and type b, where the diagnosis of an adverse drug reaction and even the identification of the drug is possible in some patients, and where, in others, the relation to a drug in the individual patient remains unclear. A combination of thorough investigation of each patient and the associated control group along with appropriate statistical methods is necessary.

Examples of such complex situations are: Adverse drug reactions with fatal outcome (IREY 1976; PORTER and JICK 1977; TÖRÖK et al. 1982) or drug-induced blood dyscrasias (BAUMGARTNER et al. 1982).

The primary evaluation (in our system at the end of the hospital stay) for such cases must be checked again by a secondary or even a further evaluation in connection with the specific characteristics of the problem studied. This final or secondary evaluation has to be independent from the causality level originally attributed (INMAN 1982). Assessing the causality of adverse drug reactions, even with standardized approaches, should remain an activity under control of physicians (VENULET 1982).

For the epidemiological situations of c) two facts seem to be important:
I) The relative frequency of the drug-induced disease to the non-drug-induced disease
II) Whether the origin of the non-drug-induced disease can be clearly established or not.

As long as the drug is the main cause of the disease, other causes may be neglected without an important epidemiological error occurring (e. g., maculopapular rash in adults) (SHAPIRO et al. 1969; STREIT 1979). If, however, the drug cause applies only to a small number of observations, the frequency is extremely difficult to determine (e. g., acute agranulocytosis, renal insufficiency).

2. Definition of Clinical Syndromes and Laboratory Findings

In any epidemiological study the definitions have to be clearly established. Serum-sickness syndrome is a good example; at least three of the symptoms described by VON PIRQUET and SCHICK (1905): exanthema, fever, arthritis, lymphadenitis, possibly leukopenia, have to be present, in our opinion, to have any degree of specificity, if small molecular drugs are the cause (HOIGNÉ 1965 a, b). If two symptoms are considered to fulfil the criteria, the incidence is several times higher and each situation of exanthema with fever will be called serum-sickness syndrome. The same is true for abnormal laboratory values without clinical symptoms. The normal and the pathological range have to be defined.

3. Time Factors in Adverse Drug Reactions

a) Events and Times of Exposure

Three types of exposure have to be distinguished:

I) The total exposure to a drug during the lifetime of the patient or an important period of life (i. e., the quantity of the drug administered). This factor may be of influence on reproduction, foetal development, teratogenicity, oncogenicity, etc. and also on a disease such as analgesic-interstitial nephritis.

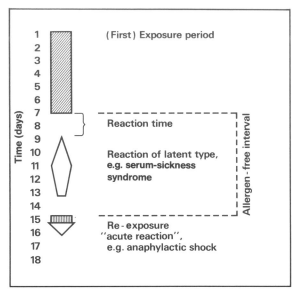

Fig. 2. Definition of time periods for allergic reactions

II) Exposure periods or treatment periods. One period is defined as the time during which a more or less continuous drug level is sustained, over days, weeks or several months. As a rule, drug allergies begin after exposure periods of at least some days, 5–7 or more. This is the (minimal) time necessary for sensitisation and the appearance of symptoms in connection with the first treatment with a specific drug. (Why exceptions to this rule occur, even in small children, cannot be explained at present.) The first exposure of a second or subsequent treatment period is especially important in elicitation of anaphylactic shock due to a drug to which the patient was sensitised, possibly without the occurrence of any symptoms, during an earlier drug exposure. The whole exposure pattern may influence sensitisation and elicitation of allergic drug reactions (Fig. 2).

III) Single applications of a drug, either as part of a treatment period or as a sporadic single dose, often used for symptomatic therapy of a discomfort, or minor disease.

Intermittent exposures have also been used with rifampicin (with 1–3 single exposures a week) and seemed to enhance markedly the otherwise extremely rare appearance of an acute thrombocytopenia. If exposure is sporadic, valuable epidemiological studies cannot usually be realised.

b) Reaction Time

This is the time between the last drug exposure and the appearance of the first symptoms, if the mechanism is considered to be allergic (Mayer 1933). Frequently there is a definite relationship between the reaction time and the type of clinical symptoms. This relationship was described by von Pirquet and Schick as early as 1905 with respect to anaphylactic shock and serum sickness due to foreign sera.

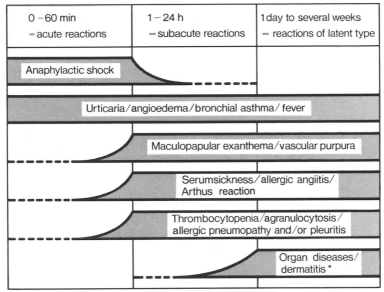

0 – 60 min	1 – 24 h	1 day to several weeks
= acute reactions	= subacute reactions	= reactions of latent type

Anaphylactic shock

Urticaria/angioedema/bronchial asthma/fever

Maculopapular exanthema/vascular purpura

Serumsickness/allergic angiitis/ Arthus reaction

Thrombocytopenia/agranulocytosis/ allergic pneumopathy and/or pleuritis

Organ diseases/ dermatitis *

* from locally applied or ingested contact allergens

Fig. 3. Time scales for different types of allergic reactions

It is valid today for the majority of the various syndromes of drug allergy (HOIGNÉ 1965 a). However, much shorter reaction times were found in allergies to small molecular drugs than in allergies to complete antigenic substances such as heterologous sera (this is due partly to the behaviour of foreign sera as long-term preparations and the fact, that the first authors used incubation time, and not reaction time, as a parameter). As a new classification we have therefore proposed three reaction times (Fig. 3; HOIGNÉ 1965 a):
0–60 min (acute reactions)
1–24 h (subacute reactions)
1 day to several weeks (reactions of latent type).
Remarkable differences of reaction times occur in connection with a first treatment or a number of treatments. Allergic reactions with short reaction times (acute allergic reactions) are often found in connection with the first dose of the second, third, etc. treatment. Subacute, or especially latent reactions occur (partly by definition) after the end of a treatment period (Figs. 2 and 3; HOIGNÉ et al. 1978).

c) Allergen-Free Interval

This term was introduced because in experimental and also in a number of human allergies, correlations exist between the reactivity and the duration of the allergen-free interval (HOIGNÉ 1965 a). If this allergen-free interval is short, perhaps only 1–2 days, the allergic reaction following the first dose of the second (or subsequent) treatment will be less severe than if the so-called allergen-free interval lasts for days or several weeks (Fig. 2). This general concept was, however, not studied prospectively (HOIGNÉ et al. 1965a).

The practical conclusion of these observations is: if a patient starts with, for example, a maculopapular exanthema due to an important drug, it is probably less dangerous to continue the treatment under close observation, than to stop treatment and to start the next application of the drug in several days or weeks. Alternatively, if the case history indicates an adverse reaction in connection with an earlier treatment period with a given drug or group of drugs, the first new application should be preceded either by a small test dose or possibly by skin or laboratory tests.

4. Frequency of Adverse Drug Reactions

General experience with allergic adverse reactions shows that most adverse reactions start during the first 3–4 weeks of treatment, and rarely after months or years (KLEIN et al. 1976). The problem is, however, difficult to study, as most drugs with common allergic reactions, such as anti-infective drugs, are seldom indicated for a duration of more than 4–6 weeks.

The time of exposure is extremely important for indications of frequencies. With various ampicillin preparations the frequency of a maculopapular rash varied from a few to 10% or more of the treated patients; these numbers are only comparable when equal exposure times are used (FRICKER 1976; SHAPIRO et al. 1969).

Frequencies of characteristic adverse drug reactions are usually compared with numbers of treatment periods rather than numbers of treated patients. In our opinion, a reaction rate of

10^{-1}–10^{-2} should be considered as high
10^{-2}–10^{-3} as intermediate
10^{-3}–10^{-4} as low
10^{-4}–10^{-5} as very low
10^{-5}–10^{-6} or less as extremely low.

The baseline risk for the same syndrome, if known, should always be indicated.

In the case of life-threatening reactions in a disease with an important indication for a particular drug, very low appearance (10^{-4}–10^{-5}), such as anaphylactic shock to penicillin, is usually acceptable (IDSØE et al. 1969). However, it is only permissible to take this type of risk after full consideration of an accurate case history, and the clinical and laboratory situation, and if the treatment possibilities are good.

For drug-induced illnesses which show the same features whether they occur with or without the heightening effect of a drug (type b situations; Table 4), JICK (1977) has proposed the following schedule:

1. The rate is "high" if the added risk of an illness experienced by users of the drug exceeds one in 200/year

2. The rate is "low" if this rate is less than one in 10,000/year; otherwise it is "intermediate".

The problem of drug-induced illness is defined in these papers by the magnitude of two risks: the added risk of illness experienced by users of a drug, and the baseline risk in the absence of the drug.

5. Degree of Importance of Adverse Drug Reactions

The severity of an adverse reaction is usually much more important than its frequency. For an effective anti-infective drug (e. g. an aminopenicillin preparation), high frequency of an exanthema (in 5%–10% of patients or 5–10,000 of 100,000 treatments) is acceptable; however, for a life-threatening reaction such as pancytopenia (in the case of chloramphenicol) observed in only about 2 of 100,000 patients treated (very low frequency), other drugs are preferred except in rare and selected indications.

We have introduced the term "degree of importance of an adverse reaction" because this considers both "actual severity" and "potential risk" in two situations: permanent damage and death. Agranulocytosis or thrombocytopenia may show no clinical symptoms at all, but if they are overlooked an infection in the former may provoke a life-threatening septicaemia and a head injury in the latter may cause an intracranial haemorrhage!

6. Outcome and Duration of Adverse Drug Reactions

In general, adverse reactions to drugs are seldom the only cause of death in patients, at least as extrapolated from the intensive hospital drug monitoring data of the Boston Collaborative Drug Surveillance Program and the Comprehensive Hospital Drug Monitoring, Bern. From analyses of the lethal situations it seems, that more of these reactions are due to pharmacologically toxic effects than to allergy (PORTER and JICK 1977; TÖRÖK et al. 1982).

Life-threatening reactions due principally or exclusively, to allergic mechanisms are: anaphylactic shock, bronchoasthmatic attack, allergic angioedema, agranulocytosis, severe thrombocytopenic purpura, pancytopenia (only exceptionally of an allergic type), Lyell syndrome and Stevens–Johnson syndrome (both of which can be caused by drug allergy), severe serum sickness or generalised allergic angiitis, severe pulmonary reactions (type of farmer's lung), allergic interstitial nephritis and allergic "benign" intracranial hypertension.

The duration of most usual allergic reactions, such as urticarial and maculopapular rashes, is limited to a few days, the exanthema seldom stays for more than 1–2 weeks. But lupus erythematosus syndrome, pancytopenia, interstitial nephritis and allergic pneumopathy (chronic interstitial) may be diseases lasting for months or years, leaving permanent damage even when treatment is possible.

II. The Drug and Drug Groups

1. Different Kinds of Drugs

The adverse reactions and diseases due to drugs vary with drug groups; some adverse reactions are quite specific to individual drugs or drug groups.

Penicillins and cephalosporins are prototypes for allergic reactions of type I by the classification of COOMBS and GELL (1963), based on the pathogenetic mechanisms. They are mostly IgE mediated. But type III and type IV reactions also occur.

Sulphonamides are usually the cause of type III or type IV allergic reactions, such as serum-sickness syndrome, or probably, the majority of maculopapular rashes.

About one-third of all adverse drug reactions are of an allergic nature, if maculopapular rashes are included in this pathogenic group (Hoigné et al. 1978). The frequency of allergic reactions is especially high with the group of antibacterial drugs.

Non-narcotic analgesics such as aspirin, other salicylates, pyrazolone derivatives, phenacetin, paracetamol, phenylbutazone, oxyphenylbutazone, indomethacin and newer analgesics, antipyretics or anti-inflammatory drugs may produce type I, II, III or IV allergic reactions. But all of them can elicit, often in patients with asthma, nonallergic attacks of bronchospasm, urticaria, angioedema and rarely, a circulatory collapse resembling anaphylactic shock. Hypotension to dipyrone (novaminsulfon), in non-asthmatic patients, probably does not have an allergic basis in most instances (Hoigné 1978). However, anaphylactic shock to amidopyrine (pyramidone), dipyrone and isopropylantipyrine can also occur.

Some of these drugs, mainly pyrazolone derivatives, may cause agranulocytosis or thrombocytopenia, or both, (type II reactions), but only in rare, or extremely rare, situations (Baumgartner et al. 1982). Digitalis and also benzodiazepines induce adverse reactions only exceptionally by an allergic mechanism (Streit 1979).

2. Method of Administration of Drug and Drug Allergic Reactions

As expected from experimental work, humans most often react to drugs applied locally to the skin, in the case of sensitisation, with an allergic contact dermatitis. Patients given a systemic treatment, with drugs administered parenterally, orally or rectally, tend to react with urticaria, maculopapular rashes, more special exanthemas, or allergic manifestations of organs or systems other than the skin. If a drug is administered systemically and a widespread allergic dermatitis follows, the patient may have been sensitised earlier by skin contact to this drug (Hoigné 1965a). Sensitisation of the delayed type (type IV), however, does not preclude a simultaneous allergic sensitivity of type I, II, or III.

E. Practical Consequences

The true value of a drug is characterised by the following formula and rules (Hoigné et al. 1978):

Usefulness	$\dfrac{\text{Efficacy} \times \text{indication}}{\text{Risk of adverse reaction}}$
Efficacy	Percentage of patients with benefit, compared with a control group; effect of the specific drug on the disease process and on symptoms
Indication	Type and degree of severity of the disease; availability of other drugs with comparable effectiveness and safety; price differences

Risk of adverse reaction   Function of the drug and disposition of the patient; basic disease and additional drugs; type and severity of adverse reaction

All three factors have to be considered: efficacy, indication and safety. The last covers the central topic of this book. If allergy tests are available, their practical value is, above all, of diagnostic and prophylactic importance.

F. Summary

This chapter is mainly concerned with the methods of epidemiology and drug monitoring, the patients' dispositions and basic diseases and different kinds of adverse drug reactions. The principal adverse reaction patterns of different drugs or drug groups and the influence of the methods of administration are mentioned. Allergic drug reactions represent only about one-third of all unwanted drug effects. The decision to use or to withdraw a drug relies mainly on a risk: benefit ratio, based on the whole situation of the individual patient.

References

Arndt K, Jick H (1976) Rates of cutaneous reactions to drugs. JAMA 235:918–923

Baumgartner A, Hoigné R, Müller U, Hess T (1982) Medikamentöse Schäden des Blutbildes. Erfahrungen aus dem Komprehensiven Spital-Drug-Monitoring Bern, 1974–1979. Schweiz med Wochenschr 112:1530–1539

Böttiger LE, Westerholm B (1973) Drug-induced blood dyscrasias in Sweden. Br med J 3:339–343

Coombs RRA, Gell PGH (1963) The classification of allergic reactions underlying disease. In: Clinical aspects of immunology. Gell PGH, Coombs RRA (eds.) Blackwell Scientific, Oxford , pp 317–337

de Weck A (1971) Acetyl-Salicylsäure: ein altes Arzneimittel in neuerem Blickwinkel. Dtsch Med Wochenschr 96:1109–1115

Dukes MNG (1978) Drug utilization studies: a perspective. In: Ducrot H, Goldberg M, Hoigné R, Middleton P (eds.) IFIP TC-4 working conference on computer aid to drug therapy and to drug monitoring, Berne. North-Holland, Amsterdam Oxford New York, pp 373–377

Dunne JF (1978) Spontaneous reporting of adverse reactions to drugs. In: Ducrot H, Goldberg M, Hoigné R, Middleton P (eds.) IFIP TC-4 working conference on computer aid to drug therapy and to drug monitoring, Berne. North-Holland, Amsterdam Oxford New York, pp 105–108

Ettlin R, Hoigné R, Bruppacher R, Müller U, Stocker F (1981) Atopy and adverse drug reactions. Int Arch Allergy 66 (Suppl. 1):93–95

Finney DJ (1974) Systematic signalling of adverse reactions to drugs. Methods Inf Med 13:1–10

Fleiss JL (1973) Statistical methods for rates and proportions. John Wiley and Sons, New York Chichester, p 142

Fricker U (1976) Exantheme bei Ampicillin- und Epicillintherapie. Medical dissertation, University of Berne

Friedman GD (1974) Primer of epidemiology. McGraw-Hill, New York

Friedman GD, Collen MF, Harris LE, Van Brunt EE, Davis LS (1971) Experience in monitoring drug reactions in outpatients. JAMA 217:567–572

Green GR, Rosenblum A (1971) Report of the penicillin study group, American Academy of Allergy. J Allergy Clin Immunol 48:331–343

Hoigné R (1965a) Arzneimittel-Allergien. Huber Berne

Hoigné R (1965b) Penicillin hypersensitivity. In: Meyler L, Peck HM (eds) Drug-induced diseases. Excerpta Medica, Amsterdam, pp 89–96

Hoigné R (1978) Monitoring of drug effects in outpatients: discussion. In: Ducrot H, Goldberg M, Hoigné R, Middleton P (eds) IFIP TC-4 working conference on computer aid to drug therapy and to drug monitoring, Berne. North-Holland, Amsterdam Oxford New York, p 97

Hoigné R, Biedermann HP, Nägeli HR (1975) INH-induzierter systemischer Lupus erythematodes (SLE): 2 Beobachtungen mit Reexpositon. Schweiz Med Wochenschr 105:1726–1729

Hoigné R, Ettlin R, Hintermann R et al. (1978) Die Auswahl antibakterieller Chemotherapeutika unter besonderer Berücksichtigung von Disposition und Grundkrankheit des Patienten. Schweiz Rundschau Med 67:1822–1828

Hoigné R, Streit C, Stocker F et al. (1981) Drug Monitoring und Epidemiologie von Arzneimittel-Nebenwirkungen. In: Borelli S, Düngemann H (eds) Fortschritte der Allergologie und Dermatologie. Klinik für Dermatologie und Allergie, Davos and I.M.P. Verlagsgesellschaft, Basel Neu Isenburg Wien, pp 169–174

Hurwitz N (1969a) Predisposing factors in adverse reactions to drugs. Br Med J 1:536–539

Hurwitz N, Wade OL (1969b) Intensive hospital monitoring of adverse reactions to drugs. Br Med J 1:531–536

Idsøe O, Guthe T, Willcox RR, de Weck AL (1969) Art und Ausmaß der Penizillinnebenwirkungen unter besonderer Berücksichtigung von 151 Todesfällen nach anaphylaktischem Schock. Schweiz Med Woschenschr 99:1190–1197, 1221–1229

Inman WH, Adelstein AM (1969) Rise and fall of asthma mortality in England and Wales in relation to use of pressurised aerosols. Lancet 2:279–285

Inman WHW (1982) Attitudes to type 1 (false positive) and type 2 (false negative) errors in assessment. In: Venulet J, Berneker GC, Ciucci AG (eds) Assessing causes of adverse drug reactions. Academic Press, London New York, pp 69–78

Irey NS (1976) Adverse drug reactions and death. A review of 827 cases. JAMA 236:575–578

Jämes D, Haller E, Rosselet G, Brooke EM, Schelling JL (1978) Fréquence des prescriptions de médicaments et de leurs effets indésirables dans un département de médecine. Schweiz Med Wochenschr 108:1270–1277

Jick H (1977) The discovery of drug-induced illness. N Engl J Med 296:481–485

Jick H, Miettinen OS, Shapiro S, Lewis GP, Siskind V, Slone D (1970) Comprehensive drug surveillance. JAMA 213:1455–1460

Karch FE, Lasagna L (1977) Toward the operational identification of adverse drug reactions. Clin Pharmacol Ther 21:247–254

Klein U, Klein M, Sturm H et al. (1976) The frequency of adverse drug reactions as dependent upon age, sex and duration of hospitalization. Int J Clin Pharmacol 13:187–195

Koch-Weser J (1968) Definition and classification of adverse drug reactions. Drug Inform Bull 2:72–78

Köhler CO, Kimbel KH (1978) Spontaneous monitoring data processing and information feedback to the physician. In: Ducrot H, Goldberg M, Hoigné R, Middleton P (eds) IFIP TC-4 working conference on computer aid to drug therapy and to drug monitoring, Berne. North-Holland, Amsterdam Oxford New York, pp 125–132

Kurland L, Annegers JF, O'Fallon W (1978) Utilization of Mayo Clinic records for population-based long-term evaluations of drug exposure. In: Ducrot H, Goldberg M, Hoigné R, Middleton P (eds) IFIP TC-4 working conference on computer aid to drug therapy and to drug monitoring, Berne. North-Holland, Amsterdam Oxford New York, pp 69–76

Lawson DH, Jick H (1976) Drug prescribing in hospitals: an international comparison. Am J Public health 66:644–648

Lee SL, Rivero I, Siegel M (1966) Activation of systemic lupus erythematosus by drugs. Arch Intern Med 117:620–626

Maronde RF, Rho J, Rucker TD (1978) Monitoring for adverse drug reactions including mutations, in outpatients. In: Ducrot H, Goldberg M, Hoigné R, Middleton P (eds) IFIP TC-4 working conference on computer aid to drug therapy and to drug monitoring, Berne. North-Holland, Amsterdam Oxford New York, pp 63–68

Mayer RL (1933) Toxicodermien. In: Marchionini A, Nasemann T (eds) Die Viruskrankheiten der Haut und die Hautsymptome bei Rickettsiosen und Bartonellosen. (Handbuch der Haut- und Geschlechtskrankheiten, vol IV/2, p 1) Springer, Berlin Heidelberg New York

McFadden ER Jr, Austen KF (1977) Asthma. In: Thorn GW, Adams RD, Braunwald E, Isselbacher KJ, Petersdorf RG (eds) Harrison's priciples of internal medicine, 8th edn. McGraw-Hill Kogakusha, Tokyo, pp 1349–1354

Meyer UA (1978) Role of genetic factors in the rational use of drugs. In: Melmon KL, Morelli HF (eds) Clinical pharmacology. Basic principles in therapeutics, 2nd edn. Macmillan, New York, pp 913–929

Miller RR (1973) Drug surveillance utilizing epidemiologic methods. A report from the Boston Collaborative Drug Surveillance Program. Am J Hosp Pharm 30:584–592

Pirquet C von, Schick B (1905) Die Serumkrankheit. Deutike, Leipzig Vienna

Porter J, Jick H (1977) Drug-related deaths among medical inpatients. JAMA 237:879–881

Rollof SL (1950) Erythema nodosum in association with sulfathiazole in children. Clinical investigation with special reference to primary tuberculosis. Acta Tuberc Scand [Suppl.] 24:1

Shapiro S, Slone D, Siskind V, Lewis GP, Jick H (1969) Drug rash with ampicillin and other penicillins. Lancet 2:969–972

Skegg DCG (1978) Use of record linkage for drug surveillance. A progress report. In: Ducrot H, Goldberg M, Hoigné R, Middleton P (eds) IFIP TC-4 working conference on computer aid to drug therapy and to drug monitoring, Berne. North-Holland, Amsterdam Oxford New York, pp 77–83

Slone D, Shapiro S, Miettinen OS, Finkle WD, Stolley PD (1979) Drug evaluation after marketing. Ann Intern Med 90:257–261

Smith JW, Johnson JE III, Cluff LE (1966a) Studies on the epidemiology of adverse drug reactions. II. An evaluation of penicillin allergy. N Engl J Med 274:998–1002

Smith JW, Seidl LG, Cluff LE (1966b) Studies on the epidemiology of adverse drug reactions. V. Clinical factors influencing susceptibility. Ann Intern Med 65:629–640

Speizer FE, Doll R, Haef P (1968) Observations on recent increase in mortality from asthma. Br Med J 1:335–339

Streit C (1979) Das komprehensive Spital-Drug Monitoring Bern in methodischer Hinsicht. A) Methodik, unter besonderer Berücksichtigung der Prüfprogramme. B) Epidemiologie der makulo-papulösen Exantheme bei erwachsenen Patienten. Medical dissertation, University of Berne

Török M, Zoppi M, Winzenried P, Marty H, Hess T, Stoller-Güleryüz D, Stucki P, Bickel MH, Stocker F, Hoigné R (1982) Drug related death among 17,285 inpatients in the division of internal medicine of two teaching hospitals in Berne, 1974–1980. In: Manell P, Johansson SG (eds) The impact of computer technology on drug information. North-Holland, Amsterdam, pp 79–84

Venulet J (1982) Concluding remarks. In: Venulet J, Berneker GC, Ciucci AG (eds) Assessing causes of adverse drug reactions. Academic Press, London New York, pp 217–221

WHO (1969) International drug monitoring. The role of the hospital. WHO Tech Rep Ser 425

CHAPTER 7

Diagnostic Procedures in Drug Allergy

J.-P. Girard and S. Zawodnik

A. Introduction

In the last decade the problem of allergic reactions to drugs has grown, owing to the daily use of more new drugs than ever. It is not unusual to investigate patients in hospital of under their own physicians who are taking ten or more different drugs a day. It is also known that the risk of developing an untoward reaction to drugs is considerably amplified when a large number of drugs is taken simultaneously.

There are many difficulties in the development of reliable diagnostic tests for durg allergy (DE WECK 1972). The fact that there is no single reliable, universally applicable test for drug allergy is not surprising since a number of different pathogenic mechanisms can lead to clinical manifestations. In addition, for most of the allergenic drugs, the antigenic determinants are unknown, and according to current ideas, new determinants appear follwing the metabolism of most drugs by liver enzymes. Some of the major difficulties in establishing adequate tests for the diagnosis of allergic reactions to drugs are given in Table 1. For these reasons, the clinical diagnosis should be based on the classification of the reaction according to the immunologic types of GELL and COOMBS (GIRARD 1972).

B. Clinical Diagnosis

The majority of symptoms from untoward reactions to drugs allow sufficient time to allow one to take a detailed history before making any decision on management. The only exception is anaphylactic shock, the diagnosis of which is usually immediately evident, implying acute therapeutic management.

A detailed history of the patient's symptoms should be carefully recorded. The following points should be scrutinized:
1. The delay between the onset of the clinical symptoms and the beginning of the therapeutic management with a specific drug
2. The periodicity of the symptoms which are often prominent a short time after the drug has been taken or injected
3. The drugs or medicines which are often taken routinely by the patient without medical prescriptions (pain killers, vitamins, sleeping pills, etc.)
4. A careful history of previous allergic reactions to drugs

The first measure, when medically possible, is to stop the administration of all drugs. Usually, clinical symptoms disappear within a few days. However, in some specific circumstances, they may persist for several weeks, for instance when there is some cross-antigenicity with chemicals or food additives.

Table 1. Difficulties in the development of adequate tests for the diagnosis of drug allergy

1. Variety of immunopathogenic mechanisms
2. Often a mixture of different types of immunologic reactions
3. Poor knowledge of antigenic determinants
4. New determinants derived from drug metabolism
5. Determinants as byproducts of drug synthesis
6. Frontier between immunologic and nonimmunologic mechanisms difficult to trace
7. Absence of information on the hapten-carrier systems in humans

Table 2. Classification of allergic reactions to drugs according to the suspected immunologic mechanism

Type	Mediators	Clinical manifestations
I	IgE (IgG)	Systemic anaphylaxis, asthma, urticaria, angio-edema
II and III	IgG, IgM, $\pm C'$	Serum sickness, vasculitis, fever, blood cytopenia, late urticaria, erythema nodosum, glomerulitis, allergic alveolitis
IV	T-lymphocytes, lymphokines	Erythrodermia, morbilliform and maculopapular rashes, drug-induced fever, lyell syndrome, contact dermatitis
Not well defined		Photosensitivity, drug-induced lupus erythematosus syndrome, hepatitis, pancytopenia

C. Immunologic Diagnosis

The table established by GELL and COOMBS is of importance when analyzing the type of immunologic reaction (Table 2). However, in this specific field of allergic reactions to drugs, there are several reactions which fail to enter into this practical but oversimplified classification. For instance:

1. Some types of vascular shock are not immunologically mediated; one exemple is the vascular shock which sometimes appears after administration of contrast media
2. In several instances, urticaria is not mediated by IgE antibodies but by IgG, thus appearing as an aborted form of serum sickness
3. Destruction of blood cells (red blood cells, platelets, leukocytes) results more often from toxic than from immunologic mechanisms
4. Isolated drug fever may be due to immune reaction of perhaps to the release of endotoxins (under antibiotic therapy), but fever can accompany all the various types of immunologic reactions
5. It is very difficult to demonstrate the relationship of lung, liver, and kidney lesions to drug-induced immunologic mechanisms
6. A mixture of symptoms belonging to several types of immunologic reaction is often present.

Table 3 illustrates the various immunologic procedures which are available for the elaboration of the diagnosis of hypersensitivity to drugs and which will be reviewed.

Table 3. Laboratory procedures for the diagnosis of allergic reactions to drugs

	IgE	IgM	IgG
A) Antibody-mediated reactions			
Passive hemagglutination	–	+ +	+ +
Radioimmunoassay	+ +	–	(+ +)
Basophil degranulation	+ +	–	–
Histamine release	+ +	–	–
Complement fixation test	–	+ +	+ +
B) Cell-mediated reactions			
In vitro stimulation of peripheral blood lymphocytes by antigen			
Release of lymphokines in vitro (MIF, LIF)			

+ + = suitable test; – = unsuitable test

D. Skin Testing

With the exception of penicillin, skin tests with drugs are usually of no value. The formation of drug antigens requires the conjugation of the drug to a macromolecule. The injection of the haptenic fraction will be dispersed rapidly from the site of injection. This is likely to be the main reason for the extremely frequent negative skin response to challenge with haptens. It seems therefore essential to prepare hapten–carrier conjugates, to improve the quality of the results. Several such experiments have been performed in our laboratory involving different drugs and carriers. A recent experiment using phenylbutazone as the offending drug will be briefly described.

I. Phenylbutazone – BSA Conjugates

For preparation of the conjugate, the method as described by OZEKI and TEJIMA (1974) was applied. Phenylbutazone (Ciba-Geigy, Basel), 3.25 mg was diluted in 10 ml phosphate buffer, pH 7.45. Bovine serum albumin (BSA) 200 mg, molecular weight 6,900 daltons (Difco, Basel), was slowly added to the haptenic solution and further incubated under constant stirring for 24 h. Free phenylbutazone molecules were separated from the conjugates by means of gel filtration on Sephadex G-25 (Pharmacia, Uppsala), using a phosphate buffer, pH 7.45. The molarity ratio of the conjugate thus obtained was 2.5. This conjugate was used for skin tests and determination of IgG antibodies with the aid of the tanned red cells hemagglutination procedure.

A group of 15 patients with a strong suspicion of allergic reaction to phenylbutazone and a group of 15 healthy control subjects were tested by means of the two procedures. The results obtained are illustrated in Table 4, which demonstrates a high percentage of positive skin tests, mainly of the immediate type, whereas all but one of the control subjects remained negative. It is important to mention that the two groups of patients were also tested with the hapten alone. Only two immediate responses were obtained among the group of allergic patients. Therefore such a procedure should be more systematically applied, especially for those drugs which frequently elicit allergic reactions.

Table 4. Results of skin and hemagglutination tests in 15 patients allergic to phenylbutazone and 15 healthy controls, with a phenylbutazone–BSA conjugate

Patients	Skin tests		Hemag-glutination test
	15 min	4–8 h	
Allergic patients	11/15	5/15	13/15
Controls	0/15	1/15	0/15

Several procedures have been described for coupling drugs to various heterologous or homologous carriers, for instance (AMOS 1976):
1. Conversion of aromatic amines to diazonium salts by treatment with nitrous acid and coupling this reagent to various side chains of proteins at alkaline pH
2. Bis-diazotized benzidine (BDE) will bind to tyrosyl, histidyl, amino, and carboxyl side chain derivates of proteins
3. Carbodiimides: substances with free aryl or alkyl groups. They are mostly used for the binding of protein to red blood cells, for serologic studies. However these reagents can also be applied to the coupling of some drugs to various carriers
4. Diisocynates which are bifunctional groups reacting with free NH_2 groups
5. Coupling of drugs with polysaccharides following conversion of hydro groups to reactive aldehydes

These coupling procedures, among many others should fulfill the following criteria.
1. Binding of the drug to the carrier should be by means of a covalent linkage to avoid dissociation
2. Alteration of the antigenic determinant should remain minimal

II. Penicillins

The penicilloyl group has been demonstrated as the major antigenic determinant of benzylpenicillin (DE WECK 1974). Coupled to polylysines, it has now been used for more than 15 years as a skin test reagent for the in vivo diagnosis of immediate allergic reactions to penicillin (penicilloyl-polylysine, PPL). According to the criteria applied to the selection of patients, the overall percentage of positive tests varies greatly from trial to trial, the lowest being around 40% and the highest 80% (DE WECK 1972; LEVINE et al. 1967; GIRARD 1973).

For several years, all of our patients with an allergic reaction to penicillin were thoroughly investigated by means of several laboratory procedures. The patients were tested between 3 months and 1 year or more following the reaction (GIRARD and CUEVAS 1975).

Results as shown in Table 5 demonstrate that testing with penicilloyl-polylysine yields a high percentage of positive skin tests in the early stage following the reaction, whereas results obtained with benzylpenicillin (BPN) are much lower, which sems to demonstrate that different determinants are involved. This is confirmed by the observation that onyl one-third of these patients react positively to both reagents.

Table 5. Laboratory diagnosis in 1047 cases of allergic reactions to penicillins

Tests	Interval between allergic reaction and investigation	
	<3 months	≤1 year
Hemagglutination (immediate)	75[a]	31[a]
Skin tests PPL	78	63
BPN	49	30
PPL+BPN	37	21
Arthus skin reaction (4–8 h)	22	11
Late skin reaction (24–48 h)	12	29
Lymphocyte stimulation	50	73

[a] Percentage of positive results

Table 6. Immunologic tests in 222 patients allergic to penicillin, having received this antibiotic a second time after the first reaction. High reactors are indicated in parentheses

Tests	Without allergic reaction (146)	With allergic reaction (76)[b]
Hemagglutination	87[a]	84[a]
Skin tests PPL	71 (21)	83 (44)
BPN	60	68 (28)
PPL+BPN	44 (10)	51 (23)
Arthus skin reaction (4–8 h)	26	21
Late skin reaction (24–48 h)	19	33
Lymphocyte stimulation	57	49

[a] Percentage of positive tests
[b] Two patients who died from anaphylactic shock are not included

Among 1,047 such patients, 222 received further doses of penicillin within a period of 1 month to 6 years following the allergic reaction. Within this second group, 76 developed a second allergic reaction (approximately one-third). These patients were again subjected to immunologic tests as illustrated in Table 6. Curiously the percentage of positive tests is not strikingly different. However, if one considers the highly reactive subjects, it appears that they are almost all segregated within the group that developed a second reaction. A second important point is the notable increase of severe anaphylactic shocks following the second administration of penicillin (no death within the group of 1,047 patients, 2 deaths within the group of 76 patients).

In a recent cooperative prospective study on the value of clinical history and skin testing with PPL and penicillin-G (GREEN et al. 1977), almost 3,000 patients were studied. Among patients with a positive history of penicillin allergy only 19%

reacted positively to PPL, 47% to penicillin-G and 25% to both reagents. The marked difference from our results could be due to the selection of patients, different origin of PPL, and differences in the concentrations used with these reagents. The concentration of PPL applied is not mentioned by GREEN et al. (1977) whereas we have been using 25, 250, or 500 mmol/ml, the highest concentration being applied when all the others gave negative results.

In our hands the routine use of PPL and BPN reagents for skin testing in cases of suspicion of an allergic reaction to penicillin is a rapid, reliable, and safe procedure which should be adopted generally. By simultaneous determination of circulating IgG antibodies, by means of the hemagglutination technique (THIEL et al. 1964), a very high proportion of patients sensitized to penicillin can be detected (GIRARD et al. 1976). There is general agreement that skin testing has to be done by first using the method of scratch or prick tests. If the response remains negative after 30 min it is recommended that one injects intradermally 0.05 ml antigen solution corresponding to one-tenth of the concentration used for scratch tests.

III. Patch Testing

The most satisfactory precedure for testing drugs which produce contact skin reactions is by patch testing. This is a safe and very sensitive procedure which allows the determination of more than 90% of cases of contact dermatitis. There are several variants of this procedure which is usually done by a dermatologist. On some occasions, the locally applied antigen may induce a generalized reaction. In most cases, the tests are performed on the back, which offers a large surface for the simultaneous application of several patches. The optimal time for reading the result is 48 h. However, some reactions may develop several days later.

This procedure is often suitable for testing nurses, physicians, pharmacists, and dentists who not infrequently develop contact sensitization following contact with various drugs, especially antibiotics, local anaesthetics, and antiseptic agents among others.

E. Laboratory Procedures for Investigating Type I Allergic Drug Reactions

Since the discovery of IgE as a specific mediator of type I allergic reactions (ISHIZAKA and ISHIZAKA 1967), several methods have been described for the measurement of total circulating IgE or specific IgE antibodies. These tests were primarily developed for the determination of allergy to agents responsible for atopic diseases (aeroallergens, molds, furs, dust, etc.). However, there are also some applications to the diagnosis of allergic reactions to drugs. Some of these procedures will be briefly described.

I. Dosage of Serum IgE

The most widely applied procedure is a radioimmunoassay technique, developed by WIDE et al. (1967) and now commercially available (RIST-Pharmacia, Upp-

Table 7. Comparative evaluation of various immunologic tests in the laboratory diagnosis of penicillin allergy

Type of reaction	Number of patients	Skin tests	IgG Ab[a]	RAST	Histamine release	Lymphocyte stimulation	MIF
Type I	16	15/16	12/16	10/16	8/16	12/6	10/16
Type II and III	10	6/10	9/10	3/10	7/10	6/10	7/10
Type IV	24	16/24	13/24	9/24	12/24	18/24	20/24

[a] Circulating antibodies to penicillin

sala). The value of quantitative determination of serum IgE in cases of drug allergy is open to question.

Under mild or isolated antigenic stimulus, the IgE level seems to be only slightly affected or, in any case, for a very short period of time. Therefore in that situation repeated measurements are of importance. Frequent increase of serum IgE has been reported by ASSEM (1972) in patients with drug allergy and, according to WIDE and JUHLIN (1971) this immunoglobulin is often raised in cases of anaphylaxis to penicillin. Considering the short half-life of IgE, several measurements of IgE during the 3–4 weeks following the drug reaction could give information about the true responsibility of the suspected drug. However, the measurement of specific IgE antibodies is much more informative.

II. Radioallergosorbent Test (RAST)

This test was developed by WIDE et al. (1967) and later extended to the determination of IgE antibodies to penicillin. The principle is rather simple. The antigen is coupled to particles such as Sephadex or paper disks which are allowed to react with the test serum. Specific antibodies will bind the antigen and the complex formed can be detected by adding a radiolabeled anti-IgE.

In type I hypersensitivity reactions, the penicillin RAST has been used by several authors to estimate the specific IgE response (ASSEM 1972; WIDE and JUHLIN 1971). Using a modification of the classical RAST which improves the sensivity of the tests, ADKINSON (1975) found an excellent correlation between the positive clinical history, skin tests with PPL, and the results of the RAST.

In a recent survey, we compared several immunologic procedures for the laboratory diagnosis of penicillin allergy in 16 patients, including skin tests, hemagglutination, histamine release, lymphocyte stimulation, and macrophage migration inhibiting factor (MIF) production in the presence of antigen (CUEVAS 1978). The results shown in Table 7 are given according to the immunologic type of reaction. In this study, the highest percentage of positive responses is obtained by means of skin tests (PPL and BPN). This emphasizes the need for several specificities to be available with the RAST since, beside the penicilloyl group, various other determinants may be involved.

These results contain, among other data, some surprising figures:
1. The frequency of IgG antibodies in all types of reaction
2. The frequent presence of IgE antibodies in types II, III, and IV reactions
3. The frequent positive nature of cell-mediated reactions in type I reactions

These observations decrease to some extent the value of tests specific for type I–IV reactions as clinical correlates. Nevertheless, the penicillin RAST offers a reliable and safe way to explore at least type I allergic reactions. An extension of that procedure to other drugs commonly responsible for allergic reactions is therefore highly desirable.

III. Basophil Degranulation Test

Basophils as target cells for the IgE-allergen complexes have been extensively used as a diagnostic tool in type I reactions. The first procedure was devized by SHELLEY and JUHLIN (1961). However the use of human basophils is a difficult task. These cells are fragile and seem to degranulate spontaneously following a slight change of pH or calcium content of the suspending fluid. Therefore, interpretation of the results has been a matter of discussion for many years. Later on, rabbit and rat, basophils were applied in an indirect test for the detection of human reagins (SHELLEY 1963; PERELMUTTER and KHERA 1969). Some results could be obtained by using pollen allergen but the tests were never seriously applied to the diagnosis of type I allergic reactions to drugs. However, there is a notable exception with the report of MONNERET-VAUTRIN et al. (1972) who showed, following some modifications of the SHELLEY's procedure, very interesting results which correlated rather well with the clinical features. Unfortunately no reports from other laboratories have been published in confirmation of these results.

Recently, an interesting simplification of the basophil degranulation test was published by BENVENISTE (1977). Human basophils are used, somehow concentrated and incubated with an antigen to which the patient is specifically sensitized. The cells are then stained with toluidine blue and the number of visible cells counted. Knowing that degranulated cells do not take up the dye, it is simple, by substracting the test cells from the number of control cells, to determine whether specific IgE antibodies were present or not on the surface of the target cells. This procedure was adapted to the diagnosis of inhaled antigens. Unfortunately, there are as yet not many published data on the possible appliation of this test to the diagnosis of allergic drug reactions.

We have tested this method in investigating 18 patients with a known hypersensitivity to penicillin by clinical and laboratory criteria, and have compared it with other procedures, i.e., skin tests and penicillin RAST. Clinically, all the patients could be classified as showing type I reactions. Six patients were excluded from the study, owing to an insufficant number of basophils, rendering the test not feasible.

The results shown in Table 8 demonstrate an excellent correlation of skin tests and RAST with the clinical diagnosis. The correlation is, however, much lower for the basophil degranulation test. Interestingly, this result improved when the test was performed several days after the clinical reaction had taken place. Such a study should be extended to other drugs in order to test its feasibility with less well-characterized antigenic determinants.

Table 8. Comparative analysis of the value of skin tests, RAST, and the basophil degranulation test in the diagnosis of type I reactions in 18 patients allergic to penicillin

Period of tests	Skin tests (PPL + BPN)	Penicillin RAST	Basophil degranulation
< 1 month	14/18	13/18	9/18
1–8 months	12/18	10/18	11/18

IV. Histamine Release from Sensitized Leukocytes

When basophils or mastocytes from atopic individuals are incubated with a specific antigen, histamine is released into the medium. A method was developed in 1968 by OSLER et al. as and assay for reaginic antibodies. To date, this test has been applied to several inhaled allergens but, to our knowledge, not to the diagnosis of drug allergy. We have a limited experience of this procedure applied to the diagnosis of allergy to penicillin (GIRARD 1973; see also Table 3). According to our experience, this procedure seems to be of value at least for penicillin allergy. The results correlate well with the skin tests and positive clinical history. However, the procedure used for the dosage of histamine is very time-consuming and no more than 2–3 tests can be performed in a single day unless costly automated procedures are introduced. A recently described method using automated analysis of histamine released from sensitized leukocytes (SIRAGANIAN 1977), could well justify a wider application of this technique.

F. In Vitro Investigation of Type II Reactions

This type of reaction is rather well documented, because the main targets are the corpuscular elements of the blood.

I. Drug-Induced Allergic Hemolysis

One of the main features of this blood dyscrasia is the presence of IgG and sometimes IgM antibodies bound to the surface of red cells. COOMBS et al. (1945) developed a sensitive method for the detection of such antibodies. In brief, red blood cells are taken from the patient with a suspected allergic reaction, thoroughly washed and incubated with a serum antiglobulin. Addition of the suspected drug improves the sensitivity of the test. Hemolysis can results from the reaction, following addition of fresh complement. By sensitizing normal human O red cells, an indirect Coombs test has been developed with the great advantage of giving a titer of the circulating antibodies, also allowing the differentiation of complete and incomplete antibodies (AMOS et al. 1968). Finally, in case of hemolytic anemia due to penicillin, the determination of circulating antibodies is another good way to confirm the responsibility of that antibiotic.

II. Drug-Induced Thrombocytopenia

Following the fundamental investigations of ACKROYD (DAUSSET et al. 1964) on Se-
dormid-induced thrombocytopenic purpura, numerous publications reported
similar effects induced by a large variety of drugs. Several methods have been devized to establish the diagnosis.

1. Inhibition of Clot Retraction

With very simple equipment, it is possible to observe the inhibition of clot retraction in the presence of the offending drug. However there are limiting factors to
the routine application of this procedure. Clot retraction requires the presence of
platelets in sufficient numbers. Frequently, the recovery of a normal platelet level
after a reaction takes 5–15 days, a time which might be sufficient to allow the antibodies to disappear.

2. Drug-Dependent Platelet Agglutination

This test requires platelet-rich plasma from a patient recovering from a drug-induced platelet lysis. Various concentrations of the suspected drug have to be used
and the mixture incubated in the presence of the patient's serum. Platelet agglutination is best determined on a siliconized slide, using a phase contrast microscope.
An indirect method using platelets from a normal donor can also be adapted. It
is, however, less sensitive and reliable (DAUSSET et al. 1964).

They are several limiting factors to the application of this technique, such as:
1. The specific antibody is often detectable in the serum for only a short period
   of time
2. The preparation of a platelet-rich plasma is a delicate operation; spontaneous
   agglutination often occurs
3. Nonimmunologic agglutination of platelets following incubation with some
   drugs can occur

3. Complement Fixation Test for Drug-Induced Thrombocytopenia

Most antigen–antibody complexes fix complement through the normal pathway.
The technique of complement fixation has been largely applied to determine the
titer of antibody (LACHMAN et al. 1973). The serum to be tested is first decomple-
mented by heat at 56 °C for 40 min and diluted in small tubes. An equal amount
of platelets, in the presence of suspected antigen, is added to each tube. Guinea pig
complement is then added. This complement fixation test is more sensitive than the
determination of platelet agglutinins and is now widely adopted.

III. Drug-Induced Agranulocytosis

1. Serologic Methods

MOESCHLIN was the first to demonstrate in 1954 the presence of drug-induced leu-
koagglutinin induced by aminopyrine (MOESCHLIN 1954). The procedure described

Table 9. Culture of lymphocytes from patients with drug-induced agranulocytosis in the presence of heterologous or autologous serum and aminopyrine

Patient	Control AB (without aminopyrine)	Activity (ct/min)	
		Serum AB (with aminopyrine)	Autologous serum (with aminopyrine)
1	360	540	1,240
2	400	700	950
3	326	390	1,625
4	630	1,020	2,030
5	475	715	890

consists in incubation of leukocyte-rich plasma from a normal donor with the patient's serum. Direct agglutination of leukocytes is then observed. Unfortunately, this procedure lacks sensivity and carries the frequent risk of false positive agglutinations. The mixed antiglobulin reaction as described by COOMBS et al. (1956) has also been applied to the determination of drug-induced leukocyte antibodies, with controversial results.

2. Lymphocyte Stimulation

This in vitro procedure was applied for several years as a diagnostic tool in drug-induced thrombocytopenia or agranulocytosis, with rather unsatisfactory results. Later on (GIRARD 1972), it was recognized that instead of using human AB serum for enrichment of the medium, the patient's own serum more often gave positive results. Such a result is illustrated in Table 9. Peripheral blood lymphocytes from patients recovering from an aminopyrine-induced agranulocytosis were washed and cultured for 5 days in the presence of the synthetic culture medium TC 199 (Difco, Basel), 20% autologous serum (as obtained at the acute stage) or AB serum and aminopyrine (40 $\mu g/10^6$ cells). H^3-Thymidine was added 12 h before harvesting the cells and the activity was determined in a well scintillation counter.

As shown in Table 9, the presence of autologous serum increases the incorporation of DNA significantly. In a large number of control cultures (SHELLEY and JUHLIN 1971), no stimulatory effect could be observed following stimulation of lymphocytes with autologous serum and aminopyrine. Similar experiments were extended to drug-induced thrombocytopenia, with significant results.

At the present time, this procedure is the most satisfactory for the determination of the offending agent. The stimulatory effect of the mixture of autologous serum and antigen is likely to be the result of antigen–antibody complexes which are known to induce cell proliferation in vitro.

G. Laboratory Procedures to Detect Serum-Sickness Syndrome (Type III)

In this type of reaction, tissue damage results from antigen–antibody complexes depositing beyond the walls of small blood vessels. The formation of complexes ac-

Table 10. Determination of immune complexes in the sera of 120 patients allergic to drugs, 50 healthy donors and 10 aspirin-induced asthma, by the C1q binding test

C1q binding test activity (%)	Aspirin-induced asthma	Controls	Drug allergy
< 4	9/10	44/50	40/120
4– 8	1/10	4/50	48/120
8–12		2/50	15/120
> 12			17/120

tivates and fixes complement, events leading to capillary dilation and afflux of leukocytes. The most frequent symptoms of serum sickness due to drugs are: fever, urticaria, arthralgia, vasculitis, and sometimes damage to the lung and kidney.

Several methods can be applied to establish, on one hand, the immunologic nature of the damage and, on the other, the etiologic agent. They are:
1. Determination of circulating immune complexes
2. Determination of complement factors or antibodies on biopsy specimens
3. Analysis of the patient's serum for the presence of circulating or precipitating antibodies

Unfortunately, most of these procedures are not readily applicable in the case of allergic reactions to drugs.

I. Determination of Immune Complexes

There are several technical procedures available. It is difficult at present to determine which is the best. For the analysis of a large group of patients exhibiting an actual allergic reaction to various drugs, immune complexes were assayed by the ^{125}C1q binding test which has shown a high degree of specificity for immune complexes in various diseases (NYDEGGER et al. 1974). Normal values of the C1q-binding test, as determined in the serum fo 50 healthy donors was $0.0 \pm 2.1\%$. Sera exceeding the normal range by more than 2 standard deviations were considered positive.

The results as illustrated in Table 10 demonstrate the absence of immune complexes in aspirin-induced asthma, whereas in 66% of the patients with allergic reactions to drugs, complexes were present, sometimes in rather high amounts. This finding is certainly not of great help in establishing the diagnosis of drug allergy. It demonstrates, however, that antigen–antibody complexes are a part of the pathogenesis of such reaction, either as contributory agents or side phenomena. These results are encouraging to those interested in tissue biopsy analysis. Complement deposits should more often be determined in small tissue biopsies, as part of the in vitro diagnosis.

II. Determination of Circulating Antibodies

This determination is currently performed in cases of allergic reactions to penicillin, using the well-established hemagglutination of penicillin-coated erythrocytes described by THIEL et al. (1964). As shown in Table 7 this determination is of great value. Appreciation of the level of antibodies is of particular importance. In our experience, an anti-penicillin antibody titer greater than 1/16 indicates with great certainty an allergic reaction to that drug (GIRARD et al. 1971).

For drugs other than penicillin, there is a need to prepare conjugates, selecting a suitable carrier, in order to obtain a complete antigen appropriate for serologic studies. Such an example is illustrated in the report of FURUYA and URASAW (1978), who prepared a phenothiazine–BSA conjugate, using various parent haptens. Specific circulating antibodies could be demonstrated in the sera of 18 psychiatric patients treated for a long period of time with these drugs. In five patients who developed allergic alveolitis to drugs (nitrofurantoin, two cases; sulfamides, two cases; penicillin, one case), hapten–BSA conjugates were prepared and used for the measurement of precipitating antibodies in double diffusion in agar. Precipitins were present in all five cases.

Therefore the procedure of preparing drug–carrier conjugates should be extended and the reagents thus obtained applied to various serologic diagnostic, procedures. In such a system, human or sheep erythrocytes are commonly used as indicator and hemagglutination has developed to a high degree of sensitivity, also allowing the identification of the class of antibody. Bacteriophages have also been used as indicators. Phage neutralization has been applied to demonstrate penicillin antibody (HAIMOVICH et al. 1967) and acetylsalicylate antibodies (AMOS et al. 1971). Phage neutralization is a particularly sensitive assay system, detecting antibody concentrations of 10^{-4} mg/ml, and certainly deserves further development.

H. Laboratory Diagnosis of Type IV Reactions or Delayed Hypersensitivity

The genesis of the term "delayed hypersensitivity" is related to the practice of skin tests with tuberculin. It is a restrictive functional term, which fails to reflect the complex phenomena of cell-mediated hypersensitivity. Restricted initially to the interaction of the effector cells with antigen, it now includes all the cooperative mechanisms existing between humoral and cell-mediated hypersensitivity.

For some time, in vitro lymphocyte transformation and later on the production of macrophage migration inhibitory factor (MIF) have been considered as in vitro correlates of delayed hypersensitivity. We now know that antigen–antibody complexes as well as T-independent antigens can stimulate lymphocyte cultures in vitro. On the other hand, MIF production results not only from T-cells but also from B-lymphocyte activation by antigen (GIRARD et al. 1976; BLOOM 1977). Therefore, no specific laboratory procedure for the measurement of delayed hypersensitivity is yet available. This partly explains the difficulties of classifying delayed hypersensitivity reactions due to drugs.

Morbilliform exanthema, fixed drug eruptions, and erythrodermia are thought to result from a cell-mediated reaction, i.e., T-lymphocytes as in contact sensitivity. However, the histologic pictures of both reactions differ in a number of features. Moreover, basophil infiltration, which is rather important in contact sensitivity, is often negligible in the tuberculin reaction. In spite of several differences between

Table 11. Stimulation of peripheral blood lymphocytes of patients allergic to penicillin with BPN, PPL, penicillin-HGG and penicillin-ovalbumin conjugates, either in the presence of AB or autologous serum. Incorporation of H^3-thymidine

Stimulatory[a] agents	Result (ct/min)		
	Patient 1	Patient 2	Patient 3
None	535	405	620
BPN (AB)	780	915	1,170
BPN (AS)	1,630	980	1,340
PPL (AB)	1,070	920	1,200
PPL (AS)	1,380	1,400	1,630
Penicillin-HGG (AB)	820	535	600
Penicillin-HGG (AS)	480	440	570
Penicillin-Ovalbumin (AB)	1,550	1,555	1,700
Penicillin-Ovalbumin (AS)	2,320	1,700	1,850

[a] AB = AB human serum; AS = autologous serum

these two types of reactions, they exhibit common features which are of importance in establishing the in vitro diagnosis.

1. Sensitized lymphocytes, when cultured in vitro in the presence of antigen, synthesize new DNA and produce lymphokines (DUMONDE et al. 1969)
2. The magnitude of the in vitro response correlates to some extent with the intensity of the skin response

For these reasons, lymphocyte transformation and leukocyte migration inhibition tests have been widely used to investigate type IV allergic drug reactions.

I. Lymphocyte Transformation Test

Peripheral blood lymphocytes, when cultured with mitogens (phytohemagglutinin, concavanalin A, or pokeweed) or specific antigens, undergo a morphological change into large blastoid cells; this corresponds to an increased synthesis of DNA.

In experimental immune responses to haptens, it has been repeatedly demonstrated that lymphocyte transformation to specific antigenic challenge is carrier specific (KABAT 1967). We do not have information about the nature of the autologous carriers in the case of allergy to drugs. Thus, in testing drugs in vitro, the usual procedure is to add a solution of the drug to the suspension of the patient's lymphocytes. Whether the cultured cells or macromolecules present in the medium function as carriers has not been determined. However, some experimental data tend to demonstrate that the nature of the carrier is far from unimportant.

Lymphocytes from patients allergic to penicillins were cultured in the presence of specific antigen or antigen conjugated with various carriers. The culture medium was enriched with normal AB human serum of autologous serum. The results, which are illustrated in Table 11, are interesting. BPN was shown to be slightly more efficient than PPL as challenging substance. However the stimulatory capacity of penicilloyl–ovalbumin was shown to be far stronger than that of the isolated haptens. It has been shown that conjugation of drugs to cell membrane proteins of lymphocytes and macrophages is strongly stimulating for drug-sensitized lymphocytes (DE WECK 1975). Results obtained with heterologous protein Carriers such as ovalbumin, bovine serum albumin, or globulin also raise the question of prior sensitization to these proteins in food.

By contrast, a complete lack of stimulation resulted from challenge with penicilloyl–HGG conjugates. In all positive experiments, the addition of autologous serum the medium improved the stimulation when compared with human AB serum. An enhancing effect of autologous serum was also shown by GIMENEZ-CAMARATA et al. (1975).

The routine application of the lymphocyte transformation test to the diagnosis of allergic reaction to drugs has been reported by several investigators (GIRARD et al. 1971; GIRARD et al. 1976; HALPERN et al. 1967; LEVENE and BAKER 1968; LING 1971) with, however, conflicting results. It is certainly difficult to explain the great variability in the percentage of positive tests reported by various investigators. The lymphocyte transformation test is not yet standardized and technical differences could well be responsible. However, summarizing results from long practice of this test appears to indicate that some conditions may interfere with the overall results obtained. These conditions are:

1. Negative responses are frequent when the test is performed within a few days of the onset of the allergic reaction
2. A negative response may result from the presence in the vascular bed of the offending drug; measurable blood levels of some drugs may persist for more than 10 days, especially in case of renal or cardiac insufficiency
3. In some clinical conditions, such as acute bacterial or viral infections, spontaneous DNA synthesis (without the presence of drug) is so high that the stimulatory effect of the added drug is negligible
4. High drug concentrations added to the suspension of lymphocytes are often inhibitory; for this reason, at least three different concentrations of the suspected drug must be used
5. Factors inhibiting cell division can be present in the serum from patients with tuberculosis, sarcoidosis, lymphomas, Hodgkin's disease, and various solid tumors

Therefore, the patient's own serum may exhibit either factors inducing blast transformation such as immune complexes, or inhibitory factors due to the features of the underlying disease. Thus, a double test using human AB serum (pool) and the patient's serum seems to be mandatory.

1. Solutions of the drug to be tested are to be prepared in phosphate buffered saline (pH 7.2), containing 20% normal human AB serum
2. When feasible, results seem to be more significant and reproducible by using hapten–protein conjugates instead of the hapten alone

Furthermore, several technical factors such as the nature and size of the tube or well in regard to the amount of cells, the percentage of added human serum, or the type of incubator are all of great importance. These factors were adequately analyzed by LING (1974) and SCHELEEKENS et al. (1968).

A final but very important point has to be mentioned. Commercial drugs contain, beside the active component several chemicals, such as coloring agents, antioxidants, and stabilizing substances which might also be potential allergens.

Drugs may contain byproducts of drug synthesis which may be reactive chemicals. One typical example was analyzed by SCHNEIDER et al. (1971). Carboxymethylcellulose (CMC) is frequently present in drug formulations. Penicillin was shown to bind to hydroxyl groups of CMC, forming conjugates which are very efficient in eliciting allergic reactions in sensitized patients. Some coloring agents, such as tartrazin, erythrosine, and carminic acid among others, are potent sensitizers and we have now collected several cases of allergic reactions which were due to these dyes and not to the pharmacologically active component.

Taking into consideration all the pitfalls and difficulties in applying the lymphocyte transformation test and assessing as precisely as possible the nature of the offending drug, we conclude that this testing procedure appears to be a reliable and a very useful tool for completing the clinical diagnosis (GIRARD 1974). This test appears to be a correlate not only of cell-mediated hypersensitivity but also frequently of humoral allergic reactions. Finally, in interpreting the results of lymphocyte transformation tests, it is important to note that this in vitro test is to be considered as an expression of immunologic response, but not necessarily of clinical manifestations due to a specific drug.

II. Leukocyte Migration Inhibition Test

This test was first described by SOBORG (1971). Now this procedure has been adapted to the measurement of either monocytes of the migration of polymorphonuclear cells as target cells. Micromethods (MIF and LIF tests) are now available (GIRARD et al. 1976), which can be adapted to analyze the effect of preformed migration inhibitory factor (MIF) (BLOOM 1977) or by immediately adding the lymphokine-inducing antigen. In essence, the technique used is a modification of that described by SOBORG and BENDIXEN (1968). Heparinized blood is allowed to sediment for 30 min in the presence of one-third its volume of 6% dextran. The leukocyte-rich layer is separated, washed, and adjusted to 10^8 cells/ml. The cell suspension is mixed with 0.5% agarose and distributed as droplets in the wells (GIRARD 1974; GIRARD et al. 1976) of a Falcon microplate (Falcon Products, Basel). Wells are filled with culture medium and antigen in appropriate concentrations. After 16 h incubation at 37 °C, the diameter of the migration area is measured with a microscope at low magnification, with an eyepiece graticule (GIRARD et al. 1976).

The migration inhibition test was applied in our laboratory for diagnosis of allergic reactions to drugs, for two main reasons:

1) The test procedure is simple, inexpensive, and the result is obtained the following day, which represents significant advantages when compared with the lymphocyte transformation test.

2) As shown by ROCKLIN et al. (1974), B-lymphocytes as well as T-cells showed the capacity to produce the inhibitory factor when put in contact with mitogens or specific antigens. Therefore, lymphokine production could result from both humoral imune reactions and cell-mediated reactions.

Experiments were performed with several drugs; however, 15 cases of penicillin allergy were thoroughly studied according to the type of immune reaction. The result shown in Table 12 demonstrates a good correlation between the leukocyte mi-

Table 12. MIF production by leucocytes from 15 patients allergic to penicillin. Comparison with the lymphocyte transformation test (LTT) and skin tests

Clinical classification	Number of patients	MIF[a]	LTT[a]	Skin tests
Anaphylactic shock	5	3/5	2/5	5/5[b]
Serum sickness	5	5/5	5/5	2/5[c]
Exanthema	5	5/5	4/5	1/5[d]

[a] Positive tests/patients tested
[b] Positive skin test at 15 min,
[c] 4–8 h, and
[d] 24–48 h

gration inhibition test and the lymphocyte transformation test. Table 12 also demonstrates that MIF production occured in typical type I reactions, such as anaphylactic shock.

J. Conclusions

The diagnosis of allergic reactions to drugs is often difficult. For instance, in the presence of a skin rash several possibilities have to be considered before admitting the possibility of an immune mechanism. Several viral and bacterial infections can lead to an erythematous or morbilliform eruption. On the other hand, drugs such as opiates, iodinated drugs, anesthetic agents, and some antibiotics have shown the property of releasing histamine from mast cells nonspecifically (ROCKOFF et al. 1970). Finally, many anti-inflammatory agents such as aspirin, mefemanic acid, indomethacin, and antipyrine, may induce nonallergic skin reactions (SAMTER and BERRYMAN 1968). This emphasizes the need for a thorough knowledge of possible side effects of drugs.

However, in many circumstances, laboratory procedures are very helpful in establishing the nature of the offending agent. This is especially true when the patient is receiving several drugs simultaneously. Interpretation of the results, however, has to be done with caution. Often, all that can be said is that an immune response to a specific drug has taken place. Furthermore, owing to the lack of absolute clinical criteria to establish the type of immune reaction involved, it is necessary to apply several tests simultaneously to the same drug.

It is not possible to rely completely on laboratory procedures to establish the etiologic diagnosis of an allergic reaction to a drug. Knowledge of the toxic and allergenic properties of drugs and a correct understanding of the immunologic mechanisms involved still remain basic requirements for the clinical immunologist.

Acknowledgements. The authors' research included in this report was supported by the Swiss National Foundation for Scientific Research (Grant 3.074.076).

References

Adkinson NF (1975) Recent developments in the use of RAST for determining hypersensitivity to penicillin. In: Evans E (ed) Advances in diagnosis of allergy. RAST, Miami

Amos HE (1976) Allergic drug reactions. Arnold, London

Amos HE, Bishop ANR, Scaman MJ, Trowell J (1968) Penicillin induced hemolytic anemia. Br Med J 3:439

Amos HE, Wilson DV, Taussig MJ, Carton SJ (1971) Hypersensitivity reactions to acetylsalicylic acid. Detection of antibodies in human sera using acetylsalicylic acid attached to proteins through the carboxyl group. Clin Exp Immunol 8:567

Assem ESK (1972) IgE and other in vitro tests in the diagnosis and follow-up of drug allergy. In: Dash CH (ed) Mechanism of drug allergy. Churchill Livingstone, Edinburgh London

Benveniste J (1977) The in vitro basophil degranulation test. In: Allergy and clinical immunology. Proceedings of the IXth International Congress of Allergology, Buenos-Aires. Excerpta Medica, Amsterdam London New York

Bloom BR (1977) Effector cells in cell-mediated immunity. In: Allergy and clinical immunology. Proceedings of the IXth International Congress of Allergology, Buenos-Aires. Excerpta Medica, Amsterdam London New York

Coombs RRA, Mourant AE, Race RR (1945) A new test for the detection of weak and incomplete Rh. agglutinins. Br J Exp Pathol 26:255

Coombs RRA, Marks J, Bedford D (1956) Mixed erythrocyte-platelet antiglobulin reaction for the detection of platelet antibodies. Br J Haematol 2:84

Cuevas M (1978) Diagnostic et prévention des allergies médicamenteuses aux pénicillines. Medical thesis, University of Geneva

Dausset J, Colombani J, Ochochi K (1964) Leucocytes and platelet agglutination. In: Ackroyd JF (ed) Immunological methods. Blackwell Scientific, Oxford

de Weck AL (1964) Penicillin allergy. Its detection by an improved technique. Nature 202:975

de Weck AL (1972) Critical evaluation of diagnostic methods in drug allergy. In: Charpin J (ed) Allergology. Excerpta Medica, Amsterdam London New York, p 23

de Weck AL (1975) Molecular mechanisms of T and B lymphocyte triggering. Int Arch Allergy Appl Immunol 49:247–257

Dumonde DC, Wolstencroft RA, Panays GS, Matthews M, Morley J, Howson WT (1969) Lymphokines, non antibody mediators of cellular immunity generated by lymphocyte activation. Nature 224:38

Furuya K, Urasawa S (1978) Demonstration of antibodies to chlorophenothiazin derivates. Int Arch Allergy Appl Immunol 57:22

Girard JP (1972) Allergic reactions to antibiotics. Helv Med Acta 36:3

Girard JP (1973) Diagnostic tests in drug allergy. In: Allergology. Proceedings of the 8th International Congress of Allergology, Tokyo, 1973. Excerpta Medica, Amsterdam London New York, p 460

Girard JP (1974) Diagnostic tests in drug allergy. In: Allergology. Proceedings of the 8th International Congress of Allergology, Tokyo, 1973. Excerpta Medica, Amsterdam London New York, p 460

Girard JP, Cuevas M (1975) Analyse clinique et immunologique de 1047 réactions allergiques à la pénicilline. Schweiz Med Wochenschr 105:953

Girard JP, Vidmar B, Laugier P (1971) Diagnostic des allergies médicamenteuses. Rev Fr Allergol 11:397

Girard JP, Cattin S, Cuevas M (1976) Immunological mechanisms and diagnosis tests in allergic drug reactions. Ann Clin Res 8:74

Gimmenez-Camarasa JM, Garcia-Calderon P, de Moraga JM (1975) Lymphocyte transformation test in fixed drug eruption. N Engl J Med 292:819

Green GR, Rosenblum AH, Sweet LC (1977) Evaluation of penicillin hypersensitivity. Value of clinical history and skin testing with PPL and penicillin G. J Allergy Clin Imunol 60:339

Haimovich J, Sela M, Dewdney JM, Batchelor FR (1967) Anti-penicilloyl antibodies: detection with penicilloylated bacteriophage and isolation with a specific immunoabsorbent. Nature 214:1369

Halpern B, Ky NT, Amache N (1967) Diagnosis of drug allergy in vitro with the lymphocyte transformation test. J Allergy 40:168

Ishizaka K, Ishizaka T (1967) Identification of IgE antibodies as a carrier of reaginic activity. J Immunol 99:1187

Kabat EA (1967) Structural conception in immunology and immunochemistry. Reinhart & Winston, New York

Lachman PJ, Hobart MJ, Aston WP (1973) In: Weir DM (ed) Handbook of experimental immunology. Blackwell Scientific, Oxford

Levene G, Baker H (1968) Drug reactions. II. Lymphocyte transformation in vitro and drug hypersensitivity. Br J Dermatol 80:415

Levine BB, Redmund AP, Voos HE, Zolov DM (1967) Prediction of penicillin allergy by immunological tests. Ann NY Acad Sci 145:298

Ling NR (1971) In vitro lymphocyte transformation, standardization of culture methods. In: Serafini U (ed) New concepts in allergy and clinical immunology. Excerpta Medica, Amsterdam London New York

Moeschlin S (1954) Weitere Beobachtungen über Immunoleukopenien und Agranulocytosen. Schweiz Med Wochenschr 84:1100

Monneret-Vautrin DA, Grillat JP, Pupil P (1972) Basophil degranulation in drug allergy. In: Dash CH, Parish WE (eds) Mechanism in drug allergy. Churchill Livingstone, Edinburgh London

Nydegger UE, Lambert P, Gerber H, Miescher PA (1974) Circulating immune complexes in the serum in systemic lupus erythematosus and in carriers of hepatitis B antigen. J Clin Invest 54:297

Osler AG, Lichtenstein LM, Levy DA (1968) In vitro study of human reaginic antibody. Adv Immunol 8:183

Ozeki S, Tejima K (1974) Drug interaction. II. Binding of some pyrazolone and pyrazolidine derivates to bovine serum albumin. Chem Pharm Bull (Tokyo) 22:1297

Perelmutter L, Khera K (1969) Rat mast cells in human reagin detection. Lancet 1:1269

Rocklin RE, MacDermott RP, Chess L, Schlossman SF, David JP (1974) Studies on mediators production by highly purified human T and B lymphocytes. J Exp Med 140:1303

Rockoff JD, Brash R, Kuhn C (1970) Contrast media as histamine liberators. Invest Radiol 5:503

Samter M, Berryman GM (1968) Drug allergy. Annu Rev Pharmacol 4:465

Scheleekens RE, Tit A, Eijsvogel VP (1968) Lymphocyte transformation in vitro. Tissue culture conditions and quantitative measurements. Clin Exp Immunol 3:571

Schneider CH, de Weck AL, Stäuble E (1971) Carboxymethylcellulose additives in penicillins and the elicitation of anaphylactic reactions. Experientia 27:167

Shelley WB (1963) Indirect basophil degranulation test for allergy to penicillin and other drugs. JAMA 184:171

Shelley WB, Juhlin L (1961) A new test for detecting anaphylactic sensitivity, the basophil reaction. Nature 191:1056

Siraganian RP (1977) Automated analysis of histamine released from leucocytes of allergic donors. In: Allergy and clinical immunology. Proceedings of the IXth International Congress Allergology, Buenos-Aires. Excerptia Medica, Amsterdam London New York

Soborg M (1971) The leucocyte migration technique for in vitro detection of cellular hypersensitivity in man. In: Bloom BR (ed) In vitro methods in cell-mediated immunity. Academic Press, New York

Soborg M, Bendixen G (1968) Human lymphocyte migration as a parameter of hypersensitivity. Acta Med Scand 98:1655

Thiel JA, Mitchell S, Parker CV (1964) The specificity of hemagglutination reaction in human and experimental penicilin hypersensitivity. J Allergy 35:399

Wide L, Juhlin L (1971) Detection of penicillin allergy of the immediate type by radioimmunoassay of reagins (IgE) to penicilloyl conjugates. Clin Allergy 1:171

Wide L, Bennich H, Johansson SGO (1967) Diagnosis of allergy by an in vitro test for allergen antibodies. Lancet 2:1105

CHAPTER 8

Prevention and Treatment of Drug Allergies

A. L. DE WECK

The problem of prevention and therapy of allergic reactions to drugs is complex and not yet satisfactorily resolved. Measures to reduce the incidence of allergic reactions to drugs may be taken at several levels, for instance by the manufacturer, the treating physician, or the patient himself.

A. Evaluation of the Allergenic Potential of Drugs

In order to induce an immune response of the antibody- or cell-mediated type, most chemotherapeutic agents, as low-molecular-weight compounds, are supposed to bind covalently to autologous proteins and cell membrane proteins, thereby forming immunogenic conjugates (see Chap. 3). Whether the binding of the allergenic drug to an autologous carrier molecule always has to be of covalent nature might be doubted; various examples in basic immunology suggest that noncovalent binding to carriers, provided it is sufficiently strong, is also capable of inducing an antibody response (GREEN et al. 1966; DE WECK 1977). Accordingly, an allergenic drug should be considered first from two angles: (a) the presence of *reactive groups* enabling covalent binding to proteins; and (b) the presence of *structures favouring attachment to cell membranes*, especially to macrophages. These considerations apply not only to the drug itself, but also to its derivatives and its metabolites. Furthermore, they apply to all *chemical contaminants* of a drug preparation; these may be either biological or chemical by-products, resulting from the process used in preparation of the drug or from the additives and preservatives deliberately added to the drug. Some examples of allergenic by-products in drug preparations are as follows:

1. *Reactive derivatives and degradation products:* benzylpenicillenic acid, benzylpenicilloic acid in aged penicillin solutions; penicillin (especially ampicillin) polymers
2. *Reactive metabolites:* phenetidin and its oxidation products in phenacetin allergy; quinones in allergy to compounds of the "para" (paraphenylenediamine) group
3. *Reactive chemical impurities as byproducts of synthesis:* acetylsalicylsalicylic acid and acetylsalicylic anhydride in aspirin
4. *Immunogenic biological impurities:* mycelial proteins in penicillins extracted from broth; *Escherichia coli* penicillin amidase in 6-aminopenicillanic acid used for synthesis of semisynthetic penicillins
5. *Additives with immunogenic potential or serving as inert carriers:* tartrazine, azo dyes, parabens; carboxymethylcellulose, starch.

Obviously, a thorough immunochemical analysis of all factors and compounds involved in the occurrence of sensitization to a given drug may in itself suggest preventive measures, such as the elimination of high-molecular-weight impurities of biological origin in penicillin allergy (BATCHELOR et al. 1967; AHLSTEDT et al. 1980), the prevention of degradation to allergenic derivatives such as penicillenic or penicilloic acids (DE WECK and EISEN 1960, LEVINE 1966; NEFTEL et al. 1981) or of the formation of allergenic polymers (DE WECK et al. 1968; DEWDNEY 1977) by appropriate storage conditions, the minimization of the formation of allergenic by-products of synthesis such as aspirin anhydride and acetylsalicylsalicylic acid in aspirin allergy (BUNDGAARD and DE WECK 1975), and the avoidance of additives potentially allergenic in themselves, such as a number of dyestuffs, or other additives (e. g., carboxymethylcellulose in penicillin preparations), and preservatives such as parabens or thimerosal.

This approach, however, has its limitations. In a number of instances, with penicillins or cephalosporins for example, chemically reactive groups responsible for the allergenic potential are also required for the desired pharmacological activity. This is why, despite 20 years intensive research and the synthesis of literally thousands of penicillin and cephalosporin derivatives, it has not been possible to my knowledge to produce totally nonimmunogenic penicillin while fully maintaining antibiotic activity. However, there are obviously differences in the degrees to which structural modifications of the basic penicillin structure affect antibiotic activity on the one hand and allergenic potential on the other.

When allergy to a drug is due not to the drug itself, but to a metabolite (e. g., phenetidin in phenacetin allergy), it could appear at first glance that not much can be done about it. However, the fact that metabolic pathways of a drug may vary from one individual to another, and also that they can sometimes be influenced by the concomitant administration of another drug or by nutritional and environmental factors, should be kept in mind by people concerned with the prevention of drug allergies. Genetic and environmental factors may well be responsible, at least in part, for regional or racial differences in the frequency of allergic reactions to some drugs.

Obviously, allergenic impurities and additives should be removed from drug preparations. To what extent the increased consciousness about high-molecular-weight impurities in penicillin preparations is responsible for the apparent decline in the incidence of severe allergic reactions to penicillin during the past years (Table 1) is not entirely clear. Other factors, such as the increased awareness of physicians and patients about penicillin allergy, have probably also played a role. Recent studies from a Swedish group, however, (KRISTOFFERSON et al. 1977; AHLSTEDT et al. 1980) suggest that significant amounts of immunogenic high-molecular-weight impurities are still present in most commercial penicillin preparations. Although high-molecular-weight impurities may undoubtedly contribute to penicillin immunogenicity and should therefore be eliminated as far as technically possible, it is my conviction, based on evidence from several lines of investigation, that even the purest penicillin obtainable will still be responsible for a significant number of allergic reactions. In a recent study (NEFTEL et al. 1981), we have shown that the immunogenicity of currently available commercial penicillins is directly related to the mode of administration: freshly dissolved and immediately injected

Table 1. Clinical cases of penicillin allergy in two different periods (Bern, Switzerland)

Main symptoms	1962–1966		1971–1976	
	n	%	n	%
Urticaria	102	33	90	39
Anaphylactic shock ⎫			8	3
Anaphylactoid symptoms ⎭	59	19	7	3
Serum-like disease	43	14	6	3
Angioneurotic edema	28	9	31	14
Generalized exanthema	25	8	65	28
Contact dermatitis	15	5	3	1
Blood dyscrasias	13	4	4	2
Generalized pruritus	6	2	7	3
Local reactions	7	2	4	2
Asthma	4	1		
Miscellaneous	9	3	6	3
Total	311		231	

penicillin solutions were not detectably immunogenic, while solutions allowed to stand for 4–24 h before administration invariably induced detectable antibenzyl-penicilloyl (anti-BPO)IgG antibodies and penicillin-sensitive lymphocytes. In fact, penicillins remain nowadays the most common cause of allergic reactions to a drug.

A problem frequently facing drug manufacturers is the assessment of potential allergenicity of a new drug. In general, considerations of pharmacological efficiency, absorption, and pharmacokinetics, as well as toxicological findings, have priority in the assessment of new drugs, all the more as accurate prediction of the allergenic potential on the basis of animal experiments is still difficult. However, increasing attention is being paid to this problem, and the endeavor to achieve low allergenicity is slowly beginning to play a role in drug development. Of course, this problem has long been recognized for those drugs primarily used for topical application and potentially inducing contact dermatitis (MAGNUSSON and KLIGMAN 1970).

B. Preventive Measures in Drug Allergy

Many drugs are given unnecessarily, and the number of adverse reactions to drugs is directly proportional to the number of courses of treatment prescribed (KLEIN et al. 1972). The administration of several drugs concurrently may also increase the risk of a reaction.

Even when specific diagnostic procedures are not available, the risk of serious allergic reaction to a drug can be minimized by:
1. Taking a careful history of previous adverse reactions to drugs, including those chemically related to the one intended for use
2. Availability of routine precautions and emergency treatment in the course of therapy with drugs known to cause immediate systemic reactions

3. Proper advice to the patient on the drugs he is receiving and on those to which
   he is believed to be allergic ("allergy pass" or tag)
4. Awareness of new clinical manifestations occurring during the course of therapy
5. Knowledge of the drugs that might cross-react immunologically with the drug
   to which the patient is demonstrably or allegedly allergic

In the penicillin series, allergy to penicillin G may be associated with allergic
reactivity to any of the semisynthetic penicillins, cephalotins or penicillamine. Recent findings suggest that the cross-reactivity for allergic reactions which are antibody-dependent rests mainly on structural similarities between penicillin and cephalosporin side chains (DE WECK and SCHNEIDER 1980), while little cross-reactivity
exists between antibodies directed against the penicillin or cephalosporin nuclei. At
the level of lymphocyte recognition and reactivity, on the other hand, cross-
reactions between penicillins and cephalosporins may be extensive (Table 2).

Other problems of cross-reactivity frequently encountered include the
aminoglycoside antibiotics (streptomycin, kanamycin, neomycin, gentamycin), the
p-aminobenzene derivatives (sulfonamides, sulfonylureas, procaine, procainamide, thiazide, carbonic anhydrase inhibitors), local anesthetics containing the p-
aminophenyl group, and iodinated contrast media.

Preventive measures also include considerations of route, mode of administration, and initial dosage. It is by now well known that a number of substances used
for depot preparations (e. g., beeswax) may act as immunological adjuvants. As
discussed above, the storage of penicillin solutions, even for a few hours, markedly
enhances their immunogenic capacity (NEFTEL et al. 1981). Oral preparations
should be preferred whenever possible, since incidence and severity of allergic
reactions, at least in the case of penicillins, appear to be markedly lower. A useful
precaution is also to initiate treatment with known allergenic drugs in the
physician's office or hospital, so that any reaction which might occur can be treated
promptly. Reducing the initial dose by giving only a fraction of a tablet or of the
intended injected therapeutic dose may provide an additional margin of safety.

C. Prevention of Allergic Reactions by Accurate Diagnosis of Drug Allergy in the Allergic Patient

Aside from measures taken by the drug manufacturer, which should lead to the
availability of pharmacologically active drugs as far as possible devoid of allergenic
potential, the physician may also contribute to a sizeable extent to the prevention
of such reactions. Besides limiting the prescription of known allergenic drugs such
as penicillin and other antibiotics to serious clinical indications, objective and reliable methods for the diagnosis of drug allergy would also be a great contribution
to prevention.

At present, the diagnostic tests available for drug allergies are still relatively unsatisfactory, with the exception of penicillin allergy. The main reasons for the difficulty encountered daily in establishing an objective diagnosis of drug allergy in
a given patient are the following:
a) The immunological mechanisms of allergic reactions to drugs are varied: therefore, an accurate diagnosis will require several types of tests.

Table 2. Cross-reactivity between some cephalorins and penicillins

IgE (RAST assay)
In 25 patients with positive RAST to the BPO group, none cross-reacts to Cefuroxim or Cefotaxim.

Lymphocyte culture Patient positive to (stimulation index > 2)	*Benzyl- penicillin*	*Ampi- cillin*	*Cefu- roxim*	*Cefo- taxim*	*Cepha- lothin*	*Cephalo- ridine*
Penicillin-allergic ($n=8$)	8	8	7	6	6	5
Normal controls ($n=5$)	0	0	0	0	0	0

RAST = radioallergosorbent test

b) In numerous instances, the immunochemical mechanisms leading to sensitization to a given drug are not precisely known; accordingly, the reagents required for performing appropriate immunological tests are not available.
c) Immunological tests indicate whether the patient has made an immunological response to the drug, but they do not have absolute predictive value about the reoccurrence of an overt clinical allergic reaction upon readministration of the drug. Tests potentially used in the diagnosis of drug allergy are as follows:
  1. Skin tests
      a) Immediate: scratch or prick, if possible with drug-polylysine conjugates
      b) Delayed: epicutaneous, with drugs or allergenic drug derivatives
  2. Detection of antibodies
      a) Hemagglutination, detecting mostly IgM and IgG
      b) RAST test, for IgE or IgG
      c) Inhibition of drug-coated bacteriophages, detecting mostly IgM and IgG
      d) Ig binding of radiolabeled drug
      e) Passive degranulation of basophils
  3. Cellular tests
      a) Lymphocyte transformation test (blasts count or ^{3}H-thymidine uptake)
      b) Macrophage migration inhibition (MIF) test
      c) Leukocyte migration inhibition (LIF) test
      d) Specific rosette tests
  Skin testing for drug allergy has a limited but still definite place in determining the risk of an allergic reaction. Such tests may be performed (a) as routine screening of patients before therapy, (b) in order to assess the significance of an alleged previous reaction to a drug, or (c) in order to identify which of several drugs has caused the allergic reaction.
  The problem with skin testing with most drugs is that the drug is usually not in a chemical form suitable for eliciting a reaction when applied to the skin of allergic patients. Either the drug, as hapten, is in a nonconjugated, monovalent form unable to elicit antibody-dependent allergic reactions, or it is structurally unrelated to the allergenic metabolite responsible for the clinical reaction. In either case, false-negative skin tests would ensue. This difficulty, however, is not present when the therapeutic agent used is a full antigen (e. g., foreign serum or insulin), or when its immunochemistry has been worked out and the corresponding multivalent con-

jugates (e. g., penicilloyl-polylysine: PPL) are available for skin testing. In such a case, there is no doubt that routine skin testing before treatment would reduce the incidence of serious allergic reactions to the drug considered.

Among the therapeutic agents for which routine skin testing prior to therapy has been recommended are xenogenic sera, enzymes, polypeptide hormones, insulin, and penicillins. In view of the considerable proportion (3%–5%) of patients in industrialized nations allegedly allergic to penicillins, and of the severity of such reactions, routine skin testing with the now commercially available PPL and minor determinant mixture (MDM) reagents should be advised (SULLIVAN et al. 1981).

Skin testing with most other drugs is usually described as unreliable, although positive immediate type reactions coinciding with the patient's history are encountered with a large variety of drugs:

ACTH	Penicillins
Insulin	Streptomycin
Asparginase	Sulfonamides
Penicillinase	Tetracyclines
Aminosalicylic acid	Vancomycin
Amphotericin B	Aminopyrine
Bacitracin	Cromolyn
Cephalosporins	Dantrolene
Clindamycin	Meprobamate
Ethambutol	Mercurial diuretics
Kanamycin	Probenecid
Lincomycin	Triamterene

Negative skin tests in such cases, however, do not permit exclusion of drug allergy.

For clinical and practical purposes, we feel that epicutaneous tests should receive more attention and credit in the diagnosis of drug allergy. Their value has probably been underestimated (AGRUP 1972; FELIX and COMAISH 1974), and could be improved still more by using the appropriate allergenic derivatives (e. g., phenetidin in phenacetin allergy; RUEGGER et al. 1973) and appropriate vehicles facilitating penetration in the skin. In penicillin allergy also, epicutaneous tests are frequently positive not only in those cases where IgE antibodies are responsible for the clinical manifestations but also, and mostly, in those clinical reactions (e. g., morbilliform exanthema) where a cell-mediated mechanism is primarily involved (Table 3). The frequent occurrence of positive reactions after epicutaneous application of the allergen in individuals or experimental animals sensitized by intramuscular injection or ingestion of the drug suggests that primary sensitization through the skin and formation of drug conjugates to skin proteins are not essential for the development of allergic contact reactions to drugs (DE WECK 1977).

Among the numerous in vitro tests proposed for diagnosis, two deserve more extensive discussion: those designed to detect specific IgE or IgG antibodies (RAST test), and those based on the presence in the blood of specifically sensitized lymphocytes.

The RAST test has for the time being been applied only to the diagnosis of penicillin allergies (WIDE and JUHLIN 1971; KRAFT et al. 1977; DE WECK 1978),

Table 3. Rcsults of epicutaneous tests with benzylpenicillin in patients with history of penicillin allergy

Main clinical symptom			Patch test with BPN (200000 units mT, 24 h)	
			+ve	−ve
Urticaria	Immediate[a]	+ve	12	7
(38 cases)	skin tests	−ve	11	8
Patch test +ve: 23/38 (60%)				
Exanthema	Immediate[a]	+ve	15	1
(56 cases)	skin tests	−ve	34	6
Patch test +ve: 49/56 (87%)				

BPN = benzylpenicillin
[a] Scratch and intradermal tests with BPO–PLL, BPN, and benzyl-penicilloic acid. For details, see DE WECK et al. (1975)

Table 4. Comparison of skin tests[a] and RAST test in patients with history of penicillin allergy

		High reactors	Low reactors	Negative
Skin test BPO–PLL				
RAST	+++	3	0	1
	++	13	0	0
	+	22	2	1
	−	39	44	47
Skin test BPN				
RAST	+++	1	2	1
	++	8	2	3
	+	9	4	12
	−	38	23	68
Skin test BPNCO				
RAST	+++	1	1	2
	++	5	4	4
	+	5	2	17
	−	21	24	85

BPO–PPL = benzylpenicilloyl-polylysine; BPN = bemylpenicillin; BPNCO = benzylpenicilloic acid
[a] For details of skin testing procedures and evaluation, see DE WECK et al. (1975)

where it is certainly quite useful. Correlation between skin tests detecting anaphylactic hypersensitivity to the major und minor determinants of penicillin allergy (Table 4) is undeniably present, especially if only highly sensitive patients are considered. On the other hand, the RAST test, like many other similar tests based on the detection of circulating antidrug antibodies, has a severe drawback: in more than 50% of the cases, the antibody level decreases within a year of the last clinical

allergic reaction to a point where the test becomes negative (KRAFT et al. 1977; DE
WECK 1978). It is not yet known why, without apparent further contact with the
drug, the antibody levels may remain high for years in some patients while they decrease massively within a few months in others.

The evaluation of anti-BPO antibodies of the IgG class, by a similar procedure
to the one used in the RAST assay, has proved of interest in the evaluation of
penicillin-induced hematological disorders, such as hemolytic anemia or leukopenia (NEFTEL et al. 1981), although anti-BPO IgG antibodies are also encountered
in asymptomatic individuals treated with high doses of penicillins. Previously described methods, such as hemagglutination or bacteriophage inhibition, are cumbersome, less reproducible, and may be considered as obsolete.

Tests based on the reactivity of peripheral blood lymphocytes are in my opinion
of greater general interest in the diagnosis of drug allergy, for the following reasons: (a) sensitive lymphocytes appear to remain detectable for years in the peripheral blood of allergic patients (DE WECK 1975); (b) lymphocytes are apparently capable of metabolizing a large number of drugs, which explains why positive
reactions may be obtained even when the drug itself and not one of its allergenic
metabolites is used for the test; and (c) such tests will detect delayed-type allergic
hypersensitivity, which is more frequently involved in allergic reactions to drugs
than antibodies. However, most test based on lymphocyte cultures in vitro are still
relatively cumbersome and expensive. It has also been disputed that they are indic-
ative of clinical allergy (SAURAT et al. 1976), since they can be positive shortly after
treatment with a drug in patients without clinical symptoms of allergy.

D. Specific Inhibition of Antibody-Mediated Reactions to Drugs

All antibody-mediated allergic reactions encompass the binding of antibodies to
antigen through the antibodies' combining sites. It is well known since Landsteiner
that an excess of monovalent free antigenic determinants (or haptens) specifically
inhibits antigen-antibody reactions in vitro. Since it has been shown that anaphylactic reactions to haptenic determinants in experimental animals in vivo may also
be inhibited by monovalent haptens (FARAH et al. 1960; OVARY and KARUSH 1960),
the application of this principle to penicillin was a logical development. After a
number of preliminary experiments (DE WECK and SCHNEIDER 1972; DE WECK and
GIRARD 1972), an extensive clinical trial has been performed, demonstrating that
a monovalent benzylpenicilloyl hapten (BPO-FLYS of Ro 6-0787) is capable of
preventing the great majority of allergic reactions to penicillin in man (DE WECK
et al. 1975). However, during the course of that trial, an unexpected finding impaired widespread use of the monovalent hapten: in 5%–10% of the allergic
patients, especially in those with a high level of sensitivity, the hapten was found
to elicit the allergic reaction, instead of inhibiting it as in the remaining 90% of
patients. Other outhors have encountered the same problem (BASOMBA et al. 1978).
Although the paradoxical elicitation of anaphylactic reactions by apparently
monovalent haptens has been encountered before in a few experimental systems
(AMKRAUT et al. 1963; FRICK et al. 1968; DE WECK et al. 1973, 1976), the mechanism
of such reactions has not been elucidated. Reactions to the monovalent benzyl-

penicilloyl hapten in man were apparently due to the development of some minor determinant or to some secondary reaction on the mast cell membrane (SCHNEIDER et al. 1979), but the precise immunochemical mechanism of this type of reaction in penicillin allergy has not yet been worked out. This state of affairs has also prevented up to now the commercial development of the monovalent hapten as preventive agent in penicillin allergy. However, the development of combined penicillin preparations in which not only the major benzylpenicilloyl, but also the minor determinants, would be prevented from interacting with their corresponding antibodies by addition of suitable monovalent haptens remains a distinct possibility. It should be pointed out however, that this mode of specific inhibition only applies to antibody-mediated allergic reactions. Clinical and experimental experience have shown that the monovalent benzylpenicilloyl hapten does not inhibit lymphocyte-induced reactions to penicillin (DE WECK 1975).

E. Symptomatic Treatment of Allergic Reactions to Drugs

The treatment of allergic reactions to drugs depends on the type of reaction involved. Successful resuscitation is possible in postanaphylactic reactions even when the reaction is severe, provided immediate and adequate treatment is given. In case of anaphylactic shock, 0.3–0.5 ml 1:1,000 aqueous epinephrine should be given subcutaneously or intravenously. If possible, a tourniquet is applied above the drug injection site or epinephrine solution injected into the site in order to delay further absorption of the drug. The patient should be observed for the various life-threatening complications of anaphylaxis (hypotension, cardiac arrest, laryngeal edema, bronchospasm) and the appropriate treatments (vasopressor agents, closed chest cardiac massage with mouth-to-mouth, nose, or mechanical ventilation, tracheotomy, aminophylline) given as needed. Antihistamines or corticosteroids can be considered at this point, but are not the medication of first choice in anaphylaxis. Recovery from anaphylaxis usually takes 15–20 min, and the patient should then be observed for the next 2–24 h depending on the severity of the reaction and whether severe hypotension has occurred, predisposing to acute tubular necrosis and other complications.

For other types of allergic reacions withdrawal of the drugs is usually sufficient, but in the case of severe serum sickness, vasculitis, interstitial nephritis, exfoliative dermatitis, or hepatitis, high-dose glucocorticoid therapy (40–100 mg prednisone daily or equivalent) is usually indicated. Prophylactic antihistamines and/or steroids may be given before using agents with a high incidence of untoward and unpredictable reactions, such as iodinated contrast media or fluorescein. Systematic premedication with glucocorticoids and/or antihistamines is probably the most efficient measure for reducing the incidence and severity of such reactions (ZWEIMAN et al. 1975).

F. Hyposensitization and Induction of Long-Lasting Immunological Tolerance to Drugs

Most attempts to achieve long-lasting desensitization to drugs in allergic patients by repeated and progressive administration of the drug have been unsuccessful, and are also quite dangerous. In special cases, however, a "rush" desensitization, in which a massive therapeutic dose is reached by progressive administration of the drug, may be justified (Reisman et al. 1962; Zolov et al. 1967; Gorevic and Levine 1981). This procedure is not without danger, has to be performed under emergency room conditions and usually has no long-term protective effects. In penicillin allergy, it may in most cases be advantageously replaced by the procedure of hapten inhibition described above (de Weck et al. 1975). Various procedures have been described to achieve rush desensitization in penicillin allergy, starting with intravenous injection of 0.1 unit/ml followed by tenfold increments at 1–2 h intervals until a full therapeutic dose is reached (van Arsdel 1978). The procedure used should vary with the level of sensitivity: in highly sensitive patients, some authors (Parker 1980) prefer to start with oral administration, starting with 1,000 units or less und giving additional amounts every 20–30 min until the oral dose has reached 50,000 units. At this point, parenteral injections with 1,000 units or less may be started, and progressively increased until the intended therapeutic dose is reached. This procedure is not without danger, and at least one death has been recorded in conjunction with attempted hyposensitization to penicillin (Grieco et al. 1964). Even in the absence of allergic symptoms, continuous monitoring of renal function and of the urinary sediment to detect glomerulonephritis, venal vasculitis, or progressive interstitial nephritis is especially important.

In addition to penicillin, hyposensitization has been accomplished to *p*-aminosalicylic acid, isoniazid, penicillamine, tetracycline, phenytoin, nitrogen mustards streptomycin, and a certain number of other drugs. A similar rush desensitization procedure is well known in therapy with xenogenic sera, such as horse antitetanus toxin serum. Another instance where desensitization is frequently required is insulin allergy with local or systemic allergic symptoms (Mattson et al. 1975). Experience shows that rush desensitization or continuation of therapy under cover of antihistamines and/or glucocorticoids is frequently successful. When continued over long periods of time, as is the case for insulin, this procedure may even lead to long-term desensitization. Usually, however, the effects of rush desensitization are only temporary. The mechanism of this type of hyposensitization may include (a) a depletion of mast cell mediators due to continued release (antianaphylactic state); (b) a consumption of drug-specific antibodies; (c) inhibition due to antigen excess, especially when presented in monovalent form ("inbuilt inhibition"); (d) high zone tolerance interfering with IgE synthesis, which is selectively impaired (Mota 1964); and (e) the production of drug-specific IgG antibody, which may act as a blocking protective antibody.

On the basis of experiments designed to achieve immunological tolerance to a number of chemically defined haptens, several new approaches potentially useful for the induction of prolonged desensitization to drugs have emerged in recent years. Characteristic for these approaches are (a) that they induce a long-lasting state of specific unresponsiveness to the hapten in animals which had already developed a full-fledged immune response, and are therefore relevant to the clinical situation, where patients are usually encountered only after they have become allergic; and (b) the specific impairment of B cells and of antibody production (B cell tolerance), while cellular immunity appears not to be affected. This form of long-lasting unresponsiveness is brought about by the injection into a sensitive animal of the hapten coupled to a so-called tolerogenic carrier. Tolerogenic carriers described so far include (a) D-aminoacid copolymer, D-glutamyl-D-lysine (KATZ et al. 1972); (b) polysaccharides such as pneumococcal polysaccharide (MITCHELL et al. 1972), levans (HOWARD and MITCHISON 1975), and dextrans (COUTINHO et al. 1974; SCHNEIDER et al. 1978); (c) homologous gammaglobulins (LEE and SEHON 1975; PALEY et al. 1975; BOREL et al. 1976); and (d) polyethyleneglycol (LEE and SEHON 1976) and polyvinylalcohol (LEE et al. 1980). Although this phenomenon was originally described for haptens without drug activity, such as dinitrophenyl (DNP), its validity for the benzylpenicilloyl determinant has been confirmed (CHIORAZZI et al. 1976; LEE and SEHON 1976). In recent years, we have also studied systematically the molecular properties required of aminoacid polymers and of dextrans as tolerogenic carriers in the penicillin system. The main conclusions of these studies (OTZ et al. 1978; SCHNEIDER et al. 1978) are that (a) a large number of aminoacid polymers and copolymers may serve as tolerogenic carriers, even with a molecular weight as low as 3,000; and (b) a D-configuration of the tolerogenic carrier is not essential, provided a high degree of hapten substitution is achieved, efficiency probably being correlated with low biodegradability.

The main practical obstacle to the clinical trial of such compounds in penicillin-allergic patients is their high efficiency in eliciting anaphylactic reactions, since they are multivalent. However, various possibilities may be visualized to overcome this difficulty (e. g., protracted administration or antianaphylactic medication).

Another potential approach to the problem of drug allergy would be the administration of drugs in such a way as to induce preferentially an immunological tolerance, possibly by the preferential induction of suppressor cells. Peroral administration of haptens is well known to favor the induction of immunological tolerance (CHASE 1946). The common experience that allergic reactions to drugs, although still possible, are much less frequent after peroral administration than after injection or topical application, may be related, at least in part, to that phenomenon.

In conclusion, although from the point of view of diagnosis and therapy, allergies to drugs are still more difficult to manage than the common allergies to protein or polysaccharide antigens, the application of immunological principles to drug allergy may open up new possibilities for its prevention and management.

References

Agrup G (1972) Patch testing in drug allergy. In: Dash CH, Jones HEH (eds) Mechanisms of drug allergy. Churchill-Livingstone, Edinburgh/ london, p 135

Ahlstedt S, Ekstroem B, Svaerd PO, Sjoeberg B, Kristofferson A, Oertengren B (1980) New aspects on antigens in penicillin allergy. CRC Crit Rev Toxicol 7:219

Amkraut AA, Rosenberg LT, Raffel S (1963) Elicitation of PCA by univalent and divalent haptens. J Immunol 91:644

Basomba A, Pelaez A, Villamanzo IG, Campos A (1978) Allergy to penicillin unsuccessfully treated with a haptenic inhibitor (Benzylpenicilloyl-N-formyllysine: BPO-Flys). A case report. Clin Allergy 8:341

Batchelor FR, Dewdney JM, Feinberg JG, Weston RD (1967) A penicilloylated protein impurity as a source of allergy to benzylpenicillin and 6-amino-penicillanic acid. Lancet 1:1175

Borel Y, Kilham L, Hyslop N, Borel H (1976) Isologous IgG-induced tolerance to benzyl-penicilloyl. Nature 261:49

Bundgaard H, de Weck AL (1975) The role of aminoreactive impurities in acetylsalicylic acid allergy. Int. Arch. Allergy Appl. Immunol 49:119

Chase MW (1946) Inhibition of experimental drug allergy by prior feeding of the sensitizing agent. Proc Soc Exp Bio Med 61:257

Chiorazzi N, Eshhar Z, Katz DH (1976) Induction of immunological tolerance to the major antigenic determinant of penicillin: a therapeutic approach to penicillin allergy, Proc Natl Acad Sci USA 72:2091

Coutinho A, Moeller G, Richter W (1974) Molecular basis of B cell activation. I. Mitogenicity of native and substitutes dextrans. Scand J Immunol 3:321

De Weck AL (1975) Molecular mechanisms of T and B lymphocyte triggering. Int Arch Allergy Appl Immunol 49:247

De Weck AL (1977a) Drug reactions. In: Samter M (ed) Immunological diseases, 2nd ed. Little, Brown & Co., Boston, p 415

De Weck AL (1977b) Immune responses to environmental antigens which act on the skin (which special reference to the role of lymphokines in contact dermatitis). Fed Proc 36:1742

De Weck AL (1978) Application du RAST dans l'allergie à la pénicilline. Med Hyg 36:118

De Weck AL, Eisen HN (1960) Some immunochemical properties of penicillenic acid, an antigenic determinant derived from penicillin. J Exp Med 112:1227

De Weck AL, Girard JP (1972) Specific inhibition of allergic reactions to penicillin in man by a monovalent hapten: II. Clinical studies. Int Arch Allergy Appl Immunol 42:798

De Weck AL, Schneider CH (1972) Specific inhibition of allergic reactions to penicillin in man by a monovalent hapten: I. Experimental immunological and toxicologic studies. Int Arch Allergy 42:789

De Weck AL, Schneider H (1980) Allergic and immunological aspects of therapy with cefotaxine and other cephalosporins. J Antimicrob Chemother 6:161

De Weck AL, Schneider CH, Gutersohn J (1968) The role of penicilloylated protein impurities, penicillin polymers and dimers in penicillin allergy. Int Arch Allergy Appl Immunol 33:535

De Weck AL, Schneider CH, Toffler O, Lazary S (1973) Inhibition of allergic reactions by monovalent haptens. In: Sehon A (ed) Mechanisms of reaginic allergy. Dekker, New York, p 323

De Weck AL, Jeunet F, Schulz KH, Louis P, Girard JP, Grilliat JP, Moneret-Vautrin D et al. (1975) Clinical trial of Ro 6-0787: a monovalent specific hapten inhibitor of penicillin allergy. Z. Immunitätsforsch 150:138

De Weck AL, Toffler O, Koleckarova M, Spengler M (1976) Theoretical basis and experimental studies on the prevention of allergic reactions to penicillins by a monovalent benzylpenicilloyl hapten. Chemotherapy 4:345

Dewdney J (1977) Immunology of the antibiotics. In: Sela M (ed) The antigens, IV. Academic Press, New York, p 74

Farah FS, Kern M, Eisen HN (1960) Specific inhibition of wheal-and-erythema responses with univalent haptens and univalent antibody fragments. J Exp Med 112:1211

Felix RH, Comaish JS (1974) The value of patch and other skin tests in drug eruptions. Lancet 1:1017

Frick OL, Nye W, Raffel S (1968) Anaphylactic reactions to univalent haptens. Immunology 14:563

Gorevic PD, Levine BB (1981) Desensitization of anaphylactic hypersensitivity specific for the penicilloate minor determinant of penicillin and carbenicillin. J Allergy clin Immunol 68:267

Green I, Paul WE, Benacerraf B (1966) The behavior of hapten-poly-L-lysine conjugates as complete antigens in genetic responders and as haptens in nonresponder guinea pigs. J Exp Med 123:859

Grieco MH, Dubin MR, Robinson JL, Schwartz MJ (1964) Penicillin hypersensitivity in patients with bacterial endocarditis. Ann Intern Med 60:204

Howard JG, Mitchison NA (1975) Immunological tolerance. Prog Allergy 18:43

Katz DH, Hamaoka R, Benacerraf B (1972) Immunological tolerance in bone marrow derived lymphocytes. I. Evidence for an intracellular mechanism of inactivation of hapten-specific precursors of antibody-forming cells. J Exp Med 136:1404

Klein U, Gikalov I, Keller M, Hoigné R (1972) "Drug monitoring" in der medizinischen Abteilung eines Regionalspitals. Schweiz Med Wochenschr 102:1083

Kraft D, Roth A, Mischer P, Pichler H, Ebner H (1977) Specific and total serum IgE measurements in the diagnosis of penicillin allergy. A long term follow-up study. Clin Allergy 7:21

Kristofferson A, Ahlstedt A, Pettersson E, Svaerd PO (1977) Antigens in penicillin allergy. I. A radioimmunoassay for detection of penicilloylated protein contaminants in penicillin preparations. Int Arch Allergy Appl Immunol 55:13

Lee WY, Sehon AH (1975) Suppression of reaginic antibody formation II. The use of adoptive transfer system for the study of immunological unresponsiveness. J Immunol 114:837

Lee WY, Sehon AH (1976) Suppression of reaginic antibody formation IV. Suppression of reaginic antibodies to penicillin in the mouse. J Immunol 117:927

Lee WY, Hubbard BA, Cripps V, Sehon AH (1980) Abrogation of the antibenzylpenicilloyl (BPO) IgE Response with BPO-polyvinyl alcohol conjugates. Int Arch Allergy Appl Immunol 63:1

Levine BB (1966) Immunochemical mechanisms of drug allergy. Ann Rev Med 17:23

Magnusson B, Kligman AM (1970) Allergic contact dermatitis in the guinea pig. Thomas, Springfield, Ill

Mattson JR, Patterson R, Roberts M (1975) Insulin therapy in patients with systemic insulin allergy. Arch Intern Med 135:818

Mitchell GF, Humphrey JH, Williamson AR (1972) B cell tolerance induced by polymeric antigens I. Comparison of the dose and epitope density requirements for inactivation of primed and unprimed B cells in vivo. Eur J Immunol 5:361

Mota I (1964) The mechanism of anaphylaxis I. Production and biological properties of "mast cell sensitizing" antibody. Immunology 7:681

Neftel KA,, Waelti M,, Spengler H,, Von Felten A,, Weitzman SA,, Buergi H,, de Weck AL (1981) Neutropenia after penicillins: Toxic or immune-mediated? Klin Wochenschr 59:877

Otz U, Schneider CH, de Weck AL, Gruden E, Gill TG (1978) Induction of immunological tolerance to the penicilloyl antigenic determinant I. Evaluation of BPO-amino acid polymers and copolymers in mice. Eur J Immunol 8:406

Ovary Z, Karush F (1960) Studies on the immunologic mechanism of anaphylaxis: I. Antibody-hapten interactions studied by passive cutaneous anaphylaxis in the guinea pig. J Immunol 84:409

Paley RS, Leskowitz S, Borel Y (1975) Effect on tolerance induction of the mode of attachment of the hapten to the carrier. J Immunol 115:1409

Parker CW (1980) Drug Allergy. In: Parker CW (ed) Clinical immunology. Saunders, Philadelphia p 1219

Reismann RE, Rose NR, Witebsky E, Arbesman C (1962) Penicillin allergy and desensitization. J Allergy Clin Immunol 33:178

Ruegger R, Spengler H, de Weck AL, Dubach UC (1973) Immunologische Aspekte der Sensibilisierung auf Phenacetin. Dtsch Med Wochenschr 98:762

Sawrat JH, Ponvert C, Burtin C, Soubrane C, Bender F, Paupe I (1976) Lymphocyte transformation, leukocyte migration, specific IgE, IgG, and IgM before, during and after penicillin treatment without adverse reaction. Acta Allergol 31:1

Schneider CH, Otz U, Gruden E (1978) Induction of immunological tolerance to the penicilloyl antigenic determinant II. Evaluation of stable and unstable penicilloyl-dextrans. Eur J Immunol 8:410

Schneider CH, Gruden E, Waelti M, Toffler O, de Weck AL, Jost R (1979) Monovalent elicitation of passive cutaneous anaphylaxis by N-1-DNCP-N-6-BPO-diaminohexane. Mol Immunol 16:269

Sullivan TJ, Wedner JH, Skatz GS, Yiecies LD, Parker CW (1981) Skin test to detect penicillin allergy. J Allergy Clin Immunol 68. 171

Van Arsdel PP Jr (1978) Adverse drug reactions. In: Middleton E Jr, Read CE, Ellis EF (eds). Allergy: principles and practice, Mosby, St. Louis, vol 2. pp 1133

Wide L, Juhlin L (1971) Detection of penicillin allergy of the immediate-type by radio-immunoassay of reagins (IgE) to penicilloyl conjugates. Clin Allergy 1:171

Zolov D, Redmond AP, Levine BB (1967) Immunological studies of desensitization in penicillin allergy. J Allergy Clin Immunol 39:107

Zweiman B, Mishkin MM, Hildreth EA (1975) An approach to the performance of contrast studies in contrast material reactive persons. Ann Intern Med 83:159

Section II:
Allergic Reactions to Specific Drugs

CHAPTER 9

Major Drugs Acting on the Central Nervous System

C. W. PARKER

A. General Anesthetics

I. Halothane

In general, the rate of allergic reactions to general anesthetics is low. However, the drug halothane (2-bromo-2-chloro-1,1,1-trifluoroethane), which was introduced into clinical pharmacologic use as a general anesthetic in 1956, has been strongly suspected of causing an allergic hepatitis. MOULT and SHERLOCK (1975) reported a series of 26 patients who developed postoperative jaundice following the use of this agent and in whom no other cause for liver disease could be found. In accord with previous reports, the clinical picture was primarily that of an acute hepatitis with hepatocellular dysfunction, developing a few days to several weeks after halothane anesthesia. Halothane-induced hepatitis usually occurs in a patient who has been exposed previously to the same agent. In MOULT and SHERLOCK's series, out of 26 patients, 24 had received halothane more than once, and 18 had had it twice within a 4-week period. The development of sensitivity may be suspected if there has been an unexplained episode of fever within 1–2 weeks following previous halothane use. Unexplained jaundice or delayed fever after a previous administration of halothane should be considered contraindications to futher use (MOULT and SHERLOCK 1975). However, while multiple exposures to halothane within the same 4-week period appear to be particularly hazardous, even in this situation the risk of jaundice is probably no greater than 1–3 in 6,000 patients.

In a study on halothane-induced hepatitis in the United States the incidence of fatal massive hepatic necrosis from any cause was 7.1 in 10,000 after multiple administrations of halothane and only 2.4 in 10,000 after multiple administrations of non-halothane anesthetics. However, this increased risk appeared to be more than offset by higher mortality for other reasons in the non-halothane group. The general enthusiasm for halothane is reflected by the fact that it is now used for more than 70% of all anesthetic procedures in the United Kingdom (DAVIES and HOLMES 1972).

Minor alterations in hepatic dysfunction also occur more commonly after halothane administration than other general anesthetics now in common use (WRIGHT et al. 1975). Nonetheless, when jaundice occurs after halothane use, the prognosis is serious. In a review by LITTLE in 1968 the mortality rate was calculated to be 35% in the 400 patients who had developed this complication. When death occurs, it is usually due to hepatic failure with coma. Obesity, early onset of jaundice after anesthesia, and associated blood coagulation abnormalities are more likely to be associated with a fatal outcome. If recovery occurs, it is almost always complete. In non-fatal cases there is diffuse hepatocellular injury resembling the pathologic picture found in acute viral hepatitis. In fatal cases there is likely to be widespread necrosis which may be particularly marked in the centrizonal areas (the central zone of the liver tubules), and resemble the lesion of acute carbon tetrachloride poisoning. Since no specific diagnostic test is available, the diagnosis is difficult to establish conclusively, because jaundice may occur postoperatively as a complication of the surgery itself.

Blood transfusions containing agents which cause viral hepatitis also produce jaundice but the incubation period is much longer. A late onset of jaundice 3 weeks or more after surgery and exposure to halothane is not characteristic of halothane-related hepatitis and suggests a diagnosis of viral hepatitis instead. Patients who have had surgery also not infrequently have been given phenothiazine drugs for symptoms such as postoperative vomiting, but the clinical picture with these agents is that of a cholestatic hepatitis. As a rule in halothane-related hepatitis evidence of cholestasis is minimal.

The possible role of allergy in halothane-induced hepatitis has been much discussed (WALTON et al. 1976). Apart from the frequent history of multiple exposures to halothane in affected individuals, perhaps the most striking indication that allergy may be involved is the report of an anesthesiologist who developed jaundice on a number of occasions after administering anesthesia with halothane. Also, jaundice occurring after halothane use is sometimes accompanied by fever and eosinophilia. Fever may be a premonitory manifestation of the liver dysfunction, usually appearing 4–6 days postoperatively, followed by onset of jaundice within the next several days. After multiple recent exposures the fever may recur within several hours. The delayed onset of symptoms in initial exposures and accelerated reactions after apparent prior sensitization is strongly suggestive of a role for allergy.

Unfortunately, attempts to demonstrate directly that an immunologic response to the drug has occurred have given variable results. PARONETTO and POPPER (1970) described positive lymphocyte transformation responses with halothane in 10 of 15 subjects with suspected halothane hepatitis. However, with one or two exceptions subsequent studies have been negative (WALTON et al. 1973). On the other hand PRICE et al. (1977) and DAVIS and WILLIAMS (1978) have reported modest but significant leukocyte migration inhibitory factor (LIF) production by halothane-stimulated lymphocytes in a high percentage of patients. EDDLESTON has reported that positive responses may sometimes be obtained by administering the drug to rabbits, allowing time for then drug to be metabolized in rabbit liver, obtaining crude liver homogenates, and using these preparations to stimulate LIF production (EDDLESTON 1980). MATHIEU et al. (1974) have reported that trifluoroacetate, a metabolite of fluorene and halothane, can be conjugated to serum proteins and used to induce delayed hypersensitivity in guinea pigs. Other immunologic alterations have been reported. According to REED and WILLIAMS (1972) mitochondrial antibodies are more frequent in halothane-induced hepatitis than in acute viral hepatitis. Atypical circulating lymphocytes which may represent lamphocytes transformed in vivo in response to antigen have also been described in this condition. Taking the results of these various studies together, one cannot state unequivocally that halothane-induced hepatitis is immunologically mediated. Nonetheless the evidence in strongly suggestive.

II. Other General Anesthetics

Methoxyfluorane, a halogenated hydrocarbon structurally related to halothane, also produces jaundice but in lower incidence, and more frequently at the time of initial exposure (ZIMMERMAN 1972). Another clinical difference of methoxyfluorane-induced from halothane-induced jaundice is that the liver dysfunction is often accompanied by defective renal concentrating capacity. Chloroform, trichlorethylene, tribromethanol, divinylether, cyclopropane, and diethylether all are capable of producing hepatic dysfunction but the available evidence strongly suggests that liver damage is due to direct toxicity rather than to an allergic mechanism.

III. Intravenous Anesthetic Agents

Intravenous anesthetic agents which have caused acute systemic reactions resembling anaphylaxis include althesin, thiopentone, suxamethonium, tubocurarine, propanidid, and methylhexitone (FISHER 1975; DUNDEE 1976; FISHER 1977). A number of these agents have been reported to produce acute increases in histamine levels although the mechanism of the increase is not clear (FISHER 1975). A role for allergy is suggested by a high frequency of previous use of the same agent which may be as high as 90% (DUNDEE 1976). Althesin produces a serious reaction in about 1 in 15,000 administrations of the drug. In a recent survey of 86 episodes of hypersensitivity to intravenous anesthetic agents althesin was responsible in 70 and thiopentone in 12, but all 4 deaths were due to thiopentone (DUNDEE 1976). While the incidence of reactions to these agents is apparently increasing, this may be due to increased reporting. Pentothal, a short-acting barbiturate given intravenously for brief general anesthesia occasionally causes acute laryngeal bronchospasm. The role of allergy in these reactions is uncertain.

B. Sedatives, Hypnotics, and Tranquillizers

I. Phenothiazines

The phenothiazines, of which chlorpromazine is the prototype, have been reported to produce a variety of clinical reactions apparently on an allergic basis including rash, eosinophilia, cholestatic jaundice, agranulocytosis, vasculitis, systemic lupus erythematosus (SLE), and hemolytic anemia (PARKER 1980a; VAN ARSDEL 1978).

Skin reactions have been reported to occur in about 5% of patients treated with chlorpromazine (BYCK 1975), although in other series the incidence is as low as 0.5% (MILLER and GREENBLATT 1976). Skin manifestations usually appear between the first and fifth week of treatment. Types of skin reactions include urticaria, maculopapular rash, petechial rash (due to vasculitis), erythema multiforme, photosensitivity dermatitis, and contact dermatitis. About 30% of individuals treated with moderate or large doses of chlorpromazine over a sustained period of time develop photosensitivity (PILLSBURY and CARO 1966). Photosensitivity may be prevented or minimized by the use of suntan preparations containing p-aminobenzoic acid. Reports of an association of chlorpromazine with SLE (BECKER 1973) are rare and if a true association exists, it must be extremely unusual.

Leukopenia is another complication of chlorpromazine (and related drug) therapy occurring in about 1 in 10,000 treated individuals (PARKER 1980a; HARTL 1973; PETZ and FUDENBERG 1976; PISCIOTTA 1973). It usually appears within the first 6 weeks of treatment. The evidence for an immunologic basis for the leukopenia is not as firm as in aminopyrine-induced agranulocytosis. The leukopenia appears to come on somewhat later during treatment with chlorpromazine than with aminopyrine, and the prognosis for complete recovery after discontinuation of the drug is not as good. Chlorpromazine-induced leukopenia is also more frequently associated with depression of circulating red cells and platelets and less precipitous fall in circulating granulocytes when a patient who has recovered completely is challenged with the drug. Serum antibodies have been difficult to demonstrate although occasionally the patient's plasma, taken during or shortly after administration of the drug, agglutinates normal polymorphonuclear leukocytes. This is presumably due to the presence both of anti-drug antibody and a reactive metabolite of the drug which is serving as the immunogen. Patients with chlorpromazine-induced granulocytopenia not infrequently have associated skin rash, fever, and hepatitis, strengthening the evidence for an allergic reaction.

Jaundice has been reported to occur in 1%–3% of all patients receiving chlorpromazine, although an incidence as high as 8% has been described (ZIMMERMAN 1972). Other phenothiazines and chlordiazepoxide produce a similar clinical syndrome. The jaundice associated with phenothiazine use is generally thought to be allergic in nature. The typical pathologic change is that of a cholestatic hepatitis, frequently with eosinophilic and lymphocyte infiltration in the periportal areas. The clinical picture is that of a cholestatic jaundice closely simulating primary biliary cirrhosis and extrahepatic biliary obstruction (ZELMAN 1959).

Clinical or laboratory evidence of marked hepatocellular damage is rare, but a mixed hepatocanicular picture is not infrequent (ZIMMERMAN 1972). Typically there is a latent period of 1–4 weeks after the start of treatment before the onset of jaundice. If jaundice does not occur within the first months of phenothiazine treatment, the likelihood that it will occur later is considerably less, although rarely jaundice appears for the first time after many months or even several years of treatment. Rash or leukopenia is present in only about 5% of patients but eosinophilia is present in about 65% (ISHAK and IREY 1972). Liver biopsy is very helpful in the differential diagnosis. The prognosis for complete recovery is good: one-third of patients recover completely within 4 weeks, another third in 4–8 weeks (ZIMMERMAN 1972). The remainder require at least several months to return to normal. Occasionally there is a prolonged course with clinical, histologic, and biochemical features typical of primary biliary cirrhosis. It is possible that this represents chlorpromazine-induced jaundice leading to true biliary cirrhosis, although the coincidental occurrence of the two forms of liver disease is equally possible.

Readministration of small doses of the drug results in prompt recurrence of jaundice, other manifestations of hepatic dysfunction, or both in approximately 50% of patients. Hyposensitization has been possible in a few individuals, either involving continued administration of the drug after a reaction has occurred or careful readministration after a period of drug withdrawal. However, further use of these drugs in the presence of a reaction is rarely justified.

II. Barbiturates

Allergic reactions to barbiturates (or, at least, reactions which are presumably allergic) are not infrequent. In a recent cooperative study sensitivity reactions were estimated to occur in 0.1%–1.0% of patients treated with phenobarbital, secobarbital, or pentobarbital (MILLER and GREENBLATT 1976). Maculopapular skin eruptions are particularly common, but there are a variety of cutaneous manifestations including fixed eruptions, urticaria, Lyell syndrome, and erythema multiforme. Localized bullous eruptions occur after suicidal doses (SCHUPPLI 1972), but probably represent a toxic rather than an allergic manifestation. Other clinical reactions to barbiturates include serum sickness, vasculitis, and drug-induced fever. It appears that any of the barbiturates can produce these manifestations. Lymphocyte transformation has been reported in response to phenobarbital in vitro in a patient with drug-induced fever (REIDENBERG and CACCESE 1975), but further substantiation is needed. The development of a radioimmunoassay for barbiturates has been described (SPECTOR et al. 1973).

In addition to various allergic of possibly allergic symptoms produced by barbiturates, barbiturates are metabolized by the cytochrome P 450 hepatic microsomal enzyme system and, by inducing these enzymes, enhance the metabolism of other drugs and presumably promote their immunogenicity. However, no direct evidence in support of this concept is available.

III. Others

Cutaneous eruptions are not infrequent to other sedatives or hypnotics such as chloral hydrate and meprobamate (GOODMAN and GILMAN 1955a, b; HARVEY 1975; SCHUPPLI 1972; VAN ARSDEL 1978; MILLER and GREENBLATT 1976), although, in contrast to the phenothiazines and chlordiazepoxide, hepatic injury is rare. Cutaneous reactions to meprobamate may be generalized or localized to the groin. A wide variety of cutaneous manifestations occur including fixed drug eruptions. Very rare but severe hypersensitivity reactions include fever, angioedema, anaphylaxis, bronchospasm, oliguria, exfoliative dermatitis, stomatitis, Stevens–Johnson syndrome, and bullous dermatitis. Meprobamate has been reported to produce aplastic anemia, but there is no evidence that an immune mechanism is involved. This drug also produces thrombocytopenia, but further study is needed to elucidate the mechanism. Reactions to chloral hydrate are rare (HARVEY 1975), although rash and granulocytopenia have been reported. Eosinophilia has been reported during chloral hydrate treatment in the absence of other overt manifestations of allergy. Chlordiazepoxide, diazepam, oxazepam, and nitrazepam are rare causes of hypersensitivity reactions (MILLER and GREENBLATT 1976; GREENBLATT and SHADER 1974), but agranulocytosis has been reported (BYCK 1975).

C. Narcotics

It is well recognized that opiates produce nonspecific skin responses when injected locally, presumably because they are nonspecific releasers of histamine and perhaps other mediators of immediate hypersensitivity (PARKER 1980a). This mechanism is supported by in vitro studies, indicating that the addition of codeine and morphine to isolated mast cells or basophils in vitro can directly stimulate histamine release (Kazimierczak and Diamant 1978).

Very large intravenous injections of opiates, particularly heroin, in addicted or nonaddicted individuals may be associated with respiratory distress and the clinical and pathologic changes of acute pulmonary edema (Rosenow 1972; Katz et al. 1972; Frand et al. 1972a; Duberstein and Kaufman 1972). Methadone and barbiturates, which are considerably different structurally from heroin, also cause pulmonary edema when given in marked overdosage (Frand et al. 1972b). The acute pulmonary edema syndrome can occur after oral overdosage with narcotics (Katz et al. 1972), so exposure via the intravenous route is not necessary. The syndrome of respiratory depression induced by heroin and other addictive drugs in usually accompanied by stupor and myosis. Occasionally the pulmonary edema has not become clinically manifest until several hours after recovery from respiratory depression, sugggesting that hypoxia per se may not be a necessary feature.

Although bronchospasm may be induced by the administration of ordinary therapeutic or larger doses of opiates, particularly in a drug abuser who also has asthma, the usual clinical and pathologic picture in the lung following an overdose of heroin is not that of acute anaphylaxis. Moreover, it has been reported that the entire clinical syndrome can be reproduced during an initial exposure to the drug (Rosenow 1972). Attempts to demonstrate IgE antibodies to opiates by cutaneous testing have not been reported but would be complicated by the nonspecific irritancy of these drugs in the skin in any case. It seems possible that the change in pulmonary function involves a combination of localized histamine release in the lung on a nonspecific basis affecting pulmonary capillary permeability, usually in combination with central respiratory depression. According to Brashear et al. (1974) intravenous injections of heroin or morphine can produce increased plasma histamine concentrations in dogs.

While it is hard to argue that acute pulmonary edema in response to heroin abuse is an immunologically mediated reaction, nonetheless there is evidence to indicate that antibody formation occurs during opiate use in humans. Ryan et al. (1972) reported that immunoglobulin levels are high in the serum of most opiate addicts in New Mexico and that many sera contained increased binding activity in the immunoglobulin fraction for radiolabeled morphine. While a subsequent study did not confirm this latter finding (Weksler et al. 1973), a radioactive marker of lower specificity was employed which may have reduced the sensitivity of the analysis for morphine-binding antibodies below the level needed for detection. It is also possible that differences in drug preparations used by addicts in different geographic areas might explain the variation in results. Transformed lymphocytes are not infrequently seen in the peripheral blood in opiate addicts, providing possible further support for an in vivo drug reaction (Sapira 1968). Nonetheless there is some evidence that the abnormality may persist after use of the drug has been stopped, so it may not be related to a continuous immunologic response as such.

The evidence for morphine immunogenicity in humans is supported by studies in experimental animals. The administration of morphine in adjuvant has been reported to produce anti-morphine antibodies in rabbits (Ringle and Herndon 1975). In addition to the opiates themselves, drug preparations obtained illegally by addicts frequently contain fillers or other contaminants. Among the substances that adulterate heroin are quinine, lactose, talc, mannitol, and baking soda. The presence of these various potentially immunogenic substances may help explain the occurrence of glomerulonephritis and the nephrotic syndrome in small proportions of the addict population. Acute transverse myelitis, progressive positive disease, and hemiparesis have been reported after intravenous heroin use (WOODS and STEWLER 1972; HALL and KARP 1973). An acute hypersensitivity reaction has been suspected but substantiation is needed.

Opiates have been observed to cause allergic contact dermatitis, although this is quite unusual. Eosinophilia is not infrequent in drug addicts.

In addition to allergic manifestations, a major role for anti-morphine antibody formation in induction of tolerance to the pharmacologic actions of narcotic agents has been suggested. There is no doubt that antibodies can partially block the effects of opiates in vivo provided moderate drug doses are used (SPECTOR et al. 1973). However, it is doubtful that the usual manifestations of opiate tolerance can be explained by this mechanism. Considering the very large quantities of opiates that can be tolerated by individuals who are chronically addicted, it would be surprising if enough antibody could be produced to neutralize the amount of drug which is present. Certainly direct evidence exists for acquired changes in tissue responsiveness to opiates in the central nervous system of chronically exposed animals in which an immune process cannot be implicated. This adaptation is apparently related to changes in receptor number and other mechanisms affecting the responding cells themselves and thus there is no need to postulate a major role for antibodies in the development of tolerance.

Regardless of the role of anti-opiate antibodies in opiate tolerance, since the first report in 1970 by SPECTOR and PARKER that morphine and related agents conjugated to proteins can be used to raise anti-morphine antibodies and develop radioimmunoassays for these agents, this approach has been widely used in the detection and experimental study of opiate addiction. Suitably chosen antibodies readily discriminate between heroin, morphine, methadone, and other drugs, which may be a source of confusion. Since peptide-forming reagents are used to conjugate the drugs to proteins in vitro prior to immunization, these observations do not bear on the immunogenicity of unconjugated opiate. However, as already discussed, unconjugated morphine is immunogenic to animals when given repeatedly in adjuvant.

Marijuana smoking can induce bronchitis, sinusitis, asthma, and rhinopharyngitis (LISKOW et al. 1971). Uveal edema has been reported to be a useful clinical sign of marijuana abuse although documentation is limited. While nonspecific irritation is probably the usual cause of respiratory symptoms, allergy to marijuana has been demonstrated in at least one patient by cutaneous testing both before and after passive transfer of her serum. This individual had a history of recurrent chest symptoms developing almost immediately after smoking cannabis cigarettes. Since passive transfer studies were done and the drug did not produce a response in the adjacent normal areas of skin, nonspecific irritancy could be eliminated as a significant factor in the cutaneous reaction. These observations suggest that marijuana is capable of producing IgE-mediated respiratory disease. Interestingly, one of the

main psychopharmacologically active agents in marijuana, δ-9-tetrahydrocannab-
inol, was shown to be an important antigen in this individual (LISKOW et al. 1971).

D. Anti-Epileptic Drugs

Hydantoins have been reported to produce a variety of known or suspected allergic
reactions including maculopapular eruptions, urticaria, exfoliative dermatitis,
vasculitis, lupus, hepatocellular jaundice, serum sickeness (GOODMAN and GILMAN
1955 b; PETZ and FUDENBERG 1976; GROB and HEROLD 1972), and thrombocytopenia. Other anti-convulsants also reported to be causes of drug-induced lupus include tridione, primidone, phenaturone, ethosuximide, and carbamazepine (HAR-
PEY 1974). Phenacetylurea (Phenurone) is perhaps the most toxic of the anti-epileptic agents. Its most serious complications are nephritis and hepatocellular jaundice.
The incidence of jaundice with this drug is about 2% (ZIMMERMAN 1972; WOOD-
BURY and FINGL 1975 a), and affected individuals have an estimated mortality rate
of 10%. Jaundice occurs in substantially lower incidence with diphenylhydantoin,
mephenytoin, trimethadione, and paramethadione. Patients with hepatitis in association with anti-convulsant therapy frequently have faver, rash, eosinophilia, or
other symptoms, suggesting that drug hypersensitivity is involved. The nephritis of
phenacetylurea toxicity takes various forms and even acute renal failure has been
described. Tridione and paradione not infrequently cause the nephrotic syndrome
(BENNET et al. 1977; ANGERVALL et al. 1972). The nephrotic syndrome may also occur with other anti-epileptic agents although this is unusual.

Systemic allergic reactions of the serum-sickness type are not infrequent during
treatment with anti-epileptic agents. Nirvanol (5,5-phenylethylhydantoin), a drug
used in the past as a sedative and hypnotic, was associated with a very high incidence of clinical manifestations strongly suggestive of drug allergy, particularly
drug-induced fever and serum sickness (BRAVERMAN and LEVIN 1963). This substance is formed when mesantoin is demethylated and may be an important intermediate in allergic reactions to mesantoin. Phenytoin also commonly produces
serum sickness, sometimes in the form of a pseudomononucleosis syndrome similar
to that of p-aminosalicylic acid hypersensitivity. In a recently described case of
phenytoin-induced serum sickness, platelet thrombi were sufficiently prominent in
the lymph node vasculature to suggest the diagnosis of thrombotic thrombocytopenic purpura (ZIDAR et al. 1975). Phenytoin- or mephenytoin-induced serum sickness may be associated with or superseded by prolonged and marked lymphadenopathy, occasionally simulating malignant lymphoma (SALZSTEIN and ACKERMAN
1959). This syndrome may also occur in the absence of an overt episode of serum
sickness.

In rare instances patients with hydantoin-induced lymphadenopathy have gone
on to develop progressive manifestations of invasive lymphoid disease with classic
manifestations of Hodgkin's disease or other forms of lymphoma at autopsy.
Whether this represents the de novo development of lymphoma or the chance association of phenytoin use with spontaneously developing lymphoma is not clear.
Certainly phenytoin is a commonly used drug and this particular complication is
rare. Nonetheless, it is of interest that phenytoin therapy may be associated with

decreased production of immunoglobulins, particularly IgA, as indicated by decreased serum levels, so it is possible that the drug is sufficiently potent as an immunosuppressive agent to interfere with normal immunologic surveillance. In a study by GROB and HEROLD (1972) decreased IgA levels were present in 5 of 20 patients who had received prolonged treatment with hydantoins. Decreased complement levels were also frequent, as were negative reactions to delayed skin testing. Other studies also suggest that phenytoin may alter immunologic responsiveness. Administration of this drug therapeutically is associated with decreased circulating lymphocyte numbers and spontaneous incorporation of tritiated thymidine into these cells in vitro (MACKINNEY and BOOKER 1972). Whether these effects explain the depression of IgA levels and alterations in delayed cutaneous sensitivity seen in vivo remains to be established. The concentrations required for in vitro effects are high and other mechanisms need to be considered.

Phenytoin use has also been associated with the development of the syndrome of angioblastic lymphadenopathy, a condition characterized by marked small blood vessel proliferation and blast transformation in the lymph nodes and other lymphoid tissues (PRUZANSKI et al. 1976; FRIZZERA et al. 1975; KREISLER et al. 1977). Angioimmunoblastic lymphadenopathy is characterized clinically by lymphadenopathy, hepatosplenomegaly, and hypergamma-globulinemia with or without dysgamma-globulinemia. Although the lesions appear benign histologically, the condition often pursues a progressive downhill course, with more than half of the patients dying within 2 years (PRUZANSKI et al. 1976). The disease usually occurs in patients over 50 years old, and there is frequently a sudden onset of symptoms. Coombs-positive hemolytic anemia and thrombocytopenia are common. Lymphocytoid plasma cells may be seen in the peripheral blood as may increased numbers of B-lymphocytes (KREISLER et al. 1977). While the cause is unknown it may represent the induction of an immune response by a drug or some other antigen in which normal mechanisms for control of lymphoid proliferation fail. This would result in a continuing immune response with encroachment or other suppressive effect by proliferating lymphocytes on normal tissues. Eventually the interference with normal lymphoid function can apparently become severe enough to cause serious disease or even death.

E. Ethanol

Ethanol produces nonspecific suppressive effects on immune resistance, probably related to a variety of factors including decreases in histamine release from mast cells, lysosomal enzyme release from neutrophils and macrophages, and leukocyte chemotaxis (ATKINSON et al. 1977). At high doses it also suppresses microbial clearing from the lung by interfering with the normal ciliary action and the cough reflex. Some alcoholic beverages contain agents such as histamine which produce acute flushing or rhinitis. However, flushing during ethanol use is more likely to be related to an inherited susceptibility to the drug, which has nothing to do with any pharmacologic impurities that alcoholic preparations might contain. This interesting symptomatic response is particularly common in Asians (SETO et al. 1978).

F. Anti-Depressive Drugs

Amitriptylene, desimpramine, and imipramine produce renal damage, agranulo-cytosis, urticaria, angioedema, rashes, pruritus, photosensitivity, and cholestatic jaundice (HAMILTON and MAHAPATRA 1972; BYCK 1975). Amitriptylene apparently is less prone to produce these manifestations than imipramine (HAMILTON and MA-HAPATRA 1972). The former has a carbon atom with a double bond in the nucleus instead of the nitrogen atom at this same position in imipramine. The jaundice is usually of the cholestatic type. Eosinophilia may be seen as may eosinophilic pneu-monitis (HAMILTON and MAHAPATRA 1972). Desipramine has been reported to pro-duce immune thrombocytopenia (HAMILTON and MAHAPATRA 1972).

The amine oxidase inhibitors or hydrazine derivatives also produce hepatic in-jury in susceptible individuals. The incidence of jaundice to iproniazid is approx-imately 1% (ZIMMERMAN 1972). Lithium produces a variety of rashes, but it is un-certain whether or not allergy is involved.

G. Stimulants and Hallucinogens

Allergic reactions to stimulatory agents such as the amphetamines appear to be rare. Nonetheless, necrotizing angiitis has been associated with methamphetamine use either alone or in combination with other drugs such as heroin or D-lysergic acid diethylamide (CITRON et al. 1970). Affected patients may be asymptomatic and the condition not identified unless detailed clinical studies are undertaken. Be-cause of the many different kinds of substances which may have been taken and the possibility of contamination, the cause of the vascular inflammation is difficult to establish and a variety of mechanisms may be involved. Some of the reactions appear to be due to hepatitis-B infection (KOFF et al. 1973) which is a known cause of vasculitis. However, in one fairly large series of patients with vasculitis associ-ated with drug abuse, hepatitis-B antigen was demonstrable in less than 30% of the patients (CITRON and PETERS 1971). It is also possible that lesions may some-times be pharmacologically induced owing to recurrent responses in small blood vessels to vasoactive agents such as methamphetamine.

H. L-Dopa

L-Dopa produces some of the same manifestations that α-methyldopa produces, including sensitization of red cells by antibody (with or without hemolytic anemia), drug fever, rash, and leukopenia, but all of these manifestations are rare. The he-molytic anemia produced by L-dopa is very rare. It appears to be of the autoim-mune type, involving Rh determinants analogous to the much more common he-molytic anemia seen with α-methyldopa therapy (WORLLEDGE 1973). L-Dopa has also been reported to produce an acute non-hemolytic anemia (ALKALAY and ZI-POLI 1977).

J. Relaxants

Mephenesin has been reported to produce eosinophilic pneumonitis (PATTERSON et al. 1974), and rarely other manifestations of hypersensitivity.

K. Analgesic Agents

Aspirin has been reported to produce clinical exacerbations in a high percentage of patients with chronic idiopathic urticaria (PARKER 1980a; WARIN 1960; YECIES and KAPLAN 1980). In addition, attacks of urticaria or angioedema may also occasionally be produced in patients without previous urticarial symptoms, apparently on a pharmacolologic idiosyncrasy basis. There also is a subgroup of patients with chronic idiopathic rhinitis or asthma who are subject to acute exacerbations of respiratory symptoms 10 min to 4 h after challenge with aspirin (PARKER 1980b). Nasal polyps are frequent in these individuals and may suggest the diagnosis. Respiratory symptoms occur in the absence of continued aspirin use, but are likely to be more marked if the drug (or other agent) that produces exacerbations is taken on a regular basis. Some physicians now deliberately challenge patients who have idiopathic asthma with aspirin in an attempt to determine whether they have the form of asthma or rhinitis associated with analgesic sensitivity (STEVENSON and MATHISON 1975). Careful supervision is necessary since the clinical symptoms may be sufficiently severe to necessitate emergency treatment. In very rare instances death has occurred during the routine pharmacologic use of aspirin in a susceptible individual.

The mechanism of these reactions is poorly understood. Other agents such as indomethacin, which interfere with prostaglandin biosynthesis but are structurally unrelated to aspirin, may produce similar symptoms. This suggests that sudden interference with the cyclooxygenase pathway may underlie the symptomatic exacerbations. Arachidonate metabolites with bronchodilator activity such as PGE_2 or prostacyclin may be present in increased amounts in these individuals as a compensatory mechanism for some underlying chronic inflammatory stimulus. When their synthesis is suddenly inhibited an acute symptomatic exacerbation occurs. Alternatively, the diminution in cyclooxygenase activity may provide extra substrate for formation of a slowly reacting substance, which is a potent bronchoconstrictor (PARKER 1973, 1979).

It appears quite possible that a hapten-mediated form of hypersensitivity is involved in a small proportion of patients with aspirin sensitivity. This is suggested by the presence in some aspirin preparations of aspiryl anhydrides which have the capability of conjugating to serum proteins and other proteins in the body, producing an aspiryl-specific immune response (DE WECK 1971). Direct evidence that antibody formation to aspiryl groups can occur has been obtained both in humans and in experimental animals, although most acute symptomatic exacerbations following aspirin use appear to involve other mechanisms. It has also been suggested that the acetyl groups of aspirin may react with circulating proteins and produce an acetyl allergy (PINCKARD et al. 1968; HAWKINS et al. 1969). However, the evidence for this mechanism is not convincing. While protein acetylation undoubtedly occurs under ordinary clinical conditions of aspirin use, the lack of structural complexity of the acetyl group probably makes it a relatively ineffective hapten, decreasing the likelihood of hypersensitivity.

Aminopyrine, indomethacin, acetoaminophen, and phenylbutazone have been reported to produce a variety of allergic manifestations affecting the skin including maculopapular and urticarial rashes, erythema multiforme, fixed drug eruptions,

Lyell syndrome, and Stevens–Johnson syndrome (PRESCOTT 1975; GOODMAN and GILMAN 1955 c; SCHUPPLI 1972; VAN ARSDEL 1978; PARKER 1980 a; GIMINEZ-CAMARASA et al. 1975). Other manifestations include anaphylaxis, serum sickness, vasculitis (phenylbutazone), hepatotoxicity (phenylbutazone), kidney disease, anemia (acetaminophen, indomethacin, phenylbutazone), thrombocytopenia (acetaminophen, phenylbutazone), and granulocytopenia (aminopyrine, indomethacin, phenylbutazone). Phenylbutazone produces a particularly diverse group of clinical reactions including liver damage with jaundice, serum sickness, salivary gland enlargement, joint pain, conjunctivitis, stomatitis, and nephritis.

The most dangerous reaction to analgesic reagents is agranulocytosis. This is particularly common with aminopyrine and its congeners and with phenylbutazone (WOODBURY and FINGL 1975 b; PRICE 1975; PARKER 1980 a; PETZ and FUDENBERG 1976). The estimated frequency of agranulocytosis in association with aminopyrine or phenylbutazone use is about 1%. Agranulocytosis may also occur in association with indomethacin use although this is somewhat less common. As a rule the granulocytopenia appears during the first 1–6 weeks of therapy. The earliest manifestations are usually those of infection owing to the markedly depressed granulocyte count and ineffective host resistance, but skin rash and other noninfectious symptoms may be present. The granulocytopenia appears to involve both peripheral destruction of leukocytes and maturational arrest at the bone marrow level. The passive transfer of serum from affected individuals into normal recipients in association with drug challenge has been reported to produce the granulocytopenia, strongly supporting a humoral immune mechanism for the granulocytopenia (MOESCHLIN and WAGNER 1952). However, not all such attempts at passive transfer have been successful, and there is no completely satisfactory in vitro assay for studying the mechanism of leukocyte destruction. Attempts to demonstrate serum antibodies in vitro in patients who have not received the drug recently are usually unsuccessful. However when blood is taken within 24–48 h after drug administration it may be possible to detect antibodies, either through their effects on granulocyte metabolism or their ability to agglutinate granulocytes (MOESCHLIN and WAGNER 1952). These effects apparently require both the presence of a circulating antibody and a metabolite of the drug formed in vivo. Drug and serum effects on granulocyte colony formation in vitro have also been reported, raising the possibility of a direct effect on granulocyte maturation (BARRETT et al. 1976).

Even with the availability of antibiotics the disease still carries a serious prognosis with death occurring in 5%–10% of affected individuals. Obviously neither aminopyrine nor phenylbutazone should be used when less toxic drugs such as aspirin produce an adequate symptomatic response. Once the diagnosis is supected, the drug should be discontinued and not readministered.

The role of immunity in anemic or thrombocytopenic reactions produced by these drugs has been less well studied, in part because of their lower frequency. Oxyphenbutazone was recently reported to be the commonest cause of drug-induced aplastic anemia in Sweden (BÖTTIGER and WESTERHOLM 1973). A positive lymphocyte transformation test has been reported in a patient with phenylbutazone-induced aplastic anemia (REIDENBERG and CACCESE 1975), suggesting an immune response to the drug and conceivably immune suppression of erythropoiesis, but further studies are needed.

Phenacetin and acetoaminophen are less prone to produce blood dyscrasias or other hypersensitivity reactions than phenylbutazone, aminopyrine, or indomethacin. However, immune thrombocytopenia has been reported during treatment with acetoaminophen, apparently due to antibody formation to a sulfated metabolite of the drug (EISNER and SHAHIDI 1972). When used in large quantities over a long period of time, phenacetin appears to cause chronic nephritis, particularly when given in combination with other analgesic agents (MACKLON et al. 1974; ANGERVALL et al. 1972). The nephritis is characterized by papillary necrosis and interstitial renal damage. It has not been reproduced experimentally in animals and there is no evidence that the renal damage is immunologically mediated. Nonetheless at least two metabolites of phenacetin, p-phenetidin and 2-hydroxy-p-phenetidin, are immunogenic in guinea pigs (FREY et al. 1974), and further studies are needed.

References

Alkalay I, Zipoli T (1977) Levodopa-induced acute non-hemolytic anemia. Ann Allergy 39:191

Angervall L, Bengtsson U, Lehmann L (1972) Renal diseases caused by drugs. In: Samter M, Parker CW (eds) International encyclopedia of pharmacology and therapeutics, Sect 75: Hypersensitivity to drugs. Pergamon, Oxford

Atkinson JP, Sullivan TJ, Kelly JP, Parker CW (1977) Stimulation by alcohols of cAMP metabolism in human lymphocytes. Possible role of cAMP in the anti-inflammatory effects of ethanol. J Clin Invest 60:284–294

Barrett AJ, Weller E, Rozengurt N, Longhurst P, Humble JG (1976) Amidopyrine agranulocytosis: drug inhibition of granulocyte colonies in the presence of patient's serum. Br Med J 2:850–851

Becker LC (1973) Allergy in systemic lupus erythematosus. Johns Hopkins Med J 133:38–44

Bennett WM, Plamp C, Porter GA (1977) Drug-related syndromes in clinical nephrology. Ann Intern Med 87:582–590

Böttiger LE, Westerhjolm B (1973) Drug-induced blood dyscrasias in Sweden. Br Med J 3:339–343

Brashear RE, Kelly MT, White AC (1974) Elevated plasma histamine after heroin and morphine. J Lab Clin Med 83:451–457

Braverman IM, Levin J (1963) Dilantin-induced serum sickness. Case report and inquiry into its mechanism. Am J Med 35:418–422

Byck R (1975) Drugs and the treatment of psychiatric disorders. In: Goodman LS, Gilman A (eds) The pharmacological basis of therapeutics, 5th edn. Macmillan, New York

Citron BP, Peters RL (1971) Angiitis in drug abusers. N Engl J Med 284:112

Citron BP, Halpern M, McCarron M et al. (1970) Necrotizing angiitis associated with drug abuse. N Engl J Med 283:1003–1011

Davies GE, Holmnes JE (1972) Drug-induced immunological effects on the liver. Br J Anaesth 44:941–945

Davis M, Williams R (1978) Drugs and the liver. In: Davies DM (ed) Textbook of adverse drug reactions. Oxford University Press, Oxford

de Weck AL (1971) Immunological effects of aspirin anhydride, a contaminant of commercial acetylsalicylic acid preparations. Int Arch Allergy Appl Immunol 41:393–418

Duberstein JL, Kaufman DM (1972) Heroin intoxication in adolescents. Pediatrics 50:746–753

Dundee JW (1976) Hypersensitivity to intravenous anaesthetic agents. Br J Anaesth 48:57–58

Eddleston ALWF (1980) Immunology and the liver. In: Parker CW (ed) Clinical immunology. Saunders, Philadelphia, pp 1009–1050

Eisner EV, Shahidi NT (1972) Immune thrombocytopenia due to a drug metabolite. N Engl J Med 287:376–381

Fisher MMcD (1975) Severe histamine mediated reactions to intravenous drugs used in anaesthesia. Anaesth Intensive Care 3:180–197

Fisher M (1977) Hypersensitivity to intravenous anaesthetic agents. Br J Anaesth 49:87–88

Frand UI, Chang SS, Williams MH Jr (1972 a) Heroin-induced pulmonary edema. Sequential studies of pulmonary function. Ann Intern Med 77:29–35

Frand UI, Chang SS, Williams MH Jr (1972 b) Methadone-induced pulmonary edema. Ann Intern Med 76:975–979

Frey JR, Geleick H, Geczy A, de Weck AL (1974) The immunogenicity of phenacetin and some of its metabolites in guinea pigs. Int Arch Allergy 46:571–583

Frizzera Gl, Moran EM, Rappaport H (1975) Angio-immunoblastic lymphadenopathy. Diagnosis and clinical course. Am J Med 59:803–818

Giminez-Camarasa JM, Garcia-Calderon P, de Moragas JM (1975) Lymphocyte transformation test in fixed drug eruption. N Engl J Med 292:819–821

Goodman LS, Gilman A (1955 a) Hypnotics and sedatives. In: Goodman LS, Gilman A (eds) The pharmacological basis of therapeutics, 2nd edn. Macmillan, New York

Goodman LS, Gilman A (1955 b) Drugs effective in convulsive disorders. In: Goodman LS, Gilman A (eds) The pharmacological basis of therapeutics, 2nd edn. Macmillan, New York

Goodman LS, Gilman A (1955 c) Analgesics and antipyretics. In: Goodman LS, Gilman A (eds) The pharmacological basis of therapeutics, 2nd edn. Macmillan, New York

Greenblatt DJ, Shader RI (1974) Benzodiazepines in clinical practice. Raven, New York

Grob PJ, Herold GE (1972) Immunological abnormalities and hydantoins. Br Med J 2:561–563

Hall JH, Karp HR (1973) Acute progressive ventral pontine disease in heroin abuse. Neurology (NY) 23:6–7

Hamilton M, Mahapatra SB (1972) Antidepressive drugs. In: Meyler L, Herxheimer A (eds) Side effects of drugs, vol 7. Excerpta Medica, Amsterdam

Harpey J-P (1974) Lupus-like syndromes induced by drugs. Ann Allergy 33:256–261

Hartl PW (1973) Drug-induced agranulocytosis. In: Girdwood RH (ed) Blood disorders due to drugs and other agents. Excerpta Medica, Amsterdam

Harvey SC (1975) Hypnotics and sedatives. In: Goodman LS, Gilman A (eds) The pharmacological basis of therapeutics, 5th edn. Macmillan, New York

Hawkins D, Pinckard RN, Crawford IP, Farr RS (1969) Structural change in human serum albumin induced by ingestion of acetyl-salicylic acid. J Clin Invest 48:536–542

Ishak KG, Irey NS (1972) Hepatic injury associated with the phenothiazines. Clinicopathologic and follow-up study of 36 patients. Arch Pathol 93:283–304

Katz S, Aberman A, Frand UI, Stein IM, Fulop M (1972) Heroin pulmonary edema. Evidence for increased pulmonary capillary permeability. Am Rev Respir Dis 106:472–474

Kazimierczak W, Diamant B (1978) Mechanisms of histamine release in anaphylactic and anaphylactoid reactions. Prog Allergy 24:295–365

Koff RS, Widrich WC, Robbins AH (1973) Necrotizing angiitis in a methamphetamine user with hepatitis B – angiographic diagnosis, five-month follow-up results and localization of bleeding site. N Engl J Med 288:945–947

Kreisler JM, Moreno E, Moneo I et al. (1977) Immunological findings in immunoblastic lymphadenopathy. A detailed case study. Clin Exp Immunol 27:497–501

Liskow B, Liss JL, Parker CW (1971) Allergy to marihuana. A case report. Ann Intern Med 75:572

Little DM (1968) Effects of halothane in liver function. In: Davis FA (ed) Clinical anesthesia: halothane. Davis, Philadelphia

Louria DB, Joselow MM, Browder AA (1972) The human toxicity of certain trace elements. Ann Intern Med 76:307–319

MacKinney AA, Booker HE (1972) Diphenylhydantoin effects on human lymphocytes in vitro and in vivo. An hypothesis to explain some drug reactions. Arch Intern Med 129:988–992

Macklon AF, Craft AW, Thompson M, Kerr DNS (1974) Aspirin and analgesic nephropathy. Br Med J 1:597–600

Mathieu A, DiPadua D, Mills J, Kahan B (1974) Experimental immunity to a metabolite of halothane and fluroxene: cutaneous delayed-type hypersensitivity. Anesthesiology 40:385–390

Miller RR, Greenblatt D (1976) Drug effects in hospitalized patients. John Wiley and Sons, New York Chichester

Moeschlin S, Wagner K (1952) Agranulocytosis due to the occurrence of leukocyte-agglutinins (pyramidon and cold agglutins). Acta Haematol (Basel) 8:29–41

Moult PJA, Sherlock S (1975) Halothane-related hepatitis. A clinical study of twenty-six cases. Q J Med 44:99–114

Parker CW (1973) Adrenergic responsiveness in asthma. In: Lichtenstein LM, Austen KF (eds) Asthma physiology immunopharmacology, and treatment. Academic Press, New York

Parker CW (1979) Prostaglandins and slow-reacting substances. J Allergy Clin Immunol 63:1–14

Parker CW (1980a) Drug allergy. In: Parker CW (ed) Clinical immunology. Saunders, Philadelphia, pp 1219–1260

Parker CW (1980b) Asthma and rhinitis. In Parker CW (ed) Clinical immunology. Saunders, Philadelphia, pp 1372–1438

Paronetto F, Popper H (1970) Lymphocyte stimulation induced by halothane in patients with hepatitis following exposure to halothane. N Engl J Med 283:277–280

Patterson R, Irons JS, Kelly JF, Mattson JR, Oh SH (1974) Pulmonary infiltrates with eosinophilia. J Allergy Clin Immunol 53:245–255

Petz LD, Fudenberg HH, (1976) Immunologic mechanisms in drug-induced cytopenias. Prog Hematol 9

Pillsbury DM, Caro WA (1966) The increasing problem of photosensitivity. Med Clin North Am 50:1295–1311

Pinckard RN, Hawkins D, Farr RS (1968) In vitro acetylation of plasma proteins, enzymes and DNA by aspirin. Nature 219:68

Pisciotta AV (1973) Immune and toxic mechanisms in drug-induced agranulocytosis. Semin Hematol 10:279–310

Prescott LF (1975) Anti-inflammatory analgesics and drugs used in the treatment of rheumatoid arthritis and gout. In: Dukes MNG (ed) Meyler's side effects of drugs, vol VIII. American Elsevier, New York

Price CD, Gibbs AR, Jones-Williams W (1977) Halothane macrophage migration inhibition test in halothane associated hepatitis. J Clin Pathol 30:312–316

Price HL (1975) General anesthetics. In: Goodman LS, Gilman A (eds) The pharmacological basis of therapeutics, 5th edn. Macmillan, New York

Pruzanski W, Sutton DMC, Pantalony D (1976) Angioimmunoblastic lymphadenopathy: an immunochemical study. Clin Immunol Immunopathol 6:62–76

Reed WD, Williams R (1972) Halothane hepatitis as seen by the physician. Br J Anaesth 44:935–940

Reidenberg MM, Caccese RW (1975) Lymphocyte transformation tests and suspected drug allergy. J Lab Clin Med 86:997–1002

Ringle DA, Herndon BL (1975) Immunologic effects of morphine administration in rabbits. J Immunol 115:876–883

Rosenow EC III (1972) The spectrum of drug-induced pulmonary disease. Ann Intern Med 77:977–991

Ryan JJ, Parker CW, Williams RC (1972) δ-globulin binding of morphine in heroin addicts. J Lab Clin Med 80:155–164

Saltzstein SL, Ackerman LV (1959) Lymphadenopathy induced by anticonvulsant drugs and minicking clinically and pathologically malignant lymphomas. Cancer 12:164–182

Sapira JD (1968) The narcotic addict as a medical patient. Am J Med 45:555–588

Schuppli R (1972) Drug-induced skin reactions. In: Samter M, Parker CW (eds) International encyclopedia of pharmacology and therapeutics, Sect 75: Hypersensitivity to drugs. Pergamon, Oxford

Seto A, Tricomi S, Goodwin D, Kolodney R, Sullivan TJ (1978) Biochemical correlates of ethanol induced flushing in Orientals. J Stud Alcohol 39:1–11

Spector S, Parker CW (1970) Morphine: radioimmunoassay. Science 168:1347–1348

Spector S, Berkowitz B, Flynn EJ, Peskar B (1973) Antibodies to morphine, barbiturates, and serotonin. Pharmacol Rev 25:281–291

Stevenson DD, Mathison DA (1975) Aeroallergen inhalation challenges in aspirin-intolerant asthmatic patients. J Allergy Clin Immunol 55:127

Van Arsdel PP Jr (1978) Adverse drug reactions. In: Middleton E Jr, Reed CE, Ellis EF (eds) Allergy: principles and practice, vol 2. Mosby, St. Louis

Walton B, Dumonde DC, Williams C et al. (1973) Lymphocyte transformation. Absence of increased responses in alleged halothane jaundice. JAMA 225:494–498

Walton B, Simpson BR, Strunin L, Doniach D, Perrin J, Appleyard AJ (1976) Unexplained hepatitis following halothane. Br Med J 1:1171–1176

Warin RP (1960) The effect of aspirin in chronic urticaria. Br J Dermatol 72:350–351

Weksler ME, Cherubin C, Kilcoyne M, Koppel G, Yoel M (1973) Absence of morphine-binding activity in serum from heroin addicts. Clin Exp Immunol 13:613–617

Woodbury DM, Fingl E (1975 a) Drugs effective in the therapy of the epilepsies. In: Goodman LS, Gilman A (eds) The pharmacological basis of therapeutics, 5th edn. Macmillan, New York

Woodbury DM, Fingl E (1975 b) Analgesic-antipyretics, anti-inflammatory agents, and drugs employed in the therapy of gout. In: Goodman LS, Gilman A (eds) The pharmacological basis of therapeutics, 5th edn. Macmillan, New York

Woods BT, Strewler GJ (1972) Hemiparesis occurring six hours after intravenous heroin injection. Neurology (NY) 22:863–866

Worlledge SM (1973) Immune hemolytic anemais. Semin Hematol 10:327

Wright R, Eade JE, Chisholm OM et al. (1975) Controlled prospective study of the effect on liver function of multiple exposures to halothane. Lancet 1:817–821

Yecies LD, Kaplan A (1980) Urticaria. In: Parker CW (ed) Clinical immunology. Saunders, Philadelphia, pp 1283–1315

Zelman S (1959) Liver cell necrosis in chlorpromazine jaundice (allergic cholangiolitis). A serial study of twenty-six needle biopsy specimens in nine patients. Am J Med 27:708–729

Zidar BL, Mendelow H, Winkelstein A, Shadduck RK (1975) Diphenylhydantoin-induced serum sickness with fibrin-platelet thrombi in lymph node microvasculature. Am J Med 58:704–708

Zimmerman HJ (1972) Drug-induced hepatic injury. In: Samter M, Parker CW (eds) International encyclopedia of pharmacology and therapeutics, Sect 75: Hypersensitivity to drugs. Pergamon, Oxford

CHAPTER 10

General and Local Anaesthetics

E. S. K. Assem

A. Hypersensitivity Reactions to Intravenous Anaesthetics

In the ensuing discussion attention will be given to acute adverse effects of those agents which are used for the induction of general anaesthesia by the intravenous (i. v.) route. The term "hypersensitivity reactions" is used in preference to "allergic reactions", contrary to the need for more precise definitions. With certain intravenous anaesthetics, e. g. thiopentone, such reactions are nearly always due to allergy but with other i. v. induction agents such as steroid anaesthetics and eugenols only a proportion (around 50% with both groups) of the reactions appear to be allergic in nature, the remainder being due to direct histamine release or some other mechanism not involving a specific immune response to the drug. It is often impossible to distinguish between truly allergic reactions and reactions of the latter type, particularly between true anaphylaxis (mediated by anaphylactic, drug-specific antibodies) and anaphylactoid reactions, where chemical mediators such as histamine are released as a result of a different abnormality (idiosyncrasy).

I. Clinical Manifestations

Clarke et al. (1978), in one review of reported reactions to intravenous anaesthetics, used the term "hypersensitivity reaction" to describe reactions resembling the effects of injected histamine. The main clinical manifestations could be grouped into four categories:
1. Cutaneous: flushing, often associated with increased vascular permeability, leading to oedema and formation of wheals
2. Cardiovasular: circulatory collapse, associated with vasodilation and tachycardia
3. Respiratory: Bronchospasm, laryngeal oedema or rarely laryngospasm
4. Abdominal: pain.

II. Predisposing Factors

The predisposing factors are similar with all intravenous anaesthetics. This was the experience of several groups, including Clarke et al. (1978) and ourselves (Assem 1977 b). The reactions were most frequent in asthmatic and allergic patients (suffering from other allergies). They were particularly frequent in those who had a previous anaesthesia within the preceding few weeks, especially if it was with the same anaesthetic.

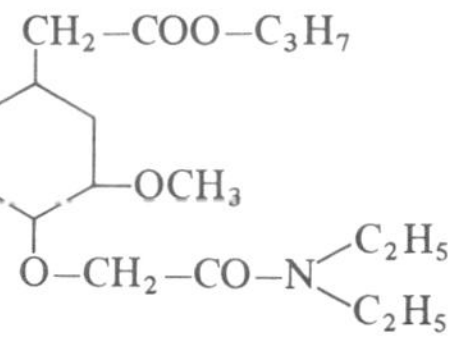

$$CH_2-COO-C_3H_7$$

$$OCH_3$$

$$O-CH_2-CO-N\begin{matrix} C_2H_5 \\ C_2H_5 \end{matrix}$$

Fig. 1. Chemical structure of propanidid, propyl-4-diethylcarbamoylmethoxy-3-methoxy-phenyl acetate

III. Relative Incidence with Various Agents

All intravenous anaesthetics appear to be capable of inducing generalised reactions of this type. CLARKE et al. (1978), reviewing their own series, and those reported by other authors, came to the conclusion that these reactions were most frequent with propanidid (Epontol, Bayer), followed by alphaxalone/alphadolone (Althesin, Glaxo), and then methohexitone. They were least frequent with thiopentone. The various groups of intravenous anaesthetics will be discussed separately, with steroid anaesthetics receiving the greatest detail. The review by WHITWAM (1978) is recommended for further reference.

1. Barbiturates

Ultrashort-acting barbiturates very rarely produce such reactions although they are the most widely used i. v. induction agents. Until a few years ago allergy to thiopentone was not thought to exist, and several textbooks dogmatically emphasised that point. However, it is clear from the work of CLARKE et al. (1975) that the case for thiopentone was overstated. The latter authors carried out a survey in Great Britain covering the period 1957–1974, during which 14 cases had been reported. They also collected 12 other cases from the literature.

Less serious reactions to barbiturates, mainly affecting the skin, occur far more frequently than the previously mentioned acute reactions.

2. Eugenols

Propanidid (Fig. 1), a eugenol and also a very short-acting drug, was introduced in the United Kingdom in 1965. CLARKE (1974), reviewed 23 incidents of acute adverse effects to this agent, and the evidence he presented suggested that allergy could undoubtedly explain at least a proportion of those incidents. Of these 11 patients had the drug on a previous occasion and acquired allergy to the drug was the likely mechanism in them.

A case of allergy to propanidid reported by DUNDEE et al. (1974) showed typical manifestations of contact dermatitis and a typical delayed hypersensitivity reaction to skin testing. Propanidid has not been much in use in the United Kingdom since 1973, when Althesin, the steroid i. v. anaesthetic, replaced it.

3. Steroid Anaesthetics

The detailed account of acute reactions to steroid anaesthetics given here does not reflect their frequency. These reactions (anaphylactic or anaphylactic-like) are not

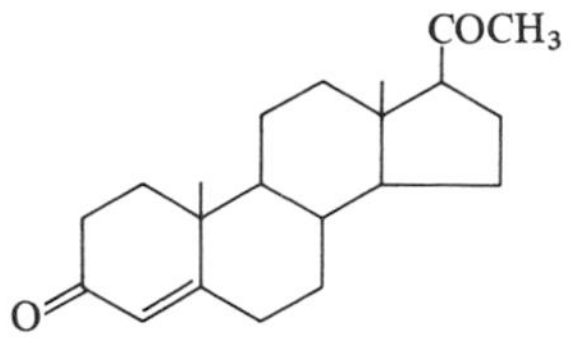

Progesterone

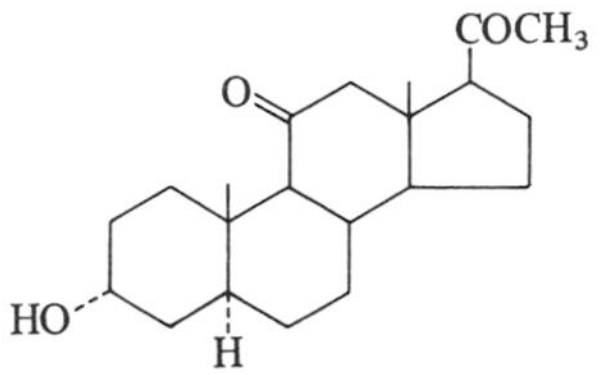

Alphaxalone

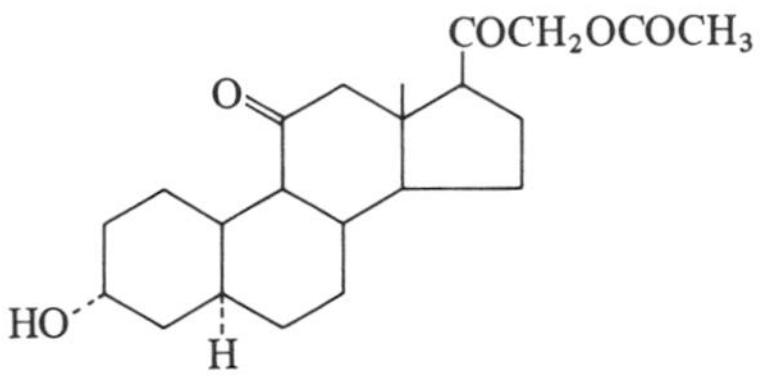

Alphadolone acetate

Fig. 2. Chemical structure of progesterone and the two structurally related intravenous steroid anaesthetics, alphaxalone and alphadolone

a pecularity of steroid anaesthetics since they occur with all intravenous anaesthetics and are even more frequent with some of them, e. g., eugenols. They also occur with various pre-anaesthetic medications.

What is special about these steroids (alphaxalone and alphadolone) is their novel effect as anaesthetics and their chemical similarity to progesterone (Fig. 2). It was SEYLE (1941) who first noted the general anaesthetic effect of progesterone, when injected in large amounts intravenously in rats. The background for the introduction of steroid anaesthetics has been reviewed by SUTTON (1972). The review by PHILLIPS (1974) of the structure–activity relationships of steroidal anaesthetics is recommended for further reference.

There have been many reports of reactions to Althesin, a mixture of two steroids, alphaxalone und alphadolone, dissolved in sodium chloride solution containing 20% polyoxyethylated castor oil (Cremophor EL). Apart from their anaesthetic effects, these steroids are weak oestrogen antagonists, but possess no other steroid properties. This preparation is a rapid and short-acting anaesthetic induction agent, it produces less cardiovascular and respiratory depression than barbiturates, and has no "hang-over" effect.

a) Incidence of Reactions

Dundee and his co-workers suggested that the incidence of reactions was less than 1 in 10,000. From sales figures the incidence of these reactions appeared to be lower than 1 in 25,000 (Dundee et al. 1974). At the time, it seemed that the large number of reported reactions was largely due to the great interest that this problem has attracted. It also appeared to follow the initiative (circulated questionnaires and published notes) taken by Dundee and Clarke (1973) and Glaxo Laboratories, the manufacturers of Althesin. The aim of the questionaires was to collect all reactions to intravenous anesthetics in the United Kingdom, with a view to determining the factors involved and the relative likelihood of reactions with the different agents available.

There is some evidence, however, that reactions to Althesin are considerably more frequent than reactions to thiopentone though the mortality, which is extremely low, may be the same (or even smaller with Althesin as suggested by some groups, e.g., Clarke et al. 1978). Evans and Keogh (1977) estimated that the frequency of adverse reactions to Althesin was 1 in 2,000, which is 15 times higher than thiopentone. In a recent circular of the Committee on Safety of Medicines (1979) it was stated that the Committee continued to receive reports of such reactions.

The Committee, however, again pointed to the possible influence of their previous warnings in previous circulars. Two other points were mentioned in that report, which are relevant to the mechanism of reactions. First, that the reaction may occur in patients previously anaesthetised uneventfully with Althesin, and second, that apart from the immediate reaction (hypotension, flushing, and bronchospasm), a milder degree of these manifestations may recur after 12 h or more. The first point is in keeping with the contention that allergy to these steroids (alphaxalone and alphadolone), and possibly to the vehicle, may occur. The second point is also in favour of an immune mechanism of reaction (allergy) being involved, with mechanisms other than immediate-type allergy (anaphylaxis) mediating the late reaction.

b) Investigation of Reactions

The problem of reactions to Althesin raised a number of questions, some of which will be discussed here. First, confirmation was needed since in some cases there was suspicion that agents other than Althesin, e. g., muscle relaxants, might have been involved. Even in those reacting to Althesin, the vehicle (Cremophor EL) was a possible "culprit".

Investigations were also needed to establish the mechanisms underlying these reactions, the most important of all questions. In some of the patients (five of the ten patients we have reported; Assem 1977 a) a history of prior exposure to Althesin without undue reaction was obtained, thus favouring the diagnosis of classic immediate allergy, i. e., a reaction presumably mediated by anaphylactic antibodies (IgE mainly, but possibly IgG subclasses as well). Furthermore, a history of other allergies, particularly atopic conditions, was commonly obtained in patients reacting to Althesin. In the patients in whom a history of previous exposure was not obtained, the acute reaction was unlikely to be due to an immune mechanism. Thus, the acute anaphylactic-like (anaphylactoid) reaction was presumably due to a different (non-immune) qualitative abnormality in the response to these agents.

Various procedures were used to answer these questions, including direct skin tests, Prausnitz–Küstner reaction, intravenous test doses and in particular the measurement of histamine release from leucocytes in vitro. We found the latter test extremely useful (ASSEM 1977a). LORENZ and DOENICKE (1978) measured plasma histamine levels in vivo, and other authors found complement studies of great value (WATKINS et al. 1978); WATKINS 1979; DYE and WATKINS 1980).

c) Role of Cremophor EL

This was the first substance to be suspected of playing a role in Althesin reactions, because of some of its already known properties, and because nobody would believe that steroids could be allergenic. Cremophor EL is a macromolecular liquid consisting of polyoxyethylated castor oil. It is a water-miscible agent, and acts as a micellophore. Thus, it is widely used as a vehicle for lipid-soluble drugs, such as propanidid. It can similarly be used with diazepam.

Cremophors are known to release histamine in dogs and possibly in cats, but not in humans and some other species (LORENZ et al. 1972). That Cremophor played a role in the anaphylactic or anaphylactic-like reactions was proved by the finding of positive skin tests (wheal and flare response) and by demonstrating leucocyte histamine release in vitro by this agent in some of the patients who reacted to Althesin or Epontol. Although in some patients the response to Cremophor EL was the only abnormality, in other patients the separate steroids (alphaxalone or alphadolone, dissolved in ethanol before dilution for testing) also gave a skin response and/or induced histamine release from their leucocytes. Examples of such reactions have been reported by KESSEL and ASSEM (1974), and ASSEM (1977a).

d) Mechanism of Reaction to Cremophor EL

α) Direct Histamine Release. In some patients a direct histamine-releasing effect (apparently not immunologically mediated and thus described as anaphylactic-like or anaphylactoid) was the presumed underlying mechanism. This was suggested by the occurrence of reactions on first exposure and by the failure to obtain evidence of reagin-mediated allergy. Regarding the lack of previous exposure, one could not completely rule out "sensitisation" to castor oil taken previously, though this seems very unlikely.

Direct histamine release may be induced with many polymer substances (PATON 1957), but the link between this finding and the abnormal release of histamine from the leucocytes of susceptible individuals with Cremophor EL (also a polymer) is yet to be disclosed. Presumably, it is either a qualitative abnormality (idiosyncrasy) or a quantitative one (extreme exaggeration of the normal), thus possibly defined as "intolerance".

The question arose as to whether a reaction to Cremophor EL would mean a potential susceptibility to other micellophores, and more importantly, as to whether Cremophor EL could be replaced by a harmless alternative. This possibility was examined in one patient who reacted to Althesin by developing airway obstruction (asthma) on the first exposure and in whom the leucocyte histamine re-

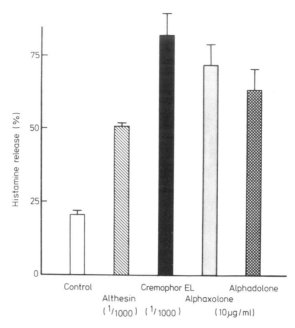

Fig. 3. Histamine release (means ± standard errors) from the leucocytes of a patient with allergy to Althesin, the steroid anaesthetic preparation, and its various components

lease test pointed to Cremophor EL as the culprit. A test dose of the latter was given i. v. in a cumulative way. Airway obstruction was obtained after this test dose, confirming this agent as the cause of the reaction. On another occasion a similar test dose of another vehicle, Cremophor RH 40 (kindly provided by Dr. A. J. Sutton, Glaxo) was given, to see if it was devoid of this risk. Unfortunately, the patient also reacted to this other agent, excluding the possibility of it being used as an alternative to Cremophor EL.

β) Allergy to Cremophor EL. Despite the suggestion that Cremophor EL may act as a histamine releaser in the majority of patients reacting to it, immediate allergy to this agent was encountered in a few patients. The strongest evidence of the latter mechanism was obtained in one patient (his own leucocyte test is shown in Fig. 3) whose serum gave a positive result in the Prausnitz–Küstner reaction.

It is not surprising that Cremophor EL is potentially allergenic since it is a macromolecular polymer. Immune responses to polymers have been well documented (Richter et al. 1978).

γ) Activation of Complement. Watkins et al. (1978) and Watkins (1979) suggested that various intravenous anaesthetic induction agents, including Althesin and thiopentone, may convert C3 to C3a (anaphylatoxin) or activate C2 without C3 intervention in susceptible individualy.

δ) Other Possible Roles of Cremophor EL. The interactions described in this section appear to be involved in Althesin reactions. Another possibility is the potential effect of Cremophor EL as an adjuvant (suggested by WATKINS 1979), potentiating the immune response. It should be added that adjuvants, and certain bacterial products, e.g., endotoxins, may potentiate the response to certain chemical mediators of inflammatory and immune reactions.

e) The Role of Steroids

In Althesin (previously known as CT 1341, Glaxo) the more active anaesthetic steroid is alphaxalone, 3α-hydroxy – 5α-pregnane – 11,20 – dione (see Fig. 2; PHILLIPPS 1974). The reason for adding the less active (possessing half the activity) anaesthetic alphadalone acetate (21-acetoxy-3α-hydroxy – 5α-pregnane-11,20-dione) was said to be the improvement of the solubility of alphaxalone. Both agents are lipid soluble, alphadolone being the more soluble. However, lipid solubility may not correlate with anaesthetic activity. A clear example of this is Δ^{16}-alphaxalone, which, though as lipid soluble as alphaxalone itself, does not possess any anaesthetic activity (RICHARDS and HESKETH 1975).

Both alphaxalone and alphadolone acetate were found to induce histamine release from the leucocytes of some of the patients who reacted to the whole preparation of Althesin (ASSEM 1977 a). In ten patients whose leucocytes gave this response, there were no significant differences in the potencies of these two steroids as "histamine releasers". Alphaxalone produced slightly more histamine release in five patients and alphadolone did so in the other five.

The mechanism of induction of histamine release by alphaxalone and alphadolone shown by the leucocyte test in susceptible individuals is not clear at present, but it appears to be like Cremophor EL. This means that it could be due either to an anaphylactic or anaphylactoid (direct histamine release) reaction. We did not find histamine release with these agents from the leucocytes of normal volunteers. We were unable to elicit a positive Prausnitz–Küstner reaction in two patients in whom a reaction occurred after a second exposure to Althesin, and in whom the vehicle did not produce any response, either in the direct skin test or in the leucocyte test.

Apart from the general tendency of the reactions to the various ingredients of Althesin to occur with repeated exposure, they also tend to occur in asthmatic and allergic patients. Thus they, like the muscle relaxants and narcotic analgesics, could be added to the list of agents to which these patients stand a higher risk of adverse effects of the types described.

f) Interactions Between Steroids and Cremophor EL

It was noted in a few patients that "interactions" between the various ingredients of Althesin occurred in the leucocyte test. A particularly remarkable and complex example is shown in Fig. 4. The complexity can be seen from the following observations, some of which appear contradictory.

a) Histamine release was induced by Cremophor EL but with neither alphaxalone nor alphadolone separately, even when their relative concentrations (as compared with a dilution of the whole preparation) were stepped up.

b) Each of these two steroids when added to Cremophor EL rather surprisingly led to a reduction in the Cremophor EL-induced histamine release, even to

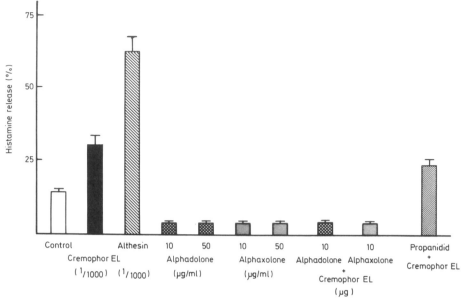

Fig. 4. Histamine release (means±standard errors) from the leucocytes of a patient with "sensitivity" to Althesin, illustrating the interaction between its components. Note the response to the entire preparation, Cremophor EL, Cremophor EL + propanidid, but not to alphadolone or alphaxalone separately even in the presence of Cremophor EL

levels well below the control value (spontaneous histamine release in the presence of the medium used, Tyrode solution).

c) When both alphaxalone and alphadolone were added to the vehicle they produced a paradoxical increase in histamine release.

These findings have, so far, been extended slightly but await further explanation.

B. Hypersensitivity Reactions to Volatile General Anaesthetics

The only documented reaction which could be due to allergy is the liver damage (hepatitis-like picture) which may be attributed to halogenated anaesthetics.

I. Halothane-Associated Liver Damage

The first well-documented case (KLATSKIN and KIMBERG 1969) was that of an anaesthetist who developed hepatitis seven times in 5 years. Each of these attacks followed his return to work and re-exposure to halothane. Jaundice was preceded by systemic manifestations which could all be explained by, or interpreted as, manifestations of an immunologically mediated reaction. These included pyrexia, myalgia and eosinophilia. Serial liver biopsies which were carried out showed hepatic cell necrosis, followed by the development of post-necrotic cirrhosis. It had to be established whether that patient was "sensitive" to halothane, because of the nature of his occupation. Thus, he was exposed to subanaesthetic doses of that agent.

These challenge tests were followed each time be fever, rigors and myalgia, which developed after 4 h. Hepatitis was shown by biopsy after 24 h.

Several other cases of hepatitis resulting from occupational exposure to halothane have been reported. Thus, there is little doubt that hepatitis may follow the inhalation of this anaesthetic. Extensive surveys of post-operative jaundice have also been carried out. A summary of the findings will be given here. Despite numerous reports in the literature of liver damage in patients who had halothane anaesthesia, there is still considerable controversy between anaesthetists and pathologists as to whether the hepatitis and halothane are causally related.

The case of the anaesthetist just mentioned points to one of the underlying factors. This patient suffered from asthma and hay fever. That this was not a mere coincidence was subsequently suggested by the high incidence of personal or family history of allergy, e. g. in the series of CARNEY and VAN DYKE (1972) 46% of all patients developing this affliction gave a history of previous allergy.

According to a number of surveys of post-operative jaundice, the majority of patients who developed jaundice after halothane administration had received that agent more than once within a short period (a few weeks).

1. Incidence

In view of the difficulty in diagnosis, the actual incidence of halothane hepatitis is hard to assess (NATIONAL HALOTHANE STUDY 1966; SIMPSON et al. 1971; DYKES et al. 1972; INMAN and MUSHIN 1974; INMAN 1978). Other causes of post-operative pyrexia and jaundice are difficult to rule out.. Furthermore, these other causes may contribute or predispose to halothane hepatitis (EDITORIAL 1980). The survey by PETERS et al. (1969) suggests that the incidence of halothane hepatitis is 0.7 in 1,000. Fatal reactions are reported to be between 1 in 6,000 and 1 in 22,000.

2. Evidence in Support of an Allergic Mechanism

The high incidence of other allergies and previous exposure, which has been mentioned previously, are suggestive of an allergic mechanism. Furthermore, the latent period before the appearance of jaundice is shorter with repeated exposure. A number of other findings which may be considered in favour of the hepatitis being due to an allergy will be discussed briefly.

a) Clinical Manifestations

Eosinophilia may develop, but the proportion of patients reported to show it varied in different surveys. Fever (post-operative) may be interpreted as indicating sensitisation to halothane (REED and WILLIAMS 1972). It should be added that, in experimental animals, fever could occur as a result of various immune mechanisms, e. g., delayed hypersensitivity, Arthus reaction or immune complexes (CLUFF and JOHNSON 1964).

b) Immunological Investigations

Antimitochondrial and microsomal antibodies (auto-antibodies) may be found. Their appearance is transient. They are said to be found more frequently than in viral hepatitis (WILLIAMS et al. 1975). Lymphocyte transformation by halothane, suggesting delayed hypersensitivity, has been reported by PARONETTO and POPPER (1970), but this was not confirmed by others (BRUCE and RAYMON 1972; SIMPSON and STRUNIN 1973; MOULT and SHERLOCK 1975). Positive macrophage and leucocyte migration inhibition tests have been reported (PRICE et al. 1977; VERGANI et al. 1978). Immune complexes, representing an alternative mechanism of immune liver damage, were demonstrated in one patient with serum-sickness-like syndrome and jaundice, apparently due to halothane (WILLIAMS et al. 1977). Metabolites of halothane were associated with these complexes.

c) Other Relevant Properties of Halogenated Anaesthetics

Since in allergy the drug, and more commonly its metabolites, act as haptens (see Chap. 1, immunological studies on certain metabolites have been carried out. The main metabolite is trifluoroacetic acid (STIER 1968; BLAKE et al. 1967). MATHIEU et al. (1974) have shown that trifluoroacetate (TFA) conjugated to serum albumin can cause delayed hypersensitivity in guinea-pigs, which can be detected by skin testing. This finding is in favour of the halothane hepatitis being due to allergy rather than to direct hepatotoxicity. Thus, it is conceivable that TFA forms covalent bonds with the hepatocyte cell membrane (or some other cell constituent), and that the halothane-induced liver damage is due to "auto-allergic" hepatitis (DONIACH et al. 1970). It is doubtful that simple dissolution of the lipid-soluble halothane into the cell lipoprotein membrane would form an adequate (or stable) conjugate, capable of initiating an immune response. The formation of highly reactive non-volatile halothane metabolites (including TFA) has been shown by radioisotope tracer techniques. These metabolites are formed rapidly, particularly after repeated exposure where increased metabolism due to enzyme induction occurs. Slow elimination of these metabolites also contributes to their cumulation, especially in the liver (COHEN and TRUDELL 1972). There is evidence that antibodies reacting with altered hepatic cell membrane (resulting from chemical conjugation with various chemicals and drugs) not only react with such membrane but also cross-react with normal cell surface antigens (SMITH et al. 1972). VERGANI et al. (1978) investigating the role of sensitisation in halothane hepatitis in humans by in vitro leucocyte migration tests, found that a "modified" liver antigen obtained from halothane-treated rabbits, was a valuable diagnostic material.

Apart from the possibility of causing an immunologically mediated liver damage, halothane and other anaesthetic agents have been shown to possess immunosuppressive properties (BRUCE and WINGARD 1971).

3. Reactions to Other Halogenated Volatile Anaesthetics

Methoxyfluorane is another fluorinated compound which is structurally related to halothane, and which has also been reported to cause hepatic necrosis. The reaction produced closely mimics halothane-induced hepatitis. Furthermore cross-reaction between these two compounds may occur (JUDSON et al. 1971). This is not surprising since they undergo similar metabolic processes.

Other halogenated anaesthetics also rarely cause jaundice due to massive liver cell necrosis, but more frequently they cause subclinical hepatocellular damage as shown by post-operative elevations in serum glutamic oxaloacetic transaminase (SGOT) levels. By contrast, non-halogenated anaesthetics have a lower incidence of such reactions (WRIGHT et al. 1975; TROWELL et al. 1975).

4. Possible Role of Idiosyncrasy in Hepatitis Associated with Halogenated Volatile Anaesthetics

Apart from the role of the metabolies as haptens, they may act as direct hepatic toxins. Idiosyncratic reactions due to the latter mechanism might be explained by the formation of an excess of toxic metabolites or normal amounts of abnormally toxic ones. For further reference the revies by DAVIS and WILLIAMS (1977), by SHERLOCK (1978) and by COHEN (1978) are recommended.

C. Allergy to Local Anaesthetics

Adverse reactions to local anaesthetics are commonly encountered in medical and dental practice, but allergy to these agents is said to be rare (ADRIANI and CAMPBELL 1956; ADRIANI 1960, 1972; DE SWARTE 1972). Most of the reactions seen are mild and transient, and further investigation is rarely needed. Among the more serious manifestations of allergy to those agents are circulatory collapse (anaphylactic shock), angioedema, local swelling occasionally leading to necrosis, widespread skin rash, asthma, fever, serum-sickness syndrome, vasculitis and contact dermatitis.

I. Structural Basis

A few words about the chemistry of local anaesthetics ought to be added, since this aspect has a bearing on the occurrence of allergic reactions to these agents. The review by BUCHI and PERLIA (1971) is recommended for further reference. All clinically useful local anaesthetics consist of three parts: 1) a hydrophilic amino group, either tertiary or secondary amine – examples of compounds with a tertiary amine are lignocaine (lidocaine) and procaine (Fig. 5) both with a diethylamino group; 2) a lipophilic aromatic residue (paraminobenzoic acid in procaine); and 3) an intermediate group (ethanol in procaine) connected to the lipophilic residue either by an ester (e. g., procaine) or amide linkage (e. g., lignocaine). The ester link is important because it is this bond that is hydrolysed by esterases during metabolic degradation in the body. Metabolites formed in this way seem to be capable of acting as haptenic groups. Thus, allergy seems to occur most frequently in response to local anaesthetics of the ester type. The allergy commonly extends (causing cross-reaction) to other substances which are chemically related to local anaesthetics, such as p-aminobenzoic acid (in preserved foods) and p-aminophenylenediamines (in hair dyes).

Knowledge of the chemistry of local anaesthetics also helps in finding possible substitutes, e.g., the replacement of an ester by an amide agent which neither cross-reacts, nor is likely to cause allergy by itself. Many other compounds have local anaesthetic properties, and may be thought of as potential alternatives, e. g., certain phenothiazine antihistamines and propranolol (the β-adrenoceptor blocker).

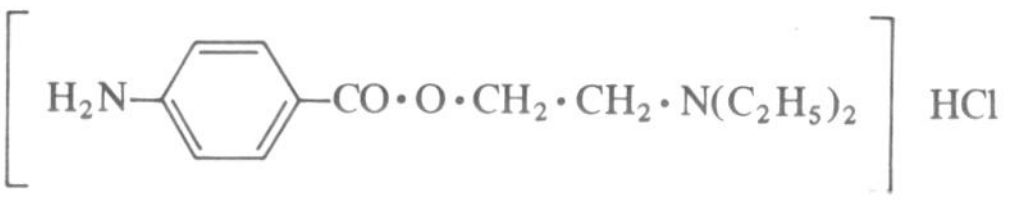

$$\left[\text{H}_2\text{N}-\langle\!\!\!\!\bigcirc\!\!\!\!\rangle-\text{CO}\cdot\text{O}\cdot\text{CH}_2\cdot\text{CH}_2\cdot\text{N}(\text{C}_2\text{H}_5)_2 \right] \text{HCl}$$

a

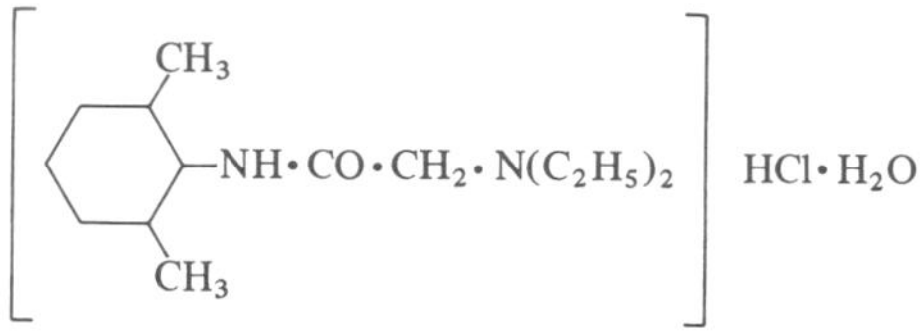

$$\mathbf{b}\quad\left[\begin{array}{c} \text{CH}_3 \\ \langle\!\!\!\!\bigcirc\!\!\!\!\rangle-\text{NH}\cdot\text{CO}\cdot\text{CH}_2\cdot\text{N}(\text{C}_2\text{H}_5)_2 \\ \text{CH}_3 \end{array} \right] \text{HCl}\cdot\text{H}_2\text{O}$$

Fig. 5. a Chemical structure of procaine hydrochloride, 2-diethylaminoethyl-4-aminobenzoate hydrochloride, an "ester" local anaesthetic. **b** Structure of lignocaine hydrochloride, *N*-diethylaminoacetyl-2,6-xylidine hydrochloride monohydrate, an "amide" local anaesthetic

However, these compounds are either irritant, or their side effects preclude their use.

II. Investigation of Reactions to Local Anaesthetics

1. Skin Tests

Skin tests are often useful. They are commonly carried out by intradermal injection, but prick, scratch and patch tests may be used (ALDRETE and JOHNSON 1969, 1970). INCAUDO et al. (1978) obtained positive results only in 5 (8%) of the 59 patients they reported. Furthermore, the information gained from the skin test results was of little value since some of these were "false positives." We had a similar experience in 18 patients with suspected acute reactions to local anaesthetics. Clearly positive results were obtained in only 2 patients, but further investigations carried out in those 18 patients cast further doubt on the validity of skin tests. These investigations are detailed in Chap. 6.

The ability of local anaesthetics to produce contact dermatitis is well known (Rothman et al. 1945; DE SWARTE 1972). Hence patch tests may be of relatively greater value than in other allergies. In fact, cross-sensitisation with *p*-aminobenzoate (used topically to prevent sunburn) was first reported in contact dermatitis studies (GAUL 1955).

In summary, the value of skin tests in suspected reactions to local anaesthetics is limited, and the situation is no different from that with the majority of drugs. Both false negatives and false positives account for their low predictive value.

2. Other In Vivo Tests

Alternative in vivo challenge tests have been proposed, such as the nasal (EYRE and NALLY 1971), and conjunctival tests, where local anaesthetics are applied locally to those mucous membranes. The subcutaneous injection of a test dose has been advocated by INCAUDO et al. (1978). We cannot see any of these tests as being either convincingly reliable or less risky than the conventional skin tests. The single case of fatal reaction to the instillation of one drop of a local anaesthetic into the con-

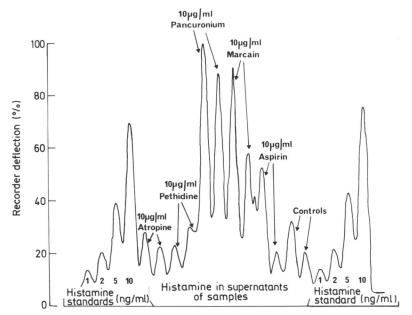

Fig. 6. Recording from spectrofluorometric assay of histamine released from the leucocytes of a patient with allergy to bupivacaine (Marcain) and pancuronium (a non-depolarising muscle relaxant)

junctival sac (ADRIANI 1972) is often quoted as a reminder of the potential risk of in vivo tests.

3. In Vitro Allergy Tests

a) Leucocyte Histamine Release Test

The leucocyte histamine release test (referred to in greater detail in Chaps. 1–7) is one of the in vitro correlates of immediate allergy which may find useful application in investigating reactions to local anaesthetics. It is of some value in detecting acute reactions, whether they are truly anaphylactic or due to direct (non-immune) histamine release (anaphylactoid). It is also more accurate (quantitative), more reliable and more predictive than skin tests, and above all it is free from risk.

We have used the leucocyte histamine release test in investigating 18 patients with suspected acute reactions to local anaesthetics. A positive result, as shown by a histamine release significantly higher with one or more of the various local anaesthetics than in the control samples, was obtained in 6 (i.e., one-third) patients (an example is shown in Fig. 6). The material used in the test consisted of a range of local anaesthetics, applied as such in different concentrations, i.e., not in any modified form. Though some of the metabolites of these agents are known, there is little information about the structure of the true allergens formed from those metabolites. Despite the proven though limited value of the leucocyte test in the diagnosis of these potentially serious reactions, the results were relatively disappointing in certain respects. Although significant histamine release could be induced, the percentage released was not high. It rarely exceeded 15% of the total leucocyte histamine content, and was rarely more than three times the histamine release in control samples (spontaneous histamine release).

The first conclusion to be drawn from those results was that much needs to be done concerning the testing material, since the histamine release was well below that obtained with the conventional allergens, such as pollen and house dust mite extracts. Secondly, the negative results in two-thirds of the patients could either be due to the poor test "allergens" used, or that the clinical diagnosis blaming the local anaesthetic for these reactions was incorrect.

As a follow-up of the latter point, four of the patients with negative leucocyte tests were re-admitted to hospital and re-exposed to the local anaesthetic (or anaesthetics) in question, under monitored observations, and taking adequate precautions. None of the four patients developed reactions under these circumstances.

Regarding the significance of histamine release from leucocytes, whether it represents a true anaphylactic reaction or direct (non-immune) histamine release as a result of an idiosyncrasy, there is no evidence to suggest that local anaesthetics may act as histamine releasers in the same way as muscle relaxants may do (this is discussed in Chap. 12). Although the latter possibility cannot be ruled out, all the indications suggest that even if that possibility proved true, it must be exceedingly rare. In none of the 18 patients we have investigated did we get a histamine release that was comparable in magnitude to that induced with muscle relaxants.

It is not totally inconceivable that in predisposed subjects, local anaesthetics may cause an anaphylactoid reaction via direct conversion of the third complement in the same way as may occur with certain anaesthetic induction agents (discussed elsewhere).

It has been suggested the local anaesthetics might have the opposite effect, namely inhibition of histamine release (Mongar and Schild 1957). This effect, if true, would to a certain extent cancel out an anaphylactic response to the drug. One of the relevant observations was that in some leucocyte experiments we noticed that histamine release was significantly lower in the presence of certain local anaesthetics, e. g., prilocaine, than in their absence (Tyrode solution was used in all experiments).

This apparent inhibitory effect which was occasionally demonstrated in spontaneous histamine release was not observed in the antigen-induced response (which was considerably higher and thus the comparison was difficult).

b) Other In Vitro Tests

In three of the patients with reactions to local anaesthetics in whom both the skin and the leucocyte histamine release tests were negative, it was thought that their reaction might have been due to an immune mechanism other than anaphylaxis. The lymphocyte transformation test was carried out in these three patients, but the results were negative.

Other authors have reported the value of the lymphocyte transformation test. Lehner (1971) reported positive results in four patients with suspected allergy to local anaesthetics, in whom the intradermal skin test was negative.

References

Adriani J (1960) The clinical pharmacology of local anaesthetics. Clin Pharmacol Ther 1:645–673

Adriani J (1972) Etiology and management of adverse reactions to local anaesthetics. Int Anesthesiol Clin 10:127–151

Adriani J, Campbell B (1956) Fatalities following topical application of local anaesthetics to mucous membranes. JAMA 162:1527–1530

Aldrete JA, Johnson DA (1969) Allergy to local anaesthetics. JAMA 207:356–357

Aldrete JA, Johnson DA (1970) Evaluation of intracutaneous testing for investigation of allergy to local anesthetic agents. Anesth Analg (Cleve) 49:173–183

Assem ESK (1977a) Examples of the correlation between the structure of certain groups of drugs and adverse effects mediated by immune and non-immune mechanisms (with particular reference to muscle relaxants and steroid anaesthetics). In: Bundgaard H, Juul P, Kofod H (eds) Drug design and adverse reactions. Copenhagan, Munksgaard, pp 209–226

Assem, ESK (1977b) Drug allergy. In: Davies DM (ed) Textbook of adverse drug reactions. Oxford University Press, Oxford, pp 380–396

Blake DA, Rozman RS, Cascorbi HF (1967) Biotransformation of fluroxene. I. Metabolism in mice and dogs in vivo. Biochem Pharmacol 16:1237–1248

Bruce DL, Raymon F (1972) Test for halothane sensitivity. N Engl J Med 286:1218–1219

Bruce DL, Wingard DW (1974) Anaesthesia and the immune response. Anesthesology 34:271–282

Buchi J, Perlia X (1971) Structure-activity relations and physicochemical properties of local anaesthetics. In: Le Chat P (ed) Local anaesthetics, vol 1. International encyclopedia of pharmacology and therapeutics, Sect 8. Pergamon, Oxford, pp 39–130

Carney FMF, Van Dyke RA (1972) Halothane hepatitis: a critical review. Anesth. Analg (Cleve) 51:135–160

Clarke RSJ (1974) The eugenols. In: Dundee JW, Wyant GM (eds) Intravenous anaesthesia. Churchill Livingstone, Edinburgh London, p 174

Clarke RSJ, Dundee JW, Garrett RT, McArdle GK, Sutton JA (1975) Adverse reactions to intravenous anaesthetics: a survey of 100 reports. Br J Anaesth 47:575–585

Clarke RSJ, Fee JH, Dundee JW (1978) Hypersensitivity reactions to intravenous anaesthetics. In: Watkins J, Ward A (eds) Adverse response to intravenous drugs. Academic Press, London, Grune & Stratton, New York, pp 41–47

Cluff LE, Johnson JE (1964) Drug fever. Prog Allergy 8:149

Cohen EN (1978) Toxicity of inhalation anaesthetic agents. Br J Anaesth 50:665–675

Cohen EN, Trudell JR (1972) Non-volatile metabolites of halothane. In: Fink PR (ed) Cellular biology and toxicity of anesthetics. Williams & Wilkins, Baltimore, pp 205–220

Committee on Safety of Medicines (1979) Current problems, No. 4

Davis M, Williams R (1977) Hepatic disorders. In: Davis DM (ed) Textbook of adverse drug reactions. Oxford University Press, Oxford, pp 146–172

De Swarte RD (1972) Drug allergy. In: Patterson R (ed) Allergic disease: diagnoses and management. Lippincott, Philadelphia, pp 393–494

Doniach D, Walker JG, Roitt IM, Berg PA (1970) "Autoallergic" hepatitis. N Engl J Med 282:86–88

Dundee JW, Clarke RSJ (1973) Idiosyncrasy to intravenous anaesthetics. Lancet 1:831

Dundee JW, Assem ESK, Gaston JM, Keilty SR, Sutton JA, Clarke RSJ, Grainger D (1974) Sensitivity to intravenous anaesthetics: a report of three cases. Br Med J 1:63–65

Dye D, Watkins J (1980) Suspected anaphylactic reaction to cremophor EL. Br Med J 2:1353–1354

Dykes MH, Gilbert J, McPeek B (1972) Halothane in the United States. Br J Anaesth 44:925–934

Editorial (1980) Editorial. The liver and halothane again. Br Med J 2:1197–1198

Evans JM, Keogh JAM (1977) Adverse reactions to intravenous induction agents. Br Med J 2:735–736

Eyre J, Nally FF (1971) Nasal test for hypersensitivity. Lancet 1:264–265

Gaul LE (1955) Cross-sensitization from para-amino-benzoate sunburn preventives. Anesthesiology 16:606–614

Incaudo G, Schatz M, Patterson R, Rosenberg M, Yamamoto F, Hamburger RN (1978) Administration of local anaesthetics to patients with a history of prior adverse reaction. J Allergy Clin Immunol 61:339–345

Inman WH (1978) Jaundice after repeated exposure to halothane: a further analysis of reports to the Committee on Safety of Medicines. Br Med J 2:1455–1456

Inman WHW, Mushin WW (1974) Jaundice after repeated exposure to halothane: an analysis of reports to the Committee on Safety of Medicines. Br Med J 1:5–10

Judson JA, De Jongh HJ, Walmsley JBW (1971) Possible cross-sensitivity between halothane and methoxyflurane: report of a case. Anesthesiology 35:527–532

Kessell J, Assem ESK (1974) Ad adverse reaction to althesin. Br J Anaesth 46:209

Klatskin G, Kimberg DV (1969) Recurrent hepatitis attributable to halothane sensitization in an anaesthetist. N Engl J Med 280:515–522

Lehner T (1971) Lignocaine hypersensitivity. Lancet 1:1245–1246

Lorenz W, Doenicke A (1978) Anaphylactoid reactions and histamine release by intravenous drugs used in surgery and anaesthesia. In: Watkins J, Ward AM (eds) Adverse response to intravenous drugs. Academic Press, London, Grune & Stratton New York, pp 83–112

Lorenz W, Doenicke A, Meyer R et al. (1972) Histamine release in man by propranidid and thiopentone: pharmacological effects and clinical consequences. Br J Anaesth 44:355–368

Mathieu A, Di Padua D, Mills J, Hahan B (1974) Experimental immunity for a metabolite of halothane and fluroxene. Anesthesiology 40:385–390

Mongar JL, Schild HO (1957) Inhibition of the anaphylactic reaction. J Physiol (Lond) 135:301–319

Moult PJA, Sherlock S (1975) Halothane-related hepatitis. A clinical study of 26 cases. Q J Med 44:99–114

National Halothane Study/NRC Report (1966) Summary of the national halothane study. Possible association between halothane anesthesia and postoperative hepatic necrosis. Report on the national halothane study of the Committee on Anesthesia, National Academy of Sciences – National Research Council. JAMA 197:775–788

Paronetto F, Popper H (1970) Lymphocyte stimulation induced by halothane in patients with hepatitis following exposure to halothane. N Engl J Med 283:277–280

Paton WDM (1957) Histamine release by compounds of simple chemical structure. Pharmacol Rev 9:269–328

Peters RL, Edmondson HA, Reynolds TB, Meister JC, Curphey TJ (1969) Hepatic necrosis associated with halothane anesthesia. Am J Med 47:748–764

Phillips GH (1974) Structure-activity relationship in steroidal anaesthetics. In: Halsy MJ, Millar RA, Sutton JA (eds) Molecular mechanisms in general anaesthesia. Churchill-Livingstone, Edinburgh London, pp 32–46

Price CD, Gibbs AR, Williams WJ (1977) Halothane macrophage migration inhibition factor test in halothane-associated hepatitis. J Clin Pathol 30:312–316

Reed WD, Williams R (1972) Halothane hepatitis as seen by the physician. Br J Anaesth 44:935–940

Richards CD, Hesketh TR (1975) Implications for theories of anaesthesia of antagonism between anaesthetic and non-anaesthetic steroids. Nature 256:179–182

Richter W, Messmer K, Hedin H, Ring J (1978) Adverse reactions to plasma substitutes: incidence and pathogenesis. In: Watkins J, Ward AM (eds) Adverse response to intravenous drugs. Academic Press, London, Grune & Stratton, New York, pp 49–70

Rothman S, Orland FJ, Flesch P (1945) Group specificity of epidermal allergy to procaine in man. J Invest Dermatol 6:191–199

Seyle H (1941) Anaesthetic effect of steroid hormones. Proc Soc exp Biol Med 46:116–121

Sherlock S (1978) Halothane hepatitis. Lancet 2:364–365

Simpson BR, Strunin L (1973) Halothane hepatitis – fact or fallacy? Proc R Soc Med 66:56–63

Simpson BR, Strunin L, Walton B (1971) The halothane dilemma: a case for the defence. Br Med J 4:96–100

Smith MGM, Golding PL, Eddleston ALWF, Mitchell CG, Kemp A, Williams R (1972) Cell-mediated immune responses in chronic liver diseases. Br Med J 1:527–530

Stier A (1968) The biotransformation of halothane. Anesthesiology 29:388–390

Sutton JA (1972) A brief history of steroid anaesthesia before althesin (CT 1341). Postgrad Med J [Suppl 2] 48:9–12

Trowell J, Peto R, Crampton Smith A (1975) Controlled trial of repeated halothane anaesthetics in patients with carcinoma of the cervix treated with radium. Lancet 1:821–824

Vergani D, Tsantoulas D, Eddleston ALWF, Davis M, Williams R (1978) Sensitization to halothane-altered liver components in severe hepatic necrosis after halothane anaesthesia. Lancet 2:801–803

Watkins J (1979) Anaphylactoid reactions to intravenous substances. Br J Anaesth 51:51–60

Watkins J, Padfield A, Alderson JD (1978) Underlying immunopathology as a cause of adverse responses to two intravenous agents. Br Med J 1:1180–1181

Whitwam JG (1978) Adverse reactions to i. v. induction agents. Br J Anaesth 50:677–687

Williams R, Davis M, Waldram R (1975) Postoperative jaundice. In: Lant T (ed) Eleventh symposium on advanced medicine. Pitman, London, p 45

Williams BD, White N, Amlot PL, Slaney J, Toseland PA (1977) Circulating immune complexes after repeated halothane anaesthesia. Br Med J 2:159–162

Wright R Eade OE, Chisholm M et al. (1975) Controlled prospective study of the effect on liver function of multiple exposures to halothane. Lancet 1:817–820

CHAPTER 11

Analgesics and Nonsteroidal Anti-Inflammatory Drugs

A. Szczeklik

A. Classification and Mode of Action of Analgesics and Nonsteroidal Anti-Inflammatory Drugs

The scarcity and high price of quinine during the last third of the nineteenth century motivated the search for synthetic antipyretics. As a result, a large number of compounds were introduced into medicine which share with cinchona the ability to produce antipyretic, analgesic, and anti-inflammatory effects (Woodbury and Fingl 1979). Of these, aspirin has become the most widely used drug in the world. Recently, there have been main reasons for the research in this area. First, the recognition of the value and the limitations of the adrenocorticosteroids for long-term therapy of inflammatory disorders. Second, the new possibilities of employing aspirin-like drugs in prevention and therapy of thromboembolic diseases.

Analgesics and anti-inflammatory drugs form a heterogeneous group which cannot be systematically classified (Miller et al. 1978). On the basis of their chemical structure, however, they can be divided into the following classes (Woodbury and Fingl 1979; Shen 1979):

1. Aspirin and the salicylates
2. Indomethacin and congeners
3. *p*-Aminophenol derivatives (paracetamol, phenacetin)
4. Pyrazolone derivatives (antipyrine, amidopyrine, noramidopyrine, phenylbutazone, oxyphenbutazone)
5. Fenamates (mefenamic acid, flufenamic acid, meclofenamic acid)
6. Substituted aryl aliphatic acids (ibuprofen, fenoprofen, ketoprofen, naproxen, diclofenac)
7. Non-acidic agents (ditazol, flumizole)
8. Other agents.

Many hypotheses have been put forward to explain the mechanism of action and therapeutic effects of nonsteroidal anti-inflammatory drugs (NSAID). In the case of salicylates, uncoupling of oxidative phosphorylation, interaction with plasma and tissue proteine, stabilization of lysosomal enzymes, and inhibition of phagocytosis are among the concepts that have been discussed (for references see Woodbury and Fingl 1979; Miller et al. 1978). It is now generally believed that the anti-inflammatory and several other effects of aspirin and related drugs are due to inhibition of prostaglandin biosynthesis.

Vane (1971), Smith and Willis (1971), and Ferreira et al. (1971) discovered that aspirin and indomethacin inhibit prostaglandin biosynthesis in lung homogenates, in platelets, and in perfused spleen. Nonsteroidal anti-inflammatory drugs

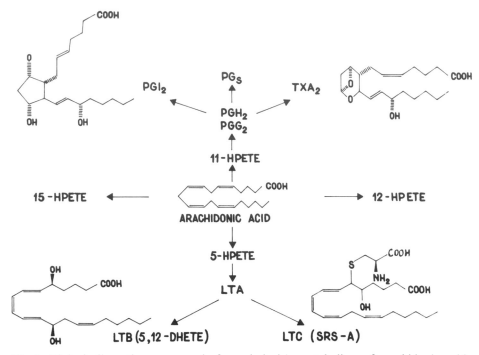

Fig. 1. Biologically active compounds formed during metabolism of arachidonic acid. Cyclooxygenation of the acid leads to formation of unstable PGG_2 and PGH_2. This step is blocked by aspirin, indomethacin, and other cyclooxygenase inhibitors. PGH_2, depending on the tissue and cofactors, is transformed into prostaglandins (PG_s), thromboxane A_2 (TXA_2), and prostacyclin (PGI_2). Other metabolic routes are controlled by specific lipoxygenases. Lipoxygenation results in formation of 12- or 15-hydroperoxy fatty acids (HPETE) which are rapidly converted into hydroxy acids (HETE). Another lipoxygenase converts arachidonic acid into leukotrienes LTA, LTB (5, 12-dihydroxyeicosotetraenoic acid, 5, 12-DHETE), and LTC (slowly reacting substance of anaphylaxis, SRS-A)

inhibit the first step of arachidonic acid transformation by the microsomal multi-enzyme system (fatty acid cyclooxygenase; FLOWER 1974), which eventually leads to formation of prostaglandins, thromboxane A_2, or prostacyclin (Fig. 1). Thus, aspirin-like drugs are cyclooxygenase inhibitors, i.e., they inhibit the conversion of arachidonic acid to an unstable endoperoxide, PGG_2. In contrast, glucocorticosteroids do not interfere with cyclooxygenase activity, but inhibit the liberation of arachidonic acid from its stores (GRYGLEWSKI et al. 1975 a; GRYGLEWSKI 1976). This action of glucocorticosteroids is mediated through the induction of intracellular biosynthesis of a phospholipase A_2 inhibitor (FLOWER and BLACKWELL 1979).

The inhibition of cyclooxygenase by NSAID occurs at concentrations (0.01–10 µg/ml) comparable to their therapeutic levels. On the contrary, much higher concentrations of these drugs are required to regulate other processes which might underly their anti-inflammatory effect, such as uncoupling of oxidative phosphorylation or inhibition of leukocyte phagocytosis. A remarkable parallelism has been

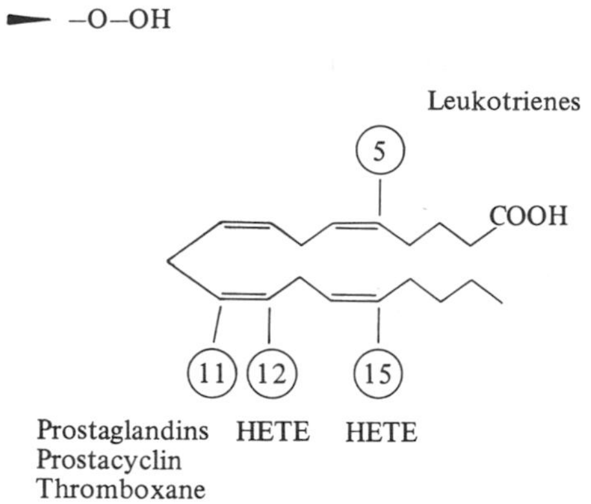

$\longmapsto$ –O–OH

Fig. 2. Oxygenation of arachidonic acid at various sites by specific enzymes (C-5, C-11, C-12, or C-15 in the molecule) leads to different compounds with potent biologic activities

observed between the structure–activity relationships for in vivo anti-inflammatory actions and in vitro cyclooxygenase inhibition for several series of NSAID (SHEN 1979). This parallelism can be further improved by taking into account binding of NSAID to the proteins, thus providing a rational approach to predicting the anti-inflammatory activity of new compounds (GRYGLEWSKI 1979).

Aspirin-like drugs, by blocking cyclooxygenase, deprive human tissues of several compounds with potent biologic activities. Of these, prostaglandins – which act predominantly locally, at the site of their synthesis – are known to modulate inflammatory reactions (VANE 1976). They are also produced in the respiratory tract and exert opposite effects there (OREHEK et al. 1975; GRYGLEWSKI et al. 1976). Prostaglandins of the E series are potent bronchodilators, while that of the F series constrict the bronchi. Thromboxane A_2, a powerful aggregator of thrombocytes, is also a bronchoconstrictor. In contrast to it, prostacyclin – a hormone produced by the arteries and released into the blood – has anti-aggregatory and vasodilating properties, but is deprived of any significant bronchial effects in healthy subjects and patients with bronchial asthma (SZCZEKLIK et al. 1978 b).

Arachidonic acid can be metabolized not only via cyclooxygenase but also via specific lipoxygenases (Fig. 2). These latter metabolic transformations lead eventually to formation of such biologically active compounds as slowly reacting substance of anaphylaxis (SRS-A or leukotriene C; BORGEAT and SAMUELSSON 1979), and hydroperoxyelicosotetraenoic acid (HETE) which appears to be chemotactic for human leukocytes. Until recently it was believed that aspirin-like drugs do not interfere with the metabolism of arachidonate via lipoxygenase pathways. However, SIEGEL et al. (1979) demonstrated that aspirin, indomethacin, and sodium salicylate block activity of a specific peroxidase which generates HETE from its precursor, a hydroperoxy acid (HPETE, 12-hydroperoxy-5,8,10,14-eicosotetraenoic acid). As the functions of HPETE and HETE become clarified in normal and pathologic processes, it may be possible to achieve a better understanding of the biochemical basis and the relative importance of these substances and the prostaglandins in the anti-inflammatory, analgesic, antipyretic, and other actions of the aspirin-like drugs.

Many NSAID may well have different or multiple mechanisms of action to inhibit the dynamic and complex inflammatory process in vivo. Fenamates have shown both cyclooxygenase inhibition and prostaglandin antagonism (Panczenko et al. 1975). Others may interfere with prostaglandin metabolism through actions on prostaglandin metabolitic enzymes, cyclonucleotide pathways, etc. Still others may exert their anti-arthritic action primarily by immunologic mechanisms which are partially or indirectly regulated by prostaglandins (Shen 1979).

B. Prevalence of Adverse Drug Reactions

The first idiosyncratic reactions to aspirin were recognized soon after its introduction into medicine, and a recent large survey (Irey 1976) listed aspirin among ten drugs most frequently involved in adverse reactions. The majority of healthy people, however, tolerate aspirin and related anti-inflammatory drugs quite well. In some common diseases (e. g., asthma, urticaria) intolerance to aspirin-like drugs is high (see Sects. C. II, IV) and constitutes a major clinical problem. But even in relatively rare types of NSAID intolerance (e. g., blood dyscrasias), the study of mechanisms involved has helped in better understanding of the ways pathologic processes run in humans.

C. Clinical Manifestations of Adverse Reactions

I. Systemic Anaphylaxis

This reaction, characterized by the appearance of a generalized flush, palpitations, weakness, dizziness, tingling of the extremities, urticaria, angioedema, and apprehension appears whithin a few minutes after administration of the drug. If not treated, the reaction may progress to respiratory distress, shock, seizures, cyanosis, coma, and death. Of the drugs discussed in this chapter, those belonging to the pyrazolone group are by far the most common cause of anaphylaxis (see Sect. C. IV. 2). Hypersensitive reactions to analgesics in patients with lupus erythematosus as well as strong reactions to aspirin-like drugs in patients with aspirin-induced asthma may also present themselves under the clinical pictures of anaphylactic shock.

II. Aspirin-Induced Asthma

1. Definition

In some patients with asthma, aspirin and several other NSAID precipitate asthmatic attacks. This is a distinct clinical syndrome. It is called aspirin-induced asthma (AIA).

2. Prevalence

Varying figures for the incidence of AIA in adults have been reported, depending on the methods used. When oral challenge studies coupled with spirometry were performed the frequency of AIA among asthmatics was 8% (McDonald et al.

1972), 12% (Harnett et al. 1978), 16% (Van Leeuven 1928), and about 25% (Stenius and Lemola 1976). Other surveys relying only on history have reported lower prevalence, e. g., 4% (Chafee and Settipane 1974). Challenge tests provide more realistic results than do methods that rely on history alone, the latter being subject to the whims of memory and communicative skills. Nevertheless, even with challenge tests, the incidence is affected by the criteria selected for the definition of the phenomenon under the study. When one study (Stenius and Lemola 1976) defined positive results as a fall in peak expiratory flow of more than 20%, a high incidence of about 25% resulted. Another study (McDonald et al. 1972) requiring a 50% decrease of forced expiratory volume in 1s (FEV_1) found only an 8% incidence.

It is generally assumed that AIA is very uncommon in children. Two recent studies, however, using oral challenge tests reported the frequency of AIA as 28% (Rachelefsky et al. 1975) and 13% (Vedenthan et al. 1977). In contrast, none of 32 children with asthma, studied by Schuhl and Pereyra (1979) developed bronchoconstriction following aspirin ingestion. These inconsistent results could be explained by differences in the populations studied. Children challenged by Schuhl and Pereyra (1979) were younger and had much higher incidence of atopy than those studied by Vedenthan et al. (1977)

Aspirin intolerance has been described in a few families (Starr 1971; Lockey et al. 1973; Von Maur et al. 1974; Delaney 1973). A family aggregation, however, appears to be very rare (Falliers 1974). In our population of 500 patients with proven AIA, we found only two cases of familial intolerance to aspirin. One was a 19-year-old male, whose only brother, also asthmatic, as known to have died after taking aspirin. The other was a 21-year-old asthmatic female, whose father had never suffered from asthma but gave a history of angioedema and urticaria without dyspnea following aspirin ingestion; this was confirmed in a challenge test.

3. Pathogenesis

Allergic mechanisms of AIA have been excluded by numerous and extensive immunologic studies (for references see Schlumberger et al. 1974). Furthermore, in aspirin-sensitive patients asthmatic attacks may be precipitated by several other analgesics with various chemical structures which make immunologic cross-reactivity most unlikely. Nonimmunologic concepts which still remain to be proved are: injury of kinin receptors by preexisting disease which results in a paradoxical stimulation of the receptor sites by aspirin (Samter and Beers 1968), activation of the complement system by aspirin (Yurchak et al. 1970), slowly progressing acetylation of body proteins by aspirin (Farr 1971), and α/β-adrenergic imbalance (Fisherman and Cohen 1974). These and other concepts have recently been thoroughly and critically reviewed by Harnett et al. (1978).

We put forward a hypothesis that, in the sensitive patients, induction of the asthmatic attacks by aspirin-like drugs is due to inhibition of prostaglandin biosynthesis in their tissues (Szczeklik et al. 1974, 1975a). The evidence that has been accumulated in favor of this hypothesis can be briefly summarized as follows:

a) Only cyclooxygenase inhibitors, i. e., analgesics which suppress the generation of prostaglandins, thromboxane A_2, and prostacyclin in vitro, induce bronchoconstriction in the sensitive patients. This statement is based on an oral challenge test in which 21 different NSAID were administered to 190 patients with AIA (SZCZEKLIK et al. 1977a; SERWOŃSKA 1979).

b) There is a good correlation between the ability of the drugs to induce bronchoconstriction in the sensitive patients and their inhibitory potency toward cyclooxygenase in vitro (SZCZEKLIK et al. 1977a).

c) Each aspirin-sensitive patient is characterized by an individual pattern of sensitivity. Thus, the degree of enzymic inhibition which is sufficient to precipitate bronchoconstriction is an individual hallmark of each patient (SZCZEKLIK et al. 1976).

d) The enzymic system generating prostaglandins of the E series (PGE) in nasal polyps of aspirin-sensitive patients has an increased sensitivity to the inhibitory action of aspirin (SZCZEKLIK et al. 1977c)

Blockade of cyclooxygenase by aspirin-like drugs in the sensitive patients can lead to adverse reactions through at least two simultaneously operating mechanisms (SZCZEKLIK et al. 1980). First, bronchi become deprived of bronchodilatory PGE and this, in turn, promotes the release of histamine. Indeed, PGE are not only bronchodilators, but stabilize histamine stores in mastocytes (WHITTLE 1977; OKAZAKI et al. 1977). In aspirin-sensitive asthmatics, aspirin challenge results in significant rise of plasma histamine (STEVENSON et al. 1976). Furthermore, aspirin-induced bronchoconstriction can be diminished or even prevented by drugs which either stabilize the mast cell membranes (BASOMBA et al. 1976; DELANEY 1976; MARTELLI and USANDIVARAS 1977) or block the H_1-receptor of histamine (SZCZEKLIK and SERWOŃSKA 1979). Second, inhibition of cyclooxygenase might lead to diversion of the arachidonic acid metabolism toward lipoxygenase products, which in turn augment (ADCOCK et al. 1978; BURKA and FLOWER 1979) the release of histamine and anaphylactic mediators. It is along these lipoxygenase pathways that novel compounds with conjugated trienes are formed, one of them being SRS-A (BORGEAT and SAMUELSSON 1979; SAMUELSSON 1979).

But why do cyclooxygenase inhibitors induce bronchoconstriction through these mechanisms only in one group of patients with asthma, and not in all asthmatics? we do not know. One explanation could be that aspirin-sensitive patients differ from other asthmatics as well as from healthy subjects by relying more on the PGE defensive mechanism than on the β-adrenergic one (SZCZEKLIK et al. 1975a; SZCZEKLIK and CZERNIAWSKA-MYSIK 1976). Another explanation is that the sensitivity of cyclooxygenase to aspirin in the bronchi of patients with AIA become partly enhanced by a specific, but unknown infectious agent (GRYGLEWSKI et al. 1977). The possibility that in certain asthmatics an abnormal mechanism exists whereby aspirin might selectively block the release of bronchodilator PEG_2 without also blocking the release of bronchoconstrictor $PFG_{2\alpha}$ (SETTIPANE et al. 1974) seems unlikely in view of recent studies (PATRONO et al. 1978).

4. Clinical Symptoms and Laboratory Findings

The sequence of symptoms and the natural history of AIA are so characteristic that a typical or "classic" case has been constructed based on a large number of clinical observations (SAMTER and BEERS 1968). Childhood and adolescence of the aspirin-intolerant patient are not distinguished by any unique characteristics. Beginning with the third or fourth decade of life, however, the typical patient (women outnumber men three to two) starts to experience intense vasomotor rhinitis. Over a period of months, chronic nasal congestion appears and physical examination reveals nasal polyps. Bronchial asthma and intolerance to aspirin develop during subsequent stages of the illness. The intolerance presents itself as a unique picture: within minutes to hours following ingestion of aspirin acute asthmatic attacks develop, often accompanied by rhinorrhea, conjunctival irritation, and flushes of the head and neck. Since many patients have taken aspirin in the past with impunity, the initial reaction is usually unexpected and, in fact, quite often not attributed to the drug. These reactions are dangerous, indeed; in a highly sensitive patient shock may develop, leading rapidly to death after ingestion of only one aspirin (300 mg).

In some patients suffering from AIA, repeated attacks of syncope occur, the incidence of which is not always easy to trace to ingestion of a drug (GIRALDO et al. 1969; KAUFMAN 1977). It has been said that loss of consciousness during an attack of asthma should always be considered highly suggestive of an "allergic" reaction to aspirin (MATTHEWS et al. 1950). In children, the classic triad of bronchial asthma, aspirin sensitivity, and nasal polyposis, described in adults, is absent (VEDENTHAN et al. 1977). Children with AIA also very rarely suffer from tartrazine sensitivity (RACHELEFSKY et al. 1975).

Tartrazine, a yellow azo dye (F. D. and C. No. 5) widely employed for coloring foods, drinks, drugs, and cosmetics, induces in some aspirin-sensitive subjects a bronchoconstriction similar to that caused by aspirin and other cyclooxygenase inhibitors. High concentrations of tartrazine are present particularly in confectionery, but significant amounts are also found in soft drinks, cakes and pastries, ice cream, preservatives, and mayonnaise (ROSENHALL 1977). Ingestion of colored food and drinks as well as colored tablets or capsules are the most common initiating causes of untoward reactions (LOCKEY 1977), but even a standard enema preparation containing a tartrazine additive may lead to bronchoconstriction and shock (TRAUTLEIN and MANN 1978). The content of tartrazine in one tablet may vary from 0.02 to 2.7 mg (SMITH and SLAVIN 1976). Tartrazine is a stable dye and is used in producing not only a bright yellow color, but also many other colors such as maroon, rust, and turquoise. It has been reported that about one-half of the patients with positive aspirin challenge tests also gave a positive tartrazine test as judged by fall in spirometric values (STENIUS and LEMOLA 1976). SAMTER and BEERS (1968), however, noticed that only 14 of 182 patients intolerant to aspirin also gave an adverse reaction to tartrazine. In a study in collaboration with S. BIANCO, P. KAMBUROFF and M. SERWOŃSKA (unpublished), including patients from Italy, Poland, and Switzerland, we found tartrazine intolerance to be rare among patients with AIA, affecting less than 10% of these patients. In contrast to aspirin-like drugs, tartrazine does not inhibit cyclooxygenase activity in sheep seminal vesicles, guinea pig lung microsomes, and human platelets (GERBER et al. 1979). Very high concentrations of tartrazine are necessary to interfere with production of prostaglandins and thromboxanes in guinea pig lungs perfused with arachidonic acid (CESERANI et al. 1978). The major metabolite of tartrazine, sulfanilic acid, has no inhibitory effect on sheep seminal vesicle cyclooxygenase (GERBER et al. 1979). It appears, therefore, that a cross-sensitivity between tartrazine and aspirin, observed sporadically in aspirin-sensitive asthmatics, is unlikely to be the basis of prostaglandin inhibition.

In AIA, skin tests with common acroollergens are usually negative, and other signs of atopy are rarely present (SAMTER and BEERS 1968). The blood eosinophil count is elevated, while both serum complement components and IgE are within normal limits (DELANEY and KAY 1976). Bronchial hyper-reactivity is characterized by vivid response to low doses of inhaled histamine, relatively good tolerance of $PGF_{2\alpha}$ (although variations among patients are great), and good response to PGE_2 (SZCZEKLIK et al. 1977 d). In contrast to FISHERMAN and COHEN (1974), we were unable to detect any changes in template bleeding time following ingestion of 40 mg aspirin in 21 patients with AIA as compared with 17 normal subjects (SZCZEKLIK et al. 1975 b). Our results are in agreement with both the clinical picture of AIA in which hemorrhagic symptoms are absent, as well as with recent findings of PATRONO et al. (1978) of unaltered susceptibility of platelet cyclooxygenase to inhibition by aspirin in vitro.

5. Diagnosis

The definitive diagnosis of aspirin hypersensitivity can be made only with oral challenge tests. These tests consist of spirometric measurements every 30 min over a period of 4 h coupled with clinical observation over the same period of time following ingestion of aspirin. The tests are begun with the smallest dose of aspirin. In our department, this is usually 20 mg. If no response occurs, the doses are gradually increased (40, 50, 100, and 300 mg) at the next challenges until the reaction becomes positive or a dose equivalent to that in 1–2 tablets is reached. In assessment of the bronchopulmonary effects of the drugs studies, a decrease in peak expiratory flow (PEF) of 16%–25% is considered positive, if accompanied by clinical symptoms of bronchial obstruction and by appearance of either rhinorrhea or lacrimation. In the absence of these symptoms, the reaction is considered only positive if fall in PEF of more than 25% is obtained. Questionable responses are unusual, but if present, they may require double-blind and randomized re-challenge with placebo. In the great majority of 500 patients with AIA tested according to this protocol in our department, the threshold dose of aspirin inducing a positive response was between 40 and 80 mg.

Uncomfortable symptoms are relieved by β_2-adrenoceptor stimulants, aminophylline, or antihistaminics. In a few patients, 50–100 mg hydrocortisone may be administered intravenously. Most patients recover from acute reaction within 2 h, but in the case of a strong reaction, a general feeling of malaise and excessive bronchial secretion might persist for a day or two.

An interesting modification of the challenge tests was developed by BIANCO and his colleagues (BIANCO et al. 1977; PASARGIKLIAN et al. 1977). In this method, instead of giving aspirin by mouth, an aerosol of lysine acetylsalicylate is administered by inhalation.

In testing for tartrazine hypersensitivity, a solution of the dye in distilled water is swallowed by the patient, followed by a close clinical observation coupled with spirometry over a period of 2–3 h. We begin testing with 0.1 mg tartrazine, the next doses being 1.0, 5.0, 10.0, 25.0, and 100.0 mg, but doses of 10 mg or less are probably sufficient.

6. Prevention and Therapy

Patients with AIA should avoid aspirin and all products containing it. The number of such products is high; over 200 of them are currently on the United States market (LEIST and BANWELL 1974). Other drugs which are absolutely contraindicated in patients with AIA, because they precipitate bronchoconstriction, and lead to life-threatening attacks (SZCZEKLIK et al. 1975 a, 1976, 1977 a, b; SERWOŃSKA 1979; SLAPKE and JÄGER 1979; VIRCHOW 1976) are as follows: indomethacin, mefenamate, flufenamate, meclofenamate, ibuprofen, fenoprofen, ketoprofen, naproxen, diclofenac, amidopyrine, noramidopyrine, phenylbutazone, flumisole, and ditazole. If necessary, patients with AIA can safely take Salicylamide, dextropropoxyphene, benzydamine, and chloroquine, even for prolonged periods (SZCZEKLIK et al. 1975 a, 1977 c; NIŻANKOWSKA and SZCZEKLIK 1979). Paracetamol can also be taken with impunity by majority of patients with AIA. It is, however, safer first to give half a tablet and observe for 2–3 h for symptoms of adverse reaction. We found such symptoms in 4 of 79 patients with AIA who were challenged with paracetamol. Similarly, phenacetin (which is metabolized in the human body to paracetamol) precipitated bronchoconstriction in 1 of 21 patients with AIA (SERWOŃSKA 1979).

When an oral challenge to tartrazine is positive, this yellow food color should be eliminated from the diet and medications containing tartrazine (SMITH and SLAVIN 1976) should be avoided.

Unfortunately, avoidance of aspirin-like drugs does not stop the disease which runs a chronic course. There is no specific therapy for this type of asthma. Disodium cromoglycate may be of help for some patients (GWIN et al. 1977; SZCZEKLIK et al. 1977 a), and we feel its therapeutic trial for 2–3 weeks is warranted in every patient with AIA. The value of a new oral cromolyn-like compound, ketotifen, which prevents aspirin-induced attacks (SZCZEKLIK et al. 1980; WUETHRICH 1979) is still unknown in the long-term therapy of this type of asthma. A substantial part of patients with AIA need corticotherapy to control their disease.

Polyposis tends to occur in both nostrils. The histologic appearance of nasal polyps of aspirin-intolerant patients is indistinguishable from nasal polyps of patients who tolerate aspirin (SAMTER 1973; MOLANEY 1977). Polypectomy does not usually control the tendency of polyps to recur, and asthma may develop with or without polypectomy.

III. Asthma Relieved by Aspirin

A few patients with bronchial asthma report that aspirin decreases their shortness of breath. Although clinicians were well aware of this phenomenon, it was only in 1978 that the first reports appeared (KORDANSKY et al. 1978; SZCZEKLIK et al. 1978 a) describing two such patients in whom not only aspirin but several other analgesics produced striking relief of airway obstruction as evidenced by spirometry and plethysmographic studies. Together with EVA NIŻANKOWSKA we have, so far, studied five such patients, aged 21–62 years. In all of them, airway obstruction was markedly reduced by aspirin and other cyclooxygenase inhibitors, i. e., indomethacin, mefenamate, and fenoprofen, but not by salicylamide and benzydamine, which do not inhibit prostaglandin biosynthesis. It is, therefore, logical to assume (SZCZEKLIK et al. 1979 a) that the pharmacologic removal of a product of arachidonic acid cyclooxygenation from the respiratory tract helped these patients to overcome their airways obstruction. Perhaps, this product was a bronchoconstrictor $PGF_{2\alpha}$, thromboxane A_2 (TXA_2), or other as yet unknown metabolite.

The number of asthmatic patients who might benefit from aspirin is not known exactly, but probably does not exceed 1% of adult asthmatics. Therapeutic trial of NSAID might seem warranted in asthma, since it could allow the steroid dose to be reduced (HUME and EDDEY 1977). Great care, however, would be necessary at the beginning of such treatment, and the initial dose of aspirin should not exceed 20–40 mg, as the same cyclooxygenase inhibitors which are so efficient in relieving bronchoconstriction in some patients, may produce bronchoconstriction in other asthmatics suffering from so-called aspirin-induced asthma.

IV. Urticaria and Angioedema

1. Intolerance to Aspirin

A few individuals react to aspirin by developing urticarial wheals and giant swellings. However, many patients with chronic urticaria from various causes develop an obvious increase in the wheals and swellings after taking aspirin. These two groups can be separated, since in the latter one dose of aspirin causes exacerbation of urticaria only while the chronic urticaria is active but does not induce any eruptions in symptomless period (WARIN 1960; MICHAËLSSON 1969). It appears that 20%–40% of patients with chronic urticaria have exacerbation of urticaria on ingesting aspirin (WARIN and SMITH 1976). A high level of salicylate in the blood of patients with chronic urticaria has been found (NOID et al. 1974). MOORE-ROBINSON and WARIN (1967) reported that 22% of patients with chronic urticaria developed a marked increase in urticaria after administration of sodium salicylate. These investigators also reported that both aspirin and sodium salicylate enhanced skin reactivity to histamine. Thus sodium salicylate derived from the parent aspirin molecule can lower the threshold of histamine-induced urticaria by different means.

It seems clear that all patients with urticaria should avoid taking aspirin in any form (KAPLAN 1978). Care should be taken also to exclude from the diet food and drug additives and colorants (e. g., benzoates, or tartrazine) to which some patients are intolerant (JUHLIN et al. 1972). Recent surveys report intolerance to tartrazine (a yellow dye widely used with foods, drinks, and drugs) as amounting to 8% (SETTIPANE et al. 1976) and 13% (DRY et al. 1979) among patients with chronic urticaria. A simple diet free of aspirin and food and drug additives leads to rapid improvement in a substantial number of patients with chronic urticaria (RUDZKI 1977).

There is a subgroup of patients who can be clearly distinguished from all the others who link their cutaneous reactions to aspirin ingestion. In this subgroup, inhibition of prostaglandin synthesis appears to play the important role in pathogenesis of the disease (SZCZEKLIK et al. 1977a; SZCZEKLIK 1980). We call this type B hypersensitivity to prostaglandin inhibitors as opposed to type A (aspirin-induced asthma). The same aspirin-like drugs that induce bronchoconstriction in type A patients (see Sect. C. II. 4) also produce angioedema associated with urticaria or rhinitis in type B patients. All the drugs causing positive reactions in both groups A and B are inhibitors of prostaglandin biosynthesis (owing to blockade of cyclooxygenase), indomethacin being the most powerful of them in this respect. It is, therefore, not surprising that of several different drugs studied by DOEGLAS (1957), indomethacin most frequently induced cutaneous reactions in patients with urticaria and hypersensitivity. A few patients have been described recently in whom both ingestion of aspirin and indomethacin led to urticaria (MATTHEWS and STAGE 1974; GRYGLEWSKI et al. 1975b).

We have studied 17 patients with type B hypersensitivity to prostaglandin inhibitors. They all had positive reactions to aspirin. Similar reactions could also be elicited by other prostaglandin inhibitors, e. g., indomethacin, fenoprofen, ibuprofen, and noramidopyrine, but not by drugs deprived of cyclooxygenase inhibitory properties, e. g., benzydamine, dextro-propoxyphene, paracetamol, or placebo (SZCZEKLIK et al. 1977a). In 12 patients, these reactions consisted of urticaria and angioedema, the latter being usually limited to the face. In 5 others, angioedema, rhinorrhea, and conjunctival injection without urticaria developed. There was a clear relationship between the dose of the drug used and the appearance and intensity of the reaction elicited. Pretreatment of one of the patients with ketotifen, a new cromolyn-like orally active drug, prevented the appearance of aspirin-induced urticaria and angioedema.

Impurities contaminating commercial aspirin preparations could be responsible for appearance of urticaria and angioedema in some patients (DE WECK 1971; BUNDGAARD and DE WECK 1975). These contaminants include acetylsalicylic anhydride, acetylsalicylic salicylic acid and cis-disalicylide. A rapid and convenient colorimetric method has been described recently for the quantitative determination of these immunogenic impurities in aspirin (BUNDGAARD 1976).

Aspirin anhydride is an extremely reactive compound prone to produce salicyloyl and aspiryl conjugates in vitro, and to induce the formation of anti-aspiryl antibodies and of contact hypersensitivity in guinea pigs and rabbits. DE WECK (1971) found antibodies directed toward these conjugates in both normal subjects and persons with aspirin-induced urticarial reactions. He has also shown that some patients with repeated urticarial reactions after ingestion of aspirin possess a high degree of skin hypersensitivity of aspiryl specificity. These well-documented studies point, therefore, to an immunologic basis of aspirin hypersensitivity in one subgroup of patients with cutaneous reactions. Impurities present in some commercial preparations of aspirin but not in others could explain why certain patients who give a clear history of aspirin-induced urticaria and angioedema show no reaction when re-challenged with aspirin (SZCZEKLIK et al. 1977a).

2. Hypersensitivity to Pyrazolone Drugs

There is a group of patients who are hypersensitive to pyrazolone analgesics, but not to the aspirin-like drugs (SZCZEKLIK et al. 1977a). These patients, more often

Table 1. Two different clinical syndromes of urticaria and/or angioedema induced by analgesics of the pyrazolone group

Characteristic features	Type B intolerance to prostaglandin inhibitors (17 patients)	Selective hypersensitivity to pyrazolone analgesics (28 patients)
Mean age (years)	41	37
Males/females	5/12	4/24
Family history of atopy	2	
Positive skin tests with common aeroallergens	1	10
Serum IgE	Normal	Often elevated
Administration of noramidopyrine	Leads to urticaria and/or angioedema	Leads to anaphylactic shock or urticaria and/or angioedema
Administration of aspirin, indomethacin, and fenamates	Leads to urticaria and/or angioedema	Causes no adverse reactions

than those with hypersensitivity to prostaglandin inhibitors, have a family history of allergic dieseases and give positive skin tests to common allergens. Their serum IgE levels are also often elevated. The untoward reactions to pyrazolone analgesics can be highly dangerous. Of 28 such patients studied by us (Czerniawska-Mysik and Szczeklik 1980), 22 developed anaphylactic shock after taking a single dose of aminophenazone of noramidopyrine, while in the remaining 6 urticaria and/or angioedema occurred. Scratch tests and/or intracutaneous tests performed with aminophenazone or noramidopyrine 2–12 months after the acute reaction were positive in all the patients. On the other hand, oral challenge tests with therapeutic doses of aspirin, indomethacin, fenamates, and paracetamol were all negative.

These clinical features permit us to distinguish clearly patients with selective hypersensitivity to pyrazolone drugs from those intolerant to prostaglandin biosynthesis inhibitors (Table 1). Noramidopyrine, therefore, can elicit urticaria and/or angioedema by two mechanisms. In one group of patients (type B hypersensitivity to prostaglandin inhibitors) its action is due to inhibition of cyclooxygenase, and similar symptoms can be evoked by other NSAID blocking the oxidation of polyunsaturated fatty acids (e. g., aspirin, indomethacin). In another group of patients, the action of noramidopyrine is not due to blockade of prostaglandin generation (aspirin and indomethacin can be taken by patients with impunity), but appears to have an immunologic basis.

V. Other Skin Reactions Produced by Analgesics

In 1894 Brocq described a special type of drug reaction which cleared up rapidly when the drug was stopped, and reappeared in the same clinical distribution when the drug was restored. The incriminated drug was antipyrine. The mechanism of fixed eruptions is unknown (Amos 1976).

The generalized form of eczema, sometimes called exfoliative dermatitis or erythrodermia has also been associated with phenylbutazone, ibuprofen, mefenamic acid, and phenacetin (see Sect. C. VIII).

VI. Liver Damage

Drug hypersensitivity may be considered a cause of hepatic damage on the basis of the following criteria: dose-related liver injury cannot by demonstrated in animals; injury to the liver occurs in a very small proportion of exposed subjects; other allergic manifestations, such as eosinophilia, fever or skin rashes, are commonly associated with hepatic necrosis (ROSENOER and TORNAY 1979). Further support for an immune mechanism is occasionally obtained by re-challenging the patient with small doses of the drug and observing hepatic injury (MADDSEY and BOITT-NOTT 1977). However, evidence is predominantly circumstantial, and direct proof is often lacking. In contrast, the number of drugs which produce a predictable and ofted dose-related response, either by direct damage to the liver cells or by interfering with bilirubin metabolism, is growing rapidly (ANONYMOUS 1979).

Many hepatotoxic reactions result from a common initiating event – the metabolic activation in the body of drugs that are chemically stable to potent alkylating or arylating agents. Paracetamol may be used as an example of this type of reaction (PRESCOTT et al. 1974); if it is taken in excess (more than 15 g) with suicidal intent, it produces a clinical, laboratory and pathologic syndrome of severe, acute, and usually fatal hepatic necrosis.

The hypersensitive and toxic mechanisms are not mutually exclusive. In some instances, a combined effect might by operating, with antigens being produced only in some subjects because of altered drug metabolism (KLATSKIN 1974). In addition, a direct toxic mechanism might also alter an immune response, exposing the cell to further injury.

A good example of a drug which has the ability to produce both dose-related toxic hepatitis and hepatic damage mediated by a hypersensitivity reaction is phenazopyridine. This is a commonly prescribed urinary analgesic used either alone (Pyridium) or in combination with an antibiotic, for example in A20 Gantrinsin, or Azotrex. Direct dose-related hepatic injury has been reported in dogs given daily doses 1.5–46 times greater than the therapeutic dose of phenazopyridine, and infants who received high doses of this drug subsequently showed evidence of hepatic dysfunction. By contrast, in a recently reported case (BADLEY 1979) the most important criteria for a diagnosis of hypersensitivity hepatitis was fulfilled: the reaction was not dose related (occurring on the fourth occasion after administration of only one tablet of phenazopyridine). Clinical symptoms included malaise, epigastric pain, and jaundice, while laboratory data showed increased serum bilirubin and aminotransferase activities. Discontinuation of the medication led to clearing up of symptoms with no residual clinical or laboratory abnormalities. Despite widespread use, phenazopyridine has been implicated in hypersensitivity hepatitis in only four patients (BADLEX 1979); the latent period varied from 10 days to about 4 h.

VII. Kidney Injury

The effect of analgesics on the kidney is particularly important because, except in certain countries, there is no strict medical control over their consumption. In 1953 SPÜHLER and ZOLLINGER focused attention on analgesics as causative agents in chronic interstitial nephritis and the weight of evidence points to phenacetin as the ingredient most likely to cause damage.

Analgesic-associated nephropathy has been established as an important cause of chronic renal disease in many parts of the world (KINCAID-SMITH 1978). Patients are usually women, over the age of 35 years, who have been taking analgesics for recurrent headache or backache. Most patients have consumed large quantities of phenacetin (1–3 kg total dose or 1 g/day for 1–3 years) along with aspirin and other drugs, but the lowest total dosage at which these drugs are nephrotoxic are unknown. Even the relatively high total doses mentioned above can be achieved, if therapeutic doses (e. g., 10 tablets/day) are consumed for a few years (GOLDBERG and MURRAY 1978).

Pathologically and clinically, analgesic-associated nephropathy is primarily a tubular–interstitial disease. The initial lesions appear to involve the renal papillae whith focal areas of necrosis, followed by scarring of the medullary interstitium and later by the changes of chronic interstitial nephritis in the cortex. The pathognomonic lesion is sclerosis of the lower urinary tract capillaries (MITHATSCH et al. 1979). Mild to moderate pyuria (1.0 g/day) is usually present, but no red cell casts are found in the sediment.

Most patients remain asymptomatic until azotemia develops. In about one-half of the patients, hypertension may be observed before the discovery of azotemia. As in other interstitial nephropathies, the earliest functional abnormality is impaired urinary concentrating capacity, with isosthenuria or hyposthenuria resistant to vasopressin. Hypochloremic metabolic acidosis is also frequently found, and intravenous urography usually reveals bilaterally contracted and scarred kidneys with distortion of the normal calyceal structures. In patients who stop analgesic ingestion azotemia improves, if the level of renal impairment was mild. Patients who continue to use analgesics almost invariably suffer progression of the renal insufficiency (GOLDBERG and MURRAY 1978).

The precise mechanism of kidney injury produced by analgesics is not known. The major metabolite of phenacetin is paracetamol, which is without nephrotoxic effects. A small proportion of phenacetin, however, is deacetylated to p-phenetidin, a potent oxidant. This substance has an affinity of the thiol groups of red cell membranes; it interferes with membrane function with resulting damage to the cells (JACOB and JANDL 1962). This oxidative tissue damage produced by phenacetin metabolites, possibly potentiated by salicylate, which is an inhibitor of glucose-6-phosphate dehydrogenase, is believed to be the reason for analgesic nephropathy. It is interesting to note that lesions similar to those which are pathognomonic for analgesic-associated nephropathy, consisting of thickening of the basement membrane of capillaries with accumulation of large amounts of lipids (MIHATSCH et al. 1979), have been described in capillaries of other human organs, though to be injured by oxidative mechanisms (GRYGLEWSKI and SZCZEKLIK 1978).

It is more difficult to postulate that kidney damage results directly from interaction of phenacetin with antibody. Claims have been made which demonstrate an antibody with phenacetin specificity, but the specific antigen determinants have not been established (for references see AMOS 1976). According to AMOS (1976) no data are available to support the concept that the kidney could be the site of allergic complex deposition with resulting type III damage.

VIII. Hypersensitivity in Lupus Erythematosus

Hypersensitive reactions to drugs are frequently observed in patients with systemic lupus erythematosus. It has become evident in recent years that NSAID are no exception to this rule.

We have found reports on eight patients whith systemic lupus erythematosus who developed adverse reactions to ibuprofen (MANDELL et al. 1976; SZCZEKLIK et al. 1977a; SONNENBLICK and ABRAHAM 1978). These reactions were characterized by sudden appearance of high fever, abdominal pain, and rash. Serum transaminases were rased in some patients. Raised concentrations of serum transaminases also seem to be common in patients with active systemic lupus erythematosus, who are receiving aspirin (SEAMAN et al. 1974). The hepatotoxic effect of aspirin in these patients may be due, not to allergic reaction but to a disturbance in aspirin transformation, resulting in the formation of a toxic metabolite (ANONYMOUS 1974).

We have seen (SZCZEKLIK et al. 1977a) a 46-year-old male with a diagnosis of lupus erythematosus in an early stage, who gave a history of adverse reaction to analgesics taken by him for arthalgia. Oral challenges with 40 mg mefenamic acid and 50 mg phenylbutazone, performed on different days were both positive. Within 1 h his temperature rose to 39 °C, erythema with pruritus appeared on the face and chest, blood pressure fell to 90/70 mm Hg and the patient complained of abdominal and back pain. With hydrocortisone and antihistamines the symptoms subsided completely within 2–3 days. Although ibuprofen was said by the patient to cause a similar reaction, the challenge was not performed. On the other hand, challenges with therapeutic doses of aspirin, indomethacin, noramidopyrine, and aminophenazone were all negative. These reactions, therefore, could not be due to inhibition of cyclooxygenase. Perhaps, similarly to many other clinical manifestations of lupus erythematosus, they resulted from formation of antigen–antibody complexes.

IX. Blood Dyscrasias

1. Agranulocytosis and Pancytopenia

The symptoms of agranulocytosis appear suddenly in a patient receiving therapeutic doses of analgesics, usually of the pyrazolone group. Of these, amidopyrine and its close congener dipyrone (Novalgin) are most often incriminated. Rare cases of pancytopenia due to phenylbutazone have also been described (GROSS and HELLRIEGEL 1976). The patient presents a history of sore throat, malaise, and fever responding poorly to antibiotics. Pharyngeal ulceration is common and cervical lymphadenopathy may be present. A pheripheral blood count discloses low leukocyte concentrations (e. g., 0.5×10^9/l) with a total absence of neutrophils. A bone marrow aspirate shows poor cellularity with an absence of granulocytes and reduced erythroid precursors and megakaryocytes. This clinical picture, after treatment, persists from 6 days up to about 4 weeks. In therapy, antibiotics and granulocyte transfusions are used, and nursing includes reverse barrier precautions. The symptoms reappear immediately on exposure to low doses of the drug. Cases have been described in which the symptoms reappeared nine times over a period of 6 years, each time owing to ingestion of combined analgesics containing pyrazolone drugs (Hennemann and Schief 1975).

Pathogenesis of the syndrome is better understood thanks to the work of Moeschlin et al. (1952) and Moeschlin (1954). In plasma and serum of patients with pyramidon- (amidopyrine)-induced agranulocytosis they found a substance which produced agglutination of the leukocytes. Administration of this substance by transfusion of the patient's blood caused an immediate and profound granulocytopenia of several hours' duration in the recipients. The conclusion was that primary peripheral destruction of leukocytes occurred which led to gradual disappearance of neutrophils from bone marrow, and in severe cases to bone marrow depletion.

In an in vitro test for leukoagglutinins, one drop of a leukocyte-rich normal plasma is mixed with three drops of the patient's serum, and the mixture incubated at 37 °C in a siliconized vessel. The cells are observed every 30 min over about 5 h. Provided that the serum is taken from the patient at the height of the reaction and the white cells are obtained from an ABO-compatible donor, agglutination should occur. If serum is taken during the convalescence period the drug must be added to the system. Moeschlin (1954) detected antibodies to leukocytes induced by sulfapyridine by taking the patient's serum and dissolving the drug in it at concentrations of 5–20 mg/100 ml serum. This serum enriched with drug agglutinated a leukocyte preparation from a normal donor.

Leukocyte agglutination tests have often been used, but the results have been difficult to interpret and widely questioned (Flandrin et al. 1971; Gross and Hellriegel 1976). Recently, two new techniques have been described. One involves inhibition of granulocyte colonies in the presence of the patient's serum (Barrett et al. 1976). Using this technique, the authors were able to show amidopyrine-dependent leukagglutinin 6 and 12 months after the acute episode of agranulocytosis. In another study (Jeannet et al. 1979) a ^{51}Cr release cytotoxicity test was used and auto-antibodies (probably induced by amidopyrine) specific for neutrophils and leukocytes were detected.

Amidopyrine agranulocytosis or pancytopenia is extremely rare and transient (Flandrin et al. 1971). Although it is an excellent antipyretic, analgesic, and antiinflammatory agent, amidopyrine should be employed only after safer drugs and other measures have proven ineffective.

2. Aspirin-Induced Thrombocytopenia

Aspirin ingestion causes significant alterations in the function of human platelets. Bleeding time becomes prolonges (Quick 1966), and the second phase of platelet aggregation is depressed (O'Brien 1968). These changes are most likely due to interference of aspirin with arachidonic acid metabolism in platelets. Thus, aspirin acetylates and inactivates cyclooxygenase (Roth et al. 1975), the enzyme which catalyzes transformation of free arachidonic acid into the endoperoxide PGH_2. The latter is subsequently converted to thromboxane A_2, a potent stimulus of platelet aggregation. The effect of aspirin on platelets is an irreversible one, and lasts for the entire platelet life time because platelets synthesize little or no new protein. Furthermore, aspirin appears also to inhibit the function of megakaryocytes in the bone marrow (SZCZEKLIK et al. 1979 b).

Although this anti-platelet action of aspirin is of little concern to healthy subjects, in some subjects suffering from a tendency to bleed (e. g., hemophilia, disorders of platelet function) it might lead to hemorrhagic diathesis or aggravate an existing one. Most unusually, however, such diatheses are due to an immune mechanism. In fact, only a few cases have been reported in which thrombocytopenia could be linked to ingestion of aspirin, and appeared to be on an immune basis (NIEWEG et al. 1963; D'ESHOUGES ct al. 1961; GARG and SARKER 1974). Petechiae developed a few hours after aspirin ingestion, and the platelet count was depressed for 6–8 days.

The inhibition of clot retraction (ACKROYD 1964) should probably be the first test in any program of investigation of suspected allergic platelet destruction. Other procedures used are documented clearly by ACKROYD (1964), who employed them in a classic investigation of thrombocytopenia following Sedormid therapy.

The in vitro platelet factor 3 immunoinjury test for antiplatelet antibody (KARPATKIN 1971) might be of diagnostic help in some cases. The most reliable method for confirmation of the diagnosis is in vivo challenge with a small amount of aspirin. This test entails a risk to the patients and should not be attempted, when any one of the in vitro tests is positive (GARG and SARKER 1974).

X. Peripheral Neuropathies

Indomethacin and chloroquine have been implicated in causing mild sensorimotor neuropathy as well as vascular myopathy. Peripheral neuropathy has been reported in patients treated with penicillamine, but less often than the myasthenic syndrome that develop in some patients treated with this drug. Paresthesiae and muscle weakness have been reported in some patients treated with phenylbutazone (ARGOV and MASTAGLIA 1979). In all these sydromes, little evidence exists that they are caused by allergic mechanisms.

References

Ackroyd JF (1964) The diagnosis of disorders of the blood due to drug hypersensitivity caused by an immune mechanism. In: Ackroyd JF (ed) Immunological methods. Blackwell, Oxford

Adcock JJ, Garland LG, Moncada S, Salmon JA (1978) The mechanism of enhancement by fatty acid hydroperoxides of anaphylactic mediator release. Prostaglandins 16:179–189

Amos HE (1976) Allergic drug reactions. Arnold, London

Anonymous (1974) Aspirin-induced hepatic injury. Ann Intern Med 80:103–105

Anonymous (1979) Liver injury, drugs, and popular poisons. Br Med J 2:574–575

Argov Z, Mastaglia (1979) Drug-induced peripheral neuropathies. Br Med M 1:663–665

Badley BWD (1979) Phenazopyridine-induced hepatitis. Br Med J 2:850

Barrett AJ, Weller E, Rozengurt N, Longhurst P, Humble JG (1976) Amidopyrine agranulocytosis: drug inhibition of granulocyte colonies in the presence of patient's serum. Br Med J 2: 850–851

Basomba A, Romar A, Villamanzo, IG, Campos A (1976) The effect of sodium cromoglycate in preventing aspirin-induced bronchospasm. Clin Allergy 6:269–275

Bianco S, Robuschi M, Petrigni C (1977) Aspirin-induced tolerance in aspirin-asthma detected by a new challenge test. IRCS Med Sci Libr Compend 5:129

Borgeat P, Samuelsson B (1979) Arachidonic acid metabolism in polymorphonuclear leukocytes. 3. Effects of ionophore – A 23187. Proc Natl Acad Sci USA 76:2148–2153

Brocq L (1894) Éruption érythèmato-pigmentée fixé due à l'antipyrine. Ann Dermatol Syphiligr 5:308–314

Bundgaard H (1976) Colorimetric analysis of immunogenic impurities in acetylsalicylic
acid. J Pharm Pharmacol 28:544–547

Bundgaard H, de Weck AL (1975) The role of aminoreactive impurities in acetylsalicylic
acid allergy. Int. Arch Allergy Appl Immunol 49:119–125

Burka JF, Flower RJ (1979) Effects of modulators of arachidonic acid metabolism on the
synthesis and release of slow-reacting substances of anaphylaxis. Br J Pharmacol 65:35–
41

Ceserani R, Colombo M, Robuschi M, Bianco S (1978) Tartrazine and prostaglandin system. Prostaglandins Med 1:499–505

Chafee FH, Settipane GA (1974) Aspirin intolerance. I. Frequency in an allergic population.
J Allergy Clin Immunol 53:193

Czerniawska-Mysik G, Szczeklik A (1980) Allergy to pyrazolone drugs. Acta Med Pol

Delaney JC (1973) Asthma, nasal polyposis and aspirin sensitivity. Ann Intern Med 79:761

Delaney JC (1976) The effect of sodium cromoglycate on analgesic-induced asthmatic
reactions. Clin Allergy 6:365–370

Delaney JC, Kay AB (1976) Complement components and IgE in patients with asthma and
aspirin idiosyncrasy. Thorax 31:425–427

D'Eshouges JR, Grigner P, Smadja A et al. (1961) Purpura thrombocytopenique aigü par
sensibilisation à l'aspirine. Nouv Rev Fr Hematol 1:609–611

de Weck AL (1971) Immunological effects of aspirin anhydride, a contaminant of commercial acetylsalicylic acid preparations. Int Arch Allergy Appl Immunol 41:393–398

Doeglas HMG (1975) Reactions to aspirin and food additives in patients with chronic urticaria, including the physical urticarias. Br J Dermatol 93:135–141

Drazen JM, Lewis RA, Wasserman SI, Orange RP, Austen FK (1979) Differential effects
of a partially purified preparation of slow-reacting substance of anaphylaxis on guinea-
pig tracheal spirals and parenchymal strips. J Clin Invest 63:1–5

Dry J, Pradalier A, Deveau A (1979) Urticaire et oedème de Quincke chroniques. Nouv
Presse Med 8:211

Falliers C (1974) Familial coincidence of asthma, aspirin intolerance and nasal polyposis.
Ann Allergy 32:65–69

Farr RS (1971) The capacity of aspirin to acetylate proteins in vitro and in vivo. In: Aldridge
WN (ed) Mechanisms of toxicity. St. Martin, New York

Ferreira SH, Moncada S, Vane JR (1971) Indomethacin and aspirin abolish prostaglandin
release from the spleen. Nature New Biol 231:237–239

Fisherman EW, Cohen GN (1974) Alpha-beta adrenergic imbalance in intrinsic-intolerance
rhinitis or asthma. Ann Allergy 33:86–101

Flandrin G, Daniel MT, Briere J, Varet B, Pestel M, Bernard J (1971) L'agranulocytose au
pyramidon, une aplasie bréve de trois lignés. Nouv Rev Fr Hematol 11:219–221

Flower RJ (1974) Drugs which inhibit prostaglandin biosynthesis. Pharmacol Rev 26:33–67

Flower RJ, Blackwell GJ (1979) Anti-inflammatory steroids induce the biosynthesis of a
phospholipase A_2 inhibitor which prevents prostaglandin generation. Nature 278:456–
459

Garg S, Sarker CR (1974) Aspirin-induced thrombocytopenia on an immune basis. Am J
Med Sci 267:129–131

Gerber JG, Payne NA, Oelz O, Nies AS, Oates JA (1979) Tartrazine and the prostaglandin
system. J Allergy Clin Immunol 63:289–294

Giraldo B, Blumenthal MN, Spink WW (1969) Aspirin intolerance and asthma. Ann Intern
Med 71:479–485

Goldberg M, Murray TG (1978) Analgesic-associated nephropathy. N Engl J Med 299:716–
717

Gross R, Hellriegel KP (1976) Arzneimittelbedingte Agranulozytosen. Blut 32:409–414

Gryglewski RJ (1976) Steroid hormones, anti-inflammatory steroids and prostaglandins. Pharmacol Res Commun 8:337–351

Gryglewski RJ (1979) Screening and assessment of potency of anti-inflammatory drugs in vitro. In: Vane JR, Ferreira SH (eds) Anti-inflammatory drugs. Handbook of experimental pharmacology, Springer-Verlag, Berlin Heidelberg New York, vol 50/2, pp 1–43

Gryglewski RJ, Szczeklik A (1978) Inhibition of prostaglandin formation by lipid peroxides in the arterial wall: hypothetical step in development of atherosclerosis. Mater Med Pol 37:338–341

Gryglewski RJ, Panczenko B, Korbut R, Grodzińska L, Ocetkiewicz A (1975a) Corticosteroids inhibit prostaglandin release from perfused lungs of sensitized guinea pigs. Prostaglandins 10:343–355

Gryglewski RJ, Szczeklik A, Czerniawska-Mysik G (1975b) Aspirin sensitivity: other drugs. Ann Intern Med 83

Gryglewski, RJ, Dembińska-Kieć, A, Grodzińska L, Panczenko B (1976) Differential generation of substances with prostaglandin-like and thromboxane-like activities by guinea pig trachea and lung strips. In: Bouhuys A (ed) Lung cells in disease. North Holland, Amsterdam Oxford New York, pp 289–307

Gryglewski RJ, Szczeklik A, Niżankowska E (1977) Aspirin-sensitive asthma: its relationship to inhibition of prostaglandin biosynthesis. NATO Adv Study Inst Ser A Life Sci 13:191–203

Gwin E, Kerby GR, Ruth WE (1977) Cromolyn sodium in the treatment of asthma associated with aspirin hypersensitivity and nasal polyps. Chest 72:148–154

Harnett JC, Spector SL, Farr RS (1978) Aspirin idiosyncrasy. In: Middleton E Jr, Reed CE, Ellis EF (eds) Allergy. Principles and practice. Mosby, St. Louis, pp 1002–1022

Hennemann HH, Schief A (1975) Rezidive von Agranulozytose. Dtsch Med Wochenschr 100:519–522

Hume M, Eddy V (1977) Treatment of chronic airways obstruction with indomethacin. Scan J Respir Dis 58:284–286

Irey NS (1976) Adverse drug reactions and death. JAMA 236:575–578

Jacob HS, Jandl JH (1962) Effects of sulfhydrol inhibition on red blood cells. J Clin Invest 41:779–790

Jeannet M, Lew D, Legendre C (1979) Amidopyrine pancytopenia: detection of leucocytotoxic antibodies by a ^{51}Cr-release test. Acta Haematol (Basel) 61:52–54

Juhlin L, Michaëlsson G, Zetterström O (1972) Urticaria and asthma induced by food-and-drug additives in patients with aspirin hypersensitivity. J Allergy Clin Immunol 50:92–98

Kaplan AP (1978) Urticaria and angioedema. In: Middleton E Jr, Reed CE, Ellis EF (eds) Allergy. Principles and practice. Mosby, St. Louis, pp 1080–1099

Karpatkin S (1971) Drug-induced thrombocytopenia. Am J Clin Sci 262:69–78

Kaufman HS (1977) Nasal polyps, syncope and asthma. Lancet 1:758

Kincaid-Smith P (1978) Analgesic nephropathy. Kidney Int 13:1–113

Klatskin G (1974) Drug-induced hepatic injury. In: Schaffner F, Sherlock S, Leevy CM (eds) The liver and its diseases. Intercontinental Medical Books, New York, pp 163–178

Kordansky D, Adkinson F, Norman PS, Rosenthal RR (1978) Asthma improved by nonsteroidal anti-inflammatory drugs. Ann Intern Med 88:508–511

Leist ER, Banwell JG (1974) Products containing aspirin. N Engl J Med 291:710–713

Lockey RF, Rucknagel DL, Vaneslow NA (1973) Familial occurrence of asthma and nasal polyps and aspirin intolerance. Ann Intern Med 78:57–63

Lockey SD (1977) Hypersensitivity to tartrazine (FD C Yellow No. 5) and other dyes and additives present in foods and pharmaceutical products. Ann Allergy 38:206–210

Maddsey WC, Boitnott JK (1977) Drug-induced chronic liver disease. Gastroenterology 72:1348–1353

Mandell B, Shen HS, Hepburn B (1976) Fever from ibuprofen in a patient with lupus erythematosus. Ann Intern Med 85–209–210

Martelli NA, Usandivaras G (1977) Inhibition of aspirin-induced bronchoconstriction by sodium cromoglycate inhalation. Thorax 32:684–690

Matthews JI, Stage D (1974) Indomethacin, aspirin and urticaria. Ann Intern Med 80:771

Matthews KP, Lowell RG, Sheldon JM (1950) The problem of aspirin allergy with a report on skin testing with salicylate containing human sera J Lab Clin Med 36:416–419

McDonald JR, Mathison DA, Stevenson DD (1972) Aspirin intolerance in asthma. J Allergy Clin Immunol 50:198–207

Michaëlsson G (1969) Chronic urticaria. Acta Derm venereol (Stockh) 49:404–416

Mihatsch MJ, Zollinger HU, Torhorst J (1979) Pathognomonic lesion of analgesic nephropathy. E Engl J Med 300:1275–1276

Miller RL, Insel PA, Melmon KL (1978) Inflammatory disorders. In: Melmon KL, Morelli WF (eds) Clinical pharmacology, 2nd edn. Macmillan, New York, pp 657–708

Moeschlin S (1954) Weitere Beobachtungen über Immunleukopenien und Agranulozytosen. Schweiz Med Wochenschr 84:1100–1103

Moeschlin S, Wagner K (1952) Agranulocytosis due to the occurrence of leukocyte agglutinins (pyramidon and cold agglutinins). Acta Haematol (Basel) 8:29–41

Molaney JR (1977) Nasal polyps, nasal polypectomy, asthma and aspirin sensitivity. J Laryngol Otol 91:837–846

Moore-Robinson M, Warin RP (1967) Effect of salicytaes in urticaria. Br Med J 4:262–266

Nieweg HO, Bouma HGD, Vries KD (1963) Hematological side effects of some antirheumatic drugs. Ann Rheum Dis 22: 440–443

Niżankowska E, Szczeklik A (1979) Keine Bedenken gegen Solosin bei Acetylsalicylsäureempfindlichen Asthmatikern. Dtsch Med Wochenschr 104:1388–1389

Noid HE, Schulze TW, Winkelmann RK (1974) Diet plan for patients with salicylate-induced urticaria. Arch Dermatol 109:666–670

O'Brien JR (1968) Effects of salicylates on human platelets. Lancet 1:779–781

Okazaki T, Ilea VS, Rosario NA, Reisman RE, Arbesman CE, Lee JB, Middleton E Jr (1977) Regulatory role of prostaglandin E in allergic histamine release with observations on responsiveness of basophil leukocytes and the effect of acetylsalicylic acid. J Allergy Clin Immunol 60:360–366

Orehek J, Douglas JS, Bouhuys A (1975) Contractile responses of the guinea pig trachea in vitro: modification by prostaglandin synthesis-inhibiting drugs. J Pharmacol Exp Ther 194:554–564

Panczenko B, Grodzińska L, Gryglewski RJ (1975) The dual action of meclofenamate or contractive response to PGF_2 in the guinea pig trachea. Pol J Phamacol Pharm 27:273–278

Pasargiklian M, Bianco S, Allegra L, Moavero NE, Petrigni C, Robuschi M, Grugni A (1977) Aspects of bronchial reactivity to prostaglandins and aspirin in asthmatic patients. Respiration 34:79–91

Patrono C, Ciabattoni G, Venuti A, Pugliese F, Schiavino D, Patriarca G (1978) Aspirin intolerance: unaltered susceptibility of platelet cyclo-oxygenase to inhibition by aspirin in vitro. J Allergy Clin Immunol 62:271–275

Prescott LF, Newton RW, Swainson CP, Wright N, Forrest ARW, Matthew H (1974) Successfull treatment of severe paracetamol overdosage with cysteamine. Lancet 1:588–592

Quick AJ (1966) Salicylates and bleeding. The aspirin tolerance test. Am J Med Sci 252:268–270

Rachelefsky GS, Carlson A, Siegel CS, Stiehm ER (1975) Aspirin intolerance in chronic childhood asthma detected by oral challenge. Pediatrics 56:443–450

Rosenhall L (1977) Hypersensitivity to analgesics, preservatives and food colorants in patients with asthma or rhinitis. Acta Univ 269:1–117

Rosenoer VM, Tornay AS (1979) Drugs and the liver. Med Clin North Am 63:405–412

Roth GJ, Stanford N, Majerus PW (1975) Acetylation of prostaglandin synthetase by aspirin. Proc Natl Acad Sci USA 72:3073–3078

Rudzki E (1977) Chronic urticaria due to aspirin and food additives (In Polish). Przegl Dermatol 64:163–166

Samter M (1973) Intolerance to aspirin. Hosp Pract 8:85–90

Samter M, Beers RJ Jr (1968) Intolerance to aspirin: clinical studies and consideration of its pathogenesis. Ann Intern Med 68:975–983

Samuelsson B (1979) Oxygenation and further transformation of polyunsaturated fatty acids. Plenary Lecture at the IVth International Prostaglandin Conference, Washington, DC, May 1979

Schlumberger HD, Löbbecke EA, Kallos P (1974) Acetylsalicylic acid intolerance. Acta Med Scand 196:451–458

Schuhl JF, Pereyra JG (1979) Oral acetylsalicylic acid (aspirin) in asthmatic children. Clin Allergy 9:83–88

Seaman WE, Ishak KG, Plotz PH (1974) Aspirin-induced hepatotoxicity in patients with systemic lupus erythematosus. Ann Intern Med 80:1–8

Serwońska M (1979) Non-acidic nonsteroidal anti-inflammatory drugs and aspirin-induced asthma (In Polish). PhD thesis, University of Cracow

Settipane GA, Chafee FH, Klein DE (1974) Aspirin intolerance. II. A prospective study in atopic and normal population. J Allergy Clin Immunol 53:200–204

Settipane GA, Chafee FH, Postman IM et al. (1976) Significance of tartrazine sensitivity in chronic urticaria of unknown etiology. J Allergy Clin Immunol 57:541–546

Shen TY (1979) Prostaglandin synthetase inhibitors. In: Vane JR, Ferreira S (eds) Anti-inflammatory drugs. Springer, Berlin Heidelberg New York (Handbook of experimental pharmacology, vol 50/2, pp 305–347)

Siegel MI, McConnel RT, Cuatrecasas P (1979) Aspirin-like drugs interfere with arachidonate metabolism by inhibition of the 12-hydroxy-5,8,10,14-eicosatetraenoic acid peroxidase activity of the lipoxygenase pathway. Proc Natl Acad Sci USA 76:3774–3778

Slapke J, Jäger L (1979) Untersuchungen zum Analgetika-Asthma. Gesellschaft Inn Med DDR 34:78–80

Smith JB, Willis AL (1971) Aspirin selectively inhibits prostaglandin production in human platlets. Nature New Biol 231:235–237

Smith LJ, Slavin RG (1976) Drugs containing tartrazine dye. J Allergy Clin Immunol 58:456–470

Sonnenblick M, Abraham AS (1978) Ibuprofen hypersensitivity in systemic lupus erythematosus. Br Med J 1:618–619

Spühler O, Zollinger HU (1953) Die chronisch-interstitielle Nephritis. Z Klin Med 151:1–50

Starr WR (1971) Familial aspirin hypersensitivity. Ann Allergy 29:498

Stenius BSM, Lemola M (1976) Hypersensitivity to acetylsalicylic acid (ASA) and tartrazine in patients with asthma. Clin Allergy 6:119–129

Stevenson DD, Arroyave CM, Bhat KN, Tan EM (1976) Oral aspirin challenge in asthmatic patients: a study of plasma histamine. Clin Allergy 6:493–506

Szczeklik A (1980) Analgesics, allergy and asthma. Br J Clin Pharacol 10:401–405

Szczeklik A, Czerniawska-Mysik G (1976) Prostaglandins and aspirin-induced asthma. Lancet 1:488

Szczeklik A, Serwońska M (1979) Inhibition by clemastine of adverse reactions to aspirin in patients with asthma and aspirin idiosyncrasy. Thorax 34:654–657

Szczeklik A, Gryglewski RJ, Czerniawska-Mysik G (1974) Is aspirin-sensitive asthma due to inhibition of prostaglandin synthesis? In: Proceedings of the Ninth European Congress of Allergy and Clinical Immunology, London, 1974, p 34

Szczeklik A, Gryglewski RJ, Czerniawska-Mysik G (1975a) Relationship of inhibition of prostaglandin biosynthesis by analgesics to asthma attacks in aspirin-sensitive patients. Br Med J 1:67–69

Szczeklik, A, Musial J, Serwońska M (1975b) The effect of aspirin on bleeding time and platelet aggregation in patients hypersensitivity to nonsteroidal anti-inflammatory drugs. Abstracts of the XIth Congress of the Polish Society of Haematologists. Gdańsk, p 64

Szczeklik A, Gryglewski RJ, Czerniawska-Mysik G, Żmuda A (1976) Aspirin-induced asthma. Hypersensitivity to fenoprofen and ibuprofen in relation to their inhibitory action to prostaglandin generation by different microsomal enzymic preparations. J Allergy Clin Immunol 58:10–18

Szczeklik A, Gryglewski RJ, Czerniawska-Mysik G (1977a) Clinical patterns of hypersensitivity to nonsteroidal anti-inflammatory drugs and their pathogenesis. J Allergy Clin Immunol 60:276–284

Szczeklik A, Gryglewski RJ, Czerniawska-Mysik G, Pieton R (1977b) Asthmatic attacks induced in aspirin-sensitive patients by diclofenac and naproxen. Br Med J 2:231–232

Szczeklik A, Gryglewski RJ, Olszewski E, Dembińska-Kieć A, Czerniawska-Mysik G (1977c) Aspirin-sensitive asthma: the effect of aspirin on the release of prostaglandins from nasal polyps. Pharmacol Res Commun 9:415–425

Szczeklik A, Niżankowska E, Niżankowski R (1977 d) Bronchial reactivity to prostaglandin F_2, E_2, and histamine in different types of asthma, Respiration 34:323–331

Szczeklik A, Gryglewski RJ, Niżankowska E (1978 a) Asthma relieved by aspirin and by other cyclo-oxygenase inhibitors. Thorax 33:664–665

Szczeklik A, Gryglewski RJ, Niżankowska E, Niżankowski R, Musia 1 (1978 b) Pulmonary and anti-platelet effects of intravenous and inhaled prostacyclin in man. Prostaglandins 16:651–660

Szczeklik A, Gryglewski RJ, Nizankowska E (1979 a) Asthma improved by nonsteroidal anti-inflammatory drugs. Ann Intern Med 90:126–127

Szczeklik A, Gryglewski RJ, Grodzińska L, Musia J, Serwońska M, Marcinkiewicz E (1979 b) Platelet aggregability, thromboxane A_2 and malonaldehyde formation following administration of aspirin to man. Throm Res 15:405–413

Szczeklik A, Czerniawska-Mysik G, Serwońska M, Kukliński P (1980) Inhibition by ketotifen of idiosyncratic reactions to aspirin. Allergy 35:421–424

Trautlein J, Mann WJ (1978) Anaphylactic shock caused by yellow dye in an enema (case report). Ann Allergy 41:28–29

Vane JR (1971) Inhibition of prostaglandin synthesis as a mechanism of action of aspirin-like drugs. Nature New Biol 231:232–235

Vane JR (1976) The mode of action of aspirin and similar compounds. J Allergy Clin Immunol 58:691–712

Van Leeuwen WS (1928) Pathognomonische Bedeutung der Überempfindlichkeit gegen Aspirin bei Asthmatikern. MMW 75:1588–1592

Vedenthan PK, Menon MM, Bell TB, Bergin D (1977) Aspirin and tartrazine oral challenge: Incidence of adverse response in chronic childhood asthma. J Allergy Clin Immunol 60:8–13

Virchow C (1976) Analgetika-Intoleranz bei Asthmatikern (Analgetika-Asthma-Syndrom). Prax Klin Pneumol 30:684–692

Von Maur K, Adkinson NF, Van Metre TE, Marsh DG, Norman PS (1974) Aspirin intolerance in a family. J Allergy Clin Immunol 54:380–395

Warin RP (1960) The effect of aspirin in chronic urticaria. Br J Dermatol 72:350–351

Warin RP, Smith RJ (1976) Challenge test battery in chronic urticaria. Br J Dermatol 94:401–406

Whittle BJR (1977) Prostaglandins and mast cell histamine release. NATO Adv Study Inst Ser Life Sci:345–351

Woodbury DM, Fingl E (1979) Analgesic-antipyretics, anti-inflammatory agents, and drugs employed in the therapy of gout. In: Goodman LS, Gillman A (eds) The pharmacological basis of therapeutics, 5th edn. Macmillan, New York, pp 325–358

Wuethrich B (1979) Protective effect of ketotifen and disodium cromoglycate against bronchoconstriction induced by aspirin, benzoic acid or tartrazine in intolerant asthmatics. Respiration 37:224–227

Yurchak WM, Wicher K, Arbesman CE (1970) Immunologi studies on aspirin. J Allergy 46:245–252

CHAPTER 12

Neuromuscular Blocking Drugs

E. S. K. Assem

A. Introduction

Muscle relaxants of this type act at the neuromuscular junction, interfering with the transmission of impulses from motor nerves to skeletal muscles, as distinct from the centrally acting muscle relaxants such as mephenesin, meprobamate, diazepam, and baclofen. In this chapter, discussion will be limited to reactions which can best be described as anaphylactic-like, and which are to a major extent not related to the normal pharmacological actions of these drugs. Reactions basically due to abnormal or deficient enzymes (e.g. enzymes involved in the metabolic degradation of various choline esters, KALOW and GUNN 1957; KALOW 1962; CLARK et al. 1968; SILK et al. 1979) will not be discussed here. However, it is the author's view that in some patients reacting in this anaphylactic-like manner to certain of these agents, particularly depolarising neuromuscular blockers such as suxamethonium, such abnormalities may coexist and thus may contribute to the intensity, manifestations and duration of the reaction. This view is based on preliminary findings in our own laboratory (ASSEM and CHONG unpublished).

The agents to be discussed consist of two chemically distinct groups, which act in pharmacologically distinct ways. The first group is that of depolarising blockers, exemplified by suxamethonium (succinylcholine, Fig. 1). The second group is that of non-depolarising agents, which act as competitive antagonists of the nicotinic effects of acetylcholine. The agents most widely used are (+)-tubocurarine, pancuronium, alcuronium, and gallamine (Fig. 1).

Two main problems face research workers in the field of adverse reactions to neuromuscular blocking drugs, particularly the non-depolarising agents. First, it is extremely difficult to distinguish between "true" anaphylaxis, i.e. reactions mediated by anaphylactic antibodies whether of the IgE class or IgG subclasses, and reactions due to direct (non-immunological) release of histamine and possibly other chemical mediators (ASSEM 1977; VERVLOET et al. 1979). The latter type of mechanism results from an abnormality which is fundamentally different from that of anaphylaxis, though the final outcome appears exactly similar in both instances. The second problem encountered in this field is that skin tests, which normally constitute the simplest and most feasible means of allergy testing, are of little or no value in the diagnosis of reactions to neuromuscular blocking drugs, particularly in the case of non-depolarising agents. This problem will be further discussed later.

Because of these difficulties in establishing the mechanism for both types of reaction, allergy, and idiosyncrasy (incidentally both are classified as "type B" adverse drug reactions, according to RAWLINS and THOMPSON's classification, 1977),

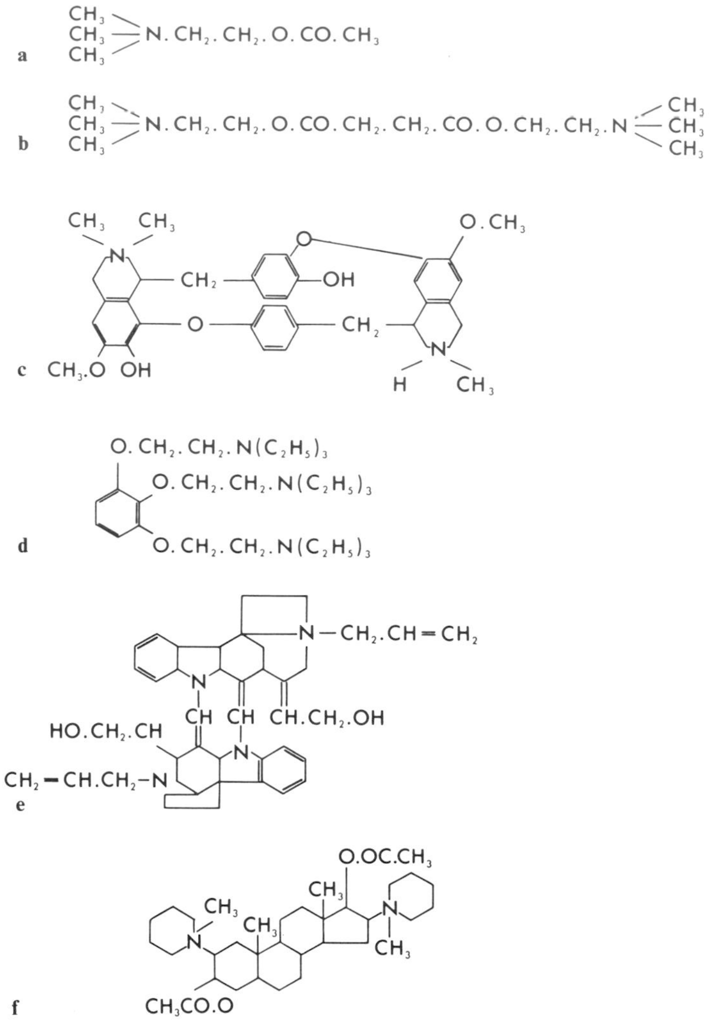

a
$$CH_3 {\textstyle>} N.CH_2.CH_2.O.CO.CH_3$$
with CH_3, CH_3, CH_3

b
$$CH_3 {\textstyle>} N.CH_2.CH_2.O.CO.CH_2.CH_2.CO.O.CH_2.CH_2.N {\textstyle<} CH_3$$
with CH_3, CH_3, CH_3 and CH_3, CH_3, CH_3

c CH$_3$.O OH

d
$$O.CH_2.CH_2.N(C_2H_5)_3$$
$$O.CH_2.CH_2.N(C_2H_5)_3$$
$$O.CH_2.CH_2.N(C_2H_5)_3$$

e
$$N-CH_2.CH=CH_2$$
$$HO.CH_2.CH$$
$$CH\ CH\ CH.CH_2.OH$$
$$CH_2=CH.CH_2-N$$

f
$$O.OC.CH_3$$
$$CH_3CO.O$$

Fig. 1 a–f. Structural formulae of **a** acetylcholine, **b** suxamethonium, **c** tubocurarine, **d** gallamine, **e** alcuronium, and **f** pancuronium

will be discussed collectively under "anaphylactic-like reactions". Many authors use the term anaphylactoid, while the terms "allergoid" and "histaminoid" are less frequently used.

B. In Vivo Diagnostic Procedures

I. Skin Tests

One of the major differences between the two groups of neuromuscular blocking drugs can be shown by skin testing. When injected intradermally, low concentrations of depolarising agents (< 100 µg/ml) produce little or no response in normal human subjects. By contrast, very low concentrations of non-depolarising agents produce wheal and flare responses in all normal individuals. Thus, skin tests are of little or no value with the latter agents, but if carried out as a carefully controlled quantitative comparison between normal and "sensitive" patients, they may prove of value in the case of depolarising blockers. In sensitive patients, a significant skin response may be obtained with a drug concentration of 0.1 µg/ml or less. However, false negative skin responses may be obtained with suxamethonium.

There is evidence to suggest that the mechanism of wheal and flare reactions to the curare-like agents is due to direct (non-immune) histamine release from mast cells in the skin (MONGAR and WHELAN 1953; PATON 1957; LORENZ et al. 1972). This view has not been challenged, although in vitro studies have cast some doubt on it, since histamine release could not be elicited with the low concentrations that brought on the strong wheal and flare responses. This may be due to the different reactivity of tissue mast cells and blood basophils. Several agents (e.g., opiates) are known to release histamine from tissue mast cells but not from blood basophils.

II. Response to an Intravenous Test Dose

Generally speaking, all the muscle relaxants discussed here have been reported to produce histamine release when injected intravenously (i.v.). This was shown by an increase in plasma histamine level (LORENZ et al. 1972). The frequency of reaction (significant increase in plasma histamine) was highest with suxamethonium (3 of 8 volunters), followed by alcuronium (alloferin, 2 of 8), and then pancuronium (1 of 7) (LORENZ and DOENICKE 1978). However, the latter authors found a poor correlation between the increase in plasma histamine levels and the incidence of clinical manifestations, e.g., such manifestations were more frequent with pancuronium than with suxamethonium. These above findings contradict the low incidence of acute (anaphylactic-like) reactions to pancuronium in practice.

The use of a small i.v. dose may be of value in assessing the potential risk of new agents, but cannot generally be advocated as a diagnostic test in patients with suspected adverse reactions, because of the risk involved. This procedure should be undertaken with appropriate precautions and in a setting where facilities for respiratory and cardiovascular resuscitation are immediately at hand. In the absence of facilities for measurement of plasma histamine levels, the diagnosis would depend on detecting significant respiratory or cardiovascular manifestations.

C. In Vitro Tests

I. Histamine Release from Leucocytes

Previous work by ASSEM (1977) had suggested that the leucocyte histamine release test was a particularly useful diagnostic tool in patients who developed reactions to muscle relaxants. In that work, it was essential to assay the histamine released by a non-biological method (i.e., not on isolated guinea-pig ileum) because of the interference by muscle relaxants with the bioassay. The assay procedure used was chemical, using an automated spectrofluorometric technique (Technicon). Good response (histamine release) was obtained with drug concentrations in the range 1–100 µg/ml. In fact, the latter concentration was usually superoptimal.

In those studies, the leucocyte test was positive in the majority of patients with clinical reactions, but rarely produced high histamine release in normal subjects, even with non-depolarising muscle relaxants which produce strong wheal and flare responses in normal subjects. Furthermore, the leucocyte test showed some drug specificity, which differed from one "sensitive" patient to another. Thus, histamine release was frequently elicited only with certain compounds but not with others, and this even occurred with members of the same pharmacological group, e.g. various non-depolarising blockers. This is unlike skin tests where all non-depolarising agents invariably produced wheal and flare responses at low drug concentrations. Not only did the leucocyte test show specificity, but more importantly it correlated with the clinical findings. When the result was negative, subsequent exposure was uneventful. Thus, the straightforward challenge of isolated patients' leucocytes fulfilled most of the desired criteria. In our own experience, these tests were not only diagnostic, specific and naturally safe (involving no risk to the patients), but were also predictive. This was best illustrated in suspected idiosyncrasy to muscle relaxants in the relatives of patients with definite reactions and in whom idiosyncrasy was a likely mechanism (Assem et al. 1981). The idiosyncrasy is presumably due to a genetically determined defect, and relatives of patients with reactions are particularly at risk. This potentially catastrophic situation can be prevented by carrying out appropriate tests, including the leucocyte histamine release test.

The distinction between normal and abnormal response in this test, is usually clear-cut, since the abnormal reaction is manifested by substantial histamine release, which is well above that elicited by in vivo challenge tests and measurement of plasma histamine levels. The risk with in vivo tests cannot be over-emphasised.

II. Passive Sensitisation Experiments

Serum from two patients whose reaction to suxamethonium appeared to be due to allergy on the basis of skin tests and leucocyte histamine release was subjected to studies for passive sensitisation of human skin fragments in vitro. No histamine release could be clearly demonstrated after such a procedure. Only a positive result would have conclusively proved that the reaction was immunologically mediated (mediated by anaphylactic antibodies). A negative result does not exclude the possibility of allergy, since passive sensitisation requires high reaginic activity of the sensitising serum, which is often difficult to demonstrate in drug allergy, for various reasons which are beyond this discussion. An important incidental finding in the work on human skin fragments was that suxamethonium did not act as a histamine releaser from mast cells in "normal" skin.

III. Lymphocyte Transformation Test

Another test for allergy diagnosis is the lymphocyte transformation test (LTT) which, if positive, would almost certainly prove such a diagnosis. The result of LTT in one of the patients in whom allergy to suxamethonium seemed very likely is shown in Fig. 2. Thymidine uptake was increased in the presence of suxamethoni-

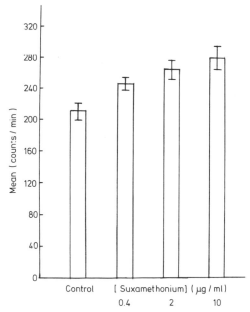

Fig. 2. Lymphocyte transformation test in a patient with "allergy" to suxamethonium (uptake of ^3H-thymidine, means $\pm$ standard errors)

um and a dose–response relationship was noticed, but the increase in thymidine uptake was not statistically significant. One of the problems which could account for the weak response is the need to add serum. We add autologous serum to tissue culture medium (10%). The presence of serum and the prolonged incubation with lymphocytes would lead to the breakdown of suxamethonium.

IV. Serum IgE Measurements

Total serum IgE in all the patients we investigated was normal (even though some had established allergy, particularly to the common inhalant allergens). Serial measurements of serum IgE in individual patients after their reaction to muscle relaxants did not show the pattern (a temporary peak after the reaction) which might have been considered compatible with the diagnosis of immediate allergy.

D. Mechanism of Reactions to Depolarising Agents (Suxamethonium)

Further studies are needed to elucidate the mechanism of these reactions. To us, it appears that depolarising agents are capable of initiating an immune response. This conclusion is based entirely on clinical grounds.

I. Clues From Case Histories and Other Clinical Findings

We had noted, particularly with suxamethonium, that the reactions in a significant proportion of the affected patients did not occur on first exposure, but occurred with subsequent exposures (Assem 1977). This suggested an immunological mechanism. The clinical manifestations were not limited to "immediate" reactions (cardiovascular collapse, asthma, acute angioedema, etc.) but often extended to rather delayed reactions, occurring 0.5–24 h after exposure, and including facial or more widespread oedema and skin rash. These could not be explained on the basis of direct (non-immune) histamine release, which is usually immediate. They are possibly due to immune mechanisms other than anaphylaxis. Complement activation (classical and alternative pathways) via immune mechanisms is likely to be involved in these reactions. However, direct (non-immune) activation of the alternative pathway by neuromuscular blocking drugs cannot be ruled out (Watkins 1979; Watkins et al. 1978).

The case history and other clinical manifestations in some of the patients with reactions to suxamethonium leaves little doubt that allergy can develop in response to the administration of this agent, which is an acetylcholine analogue. The acute reaction in these cases was therefore very likely to have been due to typical IgE-mediated anaphylaxis. Cases of similar reactions have been reported by other authors, e.g. Jerums et al. (1967), Royston and Wilkes (1978). This aspect, the immune reaction to succinylcholine is considered so fundamentally important as to warrant full consideration. The preliminary studies of Hadji and Benveniste (1980) suggest that sensitization of guinea-pigs to suxamethonium can be induced by repeated injection.

II. Immunochemical Considerations on the Nature of the Allergen

Before considering the mechanism of the assumed immunological reaction, one should mention some of the properties of suxamethonium. This compound acts like acetylcholine to produce depolarisation of the post-synaptic membrane. Like all depolarising relaxants, suxamethonium is water soluble, ionised, and relatively fat insoluble. It does not possess the three-dimensional molecular rigidity of the non-depolarising relaxants, although the presence of two positively charged terminal groups keeps the molecule in a straight chain.

Regarding the possible immune mechanisms (including anaphylaxis) which appear to be involved in the reaction of some patients to suxamethonium, I believe that one particular feature of the chemical structure appears to be relevant. This drug, as shown in Fig. 1, resembles two molecules of acetylcholine joined together. This raises the possibility of this compound acting as a bivalent allergen, however remote this possibility might be. A further implication of this hypothesis is that the endogenous neurotransmitter acetylcholine might act as a hapten, and may, therefore, be potentially capable of inhibiting this reaction.

Thus, it is the drug itself and not its metabolites which seems to trigger the reaction. The usual situation in other drug allergies is that the metabolites of the drug act as haptens. They become complete antigens only after forming polyvalent (at least bivalent) conjugates with macromolecules such as proteins. Suxamethonium, which is succinyldicholine, is rapidly metabolised by serum cholinesterase to succinylmonocholine and choline. Succinylmonocholine is broken down at a slower rate (one sixth that of succinyldicholine) to succinic acid and choline. A small proportion (10%) of suxamethonium is excreted unchanged in urine.

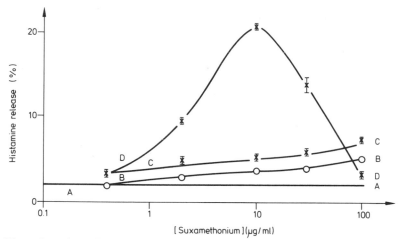

Fig. 3. Histamine release from the leucocytes of a patient with "allergy" to suxamethonium. Effect of serum (10%) on suxamethonium-induced histamine release. A = control; B = suxamethonium + normal serum; C = suxamethonium + patient's serum; D = suxamethonium alone

III. Leucocyte Histamine Release by Suxamethonium

It is quite possible that succinylmonocholine (a monovalent hapten) could react to form appropriate conjugates. However, suxamethonium itself is capable of eliciting good response in both skin and leucocyte tests, as revealed by histamine release.

1. Effect of Serum

Substantial release of histamine from basophil leucocytes could be elicited by suxamethonium in the absence of serum. The addition of serum to suxamethonium during leucocyte challenge would lead to rapid metabolism. We compared the effect of autologous serum from suxamethonium-reactive individuals with homologous serum from normal individuals (Fig. 3). The presence of normal serum in a 10% concentration completely abolished the release of histamine by suxamethonium from a patient's leucocytes. The patient's own serum had an almost identical effect. In fact, this patient's serum was found to have low cholinesterase activity, which might have accounted for the small response in the lymphocyte transformation test.

2. Dose–Response Relationships

In our patients dose–response curves were constructed in order to see if histamine release induced by neuromuscular blocking drugs could give curves similar to those obtained with typical allergens. Figure 4 shows one example. It can be seen that histamine release by suxamethonium from the leucocytes of a patient, who seemed to have developed immediate allergy to this agent following previous exposure, gave a bell-shaped curve, with drug excess producing even complete inhibition of histamine release. This inhibition, as in the case of a typical allergen, can be ex-

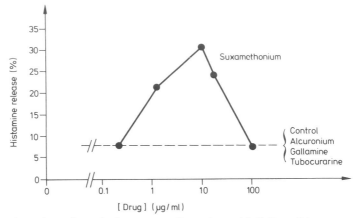

Fig. 4. Histamine release from the leucocytes of a patient with "allergy" to suxamethonium. Note the shape of the dose–response curve for suxamethonium and the lack of response to the other muscle relaxants

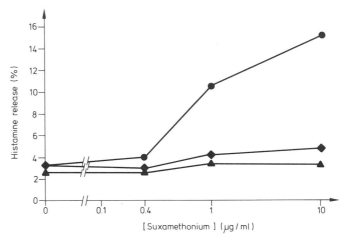

Fig. 5. Histamine release from the leucocytes of a patient with "allergy" to suxamethonium. Effect of calcium and acetylcholine on suxamethonium-induced histamine release. *Circles* = Ca^{2+}-containing Tyrode solution; *diamonds* = Ca^{2+}-free Tyrode solution; *triangles* = Ca^{2+}-containing Tyrode sulution + 5 µg/ml acetylcholine

plained by monovalent binding of the drug (allergen) to cell-fixed anaphylactic antibodies. As a result of failing to "bridge" adjacent antibody molecules, and hence failing to induce the appropriate conformational changes in the Fc region (the COOH terminal region of the heavy polypeptide chain which has a constant amino acid sequence for a given immunoglobulin class) histamine release could not be elicited.

It could be argued that inhibition by drug excess does not necessarily mean that the drug acts as a true allergen, but possibly as a histamine releaser. However, to be able to obtain complete inhibition with a histamine releaser would be very unusual.

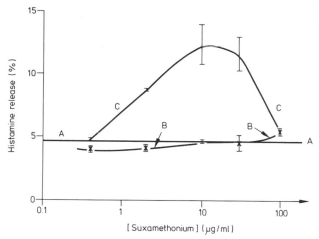

Fig. 6. Histamine release (means ± standard errors) from the leucocytes of a patient with "allergy" to suxamethonium. Effect of (+)-tubocurarine on the suxamethonium-induced histamine release. A = control; B = suxamethonium + 50 μg/ml (+)-tubocurarine; C = suxamethonium alone

3. Effect of Acetylcholine on the Response to Suxamethonium

If suxamethonium acted as a bivalent allergen, it would be expected that acetylcholine would behave at least as a weak hapten, and that it would inhibit the response (histamine release) to suxamethonium. Figure 5 shows the result of adding acetylcholine to suxamethonium. In this experiment, a low concentration of acetylcholine (5 μg/ml) completely inhibited suxamethonium-induced histamine release from the leucocytes of a patient. It should be added that the specificity of inhibition by acetylcholine was confirmed by the lack of an inhibitory effect of acetylcholine on histamine release from human leucocytes induced by other allergens.

It is of interest to see if the inhibitory effect of acetylcholine could be blocked with acetylcholine antagonists. The experiments carried out so far have shown that muscarinic antagonists such as atropine do not block the inhibitory effect of acetylcholine. The effect of nicotinic antagonists was difficult to disentangle, as explained in Sect. D.III.4.

4. Effect of Non-Depolarising Blockers on Histamine Release by Suxamethonium

Histamine release by suxamethonium was inhibited not only with acetylcholine, as mentioned above, but also with nicotinic antagonists. These findings (Fig. 6) suggest that histamine release by suxamethonium is related to its pharmacological site of action at nicotinic receptors. This may be in favour of reaction and histamine release, both being due to idiosyncrasy rather than to allergy, but it is extremely difficult to draw definite conclusions.

5. Effect of Calcium on Histamine Release

Histamine release by antigen always requires calcium. This was shown in guinea-pig and rat tissues (MONGAR and SCHILD 1958) and in human and rabbit basophil leucocytes (Lichtenstein and Osler 1964; Greaves and Mongar 1968). By contrast, direct histamine release, though calcium dependent with certain histamine releasers, may not be so with certain organic bases, e.g. compound 48/80. It certainly is not calcium dependent with some other histamine releasers, e.g. the bee venom polypeptide 401 (Assem and Atkinson 1973; Atkinson et al. 1979).

Experiments were carried out to see if suxamethonium-induced histamine release in the susceptible individuals was calcium dependent. Figure 5 shows that in the absence of calcium histamine release by suxamethonium was completely inhibited. Had it not been the case, one would have been certain that the reaction was not immunologically mediated. Thus, the calcium dependence of histamine release with suxamethonium in this patient was inconclusive, i.e., it did not contribute much to the further analysis of the mechanism, as to whether suxamethonium acts as an allergen or as a histamine releaser.

IV. Histamine Release as a Manifestation of Idiosyncrasy

Smith (1957) described cases of reactions to suxamethonium and other muscle relaxants, which occurred on the first exposure to these drugs, and therefore, could only be explained by "direct" histamine release. That many drugs or other chemicals can act as histamine releasers has been known for a long time (Paton 1957). The review by Paton (1957) included neuromuscular blocking drugs. However, the most relevant question which has not been answered so far is: why should some patients react so adversely to those agents in the absence of evidence of allergy?

As previously mentioned, a significant proportion (possibly 20%–50%) of the reactions to suxamethonium we encountered were compatible with true allergy, but the remaining cases, as well as the great majority of reactions to non-depolarising neuromuscular blockers, are almost certainly not due to allergy. However, in those patients in whom allergy seemed extremely unlikely, histamine release from basophil leucocytes could be elicited in vitro with one or more of those agents, while no such reaction has been demonstrated in normal individuals. Thus, most of the patients reacting to neuromuscular blocking drugs in an anaphylactic-like manner show histamine release from their leucocytes as an associated phenomenon. Both of these phenomena are likely to be manifestations of an underlying common abnormality.

We know very little about the underlying abnormality in those patients which renders them susceptible to acute and potentially fatal reactions. A history of asthma and allergy is frequent in those patients. The condition may be genetically determined, and any patient with a suspected family history of reaction to those agents should be investigated prior to exposure. This is the only way to prevent these potentially fatal reactions.

E. Mechanism of Reactions to Non-Depolarising Agents

I. General Structural Features Associated with Histamine Release

The release of histamine, particularly with non-depolarising blockers, can be explained by the effect of the positively charged quaternary ammonium group, in a

way similar to many simple cationic chemicals. PATON (1957) suggested the importance of the following structural features as favouring optimal histamine release:
1. Sufficient spacing between the two charged groups (present in most of these compounds, but some of them have three of these groups)
2. Substituted aromatic ring structure
3. Large bulk of these groups.

The chemical specificity of the reaction differs in different patients. Thus, a patient with idiosyncrasy may have it specifically against non-depolarising blockers, but not with depolarising agents, and vice versa. A patient with idiosyncrasy to a certain non-depolarising agent or more than one of those agents may be quite safe with yet another member of the same pharmacological group (ASSEM 1977).

Several semisynthetic derivatives of curare (e.g., methylcurare, toxiferine and diallylnortoxiferine, alcuronium) have been produced, and have been shown to be less potent as inducers of wheal and flare reactions in the skin, and of histamine release (FOLDES et al. 1961; FELDMAN 1973). Nevertheless, none of them is totally inactive as an inducer of wheal and flare reactions in the skin of everybody. Also, none of them is free from the risk of inducing reactions in susceptible individuals. Furthermore, some of those compounds which have been claimed to be virtually free from histamine releasing activity, such as alcuronium, proved to be relatively more potent in eliciting histamine release from leucocytes (ASSEM 1977).

The incidence of reaction to pancuronium was less than with other non-depolarising muscle relaxants. McDOWELL and CLARKE (1969) reported the lack of histamine release by pancuronium in guinea-pigs, cats, and humans. NANA et al. (1972) had gone further in their conclusions by suggesting that pancuronium was the best muscle relaxant for asthmatic patients. Though we agree that pancuronium is one of the safest non-depolarising agents, we have reported a few reactions to that muscle relaxant (ASSEM 1977). HEATH (1973) also reported one patient similar to ours.

II. Relation of Leucocyte Histamine Release to Skin Wheal and Flare Responses and Related Phenomena

The abnormal release of histamine from susceptible patients may or may not be related to the ability of non-depolarising muscle relaxants to elicit wheal and flare responses in the skin. It may, however, be an abnormal extension of the histamine-releasing activity of those compounds which had been demonstrated in various species, in different tissue and cell preparations (PATON 1957). In fact, the earliest reports of such an activity were concerned with a histamine-releasing effect in skeletal muscle (ALAM et al. 1939; COMROE and DRIPPS 1946).

III. Calcium Dependence of Histamine Release

We found the requirements for the idiosyncratic histamine release from leucocytes to be similar to antigen-induced response. The effect of calcium is illustrated in Figs. 7 and 8. Histamine release was completely inhibited in the absence of calcium. Work with conventional histamine releasers has not given uniform results. For example, with compound 48/80, omission of calcium blocked the histamine-releasing

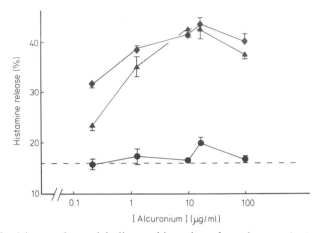

Fig. 7. Effect of calcium and acetylcholine on histamine release (means ± standard errors) by alcuronium in a patient with idiosyncrasy to non-depolarising neuromuscular blockers. *Broken line* = control; *circles* = without Ca^{2+}; *diamonds* = with Ca^{2+}; *triangles* = with Ca^{2+} and 10 μg/ml acetylcholine

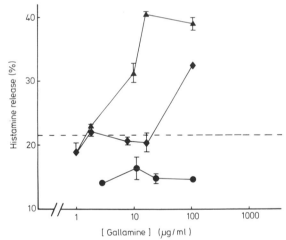

Fig. 8. Effect of calcium and acetylcholine on histamine release (means ± standard errors) by gallamine from the leucocytes of a patient with idiosyncrasy to some of the non-depolarising neuromuscular blockers. *Broken line* = control; *circles* = without Ca^{2+}; *triangles* = with Ca^{2+}; *diamonds* = with Ca^{2+} and 50 μg/ml acetylcholine

activity in rat tissues, but not from isolated rat peritoneal mast cells or guinea-pig lung. These findings suggest that compound 48/80 might release histamine by a different mechanism from antigen, though both initiate a sequence of events that produces a rather selective increase in the permeability of mast cells. For further reference regarding the role of calcium in histamine release, the review by FOREMAN et al. (1976) is recommended. The role of calcium, in the release of neurotransmitter substances and hormones reviewed by RUBIN (1970) is also recommended. Calcium is essential for stimulus–secretion coupling in various secretory processes, including histamine secretion in true anaphylactic reactions, histamine release by certain releasers, and in excitation–contraction coupling in muscles of all types.

IV. Effect of Acetylcholine on Histamine Release by Non-Depolarising Agents

The inhibitory effect of acetylcholine demonstrated with anaphylactic histamine release, particularly by suxamethonium (Fig. 5), was not so clearly demonstrated in histamine release induced by non-depolarising blockers (Figs. 7 and 8), which is usually an expression of idiosyncrasy. However, it should be born in mind when making such a comparison that both acetylcholine and succinylcholine are rapidly broken down, while non-depolarising agents generally are metabolished relatively slowly.

V. Relation Between Allergy and Idiosyncrasy

The connection between allergy, or alternative immunopathological mechanisms, and the idiosyncratic response is far from clear at present, and so is the role of genetic or acquired abnormalities in the complement system. One possible abnormality is the predisposition to C3 conversion with various drugs in the same person, leading to the production of C3a (anaphylatoxin), which in turn causes histamine release (WATKINS et al. 1978; WATKINS 1979; see also the review by WHITWAM 1978).

Although those complement factors could possibly operate in vivo, they cannot explain the abnormal response of isolated patients' leucocytes in vitro, which is shown by the substantial release of histamine that we have clearly demonstrated. The possibility that leucocyte-fixed complement components might trigger that response seems remote at present. The abnormal histamine release is due to an inherent abnormality in these cells; it resembles secretory processes and is due either to an extreme exaggeration of a normal response, or to a qualitatively abnormal response.

References

Alam M, Anrep GV, Barsoum GS, Talaat M, Wieninger E (1939) Liberation of histamine from the skeletal muscle by curare. J Physiol (Lond) 95:148–158

Assem ESK (1977) Examples of the correlation between the structure of certain groups of drugs and adverse effects mediated by immune and non-immune mechanisms (with particular reference to muscle relaxants and steroid anaesthetics). In: Bundgaard H, Juul P, Kofod H (eds) Drug design and adverse reactions. Munksgaard, Copenhagen, pp 209–226

Assem ESK, Atkinson G (1973) Histamine release by MCDP (401), a peptide from the venom of the honey bee. Br J Pharmacol 48:337–338P

Assem ESK, Frost PG, Levis RD (1981) Anaphylactic-like reaction to suxamethonium. Anaesthesia 36:405–410

Atkinson G, Ennis M, Pearce FL (1979) The effect of alkaline earth cations on the release of histamine from rat peritoneal mast cells treated with compound 48/80 and peptide 401. Br J Pharmacol 65:395–402

Clark SW, Glaubiger GA, La Du B (1968) Properties of plasma cholinesterase variants. Ann NY Acad Sci 151:710–722

Comroe JH Jr, Dripps RD (1946) The histamine-like action of curare and tubocurarine injected intracutaneously and intra-arterially in man. Anesthesiology 7:260–262

Feldman SA (1973) Muscle relaxants. Saunders, Philadelphia London

Foldes FF, Wolfson B, Sokoll M (1961) The use of toxiferine for the production of surgical relaxation. Anesthesiology 22:93–99

Foreman JC, Garland LG, Mongar JL (1976) The role of calcium in secretory processes: model studies in mast cells. In: Duncan CJ (ed) Calcium in biological systems. Society for Experimental Biology, Symposium XXX. Cambridge University Press, Cambridge, pp 193–218

Greaves MW, Mongar JL (1968) The mechanism of anaphylactic histamine release from rabbit leucocytes. Immunology 15:743–749

Hadji L, Benveniste J (1980) Experimental cardiac anaphylaxis to an anaesthetic adjuvant as a model for drug allergy. Allergol Immunopathol (Madr) 8:485–486

Jerums G, Whittingham S, Wilson P (1967) Anaphylaxis to suxamethonium. A case report. Br J Anaesth 39:73–77

Heath M (1973) Bronchospasm in an asthmatic patient following pancuronium. Anaesthesia 28:437–440

Kalow W (1962) Pharmacogenetics. Heredity and response to drugs. Saunders, Philadelphia London

Kalow W, Gunn DR (1957) The relation between dose of succinylcholine and duration of apnoea in man. J Pharmacol Exp Ther 120:203–214

Lichtenstein LM, Osler AG (1964) Studies on the mechanisms of hypersensitivity phenomena, IX. Histamine release from human leucocytes by ragweed pollen antigen. J Exp Med 120:507–530

Lorenz W, Doenicke A (1978) Anaphylactoid reactions and histamine release by intravenous drugs used in surgery and anaesthesia. In: Watkins J, Ward AM (eds) Adverse response to intravenous drugs. Academic Press, London; Grune & Stratton, New York, pp 83–112

Lorenz W, Doenicke A, Meyer R et al. (1972) Histamine release in man by propranidid and thiopentone: pharmacological effects and clinical consequences. Br J Anaesth 44:355–368

McDowell SA, Clarke RSJ (1969) A clinical comparison of pancuronium with d-tubocurarine. Anaesthesia 24:581–590

Mongar JL, Schild HO (1958) The effect of calcium and pH on the anaphylactic reactions. J Physiol (Lond) 140:272–284

Mongar JL, Whelan RF (1953) Histamine release by adrenaline and d-turbocurarine in the human subject. J Physiol (Lond) 120:146–154

Nana A, Cardan E, Leitersdorfer T (1972) Pancuronium bromide, its use in asthmatics and patients with liver disease. Anaesthesia 27:154–158

Paton WDM (1957) Histamine release by compounds of simple chemical structure. Pharmacol Rev 9:269–328

Rawlins MD, Thompson JW (1977) Pathogenesis of adverse drug reactions. In: Davies DM (ed) Textbook of adverse drug reactions. Oxford University Press, Oxford New York Toronto, pp 10–31

Royston D, Wilkes RG (1978) True anaphylaxis to suxamethonium chloride. Br J Anaesth 50:611–615

Rubin RP (1970) The role of calcium in the release of neurotransmitter substances and hormones. Pharmacol Rev 22:389–428

Silk E, King J, Whittaker M (1979) Assay of cholinesterase in clinical chemistry. Ann Clin Biochem 16:57–75

Smith NL (1957) Histamine release by suxamethonium. Anaesthesia 12:293–298

Vervloet MD, Arnaud A, Vellieux P, Kaplanski S, Charpin J (1979) Anaphylactic reactions to muscle relaxants under general anesthesia. J Allergy Clin Immunol 63:348–353

Watkins J (1979) Anaphylactoid reactions to intravenous substances. Br J Anaesth 51:51–60

Watkins J, Padfield A, Alderson JD (1978) Underlying immunopathology as a cause of adverse responses to two intravenous agents. Br Med J 1:1180–1181

Whitwam JG (1978) Adverse reactions to i.v. induction agents. Br J Anaesth 50:677–687

CHAPTER 13

Drugs Used Topically

K. E. ANDERSEN and H. I. MAIBACH

A. Epidemiology

The epidemiology of allergic reactions to topical medicaments is poorly documented. Limited information is available. A prospective normal volunteer population study from San Francisco, comprising 1158 adult volunteers (PRYSTOWSKY et al. 1979 a), showed a prevalence of positive reactions to patch tests with nickel (5.8%), neomycin (1.1%), ethylenediamine (0.43%), and benzocaine (0.17%). A survey in Copenhagen, encompassing female hospital inpatients, on a single day gave results for nickel in the same range (MENNÉ 1978).

Studies of contact dermatitis patient populations in dermatology clinics overestimate the prevalence of sensitivity of the general population to medicaments. BANDMANN et al. (1972) found 14% of 4,000 eczema patients had dermatitis from applied medicaments, equaling one-third of patiens with allergic contact dermatitis. The most frequent allergens were neomycin and benzocaine. Patients over 40 years old had medicament dermatitis more frequently than younger persons; the dermatitis was particularly frequent in departments treating stasis dermatitis and including patch tests in their management. The incidence of sensitivity to individual medicaments differed from country to country, because of variations in prescription and self-medication habits. Comparing patch test results from 163 patients with stasis dermatitis to the results from 119 patients with other eczematous conditions, DOOMS-GOOSSENS et al. (1980 a, b) found significantly more positive patch tests to medicaments in the group of stasis dermatis patients. Retesting of 50 stasis dermatitis patients 3–25 months later showed a marked decrease in the number of positive patch tests related to a reduced contact with the responsible allergens and less "irritable skin" as their dermatitis improved. We emphasize the importance of distinguishing between studies based on contact dermatitis patient populations and studies based on a normal volunteer population. The latter may aid decision making concerning the safety of consumer products intended for use by a population with normal skin.

RUDZKI and ZAKRZEWSKI (1975) calculated the "index of sensitization" for 12 topically used drugs on the basis of the occurrence of sensitivity and the number of prescriptions filled. The highest sensitization index was found for balsam of Peru and benzocaine.

The bulk of information about allergic reactions to topically used drugs comes from case reports, though two Swedish monographs; on hand dermatitis in Malmöhus County (AGRUP 1969) and irritancy reactions in patients with hand eczema (BJÖRNBERG 1968) give important information about epidemiology of contact dermatitis and the underlying mechanisms.

Predictive contact dermatitis biologic assays in the guinea pig and in human volunteers provide insight into the sensitization potential of chemicals. The techniques employed derive from the assays proposed by DRAIZE et al. (1944); an expanding literature documents modifications and standardization (MAGNUSSON and KLIGMAN 1977 a, b; KLECAK 1977; MARZULLI and MAIBACH 1977 b). It is possible to disclose sensitization potential experimentally in guinea pigs and humans to all but the weakest of allergens. These tests only disclose potential; considerable judgment must be utilized in extrapolating this to the product use situation, as many factors (dose–response relationships, type of application, vehicle, normal versus abnormal skin, acute versus chronic exposure, etc.), must be taken into consideration. Negative results with exaggerated test procedures are encouraging; positive assays do not in themselves preclude further human use without careful consideration of the benefit and risk. The investigator has many techniques to choose from and should develop considerable experience in a laboratory where these are frequently performed to choose and execute the assays prudently and interpret the results sensibly (MARZULLI and MAIBACH 1977 a).

B. Clinical Aspects of Contact Allergy

In recent years, the clinical aspect of contact allergy has broadened, as our understanding of pathogenetic mechanisms has improved, concomitant with more frequent use of patch testing. Besides the classical allergic contact dermatitis, new clinical entities representing unexpected morphology and different pathomechanisms have arisen:

1) Pigmented allergic contact dermatitis as described by OSMUNDSEN (1970 a). A similar clinical picture occurs in Asians, caused mainly by colors and fragrances (NAKAYAMA et al. 1974), and appears similar to Riehl's melanosis with pruritic pigmented skin without eczematous changes (SUGAI et al. 1977).

2) Erythema multiforme (EM) provoked by external contact with a chemical (ROED-PETERSEN 1975; DE FEO 1966). This entity will easily be missed if not considered. EM caused by ophthalmic preparations has been reported several times (GOTTSHALK and STONE 1976; RUBIN 1977; GUILL et al. 1979).

3) Noneczematous exanthemas: (SPOTT and SHELLEY 1970).

4) Contact dermatitis complicated by systemic symptoms, e. g. acute laryngeal obstruction (MAIBACH 1975 a), gastrointestinal symptoms (MATHIAS et al. 1979 b), and paresthesia (FISHER 1979).

5) Photosensitivity reactions are diagnosed with increasing frequency because dermatologists are alerted to morphology, anatomic distribution, and photopatch testing methods.

6) Contact urticaria of the immunologic or nonimmunologc nature (MAIBACH and JOHNSON 1975) occurs from numerous sources as summarized by ODOM and MAIBACH (1977). Three major etiologic subdivisions of the syndrome exist. Nonimmunologic causes (e. g., dimethylsulfoxide or histamine), immunologic (immediate hypersensitivity), and unknown (ammonium persulfate). Nonimmunologic contact urticaria has recently been investigated in more detail (LAHTI 1980). Common additives in foods and drugs as benzoic acid, sodium benzoate, sorbic acid, cinna-

mic acid, balsam of Peru, acetic acid, ethyl alcohol, butyric acid, and butyl alcohol frequently produce immediate skin reactions.

7) Subjective and objective irritation must be mentioned in this context because they constitute the major differential diagnosis, which emphasizes the importance of patch testing. Subjective irritation refers to invisible changes: burning, stinging, itching, and discomfort (MATHIAS and MAIBACH 1978).

8) Miscellaneous clinical entities include: allergic contact granulomas from zirconium (FISHER 1973), lichenoid eruptions from color developers (FRY 1965; ROED-PETERSEN and MENNÉ 1976), and contact purpura from *p*-phenylenediamine (SHMUNES 1978).

C. Immunochemical, Pharmaceutical, and Pharmacologic Aspects

The immunologic aspects of allergic reactions to contactants are complex, but our understanding of pathogenesis has improved, concomitant with the development of immunology as such. We refer the reader to POLAK's (1977) recent review on delayed hypersenitivity.

Regarding the pharmaceutical aspects of contact allergy, impurities often occur in supposedly pure compounds, making patch testing a difficult task, requiring experience to interpret test reactions and to choose substances for testing (AGRUP et al. 1969). Examples of impurities include benzocaine in sun tan preparations (Escalol 106, glyceryl PABA; FISHER 1977); formaldehyde in preservatives (DAHL-QUIST and FREGERT 1978); and low molecular weight resins in "pure" high molecular weight resins.

Of similar importance is distinguishing between allergy to tests with isolated purified substances, and allergy to tests with finished preparations. In the latter case, testing often gives false negative reactions due to too low concentration of the allergen or inhibition of the allergen by other ingredients (MAJETI and SUSKIND 1977), e. g., cinnamaldehyde sensitization inhibited by the presence of eugenol. On the other hand, testing with finished preparations, e. g. soaps and toothpaste, generally gives false positive reactions because of the occlusive patching of these primary irritants.

The value of testing with ingredients separately in a suitable concentration and vehicle is emphasized. Patch testing is the most important tool in evaluation of skin reactions to topical medicaments. The International Contact Dermatitis Research Group (ICDRG) uses a standard test tray of 20 substances, proven frequent causes of allergic contact dermatitis (RECOMMENDATION 1973). Patch test screening with the tray only supplements patch testing with suspected environmental agents. Troublesome and time-consuming correspondence with manufacturers is often necessary to reveal the composition of finished preparations and products. Medicaments constitute an exception because many countries require package labeling with all ingredients in the product.

To find a suitable concentration and vehicle for patch testing with different substances, the reader is referred to the standard dermatology textbooks, e. g., (FREGERT and HJORTH 1979; BANDMANN and DOHN 1967; FREGERT and BAND-MANN 1975; MALTEN et al. 1976; FISHER 1973; CRONIN 1980). The technical problems and pitfalls in patch testing are dealt with in these texts.

D. Diagnostic Tests

Today, patch testing is a sound, viable method for identifying allergens responsible for contact dermatitis. The technique was standardized 15 years ago by Scandinavian dermatologists (Magnusson and Hersle 1965; Magnusson et al. 1969) and subsequently expanded and popularized by the International Contact Dermatitis Research Group (ICDRG) and the North American Contact Dermatitis Research Group (NACDRG). Patch testing remains a bioassay requiring considerable experience to execute and interpret properly. Basically, a patch test implies the application to the skin of a certain amount of the suspected allergen in a suitable concentration and vehicle. The test site is occluded with an impermeable system for 24–48 h (48 h is recommended by ICDRG and NACDRG). Commercially available test units facilitate this testing. Currently the AL-Test (Imeco, Sweden), Finn Chamber (Epitest, Finland), and Silver Patch (van der Bend, Holland) are most widely used.

The patient's skin condition, vehicles, concentration of test substance, volume of test material, test site, time and the number of readings influence the result. Mistakes are easily made. Textbooks on dermatology and contact dermatitis detail the technique and pitfalls. Hjorth (1977) published a comprehensive review of diagnostic patch testing.

The risk of false positive and false negative patch test reactions is emphasized. A false negative patch test leaves the patient with his contact allergy undetected, while a false positive patch test leaves the dermatologist with the problem of interpretation. Correct interpretation can be facilitated by re-tests and or usage tests (see below in this section). The range of individual susceptibility to skin irritation makes it difficult to establish the "correct" recommended concentration for patch testing (Kligman and Leyden 1979). To compare patch test results from different investigators the ICDRG has systematized the terminology of contact dermatitis and recording of results (Wilkinson et al. 1970). The use of the following signs are recommendend: NT = not tested; ?+ = doubtful reaction; + = weak reaction (nonvesicular, slightly infiltrated or edematous); + + = strong reaction (edematous or vesicular); and + + + = extreme reaction.

The inherent risks and side effects of patch testing can be minimized by proper technique. In vitro tests (e.g., lymphocyte transformation test) demonstrate lymphocyte-mediated contact allergy in humans, (Veien and Svejgaard 1978). These tests are important research tools, but the practical clinical value for the patient at this moment is limited because of their logistic complexity.

Other test methods include open testing, where absorption of the test material is not increased by occlusion. This test minimizes occlusion-induced irritancy. The test material is applied to the patient's back or forearm as in the closed patch test. The results are read in a similar way to the closed test. A positive open test reaction can usually be regarded as a sign of allergy while negative reactions do not exclude allergy. The open test can be recommended when a high degree of sensitivity is suspected and for unknown substances.

A variant of the open patch test is the *provocative test* or *product use* test, where the patient applies a suspected topical preparation repeatedly to the forearm or cubital fossa for approximately 7 days. This is also a useful method to determine whether a patient can tolerate a certain topical preparation. Use test (provocative test) reactions are often mild even with continued application of the antigen; when neomycin in ointment and cream base was evaluated, the cream base reactions occurred earlier and were more intense (PRYSTOWSKY et al. 1979 b). The result of a provocative test is dependent on the skin area tested. Glutaraldehyde 25% in water was tolerated on the soles of six allergic subjects, while a 2.5% solution applied to the antecubital fossa gave a positive test (MAIBACH and PRYSTOWSKY 1977).

Intradermal testing is rarely indicated in practical patient-related work, but has been used for certain sensitizers such as neomycin and penicillin, which are minimally absorbed through intact skin. As a general rule, concentrations for intracutaneous tests are one-tenth to one-hundredth the dose used in the patch test.

Testing for immediate reactions has attracted attention recently, with the recognition of contact urticaria and protein dermatitis. The techniques include reading after 20 min of closed and open patch tests, prick or scratch testing, and testing of involved or uninvolved skin (MAIBACH and JOHNSON 1975; ODOM and MAIBACH 1977; HJORTH and ROED-PETERSEN 1976).

Photopatch testing uses the same principles as testing for ordinary contact dermatitis (FISHER 1973 a, p 207). (1) Patch tests are applied in duplicate under an opaque covering preventing light from reaching the test site; (2) after 24 h the covering is removed from one of the two rows of patch tests, which are subsequently irradiated from a UVA (320–400 nm wavelength) light source; (3) after 48 h, all tests are evaluated. Details of the technique are in standard textbooks (e.g., HJORTH and FREGERT 1979). The time of irradiation of the patch tests might be crucial, as found recently for photosensitivity to 6-methylcoumarin (HOLDER 1978). Only irradiation immediately after application gave a positive response. Although most reactions are UVA mediated, UVB (290–320 nm wavelength) must be considered if UVA does not produce a positive response in clinically suspected patients.

E. Anti-Psoriasis Agents

I. Tar

Tar, the oldest remedy for psoriasis is effective and relatively safe. Side effects, i.e., folliculitis and irritation, occur frequently, while carcinomas are rare. The risk of carcinoma development appears to be vehicle dependent, i.e., alcoholic tar preparations are more carcinogenic than petrolatum preparations (ZACKHEIM 1978 a). Until 1967, 13 cases of skin cancer, induced by topical tar treatment, were documented (GREITHER et al. 1967). Photosensitivity, one mechanism of action, is a phototoxic effect; photoallergy has been reported, but might be missed (STARKE and JILLSON 1961). Contact allergy to tar preparations is quite uncommon (RUDZKI and GRZYWA 1977 b). We have no quantitative epidemiology on allergy to tar.

II. Dithranol

Dithranol (anthralin, cignolin) is a mandatory irritant in psoriasis therapy. Staining of clothes, skin, nails, and hair are frequent and should be explained to patients. An unusual cutaneous anthralin-like staining of the perineum may follow use of danthrone, as a laxative. Danthrone (1,8-dihydroxyanthroquinone) is closely re lated to dithranol (1,8,9-anthracenetriol). Contact allergy has not been reported.

III. Corticosteroids

Topical Corticosteroids are the most widely used drugs in psoriasis. Contact allergy is uncommon, but should be considered in long-standing and resistant eczematous psoriasis. TEGNER (1976) reviewed the literature noting that the patch testing concentration should be higher than in the commercial product. Corticosteroid topical allergy is described in detail in Sect. L.

IV. Salicylic Acid

$$COOH$$
$$OH$$

Psoriasis preparations may contain salicylic acid, a rare sensitizer (five cases (RUDZKI and KOSLOWSKA 1976). Four of the patients used salicylic acid 2% in alcohol. They tolerated oral acetylsalicylic acid (aspirin) without causing exacerbation or relapse of the dermatitis.

V. Mechlorethamine

$$CH_3-N(CH_2CH_2Cl)_2$$

Mechlorethamine is a nitrogen mustard which is used in psoriasis. TAYLOR and HALPRIN (1972) sensitized 34 of 57 patients treated; attempts to induce immunologic tolerance were unsuccessful. A woman with mycosis fungoides developed an urticarial and anaphylactoid reaction immediately after a total body surface application of nitrogen mustard (DAUGHTERS et al. 1973). She received at least 100 applications prior to this reaction, which waned after an antihistamine injection. Immediate sensitivity to nitrogen mustard may not be rare (GRUNNET 1976).

VI. 6-Aminonicotinamide

$$H_2N \quad N$$
$$CONH_2$$

Topical application of 6-aminonicotinamide can clear psoriasis. Apparent hypersensitivity occurred in 1 of 34 patients (ZACKHEIM 1978 b), while others showed irritation. Human usage is too minimal to permit a general statement of sensitization frequency.

VII. Thioxolone

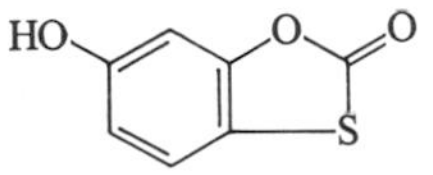

HO O O
S

Thioxolone, a benzoxathiole derivative has been used for local treatment of scalp psoriasis resulting in four cases of scalp and face dermatitis. Whether these cases were allergic or irritant was not shown (SCHOEFFINIUS 1972); this chemical sensitized one patient using it for acne treatment (WAHLBERG 1971).

VIII. 1,8,9-Triacetoxyanthracene

1,8,9-Triacetoxyanthracene is less irritating than anthralin. Delayed skin reactions have been described, and ophthalmic irritation occurs (WILKINSON 1968; BRODKIN et al. 1968).

IX. Tretinoin

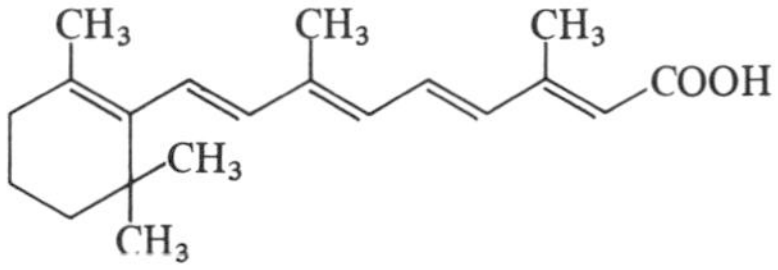

CH_3 CH_3 CH_3 COOH
CH_3
CH_3

Tretinoin, (vitamin A acid, retinoic acid,) is a counter-irritant effective in some types of acne; it is also used in psoriasis, with doubtful efficiency. Contact allergy to locally applied retinoic acid has been reported (LINDGREN et al. 1976). Patch testing with the commercial preparations containing 0.05% vitamin A acid and with vitamin A acid 0.05% in alcohol is recommended.

X. 8-Methoxypsoralen

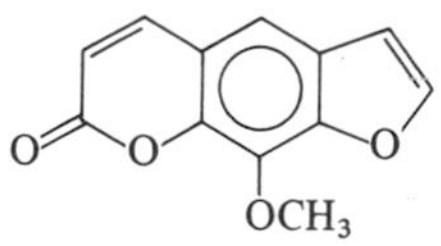

O O O
OCH_3

Treatment with 8-methoxypsoralen and UVA (PUVA) is efficient in psoriasis, but the risk of skin cancer occurring years after therapy will probably reduce the use of this approach (STERN et al. 1979). The immediate side effects from a large scale study have been reported (MELSKI 1977). Allergic reactions were not included, but recently a photoallergic dermatitis from 8-methoxypsoralen has been reported following oral administration; topical application during phototesting was positive (PLEWIG et al. 1978). Reaction occurred only with UVA: there was no photoallergy to trimethylpsoralen.

Allergic reactions from topical therapy in psoriatics create diagnostic problems, because the contact allergic lesions may look psoriasiform. Psoriasis patients have a defect in the expression of hypersensitivity (LINDHOLM et al. 1978). LINDHOLM et al. found a decreased T-lymphocyte response to stimulation with phytohemagglutinin in psoriatics.

F. Local Anesthetics

I. Benzocaine

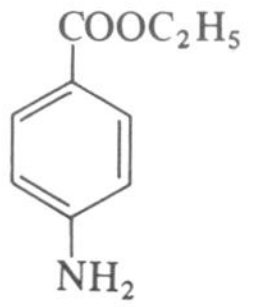

$$COOC_2H_5$$

$$NH_2$$

Benzocaine (ethyl-*p*-aminobenzoate) was for years the main culprit in allergic reactions to local anesthetics used topically. Benzocaine, derived from *p*-amino-benzoic acid (PABA), has been alleged to be a frequent sensitizer. The epidemiology of benzocaine allergy requires careful interpretation. Although it is a common cause of allergic dermatitis in dermatology clinics and a potent experimental sensitizer in guinea pigs and the human Draize test (MARZULLI and MAIBACH 1977b), testing in a normal population demonstrated a sensitization rate (0.7%) far less than with neomycin (1.1%) and nickel (5.8%) (PRYSTOWSKY et al. 1979). Whether this represents only minimal benzocaine exposure in these normals, or a discrepancy between the experimental sensitization data and actual use is not clear. Cross-reactions to other PABA derivatives often occur. The use of benzocaine topically has declined recently.

ANGELINI et al. (1975) found that 10.8% of 306 leg ulcer patients had benzocaine positive patch tests. Probably, this figure reflected a general sensitivity to substances of the "para" group and not sensitization by benzocaine itself. The "para" group contains, besides benzocaine, procaine, paraphenylenediamine, paraamino-salicylic acid, sulfanilamide, azo and aniline dyes, and PABA esters used as suntan preparations. Glyceryl PABA (Escalol 106) a widely used suntan preparation was found to be contaminated with 13% benzocaine (FISHER 1977) indicating that cross-reactions between benzocaine and glyceryl PABA (Escalol 106), might in fact be due to the presence of benzocaine in the Escalol 106. Escalol 506 (amyldimethyl PABA) and Escalol 507 (octyldimethyl PABA) do not cross react and do not contain benzocaine. Furthermore, one manufacturer of glyceryl PABA, produces commercial grade material, not producing positive patch tests in benzocaine sensitive subjects (HJORTH et al. 1978).

II. The Amide Group of Local Anesthetics

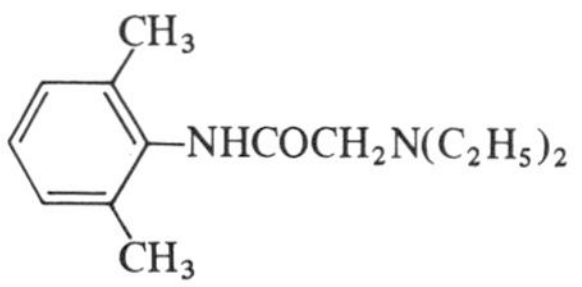

$$CH_3$$
$$-NHCOCH_2N(C_2H_5)_2$$
$$CH_3$$

Lidocaine

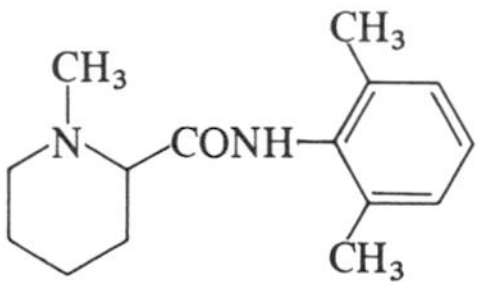

$$CH_3$$
$$N$$
$$CONH-$$
$$CH_3$$
$$CH_3$$

Mepivacaine

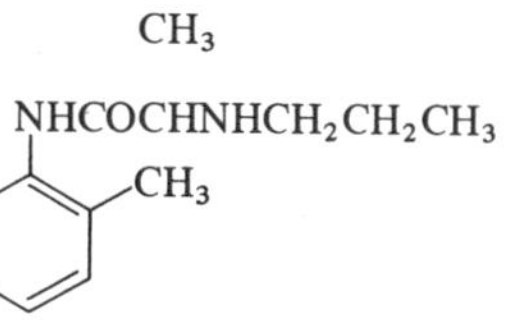

$$CH_3$$
$$NHCOCHNHCH_2CH_2CH_3$$
$$CH_3$$

Prilocaine

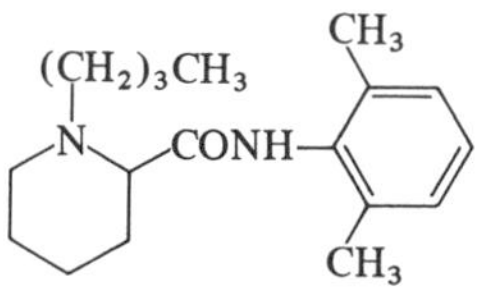

$$(CH_2)_3CH_3$$
$$N$$
$$CONH-$$
$$CH_3$$
$$CH_3$$

Bupivacaine

Cincaine structure with $O(CH_2)_3CH_3$ and $CONHCH_2CH_2N(C_2H_5)_2$, HCl

$CH_3(CH_2)_3NH-\text{⬡}-COOCH_2CH_2N(CH_3)_2$ HCl

Cincaine   Tetracaine

These local anesthetics, including lidocaine (Xylocaine), mepivacaine (Carbo-caine), Prilocaine (Citanest), and bupivacaine (Marcaine) are weak sensitizers, but allergic reactions are sporadically reported, e. g., lidocaine (TURNER 1977). Recent-ly FREGERT et al. (1979) described two patients developing lidocaine allergy after 8 and 1 month use of Xyloproct ointment (lidocaine 5%, hydrocortisone acetate); they also had positive patch tests to related amide anesthetics, both to mepivacaine, one to bupivacaine and prilocaine. A positive reaction to the chemically unrelated cincaine was interpreted as concomitant sensitivity rather than cross-sensitivity. Safe substitutes for benzocaine-sensitive patients include lidocaine, mepivacaine, prilocaine, bupivacaine, and pyrocainc (FISHER 1973 p. 312), all based on an amide structure. Lidocaine-sensitive patients may use tetracaine (pontocaine), a deriva-tive of aminobenzoic acid.

III. Propanidid

Structure with $CH_2COOCH_2CH_2CH_3$, OCH_3, and $OCH_2C-N(C_2H_5)_2$ with O

Contact allergy to propanidid, (epontol), developed from occupational exposure in an anesthetist. This compound is derived from eugenol and cross-reacts with eu-genol and balsam of Peru (SNEDDON and GLEW 1973) Another case was reported by BANDMANN and DOENICKE (1971).

IV. Proxymetacaine

Structure with $COOCH_2CH_2N(C_2H_5)_2$, NH_2, and $OCH_2CH_2CH_3$

Proparacaine

Proxymetacaine (proparacaine) in eye drops has been a contact allergen in onc patient (BANDMANN et al. 1974), and produced a scaling, fissuring dermatitis of the fingertips in an opthalmologist (MARCH and GREENWOOD 1968); cross-sensitiza-tion with other local anesthetics did not occur.

V. Falicain

$H_7C_3-O-\text{⬡}-\overset{O}{\overset{\|}{C}}-CH_2-CH_2-N\text{⬡}$

Falicain allergy reported in 28 of 70,000 dermatologic patients was mainly caused by hemorrhoidal ointments and suppositories (SCHOLZ and RICHTER 1977). It caused several cases of allergic contact dermatitis in East Germany (BEHRBOHM and LENZNER 1975).

VI. Benzamine Lactate

Benzamine lactate, used mainly as a local anesthetic, caused a generalized contact dermatitis in a patient treated for hemorrhoids. Cross-reaction to other local anesthetics did not occur (CALNAN 1975).

G. Antipruritic Agents

I. Antihistamines

Promethazine   Chlorpromazine

Many antihistamines are frequent sensitizers following topical administration. Antihistamines include ethylenediamine derivatives, aminalkyl ether derivatives, phenothiazine derivatives, and piperazine derivatives. Contact allergy to these compounds is described in Chap. 14.

II. Phenol and Resorcinol

Phenol   Resorcinol

Phenol (carbolic acid) is not a sensitizer but a deep skin penetrant producing local gangrene if not diluted. Resorcinol is used for its alleged intipruritic and anti-acne keratolytic properties. It irritates in a dose-related manner but allergic reactions occur (CARON and CALNAN 1962; KEIL 1962). Group hypersensitivity was demonstrated for some resorcinol derivatives such as resorcinol-mono-acetate and hexylresorcinol, which are metadihydroxybenzenes. The *ortho* and *para* compounds do not cross-react.

III. Menthol

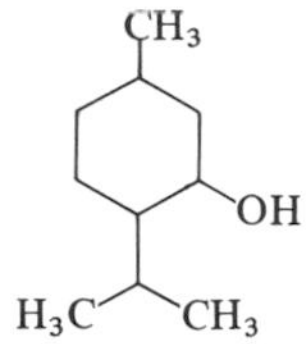

$$CH_3$$

OH

$$H_3C \qquad CH_3$$

Menthol, used because of its cooling effect, is a rare sensitizer (PAPA and SHELLEY 1964; CAMARASA and ALOMAR 1978), but has caused dermatitis, cheilitis, and stomatitis.

IV. Crotamiton

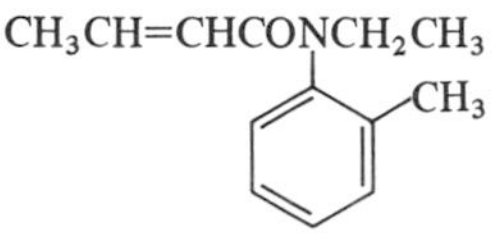

$$CH_3CH=CHCONCH_2CH_3$$
$$CH_3$$

Crotamiton (Eurax) is used as a scabicide and is antipruritic. It caused contact dermatitis in a patient with stasis dermatitis treated with Eurax ointment (VAN DIJK and MARIEN 1972). It has not sensitized in short-term exposure such as in scabies therapy.

V. Nitrofurylaminothiadazoles

Nitrofurylaminothiadazoles in antihemorrhoidal and antipruritic preparations caused perianal allergic contact dermatitis in five patients (FREGERT 1968).

VI. Oxypolyethoxydodecane

$$C_{12}H_{25}(OCH_2CH_2)_xOH$$

Oxypolyethoxydodecane, a derivative of alkyl polyethylene used as antipruritic agent in Anacal rectal ointment, caused perianal allergic contact dermatitis in a woman (CALNAN 1978).

VII. Dimethisoquin

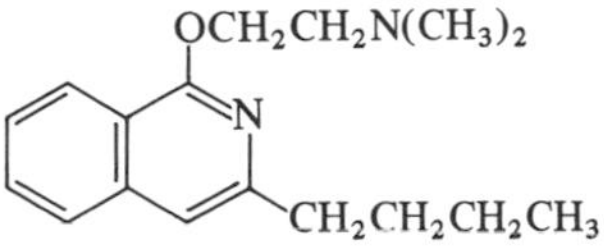

$$OCH_2CH_2N(CH_3)_2$$
N
$$CH_2CH_2CH_2CH_3$$

One case of contact allergy to dimethisoquin (Quotane hydrochloride) antipruritic ointment and lotion was reported by DALY (1952).

VIII. Zirconium Compounds

Zirconium compounds have been widely used in deodorant–antiperspirants and in topical preparations for *Rhus* dermatitis. They caused numerous cases of characteristic allergic granulomas in the skin (Shelley and Hurley 1958; Epstein 1960). Pleas from dermatologists have decreased the use of zirconium-containing preparations.

IX. Fragrances and Preservatives in Antipruritic Agents

The majority of antipruritic preparations are shake lotions, which besides having such active ingredients as have been mentioned, may contain allergenic fragrances and preservatives. Zinc oxide, often added because of its cooling effect on the skin is completely non-sensitizing but can produce black dermographia in the presence of jewelry.

H. Antiperspirants

I. Aluminum Salts

The most commonly used axillary antiperspirants contain aluminum salts, which are mild chemical irritants, but not allergens. The perfumes, preservatives and bases, however, may sensitize. Epidemiologic data on aluminum salt irritation are not generally available. If one includes subjective irritation (burning, stinging, itching, and other discomfort), more than half the population will at times note irritation. Most partially sensitive people can use these materials by either minimizing the amount applied (dose), utilizing rest periods, and avoiding use after axillary shaving, or after washing with soap and hot water. Some highly "sensitive" subjects can find no acceptable regimen and must instead use other antimicrobial deodorants. The mechanism of this subjective and objective irritation is poorly defined.

II. Formaldehyde

CH$_2$O

Formaldehyde

Hexamethylenetetramine

Formaldehyde, a potent sensitizer, is used in Europe as an antiperspirant. Hexamethylenetetramine liberates formaldehyde and is the chemical most frequently used in this type of antiperspirant. Hexamethylenetetramine is also a rubber accelerator and a urinary antiseptic (see Sect. M.IX).

III. Glutaraldehyde

$$COOH-(CH_2)_3-CH_2O$$

Glutaraldehyde (pentanedial) is an irritant, used in solution for treatment of hyperhidrosis and warts. Contact allergy has been reported (Gordon and Maibach

1969; JORDAN et al. 1972). In six glutaraldehyde-sensitive subjects a provocative use test with 25% glutaraldehyde on the soles was negative, while testing with 2.5% glutaraldehyde on the antecubital fossae provoked a severe dermatitis within 48 h (MAIBACH and PRYSTOWSKY 1977). It does not cross-react with formaldehyde (JUHLIN and HANSSON 1968; MAIBACH 1975b).

IV. Anticholinergic Agents

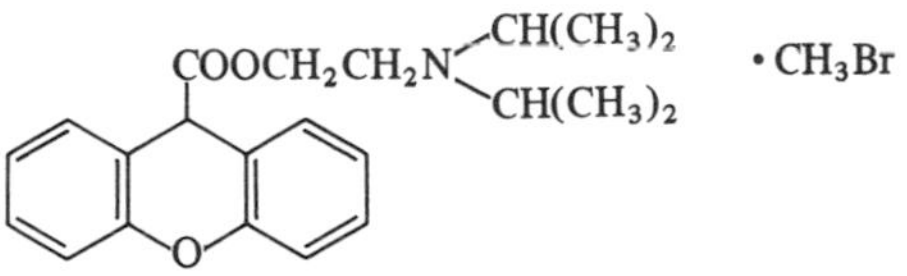

Propantheline bromide

Propantheline bromide in Ercoril Lotion has been reported as a sensitizer. AAGREN-JONSSON and MAGNUSSON (1976) found 11 positive patch tests of 14 patients with axillary dermatitis due to the product. Further, three patients reacted to trichlorocarbanilide and one to propylene glycol.

V. Zirconium Salts

The use of zirconium lactate and oxychloride in antiperspirants has been discontinued, but zirconyl hydroxychloride is still used and has not caused granulomas (FISHER 1973 p. 228).

J. Local Antibiotics and Chemotherapeutics

I. Neomycin

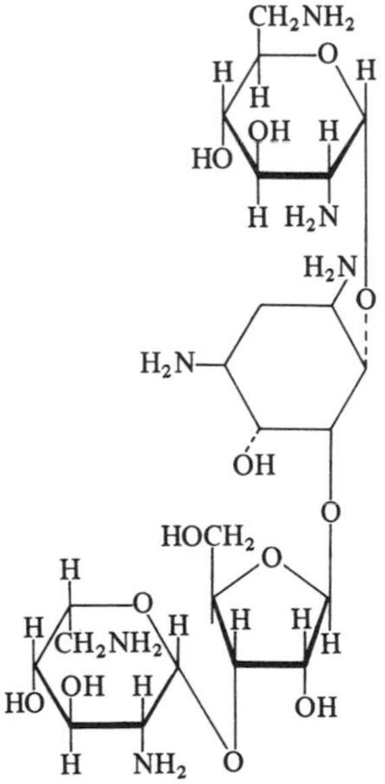

Neomycin

The most widely used topical antibiotic is neomycin. The frequency of neomycin sensitivity in the normal population in San Francisco is 1.1% (PRYSTOWSKY et al. 1979 b), while 5%–8% of eczema patients are allergic to neomycin. The diagnosis of allergic contact dermatitis to neomycin is difficult to make because the dermatitis is not vesicular or bullous; the sensitivity often appears only as an aggravation of a pre-existing dermatitis (EPSTEIN 1958 a). It is instructive to note that the therapeutic concentration of neomycin is often 0.5%, while the patch test concentration is 20% (EPSTEIN 1965).

Neomycin is a minimal penetrant through normal skin (PANZER and EPSTEIN 1970), and 20% neomycin may yield false negative patch tests. Neomycin contact allergy with negative patch tests but positive intradermal and usage tests has been reported (EPSTEIN 1980 a). Intradermal testing with a 0.1% solution is advocated by EPSTEIN (1965). Nonspecific toxic reactions may occur after intradermal testing, because neomycin acts as a histamine liberator (RAAB 1968). Controversial information exists regarding the occurrence of neomycin sensitivity in atopic subjects. EPSTEIN (1965) found that 55%–75% of neomycin-sensitive patients could be classified as atopic subjects, while WEREIDE (1970) did not confirm that result. A considerable number of his patients had stasis dermatitis of the lower leg. On the basis of the consumption of different neomycin preparations and the occurrence of neomycin sensitivity HJORTH and THOMSEN (1968) believed that neomycin in ointments was more sensitizing than neomycin in creams, powders, and lotions. Comparing neomycin in cream and ointment in a usage test in neomycin hypersensitive patients, the neomycin cream produced a faster and more intense reaction than the neomycin ointment (PRYSTOWSKY et al. 1979 b).

Kanamycin

The cross-sensitization pattern of neomycin is complex. Regular cross-sensitivity occurs between neomycin, framycetin, and paromomycin, which all contain a neosamine group (PRILÄ et al. 1967). Cross-sensitivity between neomycin and streptomycin has been reported (SIDI et al. 1958), but was not confirmed by PIRILÄ et al. (1967). Of the neomycin positive cases in Helsinki, 48% gave positive reactions to kanamycin, 36% to gentamycin, 21% to sisomycin, and 25% to tobramycin (FÖRSTRÖM and PIRILÄ 1978), while SCHORR and RIDGWAY (1977) found

65% of neomycin-sensitive patients reacting to tobramycin. Ambutyrosin (butrosin sulfate) cross-reacts with neomycin in 90% of cases.

Simultaneous sensitivity to neomycin and bacitracin has been common in Scandinavia (PIRILÄ and ROHUNKOSKI 1959) but less frequent in the Unites States (EPSTEIN and WENZEL 1963). This is explained as simultaneous sensitization because combined preparations containing these two antibiotics are extensively used in Scandinavia (PIRILÄ and WALLENIUS 1957). Because of the importance of kanamycin and gentamycin in internal medicine, the use of neomycin on the skin should be restricted.

II. Gentamycin

Gentamycin has been advocated for topical treatment because it was a non-sensitizer in prophetic patch tests, (BLACK et al. 1963). BANDMANN and MUTZECK (1973) examined 600 contact dermatitis patients and found 5% positive to neomycin sulfate, while negative to gentamycin, 0.8% positive to both, and 0.3% negative to neomycin sulfate while positive to gentamycin.

III. Penicillin

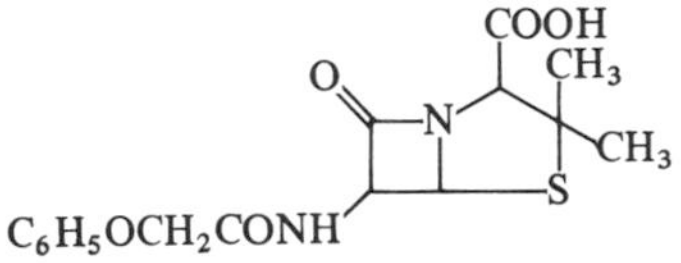

Penicillin V

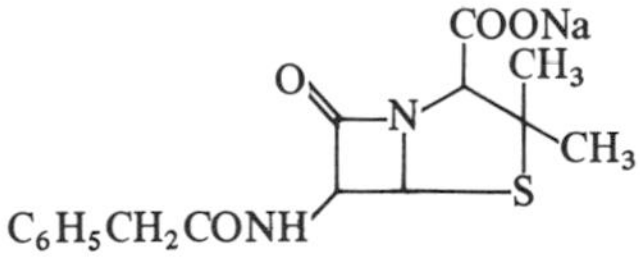

Benzylpenicillin

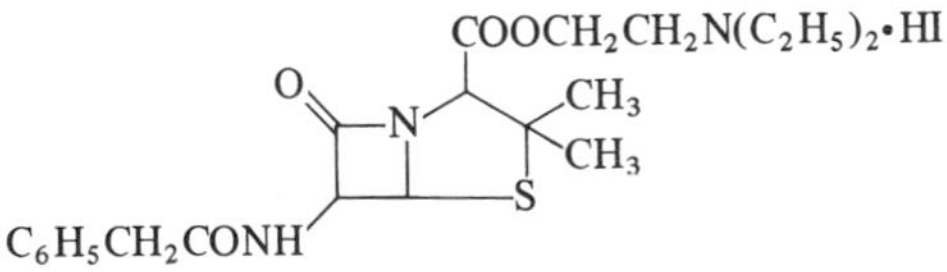

Penethamate hydroiodide

Penicillin is obsolete in local treatment in view of its high sensitization potential (DOHN 1960), but derivatives such as penethamate hydroiodide (an ester of benzylpenicillin) are used for local treatment of mastitis in cows and have caused occupational contact dermatitis in veterinary surgeons (HJORTH 1967).

IV. Chloramphenicol

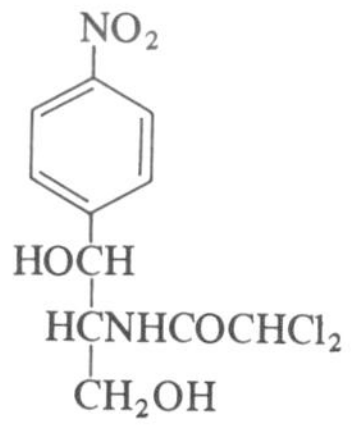

$$NO_2$$

HOCH
HCNHCOCHCl_2
CH_2OH

Chloramphenicol allergy is not uncommon (Robinson 1957), occuring in 15 of 550 patients treated topically. Cross-sensitization to 2,4-dinitrochlorobenzene has been debated but recently found not to occur (Eriksen 1978). Azidamphenicol, used as the antibiotic in a steroid–antibiotic combination cream, caused worsening of eczema under treatment in several cases, but contact allergy was only confirmed in four cases. Cross-reaction to chloramphenicol was found in all but one (Wereide 1975).

V. Bacitracin

Bacitracin sensitivity occurs not infrequently in Scandinavia together with neomycin sensitivity (Pirilä and Rouhunkoski 1959), while it has been rarely reported from United States (Binnick and Clendenning 1978). The reason for this apparent discrepancy is unexplained. Anaphylactic shock following topical application of bacitracin in an ointment has been described (Roupe and Strannegaard 1969).

VI. Polymyxin-B Sulfate

Polymyxin-B sulfate is a rare sensitizer but has been reported in one patient who had a simultaneously positive reaction to bacitracin (Van Ketel 1974).

VII. Tetracyclines

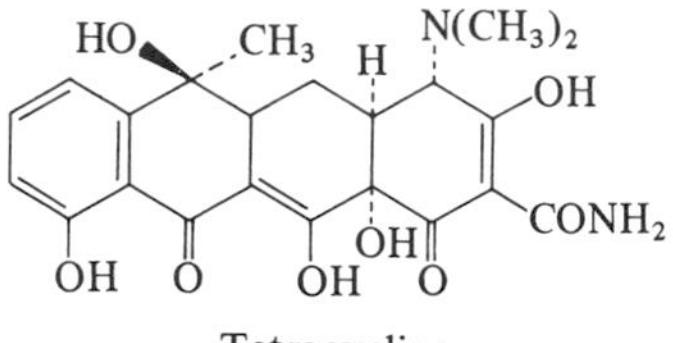

Tetracycline

Contact allergy to tetracyclines appears to be rare. Aureomycin ointment (Lederle) produced a dermatitis in a woman who applied the ointment to an area treated by dermabrasion. The patient was positive to chlortetracycline and dimethylchlortetracycline, but negative to oxytetracycline, tetracycline, and cymetycline (Calnan 1967). Bojs and Möller (1974) reported three patients with contact allergy to oxytetracycline. Cross-sensitivity to tetracyclin and methacycline was demonstrated in two of the cases.

VIII. Erythromycin

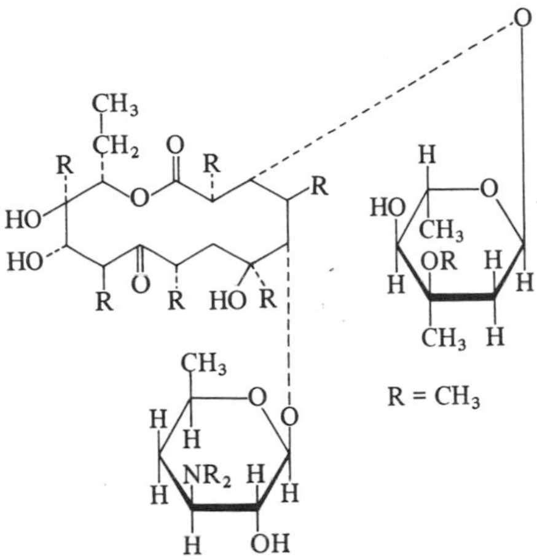

R = CH$_3$

Erythromycin sensitivity is extremely rare (FISHER 1976); few cases have been reported (VAN KETEL 1976 b). A 7-year-old girl developed urticaria after peroral administration of an erythromycin suspension. A scratch test was strongly positive, while patch testing was negative. A 52-year-old woman with a leg ulcer developed an acute allergic contact dermatitis around the ulcer caused by erythromycin stearate in petrolatum. Patch tests with 0.1, 1%, and 5% erythromycin stearate in petrolatum were positive.

IX. Sulfonamide

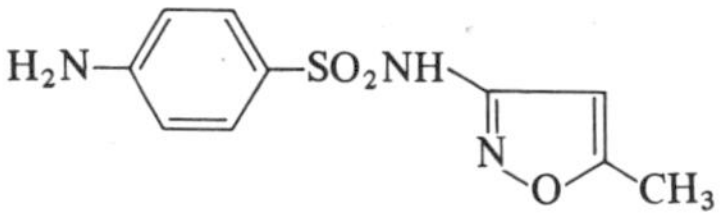

Sulfamethoxazole

Sulfonamide sensitization frequently follows repeated application to the skin (SULZBERGER et al. 1947) and cross-reactions to chemically related sulfonamides used as diuretics, oral antidiabetics, and sweetening agents occur, so subsequent systemic administration of a sulfonamide may produce eczematous contact dermatitis. Group sensitivity to sulfonamides could be traced to the common $NH_2C_6H_4SO_2$ part of the molecule (KOOIJ and VAN VLOTEN 1952). Topical sulfonamide therapy may still take place from eyedrops, suppositories, and vaginal creams, but has largely been discarded. Stevens–Johnson syndrome from ophthalmic sulfonamide has been reported (GOTTSCHALK and STONE 1976).

X. Nitrofurazone

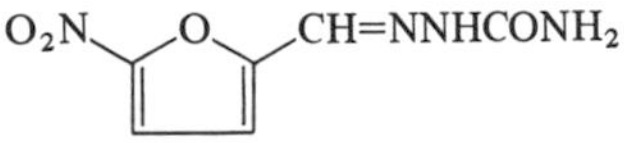

Nitrofurazone (Furacin) has over the years been used in solution or powder for leg ulcers and varicose eczema. Many cases of contact allergy occurred and subsequently descreased the dermatologic use of this drug topically (Braun and Schütz 1968). Each individual case tends to be dramatic, i.e., the extent and severity of the dermatitis is clinically striking, so that, unlike neomycin dermatitis, diagnosis presents no problem. The frequency of the dermatitis has probably been exaggerated, and may be less than that due to neomycin.

XI. Clindamycin

Clindamycin allergy has recently been described in an acne patient, who used a 1% clindamycin hydrochloride alcohol solution for 2 weeks before face itching occurred (Coskey 1978 b). Many patients receiving topical acne antimicrobial therapy develop dermatitis; it is not clear how much represents irritation rather than allergy.

XII. Sodium Fusidate

Fusidic acid

Sodium fusidate (Fucidin) allergy has been reported twice (Dave and Main 1973).

XIII. Streptomycin

Streptomycin

Streptomycin is a strong sensitizer and obsolete in topical therapy, but still presents an occupational hazard to nurses and veterinarians, because of leakage from syringes.

XIV. Virginiamycin

Contact allergy to the macrocyclic peptide, virginiamycin (Staphylomycin) has been reported (BLEUMINK and NATER 1972a, b). Cross-sensitization with pristinamycin exists. The factor M component of virginiamycin is the allergen. The eliciting patch test concentration was relatively high in one case (5%–10%), comparable to the eliciting concentration in neomycin allergy.

XV. Xanthocillin

Xanthocillin has been used in leg ulcer treatment and has caused several cases of contact allergy (HEIJER 1961).

XVI. Mafenide

Mafenide (sulfamylon), as hydrochloride and acetate is extensively used in treatment of burns, and has significantly lowered the mortality from burn wound sepsis (YAFEE and DRESSLER 1969). It was found to be a common sensitizer in studies performed in Munich, outnumbered only by benzocaine in the years from 1960 to 1965 (BANDMANN 1966). Mafenide acetate must not be used in patch testing, because patients sensitized to mafenide hydrochloride do not react to mafenide acetate (SCHREUS 1950). Cross-reactions to other related esters of *p*-aminobenzoic acid occur relatively often (BANDMANN 1967; SCHULZ 1962). Sulfonamides do not cross react with mafenide. BANDMANN and BREIT (1973) have reviewed the mafenide story.

XVII. Sulfur

Precipitated sulfur, used in many dermatologic preparations for topical treatment, is regarded as a non-sensitizing ingredient. Exceptions from this rule are reported (WILKINSON 1975; SCHNEIDER 1978).

XVIII. Halogenated Hydroxyquinolines

8–Hydroxyquinoline   Iodochlorhydroxyquin

Many related compounds exist, e.g., Vioform (5-chloro-7-iodo-8-hydroxyquinoline); Diodoquin, (5,7-diodo-8-hydroxyquinoline); Sterosan, (5-chloro-8-hydroxyquinoline), and Quinolor, a mixture of 5- and 7-chloro-8-hydroxyquinoline and 5,7-dichloro-8-hydroxyquinoline. They are widely used in topical preparations and some of them even sytemically. Contact allergy is infrequent. The 8-hydroxyquinoline part of the structure is the active component. FIEDLER et al. (1971) examined the cross-sensitivity pattern between 15 different 8-hydroxyquinolines in 9 patients sensitized to 5,7-dichloro-8-hydroxyquinoline. The degree of cross-reaction decreased in the following order: 7-chloro-8-hydroxyquinoline > 5-chloro-8-hydroxyquinoline > 8-hydroxyquinoline. Methyl substitution in the 7-position gave a positive patch test while substitution in the 5- and 2- positions gave negative tests. With halogen substitution the allergenic properties decrease in the following order: chlorinated > fluorinated > brominated > iodinated hydroxyquinolines (PEVNY and SCHELLENBERG 1971). Ten patients sensitized to Vioform were retested 2–10 years later and all showed a positive patch test at retesting, though they had avoided contact with Vioform and related substances in the meantime (KERNEKAMP and VAN KETEL 1980). Systemic administration of quinolines to sensitive patients may produce a generalized eruption (EKELUND and MÖLLER 1969; LEIFER and STEINER 1951). Three patients sensitive to halquinol (Quixalin) cross-reacted to related hydroxyquinoline compounds (ALLENBY 1965).

K. Antifungal Agents

I. Nystatin

Nystatin (mycostatin) allergy is rare and might be overlooked as a cause of contact allergy because nystatin is often associated with more commonly recognized sensitizers in broad spectrum creams and ointments. Few cases of contact allergy are reported (WASILEWSKI 1970; COSKEY 1971).

II. Variotin

Variotin (pecilocin) produced from a *Paecilomyces* fungus has caused a few cases of allergic contact dermatitis (SUNDARAVAJAN 1970; GROEN et al. 1973).

III. Undecylenic Acid

$$CH_2=CH(CH_2)_8COOH$$

Undecylenic acid (an antifungal fatty acid) is a weak sensitizer. One case of contact allergy from undecylenic acid in Desenex ointment has been reported (GELFARB and LEIDER 1960).

IV. Imidazole Derivatives

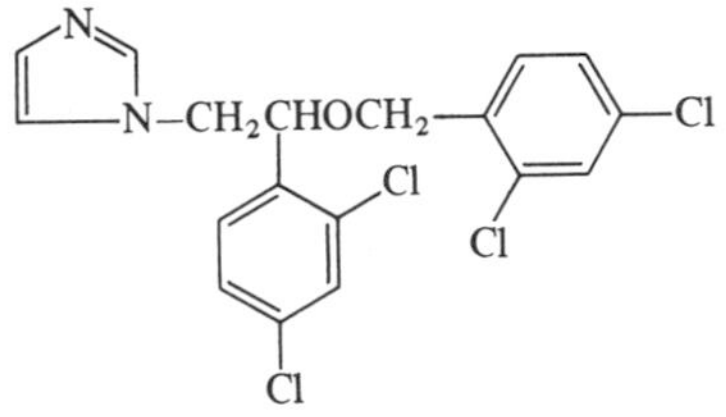

Miconazole

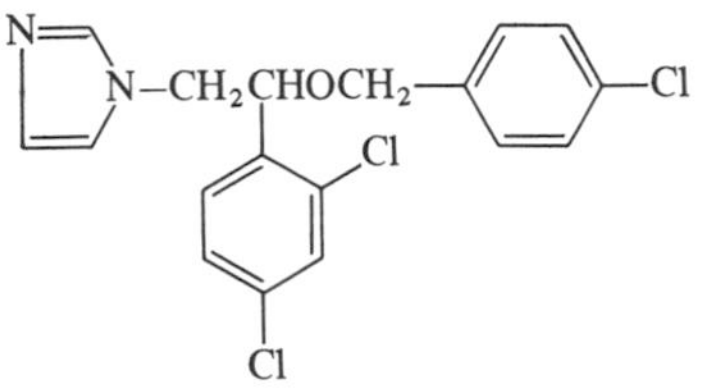

Econazole

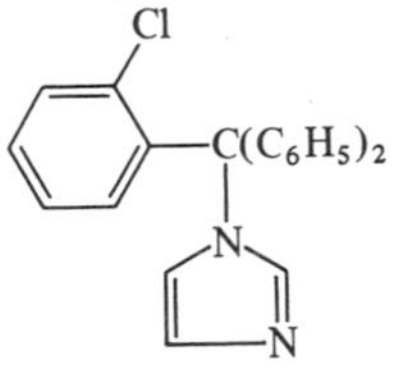

Chortrimazole

The imidazole derivatives, miconazole, econazole, and clotrimazole, are new effective antifungal agents which are known to be sensitizers; a few reports document contact allergy (DEGREEF and VERHOEVE 1975). The frequency is not known. They followed 108 patients treated locally with miconazole, finding a positive patch test to miconazole (2% in petrolatum) in one patient, worsening during treatment. Miconazole probably cross-reacts with econazole. One miconazole nitrate preparation (Micatin) was an irritant in ten patients. Three of six patch tested had positive reactions to the cream base, negative to miconazole nitrate (2% in petrolatum). The irritant reactions were most likely to occur when Micatin was applied to moist, intertriginous areas (WADE et al. 1979).

V. Tolnaftate

Tolnaftate is a weak sensitizer, with few reported cases of contact allergy (GELLIN et al. 1972).

VI. Dibenzthione

Dibenzthione (Afugin, Fungiplex) used as an antifungal agent, gave positive patch tests in two of three patients, who developed eczematous reactions to Fungiplex ointment (LIDEN and GÖRANSSON 1975). The allergenic properties depended on a product of hydrolytic decomposition, probably benzylisothiocyanate (WÜRBACH and SCHUBERT 1976).

VII. Pyrrolnitrin

Pyrrolnitrin is an antimycotic paranitro compound used in Italy and Japan. Two cases of allergic contact dermatitis to pyrrolnitrin in a cream base were reported; in one, a positive patch test to the related dinitrochlorobenzene (DNCB) was found (MENEGHINI and ANGELINI 1975).

VIII. Zinc Pyrithone

Zinc pyrithone (Zinc Omadine, Zincon, Vancide ZP) is fungicidal, bactericidal and used in antidandruff shampoos. In spite of its widespread use only few cases of contact allergy have been reported (MUSTON et al. 1979).

L. Steroids

I. Corticosteroids

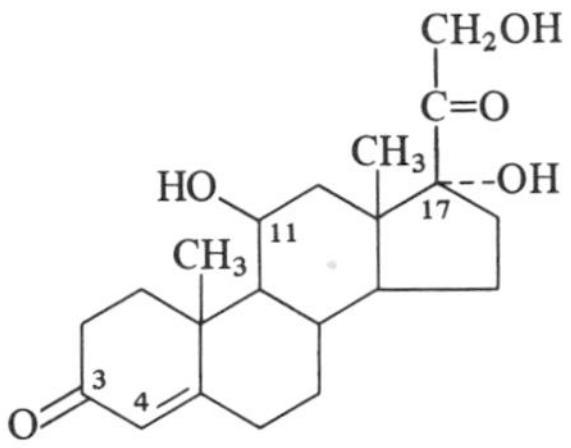

Hydrocortisone

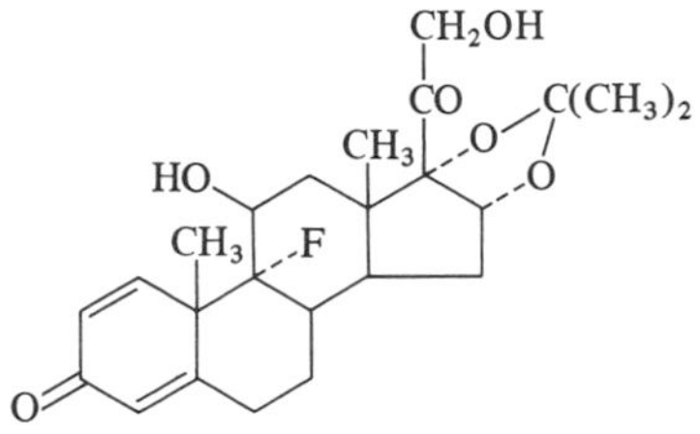

Triamcinolone acetonide

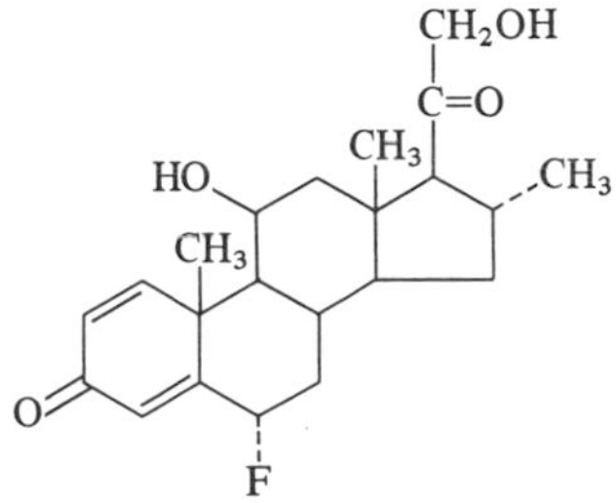

Fluocortolone

Contact allergy to topical corticosteroids appears uncommon; their sensitizing potential is probably low. However, allergy should be considered in chronic, therapy-resistant eczema. TEGNER (1976) has reviewed the literature.

Sensitivity to vehicle constituents and other ingredients such as preservatives, antibacterial agents and antifungal agents must be excluded by patch tests. A practical tool in detecting steroid allergy is patch testing with the suspected steroid in both an ointment and a cream base; if a positive reaction occurs to both patches, sensitivity to the steroid itself is probable. Another important point is the patch test concentration. With hydrocortisone a concentration fo 25% in petrolatum is recommended (ALANI and ALANI 1972). Possibly, even the fluorinated steroids should be applied in concentrations higher than those in normal use to avoid false negative reactions, caused by the anti-inflammatory effect of the steroid, which may depress the patch test reaction.

Besides hydrocortisone as an allergen, contact allergy has been reported from hydrocortisone acetate and alcohol (CHURCH 1960; EDWARDS and RUDNER 1970); methylprednisolone (COSKEY and BRYAN 1967; MATHIAS et al. 1978 b); triamcinolone acetonide (ALANI and ALANI 1972); 6α-chlorprednisone (VERMEULEN and MALTEN 1963); betamethasone valerate (ALANI and ALANI 1976 b; BUNNEY 1972); fluocortolone, fluocortolone pivalate, and fluocortolone caproate, all three ingredients in Utralan preparations (MENNÉ and ANDERSEN 1977); dexamethasone (WIEGEL 1968) halcinonide, fluocinide, and desonide (COSKEY 1978 a); budesonide (VAN HECKE and TEMMERMAN 1980); and hydrocortisone-17-butyrate (KERNEKAMP and VAN KETEL 1979). Concomitant sensitivity to various fluorinated steroids and to hydrocortisone has been described (ALANI and ALANI 1972, 1976 b), but cross-sensitivity between steroids is not the rule. Intradermal testing may be necessary in some cases to reveal an allergic reaction (MATHIAS et al. 1978 b; COMAISH 1969).

Striking a clinical balance in judgments on corticosteroid allergic contact dermatitis is difficult. This drug group provides the mainstay of current dermatologic therapy. Most dermatologists have not documented a single example, yet ALANI and ALANI (1972) quickly found 21 cases of hydrocortisone allergy in Copenhagen.

Our judgment is withheld; although contact allergy may be rare, we will not know its true or relative frequency until an energetic dermatologist performs routine patch tests on a large series. An analogy to neomycin is possible; here the allergic dermatitis is also low grade, difficult to diagnose, and rarely documented, if ever, by most practicing physicians. Yet, well-executed epidemiologic studies show a sensitization rate of 1 in 80 in a normal population.

II. Dianabol Cream

Dianabol

Dianabol cream, containing the androgenic anabolic methandrostenolone, has caused allergic contact dermatitis in five patients (SCHWARZ and STORCK 1966; PASCHOUD 1966).

III. Estrogens

Estriol   Diethylstilbestrol dipropionate

Estrogens are not frequently used topically except in vaginal and scalp preparations. FREGERT and RORSMANN (1960, 1962) described an allergic patient sensitized by a hair lotion containing diethylstilbestrol. Cross-sensitization was demonstrated to dienoestrol, hexoestrol, bisphenol A, p-benzylphenol, the monobenzylether of hydroquinone, and the benzylester of p-hydroxybenzoic acid.

M. Antiseptics and Disinfectants

A large number of antiseptics and disinfectants is available with varying physical, chemical, and toxicological properties. Many of them are used in lower concentrations as perservatives for food, cosmetics, and drugs. Consumer safety considerations precipitate constant activity in affected industries to learn about the safety of these antimicrobial agents and to develop alternatives. Regarding contact sensitization potential, 23 antimicrobial agents have been investigated using the Draize procedure on normal human subjetcs. Among the stronger skin sensitizers were mercurials, formalin, bronopol, mafenide, captan, and chloroacetamide, while propylene glycol, triclocarban, chlorinated phenolics, parabens and sorbic acid appeared to be lower grade sensitizers, and triclosan (DP 300) failed to sensitize (MARZULLI and MAIBACH 1973).

I. Quaternary Ammonium Compounds

$$\left[\bigcirc\!\!\!-CH_2-\overset{\overset{\displaystyle CH_3}{|}}{\underset{\underset{\displaystyle CH_3}{|}}{N}}-R \right]^{+} Cl^{-}$$

Benzalkonium chloride

Quaternary ammonium compounds are widely used antiseptics and disinfectants with a low sensitizing potential. Benzalkonium chloride is used as a skin disinfectant, for disinfection of instruments, and in treatment of burns, ulcers, etc. Cosmetics, deodorants, mouthwashes, and ophthalmic preparations, including contact lens solutions, may contain benzalkonium chloride.

Several case reports and patients series describe contact allergy to quaternary ammonium compounds (WAHLBERG 1962; HURIEZ et al. 1965; AFZELIUS and THULIN 1979). In the study by HURIEZ et al. (1965) a series of 71 patients cethexonium bromide was the main culprit. Cetrimonium bromide (cetrimide BP), another quaternary ammonium compound consisting of a mixture of chemicals (CRUISKSHANK 1949), caused several cases of contact allergy (MORGAN 1968).

$$[CH_3(CH_2)_{15}N(CH_3)_3]Br$$

Cetrimonium bromide

Dequaline chloride sensitivity was found in 309 of 6,000 patients in Helsinki, most of whom had leg ulcers and/or stasis dermatitis. The main allergen seemed to be 4-aminoquinaldine hydrochloride (an impurity) or dequaline chloride itself (SALO et al. 1968). HURIEZ et al. (1965) suggested that topical allergy might lead to generalized reactions from systemic administration of chemically related drugs as cholinergic agents, hypotensive drugs (e. g., tetraethylammonium chloride), neuromuscular blocking agents (e. g., decamethonium bromide), or heparin antagonists (hexadimethrine bromide). Contact urticaria and asthma from denatonium benzoate (Bitrex) used in antifrost liquids, carburettor spirits, and skin disinfectants have recently been reported in one patient (BJÖRKNER 1980). He reacted to denatonium benzoate dilutions down to 2×10^{-6} mg 1^{-1}.

Documenting allergic contact dermatitis to quaternary ammonium chloride compounds is difficult, requiring meticulous attention to detail, and should be regarded as a research project in each instance. The basic difficulty resides in the fact that these compounds have an unusual distribution of irritation with occlusive patch testing results. Björnberg (1968) noted that 70% of normal subjects reacted to benzalkonium chloride 2%; 50% to 1%; 32% to 0.5%, and 1% to 0.1%. What then is the correct contact allergy patch test concentration? We do not know. We do not doubt that contact allergy exists – only, that it is difficult to diagnose with occlusive patch testing because of the wide variation in irritant response under occlusion. At the moment we feel comfortable with the diagnosis of contact allergy to this class of compounds only when a provocative product use test is positive. (Other chemicals having this wide variation in irritancy with occlusive testing are the organic mercurials.) A thorough reexamination of contact allergy to quaternary ammonium compounds is in order. We suspect that many of the published cases refer to patch test artifacts and irritation, rather than allergy.

II. Chlorhexidine

$$Cl-\!\!\!\!\bigcirc\!\!\!\!-NHCNHCNH(CH_2)_6NHCNHCNH-\!\!\!\!\bigcirc\!\!\!\!-Cl$$
$$\qquad\quad \overset{\|}{NH}\ \overset{\|}{NH} \qquad\qquad \overset{\|}{NH}\ \overset{\|}{NH}$$

Chlorhexidine (Hibitane), another widely used antiseptic, rarely causes contact sensitivity. A few case reports document contact allergy, e.g., Wahlberg and Wennersten (1971) described a man with contact allergy and photosensitivity to chlorhexidine. Photoallergy was suspected. Ljungren and Möller (1972) reported another case with positive patch tests to chlorhexidine in alcohol or water, but negative reaction to chlorhexidine applied in petrolatum, even in high concentrations. Chlorhexidine is insoluble in hydrocarbon solvents.

III. Hexachlorophene

Hexachlorophene, a phenolic derivative, is a rare sensitizer. Fregert and Hjorth (1969) reported a sensitization index of 0.3% in 660 patients, while acute primary irritant contact dermatitis occurred more frequently (Baker et al. 1969), especially in susceptible skin such as on the scrotum. Positive patch tests believed to be cross-reactions to hexachlorophene were found in patients with allergy to tetra-chlorosalicylanilide (Wilkinson 1962; Jillson and Baughman 1963), bithionol, and dichlorophene (Epstein 1966).

IV. Dichlorophene

Dichlorophene (dichlorodihydroxydiphenylmethane, G4, cuniphen) closely related to hexachlorophene, is used in dentifrices, shampoos, antiperspirants, deodorant preparations, and over-the-counter products for athlete's foot. It is also used as an antifungal and antibacterial preservative in textiles. SCHORR (1970) reported three cases of contact allergy to dichlorophene in a skin lotion and a bandage used for stasis ulcers. Two of EPSTEIN's (1966) three patients allergic to dichlorophene were apparently sensitized by cosmetic bases. According to FISHER and TOBIN (1953) dichlorophene is a more potent sensitizer than hexachlorophene; they did not find cross-reaction between these two substances as did EPSTEIN (1966).

V. Triphenylmethane Dyes

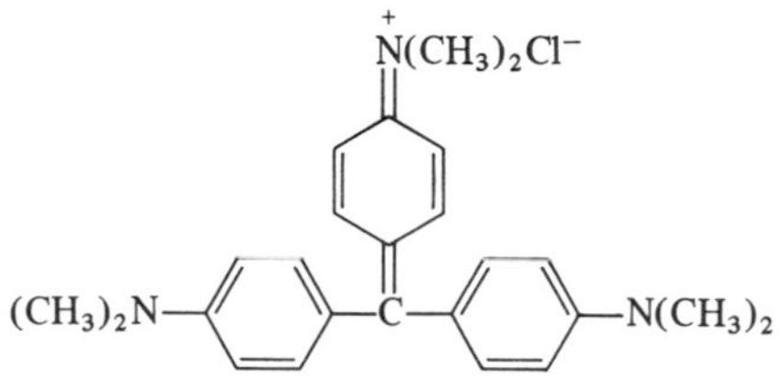

Gentian violet

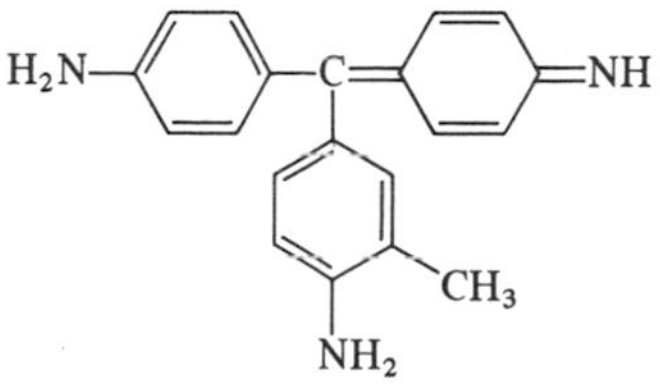

Rosaniline

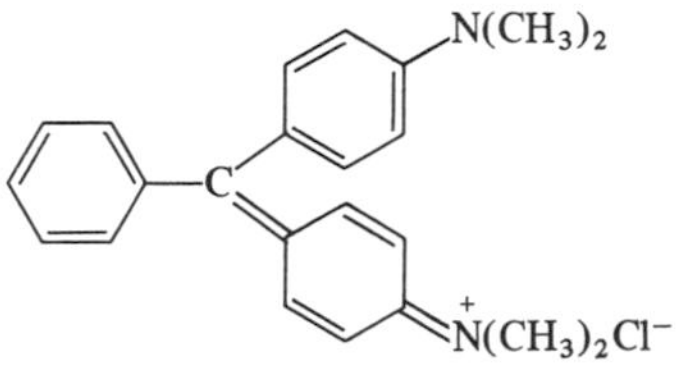

Malachite green

Triphenylmethane dyes (gentian violet, crystal violet, methyl violet, rosaniline, malachite green, brilliant green, chrysoidine, and eosin) are considered weak sensitizers. Sensitization to these dyes occurs especially when they are applied to eczematous skin. Anaphylactic reactions have been described after application of 1% gentian violet and 1% methyl green to a leg ulcer (MICHEL et al. 1958). BIELICKY and NOVAK (1969) observed 11 patients with leg eczema sensitized to brillant green. Patch tests showed the possibility of cross-sensitization between crystal violet (contained in gentian violet), brilliant green, and malachite green. The determinant group was $-N(CH_3)_2$ or $-N(C_2H_5)_2$ in the *para* position of the benzene ring. Cross-reactions are limited to substances with amino groups substituted with at least two alkyls and patch tests with triphenylmethane were negative.

VI. Acridine Dyes

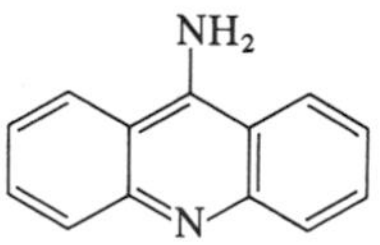

Aminacrine

Aminacrine hydrochloride 0.1% in a cream caused allergic contact dermatitis on the genitalia of one patient (WILSON 1971). Patch tests with the related substances acriflavine and proflavine were negative.

VII. Rivanol

$$CH_3-CHOH-COO^\ominus$$

Rivanol (6,9-diamino-2-ethoxyacridine lactate) another acridine derivative has been used extensively as an antibacterial agent in Europe. EPSTEIN (1958 b) found five patients allergic to Rivanol. They had negative patch tests but positive intradermal tests. Controls were negative.

VIII. Fenticlor

Fenticlor, a chlorohydroxyphenylsulfide, is used as an antiseptic and fungicide in creams, powders, vaginal creams, and pessaries. Case reports of contact allergy have been published (DUPONT 1974). Photoallergy to fenticlor and cross-sensitization between fenticlor and hexachlorophene were described by BURRY (1967).

IX. Formaldehyde

Formaldehyde is an ubiquitous and potent sensitizer, both in industry and in medicine because of its antimicrobial properties. Shampoos, soaps, lotions, ointments, powders, and dentifrices may contain formaldehyde as a preservative and many wrinkle- or crease-resistant fabrics are treated with formaldehyde resins releasing free formaldehyde. Formaldehyde is among the top ten sensitizers and is incorporated in patch test standard series recommended by the International Contact Dermatitis Research Group. Unexplainable positive patch test reactions occur frequently where no clinical relevance is found (MARCUSSEN 1959). Formaldehyde releasers used as preservatives in cosmetics and technical products are often covered by trade names or synonyms, but they are nevertheless important to recognize when tracing causes of allergic contact dermatitis from formaldehyde (DAHLQUIST and FREGERT 1978). Cream constituents as polyethylene glycols (carbowaxes, macrogols) can form formaldehyde by autooxidation. DAHLQUIST et al. (1980) found up to 51 µg formaldehyde using a fluorimetric method in 16 out of 20 corticosteroid creams. The amounts of formaldehyde are probably not high enough to sensitize, but may maintain dermatitis in previously formaldehyde-sensitized patients. The epidemiology of formalin sensitization requires reevaluation. Most early studies utilized irritant patch test concentrations. Even after an extensive study to determine the correct concentration (EPSTEIN and MAIBACH 1966), we still note low grade irritant responses in routine patch testing: the concentration required to elicit sensitization is perilously close to the irritant concentration.

X. Tetramethylthiuram Disulfide

$$(CH_3)_2N\overset{\overset{S}{\|}}{C}-SS-\overset{\overset{S}{\|}}{C}N(CH_3)_2$$

Tetramethylthiuram disulfide, a well-known sensitizer among rubber accelerators, is also a disinfectant in some soaps, wound sprays (e. g., Nobecutan), suntan preparations, and antibiotic preparations.

XI. Hexomedine

$$C_{24}H_{38}N_4O_{10}S_2$$

Hexomedine (Hexamidine), a disinfectant with a structure similar to chlorhexidine, produced allergic contact dermatitis in a female patient. Patch test with chlorhexidine was negative (VAN KETEL 1975).

XII. Iodine and Iodides

Tincture of iodine is a primary irritant and should be tested by the open method. Patch tests with iodine and potassium iodide may result in a nonspecific papulopustular reaction which must be differentiated from a contact allergic response. Patch tests with potassium iodide have been used in the diagnosis of dermatitis herpetiformis (DH) but the frequency and type of reactions expected in DH patients is neither sensitive nor specific. 1,3-diodo-2-hydroxypropane, a "white tincture of iodine" used in Denmark for first aid, caused contact dermatitis in one patient (HJORTH 1972). He had a strong positive patch test, while 20 controls were negative. Contact allergy to iodine itself may exist, but has not been documented.

XIII. Alcohols

Lower aliphatic alcohols dry and irritate the skin, but they can also sensitize, and perhaps more frequently than anticipated. In a predictive human sensitization assay 50% aqueous ethanol induced contact sensitivity in 6 of 93 volunteers. The reactivity remained for more than 2 months. Possible allergens other than ethanol itself were eliminated by gas chromatographic examination. In one subject, other short chain primary alcohols, a secondary alcohol, and acetaldehyde gave positive patch tests, suggesting an antigenic relationship (STOTTS and ELY 1977). This curious result of a high frequency ethanol sensitization has not been duplicated elsewhere in predictive testing; further studies should include biopsies and provocative product use tests. FREGERT et al. (1971) reported five patients with hypersensitivity to primary alcohols (extending from methanol to pentanol). Two of the patients also reacted positively to patch tests with gas chromatographically pure secondary alcohols (2-propanol and 2-butanol), while negative reactions occurred to tertiary alcohols. Ludwig and Hansen (1977) reported a patient with sensitivity to the secondary alcohol, isopropanol, without concomitant sensitivity to alcohols with less than three carbon atoms. The alcohol hypersensitivity cannot be ascribed to hypersensitivity to aldehydes formed in the skin. The chemicals added to denature alcool are neither potent nor frequent sensitizers, they include tartar emetic, salicylic acid, dimethylphthalate, quinine sulfate, colchicum extract, brucine, quassia, and sucrose octaacetate (Fisher 1973a, p 79).

XIV. Triclosan

Cl—⟨benzene ring⟩—O—⟨benzene ring⟩—Cl
                Cl   OH

Irgasan DP 300

Triclosan is also called Irgasan DP 300 and 2,4,4-trichloro-2-hydroxydiphenyl ether. This widely used antimicrobial agent in cosmetics, toilet soaps, and detergents caused two cases of contact allergy provoked by a deodorant and a foot powder (Roed-Petersen et al. 1975). Wahlberg (1976) included triclosan 2% in petrolatum in the standard series and found 2 sensitive among 1,100 patients tested. Compared to its widespread use, contact allergy is believed rare. In predictive contact allergy tests both in guinea pigs and in humans triclosan showed a very low sensitizing potential (Marzulli and Maibach 1973; Lachapelle and Tennstedt 1979).

XV. Triclocarban

Triclocarban or trichlorcarbanilide (TCC) has been subjected to extensive predictive testing and battery screening in dermatitis patients to disclose its dermatitis potential. It was found to be minimal. The use of this bacteriostatic agent is now restricted to bar soap. Few cases of triclocarban-associated contact dermatitis have been described after use of the chemical in antiperspirants and cosmetics (ICDRG 1978).

XVI. TEGO

$$C_{12}H_{25}-NH-CH_2-CH_2-NH-CH_2-CH_2-NH-CH_2$$
$$COOH \cdot HCl$$

TEGO (dodecylaminoethylglycine hydrochloride) is an antiseptic detergent used in hospitals, the food industry, public baths, etc., and has caused sporadic cases of contact allergy in users (Fregert and Dahlquist 1969).

XVII. Glutaraldehyde

$$COOH-(CH_2)_3-CHO$$

Besides being used in antiperspirants, glutaraldehyde (pentanedial) is used as a wart remedy and as a disinfectant in hospitals. Contact allergic reactions occur (for more detail see Sect. H).

XVIII. Mercurials

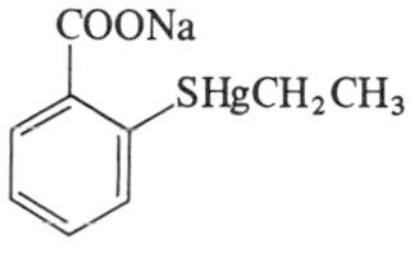

COONa
SHgCH$_2$CH$_3$

Thimerosal

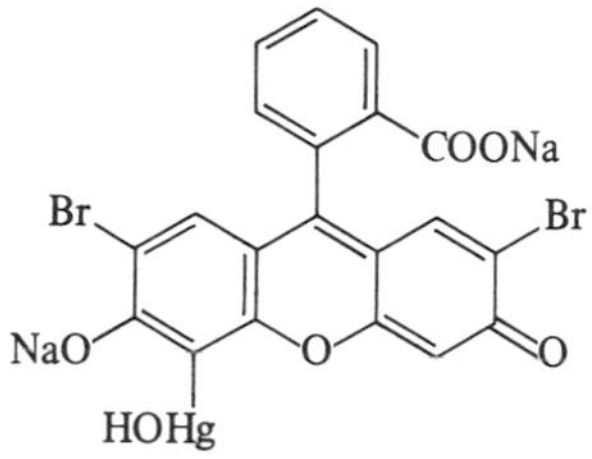

COONa
Br   Br
NaO   O   O
HOHg

Merbromin

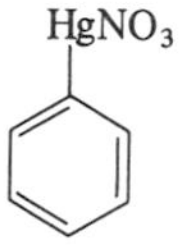

HgNO$_3$

Phenylmercuric nitrate

The organic mercurials are used as antiseptics and include merthiolate (thiomersal), mercurochrome (merbromin), metaphen (nitromersal), and mercresin (mercrocresol). They may cross-react with the inorganic mercurials as oxides and the phenylmercuric salts (FISHER 1973a, p. 109). MÖLLER (1977) found a 3.7% frequency of merthiolate allergy in a 5-year study of eczema patients with the peak incidence in the 20–30 years age group. Among healthy young military recruits he found 16% with merthiolate hypersensitivity but without eczematous reactions. He suggested that routine intracutaneous testing of young people in Sweden with merthiolate-preserved tuberculin caused the sensitization. In this study, merthiolate cross-reacted to a few other organic mercurials, but not to inorganic or metallic mercury.

There has been controversy as to whether positive patch tests to merthiolate are irritant or allergic reactions. Allergy is the most likely explanation: provocative product use tests are positive in most subjects with patch test reaction to merthiolate (MAIBACH, unpublished). Allergic reactions to merthiolate and mercurochrome may be life threatening with systemic involvement as laryngeal edema (MAIBACH 1975a; CAMARASA 1976). Patients topically sensitized to mercurials may experience "systemic flares" from mercury-containing diuretics, calomel, amalgam fillings, and cinnabar in tattoos (FISHER 1973a, p. 109).

XIX. Silver Nitrate

The extensive use of this antiseptic has not caused known contact allergic reactions.

N. Preservatives

This heterogenous group of compounds includes several antiseptics already described, creating an overlap between this and the foregoing section.

I. Parabens

HO—⟨benzene⟩—COO—R

R = —CH$_3$ = methyl paraben
             = methyl—p—hydroxybensoate

R = —CH$_2$—CH$_3$ = ethyl paraben
                     = ethyl—p—hydroxybenzoate

R = —CH$_2$—CH$_2$—CH$_3$ = propyl paraben
                             = propyl—p—hydroxybenzoate

R = —CH⟨CH$_3$ / CH$_3$⟩   = isopropyl paraben
                            = isopropyl—p—hydroxybenzoate

R = —CH$_2$—CH$_2$—CH$_2$—CH$_3$ = butyl paraben
                                   = butyl—p—droxybenzoate

R = —CH$_2$—⟨benzene⟩   = benzyl paraben
                         = benzyl—p—hydroxybenzoate

The most widely used preservatives are the parabens (esters of p-hydroxybenzoic acid) in foods, drugs, and cosmetics. Used in combination parabens have a synergistic effect. Cross-reactions between the four paraben esters: methyl-, ethyl-, propyl- and butylparaben, are common but exceptions occur. In diagnostic patch testing SCHORR (1968) found that 0.8% of tested patients were sensitized. In predictive testing using the Draize procedure in healthy volunteers MARZULLI and MAIBACH (1973) sensitized 0.3%. These results suggest that the incidence of contact sensitization in healthy persons is likely to be small, and agree with the clinical impression, that occasional cases of paraben sensitivity occur and are important to the stricken patient's welfare, but sensitization is low when the extensive use of the material is considered (FISHER et al. 1971).

Oral ingestion of parabens might induce tolerance to paraben sensitization, a mechanism reported for poison ivy, and thus explain the low incidence. Up to 0.1% parabens are permitted in foods. Systemic flare of the dermatitis in paraben-sensitive patients has been infrequently reported after oral ingestion, (MITCHELL 1971; KLEINHANS and KNOTH 1973). The most recent epidemiologic data for paraben sensitivity is published by the North American Contact Dermatitis Research Group (NACDRG), which found 3% of 1,200 dermatitis patients tested to be positive (NACDRG 1973). FISHER et al. (1971) and SCHORR (1968) assumed that repeated topical application of low concentrations of parabens in medicaments or cosmetics could cause sensitization, while HJORTH and TROLLE LASSEN (1963) stated that higher concentrations were necessary for the majority of cases. They reported a 1% incidence of paraben sensitivity, suggesting this was due to the frequent use in Denmark of topical antifungal agents containing up to 5% paraben (amycen). Cross-reactions may occur to other *para* compounds such as benzocaine, p-phenylenediamine and sulfonamides (MAUCHER 1974). Note that paraben-sensitive patients can often use paraben-preserved cosmetics on normal skin without adverse effect (FISHER 1973 b).

In the ICDRG standard series, the parabens are tested as a mixture of 3% of methyl-, ethyl-, propyl-, butyl- and benzyl-*p*-hydroxybenzoic acid, a total of 15% in petrolatum which may be irritating and enhance the occurrence of multiple false positive patch tests (angry back) (MITCHELL 1977).

The final details of the paraben story remain to be elucidated. Certainly many patients labeled as paraben allergic have instead irritant responses to the marginally irritating 15% mixture; others have angry back skin syndrome, nonspecific false positives. An epidemiologic study performed with considerable attention to confirmation of putative positives is required: the recent triclorcarbanilide study provides a model (ICDRG 1978). It is our impression that, except for high concentration (i. e., > 1%) drug use and application to leg ulcers, the parabens are rarely sensitizers. Combined with the extensive chronic toxicity data available on its systemic effects, these compounds set the standard for relative safety that new preservatives will have difficulty matching.

II. Propylene Glycol

$$CH_3CHOHCH_2OH$$

Besides its solubilizing and humectant properties, propylene glycol has antimicrobial properties, making it a useful preservative. Propylene glycol is an irritant when used under occlusion (HANNUKSELA et al. 1975). Pure propylene glycol tested as such, yielded 12.5% positive reactions in 1,556 eczema patients; only four were allergic, with positive patch tests to dilutions of propylene glycol down to 3.2% in water. In a later series HANNUKSELA and FÖRSTRÖM (1978) elicited drug exanthemas in 15 of 38 propylene glycol allergic patients after an oral challenge of 2–15 ml propylene glycol. The proper patch test concentration has not been established: 3%–10% in water is presently in favor.

The frequency and mechanism of propylene glycol sensitization requires elucidation; even the minor contaminants are suspect in the light of the observation of widely varying pH in commercial grade supplies. Many patients with positive propylene glycol patch tests lose their reactivity when retested some months later; is this spontaneous desensitization or loss of nonspecific hyperreactivity? This clinical problem produces consternation in dermatotoxicology – even after three decades of investigation (WARSHAW and HERRMANN 1952). Until the details are clarified, we are wary of branding patients propylene glycol sensitive, until they have been patch tested again some months later. When the result is positive, we follow with a provocative product use test for 7 days. The suggestion of oral challenge offers an alternate diagnostic test; we await further experience with it. Propylene glycol frequently produces subjective irritation (burning and stinging) in a dose-related fashion. This side effect occurs far more frequently than (objective) irritation and allergy.

III. Sorbic Acid

$$CH_3CH=CHCH=CHCOOH$$

This preservative is a natural product (2,4-hexadienoic acid), occurring in many berries and used in foods, cosmetics, and medicaments. According to HJORTH and TROLLE LASSEN (1962) the sensitizing index is low (0.3%), while KLASCHKA and BEIERSDORFF (1965) estimated 0.6%. Regarding allergenicity, sorbic acid compares favorably with other preservatives. Contact urticaria to sorbic acid developed on the face of a woman when she shampooed her hair. The reaction was only elicitable on intact skin of her face by open testing (RIETSCHEL 1978 b). This immediate reactivity to simple chemicals such as sorbic acid is probably more common than anticipated, though the mechanism is still unknown (LAHTI 1978).

IV. Chlorocresol and p-Chloro-m-xylenol

4—Chloro—*m*—cresol

These related chlorinated phenols are used as preservatives in betamethasone cream, electrocardiogram paste, and in over 30 over-the counter products. Contact allergic eczema does occur sporadically. The two compounds may cross-react (HJORTH and TROLLE LASSEN 1963; BURRY et al. 1975; STORRS 1975).

V. Chloracetamide

$$ClCH_2CONH_2$$

The sensitizing potential of this preservative has been established in a modified Draize test (17% of 205 volunteers) (MAIBACH 1971). The industrial exposure is widespread (e. g., wood, leather, and tanning industries, wallpaper glue, nylon spin finish, cutting oils). Chloracetamide in cosmetics and pharmaceutical preparations has caused contact allergy (NATER 1971; CALNAN 1971); of 27 contact allergic reactions to Hirudoid ointment 7 were caused by chloracetamide (SMEENK and PRINS 1972).

VI. Nordihydroguaiaretic Acid

This is an antioxidant in topical preparations. ROED-PETERSEN and HJORTH (1976) reported six cases of contact allergy with a lanolin cream containing nordihidroguaiaretic acid (NDGA) as the culprit in three cases.

VII. BHA and BHT

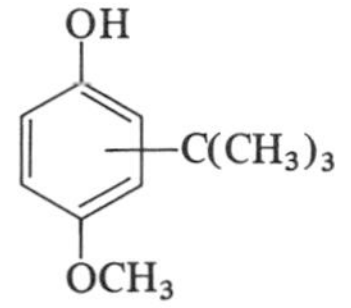

OH

—C(CH$_3$)$_3$

OCH$_3$

Butylated hydroxyanisole

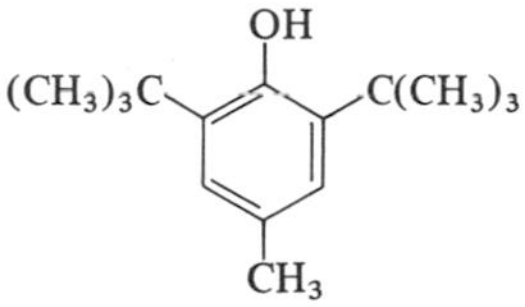

OH

(CH$_3$)$_3$C—   —C(CH$_3$)$_3$

CH$_3$

Butylated hydroxytoluene

Butylated hydroxyanisole (BHA) and butylated hydroxytoluene (BHT) are used in foods and topical preparations. MENEGHINI et al. (1971) found 1 of 360 consecutive patients positive to patch test with BHA and negative to BHT. BHA sensitivity from a miconazole nitrate cream containing 0.005% BHA has been reported (DEGREEF and VERHOEVE 1975). ROED-PETERSEN and HJORTH (1976) described 2 of 112 patients positive to BHA and/or BHT. Both had flares of dermatitis after an oral challenge.

VIII. Propyl Gallate

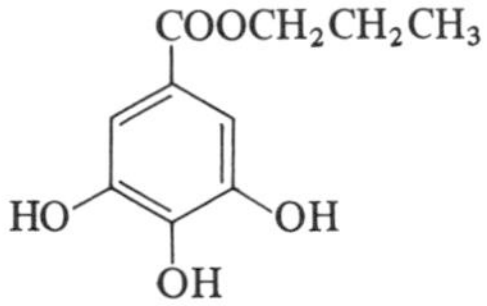

COOCH$_2$CH$_2$CH$_3$

HO—   —OH

OH

Propyl gallate was the offending agent in Alphosyl cream, causing allergic contact dermatitis in a psoriatic patient after 1.5 years use (LIDEN 1975). It appears that 1% in petrolatum is a satisfactory patch test concentration.

IX. Imidazolidinyl Urea

Germall 115 is used as an antimicrobial agent in cosmetics and has caused allergic contact dermatitis (FISHER 1975b). In a modified Draize test, Germall 115 sensitized 2 of 150 subjects (JORDAN and KING 1977). It appears as a common allergen in cosmetics (FDA 1979).

X. Other Preservatives

In a survey of cosmetic allergy SCHORR (1971) mentioned other cosmetic preservatives and antimicrobial agents: betaines, miranols (amphoteric), dimethoxane (Dioxin), and dehydroacetic acid. How often they produce allergic reactions is unknown; only a few have been reported. Dimethoxane (1.25%) sensitized 50 of 205 subjects in a Draize test (MAIBACH 1971).

O. Vitamins

I. Tretinoin

Sensitization to tretinoin (retinoic acid) has been described several times in humans without known pre-exposure (JORDAN et al. 1975) and in patients during topical treatment with the drug (LINDGREN et al. 1976; NORDQUIST and MEHR 1977; RUDZ-KI and GRZYWA 1978). Retinoic acid is an irritant, producing erythema and scaling in the majority of patients applying high concentrations of the drug.

II. Thiamine

Thiamine (vitamin B_1) is rarely used topically. Allergic contact dermatitis has been reported from occupational exposure (HJORTH 1958).

III. α-Tocopherol

α-Tocopherol (vitamin E) is an antioxidant in many pharmaceutical products and occasionally cases of allergic sensitivity are revealed. α-Tocopherol-containing deodorants have caused six reported cases of contact dermatitis (MINKIN et al. 1973; AELING et al. 1974). Severe contact urticaria occurred in siblings who had been treated with a vitamin E preparation for thermal burns (KASSEN and MITCHELL 1974).

IV. Other Vitamins

Occupational contact dermatitis to vitamin K has been described (JIRASEK and SCHWANK 1965), while allergic reactions to vitamin C and D have not been documented, in spite of their widespread use.

P. Photocontact Dermatitis

Photocontact dermatitis is subdivided into phototoxic and photoallergic reactions. Long wavelength ultraviolet light (UVA) usually constitutes the action spectrum for both types of reactions (short wavelength UVB may have an enhancing effect). Phototoxic reactions are most common; the vast majority are produced by the same compounds, which occasionally produce photoallergic reactions in sensitized individuals.

   Photoallergy is uncommon and requires an acquired altered reactivity in the subject, involving an antigen–antibody reaction. Less energy is required to elicit a photoallergic response than a phototoxic response. The clinical picture of photoallergy includes a varied morphology, usually with itching and distant flare, while the phototoxic reactions usually look like an exaggerated sunburn with a burning sensation and little itching.

   When evaluating suspected cases of photosensitivity, one should establish the action spectrum and reproduce the lesion on nonexposed skin. The distinction between phototoxicity and photoallergy is sometimes difficult. The diagnosis of photoallergy has only recently been considered and is easily missed if the physician is not prepared for it.

I. Halogenated Salicylanilides

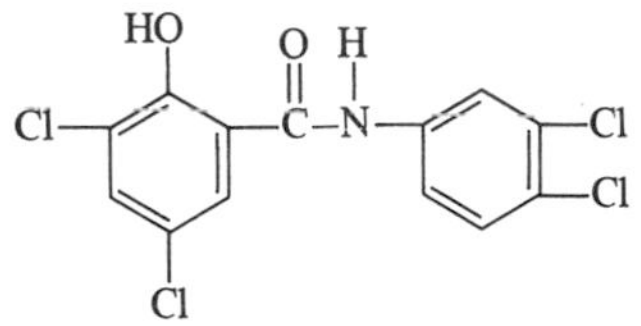

3,3',4',5—Tetrachlorosalicylanilide

The halogenated salicylanilides (tetrachlorosalicylanilide, brominated salicyl-anilides) and related compounds caused an epidemic of adverse reactions to sun-light between 1960 and 1970, when they were incorporated as antibacterials in soaps and cosmetics (WILKINSON 1961; CALNAN et al. 1961; EPSTEIN et al. 1968). After 1968 a striking reduction in numbers of patients with positive photopatch tests to these compounds has been noted (SMITH and EPSTEIN 1977), and explained partly by removal from the market of the more potent photosensitizing chemicals, partly by increased awareness by physicians.

OSMUNDSEN (1970 b) showed a varying cross-photoreaction pattern between halogenated salicylanilides and related compounds (salicylanilide, hexachloro-phene, trichlorocarbanilide, fenticlor, Jadit, 2,4-dichlorbenzylalcohol, and zinc omadine).

II. Chloro-2-phenylphenol

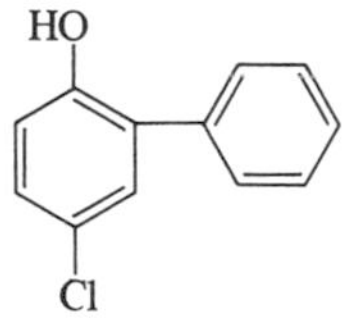

4—Chloro—2—phenylphenol

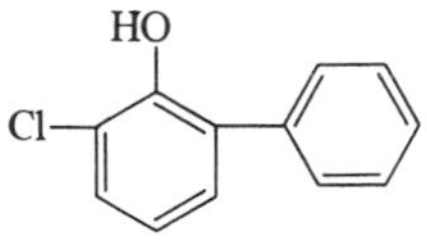

6—Chloro—2—phenylphenol

A corresponding phenolic compound Dowicide 32 (chloro-2-phenylphenol), used as a germicidal agent in a liquid soap, photosensitized four workers; cross-reaction with related compounds was not observed (ADAMS 1972).

III. Bithionol

Bithionol (2,2-thio-bis-[4,6-dichlorophenol]) is a bacteriostatic agent related to hexachlorophene. It produces both contact allergy and photocontact allergy and cross-reacts with hexachlorophene and the halogenated salicylanilides. The use of bithionol is now restricted in the United States but reactions still occur occasionally from old stock preparations (O'QUINN et al. 1967).

IV. Hexachlorophene

Hexachlorophene, widely used and described in more detail under antiseptics (Sect. M), is rarely, if at all, documented as a primary photosensitizer (O'QUINN et al. 1967; FREEMAN and KNOX 1968).

V. Fenticlor

Fenticlor (bis-2-hydroxy-5-chlorophenyl sulfide), an antifungal agent, cross-reacting with bithionol and hexachlorophene, is also a photoallergen (BURRY 1968).

VI. Multifungin

Multifungin (5-bromo-4-chlorosalicylanilide) is a photoallergenic fungicide (BURRY 1967).

VII. Jadit

Buclosamide

Jadit (buclosamide, chlorosalicylamide), used in Australia and Europe as an antifungal agent, has caused several cases of photoallergic reactions (BURRY and HUNTER 1970).

VIII. Chlorhexidine

Chlorhexidine has caused photoallergy in one case (WAHLBERG and WENNERSTEN 1971).

IX. Esters of p-Aminobenzoic Acid

p–Aminobenzoic acid   4–(Dimethylamino)benzoic acid   Glyceryl p–aminobenzoate

Paradoxically, these suntan preparations can become photosensitizers themselves (SATULSKY 1950). GOLDMAN and EPSTEIN (1969) established glyceryl-p-aminobenzoate as an ordinary contact allergen and a photosensitizer in one patient. This mechanism of photosensitization to glyceryl PABA must be differentiated from the mechanism involved when a photosensitive patient develops allergic contact dermatitis to a suntan preparation or experiences a flare of the photosensitive dermatosis (HORIO and HIGUCHI 1978). A sunburn dermatitis may enhance sensitization by increased absorption. KLIGMAN and EPSTEIN (1959) produced UV erythema and edema in 19 patients, enhancing sensitization three-fold to the monobenzylether of hydroquinone.

Recently the result of photopatch testing with PABA was shown to be vehicle dependent. A positive reaction in a photoallergic patient could be elicited by 5% PABA in alcohol but not in petrolatum (MATHIAS et al. 1978 a). A variety of other chemicals have occasionally been described as photoallergens.

X. Sulfonamides and Phenothiazines

Sulfonamides and phenothiazines are usually not intended for topical use, but accidental exposure occurs in hospital personnel and inpatients using the drugs orally. They can cause photocontact allergy, and cross-reactions between the related chemicals are seen. Related antihistamines (e. g., phenergan), used topically, may induce photoallergy.

XI. Digalloyl Trioleate

Digalloyl trioleate is a mixture of several derivatives of tannic acid and one case of photocontact allergy has been reported (SAMS 1956).

XII. Captan

Captan (Dangard, Vancide 89) is used as a fungicide on fruits and vegetables. Used as an antiseborrhoeic agent in a shampoo, it caused one case of photoallergic contact dermatitis (EPSTEIN 1968). In a human Draize test 1% Captan sensitized 4.4% of the subjects (MARZULLI and MAIBACH 1973).

XIII. Coal Tar

Crude coal tar, used because of its phototoxic properties, has caused photoallergy in a psoriatic patient (STARKE and JILLSON 1961).

XIV. 8-Methoxypsoralen

8-Methoxypsoralen and UVA (PUVA) caused photoallergic dermatitis in a psoriasis patient after 16 uneventful courses of PUVA treatment. The diagnosis of photoallergy was confirmed by reexposure to UVA and both oral and topical methoxypsoralen. UVB and UVC (< 290 nm) did not elicit the reaction and the photoallergy did not include trimethylpsoralen (PLEWIG et al. 1978).

XV. 6-Methylcoumarin

6-Methylcoumarin, a synthetic fragrance in a variety of cosmetics and toiletries, is alleged to be a potent experimental photocontact allergen but does not produce phototoxic reaction (KAIDBY and KLIGMAN 1978).

XVI. Hydrocortisone

Hydrocortisone has recently been added to the list of potential photoallergens, causing a facial photocontact dermatitis in one patient (RIETSCHEL 1978a).

Q. Vehicle Constituents

FISHER et al. (1971) introduced the vehicle tray in patch testing and thereby increased the physician's awareness of the possibility of contact allergy to vehicle ingredients. The vast majority of vehicles has not been studied in a systematic fashion; they have not been subjected to predictive testing in animals and only limited epidemiologic data exist from screening of eczema patients (HJORTH and TROLLE LASSEN 1963; HANNUKSELA et al. 1976a; IDEN and SCHROETER 1977).

Topical allergy to preservatives and antiseptics incorporated in vehicles is described in detail in Sects. M, N. In the Finish study of eczema patients over a 3-year period, perfume allergy was detected in 3.6% of the cases, sensitivity to thiomersal in 2%, to wool alcohols in 1.2%, to emulsifiers in 1%, to sorbic acid in 0.8%, and to parabens in 0.3% (HANNUKSELA et al. 1976a).

A different picture arose when the Mayo Clinic examined over 700 eczema patients over a 2-year period for sensitivity to vehicle ingredients (IDEN and SCHROETER 1977). Here, sensitivity to ethylenediamine reached 7.9%, paraben mixtures in 3.3%, dichlorophene in 2.4%, propylene glycol in 1.5%, lanolin in 1.1%, polysorbate (Tween 20) in 1%, and sorbic acid in 1%. In the Danish survey (HJORTH and TROLLE LASSEN 1963) comprising routine patch testing in 1,664 eczema patients, the main offenders among therapeutic agents were coal tar 4.3%, wood tar 4.0%, balsams 3.2%, neomycin 3.0%, balsam of Peru 2.4%, lanolin and derivatives 2.3%, and wool alcohols 1.6%. These differences between reports reflect the selection of patients, choice of vehicle tray, composition of topical drugs used in the area and patch test concentration.

I. Petrolatum

Sensitivity to this vehicle is extremely rare, but has been reported in one patient who had positive reactions to all patches in the standard series, where petrolatum was used as vehicle. Patch tests with pure white and yellow soft paraffin were positive (GRIMALT and ROMAGUERA 1978). A chronic dermatitis and hyperpigmentation from petrolatum has also been reported (MAIBACH 1978).

II. Lanolin

The general incidence of primary specific lanolin allergy is low. CLARK (1975) estimated $5.5 \pm 4.2/10^6$. Lanolin is included in the standard series of the ICDRG because of the high incidence of lanolin allergy among eczema patients. In epidemiologic studies of patients, the frequency of sensitization ranges from 1.1% (IDEN and SCHROETER 1977) to 6.0% (FISHER et al. 1971); depending upon group selection and prescription habits. Lanolin allergy is most common among leg ulcer patients.

Lanolin is a natural product from sheep fleece and consists of a complex mixture of sterols (wool alcohols), fatty alcohols, and fatty acids. The composition varies from time to time and place to place. The use of lanolin extends from topical preparations to polishes, anticorrosives, printing inks, and paper constituents. The literature on contact allergy to lanolin is extensive and has been reviewed up to 1973 by BREIT and BANDMANN (1973). HJORTH and TROLLE LASSEN (1963) described the clinical picture of lanolin allergy, emphasizing the frequent occurence of lanolin allergy in elderly women with a long history of eczema. Spread of eczema to secondary sites was common. The majority of positive patch test reactions were rather weak, with only few strong reactions. The detection of weak lanolin allergy was improved by testing with wool alcohols in a concentration of 30% in petrolatum or by adding 5% salicylic acid to the lanolin. Salicylic acid appeared to promote lanolin penetration through the skin. Antioxidants added to lanolin were shown to neutralize the allergenecity, while peroxides formed during storage appeared to accentuate the allergenecity of lanolin.

At present, because of concern over the marginal irritancy potential of the added salicylic acid in lanolin, the ICDRG recommends testing with at least two samples: 30% wool alcohol and full strength lanolin. We do not know how many lanolin allergic patients are missed by this simple and convenient test system. Until the actual allergens are chemically defined and isolated this regimen seems realistic. MORTENSEN (1979), testing with wool alcohol 30% in petrolatum, revealed 2.7% positive patch tests in 1,230 patients, while supplementary testing of 899 other eczema patients with lanolin derivatives including hydrogenated lanolin and Amerchol L 101 (mineral oil and lanolin alcohol) yielded 6.6% positive reactions.

The true frequency of lanolin allergy requires definition. We believe that lanolin allergy is uncommon on normal skin and with cosmetic usage, in contrast to the significant rate when applied to leg ulcers and other diseased skin. Because of the rarity of lanolin sensitization when applied to normal skin, we carefully verify every wool alcohol and lanolin positive patch test to ascertain that it represents allergy and not the angry skin syndrome.

The lanolin allergens are natural free fatty alcohols. Their allergenecity is increased by the simultaneous presence of detergent. Removal of the free fatty alcohols and detergent from lanolin reduced the hypersensitivity by 96% in selected lanolin-sensitive patients (CLARK et al. 1977).

Several modifications of lanolin have been tested to produce one with less sensitizing capacity. Acetylated lanolin (Modulan) was less of a sensitizer than plain lanolin (CRONIN 1966). De-waxed lanolin (Lantrol) has also been claimed to cause less sensitization than lanolin. Hydrogenated lanolin, used frequently because of its hydrophilic colorless and odorless properties, caused a higher incidence of hypersensitivity than anhydrous lanolin in Japan (SUGAI and HIGASHI 1975). A recent Belgian study (OLEFFE et al. 1978) found hydrogenated lanolin to be less sensitizing.

A patient hypersensitive to one brand of lanolin might tolerate another. Patch tests for lanolin sensitivity should be performed with wool alcohol 30% in petrolatum (EPSTEIN 1972) but it is emphasized that allergy to other lanolin derivatives might be missed, if the lanolin preparation used by the patient is not tested.

Eucerin is petrolatum with 6% wool alcohols and caused positive patch tests in 1% of 4,354 allergic contact dermatitis patients (BANDMANN 1967). Discrepancies were observed between eucerin and lanolin patch tests, explained by differences in allergen concentration

III. Emulsifiers

$$CH_3(CH_2)_{10}CH_2OSO_3Na$$
Sodium lauryl sulfate

Sodium lauryl sulfate is an emulsifier and an irritant, even in a 1% concentration, as in hydrophilic ointment (BERGSTRESSER and EAGLSTEIN 1973). Contact allergy is extremely rare but has been claimed (FOUSSEREAU et al. 1974; PRATER et al. 1978).

Common emulsifiers were tested in over 1,200 eczema patients in Finland (HANNUKSELA et al. 1976b). Allergic reactions were found in 21% of those tested, the great majority of the patients were also sensitive to other substances. The emulsifiers responsible for the positive reactions in 0.3%–0.7% of the cases were Lanette (sorbitan sesquioleate), the Spans (polyoxyethylene oxypropylene stearate), polyoxyethylene sorbitol lanolin derivative and triethanolamine stearate. Tweens were positive in only two cases. MAIBACH and CONNANT (1977) reported contact urticaria to polysorbate 60 (Tween 60). Sorbitan monolaurate in a hydrocortisone cream (Alphaderm) caused allergic contact dermatitis in a woman after treatment with Alphaderm for 1 week (FINN and FORSYTH 1975).

The synthetic emulsifiers are marketed under many different trade names which makes it difficult to evaluate emulsifier allergy. The non-ionic emulsifiers are considered weak sensitizers. Regarding translation of trade names, reference is made to the Cosmetic Ingredient Dictionary published by the Cosmetic, Toiletry and Fragrance Association Inc., 1625 Eye Street, N.W., Washington D.C. 20006.

Lanette wax or emulsifying wax consists of cetyl and stearyl alcohol with 10% sulfated esters of fatty alcohols; because of its emulsifying properties it is often used as a substitute for lanolin in creams. HJORTH and TROLLE LASSEN (1963) described hypersensitivity to Lanette wax in 0.8% of eczema patients. Concomitant sensitivity to lanette wax and to lanolin was rare.

IV. Aliphatic Alcohols

The alcohols with 8, 10, 12, and 14 carbon atoms are used mainly in detergent manufacturing, while those with longer chains are used for creams. The short chain alcohols are irritants, but the skin reactions they produce are often indistinguishable from true eczematous allergic reactions. HJORTH and TROLLE LASSEN (1963) described the wide variation in sensitivity pattern to these alcohols and emphasized the rarity of positive reactions to the higher alcohols. The high grade commercial quality of the alcohols contained a minimum of 95%–97% of the labeled substance. Impurities might be responsible for some hypersentitivity reactions, as in the case reported by SHORE and SHELLEY (1974). Urticaria-like skin reaction to cetyl and stearyl alcohol has been reported (GAUL 1969).

Few cases of allergy to glyceryl monoleate and glyceryl monostearate have been reported (HJORTH and TROLLE LASSEN 1963). Isopropyl myristate (a synthetic fatty alcohol) was an allergen in six cases reported by CALNAN (1968).

V. Polyethylene Glycol

$$H(OCH_2CH_2)_nOH$$

Polyethylene glycol (PEG) is a mixture of glycols with molecular weights ranging from 200 to 6,000 daltons. The lower molecular weights are liquids; the higher molecular weights are solids. Corbowax is a waxy polyethylene glycol with varying solidity according to the molecular weight. Polyethylene glycols are extensively used in cosmetics, detergents, shampoos, hairdressings, insect repellents, toothpastes, contraceptives, suppositories, and topical medicaments. They are also widely used in industry.

MARZULLI and MAIBACH (1974) sensitized one of 200 volunteers to a bar soap using human Draize test. Breakdown testing of the soap revealed 3% PEG 300 as the allergen. Additional challenges with 3% PEG 100, 1,000, 4,000, and 6,000 were all positive. A provocative use test with 3% polyethylene glycol was negative. BRAUN (1969) found 4% of 92 dermatologic patients to be hypersensitive to polyethylene glycol 300. The sensitivity only infrequently extended to higher molecular weight polyethylene glycols. No cross-reaction between polyethylene glycols and propylene glycol was found.

Four patients allergic to liquid polyethylene glycols in topical medications were reported by FISHER (1978). Two had immediate urticarial reactions to PEG 400 and two had delayed allergic eczematous reactions. Cross-reactions occurred between PEG 200, 300, and 400. Polyethylene glycols may form formaldehyde by autooxidation in amounts which may maintain dermatitis in patients previously sensitized to formaldehyde (Dahlquist et al. 1980).

VI. Glycerol

Glycerol is frequently used as a humectant in vehicles for topical use. Testing 420 consecutive patients, Hannuksela and Förström (1976) found 1 with a relevant positive reaction to glycerol.

VII. Propylene Glycol

Propylene glycol is described under preservatives (Sect. N.II).

VIII. Ethylenediamine Hydrochloride

$$H_2NCH_2CH_2NH_2$$

Ethylenediamine

This stabilizer is recognized as a common allergen, particularly in the United States (Fisher et al. 1971). In most cases sensitization was apparently caused by ethylenediamine in Mycolog cream. Other countries have equivalent preparations. Sensitization has followed exposure to aminophylline (Baer et al. 1959), and topical use of ethylenediamine-related antihistamines (Fisher 1973, p. 41). Cross-reactions to topical antihistamines and disodium ethylenediamine tetraacetate is not inevitable (White 1978). Adequate patch testing requires a 1% concentration of ethylenediamine; patch tests with ethylenediamine-containing medicaments give false negative results (Epstein and Maibach 1968). Industrial exposure is frequent but rarely leads to sensitization because exposure is not prolonged or intimate and normal skin is usually involved (Fisher 1973, p. 41). Sensitization by ethylenediamine in cutting oil is an exception (Crow et al. 1978).

IX. Ethylsebacate

$$C_2H_5OOC(CH_2)_8COOC_2H_5$$

Ethylsebacate is a solubilizer in haloprogin solution and cream. It may be used in cosmetics. Contact allergic reactions to this substance are rare, but have been reported (Berlin and Miller 1976; Schneider 1980).

X. Freons

$$CCl_3F$$

Freon 11

$$CCl_2F_2$$

Freon 12

$$CClF_2CClF_2$$

Freon 114

Freons (Freon 11, trichloromonofluoromethane; Freon 12, dichlorofluoro-
methane) are used as propellants in sprays. Three patients have been reported allergic to Freon 11, one of them also reacted to Freon 12. All three showed positive
reactions to ethyl chloride as well; one had an eczematous eruption on the skin after spraying for a biopsy (VAN KETEL 1976a).

R. Perfumes

Perfume allergy evaluation may be difficult. A complete perfume compound may
consist of from 3 to more than 100 basic components (FISHER 1975a), which can
be classified as: (1) natural products from flowers, plants, roots, herbs, woods, and
gums; (2) animal products and their extracts; and (3) the synthetic fragrances.

Perfume allergy evaluation is made more difficult by the fact that labeling of
perfumes with their ingredients is not required by law and the lack of cooperation
from many manufacturers to disclose the composition of their perfumes. That certain perfumes are sensitizers and photosensitizers (others are solely photosensitizers) adds to the investigator's frustration. To avoid false negative reactions, ingredient testing is necessary. FISHER (1975a) formulated an extensive list of perfume ingredients, their concentrations and the vehicles used for patch testing.
Patients with perfume dermatitis may have positive reactions to many components
of a perfume (LARSEN 1975).

The early epidemiology of perfume allergy is based on HJORTH's (1961) classic
monograph on balsam of Peru. Many perfumes contain components either identical with or cross-reacting with materials contained in balsam of Peru and other natural resins. Positive patch tests with one or more of these substances are often an
indication of perfume allergy (ROTHENBORG and HJORTH 1968). Balsam of Peru
contains 30%–40% of resins of unknown composition, while the remaining
60%–70% consists of well known chemicals: benzyl benzoate, benzyl cinnamate,
cinnamic acid, benzoic acid, vanillin, farnesol, and nerolidol. Balsam of Peru gave
positive reactions in 4.6% of males and 7.6% of females in a European epidemiologic study comprising 4,000 eczema patients (FREGERT et al. 1969). Immediate
reactions to patch tests with balsam of Peru occur (FRIIS and HJORTH 1973). The
North American Contact Dermatitis Research Group found 7.2% positive
reactions to balsam of Peru in an epidemiologic study of more than 3,000 patients
(NACDRG 1975). They did not differentiate between men and women. The high
incidence or perfume allergy is attributed to the widespread use of perfumes in cosmetics, topical preparations, and household products. Generally, the fragrance
concentration is about 0.1% but may be many times higher. Regarding the safety
of perfume and fragrance ingredients, the Research Institute of Fragrance materials Inc. (RIFM) evaluates and publishes regularly in the journal *Food and Cosmetic Toxicology*. OPDYKE (1975) has reviewed the subject.

Perfume screening trays for patch testing has been developed to increase the
sensitivity and specificity of perfume allergy detection (LARSEN 1977). In 20 per-
fume-sensitive patients examined with a screening tray of 15 fragrances, jasmin
synthetic, cinnamic alcohol, and hydroxycitronellal were the three most common
allergens. RUDZKI and GRYWA (1977a) tested 35 essential oils and 4 balsams on

450 patients. They found a poor correlation between positive reactions to essential oils and to balsam of Peru. When all four balsams (colophony, turpentine, wood tar, and balsam of Peru) were tested they revealed essential oil sensitivity in most of the sensitive patients (72 of 106).

FISHER and DOOMS-GOOSSENS (1976) suggest that sensitizing ingredients in a perfume may become hypoallergenic by interacting with other ingredients during the aging process of the perfume. Another interesting phenomenon regarding perfume allergy is the quenching phenomenon described by MAJETI and SUSKIND (1977). The sensitizing properties of cinnamaldehyde, citral, and phenylacetaldehyde were inhibited by eugenol, (+)-limonene, and phenylethylalcohol, respectively. Because of these phenomena, a provocative product use test is important in the evaluation of a patient with a suspected perfume allergy. In the use test the suspected finished product is applied openly twice daily for 5–7 days to an area of one cubital fossa and the neck or face. If it is tolerated, the patient can continue to use the product.

The fragrance contact allergy and dermatotoxicology story has just started; much work remains in identifying potential allergens, photoallergens, and phototoxins, followed by quantitating the dose responses in relation to vehicle and application method. Epidemiology in normal subjects and eczema patients is required for reasonable risk: benefit decisions. Surprising new observations, such as cinnamic aldehyde producing primary depigmentation and systemic effects, or acetylethyltetramethyl tetralin (AETT) neurotoxicity, suggests that increasingly sophisticated science should produce safer fragrances (MATHIAS et al. 1980; SPENCER et al. 1979).

S. Plant-Derived Topical Drugs

Allergic reactions to balsam of Peru are detailed under perfume allergy (Sect. R). The literature on this subject is based on HJORTH's monograph (1961).

I. 8-Methoxysporalen

8-Methoxypsoralen photoallergy has recently been reported (PLEWIG et al. 1978) and is described in the psoriasis and photocontact dermatitis sections (E and P).

II. Arnica Tincture

Arnica tincture has been used in local treatment of rheumatic complaints. BEETZ et al. (1971 b) studied 10 allergic women, finding the allergenic component in the lipid-soluble fraction. The identity of the allergen was not proven but was suspected to be either thymolmethyl ether or thymolhydroquinonedimethyl ether. HAUSEN (1978) discovered the sesquiterpene lactone, helenalin and its derivatives, as the main contact allergens in *Arnica montana*, which together with camomile belong to the family of compositae.

III. Camomile

Camomile is still used in cosmetic and topical medications. BEETZ et al. (1971a) found 3 patients of 200 unselected patients hypersensitive to a camomile chloroform extract. Only one demonstrated allergic contact dermatitis to a camomile ointment.

IV. Coumarin

Coumarin (coumarinic anhydride) and drivatives are added as a fragrance to topical preparations. Allergic contact dermatitis from coumarin derivatives was seen in a patient who had applied Jecovitol ointment to a foot ulcer (VAN KETEL 1973). The synthetic 6-methylcoumarin has caused allergic photocontact dermatitis (KAIDBY and KLIGMAN 1978).

V. Tincture of Benzoin

Benzoin tincture contains 10% benzoin in alcohol, while the compound formulation also contains 2% aloes, 8% storax, and 4% tolu balsam in alcohol. Occasionally, allergic contact dermatitis occurs to these preparations or derivatives in Arning's tincture (besides benzoin, tumenol ammonium, anthrarobin, and ether), adhesives, water repellent barrier creasms, lozenges, and cosmetics (SPOTT and SHELLEY 1970). Cross-reactions occur to balsam of Peru, storax, eugenol, vanilla, α-pinene, benzyl alcohol, and benzyl cinnamate (HJORTH 1961).

VI. Podophylin

Contact allergy to this wart remedy has not been established.

VII. Rosin (Colophony)

This natural resin is used in adhesives, e.g., adhesive tape, epilating wax, and as a tacky wax to prevent slipping (violinists, gymnasts). It is a residue after distilling oils from certain pine trees. Gum rosin and wood rosin are the two main types. They contain abietic acid which may be the sensitizer. Cross-reactions between rosin and balsam of Peru occur (FISHER 1973, p. 173; HJORTH 1961).

VIII. Gums

Other gums (plant exudates consisting of high polymer polysaccharides, some with a low nitrogen content) as karaya, acacia (gum arabic), and gum tragacanth may occasionally act as sensitizers (NILSSON 1960).

IX. Vegetable Turpentine

Vegetable turpentine was an ingredient in rubefacients such as Sloan's liniment. Allergic contact dermatitis to turpentine has been thoroughly investigated by PIRILÄ and co-workers (e.g., PIRILÄ et al. 1969).

X. Wood and Coal Tar

Wood and coal tar are described in detail in Sect. E.I. These tars are irritants but contact allergic reactions do occur. Van Andel et al. (1974) found 9% of 650 persons tested positive to wood tar; 7% reacted to coal tar. Many showed cross-reactions to balsam of Peru, colophony, and turpentine. By repeated testing of 33 tar reactors, only 20 were positive to wood tar. Juniper tar was the most active. The majority of patch test reactions to tars are irritant reactions as indicated by Rothenborg and Hjorth (1968).

XI. Propolis

Propolis (bee glue) has been used widely in folk medicine in some European countries (e.g., Denmark). It contains, among other things, well-known sensitizers such as cinnamic acid and vanillin. When a commercial propolis ointment was incorporated in the standard patch test series in a Danish dermatology department, 20 of 295 showed positive reactions (Petersen 1977).

T. Miscellaneous Agents

I. 5-Fluorouracil

This antimitotic agent is used topically for treatment of actinic keratoses and related conditions. Allergic sensitization to 5-fluorouracil was first reported by Sams (1968). Goette and Odom (1977) reported six cases of allergic contact dermatitis to 5-fluorouracil characterized by a severe pruritic eruption at the application site. Five of the six patients had two courses of treatment before allergy occurred. Intracutaneous testing proved valuable. Recently fluorouracil contact allergy with false negative patch tests and positive intradermal tests has been reported (Epstein 1980 a). In predictive testing 5-fluorouracil was unable to sensitize humans or guinea pigs (Andersen and Maibach 1979).

II. Tromantidine Hydrochloride

In treatment of herpes simplex infections, this synthetic antiviral agent is used topically. Of 240 patients treated with a 1% tromantidine ointment, 20 showed local

irritation, and contact allergy was found in 12 cases, proved by patch testing (FAN-
TA and MISCHER 1976; MISCHER and FANTA 1978).

III. Idoxuridine

Used both in eyedrops and in skin preparations for herpes infections, this antiviral
agent has caused scattered cases of allergic contact dermatitis (e.g., OSMUNDSEN
1975; VAN KETEL 1977; CALNAN 1979). Three of 45 herpes zoster patients treated
locally with idoxuridine in DMSO showed positive patch test reactions two years
later (THORMANN and WILDENHOFF 1980). DMSO (dimethylsulfoxide) used as a vehicle for idoxuridine in skin preparations, increases the penetration of idoxuridine
and might increase the risk of developing contact allergy. This mechanism of facilitating sensitization and challenge has experimental support (MAGUIRE 1974).

IV. Neutral Red

This natural dye has been used in treatment of herpes genitalis. Six cases of contact
allergy were reported (GOLDENBERG and NELSON 1975; CONANT and MAIBACH
1974).

V. Suntan Preparations

The occurrence of photoallergy to esters of p-aminobenzoic acid was described in
the discussion of photoallergic topical drugs (Sect. P.IX). Ordinary contact sensitization is more frequent, described as early as 1949 by MELTZER and BAER (1949).
Cross-reactions to other "para" compounds such as paraphenylenediamine-de-
rived hair dyes, azo and aniline dyes, local anesthetics (procaine, benzocaine), sulfonamides, and p-aminosalicylic acid occur. The spectrum of cross-reactions varies
from patient to patient (FISHER et al. 1958). FISHER (1977) has emphasized the importance of recognizing impurities in a compound as responsible for certain cross-
reactions, i.e., benzocaine in glyceryl-p-aminobenzoic acid (Escalol 106).

2,2'-Dihydroxy-4,4'-dimethoxybenzophenone

Benzophenones constitute another group of suntan preparations. Deoxybenzone and/or oxybenzone caused allergic contact dermatitis in a few patients (THOMPSON et al. 1977; PARISER 1977). A concomitant positive reaction to deoxybenzone and oxybenzone was explained as cross-sensitization or concomitant sensitization; contamination of one with the other was ruled out by chromatographic analysis in PARISER's case. THOMPSON et al. (1977) also mentioned a new suntan preparation sensitizer, cinoxate.

Sulisobenzone (2-hydroxy-4-benzophenone-5-sulfonic acid) was the allergen in a case showing immediate and delayed hypersensitivity (BAER and RAMSAY 1971; RAMSAY et al. 1972). Digalloyl trioleate has been described as a photoallergen (SAMS 1956). Many suntan preparations contain cinnamates, which may cause contact allergy and photocontact allergy (GOODMAN 1970).

Homomenthyl salicylate in a suntan preparation produced a follicular allergic contact dermatitis in two patients (RIETSCHEL and LEWIS 1978). That one investigator documented two patients in a short period suggests that many such examples may be missed by less observant physicians. Various salicylates, e.g., menthyl, benzyl, and phenyl compounds are used in suntan preparations and are sensitizers (RIETSCHEL and LEWIS 1978; KAHN 1971). The same is true of anthranilates. FISHER (1973, pp. 209–216) reviews the literature on allergic reactions to suntan preparations and lists the active ingredients in the most popular brands.

VI. Dihydroxyacetone

$$HOCH_2COCH_2OH$$

Dihydroxyacetone, a pigmenting agent, used in treatment of vitiligo, caused a severe and chronic contact dermatitis in a woman after application of a 1% solution to the neck and chest area (HARMAN 1961). Later, the same preparation was applied to vitiligous areas of the arms with no adverse effect. No patch tests were performed because of the severity of the dermatitis in the neck and chest area.

VII. Hydroquinone and Derivatives

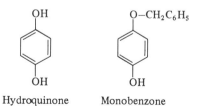

Hydroquinone   Monobenzone

Hydroquinone and the monobenzyl ether of hydroquinone are used as depigmenting agents in bleach creams and skin lighteners. The latter is a well-known sensitizer, also used in the rubber industry. FISHER (1973, p. 235) found 5% of users allergic to this compound.

Hydroquinone appears to be less of a sensitizer, but erythema, progressing to post inflammatory hyperpigmentation, occurred among the most frequently encountered adverse effects in a trial comprising 840 South African volunteers (BENT-

LEY-PHILLIPS and BAYLES 1975). A concentration of 1% in petrolatum is appropriate for patch tests. The sensitization frequency will presumably decrease with the current trend of lowering the concentration to 2% in over-the-counter preparations.

VIII. Resorcinol

Resorcinol allergic contact dermatitis is infrequent despite widespread exposure to this compound in acne remedies, hair tonics, cosmetics, and suppositories. Cross-reactions occur with resorcinol monoacetate and to a lesser degree with pyrocatechol, hydroquinone, and hexylresorcinol (CARON and CALNAN 1962; KEIL 1962).

IX. Benzoyl Peroxide

$$(C_6H_5CO)_2O_2$$

Benzoyl peroxide is used mainly in acne treatment and is an irritant. Allergic contact dermatitis to this compound is not infrequent. EAGLSTEIN (1968) reported two cases. The sensitization rate has been estimated to be 1%–2.5%. In a human maximization test, 76% became sensitized (LEYDEN and KLIGMAN 1977). Cross-reactions to benzoic acid and related compounds were not found. The drug has been advocated for treatment of chronic leg ulcers. Eight of 16 patients showed positive patch tests to 2% benzoyl peroxide after 6 weeks of leg ulcer treatment with 10% benzoyl peroxide (JENSEN et al. 1980). Patients sensitized to benzoyl peroxide may be at risk in certain occupations (e.g., baking and the plastics industry).

X. Epinephrine and Derivatives

$$
\underset{\text{Ephedrine}}{\text{HOCHCHNHCH}_3}
\qquad
\underset{\text{Phenylephrine hydrochloride}}{\text{HOCHCH}_2\text{NHCH}_3 \cdot \text{HCl}}
\qquad
\underset{\text{Echothiopate iodide}}{\left[\substack{C_2H_5O \\ C_2H_5O} P\!-\!SCH_2CH_2\overset{+}{N}(CH_3)_3 \right] I^-}
$$

Adrenergic agents are used topically in eyedrops. Allergic conjunctivitis and periorbital dermatitis developed in a man, whose glaucoma had been treated for several years with epinephrine drops (ALANI and ALANI 1976a). ROED-PETERSEN (1976) described two patients hypersensitive to metaoxedrine (phenylepinephrine), a sympathomimetic amine in Flubenisolonvalerate with metaoxedrine and lidocaine. The second patient was also sensitive to lidocaine hydrochloride. MATHIAS et al. (1979a) described a case with allergy to phenylephrine and echothiopate iodide, a cholinesterase inhibitor. Cross-reaction between epinephrine and phenylephrine was not found.

XI. Pyrazolone Compounds

$$\underset{\text{Phenylbutazone}}{\overset{\displaystyle C_6H_5}{\underset{CH_3CH_2CH_2CH_2}{\bigotimes}}}$$

Phenylbutazone

As anti-inflammatory drugs, pyrazolone preparations have been used topically for superficial phlebitis and similar inflammatory conditions. KROOK (1975) described three cases of contact allergy, one sensitive to oxyphenbutazone, the two others sensitive to phenylbutazone. Phenylbutazone did not cause cross-sensitivity to oxyphenbutazone, while cross-sensitivity the opposite way was found. VOOYS and VAN KETEL (1977) added one more case of phenylbutazone allergy, and THORMANN and KAABER (1978) recorded four, emphasizing the increased risk of developing hypersensitivity in patients with preexisting skin disorders.

XII. Bufexamac

Bufexamac (p-butoxyphenylacethydroxyamic acid) is another nonsteroidal anti-inflammatory drug used topically. SMEENK (1973) and LACHAPELLE (1975) described five cases of contact allergy.

XIII. Nitroglycerin

$$\begin{array}{l} CH_2-ONO_2 \\ CH-ONO_2 \\ CH_2-ONO_2 \end{array}$$

Nitroglycerin ointment applied frequently over large body areas in angina pectoris patients has caused allergic contact dermatitis (HENDRICKS and DEE 1979; SAUSKER and FREDERICK 1978). Sensitization developed even after previous peroral use of the drug.

XIV. Allylthiocarbamide

This compound was applied to the skin for massage purposes and 11 cases of widespread allergic contact dermatitis noted (TARNICK 1976).

XV. Heparinoid

In evaluating this drug, 1 case of contact allergy among 513 patients treated was observed (SCHÖNE 1975).

XVI. TEA–Coco Hydrolyzed Protein

This complex triethanolamine salt of the condensation product of coconut fatty acids, polypeptides, and amino acids was the culprit in a severe allergic dermatitis on the face of a young woman (EMMET and WRIGHT 1976). Patch tests were positive down to a 5% aqueous solution. This, and similar conjugates have been used for over 30 years in various cosmetic and toilet preparations, so allergic reactions are probably rare.

XVII. Metoprolol

Topically applied beta-blocking agents are used in glaucoma treatment. In 5 of 11 patients with ocular and periorbital dermatitis, a reproducible positive patch test to metoprolol 3% in water was found (VAN JOOST et al. 1979).

U. Conclusions

This is not an exhaustive review attempting to list every reference, but a survey of the current status of contact allergy to topical drugs. The bulk of the information comes from case reports which, although important to a given patient, do not provide the most valuable way of looking at drug reactions. NATER and DE GROOT (1980) give a comprehensive review of topical drug side effects, including contact allergy. The best way of looking at these reactions is to obtain epidemiologic data from patient populations (FREGERT et al. 1969; BANDMANN et al. 1972) and normal populations (PRYSTOWSKY et al. 1979 b).

Further valuable information comes from predictive testing in animals and humans, requiring considerable judgement and interpretation (MARZULLI and MAIBACH 1977 a). The most valuable thing the physician can do in dealing with government agencies and the pharmaceutical and cosmetics industries is to perform proper patch testing and report important findings. The new journal, *Contact Dermatitis*, is useful in reporting both individual cases and epidemiologic studies.

If manufacturers made available patch test guidelines (i.e., appropriate concentration and vehicle) for individual chemicals and final formulations, the physician could patch test with greater facility and frequency. Unfortunately, it seems probable that the impetus for making this information routinely available will have to be government regulation.

References

Aagren-Jonsson S, Magnusson B (1976) Sensitization to propantheline bromide, trichlorcarbanilide and propylene glycol in an antiperspirant. Contact Dermatitis 2:79–80

Adams RM (1972) Photoallergic contact dermatitis to chloro-2-phenylphenol. Arch Dermatol 106:711–714

Aeling JL, Panagotacos PJ, Andreozzi RJ (1974) Allergic contact dermatitis to vitamin E aerosol deodorant (letter). Arch Dermatol 108:579–580

Afzelius H, Thulin H (1979) Allergic reactions to benzalkonium chloride. Contact Dermatitis 5:60

Agrup G (1969) Hand eczema and other hand dematoses in south Sweden. Acta Derm Venereol (Stockh) [Suppl] 49:61

Agrup G, Fregert S, Övrum P (1969) Importance of pure chemicals in investigations of cross sensitivity. Acta Derm Venereol (Stockh) 49:417–421

Alani MD, Alani SD (1972) Allergic contact dermatitis to corticosteroids. Ann Allergy 30:181–185

Alani SD, Alani MD (1976a) Allergic contact dermatitis and conjunctivitis from epinephrine. Contact Dermatitis 2:147–150

Alani SD, Alani MD (1976b) Allergic contact dermatitis and conjunctivitis to corticosteroids. Contact Dermatitis 2:301–304

Allenby CF (1965) Skin sensitization to Remiderin and Cross sensitization to hydroxyquinoline compounds. Br Med J 2:208–209

Andersen KE, Maibach HI (1979) Predictive testing with 5-fluorouracil. Contact Dermatitis
5:404

Angelini G, Rantuccio F, Meneghini CL (1975) Contact dermatis in patients with leg ulcers.
Contact Dermatitis 1:81–87

Baer RL, Ramsay DN (1971) Polyvalent light sensitivity. Allergic contact sensitivity to
sulisobenzone (letter). Arch Dermatol 104:446–448

Baer RL, Cohen HJ, Neidorff AH (1959) Allergic eczematous sensitivity to aminophylline.
Arch Dermatol 79:647–648

Baker H, Ive FA, Lloyd MJ (1969) Primary irritant dermatitis of the scrotum due to hexachlorophene. Arch Dermatol 99:663–693

Bandmann HJ (1966) Die Kontaktallergie durch Arzneimittel. Pharm Zeit 111:1470

Bandmann HJ (1967) Kontaktekzem und Ekzematogene. MMW 109:1572–1580

Bandmann HJ, Breit R (1973) The mafenide story. Br J Dermatol 89:219–221

Bandmann HJ, Doenicke A (1971) Allergisches Kontaktekzem durch Propanidid bei einem
Anaesthesisten. Berufsdermatosen 19:106–165

Bandmann HJ, Dohn W (1967) Die Epicutantestung. Bergman, Munich

Bandmann HJ, Mutzeck E (1973) Contact allergy to gentamycin sulfate. Contact Dermatitis Newslett 13:371

Bandmann HJ, Calnan CD, Cronin E et al. (1972) Dermatitis from applied medicaments.
Arch Dermatol 106:335–337

Bandmann HJ, Breit R, Matzeck E (1974) Allergic contact dermatitis from proxymetacaine.
Contact Dermatitis Newslett 15:451

Bandmann M (1967) Zur monovalenten Kontaktallergie gegen Eucerinum anhydricum.
Thesis, University of Munich

Beetz D, Cramer HJ, Mehlhorn HC (1971a) Zur Häufigkeit der epidermalen Allergie gegenüber Kamille in kamillenhaltigen Arzneimitteln und Kosmetika. Dermatol Monatsschr
157:505–510

Beetz D, Würbach G, Cramer HJ (1971b) Allergenanalytische Untersuchungen mit Hilfe
der Dünnschichtchromatographie bei Überempfindlichkeit gegenüber Arnika-Tinctur.
Allerg Immunol (Leipz) 17:228

Behrbohm P, Lenzner M (1975) Sensitivity to Falicain (propoxypiperocainhydrochloride).
Contact Dermatitis 1:187–188

Bentley-Phillips B, Bayles MAH (1975) Cutaneous reactions to topical application of hydroquinone. S Afr Med J 49:1391–1395

Bergstresser PR, Eaglstein W (1973) Irritation by hydrophilic ointment under occlusion.
Arch Dermatol 108:218–219

Berlin AR, Miller F (1976) Allergic contact dermatitis from ethyl sebacate in haloprogin
cream. Arch Dermatol 112:1563–1564

Bielicky T, Novak M (1969) Contact group sensitization to triphenylmethane dyes. Arch
Dermatol 100:540–543

Binnick AM, Clendenning WE (1978) Bacitracin contact dermatitis. Contact Dermatitis
4:180–181

Björkner B (1980) Contact urticaria and asthma from denatonium benzoate (Bitrex®). Contact Dermatitis 6:466–471

Björnberg A (1968) Skin reactions to primary irritants in patients with hand eczema. Oscar
Isacsons Tryckeri AB, Göteborg

Black J, Calesnick B, Williams D, Weinstein MJ (1963) Pharmacology of gentamycin, a new
broad spectrum antibiotic. In: Proceedings, Symposium on antimicrobial agents and
chemotherapy. Ann Arbor, Mich. American Society for Microbiology, pp 138–147

Bleumink E, Nater JP (1972a) Allergic contact dermatitis to virginiamycin. Dermatologica
144:253–256

Bleumink E, Nater JP (1972 b) Allergic contact dermatitis to virginiamycin. Contact Dermatitis Newslett 12:337

Bojs G, Möller H (1974) Eczematous contact allergy to oxytetracycline with cross sensitivity to other tetracyclines. Berufsdermatosen 22:202–208

Braun W (1969) Kontaktallergien gegen Polyaethylenglykole. Z Hautkr 44:385–389

Braun W, Schütz R (1968) Kontaktallergie gegen Nitrofurazon (Furacin). Dtsch Med Wochenschr 93:1524–1526

Breit R, Bandmann HJ (1973) Dermatitis from lanolin. Br J Dermatol 88:414–416

Brodkin RH, Bleiberg J (1968) Ophthalmic side effects of a new topical psoriatic medication. Arch Dermatol 98:525

Bunney MH (1972) Contact dermatitis due to bethamethasone 17 valerate (betnovate). Contact Dermatitis Newslett 12:318

Burry JN (1967) Photoallergies to fentichlor and multifungin. Arch Dermatol 95:287–291

Burry JN (1968) Cross sensitivity between fentichlor and bithionol. Arch Dermatol 97:496–502

Burry JN, Hunter GA (1970) Photocontact dermatitis from jadit. Br J Dermatol 82:224–229

Burry JN, Kirk J, Reid JG, Turner T (1975) Chlorocresol sensitivity. Contact Dermatitis 1:41–42

Calnan CD (1967) Chlortetracycline sensitivity. Contact Dermatitis Newslett 1:16

Calnan CD (1968) Isopropyl myristate sensitivity. Contact Dermatitis Newslett 2:38

Calnan CD (1971) Chloracetamide dermatitis from a cosmetic. Contact Dermatitis Newslett 9:215

Calnan CD (1975) Sensitivity to benzamine lactate. Contact Dermatitis 1:56

Calnan CD (1978) Oxypolyethoxydodecane in an ointment. Contact Dermatitis 4:168

Calnan CD (1979) Allergy to idoxuridine ointment. Contact Dermatitis 5:194–195

Calnan CD (1980) Allergy to the local anaesthetic diperodon. Contact Dermatitis 6:367

Calnan CD, Harmon RRM, Wells GC (1961) Photodermatitis from soap. Br Med J 2:1266

Camarasa G (1976) Contact dermatitis from mercurochrome. Contact Dermatitis 2:120

Camarasa G, Alomar A (1978) Menthol dermatitis from cigarettes. Contact Dermatitis 4:169

Caron GA, Calnan CD (1962) Studies in contact dermatitis. XIV. Resorcin. Trans St John's Hosp Dermatol Soc 48:149–156

Church R (1960) Sensitivity to hydrocortisone acetate ointment. Br J Dermatol 72:341–344

Clark EW (1975) Estimation of the general incidence of specific lanolin allergy. J Soc Cosmet Chem 26:323–335

Clark EW, Cronin E, Wilkinson DS (1977) Lanolin with reduced sensitizing potential. Contact Dermatitis 3:69–74

Comaish S (1969) A case of hypersensitivity to corticosteroid. Br J Dermatol 81:919–925

Conant M, Maibach HI (1974) Allergic contact dermatitis due to neutral red. Arch Dermatol 109:735

Coskey RJ (1971) Contact dermatitis due to nystatin (letter). Arch Dermatol 103:228

Coskey RJ (1978 a) Contact dermatitis due to multiple corticosteroid creams. Arch Dermatol 114:115–117

Coskey RJ (1978 b) Contact dermatitis due to clindamycin. Arch Dermatol 114:446

Coskey RJ, Bryan HG (1967) Contact dermatitis due to methylprednisolone. JAMA 199:136

Cronin E (1966) Lanolin dermatitis. Br J Dermatol 78:167–174

Cronin E (1980) Contact dermatitis. Churchill Livingstone, Edinburgh London

Crow KD, Peachey RDG, Adams JE (1978) Coolant oil dermatitis due to ethylenediamine. Contact Dermatitis 4:359–361

Cruickshank CND, Squire JR (1949) Skin sensitivity to cetrimide (CTAB). Br J Ind Med 8:164–167

Dahlquist I, Fregert S (1978) Formaldehyde releasers. Contact Dermatitis 4:173

Dahlquist I, Fregert S, Gruvberger B (1980) Detection of formaldehyde in corticoid creams. Contact Dermatitis 6:494

Daly JF (1952) Contact dermatitis due to quotane. Arch Dermatol 66:393–394

Daughters D, Zackheim HS, Maibach HI (1973) Urticaria and anaphylactoid reactions after topical application of mechlorethamine. Arch Dermatol 107:429–430

Dave VK, Main RA (1973) Contact sensitivity to sodium fusidate. Contact Dermatitis Newslett 14:398

De Feo CP (1966) Erythema multiforme bullosum caused by 9-bromofluorene. Arch Dermatol 94:545–551

Degreef H, Verhoeve L (1975) Contact dermatitis to miconazole nitrate. Contact Dermatitis 1:269–270

Dooms-Goossens A, Degreef H, Parijs M, Kerkhofs L (1980 a) A retrospective study of patch test results from 163 patients with stasis dermatitis or leg ulcers I. Dermatologica 159:93–100

Dooms-Goossens A, Degreef H, Parijs M, Maertens M (1980 b) A retrospective study of patch test results from 163 patients with stasis dermatitis or leg ulcers II. Dermatologica 159:231–238

Dohn W (1960) Kontaktallergien gegen Antibiotica. Hautarzt 11:433–440

Draize JH, Woodgard G, Calvery HO (1944) Methods for the study of irritation and toxicity of substances applied topically to the skin and mucous membranes. J Pharmacol Exp Ther 82:377–390

Dupont C (1974) Fentichlor sensitivity. Contact Dermatitis Newslett 16:473

Eaglstein WH (1968) Allergic contact dermatitis to benzoyl peroxide. Arch Dermatol 97:527

Edwards M, Rudner EJ (1970) Dermatitis venenata due to hydrocortisone alcohol. Cutis 6:757–758

Ekelund A, Möller H (1969) Oral provocation in eczematous contact allergy to neomycin and hydroxyquinolines. Acta Derm Venereol (Stockh) 49:422–426

Emmett EA, Wright RC (1976) Allergic contact dermatitis from TEA-Coco hydrolyzed protein. Arch Dermatol 112:1008–1009

Epstein E (1966) Dichlorphene allergy. Ann Allergy 24:437–439

Epstein E (1972) The detection of lanolin allergy. Arch Dermatol 106:678–681

Epstein E (1980 a) Contact dermatitis to neomycin with false negative patch tests: allergy established by intradermal and usage tests. Contact Dermatitis 6:219–220

Epstein E (1980 b) Contact dermatitis to 5-fluorouracil with false negative patch tests. Contact Dermatitis 6:220–221

Epstein E, Maibach HI (1966) Formaldehyde allergy. Arch Dermatol 94:186–190

Epstein E, Maibach HI (1968) Ethylenediamine: allergic contact dermatitis. Arch Dermatol 98:476–477

Epstein JH, Wuepper KD, Maibach HI (1968) Photocontact dermatitis to halogenated salicylanilides and related compounds. Arch Dermatol 94:236–244

Epstein S (1958 a) Dermal contact dermatitis from neomycin. Observations on forty cases. Ann Allergy 16:268–280

Epstein S (1958 b) Dermal contact dermatitis, sensitivity to rivanol and gentian violet. Dermatologica 117:287–296

Epstein S (1965) Neomycin sensitivity and atopy. Dermatologica 130:280–286

Epstein S (1968) Photoallergic contact dermatitis; report of a case due to Dangard. Cutis 4:856–861

Epstein S, Wenzel FJ (1963) Sensitivity to neomycin and bacitracin, cross sensitization or coincidence? Acta Derm Venereol (Stockh) 43:1–9

Epstein WL (1960) Contribution to the pathogenesis of zirconium granulomas in man. J Invest Dermatol 34:183–188

Eriksen K (1978) Cross allergy between paranitro compounds with special reference to DNCB and chloramphenicol. Contact Dermatitis 4:29–32

Fanta D, Mischer P (1976) Contact dermatitis from tromantadine hydrochloride. Contact Dermatitis 2:282–284

FDA (1979) Cosmetic confirmed reaction study. Food and Drug Administration, Washington, DC

Fiedler H, Novak M, Schwank R (1971) Untersuchungen über Gruppensensibilisierung gegen neue Hydroxychinolin Derivate. Dermatologica 143:298–304

Finn OA, Forsyth A (1975) Contact dermatitis due to sorbitan monolaurate. Contact Dermatitis 1:318

Fisher AA (1973 a) Contact dermatitis, 2nd edn. Lea & Febiger, Philadelphia

Fisher AA (1973 b) The paraben paradox. Cutis 12:830–832

Fisher AA (1975 a) Patch testing with perfume ingredients. Contact Dermatitis 1:166–168

Fisher AA (1975 b) Allergic contact dermatitis from Germall 115, a new cosmetic preservative. Contact Dermatitis 1:126

Fisher AA (1976) The safety of topical erythromycin. Contact Dermatitis 2:43–44

Fisher AA (1977) Dermatitis due to benzocaine present in sunscreens containing glyceryl PABA (escalol 106). Contact Dermatitis 3:170–171

Fisher AA (1978) Immediate and delayed allergic contact reactions to polyethylene glycol. Contact Dermatitis 4:135–138

Fisher AA (1979) Paresthesia of the fingers accompanying dermatitis due to methylmethacrylate bone cement. Contact Dermatitis 5:56–57

Fisher AA, Dooms-Goossens A (1976) The effect of perfume "ageing" on the allergenecity of individual perfume ingredients. Contact Dermatitis 2:155–159

Fisher AA, Tobin L (1953) Sensitivity to compound G4 ("dichlorophene") in dentifrices. JAMA 15:998

Fisher AA, Pelzig A, Kanof NB (1958) The persistence of allergic eczematous sensitivity and the cross sensitivity pattern to paraphenylinediamine. J Invest Dermatol 30:9–13

Fisher AA, Pascher F, Kanof NB (1971) Allergic contact dermatitis due to ingredients of vehicles. Arch Dermatol 104:286–290

Förstrom L, Pirilä V (1978) Cross sensitivity within the neomycin group of antibiotics. Contact Dermatitis 4:312

Foussereau J, Petitjean J, Lantz JP (1974) Allergy to sodium laurylsulphate. Contact Dermatitis Newslett 15:433

Freeman RG, Knox JM (1968) The action spectrum of photocontact dermatitis: Caused by halogenated salicylanilides and related compounds. Arch Dermatol 97:130–136

Fregert S (1968) Cross sensitization among nitrofurylaminothiadazoles. Acta Derm Venereol (Stockh) 48:106–109

Fregert S (1979) Batch-consciousness in dermatologic management. Acta Derm Venereol (Stockh) 59 (Suppl 89):63–65

Fregert S, Bandmann HJ (1975) Patch testing. Springer, Berlin Heidelberg New York

Fregert S, Dahlguist I (1969) Allergic contact dermatitis from TEGO. Contact Dermatitis Newslett 5:103

Fregert S, Hjorth N (1969) Results of standard patch tests with substances abandoned. Contact Dermatitis Newslett 5:85

Fregert S, Hjorth N (1979) The principal irritants and sensitizers. In: Rook A, Wilkinson DS, Ebling FJG (eds) Textbook of dermatology, 3rd edn. Blackwell Scientific, Oxford Edinburgh

Fregert S, Rorsman H (1960) Hypersensitivity to diethylstilbestrol. Acta Derm Venereol (Stockh) 40:206–219

Fregert S, Rorsman H (1962) Hypersensitivity to diethylstilbestrol with cross sensitization to benzestrol. Acta Derm Venereol (Stockh) 42:290–293

Fregert S, Hjorth N, Magnusson B et al. (1969) Epidemiology of contact dermatitis. Trans St John's Hosp Dermatol Soc 55:17–35

Fregert S, Groth O, Gruvberger B, Magnusson B, Mobacken H, Rorsman H (1971) Hypersensitivity to secondary alcohols. Acta Derm Venereol (Stockh) 51:271–272

Fregert S, Tegner E, Thelin I (1979) Contact allergy to lidocaine. Contact Dermatitis 5:185–188

Friis B, Hjorth N (1973) Immediate reactions to patch tests with balsam of Peru. Contact Dermatitis Newslett 13:389

Fry L (1965) Skin disease from color developers. Br J Dermatol 77:456–461

Gaul LE (1969) Dermatitis from cetyl and stearyl alcohols. Arch Dermatol 99:593

Gelfarb M, Leider M (1960) Allergic eczematous contact dermatitis. Arch Dermatol 82:642–643

Gellin GA, Maibach HI, Wachs GN (1972) Contact allergy to tolnaftate. Arch Dermatol 106:715–716

Goette DK, Odom RB (1977) Allergic contact dermatitis to topical fluorouracil. Arch Dermatol 113:1050–1061

Goldenberg RL, Nelson K (1975) Dermatitis from neutral red therapy of herpes genitalis. Obstet Gynecol 46:359–360

Goldman GC, Epstein E (1969) Contact photosensitivity from sunprotective agent. Arch Dermatol 100:447–449

Goodmann TF (1970) Photodermatitis from a sunscreening agent (letter). Arch Dermatol 102:563

Gordon BI, Maibach HI (1969) Eccrine anhidrosis due to glutaraldehyde, formaldehyde and iontophoresis. J Invest Dermatol 53:436–439

Gottschalk HR, Stone OJ (1976) Stevens-Johnson syndrome from ophthalmic sulfonamide. Arch Dermatol 112:513–514

Greither A, Gisbertz C, Ippen H (1967) Teerbehandlung und Krebs. Z Hautkr 42:463–635

Grimalt F, Romaguera C (1978) Sensitivity to petrolatum. Contact Dermatitis 4:377

Groen J, Bleumink E, Nater JP (1973) Variotin sensitivity. Contact Dermatitis Newslett 15:456

Grunnet E (1976) Contact urticaria and anaphylactoid reaction induced by topical application of nitrogen mustard. Br J Dermatol 94:101–103

Guill MA, Goette DK, Knight CG, Peck CC, Lupton GP (1979) Erythema multiforme and urticaria. Arch Dermatol 115:742–743

Hannuksela M, Förström L (1976) Contact hypersensitivity to glycerol. Contact Dermatitis 2:291

Hannuksela M, Förström L (1978) Reactions to peroral propylene glycol. Contact Dermatitis 4:41–45

Hannuksela M, Pirilä V, Salo OP (1975) Skin reactions to propylene glycol. Contact Dermatitis 1:112–116

Hannuksela M, Kousa M, Pirilä V (1976a) Allergy to ingredients of vehicles. Contact Dermatitis 2:105–110

Hannuksela M, Kousa M, Pirilä V (1976b) Contact sensitivity to emulsifiers. Contact Dermatitis 2:201–204

Harman RRM (1961) Severe contact reaction to dihydroxyacetone. Trans St John's Dermatol Soc 47:157–159

Hausen BM (1978) Indentification of the allergens of *Arnica montana L.* Contact Dermatitis 4:308

Heijer A (1961) Sensitization to xanthocillin in salve. Acta Derm Venereol (Stockh) 41:201–204

Hendricks AA, Dec GW (1979) Contact dermatitis due to nitroglycerin ointment. Arch Dermatol 115:853–855

Hjorth N (1958) Contact dermatitis from vitamin B (thiamine). Relapse after ingestion of thiamine. Cross sensitization to cocarboxylase. J Invest Dermatol 30:261–264

Hjorth N (1961) Eczematous allergy to balsams. Acta Derm Venereol [Suppl] (Stockh) 41:46

Hjorth N (1967) Occupational dermatitis among veterinary surgeons caused by penethamate (benzyl-penicillin-B-diethyl-aminoethyl ester). Berufsdermatosen 15:163–175

Hjorth N (1972) Contact dermatitis from 1,3-diiodo-2-hydroxypropane. Contact Dermatitis Newslett 12:322

Hjorth N (1977) Diagnostic patch testing. In: Marzulli FN, Maibach HI (eds) Dermatotoxicology and pharmacology. John Wiley & Sons, New York Chichester, pp 341–352

Hjorth N, Fregert S (1979) Contact dermatitis. In: Rook A, Wilkinson DS, Ebling FJ (eds) Textbook of dermatology, 3rd edn. Blackwell Scientific, Oxford Edinburgh

Hjorth N, Roed-Petersen J (1976) Occupational protein contact dermatitis in food handlers. Contact Dermatitis 2:28–42

Hjorth N, Thomsen K (1968) Differences in sensitizing capacity of neomycin in creams and in ointments. Br J Dermatol 80:163–169

Hjorth N, Trolle Lassen C (1962) Skin reactions to preservatives in cream with special regard to paraben esters and sorbic acid. Am Cosmet Perf 77:43–46

Hjorth N, Trolle Lassen C (1963) Skin reactions to ointment bases. Trans St John's Hosp Dermatol Soc 49:127–140

Hjorth N, Wilkinson D, Magnusson B, Bandmann HJ, Maibach HI (1978) Glyceryl p-aminobenzoate patch testing in benzocaine-sensitive subjects. Contact Dermatitis 4:46–48

Holder R (1978) Presentation; American Academy of Dermatology, San Francisco, CA

Horio T, Higuchi T (1978) Photocontact dermatitis from p-aminobenzoic acid. Dermatologica 156:124–128

Huriez C, Agache P, Marten P, Vandaume G, Mennecier J (1965) L'Allergie aux sels d'ammonium quaternaire. Sem Hop Paris 41:2301–2304

Iden DL, Schroeter AL (1977) The vehicle tray revisited: the use of the vehicle tray in assessing allergic contact dermatitis by a 24-hour application method. Contact Dermatitis 3:122–126

International Contact Dermatitis Research Group (ICDRG) (1978) Triclocarbon – evaluation of contact dermatitis potential in man. Contact Dermatitis 4:283–288

Jensen O, Petersen SH, Vesterager L (1980) Contact sensitization to benzoyl peroxide following topical treatment of chronic leg ulcers. Contact Dermatitis 6:179–182

Jillson OF, Baughman RD (1963) Contact photodermatitis from bithionol. Arch Dermatol 88:409–418

Jirásek L, Schwank R (1965) Berufskontaktekzem durch Vitamin K. Hautarzt 16:351–353

Jordan WP, King SE (1977) Delayed hypersensitivity in females. Contact Dermatitis 3:19–26

Jordan WP, Dahl MV, Albert HL (1972) Contact dermatitis from glutaraldehyde. Arch Dermatol 105:94–95

Jordan WP, Higgins M, Dvorak J (1975) Allergic contact dermatitis to all-transretinoic acid; epicutaneous and leukocyte migration inhibition testing. Contact Dermatitis 1:306–310

Juhlin L, Hansson H (1968) Topical glutaraldehyde for plantar hyperhidrosis. Arch Dermatol 97:327–330

Kahn G (1971) Intensified contact sensitization to benzyl salicylate. Arch Dermatol 103:497–500

Kaidby KH, Kligman AM (1978) Photocontact allergy to 6-methylcoumarin. Contact Dermatitis 4:277–282

Kassen B, Mitchell JC (1974) Contact urticaria from a vitamin E preparation in two siblings. Contact Dermatitis Newslett 16:482

Keil H (1962) Group reactions in contact dermatitis due to resorcinol. Arch Dermatol 86:212–216

Kernekamp ASVW, van Ketel WG (1979) Contact allergy to hydrocortisone-17-butyrate. Contact Dermatitis 5:268–269

Kernekamp ASVW, van Ketel WG (1980) Persistence of patch test reactions to clioquinol (Vioform®) and cross-sensitization. Contact Dermatitis 6:455–460

Klaschka F, Beiersdorf HU (1965) Crux medicorum: Allergie gegen nichtdeklarierte Salbenkonservantien. MMW 107:185–188

Klecak G (1977) Identification of contact allergens: predictive tests in animals. In: Marzulli FN, Maibach HI (eds) Dermatotoxicology and pharmacology. John Wiley & Sons, New York Chichester, pp 305–339

Kleinhans D, Knoth W (1973) Paraben-kontakt Allergie mit enteraler Provokation. Z Hautkr 48:699–701

Kleinhans D, Zwissler H (1980) Anaphylaktischer Schock nach Anwendung einer benzokainhaltigen Salbe. Z Hautkr 55:945–947

Kligman AM, Epstein WL (1959) Mechanisms of hypersensitivity. Little Brown, Boston

Kligman AM, Leyden JH (1979) "Reactions" to standard patch test materials. Acta Derm Venereol (Stockh) 59 (Suppl. 89):101–103

Kooij R, Van Vloten ThJ (1952) Epidermal sensitization due to sulphonamide drugs. Dermatologica 104:151–167

Krook G (1975) Contact sensitivity to oxyphenbutazone (tanderil) and cross sensitivity to phenylbutazone (butazolidine). Contact Dermatitis 1:385–386

Lachapelle JM (1975) Contact sensitivity to bufexamac. Contact Dermatitis 1:261

Lachapelle JM, Tennstedt D (1979) Low allergenicity of triclosan. Dermatologica 158:379–383

Lahti A (1978) Skin reactions to some antimicrobial agents. Contact Dermatitis 4:302–303

Lahti A (1980) Non-immunologic contact urticaria. Acta Derm Venereol (Stockh) 60 (Suppl. 91):1–49

Larsen WG (1975) Cosmetic dermatitis due to a perfume. Contact Dermatitis 1:142–145

Larsen WG (1977) Perfume dermatitis, a study of 20 patients. Arch Dermatol 113:623–626

Leifer W, Steiner K (1951) Studies in sensitization to halogenated hydroxyquinolines and related compounds. J Invest Dermatol 17:233–240

Leyden JJ, Kligman AM (1977) Contact sensitization to benzoyl peroxide. Contact Dermatitis 3:273–275

Liden S (1975) Alphosyl sensitivity and propyl gallate. Contact Dermatitis 1:257–258

Liden S, Göransson K (1975) Contact allergy to dibenzthion. Contact Dermatitis 1:258

Lindgren S, Groth O, Molin L (1976) Allergic contact response to vitamin A acid. Contact Dermatitis 2:212–217

Lindholm L, Magnusson BL, Mobacken H (1978) Depressed nonspecific lymphocyte reactivity in psoriasis. Arch Dermatol Res 263:121–125

Ljungren B, Möller H (1972) Eczematous contact allergy to chlorhexidine. Acta Derma Venereol (Stockh) 52:308–310

Ludwig E, Hansen BM (1977) Sensitivity to isopropyl alcohol. Contact Dermatitis 3:240–244

Magnusson B, Hersle K (1965) Patch test methods. Acta Derm Venereol (Stockh) 45:257–261

Magnusson B, Kligman AM (1977a) Usefulness of guinea pig tests for detection of contact sensitizers. In: Marzulli FN, Maibach HI (eds) Dermatotoxicology and pharmacology. John Wiley & Sons, New York Chichester, pp 551–560

Magnusson B, Kligman AM (1977b) Factors affecting allergic contact sensitization. In: Marzulli FN, Maibach HI (eds) Dermatotoxicology and pharmacology. John Wiley & Sons, New York Chichester, pp 289–304

Magnusson B, Fregert S, Hjorth N, Høvding G, Pirilä V, Skog E (1969) Routine patch testing V. Acta Derm Venereol (Stockh) 49:556–563

Maguire HC (1974) Induction of delayed hypersensitivity to nitrogen mustard in the guinea pig. Br J Dermatol 91:21–26

Maibach HI (1971) Allergic sensitization potential (Draize test) in man of several preservatives. Contact Dermatitis Newslett 9:213

Maibach HI (1975a) Acute laryngeal obstruction presumed secondary to thiomersal (merthiolate) delayed hypersensitivity. Contact Dermatitis 1:221–222

Maibach HI (1975b) Glutaraldehyde cross reactions to formaldehyde. Contact Dermatitis 1:326–327

Maibach HI (1978) Chronic dermatitis and hyperpigmentation from petrolatum. Contact Dermatitis 4:62

Maibach HI, Conant M (1977) Contact urticaria to a corticosteroid cream: polysorbate 60. Contact Dermatitis 3:350–351

Maibach HI, Johnson HL (1975) Contact urticaria syndrome. Arch Dermatol 111:726–730

Maibach HI, Prystowsky SD (1977) Glutaraldehyde (pentanedial) allergic contact dermatitis. Arch Dermatol 113:170–171

Maibach HI, Akerson JM, Marzulli FN et al. (1980) Test concentrations and vehicles for dermatological testing of cosmetic ingredients. Contact Dermatitis 6:369–404

Majeti VA, Suskind RR (1977) Mechanism of cinnamaldehyde sensitization. Contact Dermatitis 3:16–18

Malten KE, Nater JP, Van Ketel WG (1976) Patch testing quidelines. Dekker & Van de Vegt, Nijmegen

March C, Greenwood MA (1968) Allergic contact dermatitis to proparacaine. Arch Ophthalmol 79:159–160

Marcussen PV (1959) Contact dermatitis due to formaldehyde in textiles, 1934–1958. Preliminary report. Acta Derm Venereol (Stockh) 39:348–356

Marzulli FN, Maibach HI (1973) Antimicrobials: experimental contact sensitization in man. J Soc Cosmet Chem 24:399–421

Marzulli FN, Maibach HI (1974) The use of graded concentrations in studying skin sensitizers: experimental contact sensitization in man. Fd Cosmet Toxicol 12:219–227

Marzulli FN, Maibach HI (1977a) Dermatotoxicology and pharmacology. John Wiley & Sons, New York Chichester

Marzulli FN, Maibach HI (1977b) Contact allergy: predictive testing in humans. In: Marzulli FN, Maibach HI (eds) Dermatolotoxicology and pharmacology. John Wiley & Sons, New York Chichester, pp 353–372

Mathias CGT, Maibach HI (1978) Dermatotoxicology monographs I. Cutaneous irritation: factors influencing the response to irritants. Clin Toxicol 13:333–346

Mathias CGT, Maibach HI, Epstein J (1978a) Allergic contact photodermatitis to para-amino-benzoic acid. Arch Dermatol 114:1165–1666

Mathias CGT, Maibach HI, Ostler HB, Conant MA, Nelson W (1978b) Delayed hypersensitivity to retrobulbar injections of methylprednisolone acetate. Am J Ophthalmol 86:816–819

Mathias CGT, Maibach HI, Irvine A, Adler W (1979a) Allergic contact dermatitis to echothiophate iodide and phenylephrine. Arch Ophthalmol 97:286–287

Mathias CGT, Caldwell TM, Maibach HI (1979b) Contact dermatitis and gastrointestinal symptoms from hydroxyethylmethacrylate. Br J Dermatol 100: 447–449

Mathias CGT, Maibach HI, Conant MA (1980) Perioral leucoderma simulating vitiligo from use of a toothpaste containing cinnamic aldehyde. Arch Dermatol 116:1172–1173

Maucher OM (1974) Beitrag zur Kreuz- oder Kopplingsallergie zur Parahydroxybenzoe-Säure-Ester. Berufsdermatosen 22:183–187

Melski JW, Tannenbaum L, Parrish JA et al. (1977) Oral methoxysalen photochemotherapy for the treatment of psoriasis. A cooperative clinical trial. J Invest Dermatol 68:328–335

Meltzer L, Baer RL (1949) Sensitization to monoglycerol paraaminobenzoate. J Invest Dermatol 12:31–38

Menné T (1978) The prevalence of nickel allergy among women. Derm Beruf Umwelt 26:123–125

Menné T, Andersen KE (1977) Allergic contact dermatitis from fluocortolone, Fluocortolone pivalate and fluocortolone caproate. Contact Dermatitis 3:337–340

Meneghini CL, Angeline G (1975) Contact dermatitis from pyrrolnitrin (an antimycotic agent). Contact Dermatitis 1:288–292

Meneghini CL, Rantuccio F, Lomuto M (1971) Additives, vehicles and active drugs of topical medicaments as causes of delayed-type allergic dermatitis. Dermatologica 143:137–147

Michel PJ, Buyer R, Delorme M (1958) Accidents généraux (cyanose, collapse cardiovasculaire) par sensibilisation á une solution aqueuse de violet de gentiane et vert de méthyle en application locale. Bull Soc Fr Dermatol Syphiligr 65:183

Minkin W, Cohen HJ, Frank SB (1973) Contact dermatitis from deodorants (letter). Arch Dermatol 107:774–775

Mitchell JC (1971) The skin and chemical additives to foods (letter). Arch Dermatol 104:329–330

Mitchell JC (1977) Multiple concomitant positive patch test reactions. Contact Dermatitis 3:315–320

Mischer P, Fanta D (1978) Das Tomantadin-Kontaktekzem. Hautarzt 29:337–339

Möller H (1977) Merthiolate allergy: a nationwide iatrogenic sensitization. Acta Derm Venereol (Stockh) 57:509–517

Morgan JK (1968) Iatrogenic epidermal sensitivity. Br J Clin Pract 22:261–264

Mortensen T (1979) Allergy to lanolin. Contact Dermatitis 5:137–139

Muston HL, Messenger AG, Byrne JPN (1979) Contact dermatitis from zinc pyrithone, an antidandruff agent. Contact Dermatitis 5:276–277

Nakayama H, Nanaoka H, Ohshiro A (1974) Allergen controlled system (ACS). Kanekara Shuppan, Tokyo

Nater JP (1971) Allergic reactions due to chloracetamide. Dermatologica 142:191–192

Nater JP, De Groot AC (1978) Drugs used on the skin. In: Dukes MNG (ed) Meyler's side effects of drugs, 9th edn. Excerpta Medica, Amsterdam London New York, pp 234–264

Nilsson DC (1960) Sources of allergenic gums. Ann Allergy 18:518–524

Nordquist BC, Mehr K (1977) Allergic contact dermatitis to retinoic acid. Contact Dermatitis 3:55–56

North American Contact Dermatitis Group (1973) Epidemiology of contact dermatitis in North America, 1972. Arch Dermatol 108:537–540

North American Contact Dermatitis Group (1975) The frequency of contact sensitivity in North America 1972–1974. Contact Dermatitis 1:277–280

Odom RB, Maibach HI (1977) Contact urticaria: a different contact dermatitis. In: Marzulli FN, Maibach HI (eds) Dermatotoxicology and pharmacology. John Wiley & Sons, New York Chichester, pp 441–453

Oleffe JA, Blondel A, Boschmans S (1978) Patch testing with lanolin. Contact Dermatitis 4:233–234

Opdyke DL (1975) The safety of fragrance materials. Br J Dermatol 93:351

O'Quinn SE, Kennedy CB, Isbell KH (1967) Contact photodermatitis due to bithionol and related compounds. JAMA 199:89–92

Osmundsen PE (1970a) Pigmented contact dermatitis. Br J Dermatol 83:296–301

Osmundsen PE (1970b) Contact photodermatitis due to tribromsalicylanilide (cross reaction pattern). Dermatologica 140:65–74

Osmundsen PE (1975) Allergic contact dermatitis from idoxuridine. Contact Dermatitis 1:251

Panzer JD, Epstein WL (1970) Percutaneous absorption following topical application of neomycin. Arch Dermatol 102:536–539

Pariser RJ (1977) Contact dermatitis to dioxybenzone. Contact Dermatitis 3:172

Papa CM, Shelley WB (1964) Menthol hypersensitivity. JAMA 189:546–548

Paschoud JM (1966) Eczéma de contact par la crème Dianabol. Dermatologica 133:125–127

Petersen HO (1977) Hypersensitivity to propolis. Contact Dermatitis 3:278

Pevny I, Schellenberg J (1971) Sensibilisierungen und Gruppensensibilisierungen durch Chinolinderivate. Hautarzt 22:13–18

Pirilä V, Rouhunkoski S (1959) On sensitization to neomycin and bacitracin. Acta Derm Venereol (Stockh) 39:470–476

Pirilä V, Wallemius T (1957) Über die ekzematöse Sensibilisierung gegen Neomycin und Bacitracin. Hautarzt 8:518

Pirilä V, Förström L, Rouhunkoski S (1967) Twelve years of sensitization to neomycin in Finland: report of 1760 cases of sensitivity to neomycin and/or bactracin. Acta Derm Venereol (Stockh) 47:419–425

Pirilä V, Kilpio O, Olkkonen A, Pirilä L, Siltanen E (1969) On the chemical nature of the eczematogens in oil of turpentine. Dermatologica 139:183–194

Plewig G, Hofmann C, Braun-Falco O (1978) Photoallergic dermatitis from 8-methoxy psoralen. Arch Dermatol Res 261:201–211

Polak L (1977) Immunological aspects of contact sensitivity. In: Marzulli FN, Maibach HI (eds) Dermatotoxicology and pharmacology. John Wiley & Sons, New York Chichester, pp 225–288

Prater E, Göring HD, Schubert H (1978) Sodium lauryl sulfate – a contact allergen. Contact Dermatitis 4:242–243

Prystowsky SD, Allen AM, Smith RW, Nonomura JH, Odom RR, Akers WA (1979a) Allergic contact hypersensitivity to nickel, neomycin, Ethylenediamine and Benzocaine. Arch Dermatol 115:959–962

Prystowsky SD, Nonomura JH, Smith RW, Allen AM (1979b) Allergic hypersensitivity to neomycin. Arch Dermatol 115:713–715

Raab WP (1968) Mast cell depleting properties of neomycin. J Invest Dermatol 50:138–140

Ramsay DL, Cohen HJ, Baer RL (1972) Allergic reaction to benzophenone. Arch Dermatol 105:906–908

Recommendation by the International Contact Dermatitis Research Group (1973) Routine patch test series, 1974. Br J Dermatol 89:437–438

Rietschel RL (1978a) Photocontact dermatitis to hydrocortisone. Contact Dermatitis 4:334–337

Rietschel RL (1978 b) Contact urticaria from synthetic cassia oil and sorbic acid limited to the face. Contact Dermatitis 4:347–349

Rietschel RL, Lewis CW (1978) Contact dermatitis to homomentyl salicylate. Arch Dermatol 114:442–443

Robinson HM (1957) Local antibiotic therapy. Proc. 11th Int Congr Dermatol. Acta Derm Venereol (Stockh) 3:108–112

Roed-Petersen J (1975) Erythema multiforme as an expression of contact dermatitis. Contact Dermatitis 1:270–271

Roed-Petersen J (1976) Contact sensitivity to metaoxedrine. Contact Dermatitis 2:235–236

Roed-Petersen J, Hjorth N (1976) Contact dermatitis from antioxidants. Hidden sensitizers in topical medications and foods. Br J Dermatol 94:233–241

Roed-Petersen J, Menné T (1976) Allergic contact dermatitis and lichen planus from black and white photographic developing. Cutis 18:699–705

Roed-Petersen J, Auken G, Hjorth N (1975) Contact sensitivity to irgasan DP 300. Contact Dermatitis 1:293–294

Rothenborg HW, Hjorth N (1968) Allergy to perfumes from toilet soaps and detergents in patients with dermatitis. Arch Dermatol 97:417–421

Roupe G, Strannegaard O (1969) Anaphylactic shock elicited by topical administration of bacitracin. Arch Dermatol 100:450–452

Rubin A (1977) Ophthalmic sulfonamide induced Stevens-Johnson syndrome. Arch Dermatol 113:235–236

Rudzki E, Grzywa Z (1977a) Balsam of Peru as screening agent for essential oils sensitivity. Dermatologica 155:115–121

Rudzki E, Grzywa Z (1977b) Occupational dermatitis partly elicited by coal tar. Contact Dermatitis 3:54

Rudzki E, Grzywa Z (1978) Dermatitis from retinoic acid. Contact Dermatitis 4:305–306

Rudzki E, Koslowska A (1976) Sensitivity to salicylic acid. Contact Dermatitis 2:178

Rudzki E, Zakrzewski Z (1975) Incidence of contact sensitivity to topically applied drugs as compared with the frequency of their prescription. Contact Dermatitis 1:249–250

Salo OP, Pirilä V, Viljanen E (1968) Sensitivity to topical dequalene. Acta Allergol 23:490–496

Sams WM (1956) Contact photodermatitis. Arch Dermatol 73:142–148

Sams WM (1968) Untoward response with topical fluorouracil. Arch Dermatol 97:14–22

Satulsky EM (1950) Photosensitization induced by monoglycerol paraaminobenzoate. Arch Dermatol 62:711–713

Sausker WF, Frederick FD (1978) Allergic contact dermatitis secondary to topical nitroglycerin. JAMA 239:1743–1744

Schneider HG (1978) Schwefelallergie. Hautarzt 29:340–342

Schneider KW (1980) Contact dermatitis due to diethyl sebacate. Contact Dermatitis 6:506–507

Schoeffinius HH (1972) Kontaktdermatitis mit erhöhter Körpertemperatur unter Behandlung von Psoriasis vulgaris capillitii mit einen Benzoxathiol-desinat. Z Hautkr 47:227–229

Schöne K (1975) Klinische Erfahrungen mit einem Haparinoid externum in hoher Wirkstoffkonzentration. Fortschr Med 93:1565–1566

Scholz A, Richter G (1977) Zur Allergie gegen Falicain (propipokain-hydrochlorol). Dermatol Monatsschr 163:966–969

Schorr WF (1968) Paraben allergy: a cause of intractable dermatitis. JAMA 204:859–862

Schorr WF (1970) Dichlorophene (G-4) allergy. Arch Dermatol 102:515–520

Schorr WF (1971) Cosmetic allergy. Arch Dermatol 104:459–466

Schorr WL, Ridgway HB (1977) Tobramycin-neomycin cross sensitivity. Contact Dermatitis 3:133–137

Schreus HT (1950) Warum und wie sensibilisiert Marfanil? Hautarzt 1:401–404

Schulz KH (1962) Chemische Struktur und allergene Wirkung. Cantor, Aulendorf

Schwarz K, Storck H (1966) Ekzematose Sensibilisierung auf Methandrostenolon in Salbenform. Dermatologica 132:73–75

Shelley WB, Hurley HJ (1958) The allergic origin of zircomium deodorant granulomas in man. Br J Dermatol 70:75–101

Shmunes E (1978) Purpuric allergic contact dermatitis to paraphenylenediamine. Contact Dermatitis 4:225–229

Shore RN, Shelley WB (1974) Contact dermatitis from stearyl alcohol and propylene glycol in fluocinonide cream. Arch Dermatol 109:397–399

Sidi E, Hincky M, Longueville R (1958) Cross sensitization between neomycin and streptomycin. J Invest Dermatol 30:225–231

Smeenk G (1973) Contact allergy to bufexamac. Dermatologica 147:334–337

Smeenk G, Prins FJ (1972) Allergic contact eczema due to chloracetamide. Dermatologica 144:108–114

Smith SZ, Epstein JH (1977) Photocontact dermatitis to halogenated salicylanilides and related compounds. Arch Dermatol 113:1372–1374

Sneddon IB, Glew RC (1973) Contact dermatitis due to propanidid in an anaesthetist. Practitioner 211:321–323

Spencer PS, Sterman AB, Horoujian D, Bischoff M (1979) Neurotoxic changes in rats exposed to the fragrance compound acetyl ethyl tetramethyl tetralin. Neurotoxicology 1:221–237

Spott DA, Shelley WB (1970) Exanthem due to contact allergen (benzoin) absorbed through skin. JAMA 214:1881–1882

Starke JC, Jillson OF (1961) Photosensitization to coal tar. A cause of psoriatic erythroderma. Arch Dermatol 84:935–936

Stern RS, Thibodeau LA, Kleinerman RA et al. (1979) Risk of cutaneous carcinoma in patients treated with oral methoxsalen photochemotherapy for psoriasis. N Engl J Med 300:809–813

Storrs F (1975) Para-chloro-meta-xylenol allergic contact dermatitis in seven individuals. Contact Dermatitis 1:211–213

Stotts J, Ely WJ (1977) Induction of human skin sensitization to ethanol. J Invest Dermatol 69:219–222

Sugai T, Higashi J (1975) Hypersensitivity to hydrogenated lanolin. Contact Dermatitis 1:146–157

Sugai T, Takahashi Y, Takagi T (1977) Pigmented cosmetic dermatitis and coal tar dye. Contact Dermatitis 3:249–256

Sulzberger NB, Kanof A, Baer RL, Lowenberg C (1947) Sensitization by topical application of sulfonamides. J Allergy Clin Immunol 18:92–103

Sundararajan V (1970) Variotin sensitivity. Contact Dermatitis Newslett 8:188

Tarnick M (1976) Hautsensibilisierungen gegen Thiosinamin (Aurinosin®) Allylthiokarbamid. Dermatol Monatsschr 162:905–908

Taylor JR, Halprin KM (1972) Topical use of mechlorethamine in the treatment of psoriasis. Arch Dermatol 106:362–364

Tegner E (1976) Contact allergy to corticosteroids. Int J Dermatol 15:530–523

Thompson G, Maibach HI, Epstein J (1977) Allergic contact dermatitis from sunscreen preparations complicating photodermatitis. Arch Dermatol 113:1252–1253

Thormann J, Kaaber K (1978) Contact sensitivity to phenylbutazone ointment (butazolidine). Contact Dermatitis 4:235–236

Thormann J, Wildenhoff KE (1980) Contact allergy to idoxuridine. Contact Dermatitis 6:170–191

Turner TW (1977) Contact dermatitis due to lignocaine. Contact Dermatitis 3:210–211

Van Andel P, Bleumink E, Nater JP (1974) The significance of positive patch tests to wood tars. Trans St John's Hosp Dermatol Soc 60:94–98

Van Dijk TJA, Marier K (1972) Allergic contact dermatitis from Eurax®. Contact Dermatitis Newslett 12:344

Van Hecke EV, Temmerman L (1980) Contact allergy to the corticosteroid budesonide. Contact Dermatitis 6:509

Van Joost Th, Middelkamp Hup J, Ros FE (1979) Dermatitis as a side-effect of long-term topical treatment with certain beta-blocking agents. Br J Dermatol 101:171–176

Van Ketel WG (1973) Allergy to coumarin and coumarin-derivatives. Contact Dermatitis Newslett 13:355

Van Ketel WG (1974) Polymyxine B sulfate and bactracin. Contact Dermatitis Newslett 15:445

Van Ketel WG (1975) Allergic contact eczema by Hexomedine®. Contact Dermatitis 1:332

Van Ketel WG (1976 a) Allergic contact dermatitis from propellants in deodorant sprays in combination with allergy to ethyl chloride. Contact Dermatitis 2:115–119

Van Ketel WG (1975 b) Immediate and delayed type allergy to erythromycin. Contact Dermatitis 2:363–364

Van Ketel WG (1977) Allergy to idoxuridine eyedrops. Contact Dermatitis 3:106

Veien NK, Svejgaard E (1978) Lymphocyte transformation in patients with cobalt dermatitis. Br J Dermatol 99:191–196

Vermeulen CW, Malten KE (1963) Contact eczeem door 6-alpha-chloorprednison en neomycine. Ned Tijdschr Geneeskd 107:548–551

Vooys RC, Van Ketel WG (1977) Allergic drug eruption from pyrazolone compounds. Contact Dermatitis 3:57–58

Wade TR, Jones HE, Artis WA (1979) Irritant and allergic reactions to topically applied Micatin® cream. Contact Dermatitis 5:168–170

Wahlberg JE (1962) Two cases of hypersensitivity to quaternary ammonium compounds. Acta Derm Venereol (Stockh) 42:230–234

Wahlberg JE (1971) Sensitization to thioxolone. Contact Dermatitis Newslett 10:222

Wahlberg JE (1976) Routine patch testing with irgasan DP 300. Contact Dermatitis 2:292

Wahlberg JE, Wennersten G (1971) Hypersensitivity and photosensitivity to chlorhexidine. Dermatologica 143:376–379

Warshaw TG, Herrmann F (1952) Studies of skin reactions to propyleneglycol. J Invest Dermatol 19:423–430

Wasilewski C (1970) Allergic contact dermatitis from nystatin. Arch Dermatol 102:216–217

Weissmann I, Wagner G, Plewig G (1980) Contact allergy to 8-methoxypsoralen. Br J Dermatol 102:113–115

Wereide K (1970) Neomycin sensitivity in atopic dermatitis and other eczematous conditions. Acta Derma Venereol (Stockh) 50:114–116

Wereide K (1975) sensitivity to azidamphenicol. Contact Dermatitis 1:271–272

White MI (1978) Contact dermatitis from ethylene diamine. Contact Dermatitis 4:291–293

Wiegel O (1968) Kontaktallergie durch Kortikosteroid-haltige Externa. Med Welt 19:828–829

Wilkinson DS (1961) Photodermatitis due to tetrachlorosalicylanilide. Br J Dermatol 73:213–219

Wilkinson DS (1962) Patch test reactions to certain halogenated salicylanilides. Br J Dermatol 74:302–306

Wilkinson DS (1968) Delayed reactions to triacetoxyanthracene. Contact Dermatitis Newslett 4:75

Wilkinson DS (1975) Sulphur sensitivity. Contact Dermatitis 1:58

Wilkinson DS, Fregert S, Magnusson B et al. (1970) Terminology of contact dermatitis. Acta Derm Venereol (Stockh) 50:287–292

Wilson HTH (1971) Dermatitis from an acridine dye. Contact Dermatitis Newslett 9:212

Würbach G, Schubert H (1976) Untersuchungen über Afugin® Allergie. Dermatol Monatsschr 162:317–322

Yaffee HS, Dressler DP (1969) Topical application of mafenide acetate. Arch Dermatol 100:277–281

Zackheim HS (1978 a) Should therapeutic coal tar preparation be available over-the-counter? Arch Dermatol 114:125–126

Zackheim HS (1978 b) Topical 6-aminonicotinanide plus oral niacinamide therapy for psoriasis. Arch Dermatol 114:1632–1638

CHAPTER 14

Antihistamines

A. A. FISHER

A. Introduction

On rare occasions the systemic administration of an antihistamine can induce allergic hypersensitivity with production of urticaria, morbilliform and scarlatiniform eruptions, erythema multiforme, photosensitivity, and anaphylactic shock. In asthmatic patients, the antihistamine may lead to bronchial obstruction with anaphylactic reactions.

Eruptions due to antihistaminic agents usually appear 6–12 h after ingestion of the exciting agent. There may be an incubation period or the dermatitis may appear after the ingestion of the first dose. The eruption is usually generalized and explosive. The lesions may resemble any of the acute drug eruptions. Skin tests are of little value in these reactions. The history of a dermatitis occurring within 12 h after the introduction of one of these agents is very suggestive that the antihistamine is the cause of the eruption. Testing by readministering the drug is justifiable only in mild dermatoses and contraindicated in severe reactions.

At the onset, it must be emphasized that although the *systemic* administration of the antihistamines rarely engenders sensitization, *topical* applications such as antihistamines not infrequently produce allergic contact sensitivity. Once the patient is sensitized by topical application of the antihistamine, an eczematous contact dermatitis may occur from the antihistamine or from immunochemically related compounds. As a rule the systemic administration of an antihistamine to which there has been topical sensitization will not only reproduce the original allergic eczematous contact dermatitis, but at times a generalized dermatitis will occur with a resulting exfoliative dermatitis (FISHER 1976b). In some instances, the "systemic" eczematous contact dermatitis is accompanied by urticarial elements.

B. The Nature and Classification of the Antihistamines

In order to manage antihistamine dermatitis, properly a knowledge of the nature and the classification of the various antihistamines is necessary. Most antihistamines are basically related at their structural core by a substituted ethylamine group, which is also present in the histamine and has the following structure: X–CH_2–CH_2–N. This portion of the molecule presumably competes with histamine for cell receptors and thus blocks the action of histamine. To this substituted core different arrangements of atoms can be added to make different antihistamines. X represents the element that links the ethylamine group to the rest of the compound. Depending on the nature of X, oxygen (O), nitrogen (N), or carbon (C), the anti-

Table 1. Classes of antihistamines

Nitrogen-linked ethylenediamines
Oxygen-linked ethanolamines
Carbon-linked alkylamines
Phenothiazine antihistamines
Cyclizines (piperazines)
Piperidines
Miscellaneous

histamine belongs to a specific class. In addition, most authorities include a miscellaneous class.

Table 1 lists the various classes of antihistamines. There are two principal reasons for becoming familiar with the various groups of antihistamines. First, it is generally agreed that if any antihistamine is not effective in a particular patient, the rest of the antihistamines in that group are not likely to be as effective as an antihistamine from a different group. This concept of choosing an antihistamine from a new group is one of the reasons certain pharmaceutical companies manufacture two different antihistamine compounds. Second, a patient who is allergic to an antihistamine in one group is very likely to be allergic to every other antihistamine in that particular group. It is therefore of paramount importance that the sensitive patient be informed what antihistamines to avoid and which can be safely used as a substitute for the sensitizing antihistamine.

The antihistamines are useful primarily in the control of certain allergic disorders. Their effect in allergic conditions is purely palliative and largely due to the suppression of symptoms attributable to the action of histamine, which is but one of the chemicals released by the antigen–antibody reaction. In addition, they may diminish capillary permeability to substances other than histamine.

Topical antihistamine preparations are used because they are slightly antipruritic and may have a mild local anesthetic effect. However, such topical antihistamines are common and potent sensitizers.

C. The Role of Tartrazine in Allergic Antihistamine Reactions

Like many other drugs, the antihistamines may be colored by various dyes which are allergenic (Lockey 1975). Tartrazine, the azo dye F. D. and C. Yellow No. 5 has been implicated as a cause of urticaria (Michaelsson and Juhlin 1973) and asthma (Juhlin et al. 1972).

Tartrazine is most likely to produce urticaria in patients with allergic hypersensitivity to aspirin and the salicylate drugs (Ros et al. 1976). It is, therefore, prudent to administer "white" antihistamines, free of dyes, to such aspirin-sensitive individuals. (The presence of color in a tablet or capsule does not necessarily imply that the F. D. and C. Yellow No. 5 is necessarily used in its manufacture, however, a "white" antihistamine is free of *all* dyes.) The antihistamines shown in Table 2 are free of all dyes.

Table 2. "White" antihistamines free of all dyes

Trade name	Generic name
Marezine	Cyclizine hydrochloride
Promethazine (Purepac)	Promethazine hydrochloride
Periactin	Cyproheptadine hydrochloride
Actidil	Triprolidine hydrochloride
Tavist	Clemastine fumarate

Table 3. Nitrogen-linked ethylenediamine antihistamines

Trade name	Generic name
Pyribenzamine	Tripelennamine hydrochloride
Histadyl	Methapyrilene hydrochloride
Fiogesic	Pyrilamine maleate
Pyma	Pyrilamine maleate
Atarax	Hydroxyzine hydrochloride
Vistaril (oral)	Hydroxyzine pamoate
Vistaril (intramuscular)	Hydroxyzine hydrochloride

D. The Nitrogen-Linked Ethylenediamines

Table 3 lists the ethylenediamine antihistamines. It should be noted that ethylenediamine hydrochloride, the parent substance of this group of histamines, a component of aminophylline and a stabilizer in the popular nystatin–neomycin sulfate–gramicidin–triamcinolone acetonide cream (Mycolog) has become such a common sensitizer that it is included in the "Screening Patch Test Series" of the North American Contact Dermatitis Research Group. Ethylenediamine hydrochloride now rivals nickel and dichromates as a "most common" sensitizer (FISHER 1973). The use of nystatin–neomycin sulfate–gramicidin–triamcinolone acetonide cream has produced so many instances of allergic contact dermatitis owing to the presence of ethylenediamine hydrochloride in the cream that its use has been forbidden at the New York Skin and Cancer Unit. [Nystatin–neomycin sulfate–gramicidin–triamcinolone acetonide *ointment* (Mycolog) is free of ethylenediamine hydrochloride.] Reports from Europe and Australia confirm the fact that ethylenediamine hydrochloride used as a stabilizer in a similar topically applied cream is a very common sensitizer.

Unless the sensitized patient is informed how to avoid ethylenediamine hydrochloride and related chemicals, the ethylenediamine-sensitive individual is not only doomed to repeated attacks of dermatitis (PROVOST and JILLSON 1967), but also to drug eruptions from the systemic administration of aminophylline and ethylenediamine-related antihistamines and from topical exposure to antihistamines derived from ethylenediamine (RAJKA and PALLIN 1964).

Table 4. Piperazine (cyclizine) antihistamines

Trade name	Generic name
Fedrazil, Mantadil	Chlorcyclizine hydrochloride
Migral	Cyclizine hydrochloride
Marezine	Cyclizine hydrochloride
Bucladin-S	Buclizine hydrochloride
Bonine antivert	Mecline hydrochloride

I. The Asthmatic Patient and Ethylenediamine Sensitivity

The following facts must be taken into consideration by the practitioner should an asthmatic patient become sensitized to ethylenediamine hydrochloride:

a) Aminophylline is composed of theophylline and ethylenediamine hydrochloride.

b) Although there are many theophylline medications without ethylenediamine that can be given orally, in an emergency there are no *injectable* aminophylline preparations that do not contain ethylenediamine hydrochloride.

c) The administration of aminophylline to an ethylenediamine-sensitive individual can produce a severe disabling systemic contact dermatitis with generalized exfoliative dermatitis (Petrozzi and Shore 1976).

II. Industrial Dermatitis due to Ethylenediamine Sensitivity

In industry ethylenediamine is used in the preparation of dyes, inhibitors, rubber accelerators, fungicides, synthetic waxes, resins, insecticides, and asphalt wetting agents. However, industrial exposure rarely leads to sensitization, probably because exposure is usually not prolonged or intimate and normal rather than abnormal skin is exposed.

1. Epoxy Resin Dermatitis

Certain polyamines such a triethylenetetramine, triethylenediamine, and ethanolamine, used as amine "curing" agents of "hardeners" in epoxy resin systems, may cross-react with ethylenediamine (van Hecke 1975). Such cross-reactions can produce epoxy resin dermatitis in ethylenediamine-sensitive individuals (Fisher 1976a).

2. Machine Worker's Dermatitis

Synthetic coolants used in factories producing pistons can produce eruptions on the hands of machine tool operators (Angelini and Meneghini 1977). In these cases, ethylenediamine sensitivity may be a major cause (Crow et al. 1978).

Table 5. The ethanolamines: oxygen-linked antihistamines

Trade name	Generic name
Ambenyl	Diphenhydramine hydrochloride
Benadryl	Diphenhydramine hydrochloride
Benylin	Diphenhydramine hydrochloride
Diphenadril	Diphenhydramine hydrochloride
Tavist	Clemastine fumarate
Clistin	Carbinoxame maleate
Dramamine	Dimenhydrinate
Decapryl	Doxylamine succinate
Rondec	Carbinoxamine maleate

III. The Relationship of the Hydroxyzines to Ethylenediamine

Although the hydroxyzine ethylenediamines, Atarax and Vistaril, are not usually classified with the ethylenediamine antihistamines it should be noted that the formula of Atarax (hydroxyzine hydrochloride) is 1-*p*-chlorobenzyhydryl-4,2 (2(2-hydroxyethoxy)ethyl)*diethylenediamine dihydrochloride*. It therefore would be prudent to avoid the use of hydroxyzine antihistamines in individuals with ethylenediamine sensitivity.

IV. The Relationship of the Piperazine (Cyclizine) Antihistamines to Ethylenediamine

The piperazine (cyclizine) antihistamines are listed in Table 4. The piperazine antihistamines, like the hydroxyzines, are closely related to the ethylenediamine antihistamines. It is felt that, since ethylenediamine is on the metabolic pathway of both piperazine and hydroxyzine, it is advisable to avoid the use of piperazine antihistamines in ethylenediamine-sensitive individuals.

Thus piperazine citrate used for the treatment of pinworms (threadworms) can produce an allergic drug eruption in ethylenediamine-sensitive individuals (BURRY 1978). Cross-reactions can occur in chemists and laboratory technicians who handle both of these chemicals (CALNAN 1975).

E. The Oxygen-Linked Ethanolamine Antihistamines

Table 5 lists these antihistamines. Of this group of antihistamines, diphenylenediamine hydrochloride has been widely used both systemically and topically for three decades. The other ethanolamines are used only systemically.

The incidence of cutaneous reactions to topically applied diphenhydramine is difficult to asses (EMMETT 1974). In one series, 12 of 117 cases of dermatitis medicamentosa seen in England, in one year were due to a lotion comprised of diphenhydramine hydrochloride and calamine (Caladryl) (VICKERS 1961). All 12 were confirmed by positive patch tests, although in 10 instances, closed patch tests were positive only when performed on areas which had undergone repeated cellophane tape strippings.

I. Systemic "Endogenic" Contact Dermatitis to Ethanolamines

Individuals who have become sensitized by topically applied diphenhydramine can acquire a "systemic" eczematous contact dermatitis when diphenhydramine or any of the other ethanolamines listed in Table 5 is ingested or injected (Fisher 1973).

It is not generally realized that dimenhydrinate (Dramamine) is an ethanolamine (the chlorotheophylline salt of the antihistaminic agent diphenhydramine). Dimenhydrinate contains between 53% and 56% diphenhydramine and therefore should not be administered to any individual with allergic hypersensitivity to the ethanolamine group of antihistamines.

II. Photoallergic Dermatitis due to Diphenhydramine

Antihistamine photodermatitis of the *systemic* administration of such ethanolamines as diphenhydramine and carbinoxamine and to topical ethanolamines are very rare (Schreiber and Naylor 1962). Although topical promethazine therapy appears to be a relatively frequent cause of photoallergic contact dermatitis a single report of photoallergy induced by topical diphenhydramine therapy was reported (Emmett 1974). The diagnosis was confirmed by photopatch testing. This diphenhydramine photoallergy appeared to differ from most other forms of photoallergy in that it was elicited by ultraviolet light in the 290–320 nm wavelength range (UVB), rather than the more usual 320–400 nm range (UVA). This finding may be related to the photochemical properties of diphenhydramine, which absorbs in the UVB, but not in the UVA, the UVB absorption being associated with a distinctive fluorescence.

F. The Phenothiazines

Although topical phenothiazine antihistamine preparations such as promethazine hydrochloride (Phenergan) cream are no longer used in the United States, such topical antihistamine preparations are still widely used in Europe. Individuals who have become sensitized by such topical phenothiazine antihistamines often suffer a flare of the dermatitis when a phenothiazine antihistamine is taken, i.e., a "systemic" eczematous contact dermatitis. In addition, many individuals acquire allergic sensitization to various phenothiazine drugs which show cross-reactions with the phenothiazine antihistamines. Table 6 lists the phenothiazine antihistamine compounds.

I. Promethazine Hydrochloride

This antihistamine is used not only in tablet form but also as suppositories. Proctitis and perianal dermatitis have occurred from the use of such suppositories in sensitized individuals. This antihistamine can also produce phototoxic and

Table 6. Phenothiazine antihistamines

Trade name	Generic name
Tacaryl hydrochloride	Methdilazine hydrochloride
Phenergan	Promethazine hydrochloride
Temaril	Trimeprazine tartrate

Table 7. Drugs which cross-react with phenothiazine antihistamines

Trade name	Generic name
Thorazine	Chlorpromazine
Compazine	Prochlorperazine
Stelazine	Trifluoperazine
Temaril	Trimepazine
Vesprin	Triflupromazine hydrochloride

photoallergic reactions (CAMARASA 1976). In France, where Phenergan cream is used extensively as a topical antipruritic agent, many instances of photocontact dermatitis occur. Photosensitivity seems to be induced primarily by contact exposure to promethazine hydrochloride cream (EPSTEIN et al. 1957). Systemic administration without topical sensitization does not appear to induce photosensitivity (CAHN and LEVY 1957).

II. Cross-Reactions Between the Phenothiazine Antihistamines and Other Phenothiazine Compounds

The phenothiazine drugs listed in Table 7 are all capable of cross-reacting with the phenothiazine antihistamines, and all of these compounds are potential photosensitizers (LEWIS and SAWICKY 1955). Often a photoallergic reaction occurs in combination with the allergic eczematous contact dermatitis. The systemic administration of the phenothiazine drugs shown in Table 7 may produce an eczematous contact dermatitis medicamentosa in individuals sensitized by such topical exposure. Cross-reactions readily take place between these phenothiazines and the related antihistamines (MITCHELL and ONGLEY 1972).

III. Exposure of Medical and Nursing Personnel to Phenothiazines

Medical and nursing personnel who inject these phenothiazine drugs or who handle phenothiazine tablets which are given to patients, and those who come into contact with the compounds in the pharmaceutical industry readily acquire allergic eczematous contact dermatitis of the hands from such exposure; the dermatitis may flare when a phenothiazine antihistamine is given (CALNAN et al. 1962). Since chlorpromazine, in particular, is excreted almost unchanged in the urine, sensitized nurses and orderlies who handle unwashed linen may experience flares.

Table 8. Phenothiazines used in veterinary medicine

Insecticides	"Fly Free Eddie"
	"Bar-Fly Feed"
Anthelmintics	"Worm Free Eddie"
	"Early Bird Wormer"

Table 9. Sources of exposure to methylene blue (a phenothiazine dye)

Urinary antiseptics
  M-B tablets, Urolene Blue, TRA tablets, Urised
Blue hair dyes
Antidotes for methemoglobinemia and cyanide poisoning
Biologic stains
Photodynamic treatment of herpes

IV. Exposure of Veterinarians and Farmers to Phenothiazines

The same phenothiazines or closely related compounds which are used as psychotropic drugs or as sedatives in humans are used by veterinarians and farmers as insecticides and anthelmintics for animals and birds. Table 8 lists the commercial phenothiazine insecticides and "wormers" used by veterinarians. Many individuals in these professions have acquired allergic contact dermatitis, photoallergic reactions, or both by spraing such phenothiazines for insect control or feeding these compounds as wormers. Such individuals must avoid using phenothiazine antihistamines because of the likelihood of producing flares of the phenothiazine dermatitis.

V. Exposure to Methylene Blue

Methylene blue is 3,7-bis-(dimethylamino)phenozathionium chloride tetramethyl thionin chloride, a phenothiazine derivative used in various ways as shown in Table 9. In one observed individual who had acquired a photosensitivity from a phenothiazine compound, the administration of methylene blue urinary antiseptic produced a flare of the photodermatitis.

Dilute mixtures of methylene blue, acid violet, and nigrosine are used as a color rinse for gray hair. Such rinses should be used with great care in those who have become sensitized to the phenothiazines.

VI. Varieties of Allergic Reactions to Phenothiazine Compounds

There are three types of allergic hypersensitivity seen with the phenothiazine drugs. These reactions are:

a) The classical allergic contact eczematous variety, in which the covered patch test reaction is positive.

b) A photoallergic reaction, in which the *covered* patch reaction is negative but becomes positive when the patch test site is exposed to sunlight or ultraviolet radiation (EPSTEIN 1960).

c) A photoallergic reaction in combination with an allergic eczematous contact sensitization, in which the patch test reaction is positive with the phenothiazine derivative alone, but a stronger response is elicited if the site is irradiated with a suberythematous dose of ultraviolet rays or exposed to strong sunlight for 20 min. The increase in intensity of an ordinary patch test reaction on exposure to light must be carefully interpreted, because it may be a nonspecific irritating effect.

If possible, controls should be used as on other positive patch test reactions. Whenever an allergen can produce both photoallergic and allergic eczematous contact hypersensitivity, the photoallergic reaction appears to be more intense. At times, phenothiazine, capable of producing photoallergic and ordinary allergic eczematous contact dermatitis, will produce a photoallergic reaction in areas exposed to light, while the same concentration of the drug that reaches the skin from systemic administration will not produce a contact dermatitis on covered areas of the body. However, in many instances both types of reactions occur simultaneously.

A unique feature of photoallergic reactions to the phenothiazines is that the wavelengths that produce the photoallergic reactions are not always identical to those absorbed by the phenothiazine drug. These drugs have a maximal absorption in the ultraviolet wavelengths below 310 nm. Having become photoallergic to them, however, the patient may also react to longer ultraviolet wavelengths and even visible light. This is called, "widening of the action spectrum".

The increased sensitivity of the skin to light sometimes persists for months. The patient sensitized to a phenothiazine, therefore, should avoid exposure to sunlight for at lest several weeks after recovering from the dermatitis. If sunlight exposure is unavoidable, a suntan preparation and protective clothing should be used to protect the involved skin, otherwise, the patient will become a "persistent light reactor". In one instance (EPSTEIN and ROWE 1957) a case of photosensitivity to Phenergan and chlorpromazine was described in which originally contact sensitivity could be demonstrated only to Phenergan; but cross-photo-sensitivity excisted at the same time, also to chlorpromazine (Thorazine).

From a study of the literature (SIDI et al. 1955; SCHREIBER and NAYLOR 1962; KIMMIG 1956) the following conclusions can be drawn:

a) In photoallergy to phenothiazine derivatives, such as Phenergan or chlorpromazine (Thorazine) both contact and photocontact sensitivity to these drugs may be found.

b) The allergen in this photoallergic reaction is different from the original drug, probably an oxidation or decomposition product.

c) Crossphoto-sensitivity between Phenergan and chlorpromazine may exist, even though plain contact sensitivity (without light) can be demonstrated only to Phenergan, and vice versa.

d) Photoallergy plays a role in only some cases of photosensitivity to phenothiazine derivatives.

Table 10. The carbon-linked alkylamine (propylamine) antihistamines

Trade name	Generic name
Chlor-trimeton	Chlorpheniramine maleate
Dimetane	Bromophenipramine maleate
Teldrin	Chlorpheniramine maleate
Polaramine	Dexchlorpheniramine maleate
Disomer	Dexbrompheniramine maleate
Histaspan	Chlorpheniramine maleate
Actidil	Triprolidine hydrochloride
Forhistal	Dimethindene Maleate

Table 11. The miscellaneous antihistamines

Trade name	Generic name
Periactin[a]	Cyproheptadine hydrochloride
Optimine[a]	Azatadine maleate
Hispril	Diphenylpyraline hydrochloride
Actidil	Triprolidine hydrochloride

[a] Periactin and Optimine may be classed as piperidine antihistamines

G. The Carbon-Linked Alkylamine (Propylamine) Antihistamines

Fortunately these carbon-linked alkylamine antihistamines (Table 10) are not used as topical agents. Allergic reactions of the "systemic" contact variety do not occur since topical sensitization has not occurred. However, urticaria and other allergic drug manifestations may occur.

H. Miscellaneous Antihistamines

Table 11 lists a number of antihistamines which are not readily incorporated into the classes discussed previously.

J. Facial Dyskinesia from the Antihistamines

Although strictly speaking facial dyskinesia following administration of the antihistamines may not be an allergic phenomenon, this unusual complication is worth noting. Granacher (1977) in a review of the literature (Thach et al. 1975; Favis 1976; Brait and Zagerman 1977; and Lavenstein and Cantor 1976) suggests that oral dyskinesia after use of antihistamine agents is rare but not unexpected.

It seems probable that the anticholinergic activity of antihistamine agents centrally alter nigrostriatal cholinergic–dopaminergic interaction and thereby produce acute and chronic oral dyskinesia. In patients with markedly severe acute dystonia induced by antihistamines, an intramuscular or intravenous trial of the centrally active cholinomimetic, physostigmine, might prove therapeutic.

References

Angelini G, Meneghini CL (1977) Dermatitis in engineers due to synthetic coolants. Contact Dermatitis 3:219–220

Brait KA, Zagerman AJ (1977) Dyskinesias after antihistamine use. N Engl J Med 296:111–114

Burry JN (1978) Ethylenediamine sensitivity with a systemic reaction to piperazine citrate. Contact Dermatitis 4:380

Cahn MM, Levy EJ (1957) Ultraviolet light factor in chlorpromazine dermatitis. Arch Dermatol 75:38–40

Calnan CD (1975) Occupational piperazine dermatitis. Contact Dermatitis 1:126

Calnan CD, Frain-Bell W, Cuthbert JW (1962) Occupational dermatitis from Chlorpromazine. Trans St John's Hosp Dermatol Soc 48:49–51

Camarasa G (1976) Contact dermatitis to phenothiazines nemactil and decentan. Contact Dermatitis 2:123

Crow KD, Peachey RDG, Adams JE (1978) Coolant oil dermatitis due to ethylenediamine. Contact Dermatitis 4:359–361

Emmett EA (1974) Diphenhydramine photoallergy. Arch Dermatol 110:249–252

Epstein JH, Brunsting LA, Petersen MC, Schwarz BE (1957) A study of photosensitivity occurring with chlorpromazine therapy. J Invest Dermatol 28:329–338

Epstein S (1960) Allergic photocontact dermatitis from promethazine (phenergan). Arch Dermatol 81:175–177

Epstein S, Rowe JR (1957) Photoallergy and photocross sensitivity to phenergan. J Invest Dermatol 29:319–323

Favis GR (1976) Facial dyskinesia related to antihistamine? N Engl J Med 294:730–732

Fisher AA (1973) Contact dermatitis, 2nd edn. Lea & Febiger, Philadelphia

Fisher AA (1976a) Epoxy resin dermatitis. Cutis 17:1027–1028, 1041

Fisher AA (1976b) Antihistamine dermatitis. Cutis 18:329–330, 336

Granacher RP (1977) Facial dyskinesia after antihistamine? N Engl J Med 296:516–518

Juhlin L, Michaelsson G, Zetterstrum O (1972) Urticaria and asthma induced by food and drug additives in patients with aspirin hypersensitivity. J Allerg Clin Immunol 50:92–98

Kimmig J (1956) Welche Bedeutung besitzen die Phenothiazine für die Behandlung von Hautkrankheiten? (Umfrage). Dermatol Wochenschr 134:1250–1252

Lavenstein BL, Cantor FK (1976) Acute dystonia: an unusual reaction to diphenhydramine. JAMA 236:291–294

Lewis GM, Sawicky HH (1955) Contact dermatitis from chlorpromazine. JAMA 157:909–910

Lockey S (1975) Reactions to hidden agents in foods and drugs can be serious. Ann Allergy 35:239–242

Michaelsson G, Juhlin L (1973) Urticaria induced by preservatives and dye additives in food and drugs. Br J Dermatol 88:525–532

Mitchell JC, Ongley R (1972) Photodermatitis presenting as universal exfoliative dermatitis ("phenothiazine contact photoallergy"). Contact Dermatitis Newslett 11:278

Petrozzi JW, Shore RN (1976) Generalized exfoliative dermatitis from ethylenediamine. Arch Dermatol 112:525–526

Provost TT, Jillson OF (1967) Ethylenediamine contact dermatitis. Arch Dermatol 96:231–234

Rajka G, Pallin O (1964) Sensitization to locally applied antistine. Acta Derm Venereol (Stockh) 44:255–256

Ros A, Juhlin L, Michaelsson G (1976) A follow up study of patients with recurrent urti-
    caria and hypersensitivity to aspirin benzoates and azo dye. Br J Dermatol 95:19–24
Schreiber MM, Naylor LZ (1962) Antihistamine photosensitivity. Arch Dermatol 86:58–62
Sidi E, Hincky M, Gervais M (1955) Allergic sensitization and photosensitization to phener-
    gan cream. J Invest Dermatol 24:345–352
Thach BT, Chase TN, Bosma JF (1975) Oral facial dyskinesia associated with prolonged
    use of antihistaminic decongestant. N Engl J Med 293:486–490
Van Hecke E (1975) Ethylenediamine sensitivity from exposure to epoxy resin hardeners
    and mycolog cream. Contact Dermatitis 1:344–348
Vickers CFH (1961) Dermatitis medicamentosa. Br Med J 1:1366–1368

CHAPTER 15

Drugs Acting on the Cardiovascular System

H. E. Amos

The development of therapeutic compounds which influence the cardiovascular system has exercised the imagination of medicinal chemists for many years. This has led to a wide variety of chemical structures being marketed as therapeutic compounds. A logical analysis of toxic reactions, based on structural activity relationships, is difficult to carry out because of this chemical hetrogeneity, but for hypersensitivity reactions each compound must be considered unique and any adverse relationships analyzed accordingly.

A. Incidence of Hypersensitivity Reactions

The overall impression of the incidence of allergic reactions to cardiovascular drugs is that it is very low. The majority of compounds do not cause hypersensitivity reaction, and, with those that do, it is a rare event.

I. Cardiac Glycosides

Adverse reactions with a possible immunological etiology have been reported for the cardiac glycosides but they are confined to damage in the skin or to the platelets. Skin reactions have been reported by Cohen and Brodsky (1940), Mosko and Taylor (1954), and Grettre and Johansson (1958). Each one of these reports cites one case, which serves to emphasize the rarity of such reactions.

Thrombocytopenia is equally rare: a total of four cases have been reported: Berger (1952), Miescher and Ritter (1953), Young et al. (1966), and Medenica et al. (1972). A single case of vasculitis but with purpuric lesions on the thigh has been reported by Brauner and Greene (1972).

II. Quinidine

Hypersensitivity reactions associated with quinidine are rare, but some of the reported cases have been extensively investigated. Practically all the immunologically induced adverse responses seem to be confined to the formed elements of the blood or to the skin.

This study was written when the author was employed by the British Industrial Biological Research Association. His current affiliation can be found in the List of Contributors.

Thrombocytopenia is a well-recognized hypersensitivity reaction, inducible by quinidine, but only about 50 cases have been reported (ROBINSON 1978). Hemolytic anemia is even more rare: one well-documented case was reported by FREEDMAN et al. (1956) and one case of agranulocytosis with marrow depression was reported by BARZEL (1967).

Cutaneous reactions are uncommon with quinidine; they are more commonly associated with the optical isomer, quinine. Drug fever either occuring alone or in combination with other symptoms is a more frequent manifestation of hypersensitivity than the cutaneous signs (STURNICK 1942), but even quinidine fever is very unusual (ABRAMS 1973).

III. Procainamide

Procainamide therapy is the most frequent cause of drug-induced lupus erythematosus. About 100 cases have so far been reported; the largest series, 44 cases, was by BLOMGREN et al. (1972), but there have been several smaller series (SIEGEL et al. 1967; HOPE and BATES 1972; SWERBRICK and GREY 1973; BAREIS 1974).

It is difficult to derive an overall figure for the incidence of procainamide-induced lupus erythematosus, mainly due to the difficulty of accurately diagnosing some of the early clinical signs which often cause the patient to stop taking the drug. But in one series more than 10% of patients taking procainamide developed severe lupus erythematosus and another 10% developed a milder form of the syndrome (FAKHRO et al. 1967). In the series by HOPE and BATES (1972) 3 out of 61 patients who had taken procainamide for more than 4 weeks were found to have the full lupus syndrome, and another 3 had some features of the condition.

Drug fever has been reported in about 11 patients but the true incidence is likely to be much higher (ROBINSON 1978). In a prospective study by KOSOWSKY et al. (1973) 5 out of the 39 patients who started treatment with procainamide developed a fever after 2–18 days.

Rashes of various types have been reported associated with procainamide, but two cases worthy of special mention are a case of generalized vasculitis reported by DOLAN (1968) and a case of digital vasculitis reported by ROSIN (1967); both could indicate some immune complex phenomena. Agranulocytosis developing after 26–78 days of treatment with the drug and not clearly dose-related has been reported in 12 cases (WANG and SCHULLER 1969; KONTTINEN and TUOMINEN 1971; HICKSON et al. 1972; HENSEN 1974).

IV. Adrenergic Neuron Blocking Agents

The treatment of hypertension by compounds which affect adrenergic neuron transmission has been the main form of therapy for many years. Consequently there are a large number of available drugs in the physician's armamentarium, but only one compound causes hypersensitivity problems – methyldopa. The Swedish Advisory Drug Reactions Committee analyzed 308 patients on methyldopa therapy between 1966 and 1975 and listed the adverse effects associated with methyldopa as shown in Table 1 (Notice from the SWEDISH ADVERSE DRUG REACTION 1977).

Table 1. Adverse reactions to methyldopa reported to the Swedish Adverse Drug Reaction Committee 1966–1975 (308 patients)

Diagnosis	Number
Fever	166
Hemolysis	67
Hepatic effects	29
Allergic reactions	23
Gastrointestinal symptoms	17
Psychic and neurological symptoms	13
Other hematological effects including positive Coombs' test	11
Other	16

It can be seen that 23 patients were reported as experiencing some type of allergic reaction, but it is likely that fever, hemolysis, and certain of the hepatic effects may also have an immunological basis.

Fever is known to occur in about 3% of all cases treated (ROBINSON 1978) but it is not a typical hypersensitivity fever. It usually runs a relapsing course with night sweats and often subsides despite continued treatment; it is also evident only during the first week of treatment.

Hemolytic anemia is a rare complication occurring in about 0.5%–3% of cases. A number of such cases have been reported (MEHROTRA and GUPTA 1971; KESSEY et al. 1973; INZOLI and ALMICI 1973).

Skin reactions, particularly papular rashes, are seen in some patients (VICTOR 1970; CORBETT 1972) and a type of seborrhoric dermatitis has been reported by CHURCH (1973). Over a 3-year period CHURCH reported 13 cases of dermatitis which cleared in the majority of patients when the drug was stopped, but when 7 of the patients were challenged with the drug it reappeared in 6 of them.

Two adverse effects attributable to a hypersensitivity mechanism are particularly serious – hepatotoxicity and myocarditis. Several cases have been reported of hepatotoxicity which may progress even on stopping the drug. TOGHILL et al. (1974) reported a series of 20 patients in whom liver damage appeared to be directly related to methyldopa administration, but other smaller series (RODMAN et al. 1976) and single case reports have also been published. The true incidence has not yet been established; KLINGER (1974) has reported an incidence of liver dysfunction in 14%–35% of treated cases and RIDDIOUGH (1977) reported an incidence of 2%–3%.

The second adverse effect is not so firmly established as hepatotoxicity. CONSTON (1974) reported a fatal case of myocarditis which he claimed was caused by a hypersensitivity reaction to methyldopa; five more fatal cases were reported by MULLICK and MCALLISTER (1977). The latter five patients all had associated hepatic lesion. The main piece of evidence cited which the authors claim suggested an immunological mechanism was that histology of the lesions showed a lymphocyte infiltration with a large number of eosinophils.

V. Hydralazine

In 1954 a series of reports were published linking hydralazine with drug-induced lupus erythematosus (Perry and Schroder 1954; Dunstan et al. 1954; Rein-hardt and Waldron 1954; Shackman et al. 1954). Since then numerous clinical studies have confirmed that hydralazine is a high risk drug for producing lupus. The incidence of hydralazine-lupus is not clearly defined; it depends on the criteria used to diagnose the disease. If the presence of antinuclear auto antibodies is taken as a diagnostic criterion, Blomgren (1973) reported an incidence of 27% in patients treated, but on follow-up only 12% of the patients developed the full syndrome. Perry (1973) reported a large series of 371 patients being treated with hydralazine in which 44 developed the full syndrome.

VI. Beta-Adrenoceptor Blocking Drugs

β-Adrenoceptor blocking drugs have recently been introduced for the treatment of cardiac arrhythmias and hypertension. There are about 12 proprietary brands available and most of these compounds have not been used sufficiently widely or for a sufficient length of time to allow any real assessment of their potential immunological hazard. Unfortunately one member of the group, practolol, has caused considerable problems which necessitated its withdrawal from circulation and, furthermore, caused concern about possible similar adverse reactions with the other β-receptor blocking compounds.

Adverse effects associated with practolol have been collectively described as the oculomucocutaneous syndrome. The incidence of the syndrome is small but the seriousness of the tissue damage has tended to overshadow this incidence. Practolol was marketed in 1970, and by the end of 1975 the drug had been used for some 300,000 patient years in the UK, and around one million worldwide. By October 1974, 164 cases were known, and in November 1977, the total had reached 915 (Nicholls 1978). The drug was withdrawn in 1976. It is now reasonably certain that none of the other β-blockers in clinical use has so far induced an oculomucocutaneous-type syndrome.

B. Clinical Aspects of the Adverse Effects

A noticeable omission from the spectrum of immunologically mediated tissue damage induced by cardiovascular drugs is anaphylaxis. There is no firm documentary evidence that any of the major drugs in current use for cardiovascular disease have either induced clinical anaphylaxis or indeed stimulated specific IgE antibodies. The main target tissue damaged by hypersensitivity reactions to these drugs is connective tissue and formed elements of the blood.

I. Drug-Induced Lupus Erythematosus

Drug-induced lupus is a major adverse effect of procainamide and hydralazine. Isolated case reports have incriminated other compounds such as reserpine, methyldopa, and quinidine, but it is not a recognized hazard of these drugs. The only other cardiovascular drug which has caused the lupus syndrome in a small number of patients is practolol (RAFTERY and DENMAN 1973).

Since the original reports by PERRY and SCHRODER (1954) and DUNSTAN et al. (1954) describing a lupus-like syndrome inducible with hydralazine, and by LADD (1962) with procainamide, much attention has been paid to the relationship of drug-induced lupus with the established clinical entity – systemic lupus erythematosus.

A number of clinical manifestations seems to be common to both diseases: fever, arthralgia, myalgia, pleuritis, pericarditis, skin rashes, and anemia. An analysis of patients with drug-induced lupus enables a number of generalizations to be drawn about the chief features of the disease.

There is, by definition, an association with drug administration, but there is no relationship between the disease and dose or duration of treatment. Clinical signs may appear as early as 2 weeks after starting treatment or be delayed for as long as 8 years (KOSOWSKY et al. 1973; BLOMGREN 1973; SIEGEL et al. 1967). Drug-induced lupus seems more common in older patients but this is probably an apparent finding reflecting the age groups of patients taking the drug. There is also no clear sex difference; this is a point of distinction between drug-induced and systemic lupus, since the latter occurs predominantly in young women.

A second difference between the two diseases is the predilection of organ involvement. Most investigators accept that drug-induced lupus rarely affects the kidney. There are, however, reports of immune complex nephritis induced by hydralazine (DAMMIN et al. 1955; ALARCON-SEGORIA et al. 1967) but it could be argued that since lupus nephritis is a comparatively late pathological manifestation, it rarely has time to develop in the drug-induced syndrome before the offending compound is withdrawn.

II. Thrombocytopenia

The two cardiovascular drugs which induce thrombocytopenia by immunological mechanisms are digitoxin and quinidine. The cardiac glycoside, responsible for the four reported cases of thrombocytopenia attributable to this group of drugs, is digitoxin; none of the other proprietary preparations of cardiac glycosides has produced similar adverse effects. An explanation for this specificity is outlined in a later section.

Considerable experimental effort has been directed toward elucidating the mechanisms by which drugs stimulate specific cytotoxic antibodies for platelets, but the fact that all reported cases of thrombocytopenia have been in patients who have tolerated treatment with the offending drug for many years still needs explanation. It is unlikely that the antigen is too weak to stimulate an antibody response except after years of repeated administration, so the possibility must exist that the antigen is suddenly created. This could occur if a change in the metabolic status of the patient consequent upon their debilitating condition altered the pattern of metabolites formed. Whatever the explanation of thrombocytopenia suddenly developing in patients on prolonged treatment with these drugs, it must be recognized as an ever-present complication of therapy.

There is usually no permanent sequela to the thrombocytopenia; it is totally reversible within a few days following removal of the drug. One reported case, however, did require a platelet transfusion to stabilize the acute phase (Moss and Castro 1973).

III. Hemolytic Anemia

Hemolytic anemia is particularly associated with quinidine and methyldopa. The one case induced by quinidine (Freedman et al. 1956) was in a 69-year-old male with a past history of syphilis who developed signs of a purpuric eruption 4 days after starting treatment. The patient was treated with adrenocorticotrophic hormone and the red blood cell count had returned to normal by day 20.

There was concern, at one stage, about a number of reports demonstrating a positive antiglobulin test in patients who had been treated for more than 6 months with methyldopa. The incidence of this finding was established at about 5%–25% of treated patients (Gillies 1974; Corbett 1972; Seedat and Vawda 1972). It was expected that these patients would subsequently exhibit immune hemolysis and clinical anemia. This, however, proved not to be; very few patients developed anemia (0.3%–5%) and then it was often precipitated by another factor such as infection.

IV. Cutaneous Manifestations

Skin rashes of various types are a recognized hazard of therapy with many drugs and those used in cardiovascular disease are no exception. The cardiac glycosides have been reported to produce urticaria, scarlatiniform eruptions, papular and vesicular lesions (Almeyda and Levantine 1973), but it is unlikely that they are all the results of immunological mechanisms.

The basis for concluding that some of the induced rashes might be immunologically mediated is the finding of a positive skin reaction to the glycoside involved and a positive provocation test. Timpanaro (1973), for example, reported a patient who developed an erythematous eruption 10 days after beginning treatment with lanatoside-C. The reaction cleared when the drug was stopped but reappeared on challenge.

One case has been reported of an allergic Type III tissue damage (Coombs and Gell 1953) manifesting as vasculitis. Grette and Johansson (1958) described a 60-year-old woman who developed generalized pruritus and epidermal bullae while taking digitalis leaf. When her therapy was changed to digitoxin, additional lesions developed which appeared as multiple oval light-brown pigmented areas with an elevated erythematous edge. These lesions could be reinduced by challenge, with either acetyl-digitoxin or lanatoside-C.

Cutaneous reactions associated with quinidine include morbilliform, scalatiniform, and urticarial eruptions (Shafter and Halpern 1958). A case of exfoliative dermatitis has been reported (Taylor and Potashnick 1951), but the patient in addition to taking quinidine was also taking penicillin, codeine sulphate, diphenhydramine, and meperidine. The causal relationship implicating quinidine was established by withdrawing the individual drugs and demonstrating clinical exacerbation with quinidine.

Occupational quinidine contact dermatitis has also been reported (FERNSTROM 1965). The patient was an employee of a pharmaceutical company and was required to grind drugs into a powder. A positive patch test to crystals of quinidine sulphate confirmed the already strong clinical evidence.

Purpuric lesions are evident in patients with thrombocytopenia induced by both quinidine and methyldopa, but papular rashes, particularly on the legs, are seen more commonly in patients taking methyldopa.

V. Specific Organ Damage Induced by Cardiovascular Drugs

1. Liver

The liver is very susceptible to toxic damage by drugs, but evidence implicating hypersensitivity mechanisms as the cause of hepatotoxicity is inconclusive. The hepatotoxic reactions seen in some cases of methyldopa therapy are causally related but the mechanism is unclear. In the series studied by TOGHILL et al. (1974), two distinct types of clinical syndrome were apparent. Most patients, 14 out of 20, had hepatitis which was clinically indistinguishable from viral hepatitis. The histological findings of the two conditions differed slightly in that there was a mixed inflammatory portal infiltrate with eosinophilia, associated with the drug-induced hepatitis.

The second syndrome resembled active chronic hepatitis, which was confirmed by demonstrating confluent areas of lobular collapse with condensation of reticulin and an intense inflammatory cell infiltrate which contained plasma cells. Many of the individual liver cells showed ballooning degeneration and the presence of Concitma bodies.

The basis for incriminating methyldopa as a causative agent is that the hepatitis syndrome is dependent upon methyldopa administration, clears up when the drug is stopped, and reappears when the drug is reintroduced. Association between the drug and the active chronic hepatitis type is less distinct; the condition may progress to cirrhosis even after the drug is stopped.

It is perhaps difficult to challenge the evidence supporting a methyldopa-induced effect for both types of hepatoxicity, but there is not sufficient data, either clinical or experimental, to indicate that the syndromes are the result of hypersensitivity mechanisms.

2. Heart

The case report by CONSTON (1974) of methyldopa-induced cardiomyopathy was of a 47-year-old male who was given methyldopa for a few days before feeling unwell. The drug was stopped, then reintroduced 2 weeks later and after approximately 70 h of treatment the patient died. At autopsy the heart was large, dilated, and had a pale, flabby, mottled myocardium. Histological examination revealed an acute inflammatory response with eosinophils.

Similar histological changes were seen in the cases reported by MULLICK and McALLISTER (1977). Since the development of myocarditis was totally unexpected in these patients and the diagnosis made only at autopsy, there were no investigations carried out to determine the etiology. Thus, a hypersensitivity reaction, al-

Table 2. Grading system for oculomucocutaneous syndrome together with cases reported at 20 November 1977

Grade	Definition	Male	Female	Total
I	Severe corneal involvement resulting in major visual impairment	46	76	122
II	Corneal involvement without visual impairment	145	178	323
III	Conjunctivity and/or xerophthalmia	137	101	238
IV	Rash only	109	95	204
V	Sclerosing peritonitis	11	12	23
VI	Hearing impairment only	5	0	5
		453	462	915

though a possibility, is unconfirmed; the myocarditis could equally be caused by a viral infection.

VI. Oculomucocutaneous Syndrome

The adverse effects associated with practolol administration have been well documented (Downie 1974) and the term "oculomucocutaneous syndrome" was an attempt to devise an all-embracing term for the pathological features. A number of organ systems are involved in the syndrome, but individual patients may have one system more obviously damaged than others.

A grading scheme for the severity of the syndrome was agreed with the Committee on Safety of Medicines for the United Kingdom (CSM) in 1977 and it is given in Table 2. A major difficulty in establishing the grading system was in determining, as far as possible, causality. There was a very real danger of attributing to practolol many side effects which occur quite coincidentally in patients receiving the drug. Nevertheless eye lesion, cutaneous manifestation, and sclerosing peritonitis have been investigated extensively and there is no doubt that they are causally related to practolol.

1. Cutaneous Manifestations

A skin rash was one of the first identifiable features of the oculomucocutaneous syndrome. Felix et al. (1974) reported a series of 21 patients with a practolol-associated rash which they call psoriasiform. The rash was most marked over bony prominances and was invariably proceeded by hyperkeratotic changes of the palms, soles, and sides of fingers. Histological changes bore no relationship with those of psoriasis. They consisted of patchy swelling, disruption of the basement membrane, and epidermal atrophy with colloid bodies migrating through the epidermis.

Although the so-called psoriasiform rash is the main "practolol rash", Assem and Banks (1973) reported lichenoid eruptions in a patient on practolol and various other types of mixed eruptions have also been reported (Felix et al. 1974). Figures generated in November 1977 indicated that the average time on practolol to development of the "practolol rash" was 19.1 months, with a range of 1–84 months (Nicholls 1978).

2. Eye Lesions

WRIGHT (1975) reported a series of 27 patients with conjunctival damage directly related to practolol therapy. Patients complained of dry gritty eyes, which on examination revealed a hyperemic conjunctiva and an irregular blood vessel pattern. In more severely affected cases, there was a subconjunctival sheet of fibrovascular tissue which contracted to produce scarring, conjunctival shrinkage, and fornix obliteration. Adhesions between the conjunctiva and cornea occurred as the condition progressed, with eventual perforation of the cornea producing permanent blindness.

The average time on practolol before symptoms appeared was about 25 months, with a range of 1–84 months (NICHOLLS 1978).

3. Sclerosing Peritonitis

Peritonitis caused by practolol was first recognized by BROWN et al. (1974). Patients presented with a history of nausea, vomiting, abdominal pain, steatorrhea, loss of weight, and in some cases an abdominal mass.

The average length of treatment with practolol prior to the development of the first symptom of sclerosing peritonitis was about 34 months (NICHOLLS 1978). A disturbing feature, however, and one which eventually led to withdrawal of the drug, was that the symptoms had been reported up to 18 months after cessation of treatment (ALLAN and CADE 1975; HALLEY and GOODMAN 1975). About 50 patients with this particular feature of the syndrome are known to the CSM, either in conjunction with other aspects of the syndrome, or as the main one.

Laparotomy findings showed that the peritoneal cavity was obliterated with gross thickening and contraction of the parietal and visceral layers of the peritoneum. The small bowel was encased in a rigid tube and usually shortened, but the adverse effect stopped at the ileocecal valve.

Peritoneal biopsies showed a nonspecific inflammatory reaction with fibrous tissue comprising layers of coarse collagen bundles interspersed with the visceral peritoneum.

4. Oral/Nasal Lesions

In WRIGHT's 27 patients, 5 had recurrent ulceration of the oral and nasal mucosa, which stopped when practolol therapy was discontinued. Although there is no argument that this is part of the oculomucocutaneous syndrome, it is not a major component.

5. Hearing Impairment

Patients on practolol have complained of deafness and tinnitus (WRIGHT 1975; McNAB-JONES et al. 1977). On examination sensorineural hearing defect could be demonstrated and this was associated with a form of secretory otitis media.

The hearing defect rarely occurred as a single entity; it was usually associated with one of the major features of the syndrome and had a mean time of onset of about 28 months.

6. Fibrotic Reactions

The main target tissues incorporated in the oculomucocutaneous syndrome are skin, conjunctiva, serosal surfaces, and peritoneum, but there are reports of fibrotic reactions affecting the lungs and liver which appear to be the result of practolol therapy. BROWN et al. (1978) reported two patients who developed biliary cirrhosis after long-term practolol administration. One of the patients also had an eczematous rash and complained of dry eyes, and the second had the typical psoriasiform rash.

Intestinal pulmonary fibrosis associated with practolol therapy has been reported (ERWTEMAN et al. 1977). The patient also had concomitant sclerosing peritonitis, but eventually died of a rapidly progressing pulmonary insufficiency. Evidence directly implicating practolol as a causative agent for the pulmonary condition is circumstantial; however, the simultaneous presence of sclerosing peritonitis does suggest that practolol may be a common etiological agent for the two conditions.

VII. Oculomucocutaneous Syndrome and β-Blocking Drugs Other than Practolol

The attendant publicity given to the tissue damage induced by practolol prompted a number of reports of similar reactions to propranolol and the so-called second generation β-blockers. Most of the reports describe a particular feature of the syndrome, but no case has yet been described which convincingly demonstrates that any of the β-blockers produce the same pattern of lesions as practolol.

1. Propranolol

Cutaneous reactions due to propranolol have ben reported by CUBEY and TAYLOR (1975), COCHRAN et al. (1976), and JENSEN et al. (1976).

JENSEN et al. (1976) reported six patients in whom cutaneous changes closely resembling those seen with practolol were produced after treatment with propranolol for about 10 months. The histology was described as slight epidermal hyperplasia, acanthosis, patchy parakeratosis and edema of the epidermis; no mention was made of colloid bodies, a feature particularly prominent in the practolol rash. Propranolol was shown to be the causative agent by demonstrating that the rash disappeared when the drug was stopped and reappeared on challenge. One of the reported patients did complain of dry eyes but no keratoconjunctivitis sicca was found using Schimer's test and no corneal lesions were detected.

It has been claimed that propranolol produces an abnormal fibroblastic response: two patients with Peyronie's disease, ostensibly due to propranolol administration, were reported by OSBORNE (1977). This alleged response has been studied more extensively by the authors who now admit that corroborative data to support the original claim have not been obtained.

A case of cheilostomatitis associated with propranolol has been reported by TANGSRUD and GOLF (1977). The symptoms subsided over a 12-week period when propranolol was changed to alprenolol but reappeared following the reintroduction of propranolol.

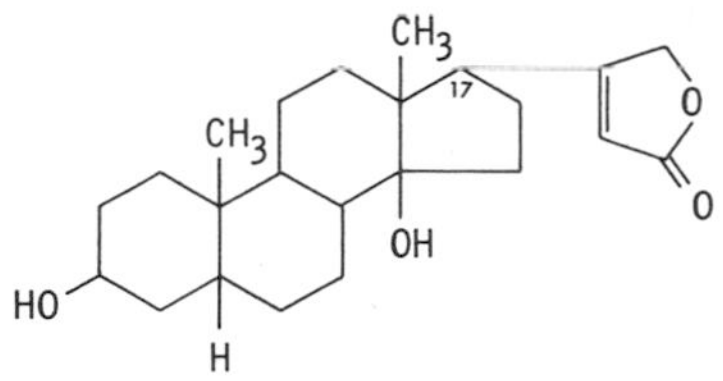

Fig. 1. Structural formula for digitoxigenin; cyclopentaperhydrophenanthrene nucleus, unsaturated lactone ring attached at C-17

2. Alprenolol

Industrial exposure to alprenolol causing contact eczema was reported by EKENVALL and FORSBECK (1978). Positive patch test reactions were demonstrated in 14 out of 32 patients with suspected contact dermatitis to alprenolol.

3. Timolol

BAXTER-SMITH et al. (1978) claimed that a 50-year-old man treated with timolol developed sclerosing peritonitis. The patient presented with small bowel obstruction and at laparotomy the gross pathological lesions were similar to those seen with practolol. Histological examination of the adhesions showed jejunal angiitis and evidence of a previous perforation. The histology was not typical of that reported for practolol; the findings were more compatible with an organizing peritonitis following a small bowel perforation. A case of dry eyes has been reported by FRAIS and BAILEY (1979): The patient complained of dryness in both eyes after 14 months of treatment with timolol which improved immediately timolol was withdrawn.

C. Immunopharmacological Aspects

I. Cardiac Glycosides

The basic structure of all the cardiac glycosides is a cyclopentaperhydrophenanthrene nucleus to which is attached an unsaturated lactone ring at C-17. This is termed the aglycone; additional attachment of sugar residues is needed to form the glycoside, as shown in Fig. 1.

Considerable attention has been paid recently to the development of radioimmunoassay techniques for detecting serum levels of glycosides and this has led to valuable information on the antigenicity of individual members of the series.

1. Digitoxin

High affinity antibodies to digitoxin can be induced in rabbits by injecting the aglycone, digitoxigenin, coupled to human serum albumen. The standard method for forming the antigen is to react digitoxigenin with succinic anhydride producing 3-*O*-succinyl digitoxigenin. This is then linked via its carboxyl end to free amine groups of human serum albumin. The coupling can be achieved either with bifunctional coupling reagents such as carbodiimide or by the mixed anhydride method (BUTLER 1978).

Antibodies formed against these conjugates are capable of binding ^{125}I-labelled succinyl digitoxinogenin tyrosine methyl-ester. This interaction can be inhibited by free digitoxin (BUTLER 1978) showing that the specificity is directed against the haptenic structure. Inhibition experiments with related glycosides, digoxin or 12-hydroxydigitoxin show that these compounds are about one-tenth as effective as inhibitors than the inducing hapten. Moreover, it has been pointed out by BUTLER and CHEN (1967) that the structure of aglycones is similar to steroid hormones and immunological cross reactivity may be expected. The steroid hormones at physiological concentration, however, fail to inhibit the reaction between digitoxigenin and its corresponding antibody (BUTLER 1978).

2. Digoxin

Formation of immunogens from digoxin can be achieved by coupling through the terminal digitoxose residues. The aglycone of digoxin is digoxigenin and the complete molecule consists of the aglycone and an additional 3-glycosidic digitoxose residue linked to the aglycone at the C-3 position. Conversion of the vicinal hydroxyl groups to aldehydes by oxidation with sodium periodate yields a dialdehyde derivative which can be linked to the free amino groups of protein. A course of injections for several months into rabbits with these conjugates produces antibodies with optimum specificity and affinity (SMITH et al. 1970; SMITH and HARBER 1973).

Immunological specificity of the rabbit antibodies has been extensively studied mainly because digoxin is the most widely used of the cardiac glycosides. Antibodies have been shown to bind tritium-labelled digoxin using both equilibrium and dextran-coated charcoal separation (STOLL et al. 1973). The formation of metabolic products which cross react in immunological systems with the parent digoxin molecule is not likely to compound an investigation of a digoxin hypersensitivity response. However, with other glycosides which contain digoxigenin, such as deslanoside, lanatoside C, α-acetyldigoxin, β-acetyldigoxin, and β-methyl-digoxin, the metabolic products may well complicate any clinical or laboratory exploration of an adverse tissue effect.

3. Gitaloxin

This glycoside 16-formylgitoxin is obtained from digitalis leaf. An immunogen can be prepared by reacting the aglycone, gitaloxigenin, with succinic anhydride to produce gitaloxigenin hemisuccinate, which can then be coupled through its carboxyl group to free amino groups of protein using carbodiimide (BUTLER 1978).

Antibodies formed in response to injecting the conjugate will bind digoxin and gitoxin; this latter compound is more effective at inhibiting the interaction between the antisera and gitaloxin than the gitaloxin itself. The reason for this is that the formyl groups are rapidly hydrolyzed after injecting the conjugate so that the antibodies formed are effectively antigitoxin (LESNE and DOLPHEN 1976).

4. Gitoxin

Gitoxin is also formed from digitalis leaf. It is a better inhibitor of the interaction between digoxin and antidigoxin sera than gitaloxin (LESNE 1972) and for the reasons already stated it will effectively inhibit the binding of specific antibodies formed in response to gitaloxigenin protein conjugates.

5. Lanatoside C

The aglycone of lanatoside C is the same as that for digoxin, i.e., digoxigenin, as it only differs from digoxin by an additional glucose and acetyl group in its terminal digitoxone. Thus, cross reactivity would be expected between compounds derived from digitalis purpura and digitalis lanata.

6. Ouabain

This compound is the glycoside of strophanthus gratus. It can be converted into an immunogen by conjugating through its glycosidic rhamnose residues to the free amino groups poly (DL-alanyl)-human serum albumen by the periodate oxidation method (SKUBITZ and SMITH 1975).

The antisera will bind ouabain and the interaction can be readily inhibited by ouabain and acetylstrophanthidin. Digoxin and digitoxin will also inhibit the reaction but are about 1/15th as effective as ouabain and endogenous steroids will not cross react at all (SMITH 1972).

7. Proscillaridin

An immunogen for proscillaridin, a squill glycoside, can be prepared in the same way as that for ouabain, and the specificity is almost exclusively directed toward proscillaridin and closely related derivatives. Digoxin, digitoxin, and ouabain have only weak cross reactivity whilst steroids are totally ineffective as inhibiting antigens (BELZ et al. 1973).

It would be reasonable to expect, from the work which has been carried out on the production of antibodies to various glycosides in animals, that antibodies would also be produced in man following therapeutic administration of the compounds. The ability of cardiac glycosides to induce antibodies in man, however, will depend upon a number of pharmacokinetic and pharmacodynamic variables, the most important being oral absorption, type of protein binding, and extent of metabolism. As a general rule, these properties are related directly to lipid solubility and inversely to polarity. The polarity of the cardiac glycosides is determined primarily by the number of hydroxyl groups attached to the steroid nucleus. It would be expected, therefore, that the conditions for antibody formation would be best satisfied by digitoxin with one OH-steroidal group rather than the other related compounds. This prediction is, in fact, comparable with clinical reports.

II. Quinidine

Quinidine consists of a quinolinic group attached through a secondary alcohol linkage to a quinuclidine ring. A methoxy side chain is attached to the quinoline

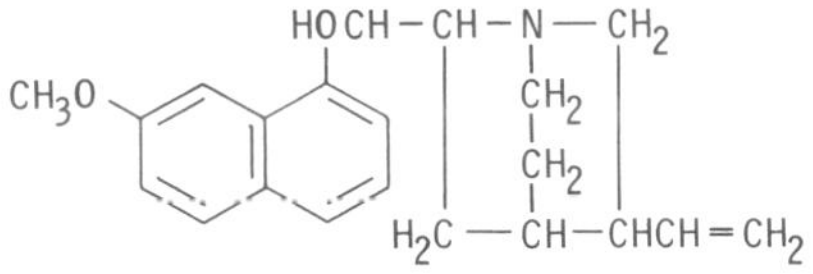

Fig. 2. Structural formula for quinidine

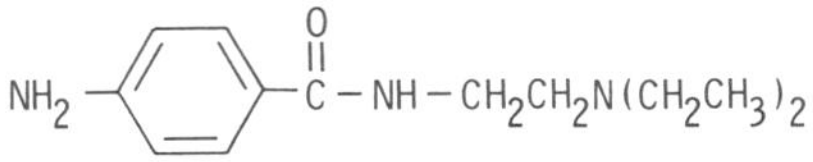

Fig. 3. Structural formula for procainamide

ring and a vinyl group to the quinuclidine, as shown in Fig. 2. Quinidine is distinguished from its isomer quinine by the steric configuration of the secondary alcohol group.

Pharmacokinetic studies show that quinidine is virtually completely absorbed after oral administration and, in the therapeutic range 3–6 µg/ml^{-1} plasma, 60% of the drug is bound to plasma albumin (CONN and LUCHI 1961).

There is very little known about the immunogenic properties of quinidine; no systematic attempt to raise antibodies to quinidine and investigate their specificity has been published. AMOS (1967, unpublished work) incubated quinidine with serum albumin to effect electrostatic interaction through the basic bridgehead nitrogen and produce an immunogenic "complex", which was then injected repeatedly into rabbits, but no antibodies with quinidine specificity were produced.

Although many of the metabolic products of quinidine are known (BRODIE et al. 1951), there is no information relating to their immunogenicity. Nevertheless, there is evidence that quinidine does induce an antibody in man as inferred from the reports of FREEDMAN et al. (1956), but the immunological specificity is not known.

III. Procainamide

Procainamide (*p*-amino-*N*(2)-diethylaminoethyl) benzamide (Fig. 3) is an anti-arrhythmic drug developed from procaine. Procaine itself has been used experimentally to abort arrhythmias in anesthesia, but it proved to be rapidly hydrolyzed to diethylaminoethanol and *p*-aminobenzoic acid and therefore unsuitable for clinical use (BRODIE et al. 1948). Of the two hydrolysis products, diethylaminoethanol proved to have the antiarrhythmic action (ROSENBERG et al. 1949), but large doses were required. Nevertheless this finding did demonstrate that the ester part of procaine was not involved in the pharmacological action. Substituting the ester linkage for the amide structure produced an effective anti-arrhythmic agent resistant to the action of nonspecific serum esterases and therefore stable in vivo.

RUSSELL and ZIFF (1968) showed that procainamide was immunogenic in rabbits, by injecting the animals with a procainamide bovine serum albumin complex

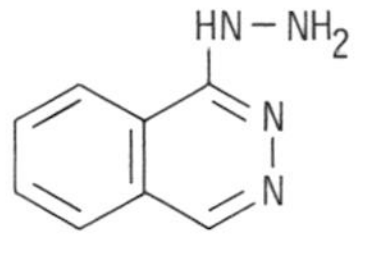

Fig. 4. Structural formula for hydralazine

produced by a diazo-likage through the amido group. Antibodies were detected by a passive hemagglutination technique in which the drug was diazotized to sheep red blood cells.

More significantly, procainamide can be complexed to DNA in vitro. BLOM-GREN and VAUGHAN (1968) showed that procainamide, in the presence of a photoactive molecule and visible light, bound to DNA to produce a highly antigenic complex. It has been postulated that such a complex may be involved in the pathogenesis of procainamide-induced lupus.

IV. Hydralazine

The structural formula of hydralazine, 1-hydrazinophthalazine, is shown in Fig. 4. The association between hydralazine therapy and a clinical state of immunological activation is well established as it is considered a high-risk drug for the induction of lupus erythematosus.

Hydralazine can also behave as an immunogen and stimulate drug-specific antibodies, but it is unclear at present whether such antibodies are causally related to the hydralazine lupus syndrome.

FRIEDMAN and HEINE (1963) reported that serum from one out of three patients with active hydralazine lupus would agglutinate sheep red blood cells coated with hydralazine; hydralazine was coupled to the cells by means of the bifunctional coupling reagent bis-diazotized benzidine. The immunological specificity of the reaction was established by demonstrating that agglutination could be inhibited by free drug but not by bovine serum albumin, ragweed pollen extract, or penicillin. FRIEDMAN and HEINE (1963) also claimed to have induced hydralazine antibodies in rabbits by injecting hydralazine in Freund's complete adjuvant.

This latter finding was not confirmed by the elegant studies of PAZ and SEIFTER (1972) who investigated the immunogenicity of complexes formed between hydralazine and various types of collagen and proteins. They reasoned that the presence of a reactive hydrazine group in hydralazine might react with the aldehydes present in collagen to form antigenic complexes. Antibodies to the collagen carrier might then be formed which could cross-react with other tissue proteins. This proposition was tested by reacting hydralazine with skin collagen, egg albumen, and serum glycoprotein using the periodate oxidation method and then injecting the characterized products into animals. They were able to demonstrate that proteins as hydralazines induced antibodies that cross-reacted with other protein hydralazines and induced antibodies with specificity for the carrier collagen/protein molecule and the hydralazine function. The injection of hydralazine without conjugation to a carrier failed to produce an antibody response.

HAHN et al. (1972) examined four patients with hydralazine lupus and found drug-specific antibodies in them all. Moreover, demonstration of the antibody correlated with the lupus syndrome, as patients treated with hydralazine, but with no clinical signs of lupus, did not have detectable hydralazine antibodies. The finding that hydralazine induces drug-specific antibodies only in association with the active lupus syndrome may not be a true reflection of its immunogenic potential.

MAYER et al. (1955) investigated the ability of hydralazine to induce contact sensitivity in guinea-pigs. They injected a number of guinea-pigs intradermally with 0.1 ml of a 0.5% aqueous solution of hydralazine at three sites on three alternate days and then challenged by injecting 0.1 ml of a 0.5% solution intradermally 16 days later. They found that the majority of guinea-pigs injected developed a typical delayed-type skin reaction on challenge. By injecting sensitized animals with compounds chemically allied to hydralazine and recording the degree of cross reactivity, the investigators were able to deduce the following:

1. Animals sensitized to hydralazine would also react with closely related hydrazinopthalazines bearing substitutions on the nitrogen ring.
2. Weaker cross reactivity was achieved with compounds bearing substitutions on the hydrazino-group.
3. The specificity of the response was not directed solely against the hydrazino-group as compounds such as phenyl-hydrazine did not cross-react.
4. No cross reaction was achieved with compounds without the phthalazine nucleus.
5. Phthalazine compounds lacking a hydrazino-group also failed to cross-react.

The conclusions drawn from these observations are that hydralazine is a potent skin sensitizer and the specificity of the response is directed against the whole of the unchanged molecule.

The therapeutic use of hydralazine does not involve topical application and there is no information available about the skin-sensitizing capacity of hydralazine to man. When given orally, in contrast to the dermal sensitivity, hydrazaline acts as a weak immunogen.

One possible explanation for the difference in antigenic potency of hydralazine when given orally as opposed to topically is that the specificity of the two immunological responses is different. The specificity of skin contact reactions, as Mayer's group have shown in guinea-pigs, is directed against the whole molecule which implies that metabolism plays no part in forming the antigenic determinant. But in man, given oral hydralazine, two unrelated observations have been made which favor a role for metabolic activation. The first is by HAHN et al. (1972) who showed that hydralazine antibodies are closely related to the drug-induced lupus syndrome and may be a necessary prerequisite for the appearance of hydralazine lupus; the second is the observation by PERRY et al. (1970) which defined a clinical relationship between the rate of hydralazine acetylation and the lupus syndrome. The metabolism of hydralazine depends on second phase acetylation which is under genetic control. The phenotype is expressed as a bimodal distribution of fast and slow acelylators and the lupus syndrome appears to be more identifiable in the slow acelylation groups.

There is an alternative explanation that could possibly account for the failure of hydralazine to induce specific antibodies except in association with hydralazine

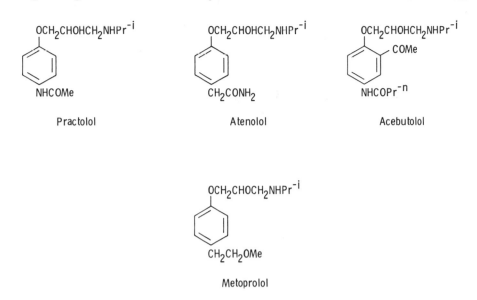

Fig. 5. Selective B_1 receptor blockers showing degree of structural homology

lupus and that depends on hydralazine acting as a tolerogen. MAYER et al. (1955) showed that guinea-pigs given hydralazine orally developed a resistance to sensitization by skin contact. This hyposensitization phenomenon was first recorded by CHASE (1946) using dinitrochlorobenzene as a sensitizer and is now known to be due to the induction of specific immunological tolerance induced by feeding the sensitizing agent. Thus, if hydralazine is a tolerogen, no antibodies would be detectable in the serum unless the tolerogenic mechanism is broken. It is conceivable that tolerance could be broken by a hydralazine-dependent mechanism which results in auto-antibody formation.

The available data are insufficient to allow a more precise speculation on which of the two explanations, if either, is the more likely. Further investigative work is needed.

V. Beta-Adrenoceptor Blocking Drugs

The structural formulae of the β-adrenoceptor blocking drugs used in clinical practice are given in Fig. 5. It can be seen that there is considerable structural homology between the various members of the group but, as stated in an earlier section, the associated adverse responses are mainly confined to one particular compound – practolol. Practolol antibodies can be raised in rabbits which can recognize two distinct domains of the practolol molecule depending upon the configuration of the haptenic determinant (GREGORY 1977, personal communication).

Determinant 1 is formed by linking through the isopropanolamine chain and
Determinant 2 is formed by linking through the *N*-acetylamino group. Practolol can be deacetylated in vitro to yield a product which can be diazotized and then

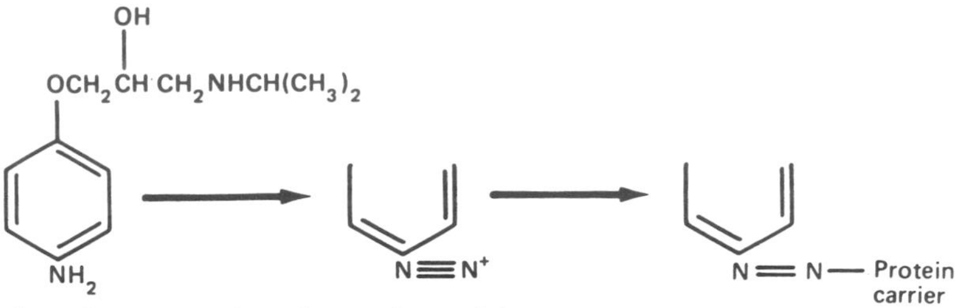

Determinant 2 – prepared from des-acetyl practolol

Fig. 6. Linkage of practolol protein carrier via isopropanolamine

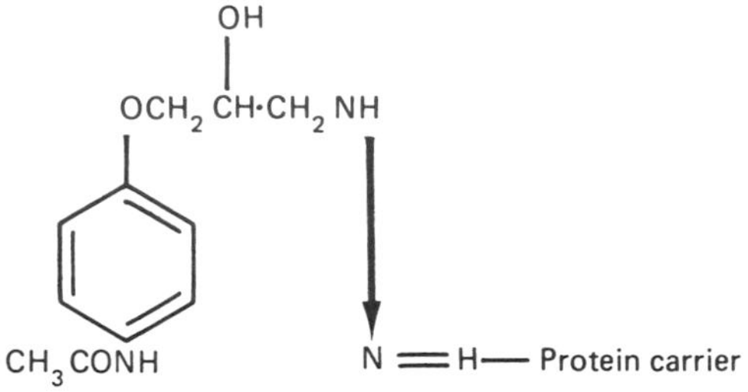

Determinant 1 – prepared from des-isopropyl practolol

Fig. 7. Linkage of practolol to protein carrier via the N-acetylamino

coupled to human serum albumin using bis-diazotized benzene, as shown in Fig. 6. Antibodies formed in response to this determinant have been shown to have specificity for the isopropanolamine side chain and the benzene ring. It is possible to synthesize the des-iso-propyl derivative of practolol to produce a primary amine which can then be coupled to protein through the exposed-NH group (Fig. 7). The specificity of antibodies formed in response to this determinant is toward the benzene ring and the N-acetylamino derivative.

Cross reactivity between the two antigens as determined in a radioimmunoassay is very low, which indicates that the benzene ring must be recognized in two halves (GREGORY 1977, personal communication). These experiments demonstrate that practolol is sufficiently antigenic to induce antibody production in experimental animals but when the two derived practolol complexes were used to examine sera from patients with the oculomucocutaneous syndrome, no antibody activity could be detected (GREGORY 1977, personal communication; AMOS 1977, unpublished work).

AMOS et al. (1977) were able to detect antibodies in patient's sera which reacted with a first-phase metabolic product(s) of practolol. Their system involved metabolizing practolol in vitro in a mixed function oxygenase system using rat and hamster liver microsomes. An affinity purified antibody to human O red cells was added to the enzyme generating system to act as a scavenger molecule for binding the metabolites. On completion of the metabolic process, human O red cells were added to the metabolic mix and allowed to react with the red cell antibody containing bound metabolites. The red cells, after thoroughly washing to remove unbound

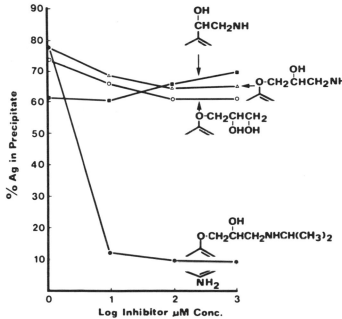

Fig. 8. Inhibition by model compounds of the response between Practolol metabolite antibody and the homologous antigen

material, were used in a passive hemagglutination assay, which showed that agglutination was achieved by sera taken from patients taking practolol but not with normal human sera.

In order to obtain information on the specificity of the response and the nature of the metabolite, Amos et al. (1978) modified the experiment by using radiolabelled human serum albumin instead of the red cell antibody. This enabled a Farr-type assay to be developed (Farr 1958), in which a number of model compounds could be tested for their ability to inhibit the reaction. Figure 8 shows the results of the inhibition studies. It can be deduced from the figure that compounds with an intact or slightly modified isopropanolamine side chain failed to inhibit the interaction of antibody with the metabolite, whereas compounds in which the N-acetyl-amino function was altered inhibited the response even though the side chain remained exposed.

Detailed metabolic studies carried out in vitro and in vivo, using hamsters, showed that two terminal metabolites were formed – desacetylpractolol and 3-hydroxy practolol (Orton and Lowery 1977). In man, however, neither of these two metabolites has been found, but deacetylation has been shown to be a minor metabolic pathway accounting for about 5%–6% of the metabolism (Reeves et al. 1978).

From the inhibition studies shown in Fig. 8 it can be seen that 3-hydroxy practolol did not inhibit the antibody interaction but desacetylpractolol did. An interpretation of this finding is that 3-hydroxy practolol is not the metabolite antigen. Whether the specificity of the antibody is directed solely against products resulting from deacetylation still remains to be demonstrated.

Table 3. In vitro metabolism of practolol by hamster liver microsomes: parallel effects on binding to microsomal protein and immune reactivity

	Biochemical results based on covalent binding of ^{14}C ring labeled practolol (Orton and Lowery 1977; Case et al. 1978)	Imunological results based on reaction of patients' sera with generated metabolites (H.R. Amos, unpublished work)
NADPH [a]	Necessary	Necessary
Enzyme induction – animal pretreatment with:		
phenobarbitone	No enhancement	No effect
20-methylcholanthrene	Reduced	Reduced
Compounds added to microsomal system:		
1,2-Epoxy-3-3-3-tricyclopropene oxide [b]	No effect	No effect
bis-(p-nitrophenyl) phosphate	Reduced	Not done
glutathione	Reduced	Reduced
sodium fluoride	Variable	Variable
desacetyl practolol	Not done	Partial inhibition
3-hydroxy practolol	Not done	No inhibition

[a] Reduced nicotinamide adenine dinucleotidephosphate
[b] Compound inhibits epoxyhydratase

In an attempt to obtain further information on the nature of the metabolite antigen formed in vitro, various modifications of the enzyme generating system were made to see if they altered the antibody activity. Table 3 shows the modifications that were used and compares their effects on the immunological reaction with those obtained by measuring the covalent binding of ^{14}C practolol with liver microsomes (Amos 1978).

These data are inconclusive but they do emphasize the importance of the N-acetyl-amino group and indicate that the direction of further work should be aimed at determining metabolic interactions involving this function.

VI. Methyldopa

Methyldopa (L-α-methyl-3-4-dihydroxy-phenylalanine) is an effective inhibitor of 1-aromatic amino acid (dopa) decarboxylase (Sourkes 1954). There is no evidence that methyldopa is an immunogen; methyldopa-specific antibodies have not been reported and there is no evidence of antibody production specific for first-phase metabolites.

D. Clinical Immunological Aspects

Hypersensitivity responses induced by cardiovascular drugs can be divided into two broad groups. There are those clinical syndromes which do not depend upon the formation of drug-specific antibodies and there are drug-antibody interactions which cause tissue damage by the mechanism outlined by COOMBS and GELL (1953). The two most important diseases associated with the former are lupus erythematosus and the oculomucocutaneous syndrome, whilst thrombocytopenia and hemolytic anemia are examples associated with the latter.

I. Drug-Induced Lupus Erythematosus

Finding antibodies which react with nuclear components of xenogenic tissue is a positive indication that a drug may be responsible for a lupus-like syndrome. Drug-induced lupus is a complex disease while the mechanism, despite detailed investigation, is still unclear.

Lupus erythematosus is thought to be generated by the expression of a genetically determined diathesis. This belief is based on statistical evaluation of family studies by ROWELL (1968), and MIESCHER and PARONETTO (1969). Studies on a similar disease found in certain strains of dogs (ORKIM 1967) supports the existence of a lupus diathesis which, if strong, will be triggered by weak stimuli and may appear to occur spontaneously, but if the predisposition is weak then stronger stimuli are required, such as a response to drugs.

It is tempting to consider drug-induced lupus as a single entity induced by multiple agents acting through a single mechanism, but this is likely to be an over-simplification.

Studies which have been carried out on hydralazine lupus have shown that in all cases antihydralazine antibodies and antinuclear antibodies can be found (HAHN et al. 1972). Moreover, antihydralazine antibodies have so far been found only in patients with the lupus syndrome – clearly hydralazine does not appear to be immunogenic unless there is a developed or developing lupus condition. Thus, a mechanism must exist for the initial induction of ANAs and those for antibodies to the drug itself. Whether drug-specific antibodies contribute to the pathogenesis of the tissue damage or whether the altered immune function in these patients predisposes to the production of anti-drug antibodies is not at all resolved.

One factor which might be of significance in this respect is the genetic variation in hydralazine metabolism. Hydralazine is primarily acetylated by hepatic acetyl transferases which exhibit genetic polymorphism. A prospective study by PERRY et al. (1970) showed that, within a group of 51 patients, two distinct acetylation phenotypes could be detected and that hydralazine lupus appeared to be confined to the group which slowly acetylated the drug. The study by PERRY et al. is the citation work for the correlation between the clinical disease and acetylation phenotypes, but a more searching investigation is needed to piece together the interaction between ANA, drug-specific antibodies and the metabolic status of the patient. Until such a study is available, the mechanism of hydralazine lupus must remain speculative.

Differences in acetylation rates have also been shown to occur with procainamide, but unlike hydralazine, the conclusion is less clear. HENNINGSEN et al. (1975) carried out a prospective study of 42 patients on long-term procainamide treatment: they were able to show that 12 patients (29%) developed a classic drug-induced lupus syndrome. The acetylation status was determined on 11 of these 12 patients, 8 proved to be slow and 3 fast acetylation. The authors concluded that there may be a reason for fast acetylators to develop procainamide-lupus, but in general it is the slow acetylation group that is more vulnerable.

The interpretation of these data has been complicated by the findings and conclusions of Davies et al. (1975), who claim that it is the rapid acetylation which predispose to the formation of ANAs and that acetyl procainamide might be the inducing stimulus for the disease process. Moreover, they point out the structural similarity between acetyl procainamide and practolol and suggest that an acetylated product might be an etiological agent in practolol-induced lupus.

Procainamide itself, as Russell and Ziff (1968) have shown, can induce drug-specific antibodies in experimental models, they also showed that similar specific antibodies, particularly of the IgM class, were present in about one-third of the population and 70% of normal dogs. Clearly, the antibodies are not related to a single disease process.

The fact that procainamide can be photocomplexed to DNA in vitro is an interesting observation. If a procainamide-DNA complex is the form of the complete antigen in vivo, then the antibodies should have limited cross reactivity with native DNA. This, indeed, appears to be the case: no antibodies to native DNA have been found in patients with procainamide-induced lupus (Blomgren and Vaughan 1970; Koffler et al. 1971). Moreover, it would be expected that, if the mechanism for procainamide lupus is centered around a drug DNA complex and no similar complex is demonstrable for hydralazine, DNA antibodies might be likely to occur in patients with hydralazine lupus. Hahn et al. (1972) and Blau (1973) have reported DNA antibodies in hydralazine-treated patients, but the data are not sufficiently definitive to be conclusive.

II. Thrombocytopenia

A number of cardiovascular drugs of different chemical structure are known to produce a reduction in the platelet count, but it is likely that the mechanism by which the thrombocytopenia is brought about is common to all the drugs which cause such an effect. The pioneering work on drug-induced thrombocytopenia was carried out by Ackroyd (1949). Ackroyd worked on Sedormid and his fundamental contention was that the specificity of the Sedormid antibody was directed against a platelet-Sedormid complex, implying that platelets contributed to the formation of the antigenic determinant. Bolton (1956) was able to show that the qualitative findings reported by Ackroyd held for quinidine.

Shulman (1963), also working with quinidine, proposed an alternative explanation to explain the mechanism. He relegates the platelets to a passive role and considers them to be specialized cells capable of adsorbing onto their surface a drug-antibody complex. This hypothesis was a deduction based on the study of a steric and kinetic model for the immunoreactants involved in platelet lysis (Shulman 1958). By varying the concentrations of the reactants in the model, Shulman was able to show that there was only stoichiometric combination between the four reactants, antibody, antigen, platelets, and complement, and that the interactions were most likely bimolecular and sequential. The most probable sequence appeared to be first an initial combination of quinidine with either antibody of platelets, followed by the formation of the complete antibody-quinidine-platelet complex, and finally complement fixation by the complex. The interesting question whether quinidine bound first to the antibody or to the platelets could not be answered by SHULMAN's data. However, when the system was mathematically modelled by HILL (1958), a model was found to fit the data, but the final equation was common to both situations.

Support for SHULMAN's hypothesis would be the in vitro demonstration of platelet damage by drug-antibody complexes or the demonstration of such complexes in the sera of patients with thrombocytopenia. Despite numerous attempts by various investigators (CRONIN 1965; AMOS 1967, unpublished work) no evidence of this type could be found.

The work of YOUNG et al. (1966) on digitoxin-induced thrombocytopenia does tend to support SHULMAN. They were able to show that digitoxin in the presence of the patient's serum concentrated about the surface of platelets and could be easily dissociated by a single saline wash. When the serum was electrophoresed on starch gel, digitoxin was found in the α-globulin fraction, a finding which would be compatible with the presence of drug-antibody complexes. The case investigated by MEDENICA et al. (1972) also had digitoxin-antibody complexes, as detected by a thrombolysis test.

An interesting fact to emerge from the studies of YOUNG et al. (1966) and MEDENICA et al. is that the thrombocytopenia is highly specific for the digitoxin glycoside. Substituted alternative glycosides did not precipitate the condition. This is surprising as it has been shown that in an animal model there is a substantial degree of cross reactivity between the glycosides. A clue to the explanation could be the apparent specialization of the target tissue – platelets. If the receptor on platelets is complementary to a functional group expressed only on digitoxin, then digitoxin complexes will be absorbed. This would be independent of the antibody cross reactivity with the other glycosides.

III. Oculomucocutaneous Syndrome

The basis for considering that the oculomucocutaneous syndrome is a hypersensitivity response induced by practolol administration is a combination of clinical observations and laboratory findings which do not easily fit any alternative explanation.

Clinical. It is now established that the syndrome as defined by ICI and accepted by the Committee on Safety of Medicines, U.K., is related solely to practolol (NICHOLLS 1978). Since none of the other β-adrenoceptor blocking drugs produces the same adverse effect, it is difficult to construct hypotheses for the syndrome which postulate some pharmacological malfunction. Moreover, extensive epidemiological studies have been carried out and they fail to demonstrate any drug interaction (NICHOLLS 1978), genetic predisposition (DICK et al. 1978), or metabolic acetylator states (REEVES et al. 1978). More pertinent to an immunological hypothesis is the finding that the tissue damage is not dose related (NICHOLLS 1978).

Failure to find a common denominator which would give some indication of a possible mechanism leads to the conclusion that the syndrome might be an idiosyncratic response to the drug.

Laboratory. The earliest findings to be reported were the presence of antinuclear antibodies in the sera and IgG deposits in the basement membrane of biopsied skin (FELIX et al. 1974). These findings would be compatible with a drug-induced lupus erythematosus but this is not considered part of the oculomucocutaneous syndrome.

Amos et al. (1975) reported the presence of a second auto-antibody which is not found in drug lupus. This antibody reacted with the intercellular ground substance of xenogenic epidermis. The immunofluorescence staining pattern was indistinguishable from the pattern considered pathognomonic for pemphigus, but it could be identified from the pemphigus antibody by its inability to bind to isolated epidermal cells. A search for auto-antibodies by BEHAN et al. (1976) revealed that patients suffering from practolol toxicity had many types of auto-antibody, but they were unable to demonstrate convincingly any associated immunological findings such as a change in the level of serum immunoglobulin or complement components.

Drug-specific antibodies demonstrated by Amos et al. (1977) were not confined to patients with the oculomucocutaneous syndrome. Figure 9 shows an analysis of the presence of the antibody in various patient groups and it can be seen that it occurred in most patients on long-term practolol, but the titer was higher in those patients with the oculomucocutaneous syndrome (Amos et al. 1978).

IV. Mechanism of Practolol-Induced Tissue Damage

In order to construct a hypothesis for the mechanism by which practolol produces such diverse pathological lesions, it is necessary to explore the two basic findings of auto-antibodies and drug-specific antibodies. An explanation for auto-antibody production was offered by ALLISON et al. (1971). They suggested that auto-antibody production is due to a breakdown of a normal suppressor function mediated by T cells. HADDEN et al. (1970) and SHERMAN et al. (1973) have shown that the function of lymphoid cells in vitro can be modified by drugs which react with adrenergic receptors. It is conceivable, therefore, that practolol could selectively interfere with lymphocyte subpopulations in vivo and alter their control function on antibody producing B cells.

This possibility was given credence for practolol by the experiments of BEHAN et al. (1976) who showed that there was a lack of skin responsiveness to candida antigens in practolol patients and a reduction in protein synthesis by lymphocytes in response to mitogen stimulation in vitro if the cells were taken from a patient with the oculomucocutaneous syndrome. Similar experiments, carried out by other workers (Amos and BRIGDEN 1976; PUGH et al. 1976), failed to demonstrate a reduction. It is unfortunate that studies to demonstrate an immunosuppressed state in practolol patients were not conclusive. Lymphocyte transformation to mitogens as a single criterion is of limited value and tests of more physiological relevance would be needed to clarify the issue.

A possible clue to the role of practolol-specific antibodies was found when a retrospective analysis of sera was carried out in a group of patients who had taken part in a challenge study. The pre- and post-challenge antibody titers for the five patients in the study are shown in Table 4. The titer at the height of the adverse

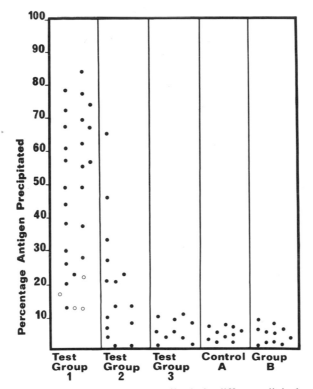

Fig. 9. Distribution of practolol metabolite antibody in different clinical groups.
Test Group 1:   Patients with the oculomucocutaneous syndrome
Test Group 2:   Patients receiving practolol but with no clinical signs
Test Group 3:   Patients with drug-induced systemic lupus erythematosus
Control Group A: Patients with either pemphigus or pemphigoid
Control Group B: Age-related individuals with no clinical manifestation of disease

effect was high, but it fell to prechallenge levels during the period when the drug was discontinued. After challenge, the titer rose steeply but only in one patient were there clinical signs of an adverse effect. This was patient 4 and it can be seen that this was the one patient with a prechallenge titer at a level found at the height of the reaction.

The question posed but not answered by these results is whether tissue damage would develop in the remaining patients if the drug was continued in the presence of a high antibody titer. On the evidence available, it is not possible to offer a plausible explanation for the mechanism based on an immunological hypothesis. Furthermore, it is unlikely that such an explanation will be forthcoming until there is a suitable animal model system developed which can be investigated.

V. Hemolytic Anemia

Immunologically induced hemolytic anemia can occur by at least three independent mechanisms typified by the drugs stibophen, penicillin, and methyldopa.

Table 4. Antibody activity in serum samples from patients with history of adverse reaction to practolol who were subsequently challenged with the drug

Case No.	Date of sampling	Type of sample [a]	Serum dilutions [b]		
			1/10	1/50	1/100
1	26 March 1975	A	77	64	46
	10 March 1976	B	26	15	10
	17 March 1976	C	74	70	63
2	24 Feb 1976	B	8.6	8.5	3.4
	3 March 1976	C	67	37	30
3	18 May 1975	A	46	30	25
	30 March 1976	B	10	8.6	6.3
	7 April 1976	C	43	35	21
4	20 April 1976	B	71	23	27
	23 April 1976	C	47	37	27
5	9 May 1975	A	60	41	36
	22 Feb 1976	B	13	7.6	6.4
	29 Feb 1976	C	71	26	32

[a] Treatment with practolol continuing or recently withdrawn; B, practolol withdrawn from date; A, prechallenge sample; C, postchallenge sample
[b] Figures are percentages of metabolite antigen precipitated by sera

1. Stibophen

Stibophen is not a cardiovascular drug, but the proposed mechanism by which stibophen induces anemia would also fit the data generated by Freedman et al. (1956) for quinidine anemia and be compatible with Shulman's "passive bystander" hypothesis for drug-induced thrombocytopenia (Shulman 1958). The essential feature of the mechanism is the formation of a drug-antibody complex which passively adheres to red cells. Complement is fixed by the complex and the cells are lysed as a result.

2. Penicillin

The major determinant of penicillin, formed via an amide linkage to proteins through an opened β-lactam ring readily induces IgM antibodies of penicilloyl specificity. This determinant can be formed by direct interaction with red cell membranes but rarely leads to hemolysis. Under certain circumstances, however, hemolysis is produced, but the antibody resonsible is usually an incomplete IgG (White et al. 1968). Specificity studies show that the binding of specific IgE antibody to penicillin-coated red cells is only partially inhibited by the penicilloyl conjugate, but it is completely inhibited by benzypenicilloyl propylamine (Levine and Redmond 1967). This latter observation suggests that the antibody specificity is directed against a benzylpenaldic group and involves functional groups contributed by the red cell membrane. Thus, the cardinal feature of the mechanism is a stable bond between the drug and cell membrane with complement fixation by antibody-antigen interaction as the final pathway leading to cell lysis.

3. Methyldopa

Methyldopa-induced hemolytic anemia is probably the most common form of hemolysis which implicates immunological mechanisms mediated by drugs. The anemia is strictly auto-allergic, as the drug does not act as an immunogen. CARSTAIRS et al. (1966) reported that patients treated with methyldopa developed a positive direct Coombs' test: 41 out of 202 patients investigated had a positive test with anti-IgG. In fact it is now accepted that about 15% of patients treated with methyldopa will at some stage become Coombs positive. Not all the positive patients, however, developed hemolytic anemia: of the 41 original patients in CARSTAIR's studies, 30 subsequently developed the condition. Specific experiments carried out by WORLLEDGE et al. (1966) showed that the antibody was not directed against a methyldopa component but reacted with the Rh group either anti-e or all cells except -D-D. The part played by the drug is to react primarily with the red cells and create or expose determinants on their surface which then stimulate auto-antibodies.

E. Conclusion

Cardiovascular pharmacology is a fruitful area of research for many pharmaceutical organizations and this is reflected in the number and variety of drugs available for medical use. It is to be expected, therefore, that the incidence of adverse effects to cardiovascular drugs should parallel this widespread usage. Until the advent of β-receptor blocking drugs, such adverse effects were of relatively minor clinical importance and the majority were not immunologically mediated. The identification, however, of the oculomucocutaneous syndrome, induced by practolol, focused attention on the complexity of drug action and on the inadequacy of systems for evaluating their safety to man. Clearly much more research is needed.

References

Abrams (1973) Quinidine fever: an unusual manifestation of quinidine allergy. Chest 64:120–122

Ackroyd JF (1949) The pathogenesis of thrombocytopenic purpura due to hypersensitivity to sedomoid (allyl-isopropyl-acetyl-carbamide). Clin Sci 7:231–247

Alarcon-Segoria D, Wakins KG, Worthington JW (1967) Clinical and experimental studies on the hydralazine syndrome and its relationship to systemic lupus erythematosus. Medicine (Baltimore) 46:1–33

Allan D, Cade D (1975) Delayed fibrinous peritonitis after practolol treatment. Br Med J 4:40

Allison AC, Denman AM, Barnes RD (1971) Co-operating and controlling functions of thymus-derived lymphocytes in relation to autoimmunity. Lancet 2:135–136

Almeyda J, Levantine A (1973) Cutaneous reactions to cardiovascular drugs. Brit J Derm 88:313–315

Amos HE (1978) Immunological aspects of practolol toxicity. Int J Immunopharmacol 1:9–16

Amos HE, Brigden WD (1976) Immunological changes and practolol. Lancet 2:1298

Amos HE, Brigden WD, McKerron RA (1975) Untoward effects associated with practolol: demonstration of antibody binding to epithetral tissue. Br Med J 1:598–600

Amos HE, Lake BG, Atkinson HAC (1977) Allergic drug reactions: an in vitro model using a mixed function oxidase complex to demonstrate antibodies with specificity for a practolol metabolite. Clin Allergy 7:423–428

Amos HE, Lake BG, Artis J (1978) Possible role of antibody specific for a practolol metabolite in the pathogenesis of oculomucocutaneous syndrome. Br Med J 1:402–404

Assem ESK, Banks RA (1973) Practolol induced drug eruption. Proc R Soc Med 66:179–181

Bareis RJ (1974) Procainamide induced lupus erythematosus. SD J Med 27:19–20

Barzel US (1967) Quinidine sulfate induced hypoplastic anaemia and agranulocytosis. JAMA 201:325–327

Baxter-Smith DC, Monypenny IJ, Darricott NJ (1978) Sclerosing peritonitis in patient on timolol (letter). Lancet 2:149

Behan PO, Behan WMH, Zacharias FJ, Nicholls JT (1976) Immunological abnormalities in patients who had the oculomucocutaneous syndrome associated with practolol therapy. Lancet 2:984–987

Belz GC, Brech WJ, Kleeberg UR, Rudolsky G, Belz G (1973) Characterization and specificity of proscillaridin antibodies. Naunyn Schmiedebergs Arch Pharmacol 279:105–114

Berger H (1952) Thrombopenic purpura following use of digitoxin. JAMA 148:282–283

Blau SP (1973) Anti DNA antibodies: specificity. Ann Intern Med 78:308–310

Blomgren SE (1973) Drug induced lupus erythematosus. Semin Hematol 10:345–354

Blomgren SE, Vaughan JH (1968) The immunogenicity of photooxidized DNA and of the photoproduct of DNA and procainamide hydrochloride. Arthritis Rheum 2:470–478

Blomgren SE, Vaughan JH (1970) Antinuclear antibody specificity in procainamide-induced lupus. Arthritis Rheum 13:308

Blomgren SE, Condemi JJ, Vaughan HJ (1972) Procainamide induced lupus erythematosus. Clinical and laboratory observations. Am J Med 52:338–348

Bolton FG (1956) Thrombocytopenic purpura due to quinidine. Blood 2:547–564

Brauner GJ, Greene MH (1972) Digitalis allergy: digoxin-induced vasculitis. Cutis 10:441–445

Brodie BB, Leif PA, Poet R (1948) Fate of procainamide in man following its intravenous administration and methods for estimation of procaine and diethylemmoethanol. J Pharmacol Exp Ther 94:359–366

Brodie BB, Baer JE, Craig LC (1951) Metabolic products of the cinchona alkaloids in human urine. J Biol Chem 188:567–581

Brown P, Baddley H, Read AE, Davies JD, McGarry J (1974) Sclerosing peritonitis – an unusual reaction to a beta-adrenergic blocking drug (practolol). Lancet 2:1477–1481

Brown PJE, Lesna M, Hamlyn AN, Record CO (1978) Primary biliary cirrhosis after long term practolol administration. Br Med J 1:1491

Butler VP Jr (1978) The immunological assay of drugs. Pharmacol Rev 29:103–184

Butler VP Jr, Chen JP (1967) Digoxin – specific antibodies. Proc Nat Acad Sci USA 57:71–78

Carstairs KC, Breckenridge A, Dollery CY, Worlledge SM (1966) Incidence of a positive direct Coombs' test in patients on alpha methyldopa. Lancet 2:133–135

Case DE, Lindup WE, Lowery C, Orton TC, Reeves PR, Whittaker SE (1978) Metabolism studies with practolol. Br J Pharmac 63:352P

Chase MW (1946) Inhibition of experimental drug allergy by prior feeding of 14 sensitizing agents. Proc Soc Exp Biol Med 61:257–260

Church R (1973) Methyldopa causing a seborrhoeic dermatitis like eruption. Br J Dermatol [Suppl] 9:10

Cochran REI, Thomason J, McQueen A, Beevers GD (1976) Skin reactions associated with propranolol. Arch Dermatol 112:1173–1174

Cohen R, Brodsky M (1940) Allergy to digitalis. J Allergy 12:69–71

Conn HL, Luchi RJ (1961) Ionic influences on quinidinealbumin interaction. J Pharmacol Exp Ther 133:76–83

Conston AS (1974) Hypersensitivity myocarditis: a fatal reaction. J Med Soc NJ 71:61

Coombs RRA, Gell GPH (1953) Classification of allergic reactions responsible for clinical hypersensitivity and disease. In: Gell PG, Coombs RRA (eds) Clinical aspects of immunology. Blackwell Scientific, Oxford, pp 575–596

Corbett AC (1972) Methyldopa in general practice. Update. J Postgrad Gen Pract 5:159–166

Cronin AE (1965) The immunology of allergic drug reactions. PhD thesis, University of Cambridge, Cambridge

Cubey RB, Taylor SH (1975) Ocular reaction to propranolol and resolution on continued treatment with a different beta-blocking drug. Br Med J 4:327–328

Dammin GJ, Nova JR, Rearden JB (1955) Hydralazine reaction: case with L.E. cells ante mortem and post mortem and pulmonary renal splenic and muscular lesions of disseminated lupus erythematosus. J Lab Clin Med 46:806–809

Davies DM, Beedie MA, Rawlings MD (1975) Antinuclear antibodies during procainamide treatment. Br Med J 3:682–683

Dick DM, Wright P, Chapman CM, Zacharias SJ, Nicholls JT (1978) Adverse reactions to practolol: some observations on the syndrome associated with practolol therapy. Lancet 2:984–987

Dolan DL (1968) Angiitis following procainamide therapy. Mo Med 65:365–366

Downie CC (1974) Adverse reactions associated with practolol, Eraldin and Eramid. ICI report to doctors and pharmacists, UK. ICI, Pharmaceuticals Division, Alderley Park, Macclesfield, Cheshire

Dunstan HR, Taylor RD, Corcovan AC, Page IH (1954) Rheumatic and febrile syndrome during prolonged hydralazine treatment. JAMA 154:23–29

Ekenvall L, Forsbeck M (1978) Contact eczema produced by beta-adrenergic blocking agent (alprenolol). Contact Dermatitis 4:190–194

Erwteman TM, Broat MCP, Van Aken WG (1977) Intestial pulmonary fibrosis: a new side effect of practolol. Br Med J 2:297–298

Fakhro AM, Ritchie RF, Lown B (1967) Lupus like syndrome induced by procainamide. Am J Cardiol 20:367–373

Farr RS (1958) A quantitative immunochemical measure of the primary interaction between I BSA and antibody. J Infect Dis 103–239

Felix RH, Ive FA, Dahl MGE (1974) Cutaneous and ocular reactions to practolol. Br Med J 4:321–324

Fernstrom AIB (1965) Occupational quinidine contact dermatitis, a concept apparently not yet described. Acta Derm Vernereol (Stockh) 45:129–134

Frais MA, Bailey TJ (1979) Ocular reactions to timolol maleate. Postgrad Med J 55:884–886

Freedman AL, Barr PS, Brody EA (1956) Haemolytic anaemia due to qunidine observations on its mechanism. Am J Med 20:806–815

Friedman H, Heine WI (1963) Demonstration of anti-hydralazine antibody in hydralazine induced lupus erythematosus. Experientia 19:10–11

Grettre J, Johansson B (1958) Digitalis allergy: review of the literature and report of a case. Cardiologia 32:374

Gillies JD (1974) A complication of alpha methyldopa therapy. Anesth Intensive Care 2:179

Hadden JW, Hadeen EM, Middleton E Jr (1970) Lymphocyte blast transoformation: detection of adrenergic receptors in human peripheral lymphocytes. J Cell Immunol 1:583–595

Hahn BJ, Sharp GC, Irvin WS et al. (1972) Immune responses to hydralazine and nuclear antigens in hydralazine induced lupus erythematosis. Ann Intern Med 76:365–374

Halley W, Goodman TDS (1975) Practolol and sclerosing peritonitis (letter). Br Med J 2:337

Henningsen NC, Cederberg A, Hanson A, Johansson BW (1975) Effect of long term treatment with procaine amide. Acta Med Scand 148:475–482

Hensen A (1974) Agranulocytosis door procainamide (Pronestyl). Ned T Geneeskd 118:624–625

Hickson B, Davidson RJ, Walker W (1972) Agranulocytosis caused by procainamide. Scott Med J 17:165–168

Hill TJ (1958) Immunoreactions involving platelets in theoretical analysis of the model. J Exp Med 107:665–690

Hope RR, Bates LA (1972) The frequency of procainamide induced systemic lupus erythematosus. Med J Aust 2:298–301

Inzoli MR, Almici C (1973) Anemia, emolitica, autoimmune in corso di terapia con alfame-tildopea. Haematologica (Pavia) 58:169–171

Jensen AH, Mikkelsen HI, Wadskov S, Sondergaard J (1976) Cutaneous reactions to pro-pranolol (Inderal). Acta Med Scand 199:363–367

Kessey EC, Pierce S, Berk MC, Bayer WL (1973) Alpha-methyldopa induced hemolytic anaemia involving auto antibody with U specificity (Abstract). Transfusion 13:360

Klinger W (1974) Arzneimittelnebenwirkungen, 2nd edn. VEB Gustav Fischer, Jena

Koffler D, Agnello V, Carr RI (1971) Anti DNA antibodies and renal lesions of patients with systemic lupus erythematosus. Transplant Proc 1:933–938

Konttinnen YP, Tuominen L (1971) Reversible procainamide induced agranulocytosis twice in one patient (letter). Lancet 2:925

Kosowsky BD, Taylor J, Lown B, Ritchie RF (1973) Long term use of procainamide fol-lowing acute myocardial infarction. Circulation 47:365–366

Ladd P (1962) Procainamide induced lupus erythematosus. N Engl J Med 267:1357–1358

Lesne M (1972) Des are radioimmunoloigique de la gitaloxine et de la gitoxine. Arch Int Pharmacol Ther 199:206–208

Lesne M, Dolphen R (1976) Development of an original radioimmunoassay for gitoxin de-rivatives. J Pharmacol (Paris) 7:619–626

Levine BB, Redmond AP (1967) Immune mechanisms of penicillin-induced Coombs' positivity in man. J Clin Invest 46:1085

Mayer RL, Eisman PC, Jaconia D (1955) Experimental sensitisation of guinea pigs to 1-hy-drazineophthalazine with a discussion on the use of guinea pigs for the forecast of clini-cal sensitisations. J Invest Dermatol 24:281–291

McNab-Jones RF, Hammond VT, Wright D, Ballantyne JC (1977) Practolol and deafness. J Laryngol Otol 91:963

Medenica R, Hatman K, Hatman V, Girrard J-P, Junet R (1972) Digitoxin induced throm-bocytopoenia. Int Arch Allergy 43:1–8

Mehrotra TN, Gupta AK (1971) Hemolytic aneamia associated with alphamethyldopa (Aldomet). Indian J Med Sci 25:550–552

Miescher PA, Paronetto F (1969) In: Miescher PA, Mitter HJ (eds) Textbook of immuno-pathology, vol 2. Grune Stratton, New York, pp 191–200

Miescher P, Ritter O (1953) Purpura thrombopenique par allergie a la digitoxine. Int Arch Allergy 4:253–257

Mosko MM, Taylor RG (1954) Digitalis allergy with demonstrable antibody. J Allergy 25:477–479

Moss RA, Castro O (1973) Platelet transfusion for quinidine-induced thrombocytopoenia. N Engl J Med 288:522–553

Mullick FG, McAllister HA (1977) Myocarditis associated with methyldopa therapy. JAMA 234:1699–1701

Nicholls JT (1978) The practolol syndrome: a retrospective analysis. In: Post-marketing sur-veillance of adverse reactions to new medicines. Medico-Pharmaceutical Forum, No 7, The Royal Society of Medicine, London

Notice from the Swedish Adverse Drug Reaction Committee, Uppsala. Nr. 26, May 1977

Orkim M (1967) Animal models (spontaneous) for human disease: experiments of nature. Arch Dermatol 95:524–526

Orton TC, Lowery C (1977) Irreversible protein binding of (C^{14}) practolol metabolite(s) to hampster liver microsomes. Br J Pharmacol 60:319–320

Osborne DR (1977) Propranolol and Peyronie's disease (letter). Lancet 2:1111

Paz MA, Seifter S (1972) Immunological studies of collagens modified by reaction with hy-dralazine. Am J Med Sci 263:281–290

Perry HM (1973) Late toxicity to hydralazine resembling systemic lupus erythematosus in rheumatoid arthritis. Am J Med 54:58–72

Perry HMJ, Schroder HA (1954) Syndrome simulating collagen disease caused by hy-dralazine (Apresoline). JAMA 6:670–673

Perry HMJ, Tame M, Carmody S (1970) Relationship of acetyl transferase activity to antinuclear antibodies and toxic symptoms in hypertensive patients treated with hy-dralazine. J Lab Clin Med 76:114–125

Pugh S, Pelton B, Raftery EB, Denman AM (1976) Abnormal lymphocyte function is secondary to drug induced autoimmunity. Ann Rheum Dis 35:344–348

Raftery EB, Denman AM (1973) Systemic lupus erythematosus syndrome induced by practolol. Br Med J 2:452–455

Reeves PR, Case DE, Jepson HT et al. (1978) Practolol metabolism in metabolism in human subjects. J Pharmacol Exp Ther 205(2):489–498

Reinhardt DJ, Waldron JM (1954) Lupus erythematosus-like syndrome complicating hydralazine (Apresoline) therapy. JAMA 155:1491–1492

Riddiough MA (1977) Preventing, detecting and managing adverse reactions of antihypertensive agents in the ambulant patient with essential hypertension. Am J Hosp Pharm 45(5):465–477

Robinson BF (1978) Drugs acting on the cardiovascular system. In: Dukes MNG (ed) Meyer's sice effects of drugs, vol 8. Excerpta Medica, Amsterdam London New York

Rodman JS, Deutsch DJ, Gutman SI (1976) Methyldopa hepatitis. Am J Med 60:941–948

Rosenberg B, Kayden HJ, Lief PA, Mark LC, Steele JM, Brodie BB (1949) Studies on diethylaminoethanol, physiological dispositions and actions on cardiac arrhythmias. J Pharmacol Exp Ter 95:18–27

Rosin JM (1967) Vasculitis following procainamide therapy. Am J Med 42:625–626

Rowell NJ (1968) Lupus erythematosus, scleroderma, dermatomyositis polyerteritis: the "collagen" or "connective-tissue" disease. In: Rook A, Wilkinson DS, Ebling FJG (eds) Textbook of dermatology. Blackwell Scientific, Oxford

Russell AS, Ziff M (1968) Natural antibodies to procainamide. Clin Exp Immunol 3:901–909

Seedat YK, Vawda EZ (1972) Direct Coombs' test and methyldopa. Lancet 1:97–98

Shackman NH, Swiller AI, Morrison M (1954) Syndrome simulating acute disseminated lupus erythematosus. JAMA 155:1492–1494

Shafter N, Halpern A (1958) The quinidine problem. Angiology 9:34–36

Sherman NA, Smith RS, Middleton E Jr (1973) Effect of adrenergic compounds aminophylline and hydrocortisone on in vitro immunoglobulin synthesis by normal peripheral blood lymphocytes. J Allergy Clin Immunol 52:13–22

Shulman NR (1958) Immunoreactions involving platelets. 1. A steric and kinetic model for formation of a complex from a human antibody, quinidine as a hapten and platelets and for fixation of complement by the complex. J Exp Med 107:691–695

Shulman NR (1963) Mechanism of blood cell damage by adsorption of antigen antibody complexes. In: Graber P, Miescher P (eds) Immunopathology. Third International Symposium. Schwabe, Stuttgart, p 338

Siegel M, Lee SL, Peresc NS (1967) The epidemiology of drug induced systemic lupus erythematosus. Arthritis Rheum 10:407–413

Skubitz KM, Smith TW (1975) Determination of antibody-hapten association kinetics. A simplified experimental approach. J Immunol 114:1369–1374

Smith TW (1972) Ouabain-specific antibodies. Immunochemical properties and reversal of Na,K activated adenosine triphosphatase inhibition. J Clin Invest 51:1583–1593

Smith TW, Harber E (1973) Classical value of the radioimmunoassay of the digitalis glycosides. Pharmacol Rev 25:219–228

Smith TW, Butler VP Jr, Haber E (1970) Characterisation of antibodies of high affinity and specificity for the digitalis glycoside digoxin. Biochemistra 9:331–337

Sourkes TL (1954) Inhibition of dihychoryphenylalanine decarborylase by derivatives of phenylalanine. Arch Biochem Biophys 51:444–456

Stoll RG, Christensen MS, Sakmar E, Blair D, Wagner JG (1973) Determination of bioavailability of digitoxin using the radioimmunoassay procedure. J Pharm Sci 62:1615–1620

Sturnick MI (1942) Quinidine sulfate induced hypoplastic anaemia and agranulocytosis. JAMA 201:325–327

Swerbrick ET, Grey IR (1973) Procainamide induced systemic lupus erythematosus. Rheumatol Rehabil 12:94–96

Tangsrud SE, Golf S (1977) Cheilostomatitis associated with propranolol treatment. Br Med J 2:1385–1386

Taylor DR, Potashnick R (1951) Quinidine-induced exfoliative dermatitis. JAMA 145:641–642

Timpanaro S (1973) Allergia alla digitale. Minerva Med 64:1334–1337

Toghill PJ, Smith PG, Benton P, Brown RC, Matthews HL (1974) Methyldopa liver damage. Br Med J 3:545–548

Victor G (1970) Clinical trial with alpha-methyldopa (Aldomet) in hypertension. Indian Heart J 22:104–108

Wang RIH, Schuller G (1969) Agranulocytosis following procainamide administration. Am Heart J 78:282–284

White JM, Brown DL, Hepner GW, Worlledge SM (1968) Penicillin induced haemolytic anaemia. Br Med J 3:26–29

Worlledge SM, Carstairs KC, Dacie JV (1966) Auto-immune haemolytic anaemia associated with alpha-methyldopa therapy. Lancet 2:135–139

Wright P (1975) Untoward affects associated with practolol administration: oculomucocutaneous syndrome. Br Med J 1:595–598

Young RC, Nachaman RL, Horowitz HI (1966) Thrombocytopoenia due to digitoxin. Am J Med 41:605–614

CHAPTER 16

Penicillins and Cephalosporins

A. L. DE WECK

A. Introduction

The penicillins and cephalosporins, collectively known as beta-lactam antibiotics, are among the most widely used and valuable antibiotics currently available. Benzylpenicillin (penicillin G) and phenoxymethylpenicillin (penicillin V) are derived from *Penicillium* molds by fermentation, while half-synthetic penicillins are derived by chemical modification of the penicillin nucleus, 6-aminopenicillanic acid (6-APA), itself obtained either by splitting the side chain from benzylpenicillin through an enzymatic process or via a chemical deacylation reaction.

The penicillins are of the general structure shown in Fig. 1; the substitution at R is designated as the side chain, while the nucleus of the penicillin molecule is constituted by the juxtaposition of a beta-lactam and a thiazolidine ring. Hundreds of penicillins have been created in the laboratory by adjoining some side chain to the penicillin nucleus. The side chains of those penicillins which have been and in part still are the most used in clinical therapy are shown in Fig. 2. The cephalosporins are chemically closely related to the penicillins in that they also possess various side chain substitutes at R1 and a beta-lactam nucleus. In this case, however, the thiazolidine ring is replaced by a six-member dihydrothiazine ring and there is a greater variation in the substitution at C3 (R2) than is the case for penicillins. The side chains present in the main cephalosporins in clinical use are represented in Fig. 3.

B. Penicillins

I. The Formation of Antigenic Determinants from Penicillins

The fact that penicillins may induce an immune response and the formation of penicillin-specific antibodies in man and in experimental animals was recognized soon after their introduction into therapy in 1943 (LYONS 1943; ROSTENBERG and WELCH 1945; WILENSKY 1946; CHU and CUTTING 1946; BROWN 1948). In the early

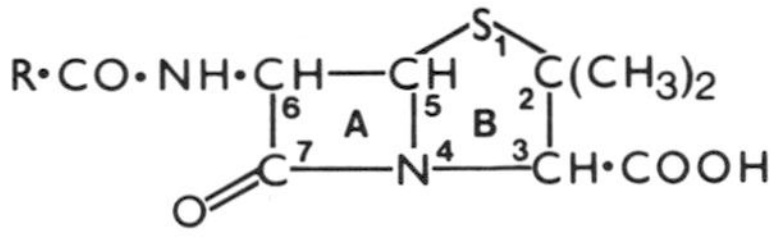

Fig. 1. Penicillin formula

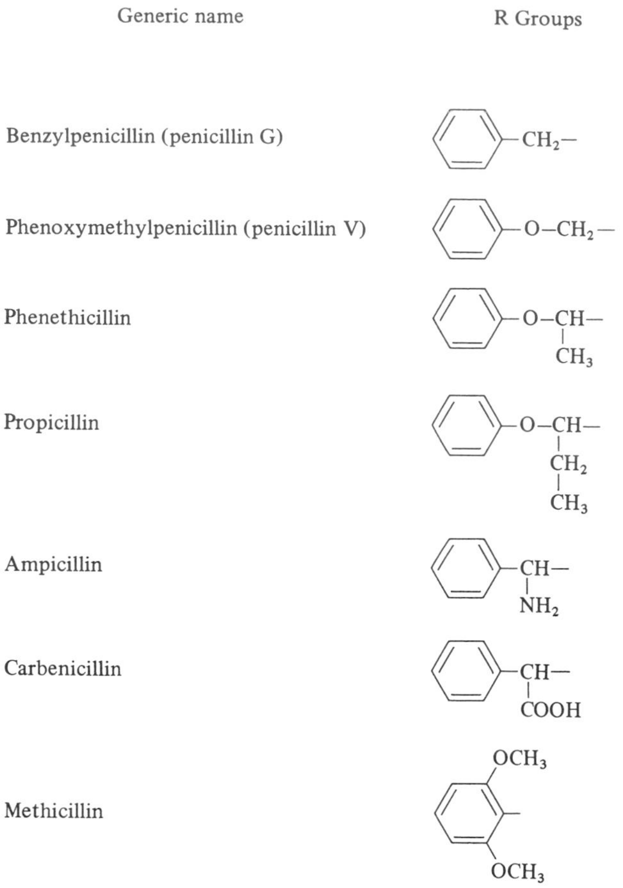

Generic name	R Groups

Benzylpenicillin (penicillin G)

$\langle\text{phenyl}\rangle-CH_2-$

Phenoxymethylpenicillin (penicillin V)

$\langle\text{phenyl}\rangle-O-CH_2-$

Phenethicillin

$\langle\text{phenyl}\rangle-O-CH-$
$\qquad\qquad\quad CH_3$

Propicillin

$\langle\text{phenyl}\rangle-O-CH-$
$\qquad\qquad\quad CH_2$
$\qquad\qquad\quad CH_3$

Ampicillin

$\langle\text{phenyl}\rangle-CH-$
$\qquad\qquad\ NH_2$

Carbenicillin

$\langle\text{phenyl}\rangle-CH-$
$\qquad\qquad\ COOH$

Methicillin

OCH_3
$\langle\text{phenyl}\rangle-$
OCH_3

Fig. 2. Side chains of various penicillins

1960s, several groups (DE WECK and EISEN 1960; LEVINE 1960a; PARKER et al. 1962a, b) studied the immunochemistry of penicillins and identified the major pathways by which penicillins may form complete immunogenic antigens and develop several structurally different antigenic determinants. However, the topic is still of interest for pharmacologists, immunochemists, and clinicians today since not all the problems pertaining to the immunogenicity of penicillins have been solved.

Penicillin allergy, because it may induce practically all possible clinical forms of allergic reactions to a drug and because the immunochemical and immunological mechanisms have been better worked out than with any other drug or group of drugs, has become a classical model of drug allergy. The study of penicillin allergy has contributed significantly to the understanding of the immune response to low-molecular-weight compounds in man and experimental animals, and also has model value in basic immunology (for reviews see LEVINE 1976; DE WECK 1978a, 1979; PARKER 1980).

Generic name	R Groups

Oxacillin

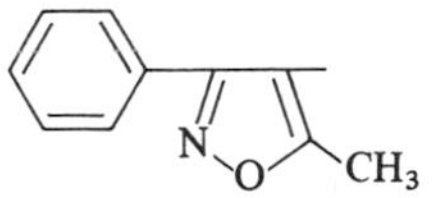

Cloxacillin

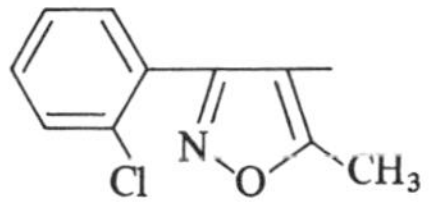

Dicloxacillin

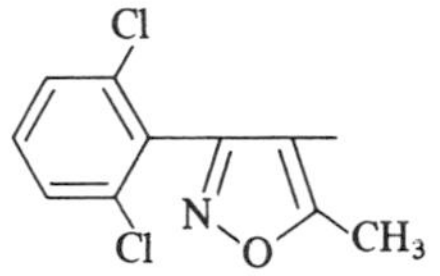

Flucloxacillin

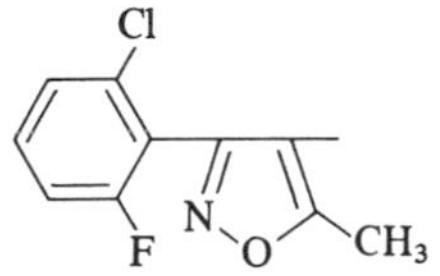

Sulfobenzylpenicillin (sulbenicillin)

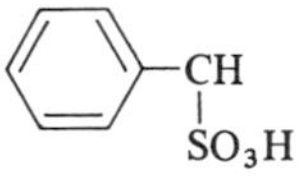

Allylthiomethylpenicillin (penicillin O) $CH_2=CH-CH_2-S-CH_2$

Fig. 2.

1. The Penicilloyl Determinant

Many antigenic determinants may derive from penicillins but most is known about the benzylpenicilloyl (BPO) determinant, a bifunctional structure comprising a nonpolar phenylacetamide and a polar thiazolidine carboxylic acid end (LEVINE 1963) (Fig. 4).

LEVINE and OVARY (1961) demonstrated that the major population of antibodies raised in rabbits by immunization with benzylpenicillin was directed against an antigenic determinant structure formed of the whole BPO group and the six-carbon lysine chain by which the BPO group is attached to a protein carrier. In other studies (PARKER et al. 1962a; DE WECK 1962a), it was shown similarly that in experimental animals and in man, most of the antibodies induced by penicillins are directed against this determinant, which was accordingly designated the major antigenic determinant of penicillin allergy.

However, this is still considered as open to question by some authors (DEWDNEY 1977) who point out that the BPO determinant may appear predominant only because the testing methods mostly used for detection of penicillin hypersensitivity (skin and serological tests) appear to be most sensitive for this type of determinant.

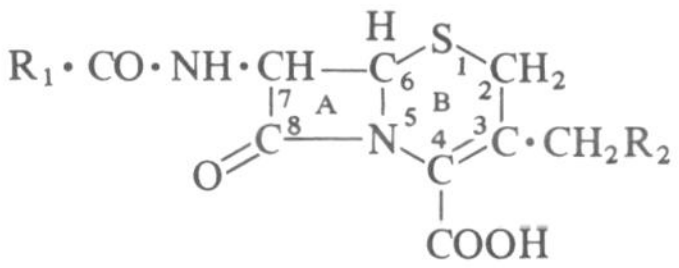

$$R_1 \cdot CO \cdot NH \cdot CH - \overset{H}{\underset{|7\ A}{C_6}} \overset{S}{\underset{|5\ B}{}} \overset{1}{\underset{}{CH_2}}$$

$$O = \overset{8}{C} - \overset{5}{N} \overset{4}{\underset{C}{}} \overset{3}{C} \cdot CH_2 R_2$$

$$COOH$$

Generic name	R_1	R_2
Cephalothin	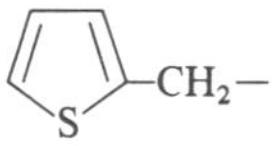 (thiophene)–CH₂–	–O–C(=O)–CH₃
Cephaloglycin	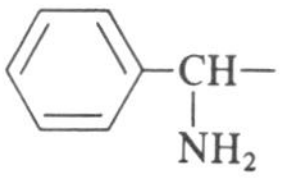 (phenyl)–CH(NH₂)–	–O–C(=O)–CH₃
Cephalexin	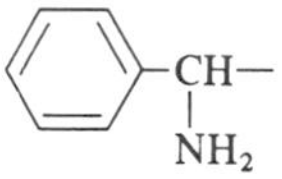 (phenyl)–CH(NH₂)–	–H
Cephapirin	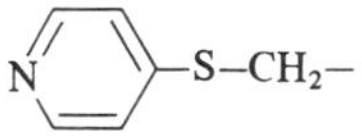 (pyridine-N)–S–CH₂–	–O–C(=O)–CH₃
Cephaloridine	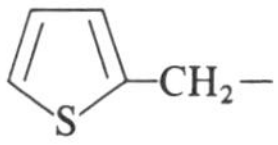 (thiophene)–CH₂–	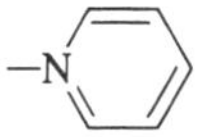 –N⁺(pyridinium)
Cefazolin	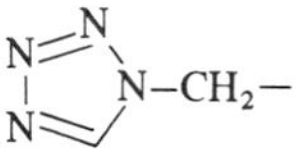 (tetrazole)N–CH₂–	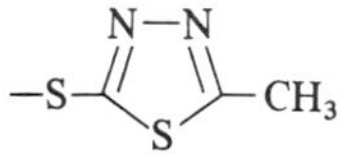 –S–(thiadiazole)–CH₃
Cephaloram	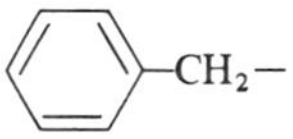 (phenyl)–CH₂–	O–C(=O)–CH₃
Cephacetrile	N≡C–	O–C(=O)–CH₃

Fig. 3. Structures of major cephalosporins. General structure (*top*): *A*, β-lactam ring; *B*, di-hydrothiazine ring; R_1, side chain

A more systematic use of reagents carrying some of the other structural determinants described below might reveals a different picture. Recent work by ASSEM and VICKERS (1975) and by EDWARDS et al. (1982) has indicated the possibility that the penicillamine and penicillanyl determinants may be more frequently involved than hitherto realized. The relatively high frequency of positive skin tests to a penicillamine-polylysine conjugate in patients allergic to penicillins (SCHNEIDER et al. 1973) points to the same conclusion.

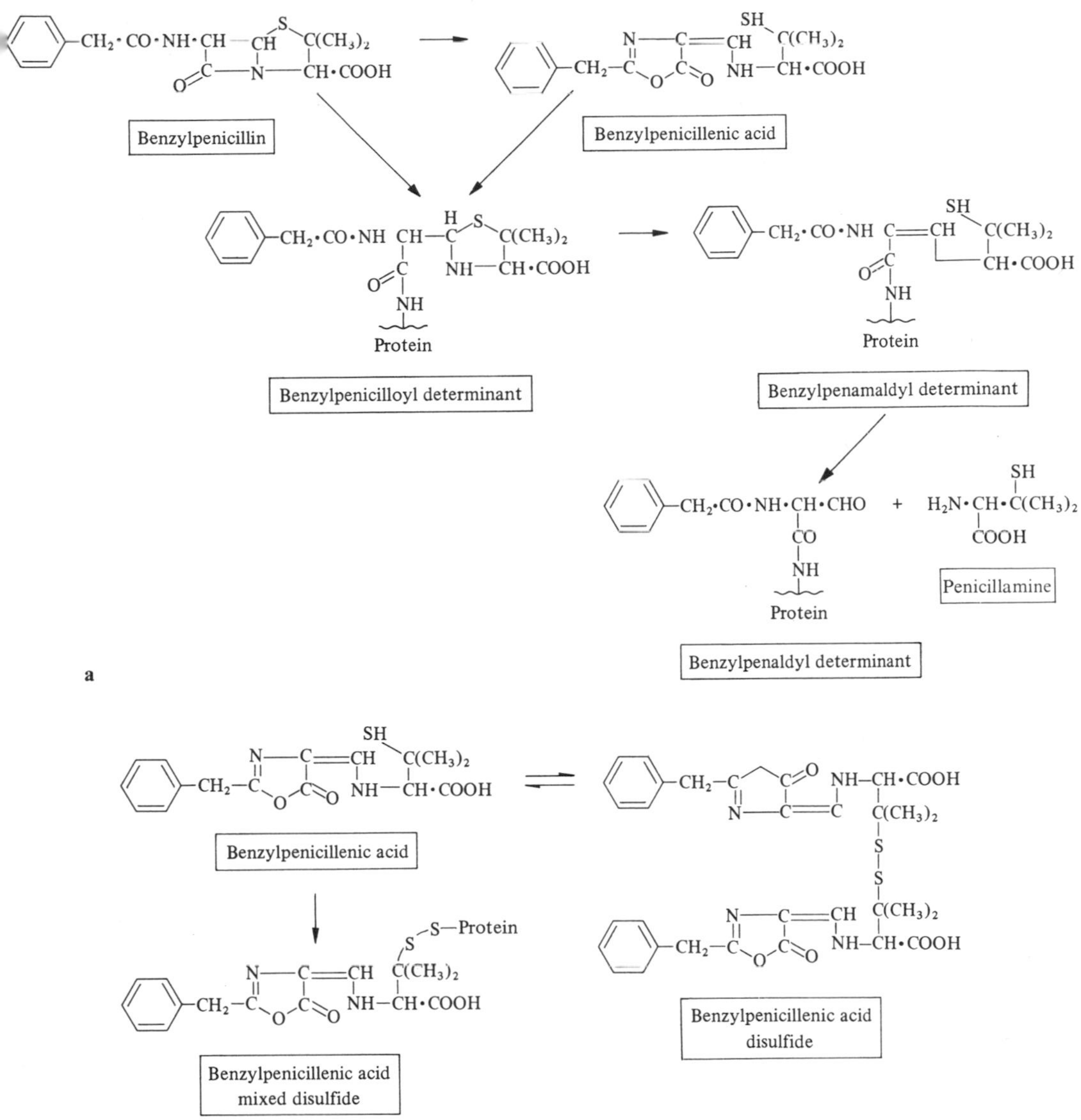

a

b   Benzylpenicillenate determinant

Fig. 4 a, b. Formation of penicilloyl, penicillenate, and other minor determinants from penicillin. **a** Routes to the formation of the penicilloyl determinant and its further degradation products. **b** Possible pathways to the formation of the benzylpenicillenate antigenic determinant

The chemical routes to the formation of the penicilloyl determinant can be multiple and have been the subject of some controversies. It has been claimed that the main source of immunogenic penicilloyl antigens leading to penicillin sensitization in therapy is the presence of penicilloylated protein impurities in most penicillin preparations. This topic is discussed extensively in Sect. I.9.

There are a number of pathways by which a BPO group may become covalently attached to a protein or polysaccharide carrier (MOLINARI et al. 1973). Direct acylation of protein amino groups by the beta-lactam carbonyl group at high pH was demonstrated by LEVINE (1962) and later also at neutral pH by BATCHELOR et al. (1965) and SCHNEIDER and DE WECK (1965, 1966 b, c). The site of such reactions on protein carriers has only recently been more directly assessed. CORRAN and WALEY (1975) have shown that [^{14}C]benzylpenicillin reacts with the N-terminal alpha amino group of insulin and at the epsilon amino group of lysine residues. With lysozyme, the site of reaction was the epsilon amino group of lysine 116. The nearby presence of negatively charged arginine residue 112 might be responsible for preferential reaction at the lysine 116 position. BPO derivatives can also be formed from benzylpenicillenic acid (DE WECK and EISEN 1960), either by direct reaction (LEVINE 1961) or via a postulated reactive intermediate thiazolidinyl oxazolone (DUDLEY et al. 1971). Penicillenic acid could also be implicated in the formation of BPO determinants by other pathways, such as benzylpenicillenic acid disulfide (SCHNEIDER and DE WECK 1970). However, the route via penicillenic acid is certainly not an obligatory one. 6-APA (BATCHELOR et al. 1965) and 2,4-dinitrophenyl 6-APA (SCHNEIDER and DE WECK 1965), which cannot rearrange to penicillenic acid, have been shown to penicilloylate proteins at neutral pH and 37 °C in vitro and to react with aminocaproic acid at the same rate as benzylpenicillin.

The controversy over the main route toward formation of the BPO determinant has not been solved by studies on stereospecificity. Several authors have found that anti-BPO antibodies are directed against a mixture of diastereoisomers (LEVINE 1960 b; LEVINE and OVARY 1961; CARON 1963; SCHNEIDER and DE WECK 1966 a, b), although some (THIEL et al. 1964) found in human sera a predominance of antibodies specific for the D-alpha-diastereoisomer, suggesting that the BPO group had been formed by the direct aminolytic route. As pointed out by SCHWARTZ (1969), specificity toward a mixture of diastereoisomers does not necessarily point out a route via penicillenic acid, since epimerization after conjugation by the direct route is also possible.

A problem still open is the rate of formation of BPO conjugates in vivo, either by direct aminolysis or by isomerization of penicillin to penicillenic acid and subsequent reaction with amino groups of proteins. These reactions are slow in aqueous solution at neutral pH and it has therefore been considered that some catalytic processes may explain the achievement of substantial penicilloylation under physiological conditions and possibly also some preferential reactions with protein carriers in vivo. Several groups have considered these questions (SCHWARTZ and WU 1966; SCHWARTZ 1968; SCHNEIDER and DE WECK 1968; BUNDGAARD 1971 a, 1972 a, b; TSUJI et al. 1975; YAMANA et al. 1975; MARTIN et al. 1976). Amines with a pKa of around 7, such as imidazole, appear to be more reactive with benzylpenicillin than amines with higher pKas, such as lysine (8.95–10.53) or glycine (9.2) (BUNDGAARD 1971, 1972 a, b). Imidazole catalyzes the formation of penicillenic acids from several penicillins, at neutral pH, through the formation of an unstable N-penicilloyl imidazole. Imidazole also catalyzes the penicilloylation of amino and hydroxyl groups by a penicillin that is incapable of forming penicillenic acid, for examle 6-ethoxycarbonyl aminopenicillanic acid (BUNDGAARD 1972 b). The mechanism proposed is that the unstable intermediate N-ethoxypenicilloyl imidazole would transfer the penicilloyl group to functional groups on proteins, thereby forming stable conjugates (BUNDGAARD 1976 a).

SCHNEIDER and DE WECK (1974) have suggested that some carrier proteins might be preferentially penicilloylated, for example due to a suitable arrangement of nucleophilic groups and histidine residues. It had been shown earlier (SCHNEIDER and DE WECK 1970) that penicillin reacts more rapidly with polyglycyl and poly-lysine side chains than with lysine alone. Some metals, such as copper (LEVINE 1960 b; CRESSMANN et al. 1966), have also been shown to catalyze penicillin hydrolysis and aminolysis in vitro and it is conceivable that such factors also play a role in vivo. The same man be true of some sugars (BUNDGAARD and LARSEN 1978; LARSEN and BUNDGAARD 1978 b). However, it will be difficult to obtain a definitive picture of the kinetics involved in the formation of penicilloyl groups on proteins and of the catalytic factors that influence rates of reactions as long as the nature of the carrier protein(s) to which penicillin binds in vivo is not known.

Only a few authors have attempted to identify penicilloylated protein conjugates formed in vivo after administration of penicillins in vivo. In the serum of patients treated with high doses of penicillin, LEVINE (1976) demonstrated the presence of penicilloylated proteins able to inhibit the agglutination of penicilloylated erythrocytes by anti-BPO antibodies. The most obvious candidate as carrier for BPO groups, under clinical conditions of penicillin administration, could be human serum albumin (HSA) (BUNDGAARD 1977 a). Indeed, penicillin therapy induces modifications in HSA (LAPRESLE and WAL 1979; WAL 1980). Accordingly, AHLSTEDT et al. (1981) have attempted to calculate the theoretical degree of substitution of HSA by BPO groups under clinical conditions and have tested experimentally the immunogenicity of BPO-HSA conjugates substituted to various degrees. The low-substituted BPO-HSA conjugates expected to be formed under in vivo conditions were found to be non- or only very poorly immunogenic in mice. From this, the authors conclude that BPO conjugates formed in vivo are unlikely to be the sensitizing molecules in penicillin allergy. They ascribe sensitization rather to highly substituted and in vitro preformed BPO-protein impurities (see Sect. I.9). In a guinea pig model, penicillin-autologous carrier protein conjugates have been shown to be immunogenic (GIRARD and CUEVAS 1975 b). The fact that the density of epitopes on the protein carrier influences the formation of antiepitope IgE has been confirmed, but the critical number of epitopes required appears to depend upon the nature of the carrier (NAKAGAWA et al. 1980).

This line of argument, however, does not take in account the recent findings that presentation of haptenic groups bound to cell membranes, in particular to membrane proteins on macrophages, are more likely to be the immunogenic signals than are soluble protein conjugates. We have shown (SPENGLER et al. 1974; DE WECK 1975) that BPO groups bind extensively to the membrane of lymphoid cells and that presentation of BPO groups on cell membranes is the decisive event for stimulating penicillin-sensitive lymphocytes.

It is only necessary to postulate rapid mechanisms of extensive substitution of some in vivo carriers by BPO groups in order to explain the prompt elicitation of anaphylactic reactions by penicillins in hypersensitive humans or animals. In this case, however, it appears more likely that the reactions may be elicited by penicillin polymers (see Sect. I.8).

2. The Penicillenate Determinant

Benzylpenicillenic acid forms readily in aqueous penicillin solutions around pH 5; it develops more slowly from penicillin solutions at neutral pH. With increasing hydrolysis of penicillin to penicilloic acid and corresponding lowering of pH, formation of penicillenic acid derivatives, with characteristic absorption at 322 nm, accelerates (DE WECK and EISEN 1960). Penicillenic acid is relatively unstable and the more stable penicillenic acid disulfide may instead be the moiety playing a role in allergic reactions to penicillins (SCHNEIDER and DE WECK 1966a; BUTLER et al. 1972). It was postulated that the formation of penicillenate determinants would occur via reaction with SH and S-S groups present on protein carriers, according to the scheme shown in Fig. 4. Recently, it has been shown that the formation of benzylpenicillenic acid from benzylpenicillin proceeds through an intermediate oxazolone-thiazolidine structure, which may be one route through which benzylpenicillenic acid reacts with proteins (DUDLEY et al. 1971).

Indeed, guinea pigs and rabbits immunized with penicillenate-protein conjugates developed antibodies specific for the oxazolone structure, as indicated by skin tests and hapten inhibition of precipitation in immunized animals (DE WECK and EISEN 1960). Hapten inhibition studies with S-(N-ethylsuccinimidyl)penicillenate in skin tests (PARKER et al. 1962a, b) and with S-(p-mercuribenzoate) benzylpenicillenate in hemagglutination studies (THIEL et al. 1964) have also demonstrated the presence of antibodies of penicillenate specificity in penicillin-sensitive humans. More recently, some studies have confirmed that IgE antibodies directed against the penicillenate antigenic determinant are indeed involved in penicillin allergy, although probably only to a minor extent (EDWARDS et al. 1982).

Benzylpenicillenic acid itself is a potent immunogen in animals and stimulates the formation of antibodies of penicilloyl specificity (BATCHELOR and DEWDNEY 1968; PORTOLES et al. 1975). It is also a potent contact sensitizer in guinea pigs (LEVINE 1960a) and elicits contact reactions in patients with penicillin-induced contact dermatitis (CARON 1963). The role of penicillenic acid in contact allergy to penicillin is probably favoured by the lower pH of the skin promoting its formation and the high concentration of sulfhydryl groups in skin proteins (SCHWARTZ 1969).

On the other hand, benzylpenicillenic acid is not able to trigger reactions due to penicilloyl antibodies, such as passive cutaneous anaphylaxis (PCA), in guinea pigs or in baboons (BATCHELOR and DEWDNEY 1968), suggesting that it does not conjugate efficiently and rapidly enough to form eliciting BPO antigens.

3. Penicilloic Acid

Benzylpenicilloic acid is the main hydrolysis product of benzylpenicillin and is able to elicit wheal and flare reactions when used in skin tests in some patients allergic to penicillins. It has therefore been considered as one of the "minor antigenic determinants" of penicillin allergy (SIEGEL and LEVINE 1964; VOSS et al. 1966) although the precise chemical nature of the determinant(s) derived from penicilloic acid has not been elucidated. The proportion of patients responding in skin test to penicilloic acid varies between 21% and 55% (Table 1).

Study of the chemical degradation pathways of penicilloic acid (LEVINE 1960b, c; SCHWARTZ 1969) (see Fig. 5) suggested that penicilloic acid interacts with

Table 1. Skin reactions to various determinants in penicillin allergy in patients with a history of penicillin allergy

	BPO		BPN		BPNCO		Penicillamine		Penicilloylamine		Penicillenate	
	N	%	N	%	N	%	N	%	N	%	N	%
GATTLEN and PETER (1976)	163/244 (66.8)		108/244 (44.2)		76/244 (31.1)		n.d.		n.d.		n.d.	
SCHNEIDER and DE WECK (1981)	idem		idem		idem		34/97 (35)[b]		15/233 (6)			
LEVINE and REDMOND (1969)	13/ 26 (50)		16/ 26 (61.5)		22/ 26 (84.6)		n.d.		19/ 26 (73.0)		n.d.	
JUHLIN et al. (1977)	14/ 35 (40)		11/ 35 (31.4)		10/ 35 (28.5)		1/35 (2)		6/35 (17.1)			
SULLIVAN et al. (1981)	358/469 (76.3)[a]		268/469 (57.1)		260/469 (55.4)		n.d.		n.d.		n.d.	
LEVINE and PRICE (1964)	11/ 15 (73.3)		4/ 15 (26.6)		n.d.		2/15 (13.3)[b]		n.d.		2/15 (13.3)	
ASSEM and VICKERS (1975)	8/ 22 (36.3)		4/ 22 (18.1)		n.d.		9/22 (40.9)[b]		n.d.		6/22 (27.2)	

BPO, benzylpenicilloyl; BPN, benzylpenicillin; BPNCO, benzylpenicilloic acid; PPL, penicillin-polylysine
[a] Among patients positive to BPN, PPL, or BPNCO
[b] Penicillamine-carrier conjugate used for test

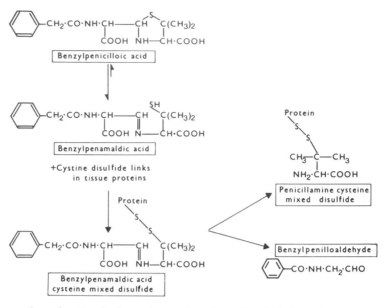

Fig. 5. Formation of antigenic determinants from benzylpenicilloic acid

cystine disulfide linkages in tissue proteins to form penicillamine conjugates through the intermediate D-penamaldic acid cysteine mixed disulfide (LEVINE 1960c; LEVINE and PRICE 1964; LEVINE and REDMOND 1969). Several degradation products of penicilloic acid possess functional groups capable of reaction with protein, such as penicillamine, penilloaldehyde, and penamaldic acid.

The specificity of reactions elicited by penicilloic acid has not yet been determined with certainty. Although such reactions certainly differ in their specificity from BPO-specific reactions, they are also inhibited quite efficiently by monovalent BPO haptens. This has been the experience for skin test reactions to penicilloic acid in man (DE WECK 1976) as well as for PCA reactions elicited by benzylpenicilloic acid in guinea pigs (DE WECK 1976; DE WECK et al. to be published).

It is still not understood how penicilloic acids could so rapidly produce in vivo the bi- or plurivalent antigens required for elicitation of anaphylactic reactions, unless the reaction rates of penicilloic acids with proteins in vivo are efficiently catalyzed (LEVINE and OVARY 1961; SCHNEIDER et al. 1973). Penicilloic acid may also act as inhibitor of reactions of BPO specificity. This has also been demonstrated in hemagglutination, precipitation, and guinea pig PCA (JOSEPHSON 1960; TORII and HORIUCHI 1961; DE WECK 1962a, b; LEVINE 1963; BATCHELOR and DEWDNEY 1968). In general, penicilloic acid is a worse inhibitor than BPO amides but markedly more efficient than benzylpenicillin.

The immunogenicity of penicilloic acids as such has not yet been definitely established. On the one hand, the fact that a selected number of penicillin-sensitive patients very strongly react to benzylpenicilloic acid, sometimes to the exclusion of other determinants (LEVINE and REDMOND 1969; GATTLEN and PETER 1976;

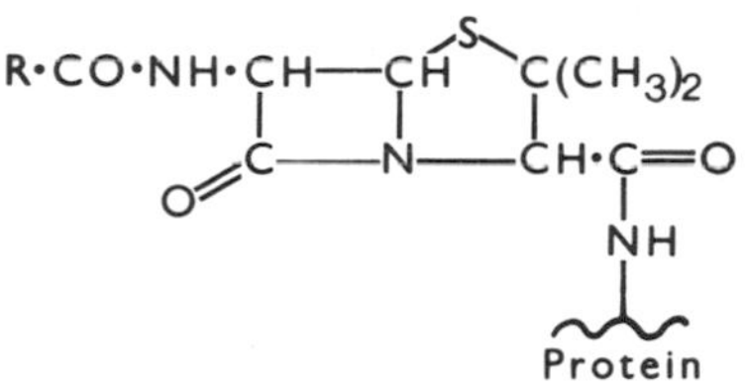

$$R \cdot CO \cdot NH \cdot CH - CH \overset{S}{\diagdown} C(CH_3)_2$$

$$O = C - N - CH \cdot C = O$$

$$NH$$

$$Protein$$

Fig. 6. The penicillanyl determinant

GOREVIC and LEVINE 1981), points to the immunogenicity and sensitizing capacity of this compound. On the other hand, several attempts to detect antibodies in rabbits immunized with benzylpenicilloic acid have been unsuccessful (JOSEPHSON 1960; DE WECK 1962 a, b).

However, in these studies, no serious attempts were made ot assess the antibodies specific for penamaldate and penicillamine determinants, which are precisely those which could be expected. Benzylpenicilloic acid, when applied to guinea pig skin, seems able through whatever immunochemical mechanism to induce contact hypersensitivity (LEVINE 1960 a).

4. The Penicillanyl Determinant

Reaction of penicilins through the C-3 carboxyl group with amino groups of proteins would lead to the formation of the penicillanyl group (Fig. 6), with an intact beta-lactam ring. This potential determinant, initially suggested by FEINBERG (1970), did not attract much attention, since it appears unlikely that such a reaction could occur under physiological conditions following the administration of penicillins. In early experimental studies, penicillanyl protein conjugates were prepared by linking the C-3 carboxyl group of benzylpenicillin to proteins via a mixed anhydride. Such conjugates raised antibodies in rabbits, which were assessed by PCA in guinea pigs and demonstrated to be of penicillanyl specificty, without cross-reaction with the penicilloyl determinant (FEINBERG 1970). Further studies by HYSLOP et al. (1974) using penicillanyl conjugates of benzylpenicillin and oxacyclin have confirmed that such conjugates may induce antibodies strongly specific for the whole penicillin molecule and different from the antibodies specific for the penicilloyl determinant. Any cross-reactions encountered have been on the basis of similarities in the side chain.

Accordingly, it has become possible to investigate in patients sensitive to penicillins whether part of the antibodies present may be of penicllanyl specificity. The recent introduction in clinical therapy of penicillins with ester groups at the C-3 position, such as pivampicillin may lead to expect action of an increased formation of such conjugates with the corresponding induction of penicillanyl-specific antibodies (DEWDNEY 1977). Upon immunization of guinea pigs by epicutaneous application of the C-3 esters of benzylpenicillin and ampicillin, the penicillanyl specificity has been shown to be the dominant specificity involved in contact hypersensitivity reactions (DEWDNEY 1977). The immunogenicity of diethylaminoethyl ester of benzylpenicillin (penethamate) for the development of clinical contact reactions had been noted by Hjörth (1967). On the other hand, pivampicillin appeared to be of low immunogenicity in rabbits and mice, from the point of view of antibodies of penicilloyl specificity (Iwata and Serizawa 1974). It remains to be seen, however, whether penicillins esterified at C-3 do not preferentially induce antibodies of penicillanyl specificity. Recently, Edwards et al. (1982) and Kraft et al. (1981) have reported that some patients do indeed possess antibodies of penicillanyl specificity demonstrated by a RAST-type immunoassay. On the other hand, no such antibodies were found in industrial workers sensitized to penicillin via professional contact.

5. The Penamaldate and Penaldate Determinants

The penamaldate and penaldate intermediates may theoretically arise either from penicilloic acids or from rearrangement of covalently bound penicilloyl groups (Fig. 5). It is not yet established whether the penamaldate group really functions as an antigenic determinant in penicillin allergy. In their study on hemagglutinating antibodies of penicillin-sensitive individuals, Thiel et al. (1964) found a serum for which the most effective inhibitor was penamaldate. It is also known that penicilloyl protein and polylysine conjugates used in skin testing may contain penamaldate groups (Levine an Ovary 1961; Parker et al. 1962 a, b) and therefore possibly detect hypersensitivity of penamaldate specificity aside from and in addition to the penicilloyl specificity. In experimental studies in guinea pigs using penamaldate and penaldate protein conjugates as immunogens, it was shown that such groups are sufficiently stable to function as antigenic determinants. However, no antibodies of penamaldate or penaldate specificities were detected with the appropriate reagents in animals immunized with BPO protein conjugates or with benzylpenicillin itself (O. Toffler, H. Bundgaard, and A. L. de Weck, unpublished results).

6. The D-Penicillamine Determinant

D-Penicillamine may arise directly from penicilloic acid or through formation of a penicillamine-cysteine mixed disulfide, following a penamaldate rearrangement (Levine 1960 c; Yemal et al. 1978). This reaction also occurs with functional derivatives of the alpha-carboxylic group of penicilloic acid (Schneider et al. 1973). The penicillamine determinant may therefore arise in vivo from any penicilloyl conjugate.

In how far skin test reactions elicited in humans by benzylpenicilloic acid or BPO-polylysine are due to antibodies of penicillamine or penamaldate specificities is not yet clear. It is noteworthy that BPO-polylysines prepared with BPO groups formylated at the thiazolidine nitrogen and which cannot undergo the penamaldate/penicillamine rearrangement are markedly less efficient in eliciting reactions (Schneider et al. 1973). This, however, may also be due to a lesser fit with anti-BPO antibodies. Skin tests with conjugates prepared with D-penicillamine linked to HSA (Levine and Price 1964) using potassium ferricyanate as oxidizing agent, or with reduced proteins to form mixed disulfides (Assem and Vickers 1975) have yielded surprisingly high proportions of positive reactions in penicillin-sensitive

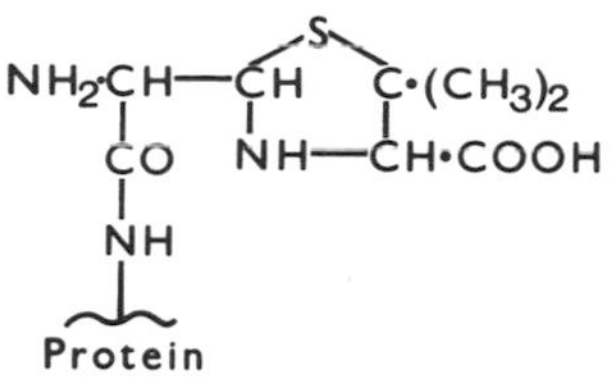

$$NH_2CH-CH \overset{S}{\underset{}{}} C\cdot(CH_3)_2$$

(structure showing the penicoyl determinant with CO, NH—CH·COOH, NH, and Protein linkage)

Fig. 7. The penicoyl determinant

patients, 13% and 41% respectively. We have obtained similar results using a stable D-penicillamine-polylysine conjugate in which the penicillamine moiety is linked to polylysine by a stable thio ether linkage (SCHNEIDER et al. 1973); the yield of positive skin reactions was as high as 35% (Table 1). Attempts to confirm the presence of antibodies of D-penicillamine specificity in penicillin-sensitive patients have been scarce and generally unsuccessful (C. H. SCHNEIDER et al., unpublished results). Recently, however, such antibodies have been detected by EDWARDS et al. (1982) in a RAST-type assay.

Experimentally, the capacity of the D-penicillamine group to act as antigenic determinant has been shown by ASSEM and VICKERS (1974), immunizing rabbits with penicillamine-disulfide protein conjugates. The immunogenicity of D-penicillamine itself, as used for treatment of Wilson's disease or in rheumatic disorders, has been demonstrated (AMOS 1973). It has also been shown that penicillamine can behave as experimental contact sensitizer in guinea pigs (LEVINE 1960a; CARON 1963).

7. The Penicoyl Derivatives

6-Aminopenicilloic acid reacts with proteins to produce the penicoyl determinant (BATCHELOR et al. 1962, 1965; MOSS 1964) (Fig. 7). However, since it has been shown that most samples of 6-APA also contain benzylpenicilloylated proteins derived from the fermentation procedure used to prepare benzylpenicillin (BATCHELOR et al. 1967; STEWART 1967), early studies claiming immunogenicity of 6-APA (DE WECK and EISEN 1960; CHISHOLM et al. 1961; STEWART 1962; WAGELIE et al. 1963) should be reevaluated. Purified 6-APA is apparently only weakly immunogenic in rabbits (DEWDNEY et al. 1971).

Since 6-APA forms the backbone and starting material for the semisynthetic penicillins but is not itself directly used as therapeutic agent, its role in penicillin allergy is probably not important, since 6-APA may be considered at most as a potential impurity in semisynthetic penicillins, although it may appear in urine after oral administration of penicillins (ENGLISH et al. 1960).

8. Penicillin Polymers

The immunological behavior of penicillin preparations may be markedly influenced by the presence of dimers, oligomers, and polymers in the penicillin preparations. It should be distinguished whether we are dealing with polymerization by internal rearrangement of the molecule or interaction between penicillin molecules carrying a free amino group, such as ampicillin.

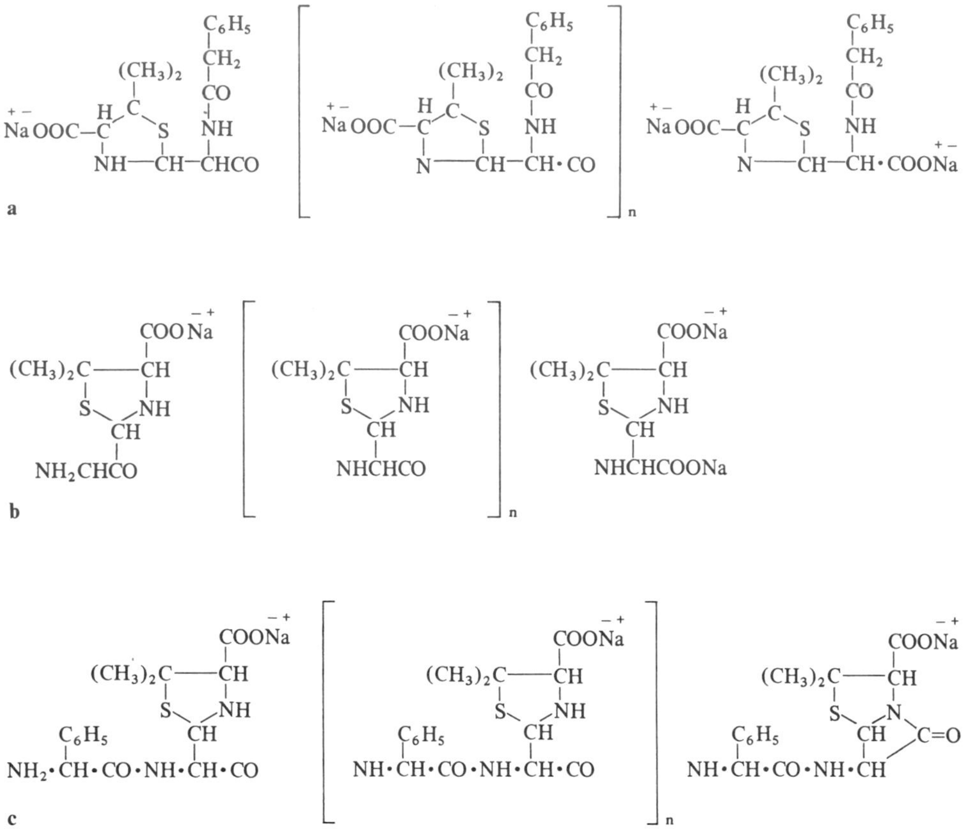

Fig. 8 a–c. Structure of benzylpenicillin, 6-APA, and ampicillin polymers. a Benzylpenicillin (SMITH and MARSHALL 1971); b 6-APA (SMITH and MARSHALL 1971); c Ampicillin (SMITH 1970; SMITH and MARSHALL 1971)

Polymerization of benzylpenicillin has been described by several authors (BATCHELOR et al. 1967; STEWART 1967 a; DE WECK et al. 1968; BUTCHER and STEWART 1969, 1970; DEWDNEY et al. 1971; SMITH et al. 1971; SMITH and MARSHALL 1971; BUNGAARD and LARSEN 1977). Polymerization probably involves hydrolysis of the beta-lactam ring to form penicilloic acid, followed by acylation of the exposed thiazolidine nitrogen by another intact penicillin molecule or a benzylpenicillenic acid derivative (STEWART 1973; SMITH and MARSHALL 1971; SCHNEIDER and DE WECK, 1970) (Fig. 8) Such polymers have been isolated by Sephadex gel chromatography (SMITH et al. 1971) or by high-pressure liquid chromatography (BUNDGAARD 1977 b). Polymers have been isolated also from other semisynthetic penicillins such as hetacillin and carbenicillin (SMITH et al. 1971), methicillin and pheneticillin (BUTCHER and STEWART 1970).

It is not clear wether polymers of that type are also separate immunogens induced by penicilloyl-protein conjugates. By incubating benzylpenicillin polymer with proteins, SHALTIEL et al. (1971) raised antibodies in rabbits which appeared to be more specific for polymer than for penicilloyl determinants.

Of great practical importance is the possible behavoir of benzylpenicillin oligomers and polymers as plurivalent antigens eliciting immediate-type anaphylactic reactions in already sensitized individuals. If such polymers, usually present in penicillin solutions (BATCHELOR et al. 1967; BUTCHER and STEWART 1969, DE WECK et al. 1968; DEWDNEY et al. 1971; MURANAKA et al. 1974) are indeed able to elicit such reactions, there is no need to explain them by rapid conjugation in vivo.

Furthermore, some measures may be visualized to prevent polymer formation in benzylpenicillin solutions. Indeed, it was shown that polymers and even small oligomers are capable of eliciting skin reactions in penicillin-sensitive individuals (BATCHELOR et al. 1967; DE WECK et al. 1968) and are also capable of eliciting PCA reactions in guinea pigs passively sensitized with IgE-like anti-BPO antibodies (MURANAKA et al. 1974, 1978; DE WECK 1976; DE WECK et al. to be published; KO-IZUMI et al. 1980; IGARASHI et al. 1978).

Beta-lactam structures possessing free amino groups, such as 6-APA or ampicillin, on the other hand are much more prone to form oligomers and polymers. (GRANT et al. 1962; BATCHELOR et al. 1967; STEWART 1967; BUTCHER and STEWART 1970; BUTCHER et al. 1971; SMITH and MARSHALL 1971; BUNDGAARD 1974). In this case, polymerization involves reaction between the free amino group of one molecule with the beta-lactam carbonyl of another molecule. The pKa of the amino group of ampicillin is about 7 and therefore available for reaction at neutral pH. BUNGAARD (1967 a, b) has studied the rate of polymerization of ampicillin at 35° and found it to be dependent upon concentration but relatively independent of pH in the range 7–9.5. Various oligomers of ampicillin could be separated by high-pressure liquid chromatography (BUNDGAARD 1978; LARSEN and BUNDGAARD 1977, 1978a). Other penicillins containing a free amino group, such as amoxicillin, epicillin, and cyclacillin, also polymerize in this way.

It is not yet entirely clear if these polymers, in particular the ampicillin polymers, are by themselves immunogenic and if they induce sensitization of a different specificity than the penicilloyl group. SHALTIEL et al. (1971) have immunized rabbits with protein conjugates of ampicillin polymers and studied the specificity of the antibodies obtained. Although extensive cross-reactivity seems to exist beween penicilloyl-specific and polymer-specific antibodies, the data were interpreted as definitely showing some polymer specificity. Immunization with polymers in rabbits and guinea pigs usually does not lead to sensitization (DEWDNEY 1977) although some success was reported in baboons by MUNRO et al. (1976) and in mice by AHLSTEDT et al. (1977). Interestingly, immunization of baboons led to strong delayed hypersensitivity reactions. One may therefore wonder whether the frequent morbilliform exanthemas observed after ampicillin therapy, which for some authors at least represent possible manifestation of delayed hypersensitivity (DE WECK 1973, 1978a, 1979) are not indeed the sign of delayed hypersensitivity to ampicillin polymers. Such interpretation may be supported by the finding that some patients having shown an exanthema to ampicillin will demonstrate lymphocyte stimulation in vitro to ampicillin polymers (DE WECK 1972). Some authors have reported that ampicillin polymers stimulate human lymphocytes in culture, but without relationship to a history of penicillin or ampicillin allergy (WEBSTER and THOMPSON 1974).

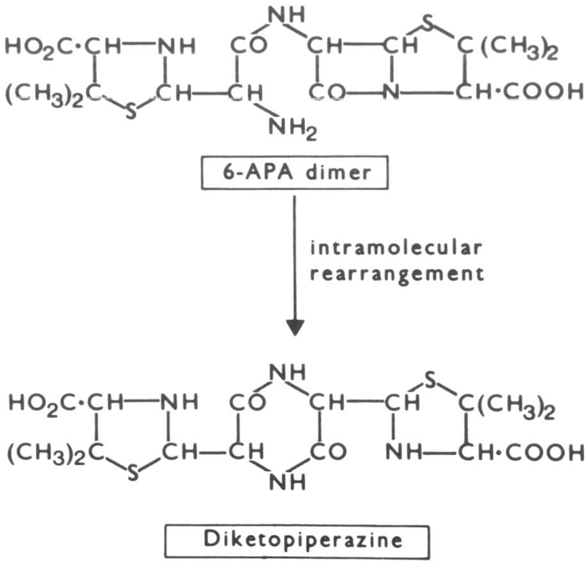

Fig. 9. Intramolecular rearrangement of 6-APA (DEWDNEY 1977)

It has repeatedly been demonstrated that ampicillin polymers are good elicitors of PCA reactions in guinea pigs passively sensitized with antipenicilloyl antibodies (DEWDNEY et al. 1971; AHLSTEDT et al. 1976; DEWDNEY 1977). In this case, the antibody specificities revealed appear to be essentially penicilloyl, since the reactions elicited by the polymers are fully inhibited by benzyl-epsilon-aminocaproic acid (DEWDNEY 1977).

In the case of 6-APA and possibly also of some other penicillin derivatives, the interaction of two molecules leading first to dimers and then to further polymerization may be interfered with by a competing intramolecular rearrangement, leading to the formation of a diketopiperazine (DEWDNEY 1977) (Fig. 9).

9. Protein Impurities

Aside from polymeric substances arising from intermolecular and intramolecular rearrangements of penicillins, proteins and polypeptides which derive from the fermentation manufacturing process have been described (BATCHELOR et al. 1967; KNUDSEN et al. 1967; STEWART 1967, 1968, 1973; BATCHELOR and DEWDNEY 1968; BUTCHER and STEWART 1969, 1970; DE WECK et al. 1968; FEINBERG 1968 a; WESTON 1968; DEWDNEY et al. 1971). During the course of fermentation of *Penicillium* moulds, protein residues become heavily penicilloylated. If carried through the extraction and purification processes, they may appear in the final product and become responsible for immunological reactions, as sensitizing antigens as well as triggering molecules for allergic reactions by sensitized individuals.

In benzylpenicillin, the presence of immunogenic protein impurities has been demonstrated by several authors (BATCHELOR et al. 1967; FEINBERG 1968a; WESTON 1968; STEWART 1967; BUTCHER and STEWART 1970; LIAKOPOULOU and

VILIM 1976; VILIM et al. 1976), although sometimes only in bulk penicillin (PREUD'HOMME and LUNEL 1969) and not in the final product. Several groups have observed the presence of high-molecular-weight impurities, probably polymers, but could not confirm their protein nature (DÜRSCH 1968; PREUD'HOMME and LUNEL 1969; MÜLLER et al. 1970; WEIDEMÜLLER and ZIEGLER 1970; WALSH et al. 1971). It is obviously technically difficult to separate polymers from protein impurities, and simple separation techniques such as chromatography on Sephadex gels cause problems because of interaction between the gels and the penicillin derivatives (SCHNEIDER and DE WECK 1967; MURANAKA et al. 1974; HYSLOP and MILLIGAN 1974).

Alkaline hydrolysis of penicillins abolishes its immunogenicity, which was considered to be an argument against protein impurities playing a role in penicillin immunogenicity (DE WECK et al. 1968) until it was observed that penicilloylated proteins are highly susceptible to alkaline hydrolysis (SCHNEIDER and DE WECK 1970) However hydrolysis of benzylpenicillin at neutral pH, catalyzed by 3,6-bis(dimethylaminoethyl)catechol, also reduces considerably the immunogenicity of benzylpenicillin in rabbits, although this conclusion has recently been disputed by AHLSTEDT et al. (1980b). In the experiments performed by this group in mice (AHLSTEDT et al. 1979), the immunogenicity of benzylpenicillin appeared directly related to the content in macromolecular impurities as determined by a radioimmunoassay. However, in guinea pigs immunized with benzylpenicillin lots of various degree of purity, the production of IgE-like antibodies of BPO specificity did not appear to depend on the impurities present (A. L. DE WECK et al., unpublished work). Clinically, it was claimed that purification of benzylpenicillin by Sephadex gel chromatography would considerably reduce the incidence of skin test reactions in penicillin-sensitive individuals (KNUDSEN et al. 1967; ROBINSON 1968; PEDERSEN-BJERGAARD 1969), which may have been due as well to the elimination of polymers. Reactivity of benzylpenicillin purified by such means was maintained in other hands (DE WECK et al. 1968). All these experiments may lead to the conclusion tht the overall immunogenicity of a sample of benzylpenicillin is the result both of the intrinsic immunogenicity of the penicillin molecule and, usually to a smaller degree, of any protein contamination. The controversy about the role of protein impurities in the immunological effects of penicillins has recently been revived by Ahlstedt's group (AHLSTEDT and KRISTOFFERSON 1979; AHLSTEDT et al. 1979). Using a concentrating step for such impurities and a sensitive radioimmunoassay, they claimed that most commercially available penicillins still contain detectable amounts of protein impurities and that elimination of such impurities woult probably reduce the incidence of allergic reactions to penicillins considerably.

There are, however, still a number of clinical arguments suggesting that patients who become sensitized to penicillins are sensitized by the penicillin molecules themselves as administered, and not by preformed impurities. If this were the case, it would be expected that sensitized patients would react not only to BPO antigens but also to the protein determinants present in high-molecular-weight residues of penicillin fermentation. Thorough experiments by MÜLLER et al. (1970) have shown that patients sensitive to penicillin usually do not respond to such mold determinants in skin and serological tests. Furthermore, recent experiments by NEFTEL et al. (1982) have shown that the mode of administration of benzylpenicillin markedly influences its immunogenicity. In 15 patients given high doses of benzylpenicillin where the solution was allowed to stand for up to 12 h before injection, all patients developed anti-BPO IgG antibodies and lymphocyte sensitivity, whereas in a similar group given high doses of benzylpenicillin dissolved immediately before injection, no apparent sensitization was observed. This strongly suggests that the derivatives occuring in solution (benzylpenicilloic and benzylpenicillenic acids) are the agents essentially responsible for sensitization, not some preformed protein impurities. In 6-APA, proteins and peptides have been isolated by dialysis, Sephadex chromatography, and ultrafiltration (BATCHELOR et al. 1967; BUTCHER and STEWART 1969, 1970; FEINBERG 1968a; WESTON 1968; OTTENS et al. 1971). The isolated proteins are potent immunogens for experimental aminals (BATCHELOR et al. 1967; BATCHELOR and DEWDNEY 1968; DEWDNEY et al. 1971). The antibodies raised appear to be specific to a large extent for the BPO group (DEWDNEY 1977), as demonstrated by inhibition with BPO-amines, but also for the protein carrier *Escherichia coli* amidase used to split the benzyl side chain from benzylpenicillin in the manufacture of 6-APA. The presence of that protein impurity probably plays a major role in the immunogenicity reported for that compound, since treatment with pronase appears to abolish it (SHALTIEL et al. 1970). Purified 6-APA appears to have almost no immunological activity (DEWDNEY 1977; DEWDNEY et al. 1971).

While 6-APA itself plays no clinical role, the amount of protein impurities surviving the manufacturing processes of semisynthetic penicillins, for which 6-APA is the base material, still represents a problem of major clinical significance. Every effort should be made to prepare semisynthetic penicillins substantially free of immunogenic protein contaminants. The determination of the amounts of protein impurities surviving the current manufacturing processes is fraught with difficulties, as pointed out by several authors (OTTENS et al. 1971; WALSH et al. 1971).

Even the method recently described by KRISTOFFERSON et al. (1977a), using first a separating and concentrating step (column chromatography) for high-molecular-weight contaminants and then a radioimmuncassay for BPO determinants, is liable to a number of misinterpretations, due to the possible presence of penicilloic acid and/or Sephadex-penicilloyl derivatives arising during the analytical procedure itself.

Penicilloylated protein impurities have been described in ampicillin (KNUDSEN et al. 1970) and the immunogenicity of ampicillin in experimental animals may be reduced by purification and/or by treatment with pronase (SHALTIEL et al. 1970). It is, however, not abolished by such measures. In our hands, ampicillin prepared by chemical cleavage of the side chain and substantially devoid of detectable protein impurities was still capable of sensitizing rabbits and of eliciting a rash in patients who had previously reacted with a similar rash to usual ampicillin (A. L. DE WECK et al., unpublished work).

In conclusion, there is no doubt that the presence of protein impurities in penicillins, which may be expected to be heavily penicilloylated and thereby very efficient in raising anti-BPO antibodies (AHLSTEDT et al. 1980a, b; NAKAGAWA et al. 1980; KRISTOFFERSON et al. 1977b) should be avoided as much as technically feasible. Whether the extremely low levels detected in current commercially available penicillins by the method of Ahlstedt (KRISTOFFERSON et al. 1980) are still playing the major role in sensitization to penicillins and in the elicitation of allergic reactions in already sensitized patients, as postulated by AHLSTEDT et al. (1979 a, 1980 a), is in our opinion still debatable.

Not to be forgotten as possibly involved are macromolecular constituents of some penicillin preparations, such as carboxymethylcellulose, which may function as multivalent carriers (SCHNEIDER et al. 1971) and have been implicated in reactions to penicillins in cattle.

10. Role of the Side Chain in Penicillin Allergy

The influence of the acyl side chain on the immunological reactivity of penicillins is felt in immunogenicity, in antibody specificity, in degradation pathways and polymerization reactions, and in overall allergenicity.

In early experiments, the side chain appeared to influence the immunogenicity of penicillins in rabbits (DE WECK 1962 b; WATSON 1962), since there were marked differences in the antibody titers obtained with different penicillins administered under similar conditions. These differences did not appear to be correlated with the rates of degradation to the respective penicillenic acids. Slightly different results were obtained later by FEINBERG (1968 b) with purified penicillins. A more complete study by WELLENSIEK (1969) did not reveal marked differences among ten penicillins with various side chains tested, among which several do not form penicillenic acids. All these studies suffered from the drawback that penicillins, in order to be detectably immunogenic for rabbits, had to be administered in complete Freund's adjuvant. Accordingly, the formation of exogenous immunogenic penicilloyl protein conjugates during the immunization procedure itself is likely and might influence the results. More relevant may be a comparison of the immunogenicity of various penicillins under conditions where the formation of IgE-like antibodies, particularly relevant for penicillin allergy, would be expected. In experiments performed in mice, AHLSTEDT and KRISTOFFERSON (1979) and AHLSTEDT et al. (1979) observed differences among various penicillins. They also pointed out the possible influence on the results of the aluminum hydroxide employed as adjuvant and the polyclonal activation due to the *Bordetella pertussis* used. When given penicillins instead of preformed penicilloyl-protein conjugates, the BPO- specific IgE response of mice is usually quite low. Genetic influences are probably also quite marked, and it may therefore be asked whether mice are a good choice of animal for such experiments.

In guinea pigs, a marked degree of immediate hypersensitivity to penicillins may be achieved by repeated immunization, together with aluminum hydroxide. Under such circumstances, marked differences could be observed in the sensitizing capacity of various penicillins (DE WECK et al. to be published) (Table 2). The side chain influences the rate of degradation to the respective penicillenic acids markedly at neutral pH and even more at pH 4.0 (DE WECK 1962 b; DUDLEY et al. 1974). On the other hand, the nature of the acyl side chain seems to have much less influence on the rates of hydrolysis (DE WECK 1962 a) or aminolysis (SCHWARTZ and WU 1966). In the presence of some catalysts, such as imidazole, the susceptibility of the beta-lactam ring to nucleophilic attack increases markedly (BUNDGAARD 1971 a, 1972 a, b). The influence of the side chain on the reactivity towards imidazole ap-

Table 2. Immunogenicity of penicillins and cephalosporins in guinea pigs[a]

	Compound itself	Conjugate with bovine gamma globulin
Benzylpenicillin	17/20 (1:200)	158/159 (>1:10,000)
Ampicillin	3/ 8 (1:20)	20/ 20 (>1:10,000)
Cephaloridin	0/ 8	not done
Cefuroxime	0/ 8	10/ 10 (>1:10,000)
Cefotaxime	0/ 8	10/ 10 (>1:10,000)

[a] Immunization with bovine gamma globulin conjugate (1 µg) or the compound itself (1 mg) in 1 mg Al (OH)$_3$ subcutaneously, repeated 5 times at 3-week intervals. Detection of antibodies by PCA using the corresponding conjugate with polylysine for intravenous challenge. The average titer of antibodies detectable by PCA is given in parentheses following the number of guinea pigs yielding positive sera in respect to the number of guinea pigs immunized

pears to be very small. The influence of the acyl side chain on the number of penicilloyl groups bound to proteins has also been studied (BATCHELOR et al. 1967). Whereas most semisynthetic penicillins in current use appear to react with amines and proteins at approximately the same rate as benzylpenicillin, ampicillin represents an exception and appears to form many fewer penicilloyl derivatives in vitro. This has been interpreted as due to the possible competition with the polymerization reaction described above (DEWDNEY 1977). It must be emphasized, however, that ampicillin also appears to be less prone to raise IgE antibodies in vivo (Table 2).

The role of the acyl side chain in the specificity of antibodies induced by penicillins in experimental animals and man has been extensively studied. Various experimental procedures, such as guinea pig PCA (TORII and HORIUCHI 1961; HORIUCHI and SHIBATA 1965), hemagglutination (DE WECK 1962b; WELLENSIEK 1969), Schulz-Dale (LOCHER et al. 1969), inactivation of hapten-modified bacteriophage (WHEELER 1971; SCHNEIDER and DE WECK 1967) and quantitative precipitation (HORIUCHI and SHIBATA 1965) have been used. Inhibition of the interaction between benzylpenicilloyl antigens and anti-BPO antibody by penicilloic acids or penicilloyl-amines carrying various side chains (DE WECK 1962a, b; HORIUCHI and SHIBATA 1965; WELLENSIEK 1969; NISHIDA et al. 1972; MUNRO et al. 1976) has been used to evaluate the role of the side chain in the combining sites of antipenicillin antibodies. In general, it may be stated that extensive cross-reactivity exists between benzylpenicillin and phenoxymethylpenicillin (penicillin V), while substitution in the alpha position of the acyl side chain with methyl or ethyl groups (pheneticillin and propicillin) or with a amino group (ampicillin) results in a very significant reduction of binding. Substitution with a carboxyl group (as in carbenicillin) has little effect. The presence of an isoxazole group, as in oxacillin, cloxacillin, dicloxacillin, and flucloxacillin results in a further diminution of cross-reactivity, but the pattern of halogen substitution in this series seems to play only a small role.

It has also been evaluated in how far antibodies directed exclusively against the side chain may be present in animals immunized with penicillin or in hypersensitive patients. The nature of the conjugates used for immunization possibly play a part in this respect. HORIUCHI and SHIBATA (1965) have reported that penicilloyl protein conjugates prepared at pH 8.5 seem to contain almost exclusively BPO groups and induce very predominantly the formation of anti-BPO antibodies. Conjugates prepared under weakly acidic conditions (pH 6.8), on the other hand, seem also to carry other groups and stimulate antibodies which appear to be more specific for the acyl side chain. By using immunosorbent techniques, ATSUMI ct al. (1967) were able to evaluate the proportion of antibodies specific only for the side chain in antisera of rabbits immunized with BPO-bovine gamma globulin (BGG). Fifty percent of the antibodies could be eluted by phenylacetic acid and phenylacetyl glycine. In guinea pigs immunized with BPO-BGG, PCA reactions can be elicited in high titer with polylysine which carries phenacetyl groups (O. TOFFLER et al., unpublished work).

Wheal and flare reactions in penicillin-sensitized patients can also be elicited by protein conjugates of phenylacetyl glycine and dimethoxybenzyl glycine (SHIBATA et al. 1968). Using conjugates prepared with various penicillins, the side chain specificity of human skin-sensitizing antibodies has also been evaluated by several groups (PARKER and THIEL 1963; VAN DELLEN et al. 1971). Exclusive or predominant side chain specificity of hypersensitivity may be responsible for the tolerance toward other penicillins of some patients who have been sensitized by penicillin G (LUTON 1964).

II. Clinical Aspects

Allergy to beta-lactam antibiotics may take almost any of the clinical forms of reaction due to drugs. Penicillin allergy has thus become a kind of universal model of drug allergy, by which mechanisms, symptoms, diagnostic tests, prevention and therapy may be studied. It would be redundant to describe here in detail the symptoms and immunological mechanisms of the various clinical reactions to penicillins, since these have been discussed at length in Chap. 3. We will therefore restrict ourselves to some remarks on the clinical reactions particularly due to penicillins.

1. Anaphylactic and Anaphylactoid Reactions

Anaphylactic reactions following administration of penicillins were described within a few years of introduction of the drug (WALDBOTT 1949; KERN and WIMBERLEY 1953; BATSON 1960; BROWN et al. 1964). In the 1950s and 1960s, anaphylactic reactions to benzylpenicillin became a major problem, since the incidence of penicillin hypersensitivity in the general population was increasing and there were no efficient means to detect individuals threatened by such a reaction. It was estimated that about 500–800 deaths from anaphylactic shock were occurring each year in the USA alone (VALENTINE 1969; BOSTON 1973), while the number or life-threatening reactions was about 10 times greater (IDSOE et al. 1968). Penicillins are responsible for about 75% of all anaphylactic deaths (DELAGE and IVEY 1972); an anaphylactic reaction occurs in about 1 in 10000 courses of treatment (IDSOE et al.

Table 3. Incidence of various forms of clinical reactions to penicillins. (Allergy Clinic, University of Bern, Switzerland)

Reaction	1962–1966 (311 cases)	1971–1976 (231 cases)
Generalized urticaria	102 (33%)	90 (39%)
Anaphylactic shock ⎫	59 (19%)	8 (3%)
Anaphylactoid symptoms ⎭		8 (3%)
Serum-like disease	43 (14%)	6 (3%)
Angioneurotic edema	28 (9%)	31 (14%)
Generalized exanthema	25 (8%)	65 (28%)
Contact eczema	15 (5%)	3 (1%)
Blood dyscrasias	13 (4%)	4 (2%)
Pruritus	6 (2%)	7 (3%)
Local reactions	7 (2%)	4 (2%)
Asthma	4 (1%)	0
Others	9 (3%)	6 (3%)

1968). Anaphylactic reactions are mainly due to intramuscular injections of benzyl-penicillin, although oral absorption was also often reported to cause such reactions (EISENSTADER and HUSSAR 1954; MAGANZINI 1957; LEVINE et al. 1960; KRAPIN 1962; BANKL and JELLINGER 1968; GEYMAN 1971; SPARK 1971). In some exquisitely sensitive individuals, merely entering a room where penicillin is being handled (KAPLAN and WEINSTEIN 1967; REISMAN and ARBESMAN 1968; MINIKIN and LYNCH 1969; ROSENBLUM 1968) or ingesting food (BIERLEIN 1956; COLEMAN and SWINE-FORD 1956) or beverages containing trace amounts of penicillin is sufficient to trigger a shock (WICHER and REISMAN 1980). Anaphylactic shock has also been reported frequently following intradermal skin testing with penicillins (DOGLIOTTI 1975) and on one occasion following a single scratch test (DOGLIOTTI 1968) or epicutaneous test (PIETZCKER and KUNER 1975).

The anaphylactoid reaction, sometimes called the Hoigné syndrome (HOIGNÉ and SHOCH 1956; HOIGNÉ 1961 a, b; HOIGNÉ and KREBS 1964), can often be distinguished clinically from true anaphylactic shock (BELL 1954; BELL et al. 1954), since it does not entail a drop in blood pressure and sets neurological and sensory disturbances in the foreground. Such reactions were observed most frequently after the injection of penicillin-procaine or microcrystalline preparations (BREDT 1965; BATCHELOR et al. 1951; UTLEY et al. 1966; GALPIN et al. 1974; MENKE and PEPPLINKHUIZER 1974; DRY et al. 1976; KRAUS and GREEN 1976; MIREL and GARNICK 1978) and are considered to be due to the toxic effects of procaine (GREEN et al. 1974) and/or to microemboli following accidental intravasal injection. Procaine, however, has also been claimed to cause true allergic reactions (FERNSTRÖM 1962). The frequency of such reactions seems to have diminished considerably with the increasing use of semisynthetic penicillins.

During the 1970s, the problem of anaphylactic shocks to beta-lactam antibiotics seems, from general experience, to have lost some of its importance, although it is certainly still present. In our own patient material, the number of anaphylactic reactions reported has certainly decreased (Table 3). However penicillin V is still, after sulfamide combinations, the most frequently prescribed antibiotic in general practice in Switzerland (SIMMEN et al. 1981)

2. Urticaria

Urticarial reactions, occurring a few minutes to a few hours after administration of penicillins, and sometimes persisting and recurring for months, even after interruption of therapy, are still the most frequent manifestations of penicillin hypersensitivity. There are no clinical or morphological characteristics which establish the diagnosis of penicillin allergy in a patient developing urticaria, and the cause may sometimes remain hidden for a long time if the source of contact with penicillin, such as milk (ZIMMERMANN 1959; WICHER et al. 1969), meat (TSCHEUNER 1972; LINDEMAYR et al. 1981), dental depots (HURLEY 1963), vaccines (PELNER 1959), or various foods is itself hidden (SIEGEL 1959; WELCH 1959; ADKINSON 1980). Accordingly, the possibility of penicillin hypersensitivity should always be considered in the differential diagnosis of any chronic recurrent urticaria. Such recurrent forms lasting for several months even after withdrawal of penicillin therapy are not rare (LEVINE et al. 1966a). Usually, a concomitant rise of BPO-specific IgG antibodies plays a "blocking" role and terminates urticaria (FELLNER et al. 1967b) or does not even let it occur.

The possible role of fungal infections in the development and/or persistence of penicillin allergic reactions has been emphasized (FEINBERG 1944; SCHUPPLI 1958, 1962; BLUM and DE WECK 1966).

3. Serum-Like Disease

The classical clinical picture of serum-like disease, with skin rash, fever, polyadenopathy, joint swellings, and glomerulopathy occurring within 9–14 days after the start of penicillin therapy, was frequently encountered in the 1950s and 1960s. For reasons which are not yet entirely clear, the frequency of such reactions seems to have diminished (Table 3). The immunopathological mechanisms of this type of reaction are still not entirely clear (ROSE et al. 1962; FELLNER and BAER 1967; FELLNER et al. 1967b); while immune complexes undeniably play a major role in the genesis of skin, joint, and kidney lesions, thereby incriminating anti-BPO IgG and/or IgM antibodies (PARKER 1975, 1980), there is no doubt that patients with serumlike disease also possess anti-BPO IgE antibodies, as detected by RAST and skin tests (DE WECK and BLUM 1965). However skin tests are usually negative during the clinical reaction itself and may become positive only several weeks after apparent clinical healing (DE WECK and BLUM 1965). The mast cell reactions due to IgE antibodies may facilitate the deposition of immune complexes (PARKER 1975).

4. Morbilliform Exanthema

Morbilliform exanthema differs markedly in morphological appearance and clinical evolution from the urticarial reaction described above. The skin lesions usually remain stable for a few days (instead of a few hours) and disappear promptly within a few days of interruption of penicillin treatment. It is not rare, however, to observe a mixture of both forms in the same patient.

Morbilliform exanthema is tending to become the most frequent form of adverse reaction to penicillins (Table 3), but it is likely that this trend represents above all the increase of rashes following ampicillin treatment (for review see ALMEYDA and LEVANTINE 1972; DEWDNEY 1980; BASS et al. 1973; BECKMANN 1971).

Although morbilliform rashes have been observed upon therapy with all penicillins, they are particularly prominent following ampicillin. In some statistics, the reported incidence of the ampicillin rash is as high as 5%–10% (ARNDT and JICK 1976; SHAPIRO et al. 1969, 1970; KERNS et al. 1973). This high incidence has led several authors to conclude that the "ampicillin rash" ist not actually a manifestation of penicillin allergy (BIERMAN et al. 1972; CROYDON et al. 1973; KERNS et al. 1973; SOKOLOFF 1977). This argument is based essentially on the following points: (a) penicillin can continue to be administered or be readministered to many of the patients who develop an ampicillin rash (ANDERSEN-LUND and BERGAN 1975; CAMPBELL and SOYKA 1977); (b) skin and serological tests for penicillin hypersensitivity are most frequently negative in such patients; and (c) the incidence of the ampicillin rash in patients with infectious mononucleosis (PATEL 1967; PULLEN et al. 1967; BROWN and KANWARE 1967; GABBERT and HOPWOOD 1968; MULROY 1973), influenza (GREGG 1973), cytomegalovirus infection (KLEMOLA 1970), leukemia (CAMERON and RICHMOND 1971) or hyperuricemia (BOSTON 1972; SHAPIRO et al. 1972; FESSEL 1972; MURPHY 1979) is so high that an immunological pathogenesis seem very unlikely. However, all these observations can be interpreted differently: (a) the possibility of continuing therapy in a patient who has developed exanthema may represent merely an instance of temporary desensitization (or antianaphylaxis) by exhaustion of the immunological reagents (antibodies or specific lymphocytes) involved in the pathogenesis of the reaction – a number of patients with exanthema to ampicillin can later be shown to be allergic to other beta-lactam antibiotics as well; (b) whereas such patients usually do not possess anti-BPO IgE antibodies detectable by skin test or RAST assay (KERNS et al. 1973; BIERMAN et al. 1972), it is not rare to obtain a positive lymphocyte transformation test with ampicillin, especially with ampicillin polymers (DE WECK 1972); and (c) it has recently been appreciated that a number of affections involving the lymphoid system may induce polyclonal activation of antibody-forming cells. This is certainly the case for infectious mononucleosis (NAZARETH et al. 1972; NORDBRING et al. 1972; MC KENZIE et al. 1976), and it is therefore possible that the frequent reactions to penicillins in such cases are related to anti-BPO antibodies or to cells temporarily stimulated by the ground disease, without the features of permanent allergy.

Still, a number of questions on ampicillin rash remain open. The role of protein impurities has been pointed out (KNUDSEN et al. 1970). Both experimentally (SHALTIEL et al. 1971; BATCHELOR and DEWDNEY 1968) and clinically (KNUDSEN et al. 1970; PARKER and RICHMOND 1976), it has been claimed that purification of ampicillin would markedly reduce the frequency of rash. However, the rash is also observed with ampicillin preparations where the side chain splitting from 6-APA has been achieved by chemical means (A. L. DE WECK, unpublished work). The role of ampicillin polymers, which are now available in isolated form (BUNDGAARD 1978), should be reinvestigated.

The immunological mechanism of the ampicillin rash also remains a controversial topic. Several authors favor the concept that such exanthemas are indeed a manifestation of immune complex deposition in the skin (CREAM and TURK 1971, AHLSTEDT et al. 1981), in which BPO-specific IgM antibodies (LEVINE et al. 1966 a) or even IgG antibodies directed against intercellular epithelial structures might play a pathogenic role (FELLNER et al. 1973). Others (DE WECK 1979) tend to believe that morbilliform exanthema is rather a manifestation of cellular, delayed-type hypersensitivity (see also FELLNER 1967, 1968, 1976; FELLNER and PRUTKIN 1970; FELLNER et al. 1969). The arguments for the one or the other view can be summarized as follows:

Morbilliform exanthema as immune complex disease:
1. Reported association between high levels of penicillin-specific IgM antibodies and exanthema (not confirmed).
2. Reports of immunoglobulin and complement components deposition in biopsies from skin lesions of penicillin-induced exanthema.

Morbilliform exanthema as manifestation of delayed hypersensitivity:
1. Frequent absence of specific IgE or other BPO-specific antibodies (IgM, IgG), negative immediate skin tests but positive epicutaneous test to benzylpenicillin and lymphocyte culture (these tests may also be positive by clinical manifestations of the immediate type, such as urticaria and anaphylactic shock).
2. Occurrence possible earlier than serum-like disease (5th instead of 9th day).
3. Can be reproduced experimentally in guinea pigs, following high-grade sensitization of the delayed type; in that case the exanthema is elicited by intravenous injection of the hapten but *not* by a hapten-protein conjugate.
4. No evidence for circulating immune complexes in patients with penicillin-induced exanthema.
5. Positive macrophage migration inhibition tests in patients with penicillin-induced exanthema (not absolute evidence of delayed hypersensitivity: immune complexes can also induce migration inhibition).

Undeniably, there are a number of patients with exanthema in whom all investigations, including skin, serological, and cellular tests, fail to detect hypersensitivity to penicillins. In such patients, the pathogenesis of the skin lesions remain mysterious. The possibility that interaction between ampicillin and lymphocytes may under some circumstances promote the formation and release of lymphokines is no more than a working hypothesis.

5. Hematologic Disorders

The best-known and probably most frequent hematologic disorder following the administration of high doses of penicillin is acute hemolytic anemia. This complication began to be described only in the early 1960s, when clinicians started to increase therapeutic doses of penicillin considerably (STRUMIA and RAYMOND 1962; SWANSON et al. 1966; DAWSON and SEGAL 1966; LAI et al. 1966; NESMITH and DAVIS 1968). For benzylpenicillin, it has been claimed that the minimum dose required is about 5–10 million units/day. In this disease, the erythrocytes become heavily loaded with BPO groups (PETZ and FUDENBERG 1966; ABRAHAM et al. 1968 b; SPATH et al. 1971). If the treated patient already possesses or concomitantly develops anti-BPO antibodies of the IgG (VAN ARSDEL and FRANZ 1963; PETZ and

FUDENBERG 1966; LEVINE and REDMOND 1967; SPATH et al. 1971) and/or IgM class (BIRD et al. 1975), the penicilloylated erythrocytes massively disappear from circulation, causing acute anemia. At this stage, a direct Coombs test may be observed. A positive direct Coombs test develops in approximately 3% of patients receiving 10–20 million units/day intravenous penicillin (ABRAHAM et al. 1968 b; PETZ 1971) but only a samll percentage actually develop hemolytic anemia (GARATTY and PETZ 1975). Other manifestations of penicillin allergy are usually absent (PARKER 1975). The mechanism of destruction of the erythrocytes does not seem to be complement-dependent intravascular hemolysis. In patients possessing anti-BPO antibodies, transfusion of ^{51}Cr-labeled penicilloylated erythrocytes confirms their reduced half-life, while such erythocytes exhibit normal decay in patients devoid of anti-BPO antibodies (LEVINE and REDMOND 1967). In most instances, the removal of BPO erythrocytes is probably due to macrophages (FRANK et al. 1977) but some instances of intravascular hemolysis with complement activation have been reported (KERR et al. 1972; RIES et al. 1975).

Another hematological manifestation of penicillin intolerance is the acute leukopenia sometimes occurring during treatment with high doses of penicillins (SPAIN and CLARKE 1946; CORCOS et al. 1964; WHITE et al. 1968; BAHMAN and KOHOUT 1973; REYES et al. 1973; COLVIN et al. 1974a; LEVENTHAL and SILKEN 1975; MARKOWITZ et al. 1975; CHU 1977; HOMAYOUNI et al. 1979; MOCK et al. 1979; WILSON et al. 1979; CARPENTER 1980). The leukopenia may develop independently from hemolytic anemia and usually affects primarily the granulocytic series (CHU 1977; WEITZMANN and STODDEL 1978). The patient recovers promptly following interruption of penicillin treatment. The mechanism of this reaction is not yet understood. Immunological studies in a number of such cases, including control patients similarly treated but not developing leukopenia, tend to implicate anti-BPO antibodies and/or penicillin-sensitive lymphocytes, which are demonstrable in such patients, but the selectivity of destruction for granulocytes is not explained (NEFTEL et al. 1981). Another recently described hematological manifestation of penicillin allergy is a coagulation disorder (ANDRASSY et al. 1976) which is clinically apparent from purpura and urogenital bleeding and appears related to some effect on platelet function (KLEIN et al. 1976; BROWN et al. 1976; CAZENAVE et al. 1976), as well as thrombocytopenia (HSI et al. 1966; BROOKS 1974; ASTER 1977).

6. Kidney and Vascular Disorders

Aside from the transient glomerulopathy due to the deposition of immune complexes in serum-like disease, as described above, several authors have described the development of interstitial nephritis during penicillin therapy (BALDWIN et al. 1968; ORCHARD and ROOKER 1974; COLVIN et al. 1974b), especially following methicillin therapy (HEWITT et al. 1961; CHESNEY and CHESNEY 1976; DITLOVE et al. 1977; GALPIN et al. 1978) but also after other penicillins (SCHRIER et al. 1966; TANNENBERG et al. 1971; GILBERT et al. 1970; PARRY et al. 1963; BURTON et al. 1974; RULEY and LISI 1974; APPEL et al. 1978). This may be accompanied by hemorrhagic ureteritis and cystitis (COOK et al. 1979; MÖLLER 1978). The immunological mechanisms of this type of reaction are not yet clear and have been much debated (MCCLUSKEY and COLVIN 1978); it is likely that both humoral and cellular immune mechanisms play a role in the pathogenesis of the disease (BORDER et al. 1974; OOI et al. 1974, 1975; APPEL 1980; LINTON et al. 1980). Acute interstitial nephritis typically occurs in patients on a prolonged course of therapy. It is characterized by the sudden onset of oliguria, renal failure, fever, rash, arthralgias, hematuria, proteinuria, and eosinophiluria. Other forms of kidney disease attributed to penicillins include angiitis and glomerulonephritis (ANDERSON 1947; SPRINGS 1951; PETERS et al. 1960), and acute renal failure with anuria has occurred after a single injection of penicillin (CARE and SQUIRE 1956). In a number of cases, localized or diffuse vasculitis has also been attributed to penicillin allergy, although the pathogenetic link has not always been evident.

7. Other Manifestations

Penicillin is a potent topical sensitizer and may cause contact dermatitis (LEVINE 1960a; FELLNER 1976): it is therefore no longer used in ointments. Several other cutaneous manifestations of penicillin allergy, such as fixed drug eruption, erythema multiforme, the Stevens-Johnson syndrome, exfoliative dermatitis, epidermal necrolysis, erythema nodosum and cutaneous necrotizing angiitis have been described (FELLNER 1976; SOTER and AUSTEN 1978; WINTRAUB et al. 1979; DE SWARTE 1972). The precise immunological mechanisms of these various forms of cutaneous reactions are usually not known.

Among pulmonary manifestations of drug allergy, therapeutic or professional (factory workers) inhalation of penicillins may lead to asthma (RUDZKI et al. 1966; DAVIES et al. 1974), while the occurrence of pulmonary infiltrates with eosinophilia has also been reported (REICHLIN et al. 1953).

The nonallergic Jarisch-Herxheimer reaction following use of penicillins has become a rare event (BUTTERLY and FISHMAN 1972; GUDJONSSON 1972; DEWDNEY 1980), while the mechanisms of isolated penicillin-induced fever (CLUFF and JOHNSON 1964; CHUSID and ATKINS 1972) are still under discussion.

III. Epidemiology and Frequency of Allergic Reactions

As already indicated above, penicillin allergy, although somewhat less prominent than in the 1960s, remains a major clinical problem. This is not only because of the relatively large proportion of the population which is estimated to be sensitized in the industrialized countries (2%–5% according to most estimates, with a range of 1%–10%; VAN ARSDEL 1965; SMITH et al. 1966), but also because the diagnosis of penicillin allergy is still today frequently established by history alone, which may be very misleading. In our experience, about 50% of patients labeled as having penicillin allergy are in fact not allergic, and 50% of the patients who are indeed sensitized are not aware of it. Under these circumstances, it is inevitable that a large number of unexpected reactions are encountered and also that a considerable number of patients are denied penicillin therapy and given some other antibiotic which is usually more toxic and more expensive and may be less efficient for that particular case.

Anaphylactic reactions occur most commonly in adults between the ages of 20 and 49 (IDSOE et al. 1968), but may also occur in infants (IDSOE 1958; MATHESON

Table 4. Incidence of penicillin (PN) allergy. (From Rudolph and Price 1973)

History of PN allergy 1969:	2382/36048 (6.6%)

Predictive value of history

	PN-treated	Allergic reactions	
		n	%
Patients with history	78	10	12.8
Patients without history	24,906	155	0.62

Incidence of reactions

	PN-treated	Allergic reactions		Anaphylactic shock	
		n	$^o/_{oo}$	n	$^o/_{oo}$
1954	19,510	116	5.95	4	(0.21)
1959	25,550	248	9.71	27	(1.06)
1964	21,922	166	7.57	10	(0.46)
1969	27,673	183	6.61	11	(0.40)

and Elegant 1955; Bierman et al. 1969; Paupe et al. 1974) and in elderly people (Idsoe et al. 1968). The real frequency of penicillin allergy is difficult to establish, since it apparently varies according to the mode of application (parenteral or per os) (Parker 1975; Herman and Jick 1979), the dose, the rhythm of injections, the thoroughness of follow-up, the reporting of adverse reactions, etc. In a comprehensive study of US venereological clinics over 20 years, Rudolph and Price (1973) found that the incidence of allergic reactions varied relatively little (Table 4).

IV. Diagnostic Tests

Since the early days of penicillin therapy, the desire of the clinician to have a simple, reliable, and rapid method of diagnosing penicillin hypersensitivity has been manifest (Boger et al. 1953; Kern and Wimberley 1953). Skin tests with penicillin alone, although sometimes positive in sensitive individuals, showed in general a poor correlation with the clinical situation and did not give the degree of reliability which the physician usually requires of a diagnostic test. With better knowledge of the immunochemical and immunological mechanisms involved in penicillin allergy, it became possible to develop a series of serological and cellular tests. Such tests, which are briefly described below, frequently make it possible to identify the immunological sensitization of the patient to penicillin (DE WECK 1971). They do not, in most cases, allow an absolute prospective statement on the risk involved in renewed penicillin treatment. Considering the variety of immuno-pathological mechanisms involved in penicillin allergy, it would be an illusion to believe that a single test may be of use for all types of reactions encountered in clinical practice. Accordingly, the diagnosis of penicillin allergy necessarily encompasses various types of tests. Some of these tests, as described below, are of no more than historical interest for penicillin allergy. Emphasis in this section will be placed on the tests currently in routine use.

1. Skin Tests

Intradermal and prick/scratch skin tests with penicillin solutions have been in use for more than 30 years (BOGER et al. 1953; TUFT et al. 1955; SIEGEL et al. 1955; SIEGEL 1962). These tests usually have a bad reputation: most clinicians consider them as unreliable, since many patients who are obviously allergic have negative skin tests and since they may be quite dangerous in some highly sensitive individuals. Nevertheless, a number of authors have recommended systematic use of such skin tests in some clinical situations and hospital conditions (ADKINSON et al. 1971; VAN DELLEN and GLEICH 1970; ADKINSON 1976), estimating that systemic screening for highly sensitive patients would help to decrease the incidence of severe allergic reactions. Others (ERFMEYER 1981) suggest a more restrictive approach, performing skin tests only when renewed administration of penicillin is mandatory, since skin tests in penicillin-allergic patients may cause anaphylactic reactions (TAO and SUNG 1958; IDSOE et al. 1968; DOGLIOTTI 1975; PIETZCKER and KUNER 1975), in some instances fatal (DOGLIOTTI 1968). However, when used appropriately, penicillin skin testing appears to be a very safe procedure (LEVINE et al. 1967; LEVINE and ZOLOV 1969).

A definite improvement in the diagnosis of penicillin allergy by skin tests has been brought about by the development of a synthetic multivalent reagent carrying BPO antigenic determinants, namely penicilloyl-polylysine (PPL) which is an optimal elicitor of immediate wheal and flare reactions in patient possessing skin-sensitizing anti-BPO antibodies (PARKER et al. 1962 a, b; DE WECK 1962 c; DE WECK and BLUM 1963; BUDD et al. 1964; LEVINE 1964; PARKER 1966). During the past 20 years, a large number of authors have reported their results from skin testing with PPL (Table 5). Most agree that PPL is a very useful reagent for the detection of penicillin hypersensitivity, although several reservations and limits have to be expressed. These may be summarized as follows:
1. Over the years, several different PPL preparations have been used, varying in their molecular size and degree of substitution with BPO groups. Since both play a role for optimal triggering of IgE-mediated reactions on mast cells (LEVINE 1966 a, b; LEVINE and REDMOND 1968; DE WECK and SCHNEIDER 1969), some of the discrepancies between published results may have occurred therefore. The manufacture of PPL has up to now involved randomly synthesized polylysine molecules, making precise chemical reproducibility difficult. A stepwise synthesized PPL reagent optimized for skin tests has recently become available (DE WECK et al. 1982).

Table 5. Retrospective skin tests with PPLs

PPL used	Author	History of PN allergy[a]		No history	
		n	%	n	%
PPL$_{\bar{n}20}$	DE WECK (1973)	108/ 146[a]	66.6	4/ 118	3.4
de Weck	GAYET (1967)	25/ 40	62.5	2/ 50	4.0
	LEONHARDI (1969)	49/ 148	66.6	0/ 80	0
	WÜTHRICH (1972)	166/ 212	78		
	GATTLEN (1976)	163/ 244	66.8		
	BASOMBA (1979)	28/ 61	45.9		
Cilligen Sigma	BROWN (1964)	396/1003	39.5		
	GROSSHANS (1978)	19/ 21	90.4		
Prepen	ADKINSON (1971)	19/ 81	23.4	9/ 163	0.5
	GREEN (1971)	73/ 352	20.7	36/ 675	5.3
	GREEN (1977)	319/1718	19	122/1319	10
	SULLIVAN (1981)	740	20.2		
Levine	LEVINE and ZOLOV (1969)	25/ 217	11.5		3
	STEMBER (1972)	9/ 64	14.0	50/ 675	7.4
Astra	JUHLIN (1977)	12/ 35	34.2	0/ 10	

[a] Interval between positive skin test to PPL and challenge with PN variable, often longer than 1 year

2. The IgE-mediated skin hypersensitivity upon which the PPL skin test rests is relatively transient in most patients if no renewed boosting contact with penicillin occurs. In some patients skin hypersensitivity markedly decreases within a few years, while other maintain positive skin tests for over 10 years. This decline was noticed many years ago (FINKE et al. 1965), and has been documented again recently by SULLIVAN et al. (1981), who observed nearly 100% positive reactions in patients tested within 3 months of their allergic reaction to penicillin, while the proportion of positive skin tests dropped to 22% when 10 years or more had elapsed since the allergic reaction and last known contact with penicillin.
3. The immediate skin test with PPL is of value primarily in detecting the presence of skin-sensitizing IgE antibodies, although possibly in some cases it detects some other anti-BPO skin sensitizing antibodies. Accordingly, allergic manifestations resulting from other immunopathological mechanisms, such as morbilliform exanthema or hematologic disorders, are usually not accompanied by positive skin tests.

Soon after the introduction of PPL to penicillin skin testing, it became obvious that some allergic patients who were negative to PPL demonstrated positive reactions when tested with penicillin itself and/or with some penicillin derivatives, such as penicilloic acid (Table 6). The increased knowledge of the immunochemical pathways of penicillin conjugation suggested such reactions to be due to so-called minor determinants (LEVINE 1965; LEVINE and REDMOND 1969). Systematic studies by several groups (GATTLEN and PETER 1976; WARRINGTON et al. 1978; SULLIVAN et al. 1981) led to the conclusion that for all practical purposes, namely the identification of the largest possible number of skin-sensitive patients, skin tests with PPL, penicillin; and penicilloic acid should be recommended. As already demon-

Table 6. Positive skin tests to $PPL_{\bar{n}20}$, BPN, and BPNCO in 244 patients with history of penicillin allergy (Bern 1971–1976)

Test positive to	Highest test concentration used	Positive	
		N	%
$PPL_{\bar{n}20}$	50×10^{-5} M scratch 25×10^{-5} M i. d.	163/244	66.8
BPN	200000 U/ml scratch 1000 U/ml i. d.	108/244	44.2
BPNCO	0.5 mg/ml i. d.	76/244	31.1
BPN ($PPL_{\bar{n}20}$ neg.)		32/244	13.1
BPNCO ($PPL_{\bar{n}20}$ and BPN neg.)		6/244	2.5
$PPL_{\bar{n}20}$ and/or BPN and/or BPNCO		201/244	82.4

strated in several prospective studies (Table 7 a and b), the prospective use of such skin tests before penicillin therapy would certainly contribute markedly to reducing the incidence of severe immediate allergic reactions, in particular of anaphylactic reactions.

The occurrence and significance of delayed reactions after intradermal injection of penicillin and penicillin derivatives in penicillin-allergic patients (REDMOND and LEVINE 1968; FELLNER et al. 1969) has not been systematically investigated, but deserves more attention. Upon epicutaneous application of benzylpenicillin, a classical delayed (24–72 h) vesicular eczematous reaction develops in patients with contact dermatitis to penicillin. However, this is also the case (although the reaction is then maculopapular rather than vesicular) for those penicillin-allergic patients manifesting an exanthematous rash and even for those displaying urticaria (Table 8). Accordingly, epicutaneous tests with benzylpenicillin or some of the other penicillins, especially ampicillin, are routinely used by us in allergy diagnosis. We have found them to be more useful than various allergy textbooks suggest.

2. Antibody Detection Techniques

a) Hemagglutination

The hemagglutination of penicillin-treated erythrocytes by sera from animals experimentally immunized with penicillins or from penicillin-allergic patients has been used as an assay since the original observation by LEY et al. (1958) that some sera could agglutinate erythrocytes incubated in vitro with benzylpenicillin. With the hemagglutination assay, it became possible to follow experimentally the development of the immune response to various penicillins (EPP 1959, 1962; HEGGIE 1960; WATSON et al. 1960, 1961; VAN ARSDEL et al. 1963a, b; DE WECK 1964; McGOVERN et al. 1964; RADERMECKER and SALMON 1966) and to assess, by hemagglutination inhibition, the specificity of the antibodies raised (DE WECK 1962a; THIEL et al. 1964). The hemagglutination assay was also of some value clinically, since it permitted detection of antipenicillin antibodies of the IgG and IgM classes,

Table 7a. Results of prospective testing with PPL in patients with positive history of PN allergy and negative skin test to PPL

PPL used	Highest concentration used for skin test	Patients challenged with PN	Patients experiencing reactions	%	Authors
Prepen	6×10^{-5} M i.d.	54	1	1.8	ADKINSON et al. (1971)
Prepen	6×10^{-5} M i.d.	169	2	1.1	WARRINGTON et al. (1979)
Prepen	6×10^{-5} M i.d.	328	3	0.9	ADKINSON (1976)
Prepen	6×10^{-5} M i.d.	346	12	3.4	GREEN et al. (1977)
Astra	1×10^{-6} M i.d.	17	0	0	JUHLIN et al. (1977)
PPL$_{\bar{n}20}$	25×10^{-5} M i.d.	16	0	0	LEONARDI and MATNER (1969)
PPL$_{\bar{n}20}$	25×10^{-5} M i.d.	6	0	0	BASOMBA et al. (1979)
Levine	1×10^{-6} M i.d.	185	1		LEVINE and ZOLOV (1969)
Levine	1×10^{-6} M i.d.	29	0 (5 exanthema)		FELLNER et al. (1971)

Table 7b. Results of prospective testing with PPL in patients with positive history of PN allergy and positive skin test to PPL

PPL used	Highest concentration used for skin test	Patients challenged with PN	Patients experiencing reactions	%	Authors
Levine	1×10^{-6} M i.d.	8	5	62	LEVINE and ZOLOV (1969)
Prepen	6×10^{-5} M i.d.	7	4	57	GREEN et al. (1971)
Prepen	6×10^{-5} M i.d.	6	4	66	GREEN et al. (1977)
Prepen	6×10^{-5} M i.d.	1	1	100	ADKINSON et al. (1971)
PPL$_{\bar{n}20}$	25×10^{-5} M i.d.	224	78[a]	35	GIRARD (1975)
PPL$_{\bar{n}20}$	25×10^{-5} M i.d.	4	1	25	BASOMBA et al. (1979)
Cilligen	6×10^{-5} M i.d.	418	30	7.1	BROWN et al. (1964)

[a] Interval between positive skin test to PPL and challenge with PN variable, sometimes longer than 1 year

which are directly involved in hematological reactions. On the other hand, correlation of hemagglutination results with the majority of clinical reactions to penicillins, due to IgE antibodies, was never very impressive (DE WECK 1971). In its most sensitive versions (LEVINE et al. 1966b, c), the hemagglutination assay was even found positive in nearly 100% of the population, suggesting that anti-BPO anti-

Table 8. Epicutaneous tests with benzylpenicillin in penicillin allergy

Clinical form of reaction	Immediate-type (20–30 min) skin tests with benzylpenicillin and/or PPL	Epicutaneous test with benzylpenicillin: 200000 U/ml (24–48 h reaction)	
		Pos.	Neg.
Urticaria (38 cases)	Positive	12	7
Epicutaneous test pos.: 23/36 (60%)	Negative	11	8
Morbilliform exanthema (56 cases)	Positive	15	1
Epicutaneous test pos.: 49/56 (87%)	Negative	34	6

bodies are present in almost everybody. In recent years, the detection of anti-BPO antibodies has been conveniently effected by more modern serological techniques such as enzyme-linked immunosorbent assay (ELISA) (DE HAAN et al. 1979) or radioimmunoassay RIA (WIDE and JUHLIN 1971; NEFTEL et al. 1981).

b) Hapten-Modified Bacteriophages

The interaction of penicillins with bacteriophages at neutral pH yields penicilloylated bacteriophages which are still able to produce lytic plaques in their target bacteria cultures (e.g., *Bacillus subtilis*). This technique was developed by HAIMOVICH et al. (1967) and used for experimental (SHALTIEL et al. 1971) as well as for clinical studies. We have also used this technique for several years (DE WECK 1971, 1972; STOFER et al. 1973) since it had the advantages of being very sensitive and of permitting the use of the same set of reagents over a number of years. With the development of ELISA and RIA assays, this technique has lost its usefulness in penicillin allergy.

c) Radioimmunoassays and Immunoenzymatic Assays

The development of an assay for BPO-specific IgE antibodies was first published by WIDE and JUHLIN (1971). In order to obtain suitable immunosorbent matrices for BPO groups, it is necessary to use either a spacer molecule or a conjugate, such as HSA (DE WECK 1978 b). This procedure is also the basis for the current commercial Phadebas assay. The usefulness of this assay for detecting BPO-specific IgE antibodies in the sera of patients putatively allergic to penicillin has been assessed by several groups (ADKINSON 1975; COUTEAUX-DUMONT et al. 1974; KRAFT and WIDE 1976; KRAFT et al. 1977; DE WECK 1978b; JUHLIN and WIDE 1979; SPATH et al. 1979; BASOMBA et al. 1979; JARISCH et al. 1981). In these studies, the percentage of correlation with positive skin tests and/or history of clinical allergy varies, but it is generally agreed that this test may be quite useful for diagnosing penicillin allergy. Its main limitation appears to be the relatively rapid decline of detectable anti-BPO IgE antibodies following contact with penicillin, a decline which is certainly more rapid than observed in skin tests. Accordingly, when patients are tested some time after their allergic reaction to penicillin, a sizeable number may still manifest skin hypersensitivity but be negative in the radioallergosorbent test (RAST). KRAFT et al. (1977) have reported that about half of the patients with positive RAST become negative within a year, and we have obtained similar results (DE WECK 1978b). Accordingly, it is our contention that the RAST alone does not suffice for investigating putative penicillin-allergic patients. IgG, IgM, and IgA antibodies against the BPO determinant can be detected by immunoenzymatic assay (DE HAAN et al. 1979) and RIA (NEFTEL et al. 1981).

d) Techniques Involving Basophils, Mast Cells, or Platelets

Basophils from patients allergic to penicillin will degranulate (SHELLEY and JUHLIN 1961; SHELLEY 1963; RESNIK and SHELLEY 1965) and release histamine (SHELLEY and COMAISH 1965; PERELMUTTER and EISEN 1970; BLOCH-MOROT et al. 1977) when challenged with penicillins or penicillin conjugates. This phenomenon has also been proposed as a passive test following sensitization by allergic serum of various targets such as rabbit basophils (SHELLEY 1963) or rat mast cells (KATZ et al. 1964; ELLIS et al. 1970). New versions of the basophil degranulation test have recently been proposed (KOROTZER and HADDAD 1970; HADDAD and KOROTZER 1971; BENVENISTE 1981), but have not yet gained wide clinical acceptance, probably because the techniques involved are still somewhat difficult.

e) Passive Transfer and Other Serological Techniques

Human skin-sensitizing antibodies from penicillin-sensitive patients can be transferred to normal individuals (WALDO and TYSON 1949; COLEMAN and SIEGEL 1956; REDMOND and LEVINE 1967), monkeys (KUNZ et al. 1966, 1967; ASSEM and SCHILD 1968), or experimental rodents (SONNTAG and MARCUS 1963; PALOMEQUE et al. 1965), although in the last case it is likely that IgG antibodies are detected, not the relevant IgE antibodies. The technique is interesting in experimental studies and its results appear roughly parallel to those of skin tests, but it is too cumbersome to be of practical use.

Additional serological techniques, such as complement consumption tests, radioimmunoprecipitation (GLEICH and STANKIEVIC 1969), fluorescence polarization (DANDLIKER et al. 1965), and variations of sandwich hemagglutination techniques (e.g., red-cell-linked antigen-antiglobulin reaction: KRAFT et al. 1976), have been used in the detection of antipenicillin antibodies, but all appear to have been supplanted by modern RIA and ELISA techniques.

3. Cellular Tests

a) Lymphocyte Transformation Test

The lymphocyte transformation test, first proposed as a morphological assessment of lymphoblast production in culture upon incubation with the antigenic drug (HEITMANN and KUWERT 1966; HALPERN et al. 1967), was soon used in its biochemical version, based on measurement of DNA synthesis and [^{3}H]thymidine uptake (ROSE et al. 1966; VISCHER 1966; EVANS 1967; FELLNER et al. 1967a; ASSEM and VICKERS 1972; SARKANY and GAYLARDE 1978; WARRINGTON and TSE 1979). Although at the beginning, probably due to technical reasons, the correlation between clinical allergy to penicillin and positive lymphocyte culture did not appear very impressive, more recent series (DE WECK 1971, 1973; DE WECK et al. 1974; GIRARD and CUEVAS 1975 a, VICKERS and ASSEM 1974; ASSEM and VICKERS 1975; WARRINGTON and TSE 1979) clearly indicate that the lymphocyte culture test may be of great interest in the diagnosis of penicillin allergy. In our experience, the main advantages of such a test are that it can also be positive in reactions which are not IgE-mediated and that allergic patients with positive lymphocyte cultures usually retain the reactivity of their peripheral blood lymphocytes over many years (memory cells). This conclusion may be somewhat weakened by the recent findings that normal, clinically nonallergic patients may also show positive lymphocyte cultures when tested shortly after penicillin treatment (LISCHKA and GOTTMANN-LÜCKERATH 1972; SAURAT et al. 1976a), especially when high therapeutic doses of penicillins have been used (NEFTEL et al. 1982). It has not yet been systematically investigated whether allergic patients would retain this reactivity longer and/or react to smaller doses. In any case, we have often found the lymphocyte culture test useful to clarify some clinical situation and we continue to use it routinely. Its main drawbacks are its cost and the time required for its completion.

b) Macrophage Migration Inhibition

Classical in vitro tests of cellular immunity, such as the macrophage migration inhibition test, have been applied in several variants to the problem of penicillin allergy (ORTIZ et al. 1974; SAURAT et al. 1976b; WARRINGTON et al. 1979). It has been found that this test does not necessarily reflect cellular hypersensitivity, since immune complexes between penicilloyl conjugates used as antigens and anti-BPO antibodies in the patient's sera also inhibit leukocyte migration. In general, this test has not gained wide acceptance, because of its relatively poor reproducibility, its technical difficulties, and the lack of quantitative evaluation.

c) Rosette-Forming Cells

Penicilloylated erythrocytes are able to form specific rosettes when incubated with leukocytes from penicillin-sensitive patients (GIRARD et al. 1975a). In this case, using mixed mononuclear populations, rosettes may be formed by lymphocytes actively carrying anti-BPO receptors as well as by mononuclear cells passively loaded with anti-BPO antibodies on their Fc receptors. The relatively low percentage of such cells in leukocytes from peripheral blood makes the search for antigen-specific rosettes rather cumbersome. This has therefore not become a routine diagnostic test.

C. Cephalosporins

The cephalosporin group of antibiotics (general structure shown in Fig. 3) are semisynthetic derivatives of 7-aminocephalosporanic acid (7-ACA): They differ from each other both in their acyl side chains at C-7 and in the substituent at the C-3 carboxyl group.

Cephalosporins are valued for their usually broader antibiotic spectrum than penicillins, but several of them are more toxic than penicillins.

Since their introduction to therapy, the question of allergic cross-reactivity between cephalosporins and penicillins has been raised, and continues to be raised for each of the new cephalosporin molecules introduced (PETZ 1971; PEVNY et al. 1973). Immunopathological reactions to cephalosporins have been reported and often confirmed by objective tests. It is, however, frequently difficult to assess whether such reactions are due to cross-reactivity on the basis of preexisting penicillin hypersensitivity or whether it is the manifestation of a de novo sensitization to cephalosporin.

I. Immunologic Aspects of Hypersensitivity to Cephalosporins

Despite chemical similarity between cephalosporins and penicillins, marked differences exist in chemical reactivity and behavior. It would be ill advised to draw analogies not based on experimental data.

1. Immunogenicity of the Cephalosporins

Several cephalosporins have been shown to be immunogenic when injected emulsified in complete Freund's adjuvant into rabbits (SCHNEIERSON et al. 1964; ABRAHAM et al. 1968 b; BUTCHER and STEWART 1969; HAMILTON et al. 1970; SPATH et al. 1971; PETERSEN and GRAHAM 1974) or mice in the form of preformed protein conjugates (MURANAKA et al. 1980). Many authors have also raised anticephalosporin antibodies in rabbits by using preformed protein conjugates (for review, see DEWDNEY 1977). In these studies, cephalothin, cephaloridine, and cefazolin have been most frequently used. The production of antibodies was assessed by hemagglutination, hemagglutination inhibition, and quantitative precipitation in agar gels (KUWAHARA et al. 1970; MINE et al. 1970), and by PCA in guinea pigs (BRANDRISS et al. 1965; BATCHELOR et al. 1966; KUWAHARA et al. 1970) or rats (MURANAKA et al. 1980).

There is also a brief report on the development of delayed hypersensitivity reactions in guinea pigs to a cephalosporin-albumin conjugate (LERNER and STANDER 1973). Little work has been reported on the elicitation of contact reactions in guinea pigs by cephalothin. Neither de novo sensitization nor cross-reactivity in animals sensitized by benzylpenicillin were achieved by the Beecham's group (BATCHELOR et al. 1966; DEWDNEY 1977), while weak and irregular sensitization was reported by SCHNEIERSON et al. (1964).

In man, allergic reactions have been in reported in patients with no prior history of penicillin allergy, leading to the assumption that cephalosporins may be immunogenic by themselves (KAPLAN and WEINSTEIN 1967; ABRAHAM et al. 1968a, b; MOLTHAN 1969; SALEH and TISCHLER 1974).

Cross-reactivities between antibodies to cephalosporins and penicillins have been observed in experimental animals (BRANDRISS et al. 1965; BATCHELOR et al. 1966; GRALNICK and MCGINNIS 1967; TADOKORO et al. 1976) and in man (ABRAHAM et al. 1968 b; GRIECO 1967; STEMBERGER et al. 1971; DELAFUENTE et al. 1979). Among 701 patients with a history of penicillin allergy, 57 (8.1%) experienced an allergic reaction upon administration of cephalosporins. Among 15,007 patients without history of penicillin allergy, only 285 (1.9%) experienced an allergic reaction to cephalosporins. Accordingly, the risk of reaction is about 4 times higher if the patient has a history of penicillin allergy (PETZ 1978). This is in agreement with the figures of other studies (THOBURN et al. 1968; MOELLERING and SWARTZ 1976) indicating an incidence of cross reactions from 5% to 16%. In individuals with histories of penicillin allergy and positive skin tests to PPL, however, the incidence of allergic reactions to cephalothin is 50% (THOBURN et al. 1966).

2. Formation of Antigenic Determinants

There is no conclusive evidence that cephalosporins, upon reaction with protein, generate a major, stable cephalosporoyl group equivalent to the penicilloyl group in penicillin allergy. On the basis of inhibition and cross reactivity studies, however, the existence of such a group is postulated by several authors. Aminolysis of cephalosporins with amino compounds leads to the formation of unstable intermediates, which decompose as a function of concentration and pH to penamaldates and penaldates (NEWTON et al. 1967; SCHWARTZ 1969; HAMILTON-MILLER and ABRAHAM 1971) (Fig. 10). There is no doubt, however, that there is an initial reaction between cephalosporins and ε-amino groups on proteins (SHIBATA et al. 1966).

In the cephalosporins, the formation of penicillenic acid equivalents appears difficult and the corresponding intermediates would generate penamaldates (Fig. 10). Furthermore, the presence of a dihydrothiazine ring instead of a thiazolidine ring makes the formation of a penicilloic acid equivalent unlikely and that of a penicillamine analogue impossible (DEWDNEY 1977).

A cephalosporoyl determinant could be introduced into proteins via routes other than direct aminolysis: if reaction occurs first at the C-3 position of the cephalosporin nucleus, it could facilitate subsequent interaction of the β-lactam ring with nucleophilic groups (SCHWARTZ 1969). The role of substituents at C-3 on the reactivity of the β-lactam ring, on aminolysis, and on the stability of the dihydrothiazine nucleus have been studied by several groups (HAMILTON-MILLER et al. 1970; HAMILTON-MILLER and ABRAHAM 1971; BUNDGAARD 1976 c, d, e). It has been shown that the substituent at C-3 may influence the stability of the dihydrothiazine nucleus and of the corresponding cephalosporoyl group, but has little effect on the rate of aminolysis. Almost nothing is known about cephalosporin equivalents of minor determinants (LEVINE 1973). The reactivity of some cephalosporins with erythrocytes is a well-known phenomenon, leading sometimes to a direct Coombs test in treated patients, especially with cephalothin. For other cephalosporins, such as cephaloridine, much higher concentrations than normal therapeutic blood levels are required in order to cause this unspecific binding of plasma proteins to red cells (KUWAHARA et al. 1970; MINE et al. 1970). Adsorption of proteins onto cephalosporin-treated erythrocytes is probably the consequence of some damage to the red cell membrane, as shown by loss of acetylcholinesterase activity (HERZ et al. 1969).

3. Role of the Side Chain in Immunological Reactivity

The acyl side chain at the C-7 position of the cephalosporins seems to play a major role in determining the specificity of antibodies raised by or reacting with cephalo-

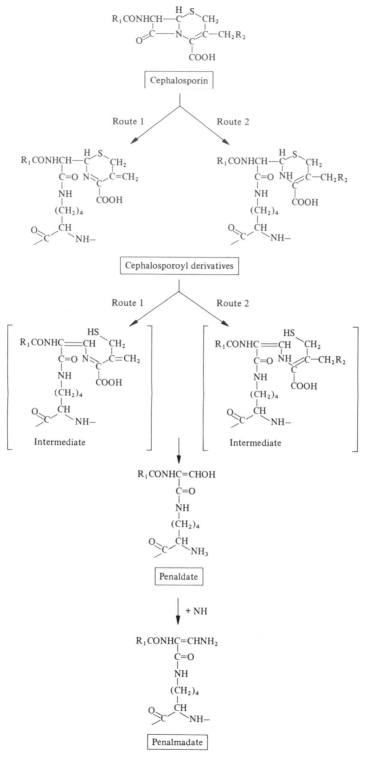

Fig. 10. Formation of antigenic determinants from cephalosporins (DEWDNEY 1977)

sporins, while the substituents at the C-3 position play no or only a very minor role (DEWDNEY 1977). This conclusion is based on a number of experimental studies, using rabbit antibodies raised against penicillins and/or cephalosporins and hemagglutination and/or guinea pig PCA inhibition (BRANDRISS et al. 1965; BATCHEFLOR et al. 1966; SHIBATA et al. 1966; HAMILTON-MILLER and ABRAHAM 1971). In general, extensive cross-reactivity was found between anti-BPO antibodies and antibodies directed against cephaloram carrying the same phenylacetyl side chain and with cephalothin and cephaloridine carrying a thiophene-2 acetic acid side chain. With cefazolin, on the other hand, carrying a tetrazolyl acetic acid side chain, there is only limited cross-reactivity with the BPO group (KUWAHARA et al. 1970; MINE et al. 1970). With the newer cephalosporins cefuroxime and cefotaxime, which carry a structurally very different side chain (Fig. 3), no cross-reactivity at all was observed with the BPO compounds using guinea pig antisera induced by the corresponding protein conjugates (SCHNEIDER and DE WECK 1981). Cephalexin seems to be a case in itself, apparently being poorly immunogenic (O'CALLAGHAN and MUGGLETON 1973; PETERSEN and GRAHAM 1974), possibly on the basis of reduced susceptibility to aminolysis (BUNDGAARD 1976a, b) or of competition reactions with the formation of polymers (DEWDNEY 1977).

In those cases where it was investigated (KUWAHARA et al. 1970), the substituents at C-3 did not appear to play a role in the antibodies' specificity.

4. Protein Impurities and Polymers

A few studies have been made on the occurrence and immunological activities of protein impurities and polymers in cephalosporin preparations. STEWART et al. (1973) reported the presence of proteins in cephalosporin C and 7-ACA, which could elicit reactions in sensitized guinea pigs. Polymerization of cephalothin and cephaloridine has also been reported (STEWART 1968; MUNRO et al. 1976; WALSH et al. 1971; O'CALLAGHAN and MUGGLETON 1973). Although some of these polymers were shown to be able to elicit PCA reactions in guinea pigs (MUNRO et al. 1976), their potential immunological role should be further evaluated.

II. Clinical Aspects

Several authors have demonstrated the occurrence of hemagglutinating IgM and/ or IgG antibodies in patients treated with cephalothin (ABRAHAM et al. 1968a, b; SPATH et al. 1971), without any evidence that such antibodies would cause harmful clinical reactions. In this, the situation resembles that with penicillin, with the exception that some cephalosporins obviously bind serum proteins to erythrocytes, a phenomenon whose immunopathological consequences are not yet entirely clear.

Skin-sensitizing antibodies detected by prick, scratch, or intradermal tests have been reported by several authors (PERKINS et al. 1965; THOBURN et al. 1968; GRIECO 1967; GIRARD 1968; VOGT 1969; LEVINE 1973; SANDERS et al. 1974; ASSEM and VICKERS 1974). In one study (PEDERSEN-BJERGAARD 1967), the reactivity could be transferred by Prausnitz-Küstner (PK) test, and of 13 sera reacting to benzylpenicillin, eight also reacted to cephalothin. There is some question, however, of whether some of the skin reactions reported with relatively high concentrations of cephalosporins may be unspecific (GRIECO 1967; SANDERS et al. 1974). In a recent study using RAST-positive sera strongly reacting with BPO antigens, we were unable to detect any cross-reactivity with the new cephalosporins cefuroxime and cefotaxime (SCHNEIDER and DE WECK 1981). However, the rate of reaction to cephalothin in patients with documented allergy to benzylpenicillin is very high (THOBURN et al. 1966); cephalosporins can therefore not be considered a uniformly safe substitute for penicillins (GREEN 1970; MOELLERING and SWARTZ 1976; MOELLERING 1975).

Clinically, immediate hypersensitivity reactions such as urticaria or even shock have been reported by several authors, usually in patients known to be allergic to penicillins (KABINS et al. 1965; PERKINS and SASLAW 1966; MERRILL et al. 1966; ROTHSCHILD and DOTY 1966; THOBURN et al. 1966; GIRARD 1968; SCHOLAND et al. 1968; BROGARD et al. 1969; LEVINE 1973; SPRUILL et al. 1974; VELASQUEZ and GOLD 1975). Maculopapular rashes (PERKINS et al. 1965; THOBURN et al. 1966; SANDERS et al. 1974) and drug fever (SANDERS et al. 1974) have also been reported.

Hematological disorders induced by the cephalosporins have been reported but the incidence of hemolytic anemia in no way parallels the occurrence of positive Coombs tests. Hemolytic anemia has been reported after cephalotin (MOLTHAN 1969; GRALNICK et al. 1972), cephalexin (FORD 1967; FORBES et al. 1972), and cephaloridine (KAPLAN and WEINSTEIN 1967) therapy. Thrombocytopenia (SHEIMAN et al. 1968; GRALNICK et al. 1972) and granulocytopenia (DAVIS et al. 1964; LEVIN et al. 1971; SILBER and DIOKNOA 1973; DICATO and ELLMANN 1975) have also been reported.

III. Epidemiology and Frequency of Allergic Reactions

The most frequent side effects of cephalosporin treatment appear to be of toxic rather than allergic nature, especially for cephaloridine, which has a marked nephrotoxicity (BOYD et al. 1973).

The true incidence of allergic sensitization due to cephalosporins alone is difficult to assess, since in most patients treated with cephalosporins, the immune status for penicillin sensitivity before treatment is not objectively known and assessed. The general clinical impression is that in patients sensitized to benzylpenicillin, overt allergic clinical reactions do not occur in more than 10%–20% of those subsequently treated with cephalosporins. The rate of adverse reactions may, however, be higher than suspected. In healthy volunteers given cephalothin and cephapirin intravenously, an unexpectedly high rate of reactions was experienced, and five patients developed skin hypersensitivity detected by skin test with PPL.

IV. Diagnostic Tests

The diagnostic of immediate-type allergy by skin tests with cephalosporins has been attempted by several groups, but, as already discussed above, does not yield very satisfactory results. Theoretically, it would be much more appropriate to use preformed conjugates of cephalosporins with polylysine. The hemagglutination

Table 9. Cross-reactivity between penicillins and cephalosporins in lymphocyte stimulation of penicillin-allergic patients[a]

Patient no	Benzylpenicillin (500 µg/ml)	Ampicillin (500 µg/ml)	Cefotaxime (100 µg/ml)	Cefuroxime (200 µg/ml)	Cephalotine (100 µg/ml)	Cephalexine (10 µg/ml)[c]	Cephaloridine (20 µg/ml)
1089	17.9	27.7	2.4	1.9	3.4	0.9c	2.3
1098	22.8	15.5	4.6	7.7	1.6	1.5	2.1
1097	11.3	3.1	2.1	2.5	2.3	1.4	1.2
1101	97.6	42.0	5.7	14.3	13.6	1.1	10.4
1100	210.5	56.2	8.6	7.0	16.0	0.8	22.4
1103	20.3	5.1	0.5	0.5	0.2	1.0	0.8
1110	3.6	4.8	3.8	4.1	6.4	1.1	3.6
1111	34.7	18.3	9.7	13.4	8.6	2.6	6.8
1066[b]	1.1	1.2	1.4	1.4	1.5	0.6	1.0

[a] Results expressed as stimulation index $\left(\dfrac{\text{cpm with drug}}{\text{cpm without drug}} \right)$

[b] Representative of non-allergic patients

[c] Inhibits lymphocyte proliferation even at low doses

reaction, although detecting anticephalosporin antibodies of the IgG and IgM classes, is probably of little clinical relevance. As already indicated above, using paper discs coated with cefuroxime- or cefotaxime-HSA conjugates, we were unable to detect specific IgE antibodies in the sera of allergic patients with high titers of anti-BPO IgE in the RAST assay (SCHNEIDER and DE WECK 1981).

Cephalosporins are also able to stimulate lymphocytes from penicillin-sensitive patients SCHNEIDER and DE WECK 1981). In this case, we observed extensive cross-reactivity among various penicillins and cephalosporins, suggesting that the lymphocyte recognition operates at the level of the nucleus rather than at that of the acyl side chain (Table 9).

D. Conclusions

The immune reactions of man and experimental animals to penicillins and cephalosporins have generated a considerable number of studies over the past 20 years. Apart from their clinical importance and relevance for antibiotic therapy, these studies have shown the model character of penicillin allergy for immunology in general. The immune response against penicillin-derived determinants remains the most frequent human response against chemically defined antigenic determinants, and its study continues to be of great help in identifying cellular and molecular events involved in the allergic process.

References

Abraham GN, Petz LD, Fudenberg HH (1980) Cephalothin hypersensitivity associated with anti-cephalothin antibodies. Int Arch Allergy Appl Immunol 34:65

Abraham GN, Petz LD, Fudenberg HH (1980b) Immunohematological cross-allergenicity between penicillin and cephalothin in humans. Clin exp Immunol 3:343

Adkinson NF Jr (1975) Recent developments in the use of RAST for determining hypersensitivity to penicillin. In: Evans R (ed) Advances in diagnosis of allergy: RAST. Symposia Specialists, Miami, p 125

Adkinson NF Jr (1976) A guide to skin testing for penicillin allergy. Med Times 104:164

Adkinson NF Jr (1980) The effects on human health of subtherapeutic use of antimicrobials animal feed. Nat Acad Sci USA 301

Adkinson NF Jr, Thompson WL, Maddrey WC, Lichtenstein LM (1973) Routine use of penicillin skin testing in an inpatient service. N Engl J Med 285:22

Ahlstedt S, Kristofferson A (1979) Experimental evidence for a decreased incidence of penicillin allergy by use of pure penicillins. Infection 7 (Suppl 5):499

Ahlstedt S, Kristofferson A, Svärd PO, Thor L, Oertengren B (1976) Ampicillin polymers as elicitors of passive cutaneous anaphylaxis. Int Arch Allergy Appl Immunol 51:131

Ahlstedt S, Kristofferson A, Svärd PO, Strannegard O (1977) Immunological properties of ampicillin polymers. Int Arch Allergy Appl Immunol 53:247

Ahlstedt S, Kristofferson A, Pettersson E (1979) Antigens in penicillin allergy. III. Antigens and antibody levels in mice treated with pure and contaminated penicillins. Int Arch Allergy Appl Immunol 58:20

Ahlstedt S, Kristofferson A, Hall E, Hall E (1980a) Antigens in penicillin allergy. V. On the relative allergenic potency of antigens carrying penicilloyl determinants derived from azidocillin, ampicillin and benzylpenicillin. Int Archs Allergy Appl Immunol 61:91

Ahlstedt S, Ekström B, Svärd PO, Sjöberg B, Kristofferson A, Oertengren B (1980b) New aspects on antigens in penicillin allergy. CRC Crit Rev Toxicol 7:219

Ahlstedt S, Bjursten LM, Hanson LA, Lidin-Janson G, Mobacken H, Belin L (1981) Evaluation of circulating immune complex-like material for development of skin reactions in connection with penicillin therapy. Int Arch Allergy Appl Immunol 64:195

Almeyda J, Levantine A (1972) Drug reactions XIX. Adverse cutaneous reactions to the penicillins – ampicillin rashes. Br J Dermatol 87:293

Amos H (1973) Diagnosis of allergic drug reactions. Int Arch Allergy Appl Immunol 45:218

Anderson-Lund BM, Bergan T (1975) Temporary skin reactions to penicillins during the acute stage of infectious mononucleosis. Scand J Infect Dis 7:21

Anderson AB (1947) Anaphylactic purpura following intramuscular penicillin therapy. Med J Australia March 8:305

Andrassy K, Scherz M, Ritz E, Walter E, Hasper B, Storch H, Wömel W (1976) Penicillin-induced coagulation disorder. Lancet 2:1039

Appel GB (1980) A decade of penicillin-related acute interstitial nephritis – more questions than answers. Clin Nephrol 13:151

Appel GB, Woda BA, Neu HC (1978) Acute interstitial nephritis associated with carbenicillin therapy. Arch Intern Med 138:1265

Arndt KA, Jick H (1976) Rates of cutaneous reactions to drugs. A report from the Boston collaborative drug surveillance program. JAMA 235:918

Assem ESK, Schild HA (1968) Detection of allergy to penicillin and other antigens by passive sensitization and histamine release from human and monkey lung. Br Med J 3:272

Assem ESK, Vickers MR (1972) Serum IgE and other in vitro tests in drug allergy. Clin Allergy 2:325

Assem ESK, Vickers MR (1974) Tests for penicillin allergy in man. II. The immunological cross-reaction between penicillins and cephalosporins. Immunology 27:255

Assem ESK, Vickers MR (1975) Investigation of the response to some haptenic determinants in penicillin allergy by skin and in vitro allergy tests. Clin Allergy 5:43

Aster RH (1977) Thrombocytopenia due to platelet loss. In: Williams WJ, Betzler E, Erslev AJ, Rundles RW (eds) Hematology. McGraw-Hill, New York

Atsumi T, Adachi M, Kinoshita Y, Kawasaki M, Horiuchi Y (1967) The heterogeneity of combining sites of anti-benzylpenicilloyl antibodies obtained from individual rabbits. Changes in combining sites of G and M antibodies during the immune response. J Immunol 101:1016

Bahman J, Kohout E (1973) Apparent penicillin-induce arrest of mature bone marrow elements. Br Med J 2:26

Baldwin DS, Levine BB, McCluskey RT, Gallo GR (1968) Renal failure and interstitial nephritis due to penicillin and methicillin. N Engl J Med 279:1254

Bankl H, Jellinger K (1968) Schocktod nach oraler Penicillineinnahme. Wien Klin Wochenschr 80:43

Basomba A, Villalmanzo IG, Campos A, Pelaez A, Burglund A (1979) IgE antibodies against penicillin as determined by Phadebas RAST. Clin Allergy 9:515

Bass JW, Crowley DM, Stelle RW, Young FSH, Harden LB (1973) Adverse effects of orally administered ampicillin. J Pediatr 83:106

Batchelor FR, Dewdney JM (1968) Some aspects of penicillin allergy. Proc R Soc Lond 61:897

Batchelor FR, Cole M, Gazzard D, Rolinson GN (1962) Penicillin-like substances in preparations of 6-aminopenicillanic acid. Nature 195:954

Batchelor FR, Dewdney JM, Gazzard D (1965) Penicillin allergy: the formation of the penicilloyl determinant. Nature 206:362

Batchelor FR, Dewdney JM, Weston RD, Wheeler AW (1966) The immunogenicity of cephalosporin derivatives and their cross reaction with penicillin. Immunology 10:21

Batchelor FR, Dewdney JM, Feinberg JG, Weston RD (1967) A penicilloylated protein impurity as a source of allergy to benzyl penicillin and 6-aminopenicillanic acid. Lancet 1:1175

Batchelor RCL, Horne GO, Rogerson HL (1951) An unusual reaction to procaine penicillin in aqueous suspension. Lancet 261:195

Batson JM (1960) Anaphylactoid reactions to oral administration of penicillin. N Engl J Med 262:590

Beckmann H (1971) Exantheme unter der Behandlung mit Ampicillin. MMW 113:1423

Bell RC (1954) Sudden death following injection of procaine penicillin. Lancet 266:13

Bell RC, Rannie I, Wynne NA (1954) Adverse reactions to procaine penicillin in cats and man. Lancet 2:62

Benveniste J (1981) The human basophil degranulation test as an vitro method for the diagnosis of allergies. Clin Allergy 2:1

Bierlein KJ (956) Repeated anaphylactic reactions in a patient highly sensitized to penicillin. A case report. Ann Allergy 14:35

Bierman CW, Van Arsdel PP Jr, Hemphill B (1969) Penicillin allergy in children: the role of immunologic tests in its diagnosis. J Allergy Clin Immunol 43:267

Bierman CW, Pierson WE, Zeitz SJ, Hoffman LS, Van Arsdel PP Jr (1972) Reactions associated with ampicillin therapy. JAMA 220:1098

Bird GWG, Wingham J, Ginstone RF, Smith AJ (1975) Acute haemolytic anemia due to IgM and IgA penicillin antibody. Lancet 2:462

Bloch-Morot E, Burtin C, Lebel B, Saurat JM, Paupe J (1977) Liberation anaphylactique d'histamine par la penicilline a partir des basophiles humains. Ann Med Nancy 16:239

Blum G, de Weck AL (1966) Über den Zusammenhang von Dermatomykosen mit der Penicillin-Überempfindlichkeit. Dermatologica 133:461

Boger WP, Sherman WB, Schiller IW et al. (1953) Allergic reactions to penicillin. A panel discussion. J Allergy 24:383

Border WA, Lehman DH, Egan JD (1974) Antitubular basement menbrane antibodies in methicillin-associated interstitial nephritis. N Engl J Med 291:381

Boston Collaborative Drug Surveillance Program (1972) Excess of ampicillin rashes associated with allopurinol or hyperuricemia. N Engl J Med 286:505

Boston Collaborative Drug Surveillance Program (1973) Drug-induced anaphylaxis: a comparative study. JAMA 224:613

Boyd JF, Butcher BT, Stewart GT (1973) The nephrotoxic effect of cephaloridine and its polymers. Int J Clin Pharmacol Biopharm 7:307

Brandriss MW, Smith JW, Steinman HG (1965) Common antigenic determinants of penicillin G, cephalothin and 6-aminopenicillanic acid in rabbits. J Immunol 94:696

Bredt J (1965) Akute nicht-allergische Reaktionen bei Anwendung von Depot-Penicillin. Dtsch Med Wochenschr 90:1559

Brogard JM, Bergoend H, Basset A (1969) Tolérance du traitement par la cephaloridine. Etude clinique et application du test de Shelley aux recherches de sensibilisation croisée entre pénicilline et céphaloridine. Nouv Presse Med 77:1539

Brooks AP (1974) Thrombocytopenia during treatment with ampicillin. Lancet 2:723

Brown BC, Price EV, Moore MB (1964) Penicilloyl-polylysine as an intradermal test of penicillin sensitivity. JAMA 189:599

Brown CH, Bradshaw MW, Natelson EA, Alfrey CP Jr, Williams CW Jr (1976) Defective platelet function following the administration of penicillin compounds. Blood 47:949

Brown EA (1948) Reactions to penicillins; a review of the literature 1943–1948. Ann Allergy 6:723

Brown GL, Kanware BS (1967) Drug rashes in glandular fever. Lancet 2:1418

Budd MA, Parker CW, Norden CW (1964) Evaluation of intradermal skin tests in penicillin hypersensitivity. JAMA 190:203

Bundgaard H (1971 a) Imidazole-catalyzed isomerization of penicillins into penicillenic acids. Tetrahedron Lett 48:4613

Bundgaard H (1971 b) Kinetic demonstration of a metastable intermediate in isomerization of penicillin to penicillenic acid in aqueous solution. J Pharm Sci 60:1273

Bundgaard H (1972 a) Penicillin allergy. Dan Tidsskr Farm 46:85

Bundgaard H (1972 b) Penicillin allergy: imidazole-catalysed formation of the penicilloyl determinant. J Pharm Pharmacol 24:985

Bundgaard H (1974) Spectrophotometric determination of ampicillin sodium in the presence of its degradation and polymerization products. J Pharm Pharmacol 26:385

Bundgaard H (1975) Chemical studies related to cephalosporin allergy. I. Kinetics of aminolysis of cephalosporins and effect of C-3 substituents on beta-lactam reactivity. Arch Pharm 3:94

Bundgaard H (1976a) Colorimetric analysis of immunogenic impurities in acetylsalicylic acid. J Pharm Pharmacol 28:544

Bundgaard H (1976b) Polymerization of penicillins: kinetics and mechanism of di- and polymerization of ampicillin in aqueous solution. Acta Pharm Suec 13:9

Bundgaard H (1976c) Hydrolysis and intramolecular aminolysis of cephalexin and cephaloglycin in aqueous solution. Arch Pharm 4:25

Bundgaard H (1976d) Hydrolysis and intramolecular aminolysis of cephalexin and cephaloglycin in aqueous solution. Arch Pharm 4:25

Bundgaard H (1976e) Chemical studies related to cephalosporin allergy. II. Competitive amine-catalyzed intra- and intermolecular aminolysis of cephalexin and cephaloglycin in aqueous solution. Acta Pharm Suec 13:299

Bundgaard H (1977) Penicillin allergy. Kinetics of penicilloylation of serum albumins by various penicillins. Acta Pharm Suec 14:391

Bundgaard H (1977a) Polymerization of penicillins. II. Kinetics and mechanism of dimerization and self-catalyzed hydrolysis of amoxycillin in aqueous solution. Acta Pharm Suec 14:47

Bundgaard H (1977b) Polymerization of penicillins. III. Structural effects influencing rate of dimerization of amino-penicillins in aqueous solution. Acta Pharm Suec 14:67

Bundgaard H (1977c) Quantitative determination of amino-penicillins in the presence of their degradation and polymerization products. Arch Pharm 5:141

Bundgaard H (1978) Impurities as factor in therapeutic equivalence of drugs: Analysis of ampicillin formulations for antigenic polymerization products. Arch Pharm 6:63

Bundgaard H, Larsen C (1977) Polymerization of penicillins. IV. Separration, isolation and characterization of ampicillin polymers formed in aqueous solution. J Chromatogr 132:51

Bundgaard H, Larsen C (1978a) Kinetics and mechanisms of the sucrose-accelerated degradation of penicillins in aqueous solution. Int J Pharm 1:95

Bundgaard H, Larsen C (1978b) Kinetics and mechanism of reaction of benzylpenicillin and ampicillin with carbohydrates and polyhydric alcohols in aqueous solution. Arch Pharm 6:184

Burton JR, Lichtenstein NS, Colvin RB (1974) Acute interstitial nephritis from oxacillin. Johns Hopkins Med J 134:58

Butcher BT, Stewart GT (1969) Immunochemical properties of macromolecular residues in beta-lactam antibiotics. Antimicrob. Agents Chemother 8:515

Butcher BT, Stewart GT (1970) Experimental studies on macromolecules from beta-lactam antibiotics. In: Stewart GT, McGovern JP (eds) Penicillin allergy. Thomas, Springfield, p 111

Butcher BT, Stanfield MK, Stewart GT, Zemelman R (1971) Antibiotic polymers: alpha-amino-benzylpenicillin (ampicillin). Mol Cryst Liq Cryst 12:321

Butler TC, Dudley KH, Johnson D (1972) Chemical studies of potential relevance to penicillin hypersensitivity: kinetics of formation and disappearance of benzylpenicillenic acid and its derivatives in solutions of benzylpenicillin. J Pharmacol Exp Ther 181:201

Butterly JM, Fishman L (1972) Jarisch-Herxheimer reaction following penicillin therapy in case of symphilitic aortitis. JAMA 148:370

Cameron SJ, Richmond J (1971) Ampicillin hypersensitivity in lymphatic leukemia. Scott Med J 16:425

Campbell AB, Soyka LF (1977) More comments on the ampicillin rash problem. Pediatrics 59:638

Caron EA (1963) The role of penicillenic acid and penicillamine in contact-type sensitivity to penicillin. Immunology 6:81

Carpenter J (1980) Neutropenia induced by semisynthetic penicillin. South Med J 73:745

Carre IJ, Squire JR (1956) Anuria ascribed to acute tubular necrosis in infancy and early childhood. Arch Dis Childh 31:512

Cazenave JP, Reimers HJ, Senyi AF, Hirsch J, Packham MA, Unstard JF (1976) Effects of penicillin G and cephalothin on platelet function in vivo. Proc Soc Exp Biol Med 152:641

Chesney RW, Chesney PJ (1976) Methicillin-associated nephritis. Clinical rarity or common entity. Clin Pediatr 15:1013

Chisholm DR, English AR, McLean NA (1961) Immunologic response of rabbits to 6-aminopenicillanic acid. J Allergy 32:333

Chu JY (1977) The mechanism of oxacillin-induced neutropenia. J Pediatr 90:668

Chu WC, Cutting WC (1946) Allergic sensitization to penicillin: experimental results. Proc Soc Exp Biol Med 63:347

Chusid MJ, Atkins E (1972) Studies on the mechanism of penicillin-induced fever. J Exp Med 136:227

Clarke HT, Johnson JR, Robinson R (1949) The chemistry of penicillin. Princeton University, Princeton

Cluff LE, Johnson JE (1964) Drug fever. Prog Allergy 8:149

Coleman M, Siegel BB (1955) Studies in penicillin hypersensitivity. II. The significance of penicillin as a contaminant. J Allergy 26:253

Coleman M, Siegel BB (1956) Studies in penicillin hypersensitivity. III. The influence of parenterally administered antihistamines on contralateral passive transfer reactions to penicillin. J Allergy 27:27

Coleman WP, Swineford O Jr (1956) Penicillin hypersensitivity: brief review and report of an extreme case. Va Med Monthly 83:6

Colvin B, Rogers M, Layton C (1974a) Benzylpenicillin-induced leukopenia: complication of treatment of bacterial endocarditis. Br Heart J 36:216

Colvin RB, Buton JR, Hyslop NE Jr (1974b) Penicillin-associated interstitial nephritis. Ann Intern Med 81:404

Cook FV, Farrar WE, Kreutner A (1979) Hemorrhagic cystitis and ureteritis and interstitial nephritis associated with administration of penicillin G. J Urol 122:110

Corcos JM, Soler-Bechara J, Mayer K, Freyberg RH, Goldstein R, Jaffe I (1964) Neutrophilic agranulocytosis during administration of penicillin. JAMA 189:265

Corran PH, Waley SJ (1975) The reaction of penicillin with proteins. Biochem J 149:357

Couteaux-Dumont C, Poncelet-Maton E, Rademecker M (1974) Immunoglobulines E et allergie a la penicilline. Rev Franc Allergol 14:71

Cream JJ, Turk JL (1971) A review of the evidence for immune complex deposition as a cause of skin disease in man. Clin Allergy 1:235

Cressman WA, Sugita ET, Doluisio JT, Niebergall PJ (1966) Complexation of penicillins and penicilloic acids by cupric ion. J Pharm Pharmacol 18:801

Croydon EAP, Wheeler AW, Grimshaw JJ, Atkins W, Cowan MA, Geddes AM, Jain S, Yassa JG, Beveridge GW, Gray JA, Murdoch JMC, Pullen H, Rowell NR, Stevenson J (1973) Prospective study of ampicillin rash. Report from a collaborative study group. Br Med J 1:7

Dandliker WB, Halbert SP, Florin MC, Alonso R, Shapiro HC (1965) Study of penicillin antibodies by fluorescence polarization and immunodiffusion. J Exp Med 122:1029

Davies RJ, Hendrick DJ, Pepys J (1974) Asthma due to inhaled chemical agents: ampicillin, benzylpenicillin, 6-aminopenicillanic acid and related substances. Clin Allergy 4:227

Davis A, Sieglman SJ, Hewitt WH (1964) Neutropenia reaction to cephalothin therapy. Antimicrob Agents Chemother 1963:272

Dawson RB, Segal BL (1966) Penicillin-induced hemolytic anemia. Arch Intern Med 118:575

De Haan P, Boorsam DM, Kalsbeck GL (1979) Penicillin hypersensitivity. Determination and classification of anti-penicillin antibodies by the enzyme-linked immunosorbent assay. Allergy 34:111

Delafuente JC, Panush RS, Caldwell JR (1979) Penicillin and cephalosporin immunogenicity in man. Ann Allergy 43:337

Delage C, Ivey NS (1972) Anaphylactic deaths: a clinicopathologic study of 43 cases. J Forensic Sci 17:525

De Swarte RD (1972) Drug allergy In: Patterson R (ed) Allergic diseases: diagnosis and management. Lippincott, Philadelphia, p 393

Dewdney JM (1977) Immunology of the antibiotics. In: Sela M (ed) The antigens, vol. IV. Academic Press, New York, p 73

Dewdney JM (1980) Pseudo-allergic reactions to antibiotics. In: Dukor P, Kallos P, Schlumberger MD, West GB (eds) PAR: Pseudo-allergic reactions, vol. 1, Karger, Basel, p 273

Dewdney JM, Smith H, Wheeler AW (1971) The formation of antigenic polymers in aqueous solutions of beta-lactam antibiotics. Immunology 21:517

de Weck AL (1962a) Studies on penicillin hypersensitivity. I. The specificity of rabbit "anti-penicillin" antibodies. Int Arch Allergy Appl Immunol 21:20

de Weck AL (1962b) Studies on penicillin hypersensitivity II. The role of the side chain in penicillin antigenicity. Int Arch Allergy Appl Immunol 21:28

de Weck AL (1962c) Etudes sur l'allergie a la penicilline. III. Nouveaux aspects immuno-chimiques. Schweiz Med Wochenschr 93:1155

de Weck AL (1964) Penicillin allergy: its detection by an improved hemagglutination technique. Nature 202:975

de Weck AL (1971) Critical evaluation of diagnostic methods in drug allergy. In: Allergology, proc. 8th Europ. congr. allergology, Int. Congr. Series 251. Excerpta Medica, Amsterdam, p 23

de Weck AL (1972) Immunochemical mechanisms in drug allergy. In: Dash CE, Jones HEH (eds) Mechanisms in drug allergy. Williams and Wilkins, Baltimore, p 3

de Weck AL (1973) Immunologische Mechanismen der allergischen Reaktion auf Antibiotika. Aktuelle Aspekte der Penicillintherapie. MMW 115:1650

de Weck AL (1975) Molecular mechanisms of T and B lymphocyte triggering. Int Arch Allergy Appl Immunol 49:247

de Weck AL (1976) Current problems in drug allergy. In: Beers RF, Bassett EG (eds) The role of immunological factors in infectious, allergic and autoimmune processes. Raven, New York, p 319

de Weck AL (1978a) Drug reactions. In: Samter M (ed) Immunological diseases, 3rd edn, Little, Brown, Boston, p 413

de Weck AL (1978b) Application du RAST dans l'allergie à la pénicilline. Med Hyg 36:118

de Weck AL (1979) Drug allergy. In Gupta S, Good RRA (eds) Cellular, molecular and clinical aspects of allergic disorders. Plenum, New York, p 355

de Weck AL, Blum G (1963) Un nouveau test cutane pour la detection de l'allergie a la penicilline. Praxis 3:67

de Weck AL, Blum G (1965) Recent clinical and immunological aspects of penicillin allergy. Int Arch Allergy Appl Immunol 27:221

de Weck AL, Eisen HN (1960) Some immunochemical properties of penicillenic acid, an antigenic determinant derived from penicillin. J Exp Med 112:1227

de Weck AL, Schneider CH (1969) Molecular and stereochemical properties required of antigens for the elicitation of allergic reactions. In Westphal O, Bock HE, Grundmann E (eds) Problems of immunological diseases. Springer, Berlin Heidelberg New York, p 32

de Weck AL, Schneider CH, Gutersohn J (1968) The role of penicilloylated protein impurities, penicillin polymers and dimers in penicillin allergy. Int Arch Allergy Appl Immunol 33:535

de Weck AL, Spengler H, Geczy AF (1974) Stimulation of penicillin-sensitive lymphocytes by antigenic determinants covalently bound to cell membranes. Monogr Allergy 8:120

Dicato MA, Ellman L (1975) Cephalothin-induced granulocytopenia. Ann Intern Med 83:671

Ditlove J, Weidmann P, Bernstein M (1977) Methicillin nephritis. Medicine 56:483

Dogliotti M (1968) An instance of fatal reaction to the penicillin scratch-test. Dermatologica 136:489

Dogliotti M (1975) Tests for penicillin allergy. Med Lett Drugs Ther 17:54

Dry J, Leynadier F, Damecour C, Pradalier A, Herman D (1976) Reaction pseudo-anaphy-lactique a la procaine-penicilline G. Nouv Presse Med 5:1401

Dudley KH, Butler TC, Johnson D (1971) Chemical studies of potential relevance to penicillin hypersensitivity: the fate of benzylpenicillenic acid in aqueous buffer solutions. J Pharmacol Exp Ther 179:505

Dudley KH, Butler TC, Johnson D (1974) Chemical studies of potential relevance to penicillin hypersensitivity: kinetic studies of methicillin, phenoxymethylpenicillin and their penicillenic acids. J Pharmacol Exp Ther 188:491

Dürsch F (1968) Search for protein contaminants in benzylpenicillin. Lancet 1:1005

Edwards RG, Spackman DA, Dewdney JM (1982) The development and use of three new radioallergosorbent tests in the diagnosis of penicillin allergy. Int Arch Allergy Appl Immunol 68:352

Eisenstader D, Hussar AE (1954) Severe anaphylactic reaction from oral penicillin. Am Pract Dig Treat 5:783

Ellis HV, Johnson AR, Moran NC (1970) Selective release of histamine from rat mast cells by several drugs. J Pharmacol Exp Ther 175:627

English AR, Huang HT, Sobin BA (1960) 6-Aminopenicillanic acid in urine after oral administration of penicillins. Proc Soc Exp Biol Med 104:405

Epp M (1959) Serological procedures for the detection of antibodies to penicillin. Science 130:1472

Epp M (1962) Penicillin antibody in maternal and cord bloods and its possible relationship to hypersensitivity. Immunology 5:287

Erfmeyer JE (1981) Adverse reactions to penicillins Ann Allergy 47:288, 294

Evans DA (1967) The lymphocyte stimulation test in penicillin hypersensitivity. J Allergy Clin Immunol 39:340

Feinberg JG (1968a) Allergy to antibiotics. I. Fact and conjecture on the sensitizing contaminants of penicillins and cephalosporins. Int Arch Allergy Appl Immunol 33:439

Feinberg JG (1968b) Allergy to antibiotics. II. Comparative immunogenicity of some penicillins. Int Arch Allergy Appl Immunol 33:444

Feinberg JG (1970) Experimental studies on penicillin allergy. In: Stewart GT, Mc Govern JP (eds) Penicillin allergy: clinical and immunologic aspects. Thomas, Springfield, p 90

Feinberg SM (1944) Penicillin allergy. On the probability of allergic reactions in fungus-sensitive individuals. J Allergy Clin Immunol 15:271

Fellner MJ (1967) Allergic cutaneous reactions to penicillin and their mechanisms. Dermatologica 135:362

Fellner MJ (1968) An immunologic study of selected penicillin reactions involving the skin. Arch Dermatol 97:503

Fellner MJ (1976) Penicillin allergy 1976: a review of reactions detection and current management. Int J Dermatol 15:497

Fellner MJ, Baer RL (1967) Immunologic studies in patients with serum sickness-like reactions following penicillin therapy. J Invest Dermatol 48:384

Fellner MJ, Prutkin L (1970) Morbilliform eruptions caused by penicillin. J Invest Dermatol 55:390

Fellner MJ, Baer RL, Ripps CS, Hirschorn K (1967a) Response of lymphocytes to penicillin: comparison with skin tests and circulating antibodies in man. Nature 216:803

Fellner MJ, Redmond AP, Levine BB, Baer RL (1967b) Immediate penicillin reactions associated with penicilloyl-specific skin-sensitizing antibodies and low titers of blocking (IgG) antibodies. J Allergy Clin Immunol 38:106

Fellner MJ, Ball EH, Allyn B, Baer RL (1969) Delayed hypersensitivity to penicillin. JAMA 210:2061

Fellner MJ, Fukuyama K, Moshell A, Klaus MV (1973) Intercellular antibodies in blood and epidermis. Br J Dermatol 89:115

Fernstrom AIB (1962) Studies on procaine allergy with reference to urticaria due to procaine penicillin treatment. Acta Derm Venerol 42:79

Fessel WJ (1972) Immunologic reactions in hyperuricemia. N Engl J Med 286:1218

Finke SR, Grieco MH, Connell JT, Smith EC, Sherman W (1965) Results of comparative skin tests with penicilloyl-polylysine and penicillin in patients with penicillin allergy. Am J Med 38:71

Foord RD (1967) A multicentre dose-response trial with cephaloridine. Postgrad Med J 43:63

Forbes CD, Mitchell R, Craig JA, McNicol GP (1972) Acute intravascular haemolysis associated with cephalexin therapy. Postgrad Med J 48:186

Frank MM, Schreiber AD, Atkinson JP (1977) Pathophysiology of immune hemolytic anemia. Ann Intern Med 87:210

Gabbert WR, Hopwood AH (1968) Ampicillin-induced rash in infectious mononucleosis. J Ky Med Ass 66:967

Galpin JE, Chow AW, Yoshikawa TT (1974) Pseudoanaphylactic reactions from inadvertent infusion of procaine penicillin G. Ann Intern Med 81:358

Galpin JE, Shinaberger JH, Stanley TM (1978) Acute interstitial nephritis due to methicillin. Am J Med 65:756

Ganier M, Lieberman P (1977) Infantile agammaglobulinemia and immediate hypersensitivity to penicillin G. JAMA 237:1852

Garratty G, Petz LD (1975) Drug-induced hemolytic anemia. Am J Med 58:398

Gattlen MC, Peter MV (1976) Allergische Reaktionen auf Penicilline und relativer Wert der diagnostischen Maßnahmen. Thesis, University of Bern

Gayet J (1967) Valeur du test cutane a la penicilloyl-polylysine pour le diagnostic biologique des allergies a la penicilline. These, Faculte de Medecine, Lyon

Geyman JP (1971) Anaphylactic reaction to oral penicillin. Calif Med 114:87

Gilbert DN, Gourley R, D'Agostino A (1970) Interstitial nephritis due to methicillin, penicillin and ampicillin. Ann Allergy 28:378

Girard JP (1968) Common antigenic determinants of penicillin G, ampicillin and the cephalosporins demonstrated in man. Int Arch Allergy Appl Immunol 33:428

Girard JP, Cuevas M (1975a) Analyse clinique et immunologique de 1047 reactions allergiques a la penicilline. Schweiz Med Wochenschr 105:953

Girard JP, Cuevas M (1975b) Immune response in the guinea pig to penicillin-autologous carrier proteins. Int Arch Allergy Appl Immunol 48:422

Gleich GJ, Stankievic RR (1969) Measurement of penicilloyl antibodies by radioimmunoprecipitation. Immunochemistry 6:85

Gorevic PD, Levine BB (1981) Desensitization of anaphylactic hypersensitivity specific for the penicilloate minor determinant of penicillin and carbenicillin. J Allergy Clin Immunol 68:267

Gralnick HR, McGinnis MH (1967) Immune cross-reactivity of penicillin and cephalothin. Nature 216:1026

Gralnick HR, McGinnis M, Halterman R (1972) Thrombocytopenia with sodium cephalothin therapy. Ann Intern Med 77:401

Grant NH, Clarke DH, Alburm HE (1962) Poly 6-aminopenicillanic acid. J Am Chem Soc 84:876

Green GR (1970) Antibiotic therapy in patients with a history of penicillin allergy. In: Stewart GT, McGovern JP (eds) Penicillin allergy: clinical and immunological aspects. Thomas, Springfield

Green GR, Rosenblum A (1971) Report of the penicillin study group, American Academy of Allergy. J Allergy Clin Immunol 48:331

Green GR, Rosenblum A, Sweet LC (1977) Evaluation of penicillin hypersensitivity: value of clinical history and skin testing with penicilloyl-polylysine and penicillin G. J Allergy Clin Immunol 60:339

Green RL, Lewis GE, Kraus SJ, Frederickson EL (1974) Elevated plasma procaine concentrations after administration of procaine penicillin G. N Engl J Med 291:223

Gregg I (1973) Ampicillin rash and influenza. Br Med J 295

Grieco MM (1967) Cross-allergenicity of the penicillins and cephalosporins. Arch Intern Med 119:141

Grosshans E, Hugues L, Samsoen M, Thierry R (1978) L'allergie aux Betalactamines. Protocole diagnostique in vivo. Correlations avec les tests in vitro (TTL et IgE specifiques). Ann Dermatol Venereol 105:609

Gudjonsson H (1972) Experiments to induce febrile Jarisch-Herxheimer reaction in syphilitic rabbits with penicillin and erythromycin. Acta Derm Venerol 52:493

Haddad ZH, Korotzer JL (1971) In vitro studies on the mechanism of penicillin and ampicillin drug reactions. Int Arch Allergy Appl Immunol 41:72

Haimovich J, Sela M, Dewdney JM, Batchelor FR (1967) Antipenicilloyl antibodies. Detection with penicilloylated bacteriophage and isolation with a specific immunoadsorbent. Nature 214:1369

Halpern B, Ky NT, Amache N (1967) Diagnosis of drug allergy in vitro with the lymphocyte transformation test. J Allergy Clin Immunol 40:168

Hamilton-Miller JMT, Newton GGF, Abraham EP (1970) Products of aminolysis and enzymatic hydrolysis of the cephalosporins. Biochem J 116:371

Heggie AD (1960) Incidence of circulating antibody to penicillin in penicillin hypersensitivity reactions. N Engl J Med 262:1160

Heitmann HJ, Kuwert E (1966) Die Lymphozytenkultur bei Penicillin-Allergie. Hautarzt 17:313

Herman R, Jick H (1979) Cutaneous reaction rates to penicillins. Oral versus parenteral. Cutis 24:232

Herz F, Kaplan E, Serdalian DA (1969) Loss of acetylcholinesterase activitiy in human erythrocytes treated with cephalothin. Acta Haematol 41:94

Hewitt WL, Finegold SM, Monzon OT (1961) Untoward side effects associated with methicillin therapy. In: Finland M, Savage GM (eds) Antimicrobial agents and chemotherapy. Braun-Brumfield, Ann Arbor, p 765

Hoigné R (1962) Allergische und pseudoallergische Reaktionen auf Penicillinpräparate. Allergy 17:521

Hoigné R (1962) Akute Nebenreaktionen auf Penicillinpräparate. Acta Med Scand 171:201

Hoigné R, Krebs A (1964) Simultaneous allergic (anaphylactic) and embolic-toxic reactions by accidental intravascular injection of procaine penicillin. Int Arch Allergy Suppl 24:48

Hoigné R, Schock K (1956) Anaphylaktischer Schock und akute nicht-allergische Reaktionen nach Procain-Penicillin. Schweiz Med Wochenschr 89:1350

Homayouni H, Gross PA, Setia U, Lynch TJ (1979) Leukopenia due to penicillin and cephalosporin homologues. Arch Intern Med 139:827

Horiuchi Y, Shibata K (1965) Immunochemical studies on the antigenic bindings of benzylpenicillin and five synthetic penicillins with proteins. Int Arch Allergy Appl Immunol 28:306

Hsi YJ, Kuo HY, Ouyang A (1966) Thrombocytopenia following administration of penicillin. Chin Med J 85:249

Hurley HJ (1963) A dental depot in penicillin hypersensitivity. Arch Dermatol 87:387

Hyslop NE, Milligan RJ (1974) Chromatography of penicillins, penicilloates, and penicilloylamides on dextran gels. Antimicrob Agents Chemother 5:617

Hylop NE, Milligan RJ, Calvert JF (1974) Antibody to penicillins: comparison of specificity of antisera to penicillanyl and penicilloyl determinants (Abstract). Fed Proc 33:785

Idsoe O (1958) Penicillin sensitivity reactions in Taiwan. Bull WHO 18:323

Idsoe G, Guthe T, Willcox RR, de Weck AL (1968) Nature and extent of penicillin side-reactions, with particular reference to fatalities from anaphylactic shock. Bull WHO 38:159

Igarashi H, Koizumi K, Muranaka M (1978) Eliciting antigenicities of benzylpenicillin, ampicillin and carbenicillin preparations examined with the reagin-mediated passive cutaneous anaphylaxis system. In Arch Allergy Appl Immunol 57:391

Iwata M, Serizawa J (1974) Immunological studies on Pivampicillin. Chemotherapy 22:388

Jarisch R, Roth A, Boltz A, Sandor I (1981) Diagnosis of penicillin allergy by means of Phadebas RAST penicilloyl G and V and skin tests. Clin Allergy 11:155

Jemal M, Hern SL, Knevel AM (1978) Demonstration of penicillamine as a product in benzylpenicillenic acid degradation in neutral media using differential pulse polarography. J Pharm Sci 67:302

Josephson AS (1960) The development of antibodies to penicillin in rabbits. J Exp Med 111:611

Juhlin L, Wide L (1979) Detection of penicillin allergy by radioallergosorbent test. Lancet 2:261

Juhlin L, Ahlstedt S, Andal L, Ekström B, Svärd PO, Wide L (1977) Antibody reactivity in penicillin-sensitive patients determined with different penicillin derivates. Int Arch Allergy Appl Immunol 54:19

Kabins SA, Eisenstein B, Cohen S (1965) Anaphylactoid reaction to an initial dose of sodium cephalothin. JAMA 193:159

Kaplan E, Weinstein L (1967) Anaphylaxis to cephaloridine in a nurse who prepared solutions of the drug. JAMA 200:75

Katz HI, Gill KA, Baxter DL, Moschella SL (1964) Indirect basophil degranulation test in penicillin allergy. JAMA 188:351

Kern RA, Wimberley NA Jr (1953) Penicillin reactions: their nature, growing importance, recognition, management and prevention. Am J Med Sci 226:357

Kerns DL, Shira JE, Go S, Summers RJ, Schwab JA, Plunket DC (1973) Ampicillin rashes in children. Am J Dis Child 125:187

Kerr RO, Cardamone J, Dalmasso AP, Kaplan ME (1972) Two mechanisms of erythrocyte destruction in penicillin-induced hemolytic anemia. N Engl J Med 287:1322

Klein KG, Parkin JD, Madaras F (1976) Studies on an acquired inhibition of factor VIII induced by penicillin allergy. Clin Exp Immunol 26:155

Klemola E (1970) Hypersensitivity reactions to ampicillin in cytomegalovirus mononucleosis. Scand J Infect Dis 2:29

Knudsen ET, Robinson OPW, Croydon EAP, Tees EC (1967) Cutaneous sensitivity to purified benzylpenicillin. Lancet 1:1184

Knudsen ET, Dewdney JM, Trafford JAP (1970) Reduction in incidence of ampicillin rash by purification of ampicillin. Br Med J 1:469

Koizumi K, Suzuki S, Fukuba S, Tadokoro K, Hirai K, Muranaka K (1980) Antigenicity of semisynthetic penicillin preparations to evoke systemic anaphylactic reactions in animal models. Allergy 35:657

Korotzer J, Haddad ZH (1970) In vitro detection of human IgE-mediated immediate hypersensitivity reactions to pollens and penicillin(s) by a modified rat mast cell degranulation technique. J Allergy Clin Immunol 45:126

Kraft D, Wide L (1976) Clinical patterns and results of radioallergosorbent test (RAST) and skin tests in penicillin allergy. Br J Dermatol 94:593

Kraft D, Wilson DV, Devey ME (1976) Penicillin allergy studies by a modified red-cell-linked antigen-antiglobulin reaction. Int Arch Allergy Appl Immunol 52:248

Kraft D, Roth A, Mischer P, Pichler H, Ebner H (1977) Specific and total serum IgE measurements in the diagnosis of penicillin allergy. A long-term follow-up study. Clin Allergy 7:21

Kraft D, Berglund A, Rumpold H, Roth A, Ebner H (1981) Radioallergosorbent test with conjugates specific for minor haptenic determinants in the diagnosis of IgE-mediated penicillin allergy in man. Clin Allergy 11:579

Krapin D (1962) Anaphylaxis with orally administered penicillin. N Engl J Med 267:820

Kraus SJ, Green RL (1976) Pseudoanaphylactic reactions with procaine penicillin. Cutis 17:765

Kristofferson A, Ahlstedt S, Pettersson E, Svärd PO (1977a) Antigens in penicillin allergy. I. A radioimmunoassay for detection of penicilloylated protein contaminants in penicillin preparations. Int Arch Allergy Appl Immunol 55:13

Kristofferson A, Ahlstedt S, Svärd PO (1977b) Antigens in penicillin allergy. II. The influence of the number of penicilloyl residues on the antigenicity of macromolecules as determined by radioimmunoassay (RIA), passive cutaneous anaphylaxis (PCA) and antibody induction. Int Arch Allergy Appl Immunol 55:23

Kristofferson A, Ahlstedt S, Hall E (1980) Antigens in penicillin allergy. IV. Induction of IgE antibody response in mice after daily treatment with contaminated but not with pure penicillin. Int Arch Allergy Appl Immunol 60:295

Kunz ML, Girard JP, Kobayashi S (1966) Penicillin hypersensitivity. 3. Immunologic studies. J Allergy Clin Immunol 37:99

Kunz ML, Reisman RE, Arbesman CE (1967) Evaluation of penicillin hypersensitivity by two newer immunological procedures. J Allergy Clin Immunol 40:135

Kuwahara S, Mine Y, Nishida M (1970) Immunogenicity of cefazolin. Antimicrob Agents Chemother 374

Lai M, Rosner F, Ritz ND (1966) Hemolytic anemia due to antibodies to penicillin. JAMA 198:483

Lapresle C, Wal JM (1979) The binding of penicillin to albumin molecules in bisalbuminemia induced by penicillin therapy. Biochim Biophys Acta 586:106

Larsen C, Bundgaard H (1977) Polymerization of penicillins. VI. Time course of formation of antigenic di- and polymerization products in aqueous ampicillin sodium solutions. Arch Pharm 5:201

Larsen C, Bundgaard H (1978a) Polymerization of penicillins. V. Separation, identification and quantitative determination of antigenic polymerization products in ampicillin sodium preparations by high-performance liquid chromatography. J Chromatogr 147:143

Larsen C, Bundgaard H (1978 b) Penicilloyl ester intermediates in glucose- und fructose-accelerated degradation of benzylpenicillin in aqueous solution. Arch Pharm 6:33

Leonhardi G, Matner T (1969) Ergebnisse von Hauttestungen mit Penicilloyl-Polylysin (PPL) auf Penicillinverträglichkeit. Hautarzt 20:21

Lerner WD, Stander M (1973) Delayed hypersensitivity to penicillin and cephalosporin in the guinea pig (abstract). Clin Res 21:63

Leventhal JM, Silken AB (1975) Oxacillin-induced neutropenia in children. J Pediatr 89:769

Levin AS, Weiner R, Fudenberg HH, Spath P, Petz L (1971) Granulocytopenia caused by anticephalothin antibodies (abstract). Clin Res 19:424

Levine BB (1960 a) Studies on the mechanism of the formation of the penicillin antigen. I. Delayed allergic cross-reactions among penicillin G and its degradation products. J Exp Med 112:1131

Levine BB (1960 b) Degradation of benzylpenicillin at pH 7.5 to D-benzyl penicilloic acid. Nature 187:939

Levine BB (1960 c) Formation of D-penicillamine-cysteine mixed disulphide by reaction of D-benzylpenicilloic acide with cysteine Nature 187:940

Levine BB (1961) Studies on the formation of the penicillin antigen. II. Some reactions of D-benzylpenicillenic acid in aqueous solution at pH 7.5. Arch Biochem Biophys 93:50

Levine BB (1962) N(a-D-penicilloyl)amines as univalent hapten inhibitors of antibody-dependent allergic reactions to penicillin. J Med Chem 5:1025

Levine BB (1963) Studies on the dimensions of the rabbit anti-benzyl penicilloyl antibody combining sites. J Exp Med 117:161

Levine BB (1964) The preparation of penicilloyl-polylysines, skin test reagents for the clinical evaluation of penicillin hypersensitivity. J Med Chem 7:675

Levine BB (1965) Immunochemical mechanisms involved in penicillin Hypersensitivity in experimental animals and in human beings. Fred Proc 24:45

Levine BB (1966 a) Immunochemical mechanisms of drug allergy. Annu Rev Med 17:23

Levine BB (1966 b) Immunologic mechanisms of penicillin allergy. A haptenic model system for the study of allergic diseases in man. N Engl J Med 275:1115

Levine BB (1973) Antigenicity and cross reactivitiy of penicillins and cephalosporins. J Infect Dis 128:364

Levine BB (1976) Immunochemical mechanisms of drug allergy. In: Miescher PA, Müller-Eberhard HJ (eds) Textbook of immunopathology, 2nd edn, Grune and Stratton, New York, p 403

Levine BB, Ovary Z (1961) Studies on the mechanisms of formation of the penicillin antigen. III. The N-(D-2a-benzylpenicilloyl) group as an antigenic determinant responsible for hypersensitivity to penicillin G. J Exp Med 114:875

Levine BB, Price VH (1964) Studies on the immunological mechanisms of penicillin allergy. II. Antigenic specificities of allergic wheal-and-flare skin responses in patients with histories of penicillin allergy. Immunology 7:542

Levine BB, Redmond A (1967) Immunochemical mechanisms of penicillin-induced Coombs positivity and hemolytic anemia in man. Int Arch Allergy Appl Immunol 21:594

Levine BB, Redmond AP (1968) The nature of the antigen-antibody complexes initiating the specific wheal-and-flare reaction in sensitized man. J Clin Invest 47:556

Levine BB, Redmond AP (1969) Minor haptenic determinant-specific reagins of penicillin hypersensitivity in man. Int Arch Allergy Appl Immunol 35:445

Levine BB, Zolov D (1969) Prediction of penicillin allergy by immunological tests. J Allergy 43:231

Levine BB, Redmond AP, Fellner MJ, Voss HE, Levytska V (1966 a) Penicillin allergy and the heterogeneous immune responses of man to benzylpenicillin. J Clin Invest 45:1895

Levine BB, Fellner MJ, Levytska V (1966 b) Benzylpenicilloyl-specific serum antibodies in man. I. Development of a sensitive hemagglutination assay method and haptenic specificities of antibodies. J Immunol 96:707

Levine BB, Fellner MJ, Levytska V, Franklin EC, Alisberg N (1966 c) Benzylpenicilloyl-specific serum antibodies in man. II. Sensitivity of the hemagglutination assay method, molecular classes of the antibodies detected and antibody titers of randomly selected patients. J Immunol 96:719

Levine BB, Redmond AP, Voss HE, Zolov DM (1967) Prediction of penicillin allergy by immunological tests. Ann NY Acad Sci 145:298

Levine MI, Perri J, Anthony JJ (1960) A fatal anaphylactic reaction to oral penicillin. H Allergy 31:487

Ley AB, Harris JP, Brinkley M, Liles B, Jack JA, Cahan A (1958) Circulating antibodies directed against penicillin. Science 127:1118

Liakopoulou A, Vilim AB (1976) Immunological properties of dialysis retentates from penicillin. Allergy 31:255

Lindemayr H, Knobler R, Kraft D, Baumgartner W (1981) Challenge of penicillin-allergic volunteers with penicillin-contaminated meat. Allergy 36:471

Linton AL, Clark WF, Driedger AA (1980) Acute interstitial nephritis due to drugs. Ann Intern Med 93:735

Lischka G, Gottmann-Lückerath L (1972) Positiver Lymphocyten-transformationstest mit Penicillin = Penicillinallergie. Arch Dermatol 243:101

Locher GW, Schneider CH, de Weck AL (1969) Hemmung allergischer Reaktionen auf Penicillin durch Penicilloyl-a-Amide und chemisch verwandter Substanzen. Z Immunitätsforsch Immunobiol 138:299

Luton EF (1964) Methicillin tolerance after penicillin G anaphylaxis. JAMA 190:39

Lyons C (1943) First reporter allergic reaction to Pn. JAMA 123:1007

Maganzini HC (1957) Anaphylactoid reactions to penicillins V and G administered orally. N Engl J Med 256:52

Markowitz SM, Rothkopf M, Holden FD (1975) Nafcillin-induced agranulocytosis. JAMA 232:1150

Martin AF, Morris JY, Page MI (1976) Intra- and intermolecular general dose catalysis in the aminolysis of benzylpenicillin. J Chem Soc 13:495

Matheson A, Elegant L (1955) Penicillin reactions in children. A study of the value of the skin test in penicillin sensitization. J Allergy 26:415

Matner T, Leonhardi G (1966) Hauttestung auf urtikarielle Penicillin-Überempfindlichkeit. Arch Klin Exp Derm 227:349

Mc Cluskey RT, Colvin RB (1978) Immunological spects of renal tubular and interstitial diseases. Annu Rev Med 29:191

McGovern JP, Dukes CD, Wagelie RG (1964) Serologic studies on penicillin hypersensitivity in human beings. Ann Allergy 22:252

McKenzie H, Parratt D, White RG (1976) IgM and IgG antibody levels to ampicillin in patients with infectious mononucleosis. Clin Exp Immunol 26:214

Menke HE, Pepplinkhuizer L (1974) Acute nonallergic reaction to aqueous procaine penicillin. Lancet I:723

Merrill SL, Davis A, Smoleus B, Finegold SM (1966) Cephalothin in serious bacterial infection. Ann Intern Med 64:1

Mine Y, Nishida M, Goto S, Kuwahara S (1970) Cefazolin, a new semisynthetic cephalosporin antibiotic. IV. Antigenicity of cefazolin and its cross reactivity with benzylpenicillin, ampicillin and cephaloridine. J Antibiot 23:195

Minikin WP, Lynch PJ (1969) Allergic reactions to penicillin in milk. JAMA 209:1089

Mirel RD, Garnick MB (1978) Skin tests, penicillin G procaine and pseudoanaphylaxis. JAMA 240:1751

Mock D, Abbot D, Choong A (1979) Penicillin-induced neutropenia. J Can Dent Assoc 7:334

Moellering RC Jr (1975) Penicillin allergy. Drug Ther Bull 13:9

Moellering RC Jr, Swartz MN (1976) Drug therapy. The newer cephalosporins. N Engl J Med 294:24

Molinari M, Schneider CH, de Weck AL, Gruden E, Pfeuti C (1973) Über pseudomonovalente penicilloyl-kohlehydrate. Z Immun Forsch 146:225

Möller NE (1978) Carbenicillin-induced haemorrhagic cystitis. Lancet 2:946

Molthan L (1969) Reactions to cephalothins in patients with hemagglutinating penicillin antibodies. (Abstract). Ann Intern Med 70:1090

Moss MO (1964) Reaction of 6-amino penicillanic acid with frequentin. Experientia 20:605

Müller E, de Weck AL, Schneider CH (1970) Die immunologische Aktivität von Rückständen aus Penicillinfermentationsmedien und ihre Bedeutung für die Penicillinallergie. Z Immunitätsforsch Immunbiol 140:18

Mulroy R (1973) Amoxycillin rash in infectious mononucleosis. Br Med J I:554

Munro AC, Dewdney JM, Smith H, Wheeler AW (1976) Antigenic properties of polymers formed by beta-lactam antibiotics. Int Arch Allergy Appl Immunol 50:192

Muranaka M, Igarashi H, Koizumi K, Okumura H, Takeda K, Suzuki S (1974) Elicitation of homologous passive cutaneous anaphylactic reactions by a benzylpenicillin preparation. J Allergy Clin Immunol 54:239

Muranaka M, Suzuki S, Koizumi K, Igarashi H, Okumura H, Takeda K, Tadekoro K, Horiuchi Y (1978) Benzylpenicillin preparations can evoke a systemic anaphylactic reaction in guinea pigs. J Allergy Clin Immunol 62:276

Muranaka M, Tadokoro K, Hirai K, Koizumi K, Fukuba S, Suzuki S (1980) IgE antibodies produced in mice instrumental in analyses of antigenicity of cephalothin preparations. Int Arch Allergy Appl Immunol 63:275

Murphy TF (1979) Ampicillin rash and hyperuricemia. Ann Intern Med 91:324

Nakagawa T, Blaser K, de Weck AL (1980) Effect of epitope density on the induction of the IgE immune response in mice. Int Arch Allergy Appl Immunol 63:212

Nazareth I, Mortimer P, McKendrick GDW (1972) Ampicillin sensitivity in infectious mononucleosis – temporary or permanent? Scand J Infect Dis 4:229

Neftel KA, Wälti M, Spengler H, von Felten A, Weitzman SA, Bürgi H, de Weck AL (1981) Neutropenia after penicillins: toxic or immune-mediated? Klin Wochenschr 59:877

Neftel KA, Wälti M, Spengler H, de Weck AL (1982) Sensitization against penicillin G in intravenous therapy is dependent on the mode of application. Lancet i:986

Nesmith LW, Davis JW (1968) Hemolytic anemia caused by penicillin. JAMA 203:81

Newton GGF, Abraham EP, Kuwabara S (1967) Preliminary observations on the formation of cephalosporoic acid. Antimicrob Agents Chemother 449

Nishida K, Kinoshita Y, Atsumi T, Shibata K, Horiuchi Y (1972) The analysis of combining sites of rabbit anti-benzylpenicilloyl antibodies. Immunochemistry 9:1195

Nordbring F, Johansson SGO, Epsmark A (1972) Raised serum levels of IgE in infectious mononucleosis. Scand J Infect Dis 4:119

O'Callaghan CH, Muggleton PW (1973) Flynn EH (ed) Cephalosporins and penicillin compounds: their chemistry and biology. Academic, New York, p 489

Ooi BS, First MR, Pesce AJ (1974) IgE levels in interstitial nephritis. Lancet I:1254

Ooi BS, Jao W, First MR (1975) Acute interstitial nephritis. A clinical and pathologic study based on renal biopsies. Am J Med 59:614

Orchard RT, Rooker G (1974) Penicillin hypersensitivity nephritis. Lancet I:689

Ortiz L, Zamacona G, Garmilla C, Arellano MT (1974) Migration inhibition test in leucocytes from patients allergic to penicillin. J Immunol 113:993

Ottens H, de Haan E, Sengers CHJ (1971) A search for high molecular impurities in penicillin G. Int Arch Allergy Clin Immunol 41:575

Palomeque FE, Fulton J, Derbes VJ (1965) Penicillin sensitivity. Arch Dermatol 92:271

Parker AC, Richmond J (1976) Reduction in incidence of rash using polymer-free ampicillin. Br Med J 1:998

Parker CW (1966) Penicilloyl-polylysines. XXII. Preparation, properties and analytical procedure, with special reference to their use in human skin testing. Meth Med Res 66:192

Parker CW (1975) Drug allergy (3 parts) N Engl J Med 292:511

Parker CW (1980) Drug allergy. In: Parker CW (ed) Clinical immunology. Saunders, Philadelphia, p 1219

Parker CW, Thiel JA (1963) Studies in human penicillin allergy: a comparison of various penicilloyl-polylysines. J Lab Clin Med 62:482

Parker CW, de Weck AL, Kern M, Eisen HN (1962a) The preparation and some properties of penicillenic acid derivatives relevant to penicillin hypersensitivity. J Exp Med 115:803

Parker CW, Shapiro J, Kern M, Eisen HN (1962b) Hypersensitivity to penicillenic acid derivates in human beings with penicillin allergy. J Exp Med 115:821

Parry MF, Ball WD, Conde JE Jr (1963) Nafcillin nephritis. JAMA 225:178

Patel BM (1967) Skin rashes with infectious mononucleosis and ampicillin. Pediatrics 40:910

Paupe J, Charlas J, Burtin C, Soubrane C (1974) Le Touze P. Etude clinique et immunologique de 140 cas d'allergie a la penicilline chez l'enfant. Arch Fr Pediadr 31:175

Pedersen-Bjergaard J (1967) Cephalothin in the treatment of penicillin-sensitive patients. Allergy 22:299

Pedersen-Bjergaard J (1969) Specific hyposensitization of patients with penicillin allergy. Allergy 24:333

Pelner L (1959) Allergic reaction to poliomyelitis vaccine probably due to penicillin. N Eng J Med 260:230

Perelmutter L, Eisen AH (1970) Studies on histamine release from leukocytes of penicillin-sensitive individuals. Int Arch Allergy 38:104

Perkins RL, Saslaw S (1966) Experiences with cephalothin. Ann Intern Med 64:13

Perkins RL, Saslaw S, Mitchell WF, Sama JT (1965) Cephalothin therapy in penicillin-allergic patients (abstract). Clin Sci Mol Med 13:415

Peters GA, Moskowitz RW, Prickman LE, Carryer HM (1960) Fatal necrotizing angiitis associated with hypersensitivity to penicillin O and iodides. J Allergy Clin Immunol 31:455

Petersen BH, Graham J (1974) Immunologic cross-reactivity of cephalexin and penicillin. J Ky Med Assoc 83:860

Petz LD (1971) Immunological reactions of humans to cephalosporins. Postgr Med J Feb Suppl:64

Petz LD (1978) Immunologic cross-reactivity between penicillins and cephalosporins: a review. J Infect Dis 137 (Suppl):74

Petz LD, Fudenberg HH (1966) Coombs-positive hemolytic anemia caused by penicillin administration. N Engl J Med 274:171

Pevny J, Hartmann K, Schöpl F (1973) Ist bei nachgewiesener Penicillin-Allergie eine Therapie mit anderen Penicillinen vertretbar? Dtsch Med Wochenschr 98:1597

Pietzcker F, Kuner V (1975) Anaphylaxie nach epikutanem Ampicillin-Test. Z Hautkr 50:437

Portoles A, Perez UT, Ramos F, Lopez R, Espinosa M (1975) Penicillin immunogenicity in the presence of different pharmaceutical adjuvants. Int J Clin Pharmacol. Biopharm 11:7

Preud'homme J, Lunel J, Penicilline G (1969) Recherche des impuretes allergisantes. Therapie 24:531

Pullen H, Wright N, McMurdoch JC (1967) Hypersensitivity reactions to antibacterial drugs in infectious mononucleosis. Lancet 2:1176

Radermecker M, Salmon J (1966) Etude de la sero-agglutination d'hematies penicillinees chez l'homme allergique et non allergique a la penicilline. Allergy 21:285

Redmond AP, Levine BB (1967) The relationship between direct immediate skin tests and passive transfer tests in man. J Allergy 39:51

Redmond AP, Levine BB (1968) Delayed skin reactions to benzylpenicillin in man. Int Arch Allergy 33:193

Reichlin S, Loveless MH, Kane EG (1953) Loeffler's syndrome following penicillin therapy. Ann Intern Med 38:113

Reisman RE, Arbesman CE (1968) Systemic allergic reactions due to the inhalation of penicillin. JAMA 203:986

Resnik SS, Shelley WB (1965) Penicillin hypersensitivity: detection by basophil response challenge. J invest Dermatol 45:269

Reyes MP, Palutke M, Lerner AM (1973) Granulocytopenia associated with carbenicillin. Am J Med 54:413

Ries CA, Rosenbaum TJ, Garratty G (1975) Penicillin-induced hemolytic anemia. JAMA 233:432

Robinson OPW (1968) Comparative cutaneous sensitivity studies in man with benzylpenicillin and its purified counterpart. Antimicrob Agents Chemother 7:550

Rose NR, Reisman RE, Witebsky E, Arbesman CE (1962) Serum sickness III. Characterization of antigens. J Allergy Clin Immunol 33:250

Rose NR, Giard JP, Kunz ML (1966) Tissue culture of lymphocytes from allergic patients. J Allergy 37:112

Rosenblum AH (1968) Penicillin allergy. A report of thirteen cases of severe reactions. J Allergy 42:309

Rostenberg A, Welch H (1945) A study of the type of hypersensitivity induced by penicillin. Am J Med Sci 210:158

Rothschild PD, Doty DB (1966) Cephalothin reaction after penicillin sensitization. JAMA 196:160

Rudolph AH, Price EV (1973) Penicillin reactions among patients in venereal disease clinics. JAMA 223:499

Rudzki E, Lukaziak B, Leszcynski W (1966) Penicillin hypersensitivity and hemagglutinating antibodies in workers at a penicillin factory. Allergy 20:206

Ruley EJ, Lisi LM (1974) Interstitial nephritis and renal failure due to ampicillin. J Pediatr 84:878

Saleh Y, Tischler E (1974) Severe anaphylactic reaction to intravenous cephaloridine in a pregnant patient. Med J Aust 2:490

Sanders WE, Johnson JE, Taggart JG (1974) Adverse reactions to cephalothin and cephapirin. Uniform occurrence on prolonged intravenous administration of high doses. N Engl J Med 290:424

Sarkany I Gaylarde PM (1978) Role of lymphocyte transformation in drug allergy. Australas J Dermatol 19:45

Saurat JH, Ponvert C, Burtin C, Soubrane C, Lebel B, Bencher F, Paupe J (1976a) Lymphocyte transformation, leukocyte migration, specific IgE, IgG and IgM before, during and after penicillin treatment without adverse reaction. Allergy 31:1

Saurat JH, Ponvert C, Lebel B, Paupe J (1976b) The penicillin antigens: presentation in the leukocyte migration test. Allergy 31:356

Schneider CH, de Weck AL (1965) A new chemical aspect of penicillin allergy: the direct reaction of penicillin with e-amino groups. Nature 208:57

Schneider CH, de Weck AL (1966a) Chemische Aspekte der Penicillinallergie: die direkte Penicilloylierung von e-Aminogruppen durch Penicilline bei pH 7,4. Helv Chim Acta 49:1695

Schneider CH, de Weck AL (1966b) Chemische Aspekte der Penicillin-Allergie: die direkte Bildung der Penicilloyl-Determinanten aus Penicillin. Helv Chim Acta 49:1707

Schneider CH, de Weck AL (1967) The reaction of benzylpenicillin with carbohydrates at neutral pH with a note on the immunogenicity of hapten polysaccharide conjugates. Immunochemistry 4:331

Schneider CH, de Weck AL (1968) Studies on the direct neutral penicilloylation of functional groups occurring on proteins. Biochim Biophys Acta 168:27

Schneider CH, de Weck AL (1970) Evaluation of intrinsic and extrinsic penicilloyl-specific immunogenicity of penicillins. The use of penicillin hydrolysis catalyzed by 3,6 bis(demethyl aminoethyl)catechol. Immunochemistry 7:157

Schneider CH, de Weck AL (1974) Imidazole and penicilloylation in penicillin allergy. J Pharm Pharmacol 26:379

Schneider CH, de Weck AL (1981) Allergy towards β-lactam antibiotics. In: Mitsuhashi S (ed) Beta-lactam antibiotics, JSSP. Springer, Berlin Heidelberg New York, p 299

Schneider CH, de Weck AL, Stauble E (1971) Carboxy-methylcellulose. Additives in penicillins and the elicitation of anaphylactic reactions. Experientia 27:167

Schneider CH, Pfeuti C, de Weck AL (1973) Aspects of formation of the D-penicillamine antigenic determinant from penicilloyl compounds. Helv Chim Acta 56:1235

Schneierson SS, Perlman E, Shore B (1964) Cephalotin antigenicity and cross-reactivity with penicillin G. Clin Med 71:1933

Scholand JF, Tennebaum JI, Cerilli GJ (1968) Anaphylaxis to cephalothin in a patient allergic to penicillin. JAMA 206:130

Schrier RW, Bulger RJ, Van Arsdel PP (1966) Nephropathy associated with penicillin and homologues. Ann Intern Med 64:116

Schuppli R (1958) Zur Frage der Überempfindlichkeit gegenüber Antibiotika, Pilzextrakten und verwandten Allergenen. Allerg Asthmaforsch 4:197

Schuppli R (1962) Über den Zusammenhang zwischen Penicillinallergien und Pilzinfektionen. Dtsch Med Wochenschr 87:333

Schwartz MH (1968) Aminolysis of benzylpenicillin by aliphatic diamines. J Pharm Sci 57:1209

Schwartz MH (1969) Chemical aspects of penicillin allergy. J Pharm Sci 58:643

Schwartz MH, Wu GM (1966) Kinetics of reactions involved in Penicillin allergy. I. Mechanism of reAction of penicillins and 6-aminopenicillanic acid with glycine in alkaline solution. J Pharm Sci 55:550

Shaltiel S, Mizrahi R, Stupp Y, Sela M (1970) Reduction in immunological manifestations of 6-aminopenicillanic acid by treatment with water-insoluble pronase. Eur J Biochem 14:509

Shaltiel S, Mizrahi R, Sela M (1971) On the immunological propterties of penicillins. Proc R Soc Lond B 179:411

Shapiro S, Siskind V, Slone D, Lewis GP, Jick H (1969) Drug rash with ampicillin and other penicillins. Lancet 2:969

Shapiro S, Slone D, Siskind V, Lewis GP, Jick H (1970) Ampicillin rashes. Lancet I:194

Shapiro S, Heinonen OP, Lawson DH (1972) Excess of ampicillin rashes associated with allopurinol or hyperuricemia. N Engl J Med 286:505

Sheiman L, Speilvogel AE, Horowitz HI (1968) Thrombocytopenia caused by cephalothin sodium. Occurrence in a penicillin-sensitive individual. JAMA 203:601

Shelley WB (1963) Indirect basophil degranulation test for allergy to penicillin and other drugs. JAMA 184:171

Shelley WB, Comaish MB (1965) New test for penicillin allergy. Fluorometric assay of histamine release. JAMA 192:36

Shelley WB, Juhlin L (1961) A new test for detecting anaphylactic sensitivity: the basophil reaction. Nature 191:1056

Shibata K, Atsumi T, Horiuchi Y, Mashimo K (1966) Immunological cross-reactivities of cephalothin and its related compounds with benzylpenicillin (penicillin G). Nature 212:419

Shibata K, Atsumi T, Horiuchi Y (1968) The heterogeneity of human anti-penicillin skin-sensitizing antibodies. Statistical analysis of wheal responses elicited with benzylpenicillin, various penicilloyl haptens and their related compounds. J Allergy 42:63

Siegel BB (1959) Hidden contact with penicillin. Bull WHO 21:703

Siegel BB (1962) Studies on penicillin hypersensitivity V. Further studies on the antigenic properties of altered penicillin. J Allergy 33:349

Siegel BB, Levine BB (1964) Antigenic specificities of skin-sensitizing antibodies in sera from patients with immediate systemic allergic reactions to penicillin. J Allergy 35:488

Siegel BB, Coleman M, Wissmann L, Sher M (1955) Studies in penicillin hypersensitivity. I. Immunologic findings in two penicillin-sensitive patients. J Allergy 26:78

Silber SS, Dioknoa A (1973) Agranulocytosis from cephalosporins. JAMA 224:1427

Simmen HP, Lüthy R, Siegenthaler W (1981) Antibiotikaeinsatz in der ambulanten Praxis. Schweiz Med Wochenschr 11:4

Smith H, Marshall AC (1971) Polymers formed by some beta-lactam antibiotics. Nature 232:45

Smith H, Dewdney JM, Wheeler AW (1971) A comparison of the amounts and the antigenicity of polymeric materials formed in aqueous solution by some beta-lactam antibiotics. Immunology 21:527

Smith JW, Johnson JE, Cluff LE (1966) Studies on the epidemiology of adverse drug reactions. II. An evaluation of penicillin allergy. N Engl J Med 274:998

Sokoloff B (1977) Ampicillin rashes. Pediatrics 59:637

Sonntag WM, Marcus S (1963) Penicillin hypersensitivity demonstrated by passive cutaneous anaphylaxis in the rat. Int Arch Allergy Allg Immunol 23:239

Soter NA, Austen KF (1978) Cutaneous necrotizing angiitis. In: Samter M (ed) Immunologic diseases, 3rd edn. Little, Brown, Boston, p 993

Spain DM, Clarke TB (1946) A case of agranulocytosis occurring during the course of penicillin therapy. Ann Intern Med 25:732

Spark RP (1971) Fatal anaphylaxis due to oral penicillin. J Clin Pathol 56:407

Spath P, Garatty G, Petz L (1971) Studies on the immune response to penicillin and cephalothin antibodies. J Immunol 107:854

Spath P, Huber H, Ludvan M, Roth A, Schwarz S, Zelger J (1979) IgE antibodies for the evaluation of hypersensitivity against penicillin. Allergy 34:405

Spengler H, de Weck AL, Geczy AF (1974) Studies on the molecular mechanisms of lymphocyte stimulation by penicillin and penicillin derivatives. In: Kissling R (ed) lymphocyte recognition and effector mechanisms. Academic, New York, p 501

Springs M (1951) Purpura and nephritis after administration of procaine penicillin. JAMA 147:1139

Spruill FG, Minette LJ, Sturner WQ (1974) Two surgical deaths associated with cephalothin. JAMA 229:440

Stember RH, Levine BB (1972) Frequency of skin reactivity to penicillin haptens in patients without histories of penicillin allergy. J Allergy Clin Immunol 49:96

Stemberger H, Kraft D, Werner HP (1971) Antigengemeinschaft zwischen Na-Penicillin-G und Cephalosporin-C-Derivaten. Z Immunitätsforsch Immunobiol 141:293

Stewart GT (1962) Cross-allergenicity of penicillin G and related substances. Lancet 1:509

Stewart GT (1967) Allergenic residues in penicillins. Lancet 1:1177

Stewart GT (1968) Protein contaminants in penicillins. Lancet 1:1088

Stewart GT (1973) Allergy to penicillins and related antibiotics: antigenic and immunochemical mechanism. Ann Rev Pharmacol Toxicol 13:309

Stofer AR, Lazary S, de Weck AL (1973) Zur Diagnostik des tödlichen anaphylaktischen Schocks auf Penicillin an der Leiche. Beitr Gerichtl Med 31:270

Strumia PV, Raimond FD (1962) Acquired hemolytic anemia and penicillin antibody: case report and review of the literature. Arch Intern Med 109:603

Sullivan TJ, Wedner JH, Shatz GS, Yecies LD, Parker CW (1981) Skin test to detect penicillin allergy. J Allergy Clin Immunol 68:171

Swanson MA, Chanmougan D, Schwartz RS (1966) Immunohemolytic anemia due to antipenicillin antibodies: report of a case. N Engl J Med 274:178

Tadokoro K, Kudo K, Nakagawa T, Suko T, Okudaira H, Igarashi H, Koizumi K, Muranaka M (1976) Studies on the drug hypersensitivity. XV. Antigenic cross reactivity of penicillins and cephalothin. Jpn J Allergy 26:249

Tannenberg AM, Wicker KJ, Rose NR (1971) Ampicillin nephropathy. JAMA 218:449

Tao J, Sung C (1958) Stillbirth caused by intradermal penicillin hypersensitivity test. Chin Med J 76:174

Thiel AJ, Mitchell S, Parker CW (1964) The specificity of hemagglutination reactions in human and experimental penicillin hypersensitivity. J Allergy 35:399

Thoburn R, Johnson JE, Cluff LE (1968) Studies on the epidemiology of adverse drug reactions. IV. Relationship of cephalothin and penicillin allergy. JAMA 198:345

Torii T, Horiuchi Y (1961) Antigenicity of penicillin and its relation to albumin binding. Nature 192:429

Tscheuner I (1972) Anaphylaktische Reaktion auf Penicillin nach Genuß von Schweinefleisch. Z Haut Geschlkrk 47:591

Tsuji A, Yamana T, Miyamoto E, Kiya E (1975) Chemical reactions involved in penicillin allergy: kinetics and mechanism of penicillin aminolysis. J Pharm Pharmacol 27:580

Tuft L, Gregory DC, Gregory I (1955) Evaluation of skin testing methods employed in the diagnosis of penicillin allergy. Am J Med Sci 230:370

Utley PM, Lucas JB, Billings TE (1966) Acute psychotic reactions to aqueous procaine penicillin. South Med J 59:1271

Valentine M (Chairman) (1979) Allergic emergencies. In: NIAID Task Force report: Asthma and other allergic diseases, Public Health Service publication 79–387. Dept Health, Education, and Welfare, Wahington DC, p 501

Van Arsdel PP Jr (1965) Allergic reactions to penicillin. JAMA 191:238

Van Arsdel PP Jr, Franz KB (1963) Nature of antibody in penicillin-induced hemolytic anemia. J Clin Invest 42:988

Van Arsdel PP Jr, O'Rourke TK, Horan JD, Kumasaka Y (1963 a) Serum hemagglutinating antibodies in penicillin allergy. JAMA 185:584

Van Arsdel PP Jr, Tobe AD, Pasnick LJ (1963 b) Association of hemagglutinating antibodies with skin sensitivity in penicillin allergy. J Allergy 34:526

Van Dellen RG, Gleich GJ (1970) Penicillin skin tests as predictive and diagnostic aids in penicillin allergy. Med Clin North Am 54:997

Van Dellen RG, Walsh WE, Peters GA (1971) Differing patterns of wheal and flare reactivity in patients allergic to penicillins. J Allergy Clin Immunol 47:230

Velasquez JL, Gold MI (1975) Anaphylactic reaction to cephalothin during anesthesia. Anesthesiology 43:476

Vickers M, Assem ESK (1974) Test for penicillin allergy in man. I. Carrier effect on response to penicilloyl conjugates. Immunology 26:425

Villim AB, Wilson WL, Hughes DW (1976) High molecular weight impurities in benzylpenicillin. J Pharm Sci 11:78

Vischer TL (1966) Lymphocyte cultures in drug hypersensitivity. Lancet 1:467

Vogt H (1969) Kreuzallergie von Cephaloridin, Cephalothin und Penicillin. Hautarzt 20:407

Voss HE, Redmond AR, Levine BB (1966) Clinical detection of the potential allergic reactor to penicillin by immunologic tests. JAMA 196:679

Wagelie RG, Dukes CD, McGovern JP (1963) Antigenicity and cross-reactivity of 6-aminopenicillanic acid and penicillin G. J Allergy Clin Immunol 34:489

Wal JM (1980) Enzymatic unmasking for antibodies of penicilloyl residues bound to albumin. Biochem Pharmacol 29:195

Waldbott GL (1949) Anaphylactic death from penicillin. JAMA 139:526

Waldo JF, Tyson JT (1949) Hypersensitivity to penicillin. Am J Med 6:396

Walsh WE, Markowitz H, Jones JD, Gleich GJ (1971) Macromolecular contaminants in penicillin and cephalosporin antibiotics. J Allergy 47:159

Warrington RJ, Tse KS (1979) Lymphocyte transformation studies in drug hypersensitivity. Can Med Assoc J 120:1089

Warrington RJ, Simons FER, Ho HW, Gorski BA, Tse KS (1978) Diagnosis of penicillin allergy by skin testing: the Manitoba experience. Can Med Assoc J 118:787

Warrington RJ, Sander PJ, Rutherford WJ (1979) Studies on migration inhibition test in penicillin hypersensitivity. Clin Exp Immunol 38:148

Watson KC (1962) Effect of various penicillin compounds on hemagglutination of penicillin-coated erythrocytes. Immunology 5:610

Watson KC, Joubert SM, Benett MA (1960) The occurrence of hemagglutinating antibody to penicillin. Immunology 3:1

Watson KC, Joubert SM, Bennett MA (1961) Some factors influencing the hemagglutination of penicillin-sensitized erythrocytes. Immunology 4:193

Webster AW, Thompson RA (1974) The ampicillin rash. Lymphocyte transformation by ampicillin polymer. Clin Exp Immunol 18:553

Weidemüller HL, Ziegler W (1970) On the proteinaceous impurity of penicillin. Arzneim Forsch 20:585

Weitzman SA, Stossel TP (1978) Drug-induced immunological neutropenia. Lancet 1:1068

Welch H (1959) Problem of antibiotics in foods. JAMA 170:139

Wellensiek HJ (1969) Immunogenicity of semisynthetic penicillins. In: Westphal O, Bock HE, Grundmann E (eds) Current problems in immunology. Springer, Berlin Heidelberg New York, p 310

Weston RD (1968) Penicilloylated protein contaminating 6-amino-penicillanic acid and benzylpenicillin. Antimicrob Agents Chemother 25:553

Wheeler AW (1971) A method for measuring different classes of human immunoglobulins specific for the penicilloyl group. Immunology 21:547

White JM, Brown DL, Hepner GW (1968) Penicillin-induced haemolytic anemia. Br Med J 3:26

Wicher K, Reisman RE (1980) Anaphylactic reaction to penicillin (or penicillin-like substance) in a soft drink. J Allergy Clin Immunol 66:155

Wicher K, Reisman RE, Arbesman CE (1969) Allergic reactions to penicillin in milk. JAMA 208:143

Wide L, Juhlin L (1971) Detection of penicillin allergy of the immediate type by radioimmunoassay of reagins (IgE) to penicilloyl conjugates. Clin Allergy 1:171

Wilensky AO (1946) Fatal delayed anaphylactic shock after penicillin. JAMA 131:1384

Wilson C, Greenhood G, Remington JS (1979) Neutropenia after consecutive treatment courses with nafcillin and piperacillin. Lancet 1:1150

Wintroub BU, Shiffman NJ, Arndt KA (1979) Adverse cutaneous reactions to drugs. In: Fitzpatrick TB (ed) Dermatology in general medicine, 2nd edn. McGraw-Hill, New York, p 555

Wüthrich B, Somazzi S (1972) Zur Klinik, Diagnose und Therapie der Penicillinallergie. Praxis 61:736

Yamana T, Tsuiji A, Miyamoto E, Kiya E (1975) Chemical aspects of penicillin allergy: imidazole-catalyzed penicilloylation. J Pharm Pharmacol 27:283

Zimmerman MC (1959) Chronic penicillin urticaria from dairy products, proved by penicillinase cures. Arch Dermatol 79:1

CHAPTER 17

Other Antibiotics

D. KRAFT

A. Introduction

In addition to the penicillins and cephalosporins, many other substances with antibiotic properties are known and widely used. Substances in this group include the tetracyclines, chloramphenicol and thiamphenicol, aminoglycosides, polymyxins, rifamycins, macrolides, lincomycins, and other miscellaneous compounds. These antibiotics are used in the systemic and topical treatment of infectious diseases. Some of these antibiotics have also been used to stimulate growth in animals; they may still be in use now and may therefore persist in the environment.

Several types of complications, but very few allergic reactions have been reported among the adverse reactions produced by these other antibiotics. In only a few cases have skin tests or laboratory investigations been carried out in order to support an immunologic etiology of the reactions observed. In general, the available data concerning drug allergies caused by this group of antibiotics are somewhat limited and further studies are required for the characterization and elucidation of the underlying mechanisms. This chapter describes the physicochemical, pharmacologic, immunochemical, and immunologic properties of the antibiotics mentioned as well as the incidence, clinical patterns, and immunologic aspects of the allergic reactions.

B. Tetracyclines

I. Physicochemical and Pharmacologic Properties

The tetracyclines are a group of antibiotics with the same basic chemical structure; they are derivatives of the naphthacene ring system. Compounds of the series differ in the composition of the side chains (Fig. 1). These antibiotics derived from different *Streptomyces* species show closely related spectra of bacteriostatic properties, with the exception of minocycline, which is very effective against most *Staphylococcus* strains resistant to other tetracyclines. Absorption, metabolism, and excretion of the different tetracyclines vary, however. After oral application, tetracycline, oxytetracycline, and chlortetracycline are absorbed to a much lesser degree than demethylchlortetracycline, methacycline, or the almost entirely absorbed minocycline. Maximum blood levels are found 2–6 h after oral intake and immediately in the case of intravenous infusion. Half-lives between 8 and 15 h were reported. The tetracyclines diffuse readily across the vascular barrier and are found in various tissues such as the liver, spleen, bone marrow, kidney, skin, and lungs as well as the peritoneal and pericardiac cavities. The tetracyclines are also able to

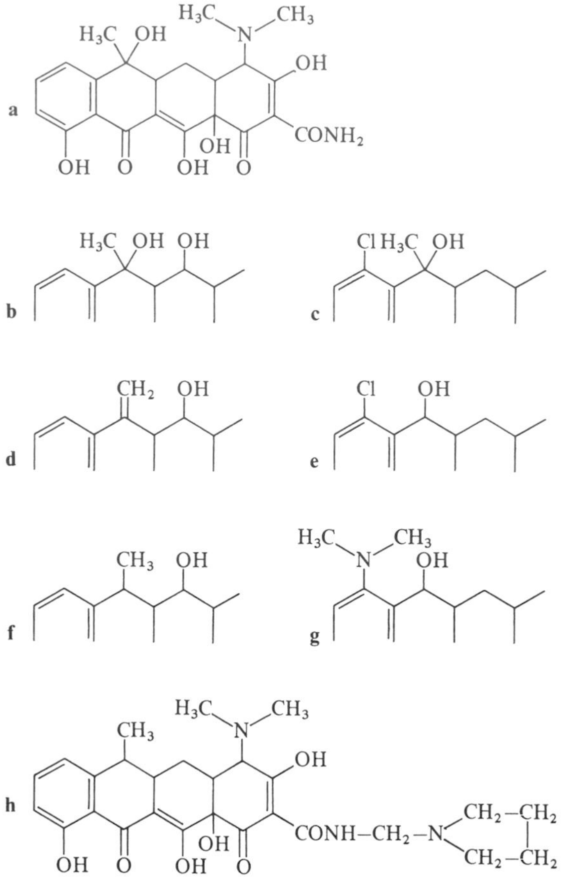

Fig. 1 a–h. Chemical structures of the tetracyclines. **a** tetracycline; **b** oxytetracycline; **c** chlortetracycline; **d** methacycline; **e** demethylchlortetracycline; **f** 6-deoxytetracycline (doxycycline); **g** minocycline; **h** roli(*N*-pyrrolidinomethyl)tetracycline

pass through the placenta and therapeutic concentrations have been described in cord blood and amniotic fluid. The binding to human plasma proteins due to hydrophobic and van der Waals forces is reported to be in the range of 40% for tetracycline and oxytetracycline, 50% for rolitetracycline, 70%–75% for demethylchlortetracycline and minocycline, and 96% for 6-deoxytetracycline. These effects may be the reason for the low clearance by glomerular filtration in the case of demethylchlortetracycline and 6-deoxytetracycline and for their characteristics as longer-acting members of the series. Excretion also occurs through the gastrointestinal tract (expecially after oral intake), the bile, saliva, sweat, and colostrum (KUCERS and BENNET 1975; OTTEN et al. 1975; SIMON and STILLE 1979).

II. Immunochemistry and Immunology

The nature of the antigenic determinants is still not properly defined, but it is widely believed that the ring system (WELSH 1955) and the substitution patterns may be important (SHELLEY and HEATON 1973). Immunogenicity studies have been carried out in different animals. QUENG et al. (1965) reported the production of antisera against oxytetracycline in rabbits. The antibodies obtained were tested by different in vitro assays. Antibodies specific to oxytetracycline were demonstrated, whereas only weakly reactive antibodies specific to the whole tetracycline series were observed. Similar results were reported by MUELLING et al. (1958) and SPEKTOROVA (1961). HOFFMANN (1970) failed to confirm the existence of differences in the immunochemical properties of the tetracyclines. Studies in humans similarly showed a cross-sensitivity pattern among the various tetracyclines (BOJS and MÖLLER 1974).

III. Clinical Aspects

Most of the side effects are of a toxic nature and manifest themselves in the bones, teeth, gastrointestinal tract, liver, kidney, the vestibular region, and the skin. Discoloration and damage to the deciduous as well as to the permanent teeth are well documented undesirable side effects of tetracycline treatment in children. Gastrointestinal disturbances such as diarrhea with nausea and vomiting have been described. Nephropathy, especially in patients with preexisting renal insufficiency, has been reported to be caused by the tetracyclines. Photoonycholysis, as well as anogenital pruritus (without any objective findings) should also be mentioned (SCHINDEL 1965; HOIGNÉ 1975).

Skin photosensitivity is a relatively frequent result of tetracycline treatment (WIEBE and MOORE 1977) and phototoxic reactions should be distinguished from photoallergic reactions (KOROSSY 1976; MORISON et al. 1979). The photosensitivity is usually phototoxic in origin and induced by drugs which accumulate in the skin and make it susceptible to sunlight exposure. By contrast, in photoallergic reactions the drug is transformed by sunlight into immunogenic substances which induce an immune response and may lead to allergic reactions by antigen–antibody or antigen–immune cell interactions. It is often impossible to distinguish with certainty between these two types of photodermatosis, which on occasion may coexist in the same patient. Phototoxic reactions may occur following the first dose of the drug and may be seen minutes to hours after exposure to light. Some wavelengths, at other times harmless, may produce clinical manifestions. Clinically, phototoxic reactions are induced mainly be tetracycline and 6-deoxytetracycline. The patterns are uniform and have the appearance of sunburn with erythema, edema, and sometimes blisters in the exposed skin areas, leading to desquamation and hyperpigmentation. An especially high incidence of this type of reaction has been reported for demethylchlortetracycline (BLANK et al. 1968; FROST et al. 1971). For other tetracyclines it may be less than 1%, at least in non-tropical countries (RAMSAY 1977). By contrast, photoallergic reactions are much more polymorphic and can appear as eczematous, urticarial, and maculopapular lesions as well as erythema and edema of the skin exposed to light. Light sensitivity after tetracycline treatment can persist if there are photoallergic manifestations. Almost all phototoxic reactions, however, tend to disappear.

Allergic reactions to tetracyclines without exposure to sunlight are uncommon, although various other clinical manifestations may be observed. Approximately

0.1%–2% of patients receiving the antibiotics and 1% of people in contact with these drugs in industry show an allergic reaction to the tetracyclines (Kleine-Natrop 1956; Weinstein and Welch 1958, 1959; Schindel 1965; Olson 1966; Moser 1966; Körössy 1976).

Several studies have even described the occurrence of anaphylactic shock after the administration of tetracyclines. Generalized circulatory failure together with other symptoms such as urticaria, angioedema, and dyspnea have been observed after short periods of latency following tetracycline treatment (Bedford 1951; Sakamoto 1956; Haas 1957; Lachmann 1959; Greenberg and Greenspan 1962; Pollen 1964; Editorial 1965; Fellner and Baer 1965; Coles et al. 1967; Furey and Tan 1969; Zelger and Seidl 1969; Singh et al. 1977). In one publication, anaphylaxis to tetracycline was reported to have occurred in a patient who had previously developed a serum-sickness-like reaction following penicillin treatment (Fellner and Baer 1965, 1966). Other clinical patterns such as urticaria, serumsickness-like reactions, maculopapular rashes, erythema exudativum multiforme, and asthma have been described as a consequence of tetracycline treatment (Peck and Feldmann 1950; Johnston and Cazort 1953; Weinstein and Welch 1958, 1959; Menon and Das 1977; Terekhova and Wushkina 1977).

Fawcett and Pepys (1976) reported the case of a patient who developed immediate bronchospasm and an urticarial reaction after ingestion of a commercial combination of three tetracyclines; no reactions could be elicited by oral challenge with the different tetracyclines, tartrazine, or the blue coating of the drug, whereas a provocation test with the commercial preparation was positive. Other clinical patterns, such as fixed drug eruptions (Kandil 1969; Delaney 1970; Csonka et al. 1971; Brown 1974; Shimizu and Shimao 1977; Pasricha and Shukla 1979), vascular purpura (Schoenfeld 1964) and a picture similar to systemic lupus erythematosus (SLE) (Sulkowski and Haserick 1964) have also been described. Contact dermatitis seems to be a very rare complication; it was, however, observed after contact with oxytetracycline (Dohn 1962; Bojs and Möller 1974) and minocycline. In the latter case subsequent oral therapy with the same drug was followed by a systemic reaction and the sensitivity was confirmed by epicutaneous tests (Shelley and Heaton 1973).

The low sensitization index has established the tetracyclines as suitable drugs for topical use and indeed the incidence of allergic reactions did not increase during and after local therapy (Bojs and Möller 1974). Tetracycline-induced immunologic blood dyscrasias are uncommon, although a few instances have been reported. A case of immune hemolytic anemia due to tetracycline administration has been described, the diagnosis being confirmed by a positive indirect Coombs test (Wenz et al. 1974). Thrombocytopenic purpura was observed in a patient receiving oxytetracycline treatment (Kounis 1975). Following withdrawal of the drug the patient recovered, the morbilliform rash disappeared, and the platelet count and bleeding time improved. Minocycline-induced acute interstitial nephritis has also been observed in one patient (Walker et al. 1979). A biopsy established the allergic nature of the reaction; immunofluorescence studies showed IgA and complement deposits along the tubular basement membrane.

Exceptional adverse reactions of undefined etiology following tetracycline administration do exist. Bean (1971) reported acneiform eruptions occurring in a male patient on two occasions after tetracycline reexposure. An allergic basis for the skin manifestation could not be demonstrated.

Benign intracranial hypertension due to tetracyclines has also been described and in a few of these individuals a tetracycline allergy seemed to be present as well (BUSINCO et al. 1968; KOCH-WESER and GILMORE 1967). The results, however, of the investigations carried out in such patients did not suggest an underlying immunologic mechanism with certainty. Some patients suffering from myasthenia gravis showed an aggravation of myasthenic symptoms shortly after tetracycline therapy (WULLEN et al. 1967; HASHIMOTO et al. 1976). There is some evidence that this may be caused by changes of the local Mg^{2+} concentration which could induce a neuromuscular block. Investigations to establish an immunologic mechanism were not carried out.

IV. Results of Diagnostic Tests

1. Skin Tests

Skin tests with various tetracycline compounds in different concentrations have been performed by many clinicians. Unfortunately, non-sensitizing conjugates of tetracyclines with small polypeptide carriers are not available. This is mainly due to our inadequate knowledge of the haptenic determinants responsible for tetracycline allergies. Therefore no effective diagnostic skin tests exist at present.

For routine skin testing, tetracycline solutions in concentrations of 0.05–0.5 mg/ml for scratch and intracutaneous tests and 10 mg/ml for patch tests have been used. Positive results were obtained in some cases of highly sensitized patients. ZELGER and SEIDL (1969) obtained a positive scratch test with oxytetracycline in a highly sensitized nurse. FELLNER and BAER (1966) reported a positive skin test of the immediate type in a penicillin- and tetracycline-sensitive patient using intracutaneous application of tetracycline. Patch tests gave positive reactions more readily, especially among medical staff and factory workers (KOROSSY 1976).

To establish IgE-mediated allergies to tetracyclines, Prausnitz-Küstner tests were performed and positive results were obtained in some cases (FELLNER and BAER 1966; LOCHMANNOVA et al. 1970).

2. Tetracycline-Specific Antibodies

A few research workers have attempted to measure serum antibodies using assays such as gel precipitation, hemagglutination, and complement fixation. These assays, however, were of limited value, because the immunoglobulins measured were not of primary importance in the genesis of the allergic symptoms. Additionally, there is evidence that not all antibody specificities can be measured. In general, a negative result does not necessarily negate tetracycline allergy, while a positive test is not necessarily definitive proof of tetracycline allergy. Up to now these tests in their present form are of no value in the diagnosis of allergic reactions to tetracyclines.

There are no reports in the literature regarding radioallergosorbent tests (RAST) in IgE-mediated tetracycline allergies. Precipitating antibodies have been demonstrated in the sera of some patients allergic to the tetracyclines (MUELLING et al. 1958; LOCHMANNOVA et al. 1970). Studies performed by HOFFMANN (1970), however, failed to confirm these results. Measurement of hemagglutinating antibodies in human sera have been published by several workers (FELLNER and BAER 1966; LOCHMANNOVA et al. 1970; WINTER and FREUND 1969; WENZ et al. 1974). Positive results were obtained in allergic as well as in nonallergic patients and no correlation between titer levels and onset of clinical patterns could be established. In contrast, the indirect basophil test has been claimed to give positive results in patients allergic to tetracyclines (SHELLEY 1965; MONERET-VAUTRIN et al. 1972).

3. Tetracycline-Specific Lymphocyte Reactivity

In hypersensitivity of the delayed type, an evaluation of in vitro lymphocyte transformation test (LTT) has been performed by many investigators (GIRARD 1974). In the case of the tetracyclines, this test, applied to the diagnosis of allergies, showed positive results in cases of contact dermatitis and maculopapular exanthemas (RIPPS et al. 1965; LAZZARO and BUZZONI 1968; REICHENBERGER and HEITMAN 1969; SARKANY 1967). Stimulation of lymphocytes was performed with tetracycline and demethylchlortetracycline without carrier molecules. Concurrence between positive results of LTT and clinical manifestations was obtained (SARKANY 1967), but considerable controversy still exists regarding the interpretation of these results. HALPERN et al. (1967) reported that the test could be used with confidence, whereas other workers do not accept this procedure as an in vitro test to detect allergy to tetracyclines.

V. Experimental Studies in Animals

The immune response to the different tetracyclines has been investigated in several animal species. Parent antibiotics as well as tetracycline–protein conjugates served as immunizing agents. Reactive antibodies to tetracycline, oxytetracycline, chlortetracycline, and demethylchlortetracycline as measured by Ouchterlony tests (SPEKTOROVA 1961; QUENG et al. 1965), have been produced. Hemagglutination assays, Schultz–Dale tests and passive cutaneous anaphylaxis (PCA) have also been carried out (QUENG et al. 1965). HOFFMANN (1970) has questioned the validity of these results. Nonspecific binding of the tetracyclines to the serum proteins (OTTEN et al. 1975), which can cause nonspecific precipitation in agar plates, might explain some of the false positive results obtained; direct histamine-releasing phenomena similarly might lead to positive PCA and Schultz–Dale tests.

VI. Conclusions Concerning Possible Pathomechanisms

With the exception of photoallergic reactions, the same clinical patterns of allergic reactions have been reported for tetracyclines as for other drugs, albeit less frequently. The low sensitization potential of tetracycline compounds might be caused by their reduced ability to bind covalently to proteins or other carrier molecules and thereby a reduced tendency to form immunogenic conjugates. The nature of the antigenic or allergic determinant (or determinants) is unknown.

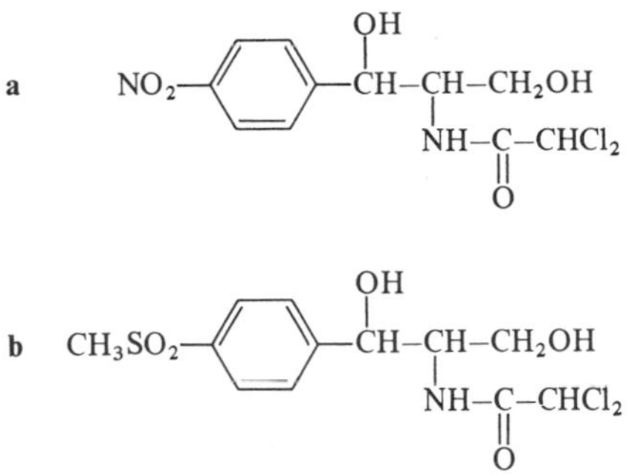

a $\quad NO_2-\langle\bigcirc\rangle-CH-CH-CH_2OH$

with substituents: OH on first CH, and NH–C(=O)–CHCl$_2$ on second CH

b $\quad CH_3SO_2-\langle\bigcirc\rangle-CH-CH-CH_2OH$

with substituents: OH on first CH, and NH–C(=O)–CHCl$_2$ on second CH

Fig. 2. Chemical structures of chloramphenicol (**a**) and thiamphenicol (**b**)

C. Chloramphenicol and Thiamphenicol

I. Physicochemical and Pharmacologic Properties

Chloramphenicol was first detected in filtrates of liquid cultures of *Streptomyces venezuelae* and is at present synthesized from *p*-nitroacetophenone. It acts effectively against a wide variety of microorganisms. Its chemical structure is characterized by the presence of a nitrobenzene group, covalently bound chlorine, an amide linkage involving a derivative of dichloroacetic acid, and a propanol moiety (Fig. 2a). Chloramphenicol is a bacteriostatic antibiotic with a potent inhibitory effect on bacterial protein synthesis. It is readily absorbed from the gastrointestinal tract, the peak value being reached within 2 h of oral intake. When it is injected intramuscularly the peak blood level is reached after approximately 2 h, whereas when it is given intravenously the peak level of the drug (in the active form) in blood is attained immediately. The half-life of active chloramphenicol is 1–3 h; however, therapeutic levels can still be detected 6–8 h later. Chloramphenicol diffuses readily into many body tissues and penetrates into the pleural and peritoneal cavities as well as the different compartments of the eye and into the cerebrospinal fluid. It may also pass through the placenta. Binding to the plasma proteins occurs to some extent (50%–60%) and is readily reversible. Chloramphenicol is rapidly conjugated with glucuronic acid in the healthy human liver and the conjugates are inactive. Active chloramphenicol is excreted by glomerular filtration only, whereas the inactive form is eliminated by tubular excretion. Only small amounts of chloramphenicol are excreted in the bile and feces, mostly in the inactive form (KUCERS and BENNET 1975; OTTEN et al. 1975; SIMON and STILLE 1979).

Thiamphenicol is the methylsulfonyl derivative of chloramphenicol (Fig. 2b). It has a similar bacteriostatic spectrum, but differs from chloramphenicol in that it is not metabolized by the liver. It is absorbed more slowly and in its active form is excreted mainly by the kidneys. There is widespread distribution and penetration into various organs.

II. Immunochemistry and Immunology

A quantitative micro-complement fixation test and the hapten inhibition method have been used for determination of the antibody binding site on the chloramphenicol molecule (HAMBURGER and DOUGLASS 1969 a). Antibodies were obtained by immunizing rabbits with chloramphenicol coupled through the nitro group to the carrier protein. Investigation of 16 compounds related to chloramphenicol, but with varying degrees of change in their structure showed that the dichloroacetamido group accounted for most of the antigenic activity of the hapten. The size of the constituent and its electronegativity might well contribute to its antigenicity. In conclusion, the major antigenic determinant seemed to be within the dichloroacetamido group, which is quite separate from the portion of the molecule responsible for antibiotic activity. Studies of the differences in immunogenicity between chloramphenicol and thiamphenicol have as yet not been carried out. Both antibiotics possess immunosuppressive properties (PETRESCU et al. 1972).

III. Clinical Aspects

A variety of side effects has been ascribed to chloramphenicol. Irritative reactions of the gastrointestinal tract with nausea, vomiting, diarrhea, and pruritus ani have been described. Dose-related phenomena such as "gray baby" syndrome (see MANTEN 1975), and reversible anemia and, most important, toxic damage to the bone marrow have also been reported. Two forms of bone marrow depression have been described (EDITORIAL 1970): (1) a common, dose-related, reversible lesion which occurs concurrently with chloramphenicol therapy and is characterized by vacuolization in erythroid and myeloid cells and by suppressed erythropoiesis; (2) a rare complication, characterized by a lack of dose–response relationship and inducing (apparently on a genetic basis) irreversible bone marrow hypoplasia or aplasia with consequent high mortality. The latter can sometimes be induced by very small amounts of chloramphenicol as reported, for instance, following the use of eyedrops (ROSENTHAL and BLACKMANN 1965; CARPENTER 1975). Jaundice, polyneuritis, optic neuropathy, and auditory disturbances are other toxic side effects of chloramphenicol therapy (for further information see MANTEN 1975).

Thiamphenicol can also be the cause of serious bone marrow damage (KEISER et al. 1972; KALTWASSER et al. 1974). The incidence of bone marrow depression, on the other hand, is lower, with an obvious dose dependence and reversibility (BECK 1975). Neurotoxicity, gastrointestinal disturbances, and alopecia are further adverse reactions to thiamphenicol (MANTEN 1975).

Hypersensitivity to chloramphenicol occurs usually after topical (RICHTER 1975) and less often after parenteral or oral intake. Besides contact dermatitis (confirmed by patch tests as being of allergic origin), the occurrence of maculopapular rashes and urticaria in association with chloramphenicol treatment has also been described (ACKER and SCHREIER 1962; KOROSSY et al. 1962; FORCK 1971; WÄTZIG and RUFFERT 1977). The immunologic nature of these reactions, however, has only been partially determined. FORCK (1971) reported two cases of urticaria, diagnosed as allergic reactions by positive scratch tests. CAHILL (1962) described a severe hemorrhagic reaction in a patient whose patch test to chloramphenicol was positive. Occasionally systemic reactions such as nausea, circulatory collapse, severe bronchospasm, and drug-induced fever were also reported (KOROSSY 1976). After oral ingestion, ACKER and SCHREIER (1962) observed that the incidence of side effects was 1.5% in 3,648 treated children. No skin tests or in vitro tests were performed, however, to confirm the allergic nature of these adverse reactions. There have been speculations that aplastic anemia and other bone marrow damage caused by chloramphenicol may be of immunologic origin (JACOTTET 1964; SCHEE-GANS et al. 1965; HAMBURGER 1966). It is difficult, however, to distinguish the immunologic response from the direct toxic action of this antibiotic, as can be seen in any patient receiving high dosages over a prolonged period of time (SCOTT et al. 1965). Chloramphenicol-specific antibodies were detected in the sera of patients in the acute phase of their disease, but convincing data about an underlying immune reactivity are still lacking. The reported hematologic disorder can also be caused by the chloramphenicol analog thiamphenicol, probably through the same mechanisms (KEISER et al. 1972).

IV. Results of Diagnostic Tests

1. Skin Tests

Skin tests of the immediate type, with 1% chloramphenicol solution as well as Prausnitz–Küstner tests have been performed, but no positive results were obtained with either method (KOROSSY et al. 1962).

Epicutaneous tests with 1% chloramphenicol ointment have been performed by various investigators and relevant results have been obtained. A sensitization occurrence of 0.18%–8.9% is reported, depending on local conditions in countries which are either in favor of or against the topical use of chloramphenicol in drops and ointments (ROBINSON et al. 1951; SCHWANK and JIRASEK 1963; EBERHARTINGER and EBNER 1966; KOROSSY et al. 1966, 1969; EBNER 1973; PEVNY and RÖCKL 1975). These results suggest a possible role for cell-mediated allergic reactions.

2. Chloramphenicol-Specific Antibodies

Investigating 1,700 routine hospital blood bank sera, WATSON and JOUBERT (1960) found 6 sera capable of agglutinating chloramphenicol-sensitized human red blood cells. None of the sera produced a positive Coombs test and 5 of 6 patients had no previous history of chloramphenicol treatment. The patient with the highest titer (1 : 128) had apparently never received any antibiotic therapy. It was suggested therefore, that sensitization had arisen by contact with an unrelated compound sharing a common determinant.

Two French reports on patients with fatal aplastic anemia stated that the sera contained agglutinating antibodies to red blood cells sensitized with chloramphenicol (JACOTTET 1964; SCHEEGANS et al. 1965). During an examination of anti-chloramphenicol antibodies in two patients, a short half-life was noted by HAMBURGER and DOUGLASS (1969 b). A relationship between the presence of antibodies to chloramphenicol and the fatal clinical course was not established.

A convenient modification of the Farr test, using chloramphenicol–[125]I-labeled human serum albumin conjugate as antigen, was described for the screening of large numbers of patients' sera for anti-chloramphenicol antibodies (ORGEL and HAMBURGER 1971). By blocking with crystalline chloramphenicol, 10 μg/ml of antibody could be detected in rabbit serum. The method described should facilitate the measurement of antibody levels in patients, both at an early phase of the disease and subsequently throughout its course.

3. Chloramphenicol-Specific Lymphocyte Reactivity

The lymphocyte transformation test has been extensively used for the detection of lymphocytes specifically allergized to drugs (Halpern et al. 1967; Rocklin and David 1971; Warrington et al. 1979). The assay, however, was found to be unsuitable for the demonstration of hypersensitivity to chloramphenicol (Dobozy et al. 1971). The reason for this lack of reactivity was attributed to the inhibition of protein synthesis by the antibiotic. Using ^{14}C-labeled histones, Dobozy et al. (1971) found that chloramphenicol had little influence on the methylation of histones and that enhanced histone methylation could be observed in the cultures of lymphocytes obtained from chloramphenicol allergic patients compared with normal controls. The overall correlation was 100% and the test was recommended as being very useful.

The old Rebuck–Crowley method of skin windows was applied to the skin of patients with allergic contact dermatitis to chloramphenicol and the influence of chloramphenicol on the cell infiltrate was studied (Pambor 1973). Eosinophils, basophils, but not mononuclear cells were observed in a higher proportion than in controls. Further application of the same method was made by Wätzig and Ruffert (1977) and details of leukocyte migration inhibition in vivo were reported. The test was positive in 16 of 17 patients with exanthemas, but negative in 5 patients with allergic contact dermatitis to chloramphenicol. The investigators concluded that this test could be of value in some cases in the demonstration of chloramphenicol allergy.

V. Experimental Studies in Animals

Antibodies to chloramphenicol were obtained by immunizing rabbits with a chloramphenicol derivative coupled to bovine gamma-globulin (Hamburger 1966). The antibodies were determined by precipitin and complement fixation tests using a chloramphenicol–rabbit serum albumin conjugate as the test antigen. Specificity of the reactions was confirmed by inhibition studies with crystalline chloramphenicol, and this hapten inhibition technique was used to explore the antibody binding to the chloramphenicol molecule (Hamburger and Douglass 1969a). The removal of the two chlorine atoms accounted for the greatest loss of antibody binding capacity. In further experiments the half-life of the antibody in the rabbit was evaluated (Hamburger and Douglass 1969b). Repeated immunization of rabbits with chloramphenicol–bovine gamma-globulin conjugates led to peak titers of antibodies to chloramphenicol which declined much more rapidly than the antibodies to the carrier protein. The authors speculated that, in rabbits, rapid clearance may be caused by cross-reaction with a tissue antigen. In another study on the antigenic sites of the chloramphenicol molecule (Hamburger and Douglass 1969c), the rabbit antibody significantly inhibited the antibiotic activity of chloramphenicol in contrast to the non-antibody globulins which were found to bind to chloramphenicol without affecting the bacteriostatic capacity.

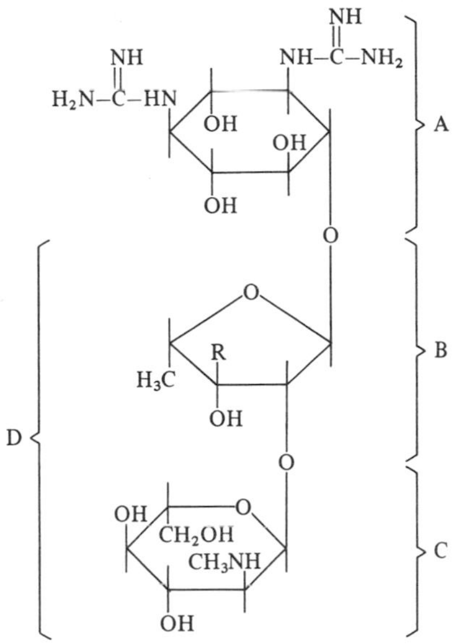

I R = –CHO
II R = –CH$_2$OH

Fig. 3. Aminoglycoside antibiotics: chemical structures of streptomycin (*I*) and dihydro-streptomycin (*II*). Ring *A* = streptidine; ring *B* = streptose; ring *C* = *N*-methyl-L-glucosamine; ring *D* = streptobiosamine

VI. Conclusions Concerning Possible Pathomechanisms

The principal side effects following chloramphenicol or thiamphenicol administration are toxic in nature, leading to bone marrow damage and subsequently to blood dyscrasias such as aplastic anemia, agranulocytosis, thrombocytopenia, and pancytopenia. The reason for this is unknown. The hypothesis that the immunologic mechanism caused aplastic anemia could not be established, although chloramphenicol-specific antibodies were found for a short period in patients who were in the acute phase of the disease. Immunization studies in animals have been carried out with protein–drug conjugates and the production of chloramphenicol-specific antibodies has been observed. The major antigenic determinant of the immune response appears to be in the dichloracetamido group. Acquired allergic contact dermatitis as well as lymphocyte reactivity in vitro indicate that chloramphenicol induces an immune response in humans mainly through the formation of specifically allergized and committed lymphocytes.

D. Aminoglycosides

I. Physicochemical and Pharmacologic Properties

The aminoglycoside antibiotics comprise several compounds with a broad spectrum of antibiotic activity and structures in which aminosugars are in glycosidic

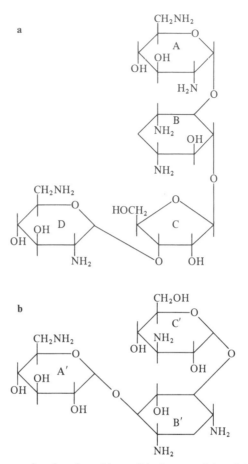

Fig. 4. Chemical structures of aminoglycoside antibiotics containing 4,5- (**a**) or 4,6- (**b**) substituted deoxystreptamine. Rings A, D = 2,6-diaminoglucose; ring A' = 6-aminoglucose; ring B = deoxystreptamine; ring C = D-ribose; ring C' = 3-aminoglucose

linkage with either streptidine or deoxystreptamine. The first group includes streptomycin and dihydrostreptomycin which differ in that the aldehyde in the streptose fragment of streptomycin is replaced by an alcohol in dihydrostreptomycin (Fig. 3). The antibiotics of the second group contain sugars linked to deoxystreptamine and differ in the substitution pattern, e.g., aminoglycosides containing a 4,5-substituted deoxystreptamine (neomycins, paromomycins, butirosins, and framycetin, Fig. 4a) or a 4,6-substituted deoxystreptamine (gentamycins, kanamycins, tobramycin, and sisomycin, Fig. 4b).

The aminoglycosides show maximal bactericidal action at a slightly alkaline pH. Because of structural similarities, the antibiotics exhibit other common properties such as a similar mode of antibacterial action and a partial or complete antimicrobial cross-resistance. The aminoglycosides are poorly absorbed from the gastrointestinal tract, but maximal serum levels are seen 1–2 h after parenteral inoculation. Binding of the antibiotics to plasma proteins is either nonexistent or found to be in the range of 4%–10% for amikacin, 14%–16% for dihydrostreptomycin and 25%–30% for streptomycin; the half-lives in the circulation are reported to be 1–2 h in the case of parenterally administered aminoglycosides. Their distribution into various organs as well as their diffusion and penetration within the organ is limited. Elimination occurs almost entirely by glomerular filtration (KUCERS and BENNET 1975; OTTEN et al. 1975; SIMON and STILLE 1979).

II. Immunochemistry and Immunology

Studies dealing with the sensitization potential of the aminoglycosides and the relationship of their chemical structure to their cross-sensitivity have been performed by various workers. Studies in guinea pigs and humans suggest that streptomycin is more immunogenic than dihydrostreptomycin (WENZEL and EPSTEIN 1964). This might be explained by the fact that covalent binding to proteins takes place via the aldehyde group in the streptose ring. Weak cross-sensitivity between these two antibiotics may be due to streptomycin impurities in dihydrostreptomycin preparations or to the existence of determinants presently unknown. According to PIRILÄ and PIRILÄ (1966), BRAUN and SCHÜTZ (1969), and SCHORR et al. (1973) both the 4,5- and the 4,6-disubstituted deoxystreptamine aminoglycosides contain aminosugars – 2,6-diaminoglucose(neosamine) or 6-aminoglucose – which seem to represent the major antigenic determinants responsible for the allergic reactions, and which apparently contribute to the pattern of complete or incomplete cross-sensitization of the deoxystreptamine-containing aminoglycosides. The deoxystreptamine ring seems to be involved only as a minor determinant, causing limited, if any, cross-sensitivity between the deoxystreptamine and the streptidine aminoglycosides (SCHORR and RIDGWAY 1977). The difficulties in drawing conclusions on the antigenic properties of the aminoglycosides are increased by the direct mast cell degranulation capacity of many of them, especially of neomycin.

III. Clinical Aspects

1. Streptomycin and Dihydrostreptomycin

Side effects of streptomycin and dihydrostreptomycin treatment are mainly toxic in nature. Toxicity to the auditory vestibular organs, nephrotoxicity, hepatotoxicity, and toxicity to the bone marrow have all been observed (RASMUSSEN 1972; HOIGNÉ 1975). There are also reports of peripheral neuritis and neuromuscular blockade, occurring presumably as a result of the potentiation of non-depolarizing anesthetics (HOIGNÉ 1975). Because of its strong ototoxicity, dihydrostreptomycin is no longer in use in the Western hemisphere.

Streptomycin, and to a much lesser extent dihydrostreptomycin, have been reported to be sensitizers in humans and also in guinea pigs (JOHN 1960; SMITH 1960; EPSTEIN and WENZEL 1962; CHUNG and CARSON 1976). There are a few reports in the literature dealing with anaphylactic shock, urticaria, and serum-sickness-like reactions in patients with tuberculosis who are receiving streptomycin therapy, or in connection with skin tests using streptomycin (ROSSEN 1948; GRUDZINSKI 1960;

HUTFIELD 1965; GIRARD and SCHWARTZ 1967; CHYREK-BOROWSKA et al. 1973). Contact dermatitis and other forms of skin reactions of the delayed type were observed in patients as well as in hospital staff with an incidence of 3%–10% (CHAKRAVARTY and SIRCAR 1961; KOROSSY 1976). Immune hemolytic anemia was recorded after streptomycin therapy (NACHMAN et al. 1962; PLA and MARTIN 1976; MARTINEZ et al. 1977). In long-term therapy, hypersensitivity reactions to the drug, as evidenced by cutaneous eruptions, drug fever, and eosinophilia, were found in about 11% of treated patients (CHAKRAVARTY and SIRCAR 1961; BERTÉ et al. 1964). In patients with contact allergy to neomycin, the systemic intake of streptomycin gave rise to eczematous and in some cases to exfoliative dermatitis (SIDI et al. 1958; FISHER 1966; CRONIN 1972).

2. Deoxystreptamine Aminoglycosides

The deoxystreptamine antibiotics show similar clinical toxicity to the streptidine aminoglycosides but there are quantitative differences regarding the frequency and severity of these effects (for details see MANTEN 1975). Gentamycin, widely used against severe bacterial infections is known to cause nephrotoxicity in patients suffering from varying degrees of renal insufficiency. Potentiation of the renal damage due to gentamycin by cephalosporins and vice versa has been reported (WADE et al. 1978). Further toxic side effects of gentamycin are auditory and vestibular disturbances and neuromuscular blockade. The same toxic effects, but more pronounced and longer lasting, were reported for the other antibiotics of this group (MANTEN 1975, 1978, 1979; SACK et al. 1978).

Allergic manifestations, such as urticaria, maculopapular rashes, and immune blood dyscrasias have been observed in 0.8% of gentamycin-treated patients (HEWITT 1974). These results were obtained in a clinical assessment of approximately 3,500 treated patients. Topical treatment with gentamycin for effective therapy or prevention of bacterial skin infections can cause allergic contact dermatitis with an associated risk of developing cross-sensitivity to kanamycin or neomycin (SCHORR et al. 1973). Hypersensitivity reactions, such as urticaria and rashes, have been noted in 0.6% of 2,789 patients evaluated for side effects of tobramycin therapy (SPEIRS 1976). Allergic reactions to kanamycin and its semisynthetic derivative, amikacin, are rather uncommon in humans. Anaphylactic shock, rashes, and eosinophilia have been observed (SACK et al. 1978). Cross-sensitization with the streptidine aminoglycosides has also been observed on occasions (KREIS 1966). Neomycin is confined primarily to topical use because of its minimal absorption after oral ingestion and the high incidence of ototoxic side effects after parenteral treatment. Contact allergy is a relatively common finding according to several reports (EPSTEIN 1956; EPSTEIN and PANZER 1971; EDITORIAL 1977).

IV. Results of Diagnostic Tests

1. Skin Tests

Reports of positive skin tests of the immediate type are rare. Using a 1% streptomycin solution, CHAKRAVARTY and SIRCAR (1961) found positive intracutaneous tests in 11.8% of 510 streptomycin-treated tuberculosis patients. Further reports on diagnostic skin tests have been published by GIRARD and SCHWARTZ (1967), ZELGER and SEIDL (1969), MAUCHER (1972), and CHYREK-BOROWSKA et al. (1973). Reports of positive skin tests of the delayed type with deoxystreptamine aminoglycosides are much more common and positive results have been obtained in patients with contact dermatitis, rashes, and drug fever. A high incidence of positive patch tests to neomycin has also been described (CALNAN and SARKANY 1958; KOOLJ 1961; BOONEN et al. 1964; MATNER 1969; PATRICK et al. 1970; EPSTEIN and PANZER 1971). Cross-sensitivity to kanamycin, gentamycin, and also to tobramycin is frequently noted in these patients (PIRILÄ and RONHUNKOSKI 1960; EDITORIAL 1977; SCHORR and RIDGWAY 1977; FÖRSTRÖM and PIRILÄ 1978). These observations are of some clinical importance since patients suffering from stasis dermatitis and leg ulcers show neomycin allergy in about 10%–34% of cases (FRAKI et al. 1979). However, the interpretation of the results of the patch tests with aminoglycosides, especially neomycin, is often complicated by the fact that they initiate a nonspecific histamine release from mast cells owing to their interactions with heparin in the mast cell granules (RAAB 1968).

2. Aminoglycoside-Specific Antibodies

The presence of antibodies to streptomycin has been demonstrated in patients with tuberculosis who are receiving streptomycin (VULLIEMOZ and FAVEZ 1964; GIRARD and SCHWARTZ 1967). Patients with adverse reactions showed higher titers of streptomycin-specific antibodies than those on streptomycin therapy without adverse reactions (GIRARD and SCHWARTZ 1967). In one case of acute immune hemolytic anemia and renal failure induced by streptomycin treatment, IgG antibodies could be demonstrated by a positive direct and indirect Coombs test (MARTINEZ et al. 1977). It was shown that these bound antibodies could fix complement to streptomycin-coated red cells. The M antigen of the erythrocytes seemed to be the most important binding site for streptomycin and the Rh system to be less important, but nevertheless still involved. The binding sites for streptomycin did not appear to be shared by the other aminoglycosides, since incubation of the red cells with kanamycin, gentamycin, and neomycin did not lead to agglutination by the patient's serum. Inhibition studies, however, using preincubation of the serum with different aminoglycosides, were not performed. Very few studies have been done to monitor the serum antibodies of patients following treatment with the other aminoglycosides. Human antibodies to neomycin-coated human erythrocytes have been described (HYSELL et al. 1975). These antibodies also reacted with red cells treated with high concentrations of gentamycin, butirosin, and kanamycin. The neamine structure seemed to be the antigenic determinant involved.

3. Aminoglycoside-Specific Lymphocyte Reactivity

Lymphocyte transformation tests have been carried out be many researchers using streptomycin (VISCHER 1966; HALPERN et al. 1967; SARKANY 1967; MATHEWS et al. 1972) and/or the other aminoglycosides (HALPERN et al. 1967; SARKANY 1967; MÜHLBERGER 1973; WARRINGTON et al. 1979). A significant proliferation response, measured by morphology or incorporation of ^3H-thymidine into DNA, could be obtained only in a limited number of cases with suspected drug allergy. In contrast, a few workers reported an excellent correlation between test results and clinical history (Sarkany 1967; Mathews et al. 1972). It is obvious that variations in methodology and patient selection may influence the results of the tests.

The direct inhibition of leukocyte migration has been used to evaluate patients with adverse reactions to neomycin (Nordquist and Rossmann 1967) and in five of seven patients significant inhibition was demonstrated.

V. Experimental Studies in Animals

Experiments were performed in animals to establish the sensitization potentials and cross-sensitivity to different aminoglycosides. After immunization of guinea pigs or rabbits with streptomycin in Freund's complete adjuvant, hemagglutinating antibodies could be detected using streptomycin-coated red cells (Wenzel and Epstein 1964; Girard and Schwartz 1967; Cronin 1967; Chung and Carson 1976). With intradermal tests, streptomycin-sensitized guinea pigs rarely showed cross-sensitization to dihydrostreptomycin or to the other aminoglycosides (paromycin, kanamycin, gentamycin) except neomycin, whereas guinea pigs sensitized to dihydrostreptomycin or to the other aminoglycosides often showed cross-sensitization to streptomycin (Chung and Carson 1976).

Immunization of rabbits with gentamycin–protein conjugates led to the production of antibodies which were used for successful monitoring of gentamycin serum levels by a radioimmunoassay (Lewis et al. 1972).

VI. Conclusions Concerning Possible Pathomechanisms

The aminoglycoside antibiotics induce mainly the production of "sensitized" lymphocytes in humans and animals and only rarely induce a humoral response. Therefore, the clinical patterns observed are more the result of allergic reactions of the delayed type than those of the immediate type. The determinants inducing an immune response appear to be mainly in the neosamine fragment of the molecule, with participation of the deoxystreptamine ring as a minor determinant. It is important to remember that some aminoglycosides exhibit anaphylactoid activity and cause direct degranulation of mast cells. Such "anaphylactoid reactions" are clinically indistinguishable from true allergic reactions and have often been misinterpreted in the past.

E. Polymyxins

I. Physicochemical and Pharmacologic Properties

The polymyxins are a group of cyclic polypeptides derived from the *Bacillus* species. In addition to various amino acids, they contain 6-methyloctanoic or 6-methylheptanoic acid (Fig. 5) and are very stable substances. Solutions of the polymyxins retain their potency during storage for several months. Only polymyxin-B

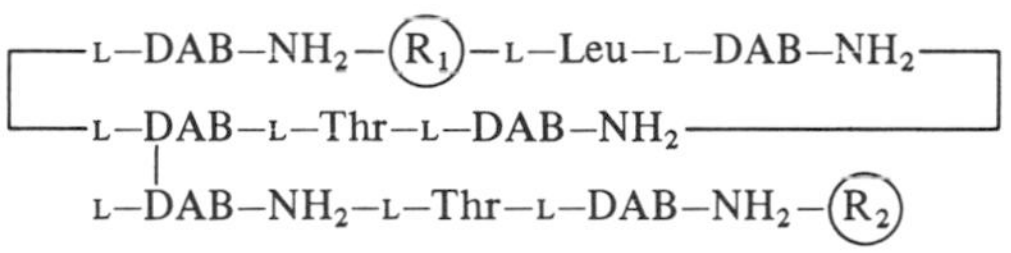

```
      ┌─L–DAB–NH₂–(R₁)–L–Leu–L–DAB–NH₂─┐
      └─L–DAB–L–Thr–L–DAB–NH₂──────────┘
           │
      L–DAB–NH₂–L–Thr–L–DAB–NH₂–(R₂)
```

(R₁)	(R₂)
I D–Phe	6–Methyloctanoyl or 6–Methylheptanoyl
II D–Leu	6–Methyloctanoyl or 6–Methylheptanoyl

Fig. 5. Polymyxin antibiotics: general structure. *DAB*=diaminobutyric acid; *Leu*=leucine; *Thr*=threonine. *I*=polymyxin-B, *II*=polymyxin-E

and polymyxin-E (chemically identical with colistin) are in clinical use because they are the least nephrotoxic compounds of the group. The antibacterial and pharmacologic porperties of polymyxin-B and polymyxin-E are almost identical. The polymyxins are strongly bactericidal, acting on the bacterial cell membrane and causing an increase in permeability, loss of essential cell constituents, and subsequent death of the microorganism. Both polymyxins are available either as sulfate or methylsulfonate. They are not absorbed from the gastrointestinal tract and have to be administered intramuscularly or intravenously for systemic use and in the form of drops or ointments for topical treatment. After parenteral injection the polymyxins are widely distributed throughout the body and readily infiltrate various organs, but are strongly protein bound. Maximal blood levels are obtained after 1–2 h and the half-life of polymyxin-B is 4 h and of polymyxin-E 2 h. The polymyxins do not reach the central nervous system, synovial-lined joint cavities, or ocular tissues unless injected locally. Excretion of parenterally administered polymyxins occurs mainly through the kidneys into the urine (KUCERS and BENNET 1975; OTTEN et al. 1975; SIMON and STILLE 1979).

II. Immunochemistry and Immunology

Immunization of rabbits with polymyxin-B–bovine serum albumin conjugates produced anti-polymyxin antibodies, as measured by direct agglutination of polymyxin-coated red blood cells (LAKIN et al. 1975a). These results and other studies in humans (LAKIN et al. 1975a, b; MÖLLER 1976) suggested a humoral response to the polymyxins, but information about antigenic determinants is as yet not available.

III. Clinical Aspects

On rare occasions, hepatotoxicity and toxic leukopenia have been observed during polymyxin-E (colistin) treatment, but a definite causal relationship has not been established. The most serious side effect of the polymyxins is their nephrotoxicity. Polymyxin-B is more nephrotoxic than polymyxin-E and the sulfate derivatives of both are more toxic than their corresponding methylsulfonates. The toxic effects are dose dependent and doses above the recommended range may be dangerous. The principal nephrotoxic effect of the polymyxins is on the epithelium of the renal convoluted tubules. The nervous system may also be damaged, leading to dizziness (progressing with increasing dosage), drowsiness, and various peripheral sensory disturbances such as numbness and paresthesias. Another serious neurotoxic effect is neuromuscular blockade, which may result in respiratory paralysis. Neurotoxic as well as nephrotoxic side effects disappear after complete excretion of the polymyxins (KUCERS and BENNET 1975; OTTEN et al. 1975; SIMON and STILLE 1979). Intrabronchial inhalation of these antibiotics as aerosols has been associated with bronchoconstriction and severe hypoxia (MARSCHKE and SARAUW 1971 a, b). The mechanism of this reaction is not clear. Polymyxin-B, on the other hand, is a well-documented nonspecific mast cell degranulating substance and may act as a direct histamine-releasing agent (LAGUNOFF and BENDITT 1960).

Other side effects such as rashes, pruritus, and fever have also been observed following polymyxin-B sulfate treatment (HOEPRICH 1970). A case with acute renal failure has also been described (BEIRNE et al. 1967) with glucosuria and eosinophilia during the oliguric stage. Renal biopsy, performed early in the course of the acute phase, revealed severe tubular damage as well as acute diffuse interstitial nephritis. Immunofluorescence studies were not carried out but the clinical and pathohistologic findings suggested that two pathogenic mechanisms existed which could have produced these symptoms. One was a direct toxic effect on the tubular cells and the other a hypersensitivity reaction resulting in interstitial nephritis.

Eczematous contact allergy due to polymyxin-B was noted on the legs of some patients with hypostatic dermatitis. Allergic reactions to many standard allergens were also noted in these patients (MÖLLER 1976). Intranasal administration of polymyxin-B led to nasal congestion, rhinorrhea, and perinasal angioedema in an acute leukemic patient who was rendered T-cell deficient for the purpose of bone marrow transplantation (LAKIN et al. 1975a). In a second patient, a generalized maculopapular eruption and fever were observed after bone marrow transplantation and attributed to polymyxin-B applied intranasally (LAKIN et al. 1975b). In both cases reaginic activity mediated by IgE antibodies against polymyxin-B was documented.

IV. Results of Diagnostic Tests

1. Skin Tests

Wheal and flare reactions to polymyxins are difficult to evaluate owing to the direct mast cell degranulating capacities of these compounds. One report stated that tests had been done with great caution and the occurrence of a positive skin test of the immediate type appears to be relevant (LAKIN et al. 1975b). In patients with stasis ulcers and dermatitis, positive patch tests have been obtained (MÖLLER 1976), but this seems to be rather uncommon.

2. Polymyxin-Specific Antibodies

Surprisingly in two patients, the existence of IgE antibodies to polymyxin-B could be confirmed by indirect hemagglutination and passive transfer tests in monkeys (LAKIN et al. 1975a, b). From these results, it was inferred that the polymyxins with a low sensitizing potential might show increased immunogenicity by way of specific IgE production in spontaneously or iatrogenic T-cell-depleted patients.

3. Polymyxin-Specific Lymphocyte Reactivity

No relevant data on polymyxin-specifically allergized lymphocytes are available at present in the literature (HALPERN et al. 1967; WARRINGTON et al. 1979).

V. Experimental Studies in Animals

Antibody formation to polymyxin-B has been reported to occur in guinea pigs following intradermal injections of the antibiotic with horse serum as adjuvant (MEL-NIKOVA 1971). This was demonstrated by skin tests with polymyxin-B in smaller amounts than those known to elicit nonspecific histamine release. Immunization of rabbits with a conjugate, prepared by the use of carbodiimide to couple polymyxin-B to bovine serum albumin, showed polymyxin-B-specific antibodies as demonstrated by passive hemagglutination with polymyxin-B-coated sheep red blood cells and hemagglutination inhibition studies using the free drug. Maximal, but not very high titers (up to 1:80), were observed after two booster injections at weekly intervals. Titers declined after 5–6 weeks to 1:10 or zero (LAKIN et al. 1975a). Antibody classes were not determined. The skin of chimpanzees was used to detect human IgE antibodies to polymyxin-B (LAKIN et al. 1975a, b). The amounts of polymyxin-B and polymyxin-B–keyhole limpet hemocyanin conjugate, appropriate for challenge without nonspecific mast cell degranulation were determined previously. Therefore, IgE antibodies appear to have been present.

VI. Conclusions Concerning Possible Pathomechanisms

The adverse reactions to the polymyxins are primarily toxic in nature. Very few of the observed adverse reactions could be shown by immunologic in vitro and in vivo tests to be of an allergic nature. Studies in animals and humans have shown, on the other hand, that under certain circumstances the polymyxins, although they have a low sensitizing potential, may stimulate specific immunoglubulin as well as lymphocytic response.

F. Rifamycins

I. Physicochemical and Pharmacologic Properties

The rifamycins comprise a group an antibiotics, originally isolated from *Streptomyces mediterranei*, which after chemical modification were marketed for clinical use as rifamycin SV, rifamide, and rifacin. At present, only the semisynthetic rifampicin is of clinical importance (Fig. 6). The rifamycins possess very potent antibiotic properties against gram-positive as well as gram-negative microorganisms and mycobacteria, especially against *Mycobacterium tuberculosis* and *M. leprae*. Rifampicin is water soluble and relatively stable in solution. It is capable of inhibiting bacterial RNA polymerase and is a strong bactericide. Bacteria can develop

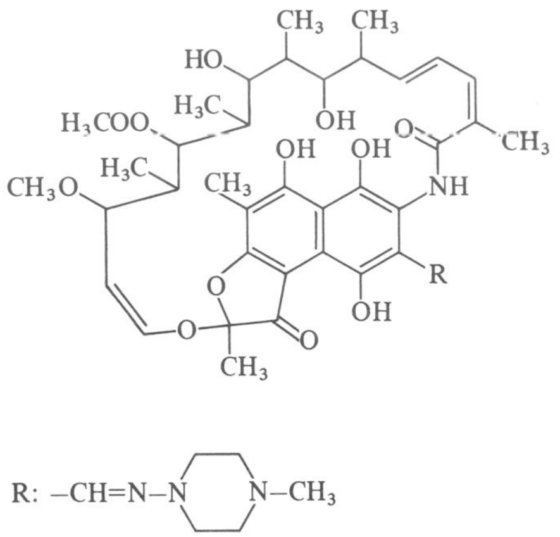

R: $-CH=N-N$⟮ ⟯$N-CH_3$

Fig. 6. Chemical structures of the rifamycin nucleus and of rifampicin ($R=$ 1-amino-4-methylpiperazine)

a resistance to rifampicin and, in order to prevent this, it should be used in combination with other antibiotics.

Rifampicin can be administered both orally or intravenously, and even when given orally, it is rapidly absorbed. Maximal serum levels are obtained within 2 h after oral intake or instantaneously following intravenous administration. About 80% of the drug is attached to plasma proteins and a half-life of 2 h has been reported. The antibiotic is widely distributed and diffuses readily into various organs. Rifampicin also has the capacity to pass through the placenta. Excretion takes place mainly via bile and only one-third is excreted through the urinary tract (KUCERS and BENNET 1975; OTTEN et al. 1975; SIMON and STILLE 1979).

II. Immunochemistry and Immunology

The immunogenic determinants responsible for the development of sensitization to rifampicin were characterized using sera from patients which contained antibodies to rifampicin (HOMBERG et al. 1973). Neither the rifampicin nucleus (rifamycin SV: R = H, Fig. 6) nor the side chain itself (1-amino-4-methylpiperazine) were able to substitute for rifampicin in the antiglobulin test, whereas extension at R (Fig. 6) as in 3-formylrifampicin-*N,N*-dimethylhydrazone, resulted in a compound which to some extent had these capacities. The results suggest that the hydrazone structure contributes significantly to the immunologic specificity of rifampicin. STEVENS et al. (1973) observed that the gel precipitation patterns of patients' sera with rifampicin–protein conjugates could be inhibited completely by rifampicin and 3-formylrifampicin SV, but only partially by rifamycin SV. This underlines the importance of the proximal end of the R side chain as an antigenic determinant. In contrast, BASSI et al. (1976) found antibodies in patients sera which cross-reacted with the rifampicin nucleus and with the chromophoric moiety of the rifamycins, but not with the side chain of rifampicin.

All these data seem to indicate that rifampicin has an immunogenic capacity, but further studies are required to confirm this unequivocally. It will be necessary to demonstrate that these results are actually caused by antibodies to rifampicin and not by other nonspecific effects (see Sect. F.IV.2).

III. Clinical Aspects

The clinically recorded adverse reaction to rifampicin suggest that its major side effects depend mainly on the treatment regimen used (BLAJCHMAN et al. 1970; POOLE et al. 1971; PUJET et al. 1974; GIRLING 1977; GIRLING and HITZE 1979).

Mild and transient reactions, occurring usually in 2%–5% of patients, have been reported regardless of whether rifampicin was given daily or intermittently. Cutaneous reactions have also been observed and consisted of flushing of the face and neck, itching, and rashes. It is interesting that a constant increase from 75 mg/day to 600–1,200 mg/day leads in most cases to complete tolerance. Other adverse reactions reported include gastrointestinal disturbances with loss of appetite, nausea, mild abdominal pain, and occasionally vomiting and diarrhea. In up to 1% of patients – most of them with abnormal liver functions – hepatitis with jaundice has been documented. In such cases, treatment has to be stopped and only resumed when liver function tests are normal again. These reactions are very rarely of a serious nature. A small number of patients, however, are unable to tolerate rifampicin treatment and administration of the drug has to be discontinued (GIRLING and HITZE 1979).

Intermittent rifamycin therapy (administered once or twice a week) rather than daily administration is much more likely to create serious complications (POOLE et al. 1971; AQUINAS et al. 1972) and in such cases an allergic reaction seems to be the basis for the complications. Occurrences of collapse and shock, shortness of breath with or without wheezing and a "flu-like" syndrome (consisting of fever, chills, headache, dizziness, and myalgias starting 1–2 h after each dose and lasting for up to 8 h) have also been described (PUJET et al. 1974; GIRLING 1977).

Potentially serious reactions have been reported by BLAJCHMAN et al. (1970), POOLE et al. (1971), AUTRAN et al. (1973), and PUJET et al. (1974) and these authors drew attention to thombocytopenia occurring when intermittent doses of rifampicin were given (GIRLING 1977). Others have observed massive hemolysis (HASSE et al. 1971; SCHUBOTHE et al. 1972; LAKSHAMINARAYAN et al. 1973; MOEHRING et al. 1974) with or without renal failure (KLEINKNECHT et al. 1972; KROENIG et al. 1972; SEUFERT 1973; CAMPESE et al. 1973; PUJET et al. 1974; MOEHRING et al. 1974; KANDRA et al. 1978; WAHL et al. 1978). The demonstration of rifampicin-specific antibodies was taken as evidence that an immunologic mechanism induced the destruction of the red blood cells and platelets, but further studies are needed to substantiate this hypothesis (see Sect. F.IV.2).

Additional side effects reported in connection with rifampicin treatment were severe exudative conjunctivitis (CAYLEY and MAJUMDAR 1976), the occurrence of the Stevens–Johnson syndrome (NYIRENDA and GILL 1977) and pemphigus vulgaris (GANGE et al. 1976). All information on adverse reactions to rifampicin has been obtained from studies of patients afflicted with tuberculosis. It is likely that similar observations will be made when patients with other diseases are treated with similar doses, but this has yet to be demonstrated.

IV. Results of Diagnostic Tests

1. Skin Tests

It is interesting to note that prick or intracutaneous tests with rifampicins or analogs were apparently carried out in very few cases, and little information is available on this subject, even in comprehensive reviews (Mattson 1973; Girling 1977). The reason for this may be the low incidence of allergic reactions, inadequate knowledge of antigenic determinants and therefore inadequate test solutions, and also the fact that chest physicians (who usually observe side effects) are not as familiar with skin testing as allergologists. Patch tests with rifampicin have, however, been carried out by some workers (Kroenig et al. 1972; Hong Kong 1975), but only negative results were recorded. In cases of thrombocytopenia with or without purpura, Prausnitz–Küstner tests have been performed and positive results reported, suggesting the existence of IgE antibodies to rifampicin (reviewed by Nessi et al. 1973, but without detailed information).

2. Rifamycin-Specific Antibodies

Circulating antibodies to rifampicin were first detected in sera from patients who had thrombocytopenia and/or a "flu-like" syndrome (Blajchman et al. 1970; Poole et al. 1971). An immunologic study, by means of the platelet complement fixation test, demonstrated antibodies of both IgG and IgM types capable of fixing complement to normal as well as patients' platelets, but only in the presence of rifampicin. The IgM antibody (but not the IgG) was able to fix complement to normal red cells in the presence of rifampicin, as observed with the antiglobulin test. Other reports have since described similar findings (Kleinknecht et al. 1972; Kroenig et al. 1972; Herrmann and Eule 1973; Virgilio 1973; Pujet et al. 1974). Acute hemolytic anemia and renal failure as a result of intermittent rifampicin treatment have also been recorded and, here also, antibodies to rifampicin were detected with the antiglobulin test (Sors et al. 1972; Schubothe and Weber 1973). Worlledge (1973) and O'Mahony (1973) established a correlation between the presence of the "flu-like" syndrome and the development of rifampicin-reactive antibodies.

These findings have been interpreted in a number of different ways. Some authors believe that hapten–antibody or antigen–antibody complexes are adsorbed onto cells and under certain circumstances lead to cell destruction. Other workers, on the other hand, claim that rifampicin can bind nonspecifically to both serum proteins and to cell surfaces (Dukor et al. 1973, Boman et al. 1973), resulting in nonimmunologically mediated antiglobulin reactions. The editors of the Stockholm Workshop Proceedings on rifampicin side effects concluded that neither the immunogenic capacity of rifampicin nor the immune origin of the so-called antirifampicin antibodies can be considered as established (Editorial 1973).

Bassi et al. (1976) have since demonstrated human IgE antibodies to rifampicin by means of histamine release from passively sensitized peritoneal mast cells. The sera were obtained from patients showing side effects to rifampicin therapy. These results seem to provide further evidence for an immunologic origin of the adverse reactions to rifampicin.

3. Rifamycin-Specific Lymphocyte Reactivity

Lymphocyte transformation tests in vitro have been carried out, but with negative results (KLEINKNECHT et al. 1972; PUJET et al. 1974). An inhibition of protein synthesis by rifampicin, similar to that observed with chloramphenicol, could explain the failure to obtain lymphocyte blast transformation (DAJANI et al. 1972).

V. Experimental Studies in Animals

Guinea pigs were immunized repeatedly with rifampicin in complete Freund's adjuvant and skin reactions after challenge were studied (DUKOR et al. 1973). There was evidence of allergic reactions of the immediate as well as of the delayed type. However, antibodies were not measured by passive cutaneous anaphylaxis or any other immunologic method. Therefore, the skin reactions observed 4 h after challenge could well have masked an incipient type of delayed hypersensitivity reaction (DEWDNEY 1977). Hence, these experiments do not establish unequivocally the immunogenicity of rifampicin.

VI. Conclusions Concerning Possible Pathomechanisms

The incidence of adverse reactions to rifamycins and especially rifampicin is low and the side effects reported are said to be mild and transient, provided the drug is administered daily. By contrast, intermittent administration or readministration after longer periods carry the risk of unpleasant, sometimes potentially dangerous reactions. It is considered possible that some of these phenomena are due to underlying immunologic mechanisms.

G. Macrolides

I. Physicochemical and Pharmacologic Properties

The macrolide antibiotics are a group of compounds which have as a nucleus a macrocyclic lactone ring to which one or more sugars are attached. These sugars are essential for the antibiotic activity. Only three of the macrolides, i.e., erythromycin, oleandomycin, and spiramycin are used in human clinical practice, while a fourth, tylosin, is used in veterinary medicine and as a food preservative in industrial canning. These are all weakly alkaline and only slightly soluble in water. Erythromycin is the most active antibiotic of this group (Fig. 7). All of them are able to inhibit bacterial protein synthesis and are characterized by their bacteriostatic qualities. The antibacterial spectrum is similar to that of benzylpenicillin.

Development of bacterial resistance, with associated cross-resistance to lincomycins, may occasionally limit the clinical use of the macrolides. The esters formed by these antibiotics are clinically important because they are more readily absorbed from the intestinal tract, but are possibly more toxic. Erythromycin is commonly administered orally as a base, stearate, or as an estolate, but it can also be administered intravenously as a lactobionate or glucoheptonate or intramuscularly as an ethylsuccinate, although such administration is rare, because the injec-

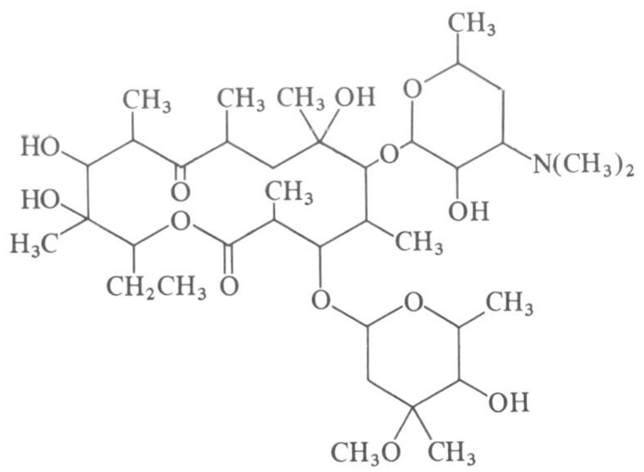

Fig. 7. Chemical structure of erythromycin

tions are painful. Maximal serum levels are obtained 1–3 h after oral and about 1 h after parenteral administration. Oleandomycin is administered orally in the form of the rapidly absorbed (but more toxic) triacetyloleandomycin, and spiramycin as a sulfate. Between 30% and 60% of the macrolides are attached to plasma proteins. The macrolides are widely distributed throughout many tissues and are retained there for long periods of time. Spiramycin produces higher and more sustained tissue concentrations than any other member of the group. Excretion occurs via the bile and feces and only partly through the kidney in the urine (KUCERS and BENNET 1975; OTTEN et al. 1975; SIMON and STILLE 1979).

II. Immunochemistry and Immunology

Clinical studies have suggested that under certain circumstances immunogenic macrolide metabolites do occur (HALPERN et al. 1967; KETEL 1976; NAIK 1976). Animal studies on the other hand, have produced inconclusive results. WHITE (1965) reported that immunization of mice resulted in the production of erythromycin-specific antibodies as proven by inhibition studies with the drug, whereas RAAB (1977) failed to produce antibodies against erythromycin in rats and guinea pigs. The maximization test (KLIGMAN 1967) also produced negative results in humans. At present, only limited information is available regarding the immunogenic determinants of macrolide antibiotics and no information pertaining to their chemical structure has been published.

III. Clinical Aspects

The macrolides can be regarded as relatively safe compounds with a very low incidence of adverse reactions. Gastrointestinal disturbances such as anorexia, nausea, vomiting, abdominal pain, and fever at times limit their use in clinical practice. Erythromycin estolate and triacetyloleandomycin are well known for their capacity to produce liver damage (GILBERT 1962). Enlargement of the liver, jaundice, elevation of alkaline phosphatase, transaminases, and direct-binding bilirubin in the serum, and blood eosinophilia have all been recorded (BRAUN 1969). Liver biopsies have demonstrated intrahepatic cholestasis and periportal cellular infiltrates of mononuclear cells and eosinophils. Discontinuation of treatment usually resulted in full recovery. The hepatic effects seen as a result of administering the two compounds mentioned, are not dose dependent and therefore have been classified as hypersensitivity reactions of the liver (SHERLOCK 1965). It is more likely, however, that these effects are due to the toxic nature of the antibiotics (BRAUN 1969).

Other types of reactions with possible allergic causes are uncommon (BENNETT 1965; BEATY and PETERSDORF 1966). In a long-term study of 20,525 patients treated with propionyl erythromycin and erythromycin estolate, the incidence of skin eruptions was found to be 0.5% (KUDER 1960). A total of 548 allergic children, most of them atopic, were treated with erythromycin ethylsuccinate and again 0.5% of children developed skin reactions (CRAWFORD and ROANE 1969). Spiramycin, given prophylactically to patients undergoing prostatectomy, produced a rash in 1 of 259 patients (MACFARLANE et al. 1968). DAVIES and PEPYS (1975) reported the occurrence of asthma and a rash in one patient after contact with spiramycin. An allergic mechanisms could not be proven by positive skin tests nor by lymphocyte transformation in vitro, but the bronchial provocation test, on the other hand, was positive.

Anaphylactic shock due to macrolides is an extremely rare event (GRATER 1962). There have been reports of urticaria (PRASAD 1960; KETEL 1976) and one report on a fixed drug eruption following erythromycin therapy (NAIK 1976). The safety of topical erythromycin treatment has been investigated in 60 patients with stasis ulcers. None of these patients showed any local irritation or contact dermatitis and this type of treatment was therefore recommended (FISHER 1976a, b). KETEL (1976), however, observed allergic contact dermatitis in one woman after topical treatment with 5% erythromycin ointment and stated that this form of therapy was not without risk, albeit small. Allergic contact dermatitis due to tylosin and spiramycin has been observed in farmers (PREYSS 1969; VELEN et al. 1980).

IV. Results of Diagnostic Tests

1. Skin Tests

Scratch as well as patch tests have been performed in a few patients suspected of allergic reactivity to macrolides. KETEL (1976) tested a 7-year-old girl with a generalized urticarial eruption following treatment with erythromycin stearate suspension. After a negative patch test, a strongly positive scratch test was obtained. In the same publication, attention was drawn to a case of eczematous eruptions after topical treatment with 5% erythromycin stearate in petrolatum; patch tests with 0.1%, 1%, and 5% erythromycin stearate ointment were positive. HALPERN et al. (1967) recorded a positive skin test of the immediate type with spiramycin in a patient with a history of allergy. PREYSS (1969) reported that epicutaneous testing with tylosin led to a positive result in a man with contact dermatitis. This patient had come into contact with tylosin while working on a poultry farm where this antibiotic was used against various poultry diseases and as a growth promotor. The results obtained highlight the fact that, under certain circumstances, macrolides possess a sensitizing potential.

2. Macrolide-Specific Antibodies

Antibodies to erythromycin in humans have not as yet been found by in vitro methods. Serologic tests have been performed by DAVIES and PEPYS (1975) who tried to find antibodies against spiramycin in a patient suffering from asthma and rash following contact with spiramycin at work, but the results were negative.

3. Macrolide-Specific Lymphocyte Reactivity

Various studies have shown that the in vitro lymphocyte transformation test is of some diagnostic value in cases of macrolide hypersensitivity. HALPERN et al. (1967) reported the induction of a lymphocyte proliferative response in vitro by spiramycin in two cases. This reactivity, combined with a typical case history and a positive scratch test to spiramycin in one case, was sufficient to demonstrate hypersensitivity. DAVIES and PEPYS (1975) as well as WARRINGTON et al. (1979), on the other hand, found no evidence of lymphocyte response in vitro in patients with rashes after erythromycin therapy or spiramycin contact.

V. Experimental Studies in Animals

Experiments have been carried out in different animal species. Immunization of mice with erythromycin in complete Freund's adjuvant has led to the production of antibodies which agglutinated erythromycin-coated red blood cells (WHITE 1965). Studies in rats and guinea pigs, however, gave no evidence of an erythromycin-specific immune response, as confirmed by skin tests (RAAB 1977).

VI. Conclusions Concerning Possible Pathomechanisms

Side effects caused by macrolides are uncommon and only a very few seem to be caused by allergic mechanisms confirmed by positive skin tests. Up to now, in vitro tests have produced only limited evidence that an immune response to these antibiotics can indeed be induced in animals as well as in humans.

H. Lincomycins

I. Physicochemical and Pharmacologic Properties

Lincomycin was isolated in 1962 from a strain of *Streptomyces lincolnensis*. It is a monobasic compound (Fig. 8) and is readily water soluble as a base or as a hydrochloride. Like its semisynthetic derivative, clindamycin (Fig. 8) it has bacteriostatic activity against most gram-positive bacteria by inhibiting bacterial protein synthesis. In their mode and range of antibacterial activity the lincomycins show great similarity to the macrolides, although no chemical relationship between the two groups of antibiotics exists. The lincomycins are used as alternate drugs to penicillin in the treatment of those patients known to have a penicillin allergy. All compounds of the series can be administered orally, intramuscularly, or intravenously. After oral administration, 20%–70% of the lincomycin (depending on whether the patient's stomach is full or empty) and 75% of the clindamycin is ab-

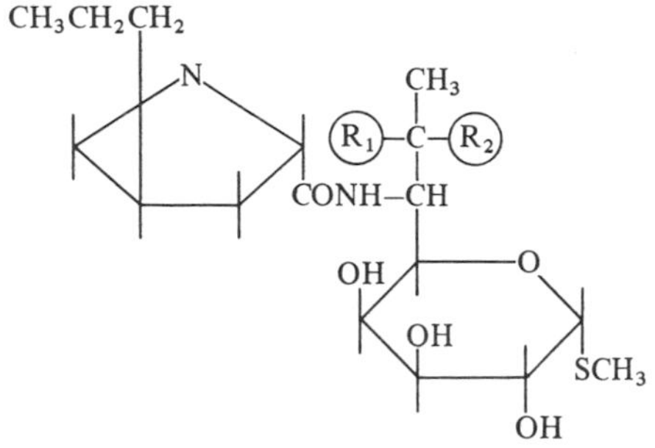

Fig. 8. Chemical structures of lincomycin (*I*) and clindamycin (*II*)

sorbed through the gastrointestinal tract and maximal blood levels are found after 1 and 4 h, respectively. Approximately 30% of lincomycin and 80% of clindamycin are attached to plasma proteins. Biologic half-lives have been reported to be 5 h for lincomycin and 2.75 h for clindamycin. Both lincomycins are widely distributed and diffuse readily into various organs and are able to pass through the placenta. Excretion occurs mainly through the urinary tract and only a small amount is excreted through the bile (KUCERS and BENNET 1975; OTTEN et al. 1975; SIMON and STILLE 1979).

II. Immunochemistry and Immunology

Studies on the immunogenicity of lincomycins have been carried out in various animal species. In mice and rabbits, different immunization schedules and different immunization routes failed to stimulate antibody formation, as shown by gel precipitation and hemagglutination tests (WHITE 1965). Similar negative results were reported by RAAB (1977), who conducted immunization experiments and skin test challenges in rats and guinea pigs. In his experiments, the maximization test according to KLIGMAN (1967) also showed negative results in humans. However, a small number of clinical observations suggest that clindamycin may well act as a sensitizing agent, especially when applied topically (COSKEY 1978; HERSTOFF 1978). The antigenic determinants are unknown.

III. Clinical Aspects

An important advantage of the lincomycins is their very low toxicity to the liver, the bone marrow, and the kidneys. Therefore, only a few adverse reactions are known. Diarrhea and severe pseudomembranous colitis have been observed after oral or parenteral treatment with either of the lincomycins. Retrospective as well as prospective studies have shown inconclusive results regarding the incidence of colitis (PITMANN et al. 1974; BASLER 1976). *Clostridium difficile* has been identified as the most probable cause of this intestinal side effect (reviewed by MANTEN 1979).

Under appropriate conditions this microorganism may become resistant to the lincomycins and become hypertrophic. It seems to be able to produce a special toxin which can cause either diarrhea or colitis, depending on the amount of toxin produced. Because of these potentially serious complications the use of the lincomycins in the treatment of various diseases has to be reevaluated.

The occurrence of anaphylactic shock (LOCHMANN et al. 1977), acute urticaria, and angioedema (WALKER 1969) have been reported and postulated to be hypersensitivity reactions. In addition, other cutaneous reactions such as rashes (GEDDES et al. 1970; MAULIDE and VILLAR 1974), and the Stevens–Johnson syndrome (FULGHUM and CATALANO 1973; MAULIDE and VILLAR 1974) have been described, but their etiology has not been defined. However, allergic contact dermatitis due to clindamycin therapy has been observed in two patients (COSKEY 1978; HERSTOFF 1978).

IV. Results of Diagnostic Tests

1. Skin Tests

Up to now, data on positive skin tests of the immediate type to lincomycin have not been reported. Positive patch tests with clindamycin have established the allergic nature of contact dermatitis in two patients (COSKEY 1978; HERSTOFF 1978).

2. Lincomycin-Specific Antibodies

Hemagglutinating antibodies to both lincomycin and clindamycin have been found in the serum of a patient with anaphylactic shock following oral administration of clindamycin (LOCHMANN et al. 1977). In the absence of other satisfactory methods, this assay seems to be useful in establishing the diagnosis of an allergic reaction to the lincomycins. The measured antibodies, however, may not be of importance in the genesis of the observed allergy.

3. Lincomycin-Specific Lymphocyte Reactivity

There are no reports in the literature concerning results obtained with in vitro lymphocyte transformation or leukocyte migration inhibition tests in patients with suspected allergy to the lincomycins.

V. Experimental Studies in Animals

Immunization experiments with lincomycins in Freund's complete adjuvant (WHITE 1965; RAAB 1977) or with lincomycin–protein conjugates (WHITE 1965) were unsuccessful; no humoral or cell-mediated response were detected in mice, rats, or guinea pigs.

VI. Conclusions Concerning Possible Pathomechanisms

Experimental studies have provided no evidence to show that the lincomycins have the ability to stimulate a specific immune response in animals, but some clinical observations have suggested the possibility of immunologically mediated adverse reactions. Further studies are required to substantiate these clinical findings.

J. Miscellaneous Antibiotics

I. Vancomycin

This antibiotic was introduced in 1956, and is derived from *Streptomyces orientalis*. It is a macromolecular glycopeptide with bactericidal activity. In spite of significant ototoxicity and nephrotoxicity, it may be a valuable drug in the treatment of endocarditis, osteomyelitis, pneumonia, or septicemia caused by gram-positive cocci which are resistant to other antibiotics. Oral vancomycin is not absorbed, and, combined with gentamycin and mystatin, has been administered to patients for bowel sterilization. Vancomycin is highly irritating to tissues; intramuscular injections are too painful to be used clinically and after intravenous administration thrombophlebitis may occur (SIMON and STILLE 1979). Vancomycin usually induces chills, fever, malaise, and rashes (GERACI 1977). Anaphylactic shock and urticarial eruptions (FRIEDBERG et al. 1968; MILLER and TAUSK 1977) as apparently allergic reactions have also been observed. At present, there is no detailed information available from animal experiments, skin tests in humans, or in vitro tests, to suggest that vancomycin is immunogenic or allergenic.

II. Spectinomycin

Spectinomycin is an aminocyclitol antibiotic. It is active against a wide range of bacteria and is used primarily in the treatment of gonorrhea. Low toxicity has been noted by several investigators (WILLCOX 1962; DUNCAN et al. 1972; SAVAGE 1973). The available information shows that some patients have noted transient dizziness, fever, headache, or local pain after intramuscular injection (SIMON and STILLE 1979). Erythematous rashes following treatment with spectinomycin have been observed in a few patients, but no other adverse reactions suggesting an allergic origin (PEDERSEN et al. 1972). Immunization experiments in guinea pigs showed no specific immune response as evaluated by skin tests in these animals (RAAB 1975).

III. Novobiocin

This drug was isolated from *Streptomyces niveus* in 1955 and is a dibasic acid. Formerly it had been used in the treatment of staphylococci-mediated infections. Since the introduction of the penicillinase-resistant penicillins, its use has been superseded by these newer drugs, which are safer and much more effective (KUCERS and BENNET 1975).

Its clinical administration was associated with many adverse reactions (reviewed by BRIDGES et al. 1957; SCHINDEL 1966). Mild gastrointestinal symptoms were common but rarely necessitated stopping treatment. Drug fever occurred frequently if treatment was given for more than one week. Eosinophilia, moderate reversible leukopenia, and maculopapular rashes have been recorded. Allergic reactions, manifested by urticaria and serum-sickness-like reactions and established by positive skin tests, have been observed. The occurrence of immunothrombocytopenic purpura in one patient has also been reported (DAY et al. 1958).

The sensitization potential of novobiocin in healthy volunteers was investigated by SHELLEY (1963). He found marked basopenia after rechallenge in one volunteer who had formerly developed a rash. In animals, immunization studies have been carried out and antibodies detected, as demonstrated by precipitation in agar gels and by hemagglutination (WHITE 1965). These results suggest that novobiocin is a drug which could induce an immune response that could result in subsequent allergic reactions. The nature of the antigenic determinants is unknown.

References

Acker R, Schreier K (1962) Erfahrungen mit der Chloramphenicolbehandlung von 3 648 Patienten einer Kinderklinik. Med Klin 57:474–479

Aquinas M, Allan WGL, Horsfall PAL et al. (1972) Adverse reactions to daily and intermittent rifampicin regimens for pulmonary tuberculosis in Hong Kong. Br Med J 1:765–771

Autran P, Kaplanski S, Dugue P, Arnaud A, Charpin J (1973) Un cas d'accident d'origine immuno-allergique avec purpura thrombocytopenigue dû à la rifampicine. Mars Med 10:845–851

Basler RSW (1976) Potential hazards of clindamycin in acne therapy. Arch Dermatol 112:383–385

Bassi L, Di Berardino L, Silvestri LG (1976) IgE antibodies in patients allergic to rifampicin. Int Arch Allergy Appl Immunol 51:390–394

Bean SF (1971) Acneiform eruption from tetracycline. Br J Dermatol 85:585–586

Beaty HN, Petersdorf RG (1966) Iatrogenic factors in infectious disease. Ann Intern Med 65:641–656

Beck EA (1975) Chloramphenicol- und Thiamphenicolschäden des Bluts. Schweiz Med Wochenschr 105:1078–1080

Bedford PD (1951) Idiosyncrasy to aureomycin. Br Med J 2:1428–1429

Beirne GJ, Hansing CE, Octaviano GN, Burus RO (1967) Acute renal failure caused by hypersensitivity to polymyxin B sulfate. JAMA 202:62–64

Bennett AH (1965) Antibiotic allergies. JAMA 194:569

Berté SJ, Di Mase ID, Christianson CS (1964) Iosoniazid para-aminosalicylic acid and streptomycin intolerance in 1,714 patients. Am Rev. Respir Dis 90:598–606

Blajchman MA, Lowry RC, Pettit JE, Stradling P (1970) Rifampicin-induced immune thrombocytopenia. Br Med J 3:24–26

Blank H, Cullen SI, Cataland PM (1968) Photosensitivity studies with demethyl-chlortetracycline and doxycycline. Arch Dermatol 97:1–2

Bojs G, Möller H (1974) Eczematous contact allergy to oxytetracycline with cross-sensitivity to other tetracyclines. Berufsdermatosen 22:202–208

Boman G, Nilsson BS, Saerens EJ (1973) Protein binding of rifampicin. Scand J Respir Dis [Suppl] 84:40–44

Boonen W, Van Waveren JW, Hogervorst A (1964) Hypersensitivity to antibiotics. Dermatologica 128:394–409

Braun P (1969) Editorial: hepatoxicity of erythromycin. J Infect Dis 119:300–306

Braun W, Schütz R (1969) Beitrag zur Gentamycin-Allergie. Hautarzt 20:108–112

Bridges RA, Berendes H, Good RA (1957) Serious reactions to novobiocin. J Pediatr 50:579

Brown ST (1974) Tetracycline balanitis: fixed drug reaction. JAMA 227:801

Businco L, Lendvai D, Cardi E (1968) Reazione allergica alla tetraciclina e sindrome della „bulging fontanel" in un bambino di quaranta giorni: sensibilizzazione attraverso il latte materno. Acta Paediatr Lat 21:834–838

Cahill KM (1962) Chloramphenicol hypersensitivity. A severe haemorrhagic reaction. Lancet 2:277–278

Calnan CD, Sarkany I (1958) Contact dermatitis from neomycin. Br J Dermatol 70:435–445

Campese VM, Marzullo F, Schena FP, Coratelli P (1973) Acute renal failure during intermittent rifampicin therapy. Nephron 10:256–260

Carpenter G (1975) Chloramphenicol eye-drops and marrow aplasia. Lancet 2:326–327

Cayley FE, Majundar SK (1976) Ocular toxicity due to rifampicin reversible. Br Med J 1:199–200

Chakravarty S, Sircar DK (1961) Allergic reactions due to streptomycin: corroboration of clinical findings with streptomycin skin tests. Acta Tuberc Scand 41:144–148

Chung CW, Carson TR (1976) Cross-sensitivity in common aminoglycoside antibiotics. Arch Dermatol 112:1101–1107

Chyrek-Borowska S, Karna T, Obrzut D (1973) Leukocyte migration inhibition tests in investigations of allergy to treptomycin. Pol Tyg Lek 28:1536–1540

Coles RB, Philips J, Nuttall JB (1967) Anaphylactoid reaction to demethyl-chlortetracycline (Ledermycin). Br Med J 2:313–314

Coskey RJ (1978) Contact dermatitis due to clindamycin. Arch Dermatol 114:446

Crawford LV, Roane J (1969) Use of erythromycin ethylsuccinate in allergic children. Ann Allergy 27:18–22

Cronin EE (1972) Contact dermatitis XVII. Reactions to contact allergens given orally or systemically. Br J Dermatol 86:104–107

Csonka GW, Rosedale N, Walkden L (1971) Balanitis due to fixed frug eruption associated with tetracycline therapy. Br J Vener Dis 47:42–44

Dajani BM, Canady MS, Thompson JS, Kasik JE (1972) Rifampicin: an immunosuppressant? Lancet 2:1094

Davies RJ, Pepys J (1975) Asthma due to enhaled chemical agents – the macrolide antibiotic spiramycin. Clin Allergy 5:99–107

Day HJ, Conrad FG, Moore JE (1958) Immunothrombocytopenia induced by novobiocin. Am J Med Sci 236:475

Delaney TJ (1970) Tetracycline-induced fixed drug eruptions. Br J Dermatol 83:357–358

Dewdney JM (1977) Immunology of the antibiotics. In: Sela M (ed) The antigens IV. Academic Press, New York San Francisco London, pp 73–245

Dobozy A, Hunyadi J, Simon H (1971) Demonstration of chloramphenicol hypersensitivity by measurement of histone methylation in lymphocyte cultures. Clin Exp Immunol 8:917–925

Dohn W (1962) Testanalytische Untersuchungen zur Frage der relativen Häufigkeit von Antibiotika-Kontaktallergien. Arzneim Forsch 12:601–606

Dukor P, Schumann G, Dietrich FM (1973) Immunological studies with rifampicin. Scand J Respir Dis [Suppl] 84:73–82

Duncan WC, Holder WR, Roberts DP, Knox JM (1972) Treatment of gonorrhoea with spectinomycin hydrochloride: comparison with standard penicillin schedules. Antimicrob Agents Chemother 1:210–214

Eberhartinger C, Ebner H (1966) Beitrag zur Kenntnis der Kontaktallergie durch Chloramphenicol. Arch Klin Exp Dermatol 224:463–470

Ebner H (1973) Kontaktallergie gegen Antibiotika. Wien Klin Wochenschr 85:203–204

Editorial (1965) Anaphylactic reaction to tetracycline. JAMA 192:992

Editorial (1970) Chloramphenicol-induced bone marrow suppression. JAMA 213:1183–1184

Editorial comments and conclusions Boman G, Nilsson BS, Saevens EJ (1973) Stockholm workshop on rifampicin 1972. Scand J Respir Dis [Suppl] 84:192–193

Editorial (1977) Topical antibiotics. Br Med J 1:1494

Epstein S (1956) Contact dermatitis from neomycin due to dermal delayed (tuberculin-type) sensitivity. Dermatologica 113:191–201

Epstein E, Panzer JD (1971) Neomycin sensitivity. Arch Dermatol 103:562

Epstein S, Wenzel FJ (1962) Cross-sensitivity to various "mycins". Arch Dermatol 86:183–194

Fawcett IW, Pepys J (1976) Allergy to a tetracycline preparation – a case report. Clin Allergy 6:301–304

Fellner MJ, Baer RC (1965) Anaphylactic reaction to tetracycline in a penicillin-allergic patient. JAMA 192:997–998

Fellner MJ, Baer RL (1966) Immunologic studies in a patient sensitive to tetracycline and penicillin. Arch Klin Exp Dermatol 224:157–167

Fisher AA (1966) Systemic eczematous "contact type" dermatitis medicamentosa. Ann Allergy 24:406–410

Fisher AA (1976 a) Erythromycin: a nonsensitizing topical antibiotic. Arch Dermatol 112:732

Fisher AA (1976 b) The safety of topical erythromycin. Contact Dermatitis 2:43–45

Förström L, Pirilä V (1978) Cross-sensitivity within the neomycin group of antibiotics. Contact Dermatitis 4:312

Forck G (1971) Häufigkeit und Bedeutung von Chloramphenicol-Allergien. Dtsch Med Wochenschr 96:161–165

Fraki JE, Peltonen L, Hopsu-Hava VK (1979) Allergy to various components of topical preparations in stasis dermatitis and leg ulcer. Contact Dermatitis 5:98–100

Friedberg CK, Rosen KM, Bienstock PA (1968) Vancomycin therapy for enterococcae and streptococcus viridans endocarditis. Arch Intern Med 122:134–138

Frost P, Weinstein GD, Gomez EC (1971) Methacycline and demeclocycline in relation to sunlight. JAMA 216:326–327

Furey WW, Tan C (1969) Anaphylactic shock due to demethylchlortetracycline. Ann Intern Med 70:357–385

Fulghum DD, Catalano PM (1973) Stevens-Johnson syndrome from clindamycin. A case report. JAMA 223:318–319

Gange RW, Rhodes EL, Edwards CO, Powell MEA (1976) Pemphigus induced by rifampicin. Br J Dermatol 95:445–448

Geddes AM, Bridgwater FAJ, Williams DN, Don J, Grimshaw GJ (1970) Clinical and bacteriological studies with clindamycin. Br Med J 2:703–704

Geraci JE (1977) Vancomycin. Mayo Clin Proc 52:631–634

Gilbert FI (1962) Cholestatic hepatitis caused by esters of erythromycin and oleandomycin. JAMA 182:1048–1051

Girard JP (1974) Diagnostic tests in drug allergy. In: Yamamura Y et al. (eds) Allergology. Excerpta Medica, Amsterdam London New York, pp 460–466

Girard JP, Schwartz H (1967) Serum hemagglutinating antibodies in streptomycin allergy. Med Pharmacol Exp 17:466–474

Girling DJ (1977) Adverse reactions to rifampicin in antituberculosis regimens. J Antimicrob Chemother 3:115–132

Girling DJ, Hitze KL (1979) Adverse reactions to rifampicin. Bull WHO 57:45–50

Grater WC (1962) Allergic reactions to oral antibacterials in hypersensitive patients. Ann Allergy 20:480–485

Greenberg M, Greenspan W (1962) Anaphylactoid reaction to demethyl-chlortetracycline hydrochloride. JAMA 181:454

Grudzinski W (1960) Death following a test injection of dihydrostreptomycin. Bull Pol med Hist Sci 13:139–140

Haas R (1957) Anaphylactoid reaction to oral tetracycline. J Maine Med Assoc 48:85–86

Halpern B, Ky NT, Amache N (1967) Diagnosis of drug allergy in vitro with the lymphocyte transformation test. J Allergy 40:168–181

Hamburger RN (1966) Chloramphenicol-specific antibody. Science 152:203–205

Hamburger RN, Douglass JH (1969 a) Chloramphenicol-specific antibody. II. Reactivity to analogues of chloramphenicol. Immunology 17:587–592

Hamburger RN, Douglass JH (1969 b) Chloramphenicol-specific antibody. III. Differential Ab decay rates to separate determinants on one antigen. Immunology 17:593–598

Hamburger RN, Douglass JH (1969 c) Chloramphenicol-specific antibody. IV. Neutralization of antibiotic effect on escherichia coli. Immunology 17:599–602

Hashimoto Y, Sasaki H, Yoshinari M, Iwatsuki K (1976) Myasthenia gravis and antibiotics. Jpn J Anesthesiol 26:143–147

Hasse W, Pohle MD, Warnecke F, Weik K (1971) Hämatologische Krise durch Rifampicin. Prax Pneumol 25:466–468

Herrmann H, Eule H (1973) Immunological and haematological investigations on patients with adverse reactions during treatment with RMP plus INH once-weekly. Scand J Respir Dis [Suppl] 84:87–93

Herstoff JK (1978) Sensitization to topical antibiotics. Arch Dermatol 114:1402

Hewitt WL (1974) Gentamycin: toxicity in perspective. Postgrad Med J [Suppl 7] 50:55–62

Hoeprich PD (1970) The polymyxins. Med Clin North Am 54:1257–1271

Hoffmann DR (1970) Model systems for the study of drug hypersensitivity. PhD thesis, California Institute of Technology, Pasadena, California. Published by Xerox University Microfilms, Ann Arbor, Michigan

Hoigné R (1975) Penicillins, cephalosporins and tetracyclines. In: Meyler's side effects of drugs, VIII. Excerpta Medica, Amsterdam London New York

Homberg JC, Pujet JC, Salmon C (1973) A study of rifampicin antigenic site. Scand J Respir Dis 84:36–39

Hong Kong Tuberculosis Treatment Services/British Medical Research Council Investigation (1975) Investigations of allergic status and blood counts in Chinese patients receiving daily or intermittent rifampicin in Hong Kong. Clin Allergy 5:189–199

Hutfield DC (1965) Streptomycin sensitization. Br J Vener Dis 41:210–212

Hysell JK, Gray JM, Hysell JW, Beck ML (1975) An antineomycin antibody interfering with ABO grouping and antibody screening. Transfusion 15:16–22

Jacottet M (1964) Panmyelophthise et anticorps antichloromycétine. Arch Fr Pediatr 21:218–221

John W (1960) Kontaktallergien gegen Antibiotika. Hautarzt 11:433–440

Johnston TG, Cazort AG (1953) Severe serum-sickness reaction with cyanosis following terramycin. Antibiot Chemother 3:481

Kaltwasser JB, Simon B, Werner E, Stille W, Becker H (1974) Untersuchungen zur Hämatotoxizität von Thiamphenicol. Arzneim Forsch 24:190–194

Kandil E (1969) Fixed drug eruption. Dermatologica 139:37–40

Kandra T, Baris I, Kolacan B (1978) Rifampicin-dependent antibodies in a patient with hepatorenal failure. Br J Dis Chest 72:67–70

Keiser G, Bolli P, Buchegger U (1972) Hämatologische Nebenwirkungen von Chloramphenicol und Thiamphenicol. Schweiz Med Wochenschr 102:1595–1598

Ketel WG van (1976) Immediate- and delayed-type allergy to erythromycin. Contact Dermatitis 2:363–364

Kleine-Natrop HE (1956) Antibiotika als berufliche Antigene in der Arzneimittelindustrie. Berufsdermatosen 4:269–276

Kleinknecht D, Homberg JC, Decroix G (1972) Acute renal failure after rifampicin. Lancet 1:1238–1239

Kligman AM (1967) The idendification of contact allergens by human assay. J Invest Dermatol 47:393–409

Koch-Weser J (1970) Adverse effects of sodium colistimethate. Ann Intern Med 72:857–859

Koch-Weser J, Gilmore EB (1967) Benign intracranial hypertension in an adult after tetracycline therapy. JAMA 200:345–347

Koolj R (1961) Allergic contact dermatitis due to neomycin: Cross-sensitivity with other antibiotics and positive patch tests with the isomeric compounds neomycin B and C and with neamine. S Afr Med J 20:406–411

Korossy S (1976) Drug allergy. In: Rajka E, Korossy S (eds) Immunological aspects of allergy and allergic diseases, vol 7. Plenum, New York London, pp 179–294

Korossy S, Vineze E, Gozony M (1962) Durch Chloramphenicolbehandlung verursachte Allergodermatosen. Allerg Asthma (Leipz) 8:228–232

Korossy S, Vincze E, Gozony M (1966) Chloramphenicol (Chlorocid)-Allergie. Z Hautkr 41:375–379

Korossy S, Vincze E, Doroszlay G, Munkácsi A (1969) Zur Revision des Allergenspektrums der in Ungarn gebräuchlichen diagnostischen Standard-Reihe für Epikutantestung. Berufsdermatosen 17:252–263

Kounis NG (1975) Oxytetracycline-induced thrombocytopenic purpura. JAMA 231:734–735

Kreis B (1966) Kanamycin toxicity in adults. Ann NY Acad Sci 132/2:957

Krönig B, Fiegel P, Weihrauch T, Hoffler D, Jahnecke J, Arndthauser A (1972) A case of severe repeated immunological reactions to intermittent rifampicin treatment. Eur J Clin Pharmacol 5:53–57

Kucers A, Bennet NMcK (1975) The use of antibiotics, 2nd edn. Heinemann, London

Kuder HV (1960) Propionyl erythromycin. A review of 20,525 case reports for side effect data. Clin Pharmacol Ther 1:604–609

Lachman SJ (1959) Anaphylactic reaction to oral chlortetracycline. Antibiot Med 6:62

Lakin JD, Grace WR, Sell KW (1975a) IgE antipolymyxin B antibody formation in a T cell-depleted bone marrow transplant patient. J Allergy 56:94–103

Lakin JD, Strong DM, Sell KW (1975b) Polymyxin B reactions, IgE antibody and T cell deficiency. Ann Intern Med 83:204–207

Lakshminarayan S, Sahn AS, Hudson LD (1973) Massive haemolysis caused by rifampicin. Br Med J 2:282–283

Langunoff D, Benditt BP (1960) Mast cell degranulation and histamine release observed in a new in vitro system. J Exp Med 112:571–580

Lazzaro C, Buzzoni A (1968) Il test della trasformazione blastica dei linfociti nell'allergia agli antibiotici. Minerva Med 59:4785–4788

Lewis JE, Nelson JC, Elder HA (1972) Radioimmunoassay of an antibiotic: gentamycin. Nature New Biol 239:214–216

Lochmann O, Kohout P, Vymola F (1977) Anaphylactic shock following the administration of clindamycin. J Hyg Epidemiol Microbiol Immunol (Praha) 21:441–447

Lochmannova J, Benis J, Lochmann O, Vymola F (1970) On the immunological reactivity of penicillin, cephalosporin and tetracycline antibiotics. J Hyg Epidemiol Microbiol Immunol (Praha) 14:201–210

MacFarlane JA, Mitchell AAB, Walsh JM, Robertson JJ (1968) Spiramycin in the prevention of post-operative staphylococcal infection. Lancet 1:1–4

Manten A (1975) Antibiotic drugs. In: Dukes MNG (ed) Meyler's side effects of drugs. Excerpta Medica, Amsterdam London New York, pp 603–647

Manten A (1978) Other antibiotics. In: Dukes MNG (ed) Side effects of drugs, annual 2. Excerpta Medica, Amsterdam London New York, pp 231–240

Manten A (1979) Other antibiotic drugs. In: Dukes MNG (ed) Side effects of drugs, annual 3. Excerpta Medica, Amsterdam London New York, pp 226–235

Marschke G, Sarauw A (1971a) Polymyxin inhalation – therapeutic hazard. Ann Intern Med 74:144–145

Marschke G, Sarauw A (1971b) Danger of polymyxin B inhalation. Ann Intern Med 74:296–297

Martinez J, Lletona L, Barbolla L, Frieyro E, Bouza E, Gilsanz F (1977) Immune haemolytic anaemia and renal failure induced by streptomycin. Br J Haematol 35:561–571

Mathews KP, Pan PM, Wells JH (1972) Experience with lymphocyte transformation tests in evaluating allergy to aminosalicylic acid, isoniazid and streptomycin. Int Arch Allergy Appl Immunol 42:653–667

Matner T (1969) Ekzematöse Sensibilisierung durch Neomycin. Hautarzt 20:446–450

Mattson K (1973) Side effects of rifamycin. A clinical study. Scand J Respir Dis 82:1–52

Maucher OM (1972) Anaphylaktische Reaktionen beim Epicutantest. Hautarzt 23:139–140

Maulide I, Villar TG (1974) Therapeutic trial with clindamycin in non-tuberculosis infections of the respiratory tract. Pneumologia (Lisbon) 5:79–82

Melnikova EA (1971) Experimental study of the sensitizing properties of the antibiotics phytobacteriomyxin and polymyxin. Antibiotiki 16:911

Menon MPS, Das AK (1977) Tetracycline asthma – a case report. Clin Allergy 7:285–290

Miller R, Tausk HC (1977) Anaphylactoid reaction to vancomycin during anesthesia. Anesth Analg (Cleve) 56:870–872

Moehring K, Asbach HW, Schubothe H, Weber S (1974) Hämolytische Krise mit akutem Nierenversagen unter Rifampicin-Behandlung. Dtsch Med Wochenschr 99:1458–1462

Möller H (1976) Eczematous contact allergy to oxytetracycline and polymyxin B. Contact Dermatitis 2:289–290

Moneret-Vautrin D, Grilliat JP, Pupil P (1972) In: Dash CH, Jones HEH (eds) Mechanisms in drug allergy. Basophil degranulation in drug allergy. Churchill Livingstone, Edinburgh London, pp 159–170

Morison WL, Parrish JA, Epstein JH (1979) Photoimmunology. Arch Dermatol 115:350–355

Moser RH (1966) Reactions to tetracycline. Clin Pharmacol Ther 7:117–132

Mühlberger F (1973) Allergie gegen Tuberkulostatika. Schweiz Med Wochenschr 103:126–131

Muelling RJ, Bevent T, Samson RF, Jenevein EP, Guillory JD (1958) Studies in human sensitivity to antibiotics. I. Testing for precipitins after reaction to antibiotics. Am J Clin Pathol 29:503–505

Nachman R, Javid J, Krauss S (1962) Streptomycin-induced hemolytic anemia. Arch Intern Med 110:187–190

Naik RPC, Singli G (1976) Bullous fixed drug eruption presumably due to erythromycin. Dermatologica 152:177–180

Nessi R, Domenichini E, Fowst G (1973) Allergic reactions during rifampicin treatment: a review of published cases. Scand J Respir Dis [Suppl] 84:15–19

Nordquist B, Rossman H (1967) Leucocytic migration in vitro as an indicator of allergy in eczematons contact dermatitis. Trans St John's Hosp Dermatol Soc 53:154–159

Nyirenda R, Gill GV (1977) Stevens-Johnson syndrome due to rifampicin. Br Med J 2:1189

Olson CA, Riley HJ Jr (1966) Complications of tetracycline therapy. J Pediatr 68:783–791

O'Mahony MG (1973) Observations on antibody reaction scores on individual patients. Scand J Respir Dis [Suppl] 84:64–72

Orgel HA, Hamburger RN (1971) Chloramphenicol antibody. V. A method for the detection of antichloramphenicol antibody in human serum. Immunology 20:233–239

Otten H, Plembel M, Siegenthaler W (1975) Antibiotika-Fibel. Antibiotika und Chemotherapie, 4th edn. Thieme, Stuttgart

Pambor M (1973) Zur Unterscheidung ekzemallergischer und toxischer Hautentzündungen im Rebuck-Test. Dermatol Monatsschr 159:806–813

Pasricha JS, Shukla SR (1979) Independent lesions of fixed eruptions due to two unrelated drugs in the same patient. Br J Dermatol 101:361–362

Patrick J, Panzer JD, Derbes VJ (1970) Neomycin sensitivity in the normal (non-atopic) individual. Arch Dermatol 102:532–535

Peck SM, Feldmann FF (1950) Sensitivity reactions to aureomycin. JAMA 142:1137–1139

Pedersen AHB, Wiesner PJ, Holmes KK, Johnson CJ, Turck M (1972) Spectinomycin and penicillin G in the treatment of gonorrhoea. A comparative evaluation. JAMA 220:205–208

Petrescu D, Marca G, Veronese M (1972) Humoral antibody production following primary and secondary immunization in rabbits treated with thiamphenicol and chloramphenicol. Antibiot Chemother 17:200–216

Pevny I, Röckl H (1975) Arzneimittelbedingte allergische Hautreaktionen vom kutan-vasculären Typ. MMW 117:9–16

Pirilä V, Pirilä L (1966) Sensitization to the neomycin group of antibiotics: patterns of cross-sensitivity as a function of polyvalent sensitization to different portions of the neomycin molecule. Acta Derm Venereol (Stockh) 46:489–496

Pirilä V, Rouhunkoski S (1960) On cross-sensitization between neomycin, bacitracin, kanamycin, and framycetin. Dermatologica 121:335–342

Pitmann FE, Pittman JC, Humphrey CD (1974) Lincomycin and pseudomembranous colitis. Lancet 1:451–452

Pla RP, Martin C (1976) Anemie hemolytique immuno-allergique liée à la streptomycine. Rev Fr Transfus Immunohematol 19:379–382

Poole G, Stradling P, Worlledge S (1971) Potentially serious side effects of high dose twice weekly rifampicin. Br Med J 3:343–347

Pollen RH (1964) Anaphylactoid reaction to orally administered demethylchlortetracycline. N Engl J Med 271:673

Prasad AS (1960) Severe urticaria following erythromycin therapy. N Engl J Med 262:139–140

Preyss JA von (1969) Allergie gegen Tylosin Tartrat. Berufsdermatosen 17:166–167

Pujet JC, Homberg JC, Decroix G (1974) Sensitivity to rifampicin: incidence, mechanisms and prevention. Br Med J 2:415–418

Queng JT, Dukes CD, McGovern JP (1965) Antigenicity of the tetracyclines. J Allergy 36:505–513

Raab W (1968) Mast cell depleting properties of neomycin. J Invest Dermatol 50:138–140

Raab W (1975) Spectinomycin. Indikationen und unerwünschte Wirkungen. Schweiz Med Wochenschr 105:1116–1123

Raab W (1977) Untersuchungen zur Frage akuter unerwünschter Wirkungen von Erythromycin, Lincomycin u. Clindamycin. Int J Clin Pharmacol 15:90–97

Ramsay CA (1977) Longwave UV radiation sensitivity induced by oxytetracycline. A case report. Clin Exp Dermatol 2:255–258

Rasmussen F (1972) Side effects of streptomycin sulphate. Scand J Respir Dis 53:35–37

Reichenberger M, Heitmann HJ (1969) Lymphocyte transformation in patients allergic to ampicillin and tetracycline. Lancet 2:491–492

Richter G (1975) Zur Kritik der externen Dermatika unter dem Aspekt ihrer allergischen Nebenwirkungen. Dermatol Monatsschr 161:384–387

Ripps CS, Fellner MJ, Hirschhorn K (1965) Response of lymphocytes to tetracycline. Lancet 1:951–952

Robinson HM Jr, Zeligman I, Shapiro A, Cohen MM (1951) Acquired contact sensitivity to chloromycetin. J Invest Dermatol 17:205–206

Rocklin RE, David JR (1971) Detection in vitro of cellular hypersensitivity to drugs. J Allergy Clin Immunol 48:276–282

Rosenthal RL, Blackman A (1965) Bone-marrow hypoplasia following use of chloramphenicol eye drops. JAMA 191:136–137

Rossen FL (1948) Streptomycin sensitivity. Anaphylactic shock with recovery following intracutaneous test. JAMA 137:1128–1130

Sack K, Freiesleben H, Zuellich B (1978) Beurteilung neuer Aminoglykosid-Antibiotika. Internist Prax 18:443–456

Sakamoto A (1956) Anaphylactoid reaction to intramuscular tetracycline hydrochloride. Report of a case. Calif Med 84:55–56

Sarkany I (1967) Lymphocyte transformation in drug hypersensitivity. Lancet 1:743–745

Savage GM (1973) Spectinomycin related to the chemotherapy of gonorrhea. Infection 1:227–228

Scheegans E, Haarschar A, Kuntzmann F (1965) Agranulocytose Mortelle après traitement au chloramphénicol. Recherche d'anticorps. Arch Fr Pediatr 22:216–219

Schindel LE (1965) Clinical side-effects of the tetracyclines. Antibiot Chemother 13:300–316

Schindel L (1966) Klinisch beobachtete Nebenwirkungen neuerer AB. Novobiocin-Polymyxin. Ther Umsch 23:341–345

Schoenfeld MR (1964) Vascular purpura caused by oxytetracyclin. JAMA 188:328–329

Schorr WF, Ridgway HB (1977) Tobramycin-neomycin cross-sensitivity. Contact Dermatitis 3:133–137

Schorr WF, Wenzel FJ, Hegedus SI (1973) Cross-sensitivity and aminoglycoside antibiotics. Arch Dermatol 107:533–539

Schubothe H, Weber S (1973) Rifampicin-dependent reactions against erythrocytes in the sera of patients receiving rifampicin therapy. Scand J Respir Dis [Suppl] 84:53–59

Schubothe H, Seufert CD, Weber S (1972) Quinine and rifampicin antibodies with hemolytic effect. Verh Dtsch Ges Inn Med 78:905–908

Schwank R, Jirasek L (1963) Kontaktallergie gegen Chloramphenicol mit besonderer Berücksichtigung der Gruppensensibilisierung. Hautarzt 14:24–30

Scott JL, Finegold SM, Belkin GA, Lawrence JS (1965) A controlled double-blind study of the hematologic toxicity of chloramphenicol. N Engl J Med 272:1137–1141

Seufert CD (1973) Acute renal failure after rifampicin therapy. Scand J Respir Dis [Suppl] 84:174–179

Shelley WB (1963) The circulating basophil as an indicator of hypersensitivity in man. Arch Dermatol 88:759–767

Shelley WB (1965) Further experiences with the indirect basophil test. Arch Dermatol 91:165–170

Shelley WB, Heaton CL (1973) Minocycline sensitivity. JAMA 224:125–126

Sherlock S (1965) Hepatic reactions to therapeutic agents. Ann Rev Pharmacol 5:429–446

Shimizu Y, Shimao S (1977) A case of minocycline-induced fixed drug eruption. J Dermatol (Tokyo) 4:73–76

Sidi E, Hincky M, Longueville R (1958) Cross-sensitization between neomycin and streptomycin. J Invest Dermatol 30:225–231

Simon C, Stille W (1979) Antibiotika – Therapie in Klinik und Praxis. Schattauer, Stuttgart New York

Singh CV, Grover V, Kamra GL (1977) Fatal anaphylactic reaction to tetracycline in the post-operative period. Anaesthesia 32:268

Smith JM (1960) Allergic reactions to anti-tuberculous drugs. Acta Allergol 15:191–195

Sors C, Sarrazin A, Homberg JC (1972) Accidents hémolytique recidivants d'origine immuno-allerque au cours d'un traitement intermittent par la refampicine. Rev Tuberc Pneumol 36:405–406

Speirs CT (1976) Tobramycin side effects; international results. Scott Med J 21:178 181

Spektorova AI (1961) Antibiotiki 6:226. Cited by Dedney JM (1977) in: Immunology of the antibiotics. In: Sela (M) ed The antigens, vol IV. Academic Press, New York London

Stevens EAM, Joniau M, Verbist L (1973) Preliminary data on immunological experiments with rifamycin conjugates. Scand J Respir Dis (Suppl.) 84:36–39

Sulkowski SR, Haserick JR (1964) Simulated systemic lupus erythematosus from degraded tetracycline. JAMA 189:152–154

Terekhova NY, Wushkina TP (1977) The syndrome of erythema exsudativum multiforme as a manifestation of drug allergy. Vestn Dermatol Venerol 10:66–68

Veien NK, Hattel T, Justesen O, Nørholm A (1980) Occupational contact dermatitis due to spiramycin and/or tylosin among farmers. Contact Dermatitis 6:410–413

Virgilio R (1973) Rifampicin-dependent antibodies during intermittent treatment. Scand J Respir Dis [Suppl] 84:83–86

Vischer TL (1966) Lymphocyte cultures in drug hypersensitivity. Lancet 2:467–469

Vulliemoz P, Favez G (1964) Propriétes antigéniques de la streptomycine. Schweiz Med Wochenschr 94:1252–1256

Wade JC, Petty BG, Conrad G, Smith CR, Liposky JJ, Ellner J, Lietman PS (1978) Cephalotin plus an aminoglycoside is more nephrotoxic than methicillin plus an aminoglycoside. Lancet 2:604–606

Wätzig V, Ruffert K (1977) Der Nachweis der Chloramphenicol-Allergie mit dem Leukozyten-Migrations-Hemmtest in der Hautkammer. Allerg Immunol (Leipz) 23:69–78

Wahl D, Menaut P, Roche G (1978) Anuric allergic tubular nephritis to rifampicin. Poumon Coeur 34:437–439

Walker WG (1969) Hypersensitivity reaction in a patient receiving lincomycin. Can Med Assoc J 101:763

Walker RG, Thomson NW, Dowling JP, Ogg CS (1979) Minocycline-induced acute interstitial nephritis. Br Med J 1:524

Warrington RJ, Tse KS (1979) Lymphocyte transformation studies in drug hypersensitivity. Can Med Assoc J 120:1089–1094

Watson KC, Joubert SM (1960) Haemagglutination of antibiotic treated cells. Nature 188:505–506

Weinstein HI, Welch H (1958/1959) Sensitivity to the tetracyclines. Antibiot Annu pp 643–646

Welsh AL (1955) Crossed fixed drug eruptions from three antibiotics. Arch Dermatol 71:521–523

Wenz B, Klein RL, Lalezari P (1974) Tetracycline-induced immune hemolytic anemia. Transfusion 14:265–269

Wenzel FJ, Epstein S (1964) Cross-sensitivity between streptomycin and dihydrostreptomycin. J Invest Dermatol 43:99–101

White GJ (1965) Nonantigenicity of lincomycin. Antimicrob Agents Chemother 398–402

Wiebe JA, Moore DE (1977) Photooxidation sensitized by tetracyclines. J Pharm Sci 66:186–189

Willcox RR (1962) Trobicin (actinospectacin) a new injectable antibiotic in the treatment of gonorrhoea. Br J Vener Dis 38:150–153

Winter V, Freund D (1969) Fluoreszenz-immunohistochemische und immunologische Studien bei einem Fall von Tetracyklin-Allergie. Hautarzt 20:74–77

Worlledge S (1973) The detection of rifampicin-dependent antibodies. Scand J Respir Dis [Suppl] 84:60–63

Wullen F, Kast G, Bruck A (1967) Über Nebenwirkungen bei Tetracyclin-Verabreichung an Myasthenikern. Dtsch Med Wochenschr 92:667

Zelger J, Seidl V (1969) Multivalente Antibiotika. Allergie mit Penicillin und Tetracyclin-Anaphylaxie. Dermatologica 139:365–373

CHAPTER 18

Other Antibacterial Drugs

M. ALEXANDER

A. Introduction

Not only antibiotics are administered in the treatment of bacterial infections; other chemotherapeutic substances used include the sulfonamides (today especially as benzyl-pyrimidine sulfonamides), nitrofurantoin, nalidixic acid, pipemidic acid, and oxolonic acid. In treatment of tuberculosis, isoniazid and ethambutol play a principal part as first choice tuberculostatics. For treatment of leprosy, sulfones and clofazimine are at our disposal. (A whole series of drugs are being tested for use in treatment of virus diseases though only a few seem to be promising.) In this chapter allergic reactions caused by the above drugs will be described and – as far as possible from the literature – discussed in regard to their physicochemical, pharmacologic, immunochemical, and immunological foundations.

B. Sulfonamides Including Benzylpyrimidine Sulfonamides

I. Physicochemical and Pharmacologic Properties

Sulfonamides are derivatives of sulfanilic acid. The first sulfonamide to be discovered was sulfanilamide, which is amphoteric and an efficient antibacterial compound. The azo group is not absolutely necessary for the chemotherapeutic effect.

$$H_2N-\underset{\text{Sulfanilamide}}{\boxed{}}-SO_2NH_2 \qquad \underset{\text{Sulfonamide}}{R_1 \cdot SO_2NH \cdot R}$$

In the human body metabolism of the sulfonamides is characterized by metaplasia and breaking-down reactions, mostly inactivating processes. It is a matter of oxidation (products of oxidation are linked to sulfuric and glucuronic acid), reduction, hydrolysis, and conjugating processes. Worth mentioning among the conjugating processes are glucoronide formation and N^4-acetylization. The most important metabolic reaction is the acetylization at the N^4-atom. Sulfonamides react bacteriostatically, taking effect only after a latency period of some hours. They inhibit the enzymatic union of para-aminobenzoic acid, which is necessary for folic acid synthesis and competitive with the pteridinic compound.

Based on their elimination half-lives, sulfonamides are classified into:
1. Short-acting ($t_{50\%} < 8$ h)
2. Medium-acting ($t_{50\%} = 8$–16 h)

3. Long-acting ($t_{50\%} = 24$–48 h)
4. Ultra-long-acting ($t_{50\%} > 48$ h).

These sulfonamides are quickly and almost completely absorbed. There are also some sulfonamides which do not dissolve readily and are hardly absorbed at all by the gastrointestinal tract. Diffusion into the different body fluids and tissues varies. The bacteriostatically efficient plasma concentration is about 50–150 mg/liter.

Generally, tissue storage is not presumed. Short-acting sulfonamides are quickly eliminated in the urine, medium-, long-, and ultra-long-acting sulfonamides distinctly more slowly. The diuretic mechanism is based mainly on glomerular filtration, partly on tubular secretion. Partial acetyl derivatives and glucuronides are excreted by the tubuli. In tubular lesions the elimination of the acetyl derivative is very slow and the high and prolonged serum concentration of total sulfonamide contains an unusually high proportion of inactive and toxic acetyl derivative. Short-acting and medium-acting sulfonamides are not reabsorbed by the kidneys. Long-acting and ultra-long-acting sulfonamides are largely reabsorbed, which is decisive for their prolonged effect.

Differences in protein binding are sometimes considerable. It lies between 50% and 99% and depends on the sulfonamide concentration. There is no connection between protein binding and elimination speed.

Benzylpyrimidine sulfonamides are based on the combination of a sulfonamide with trimethoprim or tetroxoprim. Chemically, trimethoprim is a 2,4-diamino-5-(3,4,5-trimethoxybenzyl)pyrimidine and has the following structural formula.

The left half of the formula is similar to the aminopyrimidine part of a folate molecule (tetrahydrofolate = folate).

Trimethoprim and tetroxoprim inhibit folic acid synthesis, i.e., they specifically inhibit the dihydrofolate reductase which is responsible for synthesis of folic acid. They make possible the reduction of dihydrofolic acid to tetrahydrofolic acid. The structure of purines and pyrimidines is thereby interrupted, an essential step in the synthesis of proteinic and ribonucleic acid. This inhibitory effect is selective and affects bacteria only.

After oral administration, resorption is quick and sufficient. The serum elimination half-life is about 12 h and the urine elimination half-life about 18 h. The Kidneys eliminate trimethoprim and tetroxoprim in active form in the course of which about 40%–50% of the given dose was eliminated within 24 h.

II. Immunochemistry and Immunology

Sulfonamides belong to the group of chemical compounds with replaced amino groups in paraposition at the benzol ring which can produce allergies. Admixtures of diethylcarbonate to sulfonamides may favor sensitization. On local application, for example in covering of large wound areas with sulfonamide gel, the rate of sensitization is markedly higher than in enteral application; moreover, an increased parallel allergy develops against all sulfonamides, making desensitization distinctly more difficult.

Sulfonamides are not able to bind themselves to proteins irreversibly. Therefore it is supposed that a catabolite or a metabolite is the component reacting with protein which is responsible for immunogenicity. Catabolites are developed by chemical metabolism without enzymes, metabolites by fermentative catabolism. Chemically reactive metabolites (proimmunogens) bind themselves with (tissue) protein to haptenic protein compounds. Mafenide is an aliphatic conjunction. Its amino group is not situated in paraposition to the benzol ring, but is separated from this ring by a methyl group. It is more basic than sulfonamides. Mafenide is used for the skin of burned patients in combination with sulfonamides. It often causes contact allergies. There are no cross-reactions beetween mafenide and sulfonamides (BANDMANN and BREIT 1973).

III. Clinical Aspects

The general frequency of side effects after sulfonamides is 5%. Allergic reactions against sulfonamides are common but there is a lack of exact statistics. KORTING (1980) describes toxic-allergic exanthemas in 0.3%–5% of the cases. They present predominantly on the skin and can be of different types and different degrees of severity, ranging from morbilliform, scarlatiniform, urticarial, pemphigoid, purpuric, and petechial exanthemas through erythema nodosum and Behçet's syndrome to the Stevens-Johnson syndrome and Lyell's syndrome (epidermolysis acuta toxica) (KUOKKANEN 1972; RIECHERS 1972). Especially long-acting sulfonamides and ultra-long-acting sulfonamides can cause serious allergic dermatoses (SHAW and JACOBS 1970) and also erythema multiforme gravis (BAKER 1968).

These side effects are independent of age, weight, period of clinical treatment, and urea concentration in the blood, but are more often found in women (LAWSON and JICK 1978). Mostly ist is a question of idiopathic "allergic reactions." Pyrimidine derivatives have few side effects, the hardly absorbable sulfonamides scarcely any. A syndrome similar to serum disease can appear, with fever, arthritic pains, urticaria, conjunctivitis, bronchospasms, and leukopenia. In persons previously sensitized by sulfonamides, immediate reactions of the anaphylactic type have occasionally been observed.

In about 3% of cases, sulfisoxazole causes fever, which begins immediately and develops between 7 and 10 days after application. Headaches, shivering, pruritus and exanthema can accompany the fever. KOCH-WESER et al. (1971) examined 2118 hospital patients and found allergic sideeffects after administration of sulfisoxazole in 2.8% of cases and after sulfamethoxazole in 3% of cases.

Myositis, myocarditis, and vasculitis with eosinophilia have also been observed (ELLMAN et al. 1974).

Cross-allergies to different sulfonamides can appear, but this is not the rule. The frequency of the sensitization by another sulfonamide is about 20%.

The Stevens-Johnson syndrome after application of sulfonamide eye drops has been described several times after (GOTTSCHALK and STONE 1976). MACKIE and MACKIE (1979) report a case of systemic lupus erythematosus and dermatomyositis induced by sulfacetamide eye drops. KLINGHÖFFER (1954) and DONLAN and SCUTERO (1975) each observed one case of eosinophilic pulmonary infiltration after application of a vaginal cream containing sulfonamide.

From the clinical point of view the most important side effect is renal damage. Besides the crystallizing of the sulfonamides in the renal tubules, allergic lower nephron nephrosis appears; this complication is extremely serious, but very rare. It is still not clear if it is a direct toxic effect or an idiosyncratic reaction.

Exanthemas and erythemas of very different kinds can result from allergic reactions, as can the drug fever which appears 7–9 days after commencement of therapy. There can be fever with or without exanthema, with or without arthritic pains.

Some cases of eosinophilic pneumonia have been described after sulfonamides (FEINMANN 1975; THOMAS et al. 1974; ANONYMOUS 1974). Furthermore, pathological liver changes are reported similar to those in hepatitis, sometimes with a cholestatic component which recurred after repeated application of sulfonamides (IWARSON and LUNDIN 1979; STEINBRECHER and MISCHKIN 1981).

The most dangerous reactions are purpura and agranulocytosis. They appear mostly after maximum dosage on the 10th–21st day of therapy and require immediate cessation of treatment (ASMAR et al. 1981; BRADLEY et al. 1980; KOBRINSKY and RAMSAY 1981).

In 0.05% of cases, hemolytic anemia appears after sulfadiazine. It is mostly found in negroes and in children. In some cases a sensitization phenomenon is assumed to be the cause, in other cases there is a lack of glucose-6-phosphate dehydrogenase. BÖTTIGER and WESTERHOLM (1973) observed hemolytic anemia after therapy with salicylazosulfapyridine and after a combination of the short-acting sulfonamide sulfamethizole with the long-acting sulfonamide sulfamethoxipyridazine.

Agranulocytosis occurs in 0.1% of cases after sulfadiazine and also occurs after other sulfonamides. The myelotoxic effect is demonstrated as impaired development of the myeloblasts. Granulocytopenia is not related to the applied dosage and as a rule appears after 10 days treatment. Slight passing thrombocytopenia is frequent, but serious thrombocytopenia and aplastic anemia are rare. Isolated peripheral eosinophilia can be observed, disappearing rapidly after cessation of sulfonamides. It can also appear in combination with other signs of hypersensitivity (THIRKETTLE et al. 1963; JOHNSON and KORST 1961).

COX et al. (1973) describe a case of lethal necrotizing angiitis after sulfadimethoxine therapy which took on the appearance of anaphylactoid purpura. Even after 2 years of local treatment with silver sulfadiazine cream, two patients developed leukopenia, which receded 1–2 days after stopping the cream (CHAN et al. 1976; FRASER and BEANLIEN 1979).

Long-acting sulfonamides like sulfamethoxipyridazine or sulfamethoxine are more inclined to cause allergic reactions like erythema multiforme or allergic myocarditis. Also described are syndromes like systemic lupus erythematosus, rheumatoid symptoms, edemas (for example edema of the glottis), eosinophilic pulmonary megaloblastosis, anemia, attacks of asthma, arteritides, central nervous disturbances, intrahepatic cholestasis, and esophageal ulcers (TÖNDER et al. 1974). In some of the cases of sulfonamide-induced hemocytopenia it is a question of hyporegenerative forms in which it is not quite clear if consequences of cytotoxic immune reactions and/or direct toxic effects are involved.

Photosensitivity has also been described, for example after appplication of eye ointments for staphylococcal blepharitis (FLACH 1981).

Recently, mainly benzylpyrimidine sulfonamides have been applied; in 5.9% of cases allergic reactions are described on the skin which are probably chiefly due to sulfonamide (CLARK et al. 1980; BERNSTEIN 1975).

ESPIRITU et al. (1967) describe a case of granulomatous hepatitis after administration of sulfadimethoxine (Madribon) which was connected with fever, rash, jaundice, and interstitial pneumonia. The authors trace these symptoms back to a hypersensitivity.

"Fixed genital drug eruptions" have been described after application of cotrimoxazole, sulfadiazine, sulfaphenazole, sulfadimethoxine, sulfadimidine, and sulfamethoxypyridine.

TALBOT (1980) and PASRICHA (1979) described an erythema with subsequent edema which caused vesiculae and bullae in the genital region and urethritis. GUGUÉRIN et al. (1980) report two cases of diffuse interstitial pulmonary fibrosis with fever and eosinophilia of the blood after cotrimoxazole.

PENNINGTON (1980) describes four patients ranging in age from 65 to 81 years with pseudomembranous colitis after repeated cotrimoxazole therapy for slight infections in the region of the respiratory system or of the urinary tract (BARTLE and SAIBIL 1977). A further case was observed by CAMERON and THOMAS (1977). BJARNASON and BJORNSSON (1981) report a case of esophageal ulcers after cotrimoxazole.

According to SHEEHAN (1981), at present cotrimoxazole is the most frequent cause of agranulocytosis in which there is a toxicity for the bone marrow, effected by the sulfonamide as well as by the trimethoprim (LAWSON and HENRY 1977; INMAN 1977; EVANS and TELL 1969; LASSON 1977; CHANU et al. 1981). BONE et al. (1981) and STIMMESSE et al. (1979) report cases of lethal pancytopenia after cotrimoxazole, THOREL et al. (1981) and CLAAS et al. (1979) acute thrombocytopenia.

FRIES and HIRSCHFELD (1977) observed purpura based on allergic vasculitis with arthritis at normal thrombocyte values and intact coagulation factors after cotrimoxazole in a 71-year-old man.

RICHMOND et al. (1979) report nephrotoxic effects of cotrimoxazole, and DRY et al. (1975) a case of acute tubulointerstitial nephropathy.

OGILVIE and TOGHILL (1980), describe a case of cholestatic icterus in a 70-year-old woman after cotrimoxazole. There was deterioration in the patient's condition after further treatment and complete recovery after cessation of cotrimoxazole. Similar cases were described by COLUCCI et al. (1975) and COTO et al. (1981). It is supposed that the cholestatic icterus is caused by the sulfonamide component of the drug (NAIR et al. 1980). RANSOHOFF et al. (1981) report a case of liver failure which became fatal after small doses of cotrimoxazole.

WÄHLIN and ROSMAN (1976) observed eight cases of serious skin and general reactions within 18 months after cotrimoxazole which were based on allergic reactions. BRAUN-FALCO et al. (1978) observed pustulosis acuta generalisata with distinct leukocytoclastic vasculitis in the upper corium in a 52-year-old woman who was treated with trimethoprim/sulfamethoxazole for acute bronchitis.

SMITH et al. (1980) observed two cases of interstitial nephritis after cotrimoxazole in patients with renal transplants.

Stevens-Johnson syndrome has also been described after cotrimoxazole (KIKUCHI and OKAZAKI 1978; AZINGE and GARRICK 1978; THORPE and NYSENBAUM 1978).

BRØCKNER and BOISEN report a case of acute tubulointerstitial nephritis, acute pancreatitis, fatty liver, pulmonary fibrosis, various petechial hemorrhages in the white matter of one hemisphere, and a 5-mm hemorrhage in the caudal region of the corpus callosum leading to death.

In general, hypersensitivity and gastrointestinal reactions account for two-thirds of the side effects of cotrimoxazole.

IV. Results of Diagnostic Tests

1. Skin Tests

On suspicion of a drug allergy, the first step is discontinuation of the responsible agent; a subsequent rapid regression can be taken as proof that the drug was indeed responsible. In serious hypersensitivity reactions, for example Lyell's syndrome, anaphylactic shock, thrombocytopenic purpura, periarteritis nodosa, and lupus erythematosus medicamentosus, functional tests in the sense of a provocation test are extremely dangerous and are to be avoided. In epicutaneous tests too we have to proceed with extreme care.

In every case of drug allergy we should proceed systematically, carrying out first an epicutaneous test and a friction test and then a prick test, a scratch test, and perhaps an intracutaneous test. Active substances are taken in a 1%–10% solution in physiological NaCl solution. In especially high sensitization, general reactions (including the anaphylactic shock) are yielded by the epicutaneous and intracutaneous tests. If one test is positive, other tests can mostly be dispensed with.

In anaphylactic reactions, the friction, prick, and intracutaneous tests are most easily positive; in drug fever, the epicutaneous and intracutaneous tests.

In the intracutaneous test, 0.005 ml of solution is transfused intradermally in the region of the deltoid muscle or the lower arm. The result is read after 15 min.

The scratch test or the epicutaneous test is used as a rule in testing the sulfonamides. However, false negative results are found frequently in the latter case (exception: contact allergy). Lobule tests with sulfonamides showed a positive reaction only in one-third of the patients, but all patients with serious reactions were positive (SULZBERGER et al. 1947; CRONIN 1978)

PORTER and COMAISH (1969) investigated a patient with fixed eruption due to sulfadimidine for the presence of the drug at the involved sites. Autoradiographic

studies did not reveal any evidence of preferential binding of [^{35}S] sulfadiamide:
at the site of the lesions.

2. Sulfonamide-Specific Antibodies

MOESCHLIN (1954) demonstrated leukocytic agglutinins at the peak of the sulfapyridine agranulocytosis. Addition of sulfapyridine reinforced the agglutination or
caused a new leukocytic agglutination during convalescence. MOESCHLIN also reports that the leukocytic agglutination and the enormous peripheral destruction of
the granulocytes with consequent overloading of the bone marrow are the consequence of an antigen-antibody reaction.

HAMILTON and SHEETS (1978) observed a case of thrombocytopenic purpura after sulfisoxazole which could be demonstrated by the provocation test and by the
presence of the serum factors which caused a platelet agglutination in the presence
of sulfisoxazole. Antibody investigations have not been carried out routinely in sulfonamide allergies.

3. Sulfonamide-Specific Lymphocyte Reactivity

The *lymphocyte transformation test* serves for the demonstration of mitogenic
factors in cellular allergy. When lymphocytes from sensitized patients are cultured
together with the corresponding medicamentous antigen, the result is transformation forms and mitosis formation, which can be determined autoradiographically
by fixing of radioactively DNA and RNA. Nonspecific stimulation, for example
by phytoagglutinin, is obligatory in these cases. The lymphocyte transformation
test is not used as an experienced test in sulfonamide allergies, as reliable results
cannot be expected. In the leukocyte migration inhibition test a leukocyte migration inhibiting factor (MIF) of the cellular immunity is determined. The patient's
leukocytes are packed into capillaries and allowed to migrate within a culture
chamber. HAN et al. (1969) observed a syndrome with plasmacytosis, lymphocytosis, and multiclonic gamma globulinopathy similar to serum disease. After disappearance of the hypersensitivity reaction, cultures of the patient's peripheral lymphocytes demonstrated blastic transformation with sulfapyridine and sulfisoxazole, in contrast to the controls.

V. Experimental Studies in Animals

ROBINSON et al. (1977) found no deterioration of the renal function in Wistar rats
under cotrimoxazole when they measured the blood content of urea. Neither in rats
with normal renal function nor in those with operatively produced impairment of
the kidneys was tubular necrosis found.

AOKI et al. (1974) sensitized guinea pigs by repeated cutaneous applications of
p-hydroxylaminobenzene sulfonamide (PHABSA), a photo-oxidation product of
sulfanilamide (SNA). On challenge with the substance, a marked cutaneous inflammation and an elevation of histamine level in the lesions are observed, although a single application of PHABSA to the nonsensitized animals elicits neither
of these reactions. In addition, the cutaneous changes and elevation of histamine

level induced by challenge in the sensitized animals are markedly suppressed by pretreatment with either histamine liberator or antihistamine. Thus it is presumed that PHABSA plays an important role in the photoallergic reaction caused by SNA and that one of the mediators in this process is histamine.

VI. Conclusions Concerning Possible Pathomechanisms

In some sulfonamides too (sulfamidine, sulfapyridine, and salazopyrine), it was found that there are "quick" and "slow" acetylators. After salazopyrine, cyanosis and hemolysis can occur in the slow acetylators, and might be toxic effects (MEYER and MEIER 1982).

In allergic reactions after sulfonamides, morphological signs such as anaphylactic reaction and lesions induced by immune complexes are found. In the former, more compact infiltrates of eosinophilic granulocytes are often seen, while in the latter, leukoblastic vasculitides and degenerations like polyarteriitis nodosa are prominent.

It is assumed that the hematologic side effects and those of the skin are of immunological rather than toxic etiology (FRISCH 1973).

In regard to the factors producing bone marrow damage, sulfonamides belong to the "phenothiazine type", which is marked by slow onset, initiation by high doses and long-term medication, and decrease of myelocytopoiesis in the bone marrow. The extensive disturbance of myeloid cells is probably based on a selective inhibition of DNA synthesis (LASSON 1977).

Long-acting sulfonamides are at the top of the list of drugs responsible for producing the Stevens-Johnson syndrome and Lyell's syndrome. Infections, for example by mycoplasms, herpes simplex viruses, hemolytic streptococci, salmonellae, and Epstein-Barr viruses, have been reported as additional factors (BÖTTIGER et al. 1975).

C. Nitrofurantoin

I. Physicochemical and Pharmacologic Properties

Nitrofurans are synthetic chemotherapeutics. The NO_2 group on the O_5 of the furan ring is essentially responsible for their antibacterial effect.

$$O_2N \diagdown O \diagdown R$$

The side chain R is variable. In nitrofurantoin, the therapeutically most important derivative, it is an azomethine group $(CH = N)$ with substituent.

$$O_2N \diagdown O \diagdown CH=N-N \diagdown C=O \diagup NH \quad H_2C-C=O$$

The effective optimum pH is about 5.5–6, which corresponds to the pH value of the urine. Protein binding is about 30%–40%.

Nitrofurantoin is well absorbed after oral administration but in practice it does not show measurable serum concentrations, being very quickly eliminated (about 40%) by the urine, i. e., in an unchanged form. The elimination half-life is about 20 min; tissue concentrations could not be demonstrated. Renal elimination was about 17%–20% by glomerular filtration and about 80%–85% by tubular secretion.

Nitrofurantoin acts bacteriostatically. It intervenes in protein synthesis and acts over the cytoplasmic membrane in resting as well as in dividing bacteria.

II. Immunochemistry and Immunology

Nitrofurantoin can cause type III hypersensitivity reactions, which develop when antibodies (mostly IgM or IgG) react with tissue antigens or when soluble antigen-antibody complexes are formed. These complexes are deposited on target cells in the tissues. Complement is activated and causes the accumulation of neutrophilic leukocytes which release lysosomal enzymes causing tissue damage. Prominent examples of drug reaction belonging to this category are serum disease (as general form) and Arthus phenomenon (as localized form) (WITTE and WEST 1982).

III. Clinical Aspects

Allergic reactions to nitrofurantoin can appear in 2%–4.1% of cases and are manifold, ranging from exanthema through fever reactions, allergic pulmonary infiltrations, pleuritis exsudativa allergica, and angioneurotic edema to anaphylactic shock. Sometimes cholestatic hepatitides can be seen (EGGERS and STROTHMANN 1974; KOCH-WESER et al. 1971).

Allergic exanthemas are observed in 1%–2%, fever reactions in 2% of patients treated (GROULS et al. 1970). Eosinophilia is also frequent (1%–2%), and erythema nodosum has been described (LAUBENTHAL 1969).

Cases of polyneuritis may be ascribed not to nitrofurantoin allergy, but rather to toxic influence by the metabolism (HENNING 1974). Serious neuropathic reactions can not be explained by toxic mechanisms after nitrofurantoin, especially not those after only short-term exposure or after discontinuation of the drug. RUSSEL (1971) supposes that such reactions can appear on an allergic basis too.

According to WRIGHT (1980), in the USA and Canada 5 million nitrofurantoin treatments are carried out annually. A wide spectrum of liver degenerations, including acute hepatitis with or without cholestasis, granulomatous and chronic active hepatitis, and cirrhosis, is observed (STRÖMBERG and WENGLE 1976; SHARP et al. 1980; ENGEL et al. 1975; KLEMOLA et al. 1975;; GOLDSTEIN and JANICKI 1974).

STROHSCHEER and WEGENER (1977) report two cases of granulomatous hepatitis after nitrofurantoin which were caused by hyperergy.

HATOFF et al. (1979) report a case of chronic active hepatitis in a HLA B 8–positive 27-year-old female patient after nitrofurantoin (NOLE 1981). Agranulocytoses after nitrofurantoin have also been described (PALVA und LEHMOLA 1973). In 12 of 20 patients antinucleic antibodies were seen, gammaglobulin was increased, and antibodies against smooth muscle appeared. All patients were negative to HBsAg.

Eosinophilia was not observed. In one patient pulmonary fibrosis was seen, in another pulmonary infiltrates. In one patient with chronic active hepatitis a specific lymphocytic transformation was observed within 3 months after the beginning of therapy with nitrofurantoin, in another patient the authors observed immune complexes of polyclonal IgG antibodies and autologous albumin. Some patients, all women, had HLA B 8.

ISRAEL and DIAMOND (1962) were the first to report after nitrofurantoin a case of recurrent pulmonary infiltration with eosinophilia and pleural exudate taking the course of pulmonary embolism.

GLÜCK and JANOWER (1969) describe two cases of acute pulmonary syndrome with chill, fever, tussis, dyspnea, and thoracodynia after administration of nitrofurantoin. ALLEN et al. (1969) report further cases, and DAVID et al. (1968) chronic fibrosing pulmonary degenerations. Other pulmonary reactions are reported by LEIBER (1972), TEIGELKÖTTER (1972), and PONTE (1982).

In acute cases, symptoms begin 2 h to 21 days after the first dose of nitrofurantoin. In chronic cases, the period between the beginning of nitrofurantoin administration and the appearance of pulmonary degenerations is nearly 2 years.

In subacute cases the interval from the intake of the medicament to the onset of dyspnea, tachypnea and cyanosis is up to 1 year (DELANEY et al. 1977). After discontinuation of nitrofurantoin the symptoms recede within 12–48 h in the acute form of the disease. Recovery from the chronic form takes longer and depends on the degree of irreversible lung fibrosis. Generally no therapy is necessary in the acute form, as the symptoms recede within 12–48 h after removing the drug. MORGAN (1970) recommends adrenaline, antihistaminics, and in severe cases prednisolone. When chronic forms are histologically examined, thickening of the alveolar wall and numerous infiltrating cells in the interstitium are to be seen – the same findings as in chronic interstitial fibrosis (MATTELAER 1972).

In Sweden, 921 reports of Furadantin side effects have been made. The undesirable effects of nitrofurantoin in general amount to 10%–12% of the registered drug side effects in Sweden. The two largest groups are acute pulmonary reactions (43%) and allergic reactions (42%) (HOLMBERG et al. 1980; HOLMBERG and BOMAN 1981; ISRAEL et al. 1980; LENIGER and SULZBACH 1981; MÜLLER 1974; HAINER and WHITE 1981; LÜBBERS 1969; JAMESON 1969; BACHMAN 1971; BONE et al. 1976; STRANDBERG et al. 1974; SELROOS and EDGREN 1975; HEIJER 1970; WIONTZEK 1970; NGAN et al. 1971; MÜLLER et al. 1970; MÜLLER and HOIGNÉ 1971).

The increase in cases – in absolute terms and also in relation to the number of doses-sold – is explained by permanent sensitization. In the period 1966–1976, 398 acute and 49 chronic pulmonary reactions to nitrofurantoin were registered in Sweden. Of these patients, 75% had to be admitted to hospital and 85% were female. The average age of those with acute reactions was about 59 years, of the chronic cases about 68 years. It is assumed that acute reactions are of allergic nature, chronic and hepatic reactions of toxic nature. Immediate discontinuation of the drug is necessary in either case. Chronic reactions do not follow the acute cases and acute cases do not tend to become chronic (MÜLLER 1974; HOLMBERG and BOMAN 1981).

Histologically, the acute pulmonary reaction (GELLERT 1976) lookes like interstitial pneumonia. Wagner (1971) describes the case of a 76-year-old female patient who was suffering from chronic interstitial pneumonia after nitrofurantoin but reacted with fever to an exposure test. Radiologically, in Wagner's case, there was not only accompanying cellular infiltration or fibrosis, but also alveolar degenerations such as edema.

Erythema nodosum with symptoms like serum disease has also been described after nitrofurantoin (CHRISHOLM and HEPNER 1981). FLECK (1981) describes five patients with SLE-like syndrome associated with nitrofurantoin who had been on nitrofurantoin therapy for more than a year. They all had abrupt elevations of serum IgG and antinuclear, antithyroid, and anti-smooth muscle antibodies, which returned to normal levels when nitrofurantoin was stopped.

IV. Results of Diagnostic Tests

1. Skin Tests

TYKAL and WILMS (1972) describe anaphylactic shock after repeated administration of Furadantin. The allergic reaction is explained by the increase in reagins demonstrated with a specific skin test (Prausnitz-Küster).

The Prausnitz-Küster test serves to demonstrate the presence of an allergy of the spontaneous type to a certain antigen. This reaction is regulated by the IgE sensitizing of the skin and develops within minutes after exposure to the antigen. Plasma from an allergic patient is infused and then a prick test carried out in the same skin region. There is no danger of anaphylaxis but the risk of hepatitis exists, and therefore this test is rarely employed today (RUSSEL and LESSOF 1971).

The epicutaneous test can be used as an experienced test, but its results are very weak.

LAUBSTEIN and NIEDERGESÄSS (1970) report on 24 patients with nitrofurazone sensitization. Except in one case continuation of the sensitization for 4 years could be demonstrated. The latency periods up to the manifestation of a contact allergy, were between a few weeks and 4 years. In epicutaneous tests with Nifucin, delayed reactions were seen relatively often. Group reactions against other nitrofuranes were not observed in patients sensitized by Nifucin.

2. Nitrofurantoin-Specific Antibodies

Liver toxicity after nitrofurantoin is especially serious in women. It is often connected with the appearance of autoantibodies (antinucleic factors) and hyperglobulinemia and shows no relation to the daily dosage.

In investigation of 33 controls and 18 patients with hypersensitivity with the test enzyme-linked immunoabsorbed assay to nitrofurantoin BÄCK et al. (1977) were not able to demonstrate IgE antibodies against nitrofurantoin in any case; however most of the hypersensitive patients and also the controls had specific IgG antibodies. These antibody titers were higher in the hypersensitive patients. Some patients have been shown to have increased BSR, polyclonal hypergamma-globulinemia and IgG antinucleic antibodies and a positive LE latex test simultaneously with the acute pulmonary syndrome after nitrofurantoin (SELROOS and EDGREN 1975; TEPPO et al. 1976; LUNDGREN et al. 1975; BÄCK et al. 1974).

However, there is no evidence for a specific humoral antibody reaction to nitrofurantoin in the acute pulmonary syndrome (GELLER et al. 1976; PEARSALL et al. 1974). Experienced antibody tests are not carried out with nitrofurantoin. TEPPO et al. (1976), in immune electrophoresis of ten patients of whom eight had been treated with nitrofurantoin, observed an enlarged albumin fraction to the cathode which disappeared in five cases after cessation of treatment. Most of the patients had polyclonally increased IgG und IgA levels and decreased albumin values. IgM, C3, and C4 were normal. Antinucleic activity of the IgG type was seen in nine patients. The phenomenon was the consequence of immune complexes between IgG and albumins. The activity similar to that of antibodies of IgG was directed to autologous and isologous albumin.

3. Nitrofurantoin-Specific Lymphocyte Reactivity

SPIELBERG et al. (1981) used human lymphocytes in order to investigate the biochemical base of the nitrofurantoin reactions. By means of trypan blue it was observed that the drug itself does not damage the cells. In the presence of a drug-activating system from mice liver microsomes, however, nitrofurantoin metabolites caused a toxicity dependent on the dose in lymphocytes. An inhibition of the enzyme epoxide hydrolase did not increase the toxicity; the metabolite was probably not furanepoxide. The binding of reacting metabolites on the macromolecules can cause direct cell death or secondary immunological reaction in vivo, working like haptens. The metabolite causes a decrease of the glutathionine concentration dependent on the dosage. Cells from one patient with a lack of glutathione synthetase showed a distinctly increased nitrofurantoin toxicity. The findings speak for the facts that glutathionine plays a leading part in protection against nitrofurantoin damage and that in patients with allergic reactions to nitrofurantoin, investigation of lymphocyte toxicity and glutathionine metabolism can contribute to clarifying the biochemical and genetic foundations of this drug hypersensitivity.

BÄCK et al. (1977) found the lymphocyte transformation test positive in ten of 18 patients hypersensitive to nitrofurantoin. PEARSELL et al. (1974) observed lymphocyte hypersensitivity and a lymphocyte migratory inhibitory factor in one patient who had an acute pulmonary syndrome with simultaneous skin allergy after nitrofurantoin. This hypersensitivity was seen for 2½ years and a participation of the T-lymphocytes rather than of the B-lymphocytes in the hypersensitivity is supposed. The authors suppose that a cellular mechanism is responsible for the hypersensitivity to nitrofurantoin.

GOLDSTEIN and JANICKI (1974) have the opinion that after nitrofurantoin, acute pulmonary reactions can be connected with the presence of a specific cellular reaction to the drug even there is no specific antibody reaction.

Experienced lymphocyte transformation tests are not as a rule carried out for nitrofurantoin.

V. Experimental Studies in Animals

KLEINT and VON BAEHR (1970) observed one case of drug fever after nitrofurantoin. The serum of this patient produced a distinct pyrogenic reaction in rabbits, in contrast to the control animals and those which had received serum from patients treated with nitrofurantoin.

VI. Conclusions Concerning Possible Pathomechanisms

The positive findings concerning specific IgG antibodies especially the results of the lymphocyte reactions, speak for an allergic pathogenesis of the nitrofurantoin reactions.

In acute eosinophilic pulmonary reactions after nitrofurantoin there is an interval between application of the drug and appearance of the reaction. A peripheral eosinophilia is shown. Histologically it is a matter of eosinophilic infiltration with edema and perivasculitis in the lungs. Observations supporting an allergic genesis are:
1. Fever and eosinophilia during the acute stage
2. Reproduction of the whole syndrome within hours after administration of the drug to hypersensitive subjects
3. Deceleration of pulmonary infiltration after discontinuation of the drug.

Because these phenomena are also observed in other acute pulmonary reactions caused by antigen-antibody complexes, it is supposed that nitrofurantoin acts similarly, although GOLDSTEIN and JANICKI (1974) had no success in demonstrating the specific antibody. In contrast, PEARSELL et al. (1974) assume that pathogenesis is based on hypersensitivity of the prolonged type (cell-bound immune response).

HEIJER (1970) holds the opinion that in the nitrofurantoin lung the allergic reaction corresponds most closely to the Arthus phenomenon. The increased LDH concentrations in these patients also speak for this.

D. Nalidixic, Pipemidic, and Oxolonic Acids

I. Physicochemical and Pharmacologic Properties

Nalidixic acid

Nalidixic acid is 1-ethyl-7 methyl-1,8-naphthyridine-4-one-3-carbonic acid ($C_{12}H_{12}N_2O$). It acts bacteriostatically and its optimal pH is 4.5–7.0. Solutions should not be kept in the refrigerator for more than 4 weeks. Eighty percent of orally administered nalidixic acid is absorbed. The half-life is 1 ½–2 h and the protein binding of the serum 70%–94%; 60%–80% is excreted by the kidneys, but only 20% of the dose is excreted in microbiologically active form, the rest being ineffective glucuronides and 3,7-dicarbonic acid. The antibacterial effect is limited to proliferating germs and the therapeutic action is based on inhibition of DNA replication.

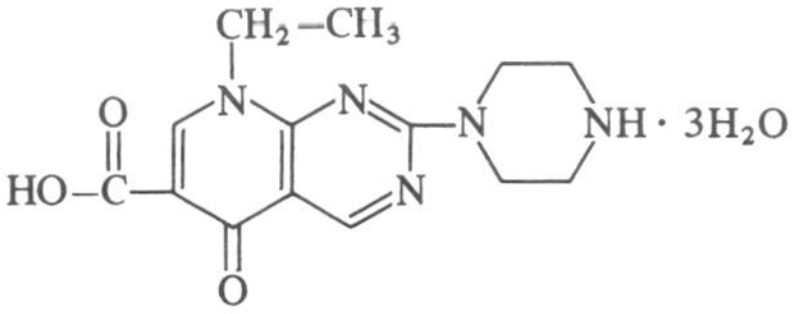

Pipemidic acid

Three to six hours after oral administration of 400 mg pipemidic acid there are concentrations of 200–800 µg/ml in the urine. Fifty to eighty percent of the dose is excreted in the urine as unchanged pipemidic acid. Metabolites (acetyl-pipemidic acid, formylpipemidic acid and oxopyremidic acid) occur only in small quantities and have less antibacterial activity than pipemidic acid. About 25% of the given dose is excreted in the feces. Penetration into the tissues is insignificant. Protein binding in the serum is 20%–30%.

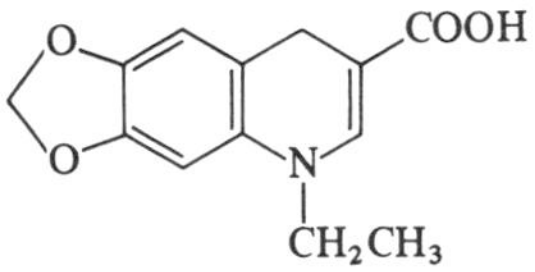

Oxolonic acid

Oxolonic acid is in vitro more efficient than nalidixic acid. The therapeutic mechanism is in this case too thought to be inhibition of bacterial DNA synthesis. The optimal action is in the range of pH 6.5–8. The half-life in serum is 2½–3 h. After oral administration of 4×240 mg oxolonic acid to human subjects, serum concentrations of 1.8 µg/ml and average 24-h-urine concentrations of 40 µg/ml are reached.

II. Immunochemistry and Immunology

In photoallergic reactions, light seems to promote the photochemical reaction between the agents and the proteins of the skin, so that complete antigens with immunogenic effect develop more quickly and to a greater degree. Thereby humorally mediated immediate reactions and/or hypersensitivity reactions of the delayed type occur. As a rule, a photoallergic reaction is caused by a lesser exposure to light than is a phototoxic response. In addition, light rays with a wavelength of 320–400 nm are more photoallergic than pure ultraviolet rays. The range of wavelength effective for these three medicaments is 290–400 nm.

Morphologically, the changes in photoallergic reactions resemble severe sunburn, with edema, papules, red maculae, vesicles, urticarial reactions, and the histological signs of a humorally and/or cell-mediated immunity.

III. Clinical Aspects

Allergic reactions (exanthemas, photosensitization, pruritus, eosinophilia, fever, reversible leukopenia, and occasionally hemolytic anemia) are described after administration of nalidixic acid and pipemidic acid. Excessive exposure to sunlight and ultraviolet light should be avoided during therapy with these drugs (BAES 1968; BIRKETT et al. 1969; RAMSAY 1973; BREHM and KORTING 1970; LOUIS et al. 1973; BURRY 1974; RAMSAY and OBRESKOVA 1974; BOISVERT and BARBEAU 1981).

More than 40 cases of bullous exanthema after nalidixic acid have been observed, mostly involving women of middle age and children. The porphyrin levels were in all cases within the normal range. Blistering began usually 3–21 days (up to 2 months) after the first administration, and relapsed at intervals even without further intake of the drug. The skin eruptions were on the parts of the body permanently exposed to light.

Occasionally, hemolytic crises are described in patients with deficiency of glucose-6-phosphate dehydrogenase under therapy with nalidixic acid. In rare cases, thrombocytopenic purpura or hemorrhagic enteritis has been observed (TRAUTMANN and OPITZ 1973). Arthralgia is sometimes described after nalidixic acid, and is thought to be of allergic origin. The joint involvement is occasionally associated with exanthema or fever (BAILEY et al. 1972). RUBINSTEIN (1979) describes a case of drug-induced lupus erythematosus after nalidixic acid.

FRASER and HARROWER (1977) observed an otherwise healthy patient with convulsions after nalidixic acid and interpreted this symptom as an idiosyncrasy. DEONNA and GUIGNARD (1974) report two cases of intracranial hypertension after nalidixic acid in infants, and GOLL and ROHWEDDER (1971) observed acute meningeal hydrops and respiratory emergency in infants under 8 weeks of age.

GOPINATHAN (1973) thinks that the intracranial hypertension during nalidixic acid therapy is due to decreased absorption of cerebrospinal fluid. The range of side effects after oxolonic acid seems to be wider on the whole than after nalidixic acid; nausea, vomiting, diarrhoea, spasms of the stomach, cardiopulmonary and neurological symptoms, and insomnia are prominent (SIMON and CHERMAT 1977). Other less frequent adverse reactions to oxolonic acid are fever, rash, photosensitivity, palpitations, and a sense of tightness in the chest (SILVERMAN 1981). Oxolonic acid should be given with food or antacids to minimize its side effects.

IV. Results of Diagnostic Tests

1. Skin Tests

Skin tests are not important in allergy to nalidixic, pipemidic, oxolonic acids.

RAMSAY (1973) made photopatch tests in three of seven patients with photosensitivity after nalidixic acid. All three were negative.

LOUIS et al. (1973) got negative results from provocation tests with the xenon high-pressure lamp and epicutaneous light exposure tests without and with detachment of the stratum corneum in patients with bullous photodermatitis after nalidixic acid. However, they were able to demonstrate the phototoxicity of nalidixic acid by means of the Daniels candida test.

2. Nalidixic, Pipemidic and Oxolonic Acid-Specific Antibodies

BREHM and KORTING (1970) had a positive consumption test with cutis extract, but consumption tests with epidermis, vessels, and thymic nuclei were negative. The consumption test by Steffen demonstrates incomplete antibodies. Therefore there is evidence that the bullous nalidixic acid reaction of the skin is an allergic phenomenon with incomplete antibodies against cutis. Routine demonstration of antibodies against nalidixic, pipemidic, and oxolonic acids are not usual.

3. Nalidixic, Pipemidic and Oxolonic Acid-Specific Lymphocyte Reactions

BREHM et al. (1970) demonstrated fluorescence in the stratum granulosum by means of immunofluorescent examination of a skin biopsy in a patient with bullous reaction of the skin after nalidixic acid.

Routine lymphocyte transformation tests for nalidixic, pipemidic, and oxolonic acids are not usual, but may be helpful if more than one potential sensitizing medicament has been given. The clinical impression that phototoxic reactions to nalidixic acid are not related to specific antibodies is supported by negative lymphocyte transformation tests (ALEXANDER and FORMAN 1971).

V. Experimental Studies in Animals

A search through the literature has revealed no reports of experimental studies in animals concerning allergy to nalidixic, pipemidic or oxolonic acid.

VI. Conclusions Concerning Possible Pathomechanisms

Regarding the skin changes after administration of nalidixic or pipemidic acid, the following points speak for photoallergic processes:
1. Only a few people are affected.
2. There is an interval between the first intake of the drug and the appearance of skin reactions.
3. Skin reactions disappear very slowly.
4. Even with lower doses there are bullous reactions (WOLF 1981).

The demonstration of immunofluorescence in the stratum granulosum and the positive consumption test with cutis extract, also indicate allergic events, but the investigations by ALEXANDER and FORMAN (1971) and also LOUIS et al. (1973) speak rather for phototoxic reactions.

The histological changes are compatible with photoallergic as well as phototoxic reactions (BRAUNER 1975).

BREHM and KORTING (1970) express the opinion that the bullous skin changes after nalidixic acid and pipemidic acid are of mixed photoallergic and phototoxic origin. The above-mentioned points speak for a photoallergic reaction: indications of phototoxicity are the morphological picture of an "intensified sunburn reaction" and the sharply-defined localization to body parts exposed to light.

E. Isoniazid

I. Physicochemical and Pharmacologic Properties

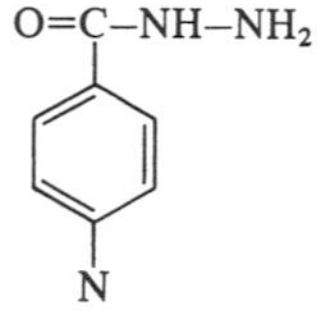

O=C–NH–NH$_2$

Isoniazid

Isoniazid has a tuberculocid effect on proliferating microorganisms, and the tuberculous bacteria become less acid-proof. Isoniazid diffuses in the cells and reaches the intracellular germs. It penetrates the bacterium cell and interacts with its metabolism, especially the lipid metabolism, and inhibits the synthesis of DNA, RNA, and proteins. Isoniazid diffuses well in the tissues, the pleura, the peritoneum, and the meninges and in tuberculous foci. The blood concentration is dependent on the degree of transformation of the biologically active isoniazid into the 100–500 times less effective acetyl derivative. The acetylation differs greatly between single subjects and populations, for individual and racial reasons. Patients are divided into three groups, depending on the serum concentration of isoniazid 6 h after oral administration of 4 mg/kg:
1. Slow inactivators (>0.8 µg/ml)
2. Intermediate inactivators (0.2–0.8 µg/ml)
3. Rapid inactivators (0.15–0.2 µg/ml).

II. Immunochemistry and Immunology

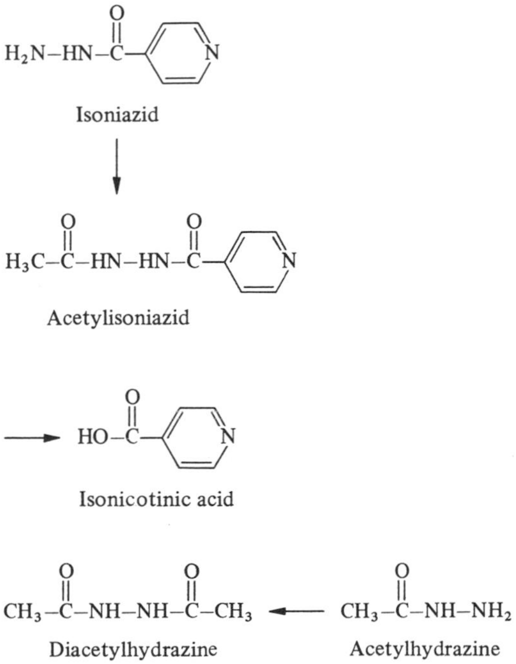

H$_2$N–HN–C–

Isoniazid

H$_3$C–C–HN–HN–C–

Acetylisoniazid

HO–C–

Isonicotinic acid

CH$_3$–C–NH–NH–C–CH$_3$ ← CH$_3$–C–NH–NH$_2$

Diacetylhydrazine   Acetylhydrazine

Metabolism of isoniazid. (Modified after ELLARD and GAMMON 1976; MITCHEL et al. 1976)

Investigations of MITCHEL et al. (1976) showed that the hepatotoxicity of isoniazid is due to its metabolite acetylhydrazin. Acetylhydrazin develops after the acetylation of isoniazid into acetylisoniazid and the following hydrolysis of acetylisoniazid to isonicotinic acid. MITCHEL postulates that rapid inactivators have a higher risk to develop liver damage than slow inactivators.

III. Clinical Aspects

Side effects are seen in 5.4% of cases after therapy with isoniazid. In 2% of the cases there are exanthemas, in 1.2% fever, in 0.6% jaundice, and in 0.2% peripheral neuritis (DAVIS and STOLER 1977).

Allergic reactions are rare. Polyneuropathy is not caused by hypersensitivity, and can be prevented and if need be treated by administration of vitamin B_6. In cases of existing liver damage isoniazid may be an additional burden, because it is metabolized in this organ. Some cases of liver damage by isoniazid are clinically difficult to differentiate from virus hepatitis (GARIBALDI et al. 1972; THOMAS et al. 1979).

There are two forms of liver damage after isoniazid:
1. Slight reversible elevations in SGOT and SGPT levels occur in 10% of cases.
2. Hypersensitivity reactions occur in 1% of cases. They are characterized by fever, necrosis of the liver, and sometimes rashes and occur 2–6 weeks after initiation of treatment. The total leukocyte count is high in most cases.

HYDE (1972) points out that patients who receive very high doses of isoniazid (16 mg/kg/day) had five times as many reactions as patiens receiving the standard doses (300 mg/day or 5 mg/kg/day). WEIL (1976) also recommends doses of 5 mg/kg/day in order to avoid complications.

Liver damage after isoniazid is not predictable and belongs to the cytotoxic type (PAUMGARTNER and PAUMGARTNER 1980). Elderly women, alcohol addicts (especially those with daily alcohol intake), and patients with diseases of the liver or gallbladder run a higher risk of liver damage from isoniazid (DASH et al. 1980; MYLES 1980; ELLARD et al. 1981; LE GUILLOU et al. 1981; PESSAYRE et al. 1977; THOMPSON 1978; GRAHAM and DUNDAS 1979; ATUK et al. 1977; WEISE et al. 1976; BYRD et al. 1979; LABAYLE et al. 1979; GROOPMAN et al. 1978; GRÖNHAGEN-RISKA et al. 1978; KOPANOFF et al. 1978; LINNA and UHARI 1980; MADDREY and BOITNOTT 1977; BRUNO and OBER 1968; RISKA 1976).

Fever after administration of isoniazid is seen mostly in patients receiving several drugs. It begins on the 9th–47th day of isoniazid therapy (DASTA et al. 1979; JACOBS et al. 1977; BHANDARI 1977).

THOMPSON (1969) successfully desensitized 22 patients with hypersensitivity to antituberculous drugs by using corticosteroids, without interruption of chemotherapy. No adverse effects on the response to their disease were noted in patients with tuberculosis, nor did deterioration in atypical diseases occur. It is stressed that rapid suppression of such allergic reactions depends on the promptness with which steroids are administered. The syndrome of algodystrophia (pains, vasomotor disorders, and trophic alterations on the upper and occasionally the lower extremities resembling Sudeck's syndrome) after administration of isoniazid has been described (KAISER 1976; GEMPERLI 1969; LEQUESNE 1967). Acute arthritis after isoniazid has also been reported (PERIMAN and VENKATARAMANI 1975; SASLAW and KLAINER 1969; MERLIN et al. 1974; TIZES et al. 1971; KESTER and HAVEN 1971; HABER and OSBORNE 1959). Structurally isoniazid resembles, some monooxidase inhibitors, and as with these inhibitors it is possible that the administration of isoniazid together with consumption of cheese leads to tachycardia and hypertension as a result of interactions (LEJONC et al. 1980; MORGAN 1980; SMITH and DURACK 1978).

Isoniazid is a potent inhibitor of histaminase, and if taken together with tuna or other fishes or cheese, it may give rise to symptoms corresponding to histamine intoxication (URAGODA 1980; URAGODA and KOTTEGODA 1977; URAGODA and LODHA 1979).

IPPEN (1978) reports the case of a 20-year-old nurse who got contact exzema because of an ulcerative BCG reaction when she was treated with isoniazid styli.

ROSIN and KING (1982) describe the case of a 75-year-old man with exfoliative dermatitis which began 8 days after the commencement of 300 mg isoniazid daily.

BOMB et al. (1976) report a case of Stevens-Johnson syndrome caused by isoniazid which deared up completely after discontinuation of the drug and corticosteroid therapy. There was recurrence of the skin rash after a test dose of isoniazid, proving that this medicament was the offending agent.

TILIAKOS et al. (1980) report a case of severe hemorrhagic cystitis after isoniazid in a 22-year-old slow inactivator. Symptomatic and laboratory recovery followed discontinuation of isoniazid. Oral isoniazid and bladder irrigation with urine containing isoniazid metabolites reproduced the syndrome, but oral acetylisoniazid and bladder irrigation with isoniazid solution did not.

In 85% of cases, isoniazid hepatitis heals in 1–3 weeks (BARTMANN 1977). STUART and ROBERTS (1976) describe a case of disseminated coagulopathy in connection with isoniazid hepatitis.

BLACK et al. (1975) analyzed 114 cases of hepatitis after isoniazid prophylaxis in 13 838 patients. Thirteen patients died, six in one city (FARER 1976). ISRAEL (1975) holds the opinion that isoniazid should be given only for treatment, not for prophylaxis.

DOLD and REICHENMILLER (1969) saw elevations of liver-specific enzymes, especially under the combination of isoniazid and antiepileptic drugs (diphenylhydantoin or carbamazepine). GREENBERG et al. (1972) describe a case of severe lupus erythematosus with tamponade of the pericardium after administration of isoniazid.

HONEYCUTT and HULDIN (1963) pointed out that after isoniazid there occur morbilliform or maculopapular exanthemas, which only in rare cases proceed to dermatitis herpetiformis but are often combined with fever, swollen lymph nodes, eosinophilia, and icterus. In some cases there are hypersensitivity reactions which resemble systemic lupus erythematosus. In general, hypersensitivity reactions after isoniazid may present as fever, hepatitis, and morbilliform, maculopapular, purpura-like, and urticarial exanthemas (FELLNER 1970). Hematologic reactions (agranulocytosis, eosinophilia, thrombocytopenia, and anemia) may also occur.

Among others, HORVÁTTH and TENGELYI (1970) report a case of anaphylactic reaction of the bone marrow after isoniazid in a 51-year-old woman. The drug was withdrawn after the first symptoms and irreversible damage was avoided.

Vasculitis with antinuclear antibodies recedes after discontinuation of therapy.

IV. Results of Diagnostic Tests

1. Skin Tests

Individual cases of contact dermatitis, e. g., involving nurses, have been described. In these cases the epicutaneous test may show a group allergy to aromatic hydrazine derivates. HERMANN et al. (1969) report the case of a 37-year-old nurse with severe drug exanthema after intake of 100 mg isoniazid. The epicutaneous test was positive against several aromatic hydrazine compounds, possessing a free aromatic hydrazine component but with different aromatic rings. The authors decided that this group allergy is due mainly to the free hydrazine residue of isoniazid and similar compounds.

In IPPEN's (1978) case of contact eczema, the epicutaneous test, with isoniazid as substance or as pulverized tablets (from several manufacturers), showed in all instances definite eczema reactions which exceeded the test areas and required local treatment with corticosteroids. WANG and SCHMID (1974) report the case of a patient with occupational allergy to isoniazid. Beside the allergic reaction of the immediate type (asthma bronchiale) there was a latent sensitization of the delayed reaction type (eczema reaction). This latent sensitization was manifested in a circumscribed area by the epicutaneous test. Reexposure to the allergen led to an asthmatic spasm of the bronchi and to recrudescence of the eczematous cutaneous efflorescences when it was inhaled.

2. Isoniazid-Specific Antibodies

In a few cases there was intravasal hemolysis after administration of isoniazid. FREEDMAN and LINN (1978) describe a positive direct antiglobulin test in such a case of hemolytic anaemia after isoniazid. The antibody was bound to IgG-complement-fixing antibodies and reacted best at 37 °C with the antiglobulin technique and only with cells previously sensitized with isoniazid. Sometimes antinuclear antibodies develop during treatment with isoniazid (ALARCÓN-SEGOVIA 1973; ROTH-FIELD et al. 1978).

MITCHELL et al. (1975) made a blind, prospective evaluation in 358 psychiatric patients during 1 year of tuberculosis prevention with isoniazid. Most of the patients who developed abnormal serum transaminases recovered completely while continuing their isoniazid therapy. No serum antibodies against isoniazid could be demonstrated and no correlation was found between the presence of antinuclear antibodies or elevated isoniazid plasma concentrations and the occurrence of hepatic injury. These data support the view that hepatotoxic metabolites of isoniazid may be responsible for the liver damage.

3. Isoniazid-Specific Lymphocyte Reactivity

WARRINGTON et al. (1978) found that the lymphocyte transformation test was positive after stimulation with isoniazid, isonicotinic acid, and conjugates of these compounds in 95% of patients who developed isoniazid hepatitis. Healthy controls and isoniazid patients who did not develop liver damage showed a negative test. There was no correlation between the degree of lymphocyte transformation and the severity of liver damage. The appearance of liver damage after isoniazid seems to depend on the presence of cellular hypersensitivity to this medicament.

WARRINGTON and OLIVIER (1979) examined the release of lymphotoxin from the lymphocytes of the peripheral blood in patients with hepatitis after isoniazid. In five of six cases there was support of release of lymphotoxin after stimulation of these lymphocytes with isoniazid or isonicotinic acid conjugated with human serum albumin. BAKER et al. (1974) had positive results from the macrophage migration inhibition test in only two of six patients after clinical hypersensitivity to isoniazid.

REIDENBERG and CACCESE (1975) found a positive lymphocyte transformation test in presumed isoniazid allergy. MATHEWS et al. (1971) also found positive lymphocyte transformation tests after isoniazid allergy, especially when the reaction appeared within the first 6 weeks after commencement of therapy and when there was eosinophilia. Positive lymphocyte transformation tests were not significantly associated with fever, personal or familial history of atopy, or allergies to other drugs.

ASSEM et al. (1969) describe a patient with jaundice and manifestations of generalized allergic reaction. The lymphocyte transformation test provided evidence of allergy to isoniazid. WARRINGTON et al. (1981) have the opinion that the lymphocyte transformation test is of predictive value in the diagnosis of isoniazid-associated hepatitis.

DOVE et al. (1972) were not able to demonstrate transformation of lymphocytes in 14 patients with isoniazid-associated hepatitis. PAUW (1979) found a statistically significant reduction of T-lymphocytes and increase of B-lymphocytes during the administration of isoniazid; after the therapy the T-lymphocytes increased and the B-lymphocytes decreased.

V. Experimental Studies in Animals

Studies in animals and in vitro showed isoniazid to be a very strong inhibitor of diphenylhydantoin metabolism (KUTT et al. 1970). SNODGRASS et al. (1974) did not find necrosis of the liver in rats after treatment with isoniazid or hydrazine, but single cell necrosis did appear after acetylisoniazid and acetylhydrazine.

VI. Conclusions Concerning Possible Pathomechanisms

There is evidence that the severe hypersensitivity reactions after isoniazid, characterized by fever, liver necrosis, and sometimes exanthema, occur mainly in rapid inactivators and are based on the accumulation of the metabolites acetylhydrazine and acetylisoniazid (MITCHELL 1976; BROWN 1976; ELLARD et al. 1978; ELLARD et al. 1981; MYLES 1980).

On the other hand, functional liver damage with elevation of serum transaminases and bilirubin levels during therapy with the combination of isoniazid and rifampicin is observed more often in slow inactivators, in whom rifampicin activates the enzyme system, which disintegrates the drugs. Therefore in these cases there is an elevated hepatotoxicity of isoniazid due to the increased appearance of reactive intermediates (VON OLDERSHAUSEN et al. 1978; SMITH 1979; SMITH et al. 1972; PESSAYRE et al. 1977; VON OLDERSHAUSEN 1976; DENGLER and EICHELBAUM 1977; MUSCH et al. 1982). Admittedly, some of these studies were carried out with relatively high doses of isoniazid (10 mg/kg/day).

F. Ethambutol

I. Physicochemical and Pharmacologic Properties

$$\left(\begin{array}{c} CH_3-CH_2-C-CH_2OH \\ | \\ NH_2 \\ | \\ CH_2 \\ | \\ CH_2 \\ | \\ NH_2 \\ | \\ CH_3-CH_2-CH \end{array}\right) 2\,Cl$$

Ethambutol

The main tuberculostatic effect of ethambutol is on proliferating, not on resting germs. Ethambutol causes a degenerative metabolism in the mycobacteriae, particularly involving the phosphate fraction. The cell division of the germs is suppressed and their vitality reduced.

Eighty percent of an oral dose of ethambutol is absorbed from the bowel. Serum concentrations of 2–5 µg/ml are reached 2–3 h after administration of 25 mg ethambutol/kg body wt. There is good diffusibility into the cerebrospinal fluid. The half-life in serum amounts to 4 h. Fifteen percent of a dose of ethambutol is metabolized in the liver; 80% is filtered in the glomerula (MELLIN and WAUBKE 1978).

II. Immunochemistry and Immunology

Immunoallergologic examinations (tuberculinallergometry, hemagglutinating antibodies) did not show any changes due to ethambutol.

III. Clinical Aspects

The ocular symptoms which occur during ethambutol treatment are not allergic, but toxic (PAN and WAHL 1974). Allergic reactions (fever, tachycardia, exanthemas, and anaphylactic shock) and leukopenia are described sporadically. Of all patients, 0.5% develop a rash, 0.3% drug fever. Pruritus, arthralgia, headache, disorientation, and possibly hallucinations also occur. Anaphylaxia and leukopenia are rare. In some cases there are erythema, pruritus, exanthema, and purpura with epistaxis and gingival hemorrhage (PASRICHA et al. 1977; JESIOTR 1979).

SCHULZ and THEISEN (1971) describe a case of drug exanthema, which was proved by exposure. Such occurrences are still very rare.

MÜHLBERGER (1973) saw a case of granulocytopenia in which the patient made a full recovery. HAEGI (1975) observed a reproducible drug fever after treatment with ethambutol. He saw thrombocytopenia and pancytopenia only with the combination of ethambutol and rifampicin.

KONNO et al. (1968) saw three cases of drug exanthema among 81 patients treated with ethambutol. One patient was successfully desensitized, starting from small doses of ethambutol, and the full dosage could eventually be given again.

IV. Results of Diagnostic Tests

1. Skin Tests

Skin tests have no essential practical importance in allergy to ethambutol.

2. Ethambutol-Specific Antibodies

DJAWARI (1978) reports the case of a 22-year-old man with visceral lupus erythematosus who had an exacerbation, when treated with ethambutol. After withdrawing the drug the clinical symptoms improved quickly and the dermatological changes declined rapidly.

GRENNAN amd STURROCK (1976) describe the case of a 9-year-old boy who was treated with rifampicin and ethambutol. He developed polyarthritis, rash, and hepatitis in association with antinative DNA antibodies and positive nuclear factor.

3. Ethambutol-Specific Lymphocyte Reactivity

Lymphocyte reactivity has no essential practical importance in allergy to ethambutol.

V. Experimental Studies in Animals

Trentini et al. (1974) observed loss of fertility and regressive changes in the testes in albino rats after 1 year of therapy with ethambutol. This phenomenon may be due to the chemical nature of the dextrogyrate isomer of ethambutol or to the accumulation of the medicament in the organism.

Real allergic reactions after treatment with ethambutol are rare.

VI. Conclusions Concerning Possible Pathomechanisms

Defects in vision after ethambutol are due to axial retrobulbar neuritis with a central scotoma and to periaxial retrobulbar neuritis with a partial concentric defect of the visual field (Mellin and Waubke 1978). This syndrome is caused by toxic, not allergic pathomechanisms.

Allergic side effects after treatment with ethambutol are extremely rare.

G. Sulfones

I. Physicochemical and Pharmacologic Properties

4,4–Diaminodiphenyl sulfone

Sulfones are applied especially to the therapy of leprosy. They penetrate the bacterial cells easily and act as antimetabolites against para-aminobenzoic acid in folate synthesis.

Diaminodiphenylsulfone is adsorbed after oral administration and distributed to the tissues of the body. Peak concentrations in serum occur 4–6 h after oral administration. The therapeutic range of serum concentrations is 1–10 µg/ml, and these concentrations are reached with the administration of 2×400 mg/week. The half-life lies between 18 and 31 h. Protein binding is 70%–80%. Maximal blood concentrations are reached within a few days as the result of accumulation.

Diaminodiphenylsulfone passes through the enterohepatic circulation and is metabolized and acetylated to glucuronide and sulfate in the liver.

Diaminodiphenylsulfone and its metabolites are excreted in the urine in the range of 70%–80% of the oral dose; 90% are excreted within 5 days.

II. Immunochemistry and Immunology

Eighty percent of diaminodiphenylsulfone is found in the blood in the free form and 20% as a water-soluble derivative.

The sulfones are powerful biological antioxidants, and can replace vitamin E biologically in white rats fed prooxidant diets. They have hepatic enzymatic inductive activity in white rats, as determined in barbiturate sleep (BERGEL 1981).

III. Clinical Aspects

Hemolytic anemia, rash, and liver damage may occur even with normal doses. In cases of overdosage, headache, vomiting, insomnia, and tachycardia are possible. Reactions may occur in leprosy with or without therapy. In lepromatous leprosy there is erythema nodosum, fever, and in some cases severe malaise. In tuberculoid leprosy the pain increases. About 50% of the treated patients with lepromatous leprosy show erythema nodosum within the 1st year, lasting for 2 weeks. As a rule, therapy with sulfones in combination with clofazimine may be continued in spite of the erythema nodosum. Analgetics, corticosteroids, and thalidomide are suitable for the treatment of leprosy reactions (REA and LEVAN 1975).

Considering the great number of sulfone treatments all over the world, severe toxic reactions are seldom observed or seldom reported. The essential side effects are hemolysis, agranulocytosis, dermatitis, hepatitis, psychoses, and occassionally severe hypalbuminemia. In addition, in the initial stages of treatment of lepromatous leprosy a syndrome has been described which resembles infectious mononucleosis with exfoliative dermatitis and eosinophilia ("DDS syndrome"). Though most of the patients with this syndrome have survived, at least three fatal cases have been reported, in one of which histology showed the picture of erythema multiforme. Most authors believe this syndrome to be due to an extremely severe hypersensitivity reaction to sulfones (FREY et al. 1981). Drug fever and rashes are also reported after sulfones.

KINGHAM et al. 1979, saw two cases of severe hypalbuminemia during the treatment of dermatitis herpetiformis with diaminodiphenylsulfone. The patients were treated for 3 and 11 months respectively, and in both cases the symptoms receded completely after discontinuation of sulfone therapy. Hemolytic anemia after sulfones depends on a deficit of glucose-6-phosphate dehydrogenase and on the dose, being found mainly with daily doses of more than 50 mg (MENEZES et al. 1981). This side effect does not seem to be of allergic origin.

IV. Results of Diagnostic Tests

1. Skin Tests

Skin tests have no great importance in relation to sulfone allergy.

2. Sulfone-Specific Antibodies

The thrombocyte agglutination test in vitro is a diagnostic measure in cases of thrombocytopenia after administration of sulfones.

3. Sulfone-Specific Lymphocyte Reactivity

Some patients with lepromatous leprosy have a deficiency of T-lymphocytes in their blood, which could be activated to serve an immunosuppressive function.

Whether this anomaly may predispose them to hypersensitivity reactions in the sense of the DDS syndrome is a subject of speculation.

V. Experimental Studies in Animals

A search of the literature has revealed no experimental studies concerning sulfone allergy in animals.

VI. Conclusions Concerning Possible Pathomechanisms

The DDS syndrome, which starts 5–6 weeks after the commencement of therapy, is probably a hypersensitivity reaction. It consists of dermatitis, hepatitis, swelling of the lymph nodes, and an increase in the mononuclear cells of the peripheral blood.

H. Clofazimine

I. Physicochemical and Pharmacologic Properties

Clofazimine

Clofazimine is chemically 3-(*p*-chloro-anilino)-10-(*p*-chlorophenyl)-1, 10-dihydro-2-(isopropylimino)-phenazine (=clofazimine).

It acts against *Mycobacterium leprae* and is also effective in the prevention and treatment of leprosy reactions. It also works in cases of sulfone resistance.

Seventy percent of clofazimine is absorbed from the gut when it is given as a microcrystalline suspension in an oily preparation. Clofazimine is well soluble in lipoids and is taken up from the adipose and the macrophages of the reticuloendothelial system. Clofazimine diffuses into liver, gallbladder, small intestine, muscle, bone, and skin. It remains in the body for a long time and is excreted very slowly; the half-life in humans after oral administration is at least 70 days. Only 0.1% of the given dose is excreted in the urine within 24 h.

II. Immunochemistry and Immunology

The leprosy reactions may be differentiated into type I (with cellular immunity) and type II (without cellular immunity), which is found in lepromatous leprosy and takes the course of erythema nodosum.

In a type I reaction the antileprosy therapy is interrupted; corticosteroids can be given. In the case of type II reaction the therapy should be continued. Corticosteroids, thalidomide, and clofazimine are all effective.

III. Clinical Aspects

The most frequent side effect is pink to black dyschromia of the skin, especially on the parts of the body exposed to light. Perspiration, hair, urine, and stools may also be colored. General dryness of the skin, pruritus, phototoxicity, acneiform changes and nonspecific exanthemas are also observed (BROWNE et al. 1981; PETTIT 1978; JOPLING 1976).

MASON et al. (1977) report a case of eosinophilic enteritis in a 29-year-old woman after 3 years of clofazimine therapy at 600 mg daily. At laparotomy there was nodular thickening of the upper ileum with black-brown pigmentation of the ileal wall, mesentery, and mesenteric lymph nodes. Ileal biopsy showed eosinophilic enteritis.

ÖHMAN and WAHLBERG (1975) and WÅLINDER et al. (1976) report slight changes of the cornea in 10 of 26 patients under therapy with clofazimine. This condition improves within 2 months after cessation of therapy. McDOUGALL et al. (1980) describe the case of a male patient aged 68 years who received clofazimine for 11 months. He was admitted to the hospital with severe abdominal pain and laparotomy revealed infarction of the spleen. Histopathological examination of spleen, duodenal biopsy tissue, and lymph nodes showed massive accumulation of crystals.

DESIKAN et al. (1975) present the autopsy findings of a young person suffering from intractable leprosy reaction treated for 4 months with clofazimine in a dose of 300 mg daily. A generalized yellow coloration of fatty tissue, brick-red tinting of muscle and viscera, and extreme congestion and edema of the mucosa of the small intestine were found and considered not to be of infectious origin. Deposits of clofazimine crystals were found in the intestinal mucosa.

IV. Results of Diagnostic Tests

1. Skin Tests

Skin tests are not very important in relation to clofazimine allergy.

2. Clofazimine-Specific Antibodies

The type I leprosy reaction is the consequence of changes in the cellular immunity, and the type II reaction is probably due to the formation of immune-complexes. Corticosteroids and clofazimine are effective against both types, thalidomide only against type II.

3. Clofazimine-Specific Lymphocyte Reactivity

JOPLING (1976) found clofazimine crystals in lymph nodes 4 years after the end of clofazimine therapy. The capacity for phagocytosis is improved by clofazimine.

Dubey et al. (1981) examined 123 cases of leprosy (41 newly ill patients, 18 with leprosy reactions, and 64 under therapy with diaminodiphenylsulfone or clofazimine) for cellular immunity (measured from the percentage of blasts), which proved to be low, especially in lepromatous leprosy. Under therapy there was an increase of blasts, more marked with clofazimine, than with diaminodiphenylsulfone.

Brandt and Svensson (1973) were not able to demonstrate stimulation of macrophages with clofazimine in vitro. Cline (1970) showed in vitro that clofazimine potentiates the killing of *Listeria* by macrophages. Berghem et al. (1977) were not able to produce a stimulation of reticuloendothelial system phagocytosis in vivo in five healthy women.

V. Experimental Studies in Animals

There are no reports in the literature on experimental studies concerning allergy to clofazimine in animals.

VI. Conclusions Concerning Possible Pathomechanisms

Allergic side effects of clofazimine are rare.

Clofazimine is able to stimulate cellular immunity. The pathogenetic mechanisms of this stimulation are not yet clear.

References

Alarcón-Segovia D (1973) Isoniazid, antinuclear antibodies and SLE. Chest 63:299

Alexander S, Forman L (1971) Which of the drugs caused the rash? Or the value of the lymphocyte transformation test in eruptions caused by nalidixic acid. Br J Dermatol 84:429

Allen RW, Hold AH, Brown MG (1968) Acute pulmonary sensitivity to nitrofurantoin. J Roentgenol 104:784

Anonymous (1974) Sulphasalazine-induced lung disease. Lancet I:504

Aoki K, Shimotoge M, Saito T (1974) Studies on photosensitivity caused by sulfa drugs. J Dermatol (Tokyo) I:99

Asmar B, Maqbool S, Dajani AS (1981) Hematologic abnormalities after oral trimethoprim-sulfamethoxazole therapy in children. Am J Dis Child 135:1100

Assem ESK, Ndoping N, Nicholson H, Wade JR (1969) Liver damage and isoniazid allergy. Clin Exp Immunol 5:439

Atuk NO, Hart AD, Hunt E (1977) Close monitoring is essential during isoniazid prophylaxis. South Med J 70:156

Azinge NO, Garrick GA (1978) Stevens-Johnson syndrome (erythema multiforme) following ingestion of trimethoprim-sulfamethoxazole on two separate occasions in the same person. A case report. J Allergy Clin Immunol 62:125

Bachmann A (1971) Lunge und Nitrofurantoin. DMW 96:1731

Bäck O, Lundgren R, Wiman LG (1974) Nitrofurantoin-induced pulmonary fibrosis and lupus syndrome. Lancet I:930

Bäck O, Lidén S, Ahlsted S (1977) Adverse reactions to nitrofurantoin in relation to cellular and humoral immune responses. Clin Exp Immunol 28:400

Baes H (1968) Photosensitivity caused by nalidixic acid. Dermatologica 136:61

Bailey RR, Natale R, Linton AL (1972) Nalidixic acid arthralgia. Can Med Assoc J 107:604

Baker H (1968) Drug reactions IV – Erythema multiforme gravis and long-acting sulphonamides. Br J Dermatol 80:844

Baker JT, Pioli E, Williams WJ (1974) In-vitro detection of hypersensitivity to antituberculous drugs. Lancet II:967

Bandmann HJ, Breit R (1973) The mafenide story. Br J Dermatol 89:219

Bartle WR, Saibil FG (1977) Antibiotic-associated pseudomembranous colitis. Can med Assoc J 116:162

Bartmann K (1977) Die Ermittlung von Nebenwirkungen bei chronischer Arzneitherapie am Beispiel der hepatotoxischen Wirkung von Isoniazid und Rifampicin. Verh Dtsch Ges Inn Med 83:1518

Bergel M (1981) Mechanism of action of sulfones. Int J Lepr 49:89

Berghem L, Lahnborg G, Schildt B (1977) does clofazimine (Lampren) affect the macro- and microphage function in man? J Reticuloendothel Soc 21:171

Bernstein LS (1975) Adverse reactions to trimethoprim-sulfamethoxazole, with particular reference to long-term therapy. Can Med Assoc J 112:96

Bhandari B (1977) Isoniazid hepatotoxicity – report of two cases. Indian Pediatr 14:859

Birkett DA, Garretts M, Stevenson CJ (1969) Phototoxic bullous eruptions due to nalidixic acid. Br J Dermatol 81:342

Bjarnason I, Bjornsson S (1981) Oesophageal ulcers. An adverse reaction to co-trimoxazole. Acta Med Scand 209:431

Black M, Mitchell JR, Hyman PhD, Ishak KG, Eple GR (1975) Isoniazid-associated hepatitis in 114 patients. Gastroenterology 69:289

Böttiger IE, Westerholm B (1973) Acquired haemolytic anaemia. Acta Med Scand 193:227

Böttiger LE, Strandberg I, Westerholm B (1975) Drug-induced febrile mucocutaneous syndrome. Acta Med Scand 198:229

Boice J, Fraumeni JF (1980) Late effects following isoniazid therapy. Am J Public Health 70:987

Boisvert A, Barbeau G (1981) Nalidixic acid-induced photodermatitis after minimal sun exposure. Drug Intell Clin Pharmacol 15:126

Bomb BS, Purohit SD, Bedi HK (1976) Stevens-Johnson syndrome caused by isoniazid. Tubercle 57:229

Bone RC, Wolfe J, Sobonya RE, Kerby GR, Stechschulte D, Ruth WE, Welch M (1976) Desquamative interstitial pneumonia following long-term nitrofurantoin therapy. Am J Med 60:697

Borgstein A, Tozer RA (1974) Infectious mononuculceosis and megaloblastic anaemia associated with daraprim and bactrim. Cent Afr J Med 20:185

Bradley PP, Warden G, Maxwell JG, Rothstein G (1980) Neutropenia and thrombocytopenia in renal allograft recipients treated with trimethoprim-sulfametoxazole. Ann Intern Med 93:560

Brandt L, Svensson B (1973) Stimulation of macrophage phagocytosis by clofazimine. Scand J Haematol 10:261

Brauner GJ (1975) Bullous photoreaction to nalidixic acid. Am J Med 58

Braun-Falco O, Luderschmidt Ch,, Maciejewski W, Scherer R (1978) Pustulosis acuta generalisata. Hautarzt 29:371

Brehm G, Korting GW (1970) Bullöse Hautreaktion auf Nalidixinsäure. Med Weld 11:423

Brøckner J, Boisen E (1978) Fatal multisystem toxicity after Co-trimoxazole. Lancet I:831

Brown A (1976) Risks of isoniazid therapy. Ann Intern Med 85:828

Browne SG, Harman DJ, Waudby H, McDougall AC (1981) Clofazimine (Lamprene, B 663) in the treatment of lepromatous leprosy in the United Kingdom. Int J Lepr 49:167

Bruno MS, Ober WB (1968) Acute fulminant hepatic failure with bilateral tuberculous cavitation. NY State J Med 68:2934

Burry JN (1974) Persistent phototoxicity due to nalidixic acid. Arch Dermatol 109:263

Byrd RB, Horn BR, Solomon DA, Griggs GA (1979) Toxic effects of isoniazid in tuberculosis chemoprophylaxis. Role of biochemical monitoring in 1,000 patients. JAMA 241:1239

Cameron A, Thomas M (1977) Pseudomembranous colitis and co-trimoxazole. Br Med JJ I:1321

Chan CK, Jarrett F, Moylan JA (1976) Acute leukopenia as an allergic reaction to silver sulfadiazine in burn patients. J Trauma 16:395

Chan M, Beale D, Moorhead J (1980) Acute megaloblastosis due to cotrimoxazole. Br J Clin Pract 34:187

Chanu B, Kernbaum S, Uzzan B, Faille A, Blasetti A, Rouffy J (1981) Aplasie médullaire au sulfaméthoxazole-triméthoprime. Démonstration d'un mécanisme allergique. Nouv Presse Med 10:3496

Chrisholm J, Hepner M (1981) Nitrofurantoin induced erythema nodosum. J Natl Med Assoc 73:59

Claas FHJ, van der Meer JW, Langerak J (1979) Immunological effect of co-trimoxazole on platelets. Br Med J 13::898

Clark AJL, Mouchizadeh J, Faunch R, McMichael HB (1980) Trimethoprim alone. Lancet I:1030

Cline JM (1970) Drug potentiation of macrophage function. Infect Immun II:601

Colucci CF, Lo Cicero M (1975) Hepatic necrosis and trimethoprim-sulfamethoxazole. JAMA 233:952

Coto H, McGowan W, Pierce E, Thomas E (1981) Intrahepatic cholestasis due to trimethoprim-sulfamethoxazole. South Med J 74:897

Cox J, de Moerloose J, Humbert J, Paunier L (1973) Fatal necrotizing angiitis after sulfadimethoxine therapy presenting as anaphylactoid purpura. Virchows Arch [Pathol Anat] 359:97

Cronin E (1978) Kutane Reaktionen auf Kontaktallergene. Z Hautkr 53:362

Dash LA, Comstock GW, Flynn J-PG (1980) Isoniazid preventive therapy. Retrospect and prospect. Am Rev. Respir Dis 121:1039

Dasta J, Prior J, Kurzrok St (1979) Isoniazid-induced fever. Chest 75:196

David RB, Andersen HA, Stickler GB (1968) Nitrofurantoin sensitivity – report of a child with cronic inflammatory lung disease. Am J Dis Child 116:418

Davis RS, Stoler BS (1977) Febrile reactions to INH. N Engl J Med 297::337

Delaney RA, Miller DA, Gerbino PP (1977) Adverse effects resulting from nitrofurantoin administration. Am J Pharmacol 149, 26 (1977)

Dengler HJ, Eichelbaum M (1977) Polymorphismen und Defekte des Arzneimittelstoffwechsels als Ursache toxischer Reaktionen. Arzneim Forsch 27:1836

Deonna T, Guignard JP (1974) Acute intracranial hypertension after nalidixic acid administration. Arch Dis Child 49:743

Desikan KV, Ramanujam K, Ramu G, Balakrishnan S (1975) Autopsy findings in a case of lepromatous leprosy treated with clofazimine. Lepr Rev 46:117

Djawari D (1978) Zur Problematik des medikamentös-induzierten Lupus erythematodes. Z Hautkr 53:180

Dold U, Reichenmiller HE (1969) Akute Leberzellschädigung beim Menschen durch gleichzeitige Gabe von Isonikotinsäurehydrazid und Antiepileptika (Diphenylhydantoin oder Carbamazepin). Med Welt 1:48

Donlan CJ, Scutero JV (1975) Transient eosinophilic pneumonia secondary to use of a vaginal cream. Chest 67:232

Dove JT, Chaparas SD, Hedrick SR (1972) Failure to demonstrate transformation of lymphocytes of patients with isoniazid-associated hepatitis. Am Rev Respir Dis 106:485

Dry J, Leynadier F, Herman D, Pradalier A (1975) L'association sulfaméthoxazole-triméthoprine (cotrimoxazole). Nouv Presse Med 4:36

Dubey GK, Joglekar VK, Hardas UD, Chaubey BS (1981) A study of cell mediated immunity in leprosy. Lepr India 53:197

Eggers B, Strothmann G (1974) Febriles Exanthem nach Nitrofurantoin-Einnahme. Z Hautkr 49:704

Ellard GA, Gammon PT (1976) Pharmacokinetics of isoniazid metabolism in man. J Pharm Biopharm 4:83

Ellard G, Mitchison D, Girling D, Nunn A, Fox W (1978) The hepatic toxicity of isoniazid among rapid and slow acetylators of the drug. Am Rev Respir Dis 118:628

Ellard GA, Girling DJ, Nunn AJ (1981) The hepatotoxicity of isoniazid among the three acetylator phenotypes. Am Rev Respir Dis 123:568

Ellman L, Miller L, Rappeport J (1974) Leukopheresis therapy of a hypereosinophilic disorder. JAMA 230:1004

Engel JJ, Vogt TR, Wilson DE (1975) Cholestatic hepatitis after administration of furan derivatives. Arch Int Med 135:733

Epstein JH (1972) Photoallergy. Arch Dermatol 106:741

Espiritu CR, Kim TS, Levine RA (1967) Sulfadimethoxine hypersensitivity. JAMA 202:985

Evans DIK, Tell R (1969) Agranulocytosis after trimethoprim and sulphamethoxazole. Br Med J I:578

Farer LS (1976) Isoniazid and liver injury. Ann Intern Med 84:753

Feinmann L (1975) Lung parenchymal changes due to ingested substances. Drug-induced lung disease: pulmonary eosinophilia and sulphonamides. Proc R Soc Med 68:440

Fellner MJ (1970) Nebenwirkungen durch Isonicotinsäurehydrazid. Hautarzt 21:320

Flach A (1981) Photosensitivity to sulfisoxazole ointment. Arch Ophthalmol 99:609

Fleck R (1981) Nitrofurantoin toxicity. Pa Med 84:36

Fraser AG, Harrower ADB (1977) Convulsions and hyperglycaemia associated with nalidixic acid. Br Med J II:1518

Fraser GL, Beaulieu JT (1979) Leukopenia secondary to sulfadiazine silver. JAMA 241:1928

Freedman J, Linn F (1978) An immunohematologic complication of isoniazid. Vox Sang (Toronto) 35:126

Frey H, Gershon A, Borkowsky W, Bullock W (1981) Fatal Reaction to dapsone during treatment of leprosy. Ann Intern Med 94:777

Friess G, Hirschfeld E (1977) Allergische Vaskulitis mit Arthritis durch Bactrim-Allergie. MMW 119:959

Frisch J (1973) Clinical experience with adverse reactions to trimethoprim-sulfamethoxazole. J Infect Dis [Suppl] 128:607

Garibaldi R, Drusin R, Ferebee S, Gregg M (1972) Isoniazid-associated hepatitis. Am Rev Respir Dis 106:357

Geller M, Dickie HA, Kass DA, Hafez GR, Gillespi JJ (1976) The histopathology of acute nitrofurantoin-associated pneumonitis. Ann Allergy 37:275

Gemperli R (1969) Beitrag zur isoniazid-induzierten fibrosierenden Arthropathie (Algodystrophie). Schw Med Wochenschr 99:1762

Girdwood RH (1976) The nature of possible adverse reactions to co-trimoxazole. Scand J Infect Dis [Suppl] 10

Glueck MA, Janower ML (1969) Nitrofurantoin lung disease clues to pathogenesis. Am J Roentgenol 107:818

Goldstein LI (1974) Hepatic injury associated with nitrofurantoin therapy. Am J Dig Dis 19:987

Goldstein RA, Janicki BW (1974) Immunologic studies in nitrofurantoin induced pulmonary disease. Med Ann Dist Columbia 43:115

Goll U, Rohwedder HJ (1971) Über das Vorkommen schwerer Nebenwirkungen bei jungen Kindern unter der Behandlung mit Nalidixinsäure. Monatsschr Kinderheilkd 119:442

Goodman Gilman A, Goodman LS, Gilman A (1980) The pharmacological basis of therapeutics. Macmillan, New York

Gopinathan KP, Saroja D (1973) Transduction of isoniazid susceptibility-resistance and streptomycin resistance in mycobacteria. Antimicrob Agents Chemother 4:643–645

Gopinathan KP (1973) Protein synthesis in mycobacterium tuberculosis H 37 Ru and the effect of streptomycin in streptomycin-susceptible and -resistant strains. Antimicrob Agents Chemother 4:205

Gottschalk H, Stone O (1976) Stevens-Johnson syndrome from ophthalmic sulfonamide. Arch Dermatol 112:513

Graham WGB, Dundas GR (1979) Isoniazid-related liver disease occurrence with portal hypertension, hypoalbuminemia and hypersplenism. JAMA 1242:353

Greenberg J, Usar MC, Lutcher CL (1972) Drug-induced systemic lupus erythematosus. JAMA 222:191

Grennan DM, Sturrock (1976) Polyarthritis, hepatitis and anti-native DNA antibodies after treatment with ethambutol and rifampicin. Tubercle 57:259

Grönhagen-Riska C, Hellström P, Fröseth B (1978) Predisposing factors in hepatitis induced by isoniazid-rifampicin treatment of tuberculosis. Am Rev Respir Dis 118:461

Groopman JE, Soloff L, Tessler S (1978) Hepatitis from isoniazid and rifampin. N Engl J Med 298:1316

Grouls V, Auer S, Steffel K, Bartsch WM (1970) Kasuistischer Beitrag zum sogenannten Nitrofurantoin-Fieber. Med Welt 15:701

Guerin JC, Chevalier JP, Kofmann J, Biot N, Bruinet JL, Kalb JC, Perrin-Fayolle M (1980) Pneumopathies interstitielles médicamenteuses après traitement par le cotrimoxazole. Deux observations. Nouv Presse Med 9:2347

Haber LC, Baer RL (1972) Pathogenic mechanisms of drug induced photosensitivity. J Invest Dermatol 58:327

Haber E, Osborne LRK (1959) Icterus and febrile reactions in response to isonicotinic acid hydrazine. Report of two cases and review of the literature. N Engl J Med 260:417

Haegi V (1975) Neuere Gesichtspunkte zur Tuberkulosetherapie. Schweiz Med Wochenschr 105:245

Hainer BL, White AA (1981) Nitrofurantoin pulmonary toxicity. J Fam Pract 13:817

Hamilton HE, Sheets RF (1978) Sulfisoxazole-induced thrombocytopenic purpura. Immunologic mechanism as cause. JAMA 239:2586

Han T, Prem L, Sokal JE (1969) Sulfapyridine-induced serum-sickness-like syndrome associated with plasmacytosis, lymphocytosis and multiclonal gamma-globulino pathy. N Engl J Med 280:547

Hatoff DE, Cohen M, Schweigert BF, Talbert WM (1979) Nitrofurantoin: another cause of drug-induced chronic active hepatitis? A report of a patient with HLA-B8 antigen. Am J Med 67:117

Haven E, Geerts J (1967) Photosensitivity caused by nolidixic acid (in Flemish). Arch Belg Dermatol Syph 23:421

Heijer A (1970) Pleuro-pulmonary allergic reaction to nitrofurantoin. Acta Allerg (Kbh) 25:63

Henning K (1974) Tetraplegie durch Nitrofurantoin-Medikation. Dtsch Med Wochenschr 99:1140

Herrmann W, Lischka G, Lückerath I (1969) Kontaktdermatitis and Arzneiexanthem bei beruflich erworbener Überempfindlichkeit gegen Isonikotinsäure-Hydrazid. Berufsdermatosen 17:13

Holmberg L, Boman G (1981) Pulmonary reactions to nitrofurantoin. Eur J Respir Dis 62:180

Holmberg L, Boman G, Böttcher L, Eriksson B, Spross R, Wessling A (1980) Adverse reactions to nitrofurantoin. Am J Med 69:733

Honeycutt WM, Huldin DH (1963) Reactions to isoniazid. Arch Dermatol 88:190

Horvátth I, Tengelyi W (1970) Anaphylaktische Knochenmarkkrise als Folge einer Isoniazid-Behandlung. Folia Haematol (Leipz) 93:419

Hyde L (1972) Hypersensitivity reaction and liver toxicity attributed to isoniazid. Am Rev Respir Dis 106:281

Inman WHW (1977) Fatal agranulocytosis attributed to co-trimoxazole therapy. Br Med J II:639

Ippen H (1978) Kontaktekzem durch Isonicotinsäurehydrazid. Derm Beruf Umwelt 26:57

Israel HL (1975) Isoniazid-associated hepatitis. Gastroenterology 69:539

Israel H, Diamond P (1962) Recurrent pulmonary infiltration and pleural effusion due to nitrofurantoin sensitivity. N Engl J Med 266:1024

Israel KS, Brashear RE, Sharma HM, Yum MN, Glove JL (1973) Pulmonary fibrosis and nitrofurantoin. Am Rev Respir Dis 108:353

Israel R, Gross R, Bomba P (1980) Adult respiratory distress syndrome associated with acute nitrofurantoin toxicity. Respiration 39:318

Iwarson S, Lundin P (1979) Multiple attacks of jaundice associated with repeated sulfonamid treatment. Acta Med Scand 206:219

Jacobs NF, Sumner E, Thompson MD (1977) Spiking fever from isoniazid simulating a septic process. JAMA 238:1759

Jameson S (1969) Allergic pulmonary complications during treatment with nitrofurantoin. Scand J Urol Nephrol 3:50

Johnson FO, Korst DR (1961) Pancytopenia associated with sulfamethoxypyridazine administration. JAMA 175:967

Jopling WH (1976) Complications of treatment with clofazimine (Lamprene: B 663). Lepr Rev 47:1

Kaiser H (1976) Medikamentös ausgelöste Algodystrophien. Verh Dtsch Ges Rheumatol 4:358

Kester NM, Haven S (1971) Isoniazid hepatotoxicity fact of fantasy. JAMA 217:699

Kikuchi S, Okazaki T (1978) Stevens-Johnson syndrome due to co-trimoxazole. Lancet II:580

Kingham JGC, Swain P, Swarbrick ET, Walker JG, Dawson AM (1979) Dapsone and severe hypoalbuminemia: a report of two cases. Lancet 2:662

Kleint V, van Baehr R (1970) Arzneimittelfieber nach Nifurantin. Z Gesamte Inn Med 25:194

Klemola H, Penttilä O, Runeberg L, Tallqvist G (1975) Anicteric liver damage during nitrofurantoin medication. Scand J Gastroenterol 10:501

Klinghöffer J (1954) Löfflers syndrome following use of a vaginal cream. Ann Intern Med 40:343

Kobrinsky N, Ramsay N (1981) Acute megaloblastic anemia induced by high-dose trimethoprim-sulfamethoxazole. Ann Intern Med 94:780

Koch-Weser J, Sidel VW, Dexter M, Parish C, Finer DC, Kanarek P (1971) Adverse reactions to sulfisoxazole, sulfamethoxazole, and nitrofurantoin. Arch Intern Med 128:399

Konno K, Oizumi K, Shimizu Y, Hayshi I (1968) Sensitivity test and side effects of ethambutol. Sci Rep Res Inst Tohoku Univ [Med] 15:51

Kopanoff D, Snider D, Caras G (1978) Isoniazid-related hepatitis. Am Rev Respir Dis 117:991

Korting GW (1980) Dermatologie in Praxis und Klinik für die fachärztliche Weiterbildung. Thieme, Stuttgart

Kuokkanen K (1972) A series of 464 cases in the Department of Dermatology, University of Turku, Finland, during 1966–1970. Acta Allergol (Kbh) 27:407

Kutt H, Brennan R, Dehejia H, Verebely K (1970) Diphenylhydantoin intoxication. A complication of isoniazid therapy. Am Rev Respir Dis 101:377

Labayle D, Lenoir C, Buffet C, Chaput JC, Etienne P (1979) Aktive H. durch Medikamente nach Oxyphenisatin α-Methyldopa und Isoniazid. Nouv Presse Med 8:2013

Languillon J (1980) Conception actuelles du traitement de la maladie de Hansen. Acta Leprol (Geneve) p 49

Lasson U (1977) Agranulozytose in Zusammenhang mit Cotrimoxazol bei einem siebenjährigen Kind. DMW 102:1287

Laubenthal F (1969) Nitrofurantoin-Fieber. DMW 94:2523

Laubstein H, Niedergesäss G (1970) Untersuchungen über Gruppensensibilisierungen bei Nitrofuranderivaten. Dermatol Monatsschr 156:1

Lawson DH, Henry DA (1977) Fatal agranulocytosis attributed to co-trimoxazole therapy. Br Med J II:316

Lawson DH, Hick H (1978) Adverse reactions to co-trimoxazole in hospitalized medical patients. Am J Med Sci 275:53

Le Blanc C, Bricard H, Levrot A, Leroy G, Trovero C, Quesnel J (1981) Pancytopénie au triméthoprime-sulfaméthoxazole. Anesth Anal (Paris) 38:281

Le Guillou M, L'Henaff F, Boisseau M, Castaing Y, Bourdalle-Badie Ch (1981) Insuffisance hépatique aigue réversible après traitement par l' association isoniazide-rifampicine. Sem Hop Paris 57:1199

Leiber B (1972) Nitrofurantoin-Syndrom. Monatsschr Kinderheilkd 120:398

Lejone J, Gusmini D, Brochard P (1979) Isoniazid and reaction to cheese. Ann Intern Med 91:793

Lejone JL, Schaeffer A, Brochard P, Portos JL (1980) Hypertension artérielle paroxystique provoquée sous isoniazide par l'ingestion de gruyère: deux cas. Ann Med Interne (Paris) 131:346

Leniger B, Sulzbeck H (1981) Pulmonales Nitrofurantoin-Syndrom. Fortschr Med 23:1092

Lequesne M (1967) L'algo-dystrophie d'origine chimiothérapique. Pseudo-rhumatisme de l'isoniazide, de l'éthionamide, du phénobarbital et de l'iode radioactif. Sem Hop Paris 43:2581

Linna O, Uhari M (1980) Hepatotoxicity of rifampicin and isoniacid in children treated for tuberculosis. Eur J Pediatr 134:227

Louis P, Wiskemann A, Schulz KH (1973) Bullöse Photodermatitis durch Nalidixinsäure. Hautarzt 24:445

Lübbers P (1969) Nitrofurantoin-Fieber. DMW 94:1922

Lundgren R, Bäck O, Wiman LG (1975) Pulmonary lesions and autoimmune reactions after long-term nitrofurantoin treatment. Scand Respir Dis 56:208

Lynn KL, Little PJ (1976) Reaction to trimoxazole. NZ Med J 377:78

Mackie BS, Mackie LE (1979) Systemic lupus erythematosus-dermatomyositis induced by sulphacetamide eye drops. Aust J Dermatol 20:49

Maddrey W, Boitnott J (1977) Drug-induced chronic liver disease. Gastroenterology 72:1348

Mandal BK, Stevenson J (1970) Haemolytic crisis produced by nalidixic acid. Lancet I:614

Mason GH, Ellis-Pegler RB, Arthur JF (1977) Clofazimine and eosinophilic enteritis. Lepr Rev 48:175

Mathews KP, Pan PM, Wells JH (1971) Experience with lymphocyte transformation tests in the evaluation of allergy to aminosalicylic acid, isoniazid, and streptomycin. Allergy 47:105

Mattelaer JJ (1972) Nitrofurantoin-Fieber. Acta Urol Belg 40:667

McDougall AC, Horsfall WR, Hede JE, Chaplin AJ (1980) Splenic infarction and tissue accumulation of crystals associated with the use of clofazimine (Lamprene; B 663) in the treatment of pyoderma gangrenosum. Br J Dermatol 102:227

McQueen CA (1978) Human lymphocyte N. acetyltransferase and the isoniazid acetylation polymorphism. Dissertation Abstr. Intern B 39, 6, 2659

Müller U, Hoignè R (1971) Lunge und Nitrofurantoin. Dtsch Med Wochenschr 96:955

Müller U, Abbühl K, Bisig J, Baumgartner H, Mühlberger F, Scherrer M, Hoigné R (1970) Überempfindlichkeitsreaktionen der Lungen auf Nitrofurantoin. Helv Med Acta [Suppl] 50:131

Müller U, Abbühl K, Bisig J, Baumgartner H, Mühlberger F, Scherrer M, Hoignè R (1970) Überempfindlichkeitsreaktionen der Lunge auf Nitrofurantoin. Schweiz Med Wochenschr 100:2206

Müller W (1974) Pulmonary reactions to furantoin. Radiol Clin Bio 43:540

Murray HW, Mann JJ (1975) Goalpost fever. Ann Intern Med 83:84

Musch E, Eichelbaum M, Weny I, von Sussen W, Ochs H, Castro-Parra M, Denyler HJ (1982) Hepatotoxizität der tuberkulostatischen Kombination INH + RMP + EMB in Beziehung zum Arzneistoffwechsel der Leber. Med Welt 33:911

Myles RK (1980) Isoniazid hepatotoxicity and acetylation during tuberculosis chemoprophylaxis. Am Rev Respir Dis 122:505

Nair SS, Kaplan JM, Levine LH, Geraci K (1980) Trimethoprim-sulfamethoxazole-induced intrahepatic cholestasis. Ann Intern Med 92:511

Nair V, Le Brun M, Kass I (1980) Peripheral neuropathy associated with ethambutol. Chest 77:98

Ngan H, Millard RJ, Lant AF, Trapnell DH (1971) Nitrofurantoin lung. Br J Radiol 44:21

Nolet HA (1981) Hepatitis caused by Nitrofurantoine often ignored. Ned. Tydschr Geneesk 125:59

Ockner RK (1979) Drug-induced liver disease. West J Med 131:36

Öhman L, Wahlberg I (1975) Ocular side-effects of clofazimine. Lancet II:933

Ogilvie AL, Toghill PJ (1980) Cholestatic jaundice due to co-trimoxazole. Postgrad Med J 56:202

von Oldershausen HF (1976) Hepatitis-ähnliche Leberveränderungen durch Infektionen, Intoxikationen und Arzneimittel. Verh Dtsch Ges Inn Med 82:106

von Oldershausen H, Musch E, Rudolf G, Gieraths A, Schunter C (1978) Zur Pharmakokinetik und klinischen Bedeutung der Interaktionen von Rifampicin mit Phenprocoumon und Isoniazid. Verh Dtsch Ges Inn Med 84:1468

Palva IP, Lehmola U (1973) Agranulocytosis caused by nitrofurantoin. Acta Med Scand 194:575

Pasricha J (1979) Drugs causing fixed eruptions. Br J Dermatol 100:183

Pasricha JS, Amrinder Ph, Kanwar J (1977) Skin eruption caused by ethambutol. Arch Dermatol 113:1122

Pau H, Wahl M (1974) Myambutol-Schädigung des Auges. Ber Dtsch Ophthalmol Ges 72:176

Paumgartner G, Paumgartner D (1980) Schäden an Leber und Gallenwegen durch medikamentöse Langzeittherapie. MMW 122:1223

Pauw FH (1979) Effects of oral isoniazid on human lymphocytes. Kidney Int 16:90

Pearsall HR, Ewalt J, Tsoi MS, Sumida S, Backus D, Winterbauer RH, Webb DR, Hones H (1974) Nitrofurantoin lung sensitivity: report of a case with prolonged nitrofurantoin lymphocyte sensitivity and interaction of nitrofurantoin-stimulated lymphocytes with alveolar cells. J Lab Clin Med 83:728

Pennington C (1980) Trimethoprim-sulfamethoxazole. N Engl J Med 303:1533

Periman Ph, Venkataramani TK (1975) Acute arthritis induced by isoniazid. Ann Intern Med 83:667

Pessayre D, Bentata M, Degott C, Nouel O, Miguet JP, Rueff B, Benhamou JP (1977) Isoniazid-Rifampin fulminant hepatitis. A possible consequence of the enhancement of isoniazid hepatotoxicity by enzyme induction. Gastroenterology 72:284

Pettit JH (1978) Clofazimine pigmentation. Int J Lepr 46:227

Ponte CD (1982) A suspected case of nitrofurantoin pneumonitis. Drug Intell Clin Pharm 16:63

Porter DI, Comaish S (969) Fixed drug eruption: an autoradiographic study of exchange grafts. Br J Dermatol 81:171

Radenbach K (1973) Zum gegenwärtigen Stand der antituberkulösen Chemotherapie. Internist 14:100

Ramsay CA (1973) Photosensitivity from nalidixic acid (abridged). Proc R Soc Med 6:747

Ramsay C, Obreshkova E (1974) Photosensitivity from nalidixic acid. Br J Dermatol 91:523

Ransohoff D (1981) Terminal Hepatic failure following a small dose of sulfamethoxazole-trimethoprim. Gastroenterology 80:816

Ransohoff DF, Jacobs G (1981) Terminal Hepatic Failure Following a Small Dose of Sulfamethoxazole-Trimethoprim. Gastroenterology 80:816

Rao KG (1974) Pseudotumor cerebri associated with nalidixic acid. Urology 4:204

Rea TH, Levan NE (1975) Erythema nodosum leprosum in a general hospital. Arch Dermatol 3:1575

Reidenberg KG, Caccese (1975) Lymphocyte transformation tests and suspected drug allergy. J Lab Clin Med 86:204

Richmond J, Whitworth JA, Fairley KF, Kincaid-Smith P (1979) Co-trimoxazole nephrotoxicity. Lancet I:493

Riechers F (1972) Arzneimittelunverträglichkeit nach Sulfamethoxypyridazin (Depovernil) im Sinne eines Lyell-Syndroms. Z Aerztl Fortbild (Jena) 66:552

Riska N (1976) L'hepatite chez les sujets des groupes traites par L'isoniazide et chez ceux d'un groupe temoin. Bull Int Union Tuberc 51:203

Robinson MF, Campbell GR, Craswell PW (1977) Co-Trimoxazole in chronic renal failure – a controlled experiment in Wistar rats. Clin Toxicol 10:411

Rosin MA, King LE (1982) Isoniazid-induced exfoliative dermatitis. South Med J 75:81

Rothfield N, Bierer W, Garfield J (1978) Isoniazid induction of antinuclear antibodies. Ann Intern Med 88:650

Rubinstein A (1979) LE like disease caused by nalidixin acid. N Engl J Med 301:1288

Russell A, Lessof M (1971) Hypersensitivity to drugs. Clin Allergy 1:179

Salter A (1973) The toxicity profile of trimethoprim-sulfamethoxazole after four years of widerspread use. Med J Aust [Spec Suppl] I:70

Saslaw S, Klainer AS (1969) Rheumatoid syndrome during isoniazid therapy. Am Rev Respir Dis 100:221

Scheuer PJ, Lal L, Summerfield JA, Sherlock S (1974) Rifampicin hepatitis. A clinical and histological study. Lancet I:421

Schulz V, Theisen H (1971) Allergische Reaktionen nach Therapie mit dem Tuberkulostatikum Myambutol. Med Welt 3:114

Seidell M (1970) Isoniazid induced life threatening neurologic reaction in an allergic individual. Ann Allergy 28:276

Selroos O, Edgren J (1975) Lupus-like syndrome associated with pulmonary reaction to nitrofurantoin. Acta Med Scand 197:125

Shah V, Joshi M (1980) Alleviation of isoniazid (INH) induced malformations in chick embryos by amino acids. Indian J Exp Biol 18:1097

Sharma GS, Gupta PK, Jain NK, Shanker A, Nanawati V (1979) Toxic psychosis to isoniazid and ethionamide in a patient with pulmonary tuberculosis. Tubercle 60:171

Sharp JR, Ishak KG, Zimmermann HJ (1980) Chronic active hepatitis and severe hepatic necrosis associated with nitrofurantoin. Ann Intern Med 92:14

Shaw D, Jacobs R (1970) Simultaneous occurrence of toxic hepatitis and Stevens-Johnson syndrome following therapy with sulfisoxazole and sulfamethoxazole. Johns Hopkins Med J 126:130

Sheehan J (1981) Trimethoprim-associated marrow toxicity. Lancet 2:692

Silverman HM (1981) Potential effects of medications at work III. Occup Health Saf 50:26

Simon P, Chermat R (1977) Isomnie imputable á l'acide oxolinique. Nouv Presse Med 6:3754

Smith D (1979) INH therapy: benefits versus risks. Neurology 29:1437

Smith E, Light J, Filo R, Yum MN (1980) Interstitial nephritis caused by trimethoprim-sulfamethoxazole in renal transplant recipients. JAMA 244:360

Smith H, Tyrrell WF, Gow A, Allan GW, Lees AW (1972) Hepatotoxicity in rifampin-isoniazid treated patients related to their rate of isoniazid inactivation. Chest 61:587

Smith K, Durack D (1978) Isoniazid and reaction to cheese. Ann Intern Med 88:520

Snodgrass W, Potter WZ, Timbrell J, Jollow DJ, Mitchell JR (1974) Possible mechanism of isoniazid-related hepatic injury. Clin Res 22:323

Spielberg S, Gordon G (1981) Nitrofurantoin cytotoxicity. J Clin Invest 67:37

Steinbrecher U, Mishkin S (1981) Sulfamethoxazole-induced hepatic injury. Dig Dis Sci 26/8:756

Stimmesse B, Daoudal P, Boillot A, Bald P, Rozenbaum A, Barale F (1979) Pancytopénie mortelle survenue au cours d'un traitement par sulfaméthoxazole-triméthoprime. Anesth Analg (Paris) 36:565

Strandberg I, Wengle B, Fagrell B (1974) Chronic interstitial pneumonitis with fibrosis during long-term treatment with nitrofurantoin. Acta Med Scand 196:483

Strömberg A, Wengle B (1976) Chronic active hepatitis induced by nitrofurantoin. Br Med J II:174

Strohscheer H, Wegener HH (1977) Nitrofurantoin-induzierte granulomatöse Hepatitis. MMW 119:1535 Stuart JJ, Roberts HR (1976) Isoniazid and disseminated intravascular coagulation. Ann Intern Med 84:490

Sulzberger M, Kunof A, Baer R, Lowenberg C (1947) Sensitisation by topical application of sulfonamides. Allergy 18:92

Talbot M (1980) Fixed genital drug eruption. Practitioner 224:823

Teigelkötter P (1972) Chronische Lungenveränderungen nach Nitrofurantoin-Medikation. Fortschr Geb Röntgenstr Nuklearmed 117:526

Teppo AM, Haltia K, Wager O (1976) Immunoelectrophoretic tailing of albumin line due to albumin-IgG antibody complexes: a side effect of nitrofurantoin treatment. Scand J Immunol 5:249

Thirkettle JL, Gough KR, Read AE (1963) Agranulocytosis associated with sulphasalazine (salazopyrin) therapy. Lancet I:1395

Thomas P, Seaton A, Edwards J (1974) Respiratory disease due to sulphasalazine. Clin Allergy 4:41

Thomas P, Mozes M, Jonasson O (1979) Hepatic dysfunction during isoniazid chemoprophylaxis in renal allograft recipients. Arch Surg 114:597

Thompson JE (1969) The management of hypersensitivity reactions to antituberculosis drugs. Med J Aust 2:1058

Thompson JE (1978) How safe is isoniazid? Med J Aust I:165

Thorel JB, Daragon A, Machon N, Courtois H (1981) Thrombopénie aigue au cotrimoxazole rôle facilitant du phénobarbital. Sem Hop Paris 57:914

Thorpe JAC, Nysenbaum A (1978) Co-trimoxazole fatality. Lancet II:276

Tiliakos N, Morales AR, Tsoukalas S (1980) Isoniazid (INH) cystitis. Bol Asoc Med PR 72:527

Tizes R, Hayden ChH, Perrin P (1971) Screening for prevention of isoniazid-associated liver disease. JAMA 218:1703

Tönder M, Nordöy A Elgjo K (1974) Sulfonamide-induced chronic liver disease. Scand J Gastroenterol 9:93

Trautmann A, Opitz K (1973) Hämorhhagische Enteritis mit Perforationsgefahr nach Nalidixinsäure-Anwendung. DMW 98:2423

Trentini GP, Botticelli A, Barbolini G (1974) Testicular lesions in rats created for one year with ethambutol in low doses. Virchows Arch [Pathol Anat] 362:311

Tykal P, Wilms H (1972) Anaphylaktischer Schock nach oraler Gabe von Nitrofurantoin und Nachweis von Reaginen durch heterologen Intrakutan-Test (Prausnitz-Küstner). DMW 97:256

Uragoda CG (1980) Histamine poisoning in tuberculous patients after ingestion of tuna fish. Am Rev Respir Dis 12:157

Uragoda CG, Kottegoda SR (1977) Adverse reactions to isoniazid on ingestion of fish with a high histamine content. Tubercle 58:83

Uragoda CG, Lodha SC (1979) Histamine intoxication in a tuberculous patient after ingestion of cheese. Tubercle 60:59

Wählin A, Rosman N (1976) Skin manifestations with vasculitis due to co-trimoxazole. Lancet II:1415

Wagner A (1971) Chronische interstitielle Pneumonie mit Lungenfibrose durch Nitrofurantoin-Langzeittherapie. Med Klin 66:1808

Wålinder PE, Gip L, Stempa M (1976) Corneal changes in patients treated with clofazimine. Br J Ophthalmol 60:526

Wang I, Schmid GH (1974) Asthma bronchiale und epicutane Sensibilisierung durch berufsbedingten Kontakt mit Isonicotinsäurehydrazid. Z Hautkr 49:803

Warrington RJ, Olivier SL (1979) Lymphocyte-mediated cytotoxicity in isoniazid-associated hepatitis. Clin Exp Immunol 38:561

Warrington RJ, Tse KS, Gorski BA, Schwenk R, Sehon AH (1978) Evaluation of isoniazid-associated hepatitis by immunological tests. Clin Exp Immunol 32:97

Weil J (1976) Hépatotoxicité de l'Isoniazide. Med Chir Dig 5:349

Weise L, Renger F, Krebs A, Steinbrück P (1976) Über die Häufigkeit und Manifestationsform von Leberschädigungen unter INH-Therapie. Z Gesamte Inn Med 31:328

Wilcox JB (1981) Phenytoin intoxication and cotrimoxazole. NZ Med J 94:235

Wiontzek H (1970) Pulmonale Erscheinungen als Ausdruck einer Nitrofurantoin-Allergie. Prax Pneumol 24:20

Witte KW, West DP (1982) Immunology of adverse drug reactions. Pharmacotherapy 2:54

Wolf A (1981) Bullöse Hautveränderungen durch Nalidixinsäure (Nogram). Z Hautkr 56:109

Wright R (1980) Drug-induced chronic hepatitis. Springer Semin Immunophathol 3:331

Yawalkar SJ, Vischer W (1978) Lamprene (clofazimine) in leprosy. Basic Information Pharma Division Ciba-Geigy, Basel

CHAPTER 19

Antifungal, Anthelmintic, and Antiprotozoal Drugs

J. DEWDNEY

A. Introduction

Adverse reactions to drugs used in the treatment of infections caused by fungi, helminths, and protozoa have been well documented, but drug-specific allergic complications during therapy are relatively uncommon (DUKES 1975, 1977, 1978). An evaluation of clinical reactions to these drugs is not however, without interest as it illustrates many of the fundamental problems in the diagnosis of drug-induced allergy.

The unambiguous demonstration, in presumptive allergic reactions, of immunochemical specificity determined by drug-derived haptenic structures, is absent in the majority of cases, with the exception of some instances of contact allergic dermatitis induced by antifungal agents applied topically. In this chapter immunochemical specificity is discussed also in relation to the antibodies responsible for quinine-induced thrombocytopenia and levamisole-induced anti-leucocyte antibodies in agranulocytosis.

In a broader perspective, the relationship between the development of immunological disorders and immunostimulant therapy must also be debated with respect to levamisole and to a lesser extent, to the benzimidazole anthelmintics, although in normal anthelmintic therapy the immunologically based side effects of these drugs are not apparent.

The evaluation of drug-induced allergic reactions is complicated by difficulty in distinguishing clinical signs and symptoms arising from the consequences of antigen-antibody interactions, from allergomimetic reactions in which identical biological pathways may be activated. The anthelmintic drug, diethylcarbamazine provides an example. Reactions to this drug, overtly allergic in appearance, are more likely a consequence of host reactions to products liberated from killed microfilaria than to any drug-specific allergic mechanism.

Polypharmacy and combination products also make evaluation of drug-induced allergic reactions difficult, and this is illustrated in this chapter most appropriately by the antifungal drugs, where for effective therapy it is frequently necessary to prescribe one or more active drugs. Where these are formulated in combination products together with a variety of excipients, solvents and bases, as in topical antifungal agents, it is essential to consider the role played in any allergic reactions by these far from inert additives.

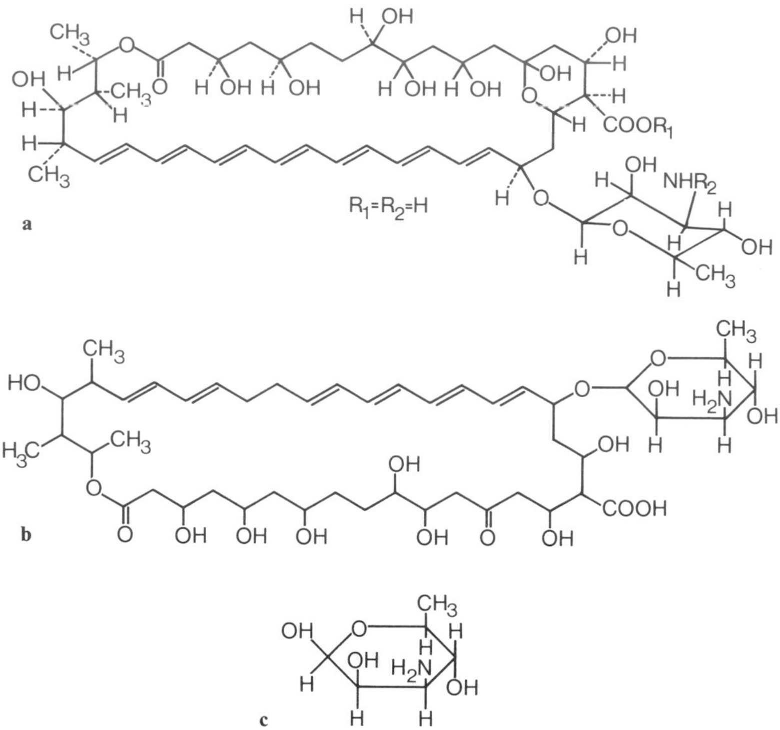

Fig. 1. Polyene antibiotics: **a** amphotericin B; **b** nystatin; **c** mycosamine

B. Antifungal Drugs

I. Systemic Agents

Although adverse reactions to systemically administered antifungal drugs are relatively common, allergic reactions are rare. The polyene antibiotics, amphotericin B and nystatin, each derived from a *Streptomyces* species, have found a valuable place in the treatment of systemic mycoses (Fig. 1). Generalised pruritic maculopapular rashes and eosinophilia have been reported during therapy with amphotericin B but these are infrequent (LORBER et al. 1976). In some cases, it has been shown that a single low dose of amphotericin B can provoke reappearance of rash and eosinophilia after a period of drug withdrawal. The ability to provoke a reaction with a low challenge dose in a patient who has previously experienced a drug reaction is regarded as one of the criteria for a diagnosis of allergic hypersensitivity to the drug. However, in the case of amphotericin B there may be some other explanation. This drug can give rise to a syndrome which may mimic a true allergic reaction (UTZ et al. 1964; MURRAY 1974; BENNETT 1974; KATZ and CASSILETH 1977). It comprises hyperthermia, hypotension and muscle rigors and it can result even from slow intravenous infusion of the drug. The syndrome has been provoked again in patients after a period off the drug and by very low doses. This is most likely a toxic reaction, possibly related to the ability of polyene antibiotics

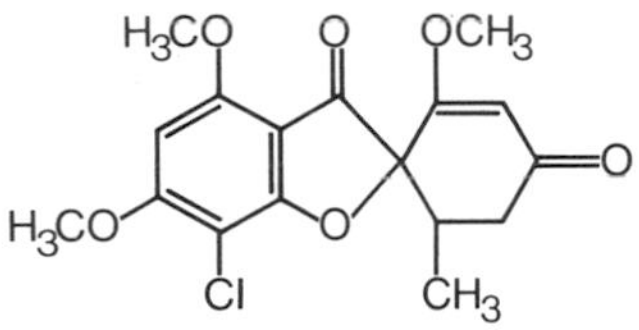

Fig. 2. Polycyclic antibiotics: griseofulvin

to bind, not only to ergosterol, the principal membrane sterol of fungi, but also to mammalian cell membranes (KINSKY 1970). The consequences of membrane perturbation could be responsible for the toxic effect of these drugs and also, as recently shown for amphotericin B methyl ester, for their adjuvant properties (LITTLE et al. 1978).

Other polyene antibiotics are in clinical use but no confirmed allergic reactions have been reported.

The polycyclic antibiotic, griseofulvin, is derived from *Penicillium griseofulvum* and is perhaps the most important agent in the systemic treatment of dermatophyte infections (Fig. 2). It is used orally for the treatment of superficial fungal infections of nails, hair, and skin, increasing the resistance of keratin to infection. Side effects of therapy are usually mild; most common are nausea, diarrhoea and headaches (SWARTZ 1962).

Adverse reactions of suspected allergic aetiology have been reported occasionally. O'DRISCOLL (1963) reported a near fatal reaction in a penicillin allergic patient involving dyspnoea and urticaria. It seems unlikely that cross allergenicity with penicillin-derived antigens explains this case as the range of allergenic determinants responsible for penicillin allergy does not normally include *Penicillium* mould protein derivatives. An equally severe reaction has been reported by STEAGALL (1963) in a patient with underlying chronic arthritis with signs of systemic lupus erythematosus who also had previously reacted to penicillin with joint pains, erythema and generalised weakness. Fever, chills and joint pains characterised the patient's reaction to griseofulvin during therapy and after a single 250 mg provocation dose. Some form of activation or exacerbation of autoimmune disease might explain this particular reaction more readily than hypersensitivity, Urticaria and other rashes have been recorded. PÖHLER and MICHALSKI (1972) described a severe urticarial rash in a patient on griseofulvin therapy. The lymphocyte tranformation test was positive with griseofulvin; 54% of cells in culture were judged to be blast forms compared with 11% in controls. Care should however be taken in interpreting this as evidence of the presence of drug-specific memory cells in view of the colchicine-like effect of griseofulvin, which might lead to difficulties in evaluating cell morphology in this test (PAGET and WALPOLE 1958). Others have reported rashes, mostly urticarial, vasculitis and serum-sickness-like reactions (MEINHOF 1965; WEINSTEIN 1970; GOTZ and REICHENBERGER 1972). In none is there firm evidence of an allergic aetiology.

CHANG (1965) reported a case of cold urticaria and photosensitisation to griseofulvin, in which an attempt was made to demonstrate the presence of griseofulvin-specific antibodies. Positive reactions were obtained using rabbit passive cutaneous anaphylaxis in which a latent period of 4 h was allowed to elapse be-

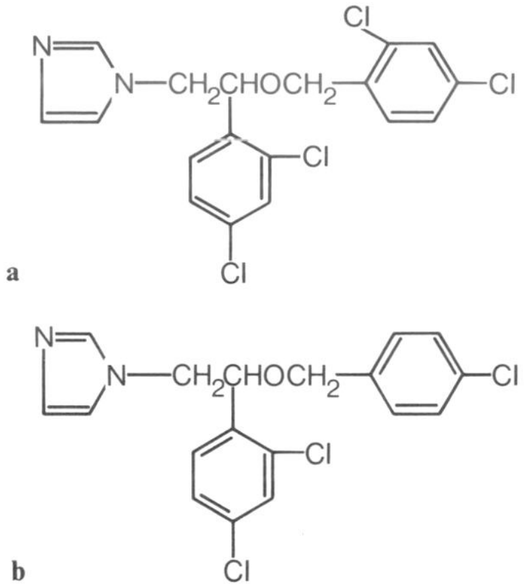

Fig. 3. Imidazole antifungal agents. **a** miconazole; **b** econazole

tween the intradermal injection of the patient's serum and intravenous challenge with 0.1% griseofulvin in a saturated alcoholic solution. Whereas sites injected with control serum failed to react, at those injected with the patient's serum, wheals rapidly developed. There appeared to be no significant difference between serum sites chilled by ice, and those at room temperature. It is extremely rare to be able to demonstrate drug-specific antibodies in this test, and confirmation is necessary before the result can be taken as firm evidence of the antigenicity of griseofulvin. SAVAGE (1977) reported a fixed drug eruption in a patient treated with griseofulvin. Provocation with a single dose caused reappearance of this reaction within 30 min. Overall, although clinical data indicates that griseofulvin might give rise rarely to allergic reactions, no convincing evidence is available and judgement should be withheld on its possible allergenicity.

Some rashes have been reported during therapy of systemic mycoses with 5-fluorocytosine but it is not thought that these are allergic in origin (DOEGLAS 1978)

The imidazoles have found a place in the treatment of fungal infections and are used both topically and systemically (Fig. 3). Rashes and pruritis have been reported following the systemic use of miconazole nitrate, 1-[2,4-dichloro-β-(2,4-dichlorobenzyloxy)phenethyl]imidazole nitrate (STEVENS et al. 1975; MARMION et al. 1976; FISCHER et al. 1977; WADE et al. 1977). Confirmation of an anaphylactic reaction by skin prick test was reported by STUCHLIK (1975); perhaps therefore miconazole is capable of stimulating an IgE antibody response but confirmation has yet to be obtained. Generalised skin rashes have been reported during oral therapy with the related drug, clotrimazole, diphenyl-(2-chlorophenyl)-1-imidazolyl methane, but these reactions are rare and are of unknown aetiology (HIRSH and DEDES 1974; CARTWRIGHT 1974).

II. Topical Agents

Antifungal drugs are frequently administered by topical application to control superficial infections of the skin. It is important to remember that products formu-

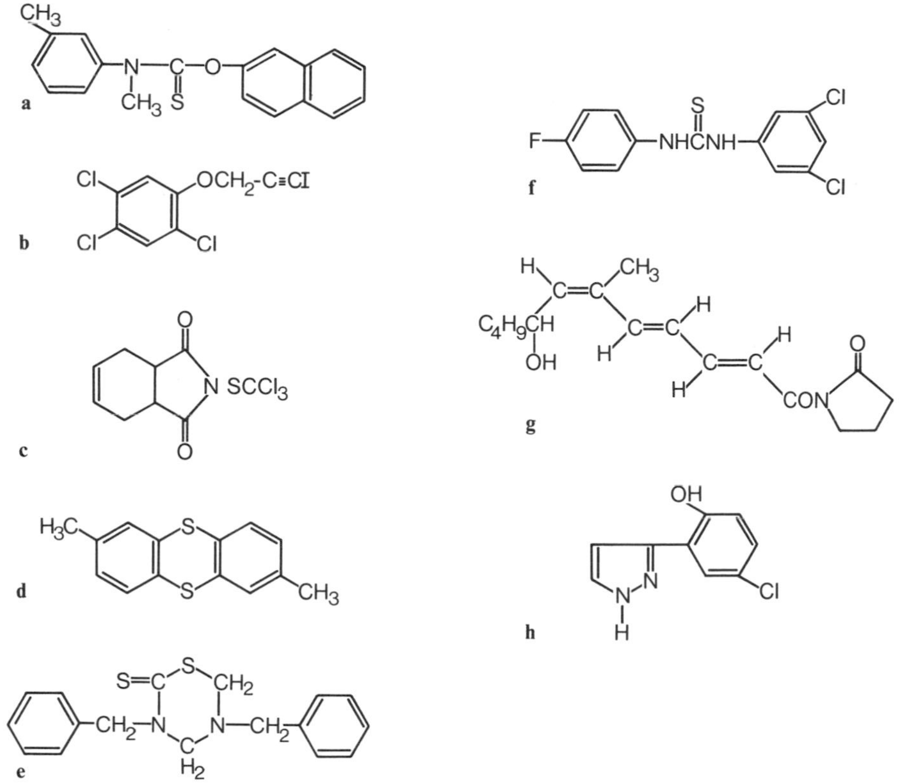

Fig. 4a–h. Topical antifungal agents: active moieties. **a** tolnaftate; **b** haloprogin; **c** chlordantoin; **d** mesulphen; **e** dibenzthione; **f** fluonilid; **g** pecilocin; **h** mycanodin

lated for this use may contain more than one active ingredient, together with excipients and other additives. Evaluation of the allergenic potential of antifungal drugs must therefore also include consideration of the sensitising capacity of these other substances.

Sensitisation to modern antifungal drugs is not a common experience. It has been reported, and confirmed by adequately controlled patch tests, to tolnaftate (GELLIN et al. 1972; EMMETT and MARRS 1973), to the polyene antibiotic, pecilocin (SUNDERARAJAN 1970; GROEN et al. 1973; NØRGAARD 1977), chlordantoin (EPSTEIN 1966), haloprogin (RUDOLPH 1975; STURDE 1975; HOLLANDER 1977) and to fluonilid (VAN HECKE 1969), but cases are sufficiently unusual for even individual case reports to be noted (Fig. 4).

Contact allergic reactions to the imidazoles are also rare. DEGREEF et al. (1975) report one such case during treatment with miconazole and both allergic exanthema and irritation have been reported during therapy with the closely related drug, econazole, 1-[2,4-dichloro-β-β-(4-chlorobenzyloxy)phenethyl]imidazole nitrate (HEMPEL 1975; PEIOS 1975; SCHERWITZ 1977). Clotrimazole, diphenyl-(2-chlorophenyl)-1-imidazolyl methane, has been extensively tested in volunteers and its allergenic potential is very low (WEUTA 1972; FREIS 1972; WAHLBERG 1974, 1976;

this appears to be borne out in clinical use where mild irritant reactions can occur on topical application, but only one case of sensitisation has been reported (HALL-SMITH 1974; THORNES 1977; ROLLER 1978).

In view of the relative ease with which low molecular weight chemical substances can sensitise human skin if applied frequently over a period of time, this low level of sensitisation must reflect the value of predictive testing of topical agents in volunteers and in patients by methods now well established (DRAIZE 1959; KLIGMAN 1966 a, b).

The older antifungal agent, phenylmercuric borate, used still in the control of athlete's foot, is a more common and more potent skin sensitiser. In a trial reported by BANDMANN (1966) more than 10% of patients developed contact allergic dermatitis, and cross-reactions with other mercury compounds can occur.

Amphotericin B and nystatin are also available as topical treatments for candidiasis, alone or in combination with steroids and other antibiotics. Allergic contact reactions have been described following application to skin or mucous membranes, of combination products containing nystatin (WASILEWSKI 1970, 1971; COSKEY 1971 a, b) but there is some difficulty in the identification of the major allergen or allergens. Mycolog cream is one such example. It is a combination of nystatin, neomycin sulphate, gramicidin and triamcinolone acetonide; ethylenediamine may also be present as a stabiliser. It thus contains several known skin sensitisers and the role of nystatin in this respect is difficult to assess. Neomycin is a recognised contact allergen (for review see DEWDNEY 1977), as also is ethylenediamine (PROVOST and JILLSON 1967; EPSTEIN and MAIBACH 1968; FISHER et al. 1971; WILKINSON 1972; WHITE et al. 1978). The data of FOUSSEREAU et al. (1971) in fact suggest that ethylenediamine may be the major allergen in Mycolog cream, as when formulated without it, Mycolog is a rare sensitiser, and this would be line with views of FISHER et al. (1971), who claim ethylenediamine to be one of the most common skin sensitisers. Triamcinolone cannot be regarded as totally blameless as allergic reactions have been recorded to it and to other corticosteroids (BURCKHARDT 1959; BANDMANN et al. 1966; TEGNER 1976), but it is more commmon for these agents to suppress contact allergic reactions to other components in a multidrug formulation (WASILEWSKI 1970; COSKEY 1971 a, b; FISHER et al. 1971).

The status of nystatin as a contact sensitiser is therefore not clear. Patch test procedures have shown that it can sensitise human skin. WASILEWSKI (1970, 1971) and COSKEY (1971 a, b) have recorded strong patch test reactions, maximal 96 h after application, to nystatin, and KANDIL (1969), in an analysis of a fixed drug eruption to a combination product containing nystatin, amphotericin B and tetracycline, found that nystatin not only gave positive patch tests but was also able to provoke a fixed drug eruption when used to challenge the patient. In consideration of the pattern of cross-sensitization in this patient, KANDIL (1969) suggests that a structure common to both amphotericin B and nystatin, the amino sugar, mycosamine (Fig. 1) could be a possible allergenic determinant, but this has not been shown experimentally.

Sensitisation to the topical antifungal agent, Mycanodin is difficult to quantitate. The active antifungal is 3-(2-hydroxy-5-chlorophenyl)pyrazole and this can cause contact allergic dermatitis and photoallergic reactions (Fig. 4; BURCKHARDT et al. 1968). The same authors showed, however, that an antihistamine co-formua Cl—⟨benzene, OH⟩—$CONHC_4H_9$

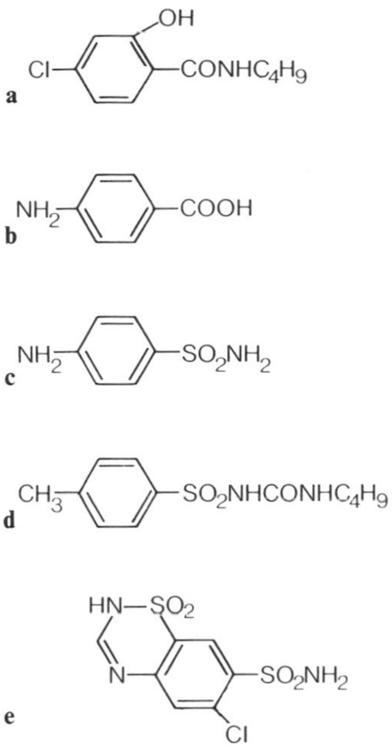

b NH_2—⟨benzene⟩—$COOH$

c NH_2—⟨benzene⟩—SO_2NH_2

d CH_3—⟨benzene⟩—$SO_2NHCONHC_4H_9$

e $HN—SO_2$ ... N—⟨benzene, Cl⟩—SO_2NH_2

Fig. 5a–e. Structures illustrating the cross-photoallergenicity of buclosamide. **a** buclosamide; **b** *p*-aminobenzoic acid; **c** sulphanilamide; **d** tolbutamide; **e** chlorothiazide

lated with the pyrazole in Mycanodin can also be responsible for sensitisation. Tineafax ointment, a popular combination product has several ingredients which have been implicated in allergic sensitisation; mesulphen (Fig. 4) appears to be responsible in several cases (VAN KETEL 1967; BURRY 1969).

The drug-metabolising properties of skin are considerable. It is reasonable therefore to expect that not only the parent compound, but also its metabolic product, or breakdown product might be responsible for sensitisation. An example seems to be provided by the thiadiazine antifungal and skin-care agent, dibenzthione. While there is evidence that dibenzthione itself can sensitise skin, it has been shown that a hydrolytic product of this compound, benzisothiocyanate, may also be responsible for some cases of sensitisation (BEHRBOHM and ZSCHUNKE 1965; WURBACH and SCHUBERT 1976).

Photoallergic dermatitis is a not uncommon complication of the use of an antifungal sulphonamide derivative, buclosamide (4-chloro-2-hydroxybenzoic acid *N*-*n*-butylamide (Fig. 5a; IPPEN 1961, FREGERT and MÖLLER 1964; JUNG and SCHWARZ 1964, 1965; JUNG et al. 1968; BURRY 1969, 1970; BURRY and HUNTER 1970; NURSE 1973). JUNG and SCHWARZ (1965) showed that patients sensitive to buclosamide gave photopatch test reactions to *p*-aminobenzoic acid, (Fig. 5b), to sulphanilamide and to some sulphonamide derivatives including the antidiabetic compounds related to tolbutamide (Fig. 5d)) and to the thiazide diuretics (Fig. 5e). BURRY (1970) and BURRY and HUNTER (1970) confirmed the cross-reactivity with *p*-aminobenzoic acid and the thiazides, but failed to show the same breadth of cross-sensitivity as shown by JUNG and SCHWARZ. It is possible that differences in

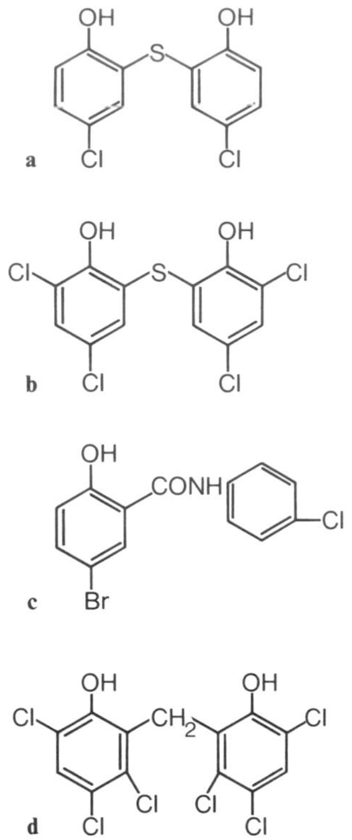

Fig. 6a–d. Antifungal agents associated with photosensitization. **a** fentichlor; **b** bithionol; **c** multifungin; **d** hexachlorophene

the light source, both in terms of wavelength and intensity, could be responsible for these differences. In a later study, these workers (JUNG et al. 1968) showed that in vitro irradiation of a complex of buclosamide and albumin provides an effective antigen for use in the lymphocyte transformation test; in ten patients who had experienced photoallergic reactions to buclosamide, lymphocyte transformation was recorded.

FREGERT and MÖLLER (1964) tested a number of close chemical analogues in buclosamide-sensitive patients. The results indicate that, in addition to the essential role of the benzoic acid amide group, the hydroxyl attached to C-2 of the aromatic ring, the pattern of halogen substitution and the length of the aliphatic chain are determining features in cross-reactivity. Of equal importance, this study underlines again the value of patch testing in cross-sensitization studies.

Some attention has been paid to the identification of a possible photodegradation product of buclosamide which could be responsible for sensitisation. BURCKHARDT et al. (1957) and BURCKHARDT and SUTTER (1963) point to a possible role of hydroxylaminobenzenesulphonamide, a photodegradation product of sulphanilamide, but it can only offer a partial explanation, and the chemical structure causing cross-reactions with thiazide derivatives is not known (BAER and HARBER 1961).

Photosensitisation has also been recorded in relation to the topical application of halogenated phenol antifungal agents (Fig. 6) bis(2-hydroxy-5-chlorophenyl) sulphide (Fenticlor, Fig. 6a) and 5-bromo-4'-chlorosalicylanilide (Multifungin, Fig. 6c; JILLSON and BAUGHMAN 1963; BURRY 1967).

These antifungal agents are structurally related to the germicidal agent hexachlorophene (Fig. 6d) and photodermatitis has been recorded, although rarely, for this agent also. They are also structurally related to bis(2-hydroxy-3,5-dichlorophenyl) sulphide, Bithionol (Fig. 6b), a potent sensitiser (WILKINSON 1961), and cross-sensitization between these agents has been found (BAUGHMAN 1964; BURRY 1967). It would seem therefore that these antifungal drugs should be used with care, particularly on exposed parts of the body and in countries where the level of sunlight is high.

It has been observed earlier, that additives can be responsible for allergic sensitisation (FISHER et al. 1971) and the case of ethylenediamine was used to illustrate the point. A further example, although it must be very rare in view of its widespread use in cosmetics and in food flavourings, is diethyl sebacate, a solubilising agent shown to be responsible for allergic sensitisation during the use of Halotex cream, the active ingredient of which is haloprogin (MOSS 1974; BERLIN and MILLER 1976).

In summary, allergic complications during antifungal therapy are not common. Recognition of contact allergic dermatitis and photoallergic dermatitis is important, not only because the resulting skin condition can confuse assessment of the clinical efficacy of a topically applied antifungal agent and lead to drug continuation when withdrawal might be the more appropriate course of action, but also because of the widespread use of certain chemicals contained in antifungal preparations in non-medicinal products.

C. Anthelmintic Drugs

Allergic reactions to anthelmintic drugs used in human and veterinary medicine are not common and only rarely cause difficulties in therapy.

I. Piperazines

The piperazine salts are widely used to treat ascaris and pinworm infections (Fig. 7), and although they have proved to be generally safe, some allergic problems have been noted. Urticaria has been reported (RACHELSON and FERGUSON 1955; HILL 1957; URELES 1958; BUTLER 1968). The latter report refers to a patient in whom a generalised erythematous, pruritic rash developed during an initial course of therapy. Provocation challenge with a single dose of piperazine given some time after the initial therapy had been discontinued caused a reappearance of rash and a shock syndrome developed. Piperazine-induced rashes have been reported and patch testing has been used with some success to implicate piperazines, although concentrations of piperazine in excess of 5% proved irritant on the skin and therefore inappropriate for use in these tests (FREGERT 1967; McCULLAGH 1968; CALNAN 1975; RUDZKI and GRZYWA 1977).

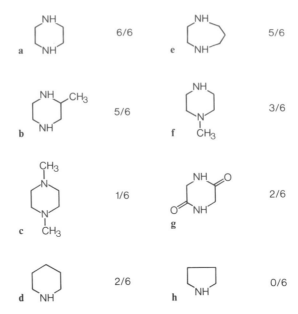

Fig. 7a–h. Cross-sensitization with piperazine derivatives in contact allergic dermatitis, expressed as the quotient: number of patients responding to patch test/number of patients tested. **a** piperazine; **b** homopiperazine; **c** 2-methylpiperazine; **d** N-methylpiperazine; **e** N,N-dimethylpiperazine; **f** dioxopiperazine; **g** piperidine; **h** pyrrolidine. (Foussereau and Benezra 1967)

Some information is available on possible antigenic determinants involved in contact dermatitis to piperazines. Foussereau and Benezra (1967) had the opportunity of evaluating six members of the nursing staff of a hospital who presented with allergic symptoms induced by a combination product of piperazine, theophylline and p-aminobenzoic acid. Patch tests performed with piperazine, homopiperazine, and 2-methylpiperazine were all positive. Modification of the ring amino group at either C-1 or C-4 of piperazine, or introduction of 2,5-dioxo into the ring resulted in a lower incidence of positive patch test. Thus, N-methylpiperazine, N,N'-dimethylpiperazine, dioxopiperazine and piperidine were significantly less antigenic, and pyrrolidine gave no reactions (Fig. 7).

The antigenic properties of piperazine were also confirmed in a study reported by McCullagh (1968) who investigated a syndrome of cough, dyspnoea and excess sputum production in men employed in a factory in Australia making a piperazine-based sheep drench. In an investigation of four of the workers, it was noted that the dyspnoea occurred some hours after exposure to piperazine, both under conditions of factory exposure and following deliberate provocation testing. Pepys et al. (1972) were able to evaluate two such patients. Provocation testing by exposure to a piperazine-lactose dust resulted in respiratory dysfunction as measured by a fall in FEV_1, the forced expiratory volume in litres over 1 s. A significant change in FEV_1 was recorded at 4 h and was maximal at 11 h when levels were only 50% of predicted values. Total IgE immunoglobulin was normal in these patients.

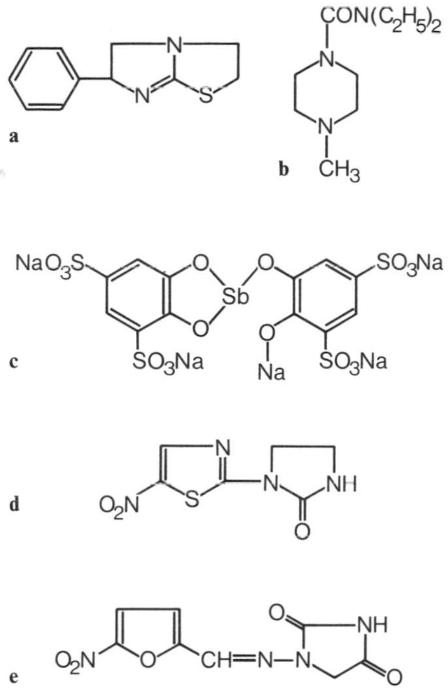

Fig. 8a–e. Anthelmintic drugs. **a** levamisole; **b** diethylcarbamazine; **c** stibophen; **d** niridazole; **e** nitrofurantoin

One patient reported by PEPYS et al. (1972) gave an immediate wheal and flare response to prick tests with piperazine, but that is the only reported evidence of an IgE-mediated response.

Piperazine salts seem therefore to be capable of forming antigenic determinants and thus taking part in immunologically mediated adverse reactions, at least under certain circumstances such as occupational exposure. Under conditions of normal anthelmintic therapy such problems are minimal.

II. Benzimidazole and Imidazothiazoles

The benzimidazole anthelmintics, for example thiabendazole, cambendazole, parbendazole and mebendazole, owe their value to their broad spectrum of activity against nematodes. Although rashes (BELCHER et al. 1975; BERTHOUD and BERTHOUD 1975) and a rare case of epidermal desquamation and bullous erythema multiforme (ROBINSON and SAMORODIN 1976) have been reported, there is no evidence that these were allergic in nature and it is possible that such adverse reactions as do occur could be a consequence of the immunostimulant properties of this series of drugs (LUNDY and LOVETT 1976; LOVETT and LUNDY 1977). Perhaps such properties also provide an explanation for some of the side effects of the imidazothiazole anthelmintic, levamisole (Fig. 8 a). It should be noted that, under normal dosage regimens used in anthelmintic therapy, neither tetramisole, nor its (−)-isomer, levamisole has been responsible for confirmed allergic side effects.

However, under different conditions of therapy, as for example high dose continuous or intermittent therapy of rheumatoid arthritis or malignant disease, in which conditions attempts are now being made to utilise the immunostimulant properties of levamisole and tetramisole (RAVE et al. 1978) serious adverse reactions have been recorded and some of these may prove to be allergic in origin. It is not appropriate to the aims of this chapter to document these fully but brief comment is justified. The most serious side effect seems to be agranulocytosis (for review see SYMOENS 1977), and in some investigations drug-dependent anti-leucocyte antibodies have been found during the acute phase (ROSENTHAL et al. 1976; GRABER et al. 1976; SKINNIDER and RIEDER 1977; PARKINSON et al. 1977; TEERENHOVI et al. 1978). However, the apparent demonstration of anti-leucocyte antibodies under the conditions of these tests, in which normal leucocytes are agglutinated in the presence of the patient's serum and the drug levamisole, must be interpreted with caution. HARTL (1973) has reviewed the general topic of drug-induced agranulocytosis and has analysed carefully the possible difficulties arising in interpretation of leucocyte agglutination tests; most important are false positive results due to iso- and auto-antibodies and paraproteins. He also notes that serological findings do not correlate with provocation testing, and that leucocyte agglutination and changes in complement components occur only during the acute phase of agranulocytosis.

The demonstration of leucocyte agglutination cannot therefore be taken as evidence of the ability of levamisole, or a metabolic product of it, to act as a hapten capable of conjugation to host macromolecules and able to stimulate drug-specific antibodies. Perhaps the view of EPSTEIN et al. (1977) that the immunostimulatory properties of levamisole are responsible for a boost in pre-existing anti-leucocyte antibodies in these patients provides a partial explanation.

On the other hand, there is other evidence that levamisole may be capable of acting as a hapten. TURK and PARKER (1979) have shown that levamisole is a potent, though capricious, sensitiser when given by the intradermal route to guinea-pigs. Sensitisation was associated with marked T-cell proliferation in draining lymph nodes. An allergic aetiology might therefore be considered to explain the rashes which develop on levamisole therapy. Some of these are frankly urticarial (TRABERT et al. 1976; for review see SYMOENS 1977) and the claim has been made that they may be associated with specific IgE production (THORNES 1977). Unfortunately, this conclusion was based on data obtained using the indirect rat mast cell technique, a difficult and unreliable test system. It was of interest that the activity observed in this system was coincident with restoration of T-lymphocyte activity in the patients. YUST et al. (1977) also claimed to have obtained positive results in the indirect rat mast cell degranulation test with serum from a patient who suffered a febrile reaction while being treated with levamisole; the authors implicated IgE antibody in this adverse reaction.

SECHER et al. (1978) report the appearance of the granular deposition of IgG and C3 at dermal-epidermal junctions in a patient who experienced a pruritic rash when being treated with levamisole; a provocation dose of levamisole resulted in further complex deposition. The authors comment on the possibility that these complexes were related more to the patient's underlying disease, rheumatoid arthritis, than to drug-specific complexes but on balance, they believe that they were in fact due to levamisole-specific antibodies. The view was strengthened by the finding that the patient's leucocytes, exposed in vitro to levamisole at doses above 0.1 µg/ml released 18%–36% of total histamine, and prick test reactions, albeit very weak ones, were obtained.

Although presumptive evidence is growing, the question of the true allergenicity and antigenicity of levamisole must remain unanswered pending more detailed investigations and it remains to be be established whether side effects similar to those reported here are ever seen in the use of this drug in anthelmintic therapy.

III. Diethylcarbamazine

The use of the anthelmintic drug, diethylcarbamazine (Fig. 8 b) in onchocerciasis has underlined a further type of adverse reaction which may mimic allergic effects but which is in all probability of different aetiology. Thus anaphylactoid reactions have been described in humans and animals treated with diethylcarbamazine. These reactions are thought to be due to toxic effects consequent upon the mobilisation and death of microfilaria, a mechanism described first by JARISCH and HERXHEIMER with respect to the release of antigens in syphilitic patients treated with mercury (SEAH 1974; ROUGEMONT et al. 1976; BRYCESON et al. 1977; KLOUSIA et al. 1977; ZYMET 1977).

Some support for this aetiology is given by observation that the incidence of side effects to diethylcarbamazine is related to the worm burden of the patient (CIFERRI and KESSEL 1967). These reactions can be very severe and represent a real therapeutic hazard, but it is not appropriate to consider them further here. It is worth noting, however, that diethylcarbamazine is not alone in causing this reaction. Other drugs used in the treatment on onchocerciasis, such as suramin, bithionol and fenthion may result in similar effects. Diethylcarbamazine is also a pharmacologically active drug which has some nicotine-like properties and mimics the effects of acetylcholine at autonomic ganglia (FORBES 1972). These properties have, in fact, been evaluated to establish any anti-allergy effects diethylcarbamazine might have, but nicotine-like effects could also result in a confusing overall pattern of adverse reactions to this drug.

A case of disseminated intravascular coagulation has been described following repeated therapy with the antischistosomal anthelmintic, Stibophen, a trivalent antimony compound, (Fig. 8 c) (WEISS et al. 1972) and an occasional haemolytic anaemia or thrombocytopenia (HARRIS 1956; KAHN and BROD 1961; DE TORREGROSA et al. 1963). In the former case, there was a weakly positive direct Coombs test and the patient's serum agglutinated both normal and the patient's red blood cells in the presence of Stibophen. In most instances, Stibophen-induced haemolytic anaemia appears to be associated with IgM antibody (VAN ARSDEL 1978).

Another anthelmintic used in the treatment of *Schistosoma* infections, niridazole (Fig. 8 d) is reported to cause pulmonary tissue eosinophilia and an increase in blood eosinophil counts (FARID et al. 1973). The structural relationship of this nitrothiazole to nitrofurantoin, (Fig. 8 e) another drug causing pulmonary eosinophilia, should be noted (ELMES 1975; ROSENOW 1976).

In summary, although allergic reactions are not a major problem in the treatment of helminth infections, and only the Herxheimer reaction caused by diethylcarbamazine is of clinical importance, anthelmintics can, under rather special circumstances, give rise to immunological problems. Piperazine salts are able to stimulate specific immune responses provided the challenge is sufficient, that is, under conditions of occupational exposure, and the imidazothiazole anthelmintics have a spectrum of activity relating to immunological function, which can be beneficial or harmful to the patient.

D. Antiprotozoal Drugs

I. Introduction

The main interest from an immunological point of view in antiprotozoal drugs lies in the possible aetiology of quinine-induced thrombocytopenia. There are very few reports describing allergic reactions to other antiprotozoal drugs. Questions have been raised about the safety of metronidazole, an effective treatment for amoebiasis and giardiasis, as well as of trichomonas infections, but these are related to neurotoxicological problems and the unresolved question of the carcinogenic potential of this compound. BAINES (1978) in a recent review gives no indications of any allergic reactions experienced with its use and this is probably true also of other nitroimidazoles used as antiprotozoal drugs.

The halogenated hydroxyquinoline group of amoebicidal drugs has also received attention, owing to its propensity to cause, under certain rather limited conditions, subacute myelo-optic neuropathy, but there is no suggestion that this is immunologically mediated (ROLLO 1975). Similarly side effects of emetine and of the drugs active against trypanosomes (for example, suramin) and the aromatic diamidines are not of allergic aetiology. It is worth recording, however, that the aromatic diamidines, both stilbamidine and pentamidine, are histamine releasers and pseudoallergic reactions might be experienced with their use. Organic arsenicals, occasionally used to treat trypanosomes, may give rise to allergic complications such as bullous exanthemas, allergic vasculitis and exfoliative dermatitis (SCHUPPLI 1972; FELIX and STEVENSON 1977); their use is, however, diminishing.

II. Quinine

Quinine (Fig. 9) is probably the oldest effective therapeutic agent for the prophylaxis and therapy of *Plasmodium* infections and, although now largely superseded for routine use, it is of considerable value in the treatment of chloroquine-resistant *P. falciparum*, for which it is used in combination with other antimalarials. The main side effects of quinine therapy comprise a syndrome of classical cinchonism, i.e., tinnitus, vision defects, nausea, headache and gastrointestinal effects, but immunologically the much rarer complication, drug-induced thrombocytopenia is of more interest.

Quinine was the first drug to be implicated in a drug-induced cytopenia (VIPAM 1865) but it was not until 1948 that the first evidence began to accumulate pointing to an immunological aetiology (GRANDJEAN 1948). This paper reported that the addition of quinine to platelet-rich plasma taken from patients who had recovered from thrombocytopenia induced by quinine, caused platelet lysis. Since that date, confirmation has been obtained that quinine, and its stereoisomer, quinidine, can

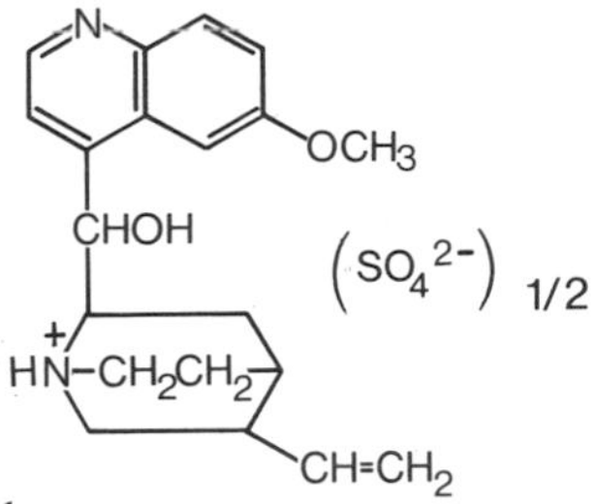

Fig. 9. Structure of quinine sulphate

give rise to thrombocytopenia, although not all reports refer to quinine used in antimalarial therapy. STEINKAMP et al. (1955) review early references and other cases have been reported (BOLTON 1956; BOLTON and DAMESLEK 1956; KISSMEYER-NIELSEN 1956; MAUER et al. 1957; WEINTRAUB et al. 1962; ADNER et al. 1967; BELKIN 1967; IIELMLY et al. 1967; VAN DER WEERDT 1967; BURGESS et al. 1969; POLASEK and DUCKERT 1971; ALBERTINI et al. 1972; EISNER and KORBITZ 1972).

In spite of extensive investigation, and the development of alternative in vitro assays to measure both the putative antibody and platelet dysfunction and damage, the mechanism of the thrombocytopenia is not clear. Excellent reviews of this topic have been published (SHULMAN 1958, 1963, 1964; DISCOMBE 1972; MCVIE 1973; NIEWEG et al. 1973; VAN ARSDEL 1978). It seems certain that a serum factor is present in drug-induced thrombocytopenia patients during the acute phase and occasionally for several months after. In vitro, in the presence of quinine and normal platelets, this serum factor can fix complement, agglutinate and lyse platelets and reduce platelet clot retraction. Serum fractionation and adsorption studies indicate that the fraction responsible is an IgG immunoglobulin (SHULMAN 1963; ADNER et al. 1967) although occasional reports implicate IgM (EISNER and KORBITZ 1972; DISCOMBE 1972). The difficulty arises in the definition of the specificity of this immunoglobulin. There are features which militate against the view that they are specific for drug-derived determinants, and equally other features are not persuasive that specificity is directed against the normal platelet. The arguments and the experimental data on these points are well reviewed by SHULMAN (1958, 1963, 1964) and MCVIE (1973).

NIEWEG et al. (1973) in re-examining the problem of the specificity of drug-dependent antibodies in thrombocytopenia have presented data which suggest that the specificity is determined, not by the chemical structure of the drug, but by its action on the platelet membrane. Thus, they find that a number of drugs, all characterised by an ability to inhibit platelet membrane SH groups, such as quinine, naphthoquinone, acetylsalicyclic acid and p-chloromercuribenzenesulphonic acid, can substitute for the initiating, responsible drug. They concluded therefore that antibodies were formed with specificity for selectively damaged platelet membranes, "spoiled membrane allergy", thus providing an explanation of why the antibodies fail to react in vitro with normal platelets in the absence of the drug and why they are clearly not drug specific in the conventional sense.

On the other hand, there is quite extensive evidence to suggest a greater degree of drug specificity than implied by this study, even to the extent of failure of cross-reactivity between quinine and quinidine, which differ only in their stereochemistry (Dawson and Garbade 1930; Bolton and Young 1953; Larson 1953; Barkham and Tocantins 1954; Weisfuse et al. 1954; Steinkamp et al. 1955; Bolton 1956; Freedman et al. 1956; Kissmeyer-Nielsen 1956). Further examination is therefore still required.

The immunological mechanism of platelet destruction is also poorly understood. Most workers favour the "innocent bystander" aetiology, in which it is assumed that the platelet is damaged by adsorption on to it of antigen-antibody complexes and subsequent complement fixation (Shulman 1963, 1964; Miescher and Pepper 1968; Van Arsdel 1978). There is some additional evidence that quinine can be antigenic and allergenic in humans. Contact dermatitis has been described (Burgess and Usher 1930; Ford 1934; Urbach and Gottlieb 1946; Calnan and Caron 1961) and in some cases, patch testing has been used to establish an allergic aetiology. However, in a recent study of skin problems in a factory processing quinine, Hardie et al. (1978) concluded that the main problem was an irritant dermatitis; affected workers were, with rare exceptions, patch test negative. One worker had a severe photoallergic reaction similar to that previously described by Calnan (1974), Frain Bell et al. (1975) and Johnson et al. (1975).

It is not clear whether quinine-induced fever, reported as a rare complication of quinine therapy of malaria (Schlutz et al. 1973) is immunologically mediated; the only evidence in support of this aetiology is that fever recurs on provocation testing. In this respect quinine behaves similarly to its (+)-stereoisomer, quinidine (Foley and Parada 1966).

III. Other Antimalarial Drugs

The quinoline group of antimalarial drugs include several acridines and 4-amino-quinolines. Quinacrine has now been largely replaced by chloroquine, the most generally used of this group in malaria, and also used to treat giardiasis and amoebiasis. Chlorquinine and the related drugs, amodiaquine and hydroxychloroquine have not been associated with allergic side effects other than brief reports of photoallergic dermatitis (Giglioli et al. 1967). The well-recognised primaquine sensitivity, a haemolytic anaemia, is not allergic in origin; it occurs only in patients deficient in glucose-6-phosphate dehydrogenase. Although the biguanides and deaminopyrimidines, such as proguanil and pyrimethamine, when used as antimalarial drugs can cause pancytopenias, again there is no evidence of an immunological aetiology.

In summary, allergic reactions are not a problem in treatment of protozoal infections. The aetiology of quinine-induced thrombocytopenia remains a fascinating immunological problem for future study.

References

Adner MM, Altstatt LB, Conrad ME (1967) The possible role of quinine in the hemolysis of malaria. Clin Res 15:302
Albertini F, Nizet F, Vergoz A (1972) Epistaxis grave par allergie à la quinine. Ann Otolaryngol Chir Cervicofac 89:63–68

Baer RL, Harber LC (1961) Photosensitivity to drugs. Arch Dermatol 83:7–14

Baines EJ (1978) Metronidazole: its past, present and future. J Antimicrob Chemother [Suppl C] 4:97–111

Bandmann H-J (1966) Die Kontaktallergie durch Arzneimittel. Pharm Zeitung 40:1470

Bandmann H-J, Huber-Riffeser G, Woyton A (1966) Kontaktallergie gegen Triamcinolona-cetonid. Hautarzt 17:183–185

Barkham P, Tocantins LM (1954) Observations on the thrombocytopenia due to hypersensitivity to quinidine. Blood 9:134–143

Baughman RD (1964) Contact photodermatitis from bithionol. Arch Dermatol 90:153

Behrbohm P, Zschunke E (1965) Allergisches Ekzem durch das Antimykotikum „Afungin" (Dibenzthion). Dermatol Wochenschr 151:1447–1453

Belcher DW, Wurapa FK, Ward WB (1975) Failure of thiabendazole and metronidazole in the treatment and suppression of Guinea worm disease. Am J Trop Med Hyg 24:444–446

Belkin GA (1967) Cocktail purpura: an unusual case of quinine sensitivity. Ann Intern Med 66:583–86

Bennett JE (1974) Chemotherapy of systemic mycoses. N Engl J Med 290:30–32

Berlin AR, Miller F (1976) Allergic contact dermatitis from ethyl sebacate in haloprogin cream. Arch Dermatol 112:1563–1564

Berthoud F, Berthoud S (1975) A propos de 18 cas d'anguillulose diagnostiques à Genève. Schweiz Med Wochenschr 105:1110–1115

Bolton FG (1956) Thrombocytopenic purpura due to quinidine. II. Serologic mechanisms. Blood 11:547–564

Bolton FG, Dameshek W (1956) Thrombocytopenic purpura due to quinidine. I. Clinical studies. Blood 11:527–546

Bolton FG, Young RV (1953) Observations on cases of thrombocytopenic purpura due to quinine, sulphamezathine and quinidine. J Clin Pathol 6:320–323

Bryceson ADM, Warrell DA, Pope HM (1977) Dangerous reactions to treatment of onchocerciasis with diethylcarbamazine. Br Med J 1:742–744

Burckhardt W (1959) Kontaktekzem durch Hydrocortison. Hautarzt 10:42–43

Burckhardt W, Sutter T (1963) Photoallergische Arzneiexantheme durch Hydrochlorothiazid. Z Hautkr 34:105–108

Burckhardt W, Schwarz-Speck K; Schwarz-Speck M (1957) Photoallergische Ekzeme durch Nadisan. Schweiz Med Wochenschr 87:954

Burckhardt W, Mahler F, Schwarz-Speck M (1968) Photoallergische Ekzeme durch Mycanodin. Dermatologica 137:208–215

Burgess JF, Usher H (1930) On hypersensitiveness to quinine. Can Med Assoc J 23:45–48

Burgess MA, Hirsh J, de Gruchy CG (1969) Acute thrombocytopenic purpura due to quinine sensitivity. Med J Aust 56:453–456

Burry JN (1967) Photoallergies to fenticlor and multifungin. Arch Dermatol 95:287–291

Burry JN (1969) The value of patch testing: a review of 363 cases of allergic contact dermatitis. Med J Aust 14:1226–1231

Burry JN (1970) Persistent light reactions from buclosamide. Arch Dermatol 101:95–97

Burry JN, Hunter GA (1970) Photo contact dermatitis from jadit. Br J Dermatol 82:224–229

Butler JBM (1968) Allergic reactions to piperazine. Med J Aust 1:676

Calnan CD (1974) Photodermatitis and quinine sensitivity. Contact Dermatitis 4:58

Calnan CD (1975) Occupational piperazine dermatitis. Contact Dermatitis 1:126

Calnan CD, Caron GA (1961) Quinine sensitivity. Br Med J 2:1750–1751

Cartwright RY (1974) Clotrimazole in the treatment of acute and "resistant" vaginal candidiasis. Postgrad Med J [Suppl 1] 50:90–92

Chang TW (1965) Cold urticaria and photosensitivity due to griseofulvin. JAMA 193:848–850

Ciferri FE, Kessel JF (1967) Relation of age, sex and microfilaria density to treatment of sub-periodic filariasis with diethylcarbamazine. Am J Trop Med Hyg 16:321–328

Coskey RJ (1971 a) Contact dermatitis due to nystatin. Arch Dermatol 103:228

Coskey RJ (1971 b) Allergic contact dermatitis from nystatin. Arch Dermatol 104:438

Dawson WT, Garbade FA (1930) Idiosyncrasy to quinine, cinchonidine and ethylhydrocu-preine. J Pharmacol Exp Ther 39:417–424

Degreef H, Verhoeve L, von Cutsem J (1975) Miconazole nitrate in the treatment of dermat-omycoses. Dermatologica 150:103–110

de Torregrosa MVVDA, Rodriguez-Rosado AL, Montilla E (1963) Hemolytic anemia sec-ondary to stibophen therapy. JAMA 186:598–599

Dewdney JM (1977) In: Sela M (ed) The antigens IV. Academic Press, New York London, p 139

Discombe G (1972) In: Samter M, Parker CW (eds) Hypersensitivity to drugs, vol. 1. Per-gamon, Oxford New York, p 173

Doeglas HMG (1978) In: Dukes MNG (ed) Side effects of drugs, annual 2. Excerpta Medi-ca, Amsterdam London New York, p 241

Draize JH (1959) In: Appraisal of the safety of chemicals in foods, drugs and cosmetics. As-sociation of Food and Drug Officials of the US, Austin, Texas, p 46

Dukes MNG (1975) In: Dukes MNG (ed) Meyler's side effects of drugs, VIII. Excerpta Medica, Amsterdam London New York

Dukes MNG (1977) In: Dukes MNG (ed) Side effects of drugs, annual 1. Excerpta Medica, Amsterdam London New York

Dukes MNG (1978) In: Dukes MNG (ed) Side effects of drugs, annual 2. Excerpta Medica, Amsterdam London New York

Eisner EV, Korbitz BC (1972) Quinine-induced thrombocytopenic purpura due to an IgM and an IgG antibody. Transfusion 12:317–321

Elmes PC (1975) In: Dukes MNG (ed) Meyler's side effects of drugs, VIII. Excerpta Medica, Amsterdam London New York

Emmett EA, Marrs JM (1973) Allergic contact dermatitis from tolnaftate. Arch Dermatol 108:98–99

Epstein E (1966) Allergic dermatitis from chlordantoin vaginal cream. Obstet Gynecol 27:369–370

Epstein E, Maibach HI (1968) Ethylenediamine allergic contact dermatitis. Arch Dermatol 98:476–477

Epstein WV, Michalski JP, Talal N (1977) Corticosteroids in levamisole-induced agranulo-cytosis. Lancet 2:8031:245

Farid Z, Bassily S, Hassan A (1973) Drug induced respiratory disorders. Br Med J 2:661–662

Felix RH, Stevenson CJ (1977) In: Davies DM (ed) Textbook of adverse drug reactions. Ox-ford University Press, Oxford

Fischer TJ, Klein RB, Kershnar HE, Borut TC, Stiehm ER (1977) Miconazole in the treat-ment of chronic mucocutaneous candidiasis: a preliminary report. J Pediatr 91:815–819

Fisher AA, Pascher F, Kanof NB (1971) Allergic contact dermatitis due to ingredients of vehicles. Arch Dermatol 104:286–290

Foley RE, Parada EA (1966) Drug fever of quinidine. Lahey Clin Found Bull 15:49–52

Forbes LS (1972) Toxicological and pharmacological relations between levamisole, pyrantel and diethylcarbamazine and their significance in helminth chemotherapy. Southeast Asian J Trop Med Public Health 3:235–241

Ford WK (1934) Drug eruption due to quinine, recurring following use of contraceptive. JAMA 103:483

Foussereau J, Benezra C (1967) Données nouvelles sur l'allergie de groupe a la pipérazine. Bull Soc Fr Dermatol Syphiligr 74:45–48

Foussereau J, Limam-Mestini S, Khochnevis A, Basset A (1971) L'allergie à l'association thérapeutique locale 'nystatine, néomycine et acétonide de triamcinolone'. Bull Soc Fr Dermatol Syphiligr 78:457–459

Frain Bell W, Johnson BE, Gardiner JM, Zaynoun S (1975) A study of persistent light reac-tion in quindoxin and quinine photosensitivity. Br J Dermatol [Suppl 11] 93:21

Freedman AL, Brody EA, Barr PS (1956) Immunothrombocytopenic purpura due to quinidine. Report of four new cases with special observations on patch testing. J Lab Clin Med 48:205

Fregert S (1967) Exacerbation of dermatitis by perorally administered piperazine derivative in a piperazine sensitized man. Contact Dermatitis Newslett 1:13

Fregert S, Möller H (1964) Photo cross-sensitization among halogenhydroxybenzoic acid derivatives. J Invest Dermatol 43:271–274

Freis A (1972) The tolerance of clotrimazole on topical application. Drugs Made Ger 15:120–121

Gellin GA, Maibach HI, Wachs GN (1972) Contact allergy to tolnaftate. Arch Dermatol 106:715–716

Giglioli G, Dyrting AE, Rutten FJ, Gentle GHK (1967) Photo-allergic dermatitis during a chloroquinized salt anti-malaria campaign in Guyana. Trans R Soc Trop Med Hyg 61:313–330

Gotz H, Reichenberger M (1972) Ergebnisse einer Fragebogenaktion bei 1670 Dermatologen der Bundesrepublik Deutschland über Nebenwirkungen bei der Griseofulvintherapie. Hautarzt 23:485–492

Graber H, Takacs L, Vedrödy K (1976) Agranulocytosis due to levamisole. Lancet 2:1248

Grandjean LC (1948) A case of purpura haemorrhagica after administration of quinine with specific thrombocytolysis demonstrated in vitro. Acta Med Scand [Suppl 213] 131:165–170

Groen J, Bleumink E, Nater JP (1973) Variotin sensitivity. Contact Dermatitis Newslett 15:456

Hall-Smith P (1974) Dermatomycoses: a brief history of therapy and initial results with clotrimazole. Postgrad Med J [Suppl 1] 50:70–72

Hardie RA, Savin JA, White DA, Pumford S (1978) Quinine dermatitis investigation of factory outbreak. Contact Dermatitis 4:121–124

Harris JW (1956) Studies on the mechanism of a drug-induced hemolytic anemia. J Lab Clin Med 47:760

Hartl PW (1973) In: Girwood RH (ed) Blood disorders due to drugs and other agents. Excerpta Medica, Amsterdam London New York

Helmly RB, Bergin JJ, Shulman NR (1967) Quinine-induced purpura. Arch Intern Med 120:59–62

Hempel M (1975) Klinische Erfahrungen in der lokalen Behandlung von Dermatomykosen mit Econazol-Hautmilch. Mykosen 18:213–219

Hill BHR (1957) An acute urticarial reaction to piperazine citrate. NZ Med J 56:572

Hirsch HA, Dedes M (1974) Local and systemic treatment of vaginal candidiasis. Postgrad Med J [Suppl 1] 50:83–84

Hollander A (1977) Neues aus der amerikanischen Dermatologie. Hautarzt 28:224–230

Ippen H (1961) Photoallergische Ekzeme durch das Antimykotikum 4-chlor-2-hydroxybenzoesaure-N-n-butylamid (Jadit). Z Hautkr 31:185–187

Jillson OF, Baughman RD (1963) Contact photodermatitis from bithionol. Arch Dermatol 88:409

Johnson BE, Zaynoun S, Gardiner JM, Frain Bell W (1975) A study of persistent light reaction in quindoxin and quinine photosensitivity. Br J Dermatol [Suppl 11] 93:21–22

Jung EG, Schwarz K (1964) Photoallergisches Jadit-Ekzem. Dermatologica 129:401

Jung EG, Schwarz K (1965) Photoallergy to "jadit" with photo cross-reactions to derivatives of sulphanilamide. Int Arch Allergy Appl Immunol 27:313–317

Jung EG, Dummler U, Immich H (1968) Photoallergie durch 4-chlor-2-hydroxy-benzoesäure-n-butylamid. Arch Klin Exp Dermatol 232:403–412

Kahn HR, Brod RC (1961) Thrombocytopenia due to stibophen. Arch Intern Med 108:496

Kandil E (1969) Fixed drug eruption. Dermatologica 139:37–40

Katz ME, Cassileth PA (1977) Disseminated candidiasis in a patient with acute leukemia, successful treatment with miconazole. JAMA 237:1124–1125

Kinsky SC (1970) Antibiotic interaction with model membranes. Annu Rev Pharmacol 10:119

Kissmeyer-Nielsen F (1956) Thrombocytopenic purpura following quinine medication. An immunological study. Acta Med Scand 154:289–298

Kligman AM (1966a) The identification of contact allergens by human assay. III. The maximization test: a procedure for screening and rating contact sensitizers. J Invest Dermatol 47:393–409

Kligman AM (1966b) The identification of contact allergens by human assay. I. A critique of standard methods. J Invest Dermatol 47:369–374

Klousia JW, McClennan BL, Semerjian HS (1977) Clyluria: a case report and brief literature review. J Urol 117:393–394

Larson RK (1953) The mechanism of quinidine purpura. Blood 8:16–25

Little JR, Plut EJ, Kotler-Brajtburg J, Medoff G, Kobayashi GS (1978) Relationship between the antibiotic and immunoadjuvant effects of amphotericin B methyl ester. Immunochemistry 15:219–224

Lorber B, Cutler C, Barry WE (1976) Allergic rash due to amphotericin B. Ann Intern Med 84:54

Lovett EJ, Lundy J (1977) The effect of thiabendazole in a mixed leukocyte culture. Transplantation 24:93–97

Lundy J, Lovett EJ (1976) Thiabendazole: a new immunopotentiator effective in therapy of murine fibrosarcoma. Surg Forum 27:132–134

Marmion LC, Desser KB, Lilly RB, Stevens DA (1976) Reversible thrombocytosis and anemia due to miconazole therapy. Antimicrob Agents Chemother 10:447–449

Mauer AM, Devaux W, Lahey ME (1957) Neonatal and maternal thrombocytopenic purpura due to quinine. Pediatrics 19:84–87

McCullagh SF (1968) Allergenicity of piperazine: a study in environmental aetiology. Br J Ind Med 25:319–325

McVie JG (1973) In: Girdwood RH (ed) Blood disorders due to drugs and other agents. Excerpta Medica, Amsterdam London New York

Meinhof W (1965) Ergebnisse der langfristigen Behandlung von Nagelmykosen mit Griseofulvin. Z Hautkr 19:399–408

Miescher P, Pepper JJ (1968) Drug-induced allergic blood dyscrasias. In: Meyler L, Peck HM (eds) Textbook of immunopathology, vol. 1. Excerpta Medica, Amsterdam London New York, p 277

Moss HV (1974) Allergic contact dermatitis due to halotex solution. Arch Dermatol 109:572

Murray HW (1974) Allergic reactions to amphotericin B. N Engl J Med 290:693

Nieweg HO, Stijnen PJ, van der Schans GS, Bos-Van Zwol F (1973) Drugs and thrombocytes. Proc Eur Soc Study Drug Toxicol 14:101–109

Nørgaard O (1977) Pecilocinum-Allergie. Hautarzt 28:35–36

Nurse DS (1973) Allergic contact sensitivity to jadit. Med J Aust 1:651–652

O'Driscoll BJ (1963) Allergy to griseofulvin. Br Med J 24:503

Paget GE, Walpole AL (1958) Some cytological effects of griseofulvin. Nature 182:1320

Parkinson DR, Jerry LM, Shibata HR et al. (1977) Complications of cancer immunotherapy with levamisole. Lancet 1:1129–1132

Peios E (1975) Lokalbehandlung von Soor-Kolpitis mit Econazol Erfahrungsbericht. Praxis 64:1261–1262

Pepys J, Pickering CAC, Loudon HWG (1972) Asthma due to inhaled chemical agents – piperazine dihydrochloride. Clin Allergy 2:189–196

Pöhler H, Michalski H (1972) Allergisches Exanthem nach Griseofulvin. Dermatol Monatsschr 158:385–390

Polasek J, Duckert F (1971) Diagnosis of quinine hypersensitivity, use of platelet factor 3 and acid phosphatase availability tests. Acta Haematol (Basel) 45:356–364

Provost TT, Jillson OF (1967) Ethylenediamine contact dermatitis. Arch Dermatol 96:231–234

Rachelson MH, Ferguson WR (1955) Piperazine in the treatment of enterobiasis. Am J Dis Child 89:346

Rave O, Albrecht JH, Vorlaender KO (1978) Ergebnisse und Risiken der Behandlung mit Tetraimidazol. Z Rheumatol 37:12–16

Robinson HM, Samorodin CS (1976) Thiabendazole-induced toxic epidermal necrolysis. Arch Dermatol 112:1757–1760

Roller JA (1978) Contact allergy to clotrimazole. Br Med J 2:737

Rollo IM (1975) In: Dukes MNG (ed) Meyler's side effects of drugs, VIII. Excerpta Medica, Amsterdam London New York, p 659

Rosenow E (1976) In: Kirkpatrick CH, Reynolds HY (eds) Immunologic and infectious reactions in the lung. Dekker, New York Basel, p 261

Rosenthal M, Trabert U, Müller W (1976) Leucocytotoxic effect of levamisole. Lancet 2:369

Rougemont A, Boisson ME, Silva GDA, Zander N (1976) Un essai de traitement collectif par la diethylcarbamazine dans un village d'hyperendemie onchocerquienne de la region de Bamako (Mali). Bull WHO 54:403–410

Rudolph RI (1975) Allergic contact dermatitis caused by haloprogin. Arch Dermatol 111:1487–1488

Rudzki E, Grzywa Z (1977) Occupational piperazine dermatitis. Contact Dermatitis 3:216

Savage J (1977) Fixed drug eruption to griseofulvin. Br J Dermatol 97:107–108

Scherwitz C (1977) Klinische Prüfung von Econazole Haut-Milch und -Creme bei Hautmykosen. Z Hautkr 52:117–125

Schlutz M, Zinneman HH, Hall WH (1973) Drug fever caused by quinine and quinidine. Minn Med 56:668–670

Schuppli R (1972) In: Samter M, Parker CW (eds) Hypersensitivity to drugs, 1. Pergammon, Oxford New York, p 205

Seah SKK (1974) Onchocerciasis in Canada. Can Med Assoc J 110:665–668

Secher L, Permin H, Skov PS, Ullman S, Halberg P (1978) Levamisole-induced hypersensitivity. Acta Derm Venereol (Stockh) 58:372–373

Shulman NR (1958) Immunoreaction involving platelets. J Exp Med 107:665–690

Shulman NR (1963) Mechanism of blood cell damage by adsorption of antigen-antibody complexes. In: Graber P, Miescher P (eds) Third international symposium of immunopathology, Basel, Switzerland. Schwabe, Basel Stuttgart, pp 338–352

Shulman NR (1964) A mechanism of cell destruction in individuals sensitized to foreign antigens and its implications in autoimmunity. Ann Intern Med 60:506–521

Skinnider LF, Rieder M (1977) Effect of levamisole on chronic lymphocytic leukaemic lymphocytes. Lancet 2/8044:932–933

Steagall RW (1963) Severe reaction to griseofulvin. Arch Dermatol 88:218–219

Steinkamp R, Moore CV, Doubek WG (1955) Thrombocytopenic purpura caused by hypersensitivity to quinine. J Lab Clin Med 45:18–29

Stevens DA, Levine HB, Deresinki SC (1975) Miconazole therapy of human coccidioidomycosis. Am Rev Respir Dis 111:950

Stuchlik S (1975) Über die Behandlung von Soor-Mykosen bei Leukemie-Patienten mit parenteral applizierbarem Miconazol. Med Welt 26:1255–1256

Sturde HC (1975) Klinische Untersuchungen über die antimyzetische und antibakterielle Wirkung von Haloprogin. Mykosen 18:467–478

Sundararajan V (1970) Variotin sensitivity. Contact Dermatitis Newslett 8:188

Swartz JH (1962) Current concepts in therapy: infections caused by dermatophytes. N Engl J Med 267:1359–1361

Symoens J (1977) In: Willoughby DA, Wood C (eds) Levamisole in rheumatoid arthritis, forum on immunotherapy 1, No. 2, 7. Royal Society of Medicine, London

Teerenhovi L, Heinonen E, Gröhn P, Klefström P, Maija M, Tiilikainen A (1978) High frequency of agranulocytosis in breast-cancer patients treated with levamisole. Lancet 2/8081:151–152

Tegner E (1976) Contact allergy to corticosteroids. Int J Dermatol 15:520–523

Thornes RD (1977) Febrile side-effects. Lancet 2/8028:90

Trabert U, Rosenthal M, Müller W (1976) Therapie entzündlich-rheumatischer Krankheiten mit Levamisol einer immunodulierenden Substanz. Schweiz Med Wochenschr 106:1293–1301

Turk J, Parker D (1979) Sensitization of guinea pigs to levamisole. Int Arch Allergy Appl Immunol 58:237–240

Urbach E, Gottlieb PM (1946) Allergy, 2nd edn. Heinemann, London, p 701

Ureles AL (1958) Clinical case history, two case histories of serum sickness-like reaction following piperazine citrate (antepar). Antibiot Med 5:585–586

Utz JP, Bennett JE, Brandriss MW (1964) Amphotericin B toxicity. Combined clinical staff conference at the National Institutes of Health. Ann Intern Med 61:334–354

Van Arsdel P (1978) In: Middleton E, Reed CE, Ellis EF (eds) Allergy. Principles and practice, 2. Mosby, St. Louis, p 1133

Van der Weerdt ChM (1967) Thrombocytopenia due to quinidine or quinine: report on a series of 28 patients. Vox Sang (Basel) 12:265–272

Van Hecke E (1969) Contact allergy to the topical antimycotic fluoro-4-dichloro-3,5'-thio-carbanilid. Dermatologica 138:480–482

Van Ketel WG (1967) Allergic dermatitis caused by tineafax ointment. Dermatologica 135:121–125

Vipan WH (1865) Quinine as a cause of purpura. Lancet 2:37

Wade TR, Jones HE, Chanda J (1977) Efficacy of parenteral miconazole therapy in mycotic infection. Clin Res 25:287A

Wahlberg JE (1974) Irritation threshold, tolerance and cross-reactions with clotrimaxole applied to skin. Postgrad Med J [July Suppl] 50:53–54

Wahlberg JE (1976) Clotrimazole (canesten) – results of patch-test trials on local tolerance. MMW [Suppl 1] 118:76–77

Wasilewski C (1970) Allergic contact dermatitis from nystatin. Arch Dermatol 102:216–217

Wasilewski C (1971) Allergic contact dermatitis from nystatin. Arch Dermatol 104:437

Weinstein L (1970) In: Goodman L, Gilman A (eds) The pharmacological basis of therapeutics, antifungal agents, 4th edn. Macmillan, London, p 1299

Weintraub RM, Pechet L, Alexander B (1962) Rapid diagnosis of drug-induced thrombocytopenic purpura. JAMA 180:528–532

Weisfuse L, Spear PW, Sass M (1954) Quinidine-induced thrombocytopenic purpura. Am J Med 17:414–422

Weiss HJ, Berger RE, Tice AD, Phillips LL (1972) Fatal disseminated intravascular coagulation and hemolytic anemia following stibophen therapy: a Study of basic mechanisms. Am J Med Sci 264:375–384

Weuta H (1972) Clotrimazole cream and solution – clinical investigation in an open study. Drugs Made Ger 15:126–132

White M, Douglas WS, Main RA (1978) Contact dermatitis attributed to ethylenediamine. Br Med J 1:415–416

Wilkinson DS (1961) Photodermatitis due to tetrachlorsalicylanilide. Br J Dermatol 73:213

Wilkinson DS (1972) Sensitivity to pharmaceutical additives. In: Dash CH, Jones HEH (eds) Mechanisms in drug allergy. Churchill Livingstone, Edinburgh London

Wurbach G, Schubert H (1976) Untersuchungen über die Afungin-Allergie. Dermatol Monatsschr 162:317–322

Yust I, Vardinon N, Fiersteter E, Avramov LA (1977) Levamisole-induced allergy. Lancet 2:457

Zymet CL (1977) A shock syndrome related to administration of diethylcarbamazine citrate, producing electrocardiographic changes in a dog with microfilariae of dirofilaria immitis. Vet Med Smal Anim Clin 72:1848–1852

CHAPTER 20

Solutions and Emulsions Used for Intravenous Infusions

W. RICHTER and H. HEDIN

A. Introduction

Intravenous infusions are widely employed in clinical therapy. This is illustrated by the fact that in the United States alone, 100 million infusions were administered during 1974 (SCHINDEL 1977). Intravenous infusions comprise colloid solutions employed as plasma substitutes such as plasma protein fractions, dextran, gelatin derivatives, hydroxyethylstarch, and polyvinylpyrrolidone. Further, agents used for parenteral nutrition such as various sugars, amino acid mixtures, and fat emulsions are of importance. The clinical usefulness of intravenous infusions is well established, but there always exists a certain risk of adverse reactions. They may arise locally from the injection trauma (thrombophlebitis, sepsis, catheter embolism), be due to microbial, pyrogenic, particulate, and chemical contamination of the solution (GUYNN et al. 1973; DUMA 1976), or manifest themselves as anaphylactoid reactions. That even today there remains the risk of contamination is exemplified by the need to recall 43 million infusion units in the United States in 1965–1975 because of contamination. This recall was associated with 54 deaths and 410 injuries (SCHINDEL 1977). Apart from contamination problems, anaphylactoid reactions represent the major problem today. This chapter will deal with the incidence and the clinical and immunologic aspects of anaphylactoid reactions to infusion solutions and emulsions. To facilitate understanding of the immunobiologic properties of the various agents, a short description of their physicochemical properties and of the manufacturing process is also given.

B. Plasma Substitutes

I. Historical

The first plasma substitute introduced was gelatin and HOGAN (1915) proved the clinical usefulness of such solutions. BAYLISS (1916) discovered gum arabic (acacia) a colloid of plant origin and prepared from it gum saline, which, following successful clinical trials (HURWITZ 1917) was used extensively as plasma expander during the World War I. Interest in plasma substitutes subsided between the World Wars for several reasons: high frequency of adverse reactions, introduction of blood transfusions, and greater safety of salt solutions. To eliminate adverse reactions, use of completely synthetic agents seemed promising. Polyvinylpyrrolidone (PVP) was chosen as a synthetic plasma substitute (HECHT and WEESE 1943), which could be infused in large quantities apparently without adverse effects. However, since

PVP is not metabolized, storage and potential oncogenicity discouraged its further clinical use.

Dextran, a partially hydrolyzed and purified bacterial polysaccharide, was introduced as plasma substitute during World War II (GRÖNWALL and INGELMAN 1944) in Sweden and has since found widespread clinical use (INGELMAN et al. 1969). Complete elimination of dextran is effected by the kidney filter and by dextranase degradation in the tissues. In attempts to produce another plasma substitute with good volume expansion and optimal pharmaceutical properties, a group of workers developed an expander based on hydroxyethylstarch (HES) (WIEDERSHEIM 1957; THOMPSON 1978). It has properties roughly comparable to those of dextran. However, a certain percentage of HES is not degraded and is retained in the body (LINDBLAD and FALK 1976; BOON et al. 1976). Its final position as a plasma substitute has not yet been evaluated.

A number of other colloids have also been used or proposed as potential expanders, but have not found clinical application because of various types of severe adverse reactions. One example is Alginon which is prepared by polymerization of sodium alginate (TOMODA and INOKUCHI 1959). Further, the following colloids have been studied (THOMPSON 1960): methylcellulose, pectin, hemoglobin, modified human globin, isinglass, bovine serum albumin, polyvinyl alcohol, and starch.

In experimentel animals, methylcellulose injection leads to hypertension, due to extensive methylcellulose thesaurosis of the glomerular endothelium (HALL and HALL 1961). Comparable hypertension and nephrotoxicity have been produced by injection of polyvinyl alcohol (HALL and HALL 1965). The pathogenic effects depended more on molecular size than on chemical structure. Similarly, dogs and rabbits injected with pectin showed atheromatous changes and thesaurosis with foam cellular storage phenomena in spleen, liver, and kidneys (HUEPER 1942).

II. General Physicochemical Properties

Plasma proteins such as albumin and each of the defined globulins are of uniform molecular size and therefore represent monodisperse or monomolecular colloids. In contrast, all other colloidal plasma substitutes contain distributions of molecules of varying size and are consequently polydisperse or polymolecular colloids. They require characterization by an average molecular weight, which can be defined either as a weight average, $\bar{M}_w$, or as a number average $\bar{M}_n$. $\bar{M}_w$ is generally determined by light scattering and $\bar{M}_n$ by osmometry or end group determination. Modern techniques permit complete characterization of molecular weight distributions of colloids and both $\bar{M}_w$ and $\bar{M}_n$ can be measured by automated gel permeation chromatography (ARTURSON and GRANATH 1972; NILSSON and NILSSON 1974). For monodisperse macromolecules $\bar{M}_w$ and $\bar{M}_n$ are identical, whereas $\bar{M}_w$ always is higher than $\bar{M}_n$ for polydisperse macromolecules. The wider the molecular weight distribution, i.e., the degree of polydispersity, the greater is the ratio of $\bar{M}_w$ to $\bar{M}_n$.

III. General Clinical Aspects

Anaphylactoid reactions to plasma substitutes present a similar clinical picture, ranging from mild skin manifestations to severe circulatory shock (SCHÖNING and

Table 1. Severity scale for quantification of intensity of anaphylactoid reactions (RING and MESSMER 1977)

Grade	Symptoms
I	Skin symptoms and/or mild fever reaction
II	Measurable, but not life-threatening cardiovascular reaction (tachycardia, hypotension), Gastrointestinal disturbance (nausea), Respiratory disturbance
III	Shock, life-threatening spasm of smooth muscles (bronchi, uterus)
IV	Cardiac and/or respiratory arrest

KOCH 1975; RING and MESSMER 1977). The reactions may be graded into four categories according to severity (Table 1). Mild reactions are characterized by one or more of the following symptoms: flush, erythema, pruritus, urticaria, nausea, localized edema, conjunctivitis, slight respiratory distress, lumbar pain, and fever. In moderate and severe reactions, arterial hypotension, vomiting, and bronchospasm are observed in addition to the previously mentioned symptoms. In the most severe reactions, occurring after infusion of a few milliliters of solution, a rapid fall of blood pressure to unmeasurable values is seen. This may be accompanied by cardiac and/or respiratory arrest. When anaphylactoid signs are observed, the infusion should immediately be discontinued. Mild reactions do not require further therapy. Severe reactions need adequate shock treatment and are then generally reversible (RING and MESSMER 1976). However, rare cases with lethal outcome have been reported, mostly in old and decrepit patients. No late adverse effects have been reported in the literature.

IV. Incidence

In recent years an increase of the number of reported anaphylactoid reactions induced by plasma substitutes has been observed. A similar increase is also apparent for reactions to many other drugs (FISHER 1975; FURHOFF 1977). These higher figures may reflect either a true increase in incidence or greater reporting. Evidence for the latter has been provided by BÖTTIGER et al. (1979).

In an attempt to estimate the incidence of anaphylactoid reactions to plasma substitutes a prospective multicenter study was performed during 1975 (RING and MESSMER 1977). A total of 31 hospitals participated and all colloidal volume substitutes in clinical use in the Federal Republic of Germany were included. Altogether 69 anaphylactoid reactions were reported upon infusion of 200,906 units (Tables 2 and 3). It is seen from Tables 2 and 3 that all plasma substitutes carry the risk of both mild and severe anaphylactoid reactions. The overall incidence was 0.033%, based on units infused, with a range varying from 0.01% for plasma protein solutions to 0.1% for gelatin derivatives. With regard to dextran reactions, dextran 60/75 showed a statistically significant higher incidence (0.069%) compared with the low molecular weight dextran 40 (0.007%).

SCHÖNING and KOCH (1975) performed a randomized study on the incidence of anaphylactoid reactions to five plasma substitutes in orthopedic patients. Each

Table 2. Incidence of anaphylactoid reactions caused by colloid volume substitutes. (Ring and Messmer 1977)

Colloid	Infusions registered (1975)	Anaphyl- actoid reactions	Incidence
Plasma protein:			
Serum solutions	25,582	5	0.019
Human serum albumin	60,048	7	0.011
Total	85,630	12	0.014
Dextran[a]			
Dextran 60/75	34,621	24	0.069
Dextran 40	51,261	4	0.007
Total	85,882	28	0.032
Gelatin:			
Urea-linked gelatin	6,151	9	0.146
Oxypolygelatin	810	2	0.247
Modified fluid gelatin	6,028	4	0.066
Total	12,989	15	0.115
Starch:			
Hydroxyethyl starch	16,405	14	0.085
Total	200,906	69	0.033

[a] Includes dextran from five manufacturers

Table 3. Severity of 69 anaphylactoid reactions after infusion of colloid volume substitutes. (Ring and Messmer 1977)

Colloid	Severity grade				
	I	II	III	IV	III and IV
Serum solutions	1	3	1	–	1
Human serum albumin	2	3	1	1	2
Dextran 60/75	7	11	5	1	6
Dextran 40	2	1	–	1	1
Urea-linked gelatin	4	2	3	–	3
Oxypolygelatin	–	1	1	–	1
Modified fluid gelatin	1	2	1	–	1
Hydroxyethyl starch	5	8	1	–	1

individual received 500 ml colloid solution at a flow rate of 25–30 ml/min. In a total of 750 patients, 107 adverse reactions were observed (14.3%). The majority were mild reactions characterized by skin manifestations. Twelve of the reactions were classified as severe. Nine of the latter occurred in connection with Haemaccel infusion two with Gelifundol-S, and one with Macrodex. The total incidence of anaphylactoid reactions was 21.3% to gelatin derivatives, 4.7% to dextran 60, and 2.7% to hydroxyethylstarch (HES). The rate of severe reactions to individual prep-arations was as follows: 6% for Haemaccel, 1.3% for Gelifundol-S, 0.6% for Macrodex, and less than 0.67% for Plasmagel. The greater overall incidence in the study of SCHÖNING and KOCH (1975) as compared with that of RING and MESSMER (1977) may reflect the type of patient selected, the very rapid infusion, the careful observation of skin manifestations, and the definition of severe reactions by the former group.

TSCHIRREN et al. (1973/1974) state that the rate of allergic reactions to modified fluid gelatin is about 0.1%. They found 14 allergic episodes in 9,290 patients treated with 12,618 units of 500 ml Physiogel, corresponding to an incidence of 0.15% per patient and 0.11% per unit infused. In a later report from the same authors (LUNDSGAARD-HANSEN and TSCHIRREN 1980) the incidence of reactions to modified fluid gelatin was 0.064% (66 incidents in 102,787 units infused). When graded according to severity (Table 1) 67% of reactions were classified as grade I, 21% as grade II, 10% as grade III, and 2% as grade IV. The grade IV reactions had a lethal outcome. Concerning oxypolygelatin a reaction rate of 39 in 3,600 = 1.08% (SCHMIDT and PFLÜGER 1971) and of 58 in 707 = 8.2% (SCHMIDT and RIEBER 1980) has been reported. Haemaccel has caused fatal reactions (FREEMAN 1979), but recently an improved preparation is claimed to cause only mild reactions (SCHÖNING and LORENZ 1981; SCHÖNING et al. 1982). LANGREHR et al. (1975) observed an incidence of anaphylactoid reactions to gelatin preparations of 1 in 359, and to dextran of 1 in 997.

BEEZ and DIETL (1979) have compared the units of dextran 75 (Longasteril) and HES (Plasmasteril) sold during the period January 1974–June 1977 with the reported number of anaphylactoid reactions. The frequency of severe anaphylactoid reactions (grades III and IV) amounted to 19 in 458,924 = 0.0041% for dextran 75 and 2 in 550,350 = 0.0004% for HES. In two studies from Sweden (BAUER and ÖSTLING 1970; CARLSSON et al. 1972) the combined average incidence of dextran reactions per patient was 15 in 15,312 = 0.1%. FURHOFF (1977) reported an incidence for dextran 70 (Macrodex) of 0.04% based on units infused. This figure is in agreement with the above incidence per patient, since two to three 500-ml bottles are usually given to each individual. Recently, an incidence of 22 reactions to Dextran 70 in 1993 patients = 1.1% has been reported in a multicenter study (GRUBER et al. 1980). In a further study the calculated incidence of severe dextran reactions per patient was found to be 0.037%–0.05% (LJUNGSTRÖM et al. 1983a).

To summarize, the incidence of anaphylactoid reactions to plasma substitutes is low. For comparison, it is less than that to blood, ranging from 1%–6% (MOLLISON 1972; KAARS-SIJPESTEIJN and HUIZINGA 1975; SILVER 1976).

C. Plasma Protein Fractions

I. Physicochemical and Pharmaceutical Aspects

Among the colloids prepared from human blood and used for plasma volume expansion, human serum albumin (HSA) and plasma protein fractions (PPF) are the most important products. HSA is a monodisperse, relatively symmetrical protein with a calculated molecular weight between 66,300 and 69,000 daltons, prepared from plasma by fractionation (for review, see TULLIS 1977). PPF is a solution of plasma proteins containing about 85% albumin and 15% globulins of which the thermolabile fraction has been removed by salt precipitation. Both HSA and PPF solutions are pasteurized at 60 °C for 10 h to inactivate hepatitis virus. Upon storage, a certain amount of aggregates is formed. Stabilizers such as sodium acetyl-tryptophanate and sodium caprylate are therefore mixed with plasma protein solutions intended for clinical use in order to minimize formation of aggregates (Roelands et al. 1974). The commercial HSA preparations are available as 5%, 20%, and 25% solutions with a balanced electrolyte content (e.g., Human Albumin Kabi, Behringwerke and -Biotest, Albuminar, Albumisol, Albuspan, and Albutein). They are stable to cold storage with a shelf-life of 2–5 years. PPF is available as 5% solution with a balanced electrolyte content (Plasmanate, Plasmatein, Plasmaplex, Protenate, Sekretin, Biseko).

II. Immunochemistry and Immunology

HSA is a globular protein consisting of a single folded polypeptide chain of 584 amino acids (Behrens et al. 1975). Its antigenic structure has been studied by comparative determinant analysis and the presence of at least six different antigenic determinants could be established (Bauer 1974). It could also be shown that two of the determinants are shared only by primates, whereas the remaining four are common to other mammalian albumins as well. There was no human species-specific determinant demonstrable. Owing to genetic variation, HSA of slightly different structure occurs in low frequency in normal human populations. Twenty different monomeric (Weitkamp et al. 1973) and three dimeric variants (Weitkamp et al. 1972) have been described. Albumin B, the most common European variant, has a frequency of less than 1 in 1,000. Since the percentage of allotypic determinants in pooled HSA is extremely low, HSA is practically devoid of immunogenic properties. In animal experiments it has, however, been shown that the immunogenicity of HSA is markedly increased by the presence of aggregates (Ring 1978a). This may be due to generation of new conformational determinants.

III. Clinical Aspects

Several reports on anaphylactoid reactions to HSA and PPF are found in the literature (Harrison et al. 1971; Bland et al. 1972; Ring et al. 1975a; Isbister and Biggs 1976; McMillin et al. 1978; Alving et al. 1978; Ring et al. 1979).

With regard to the onset in time, "early" and "late" reactions to HSA can be distinguished (Ring et al. 1974). Early reactions appear soon after or up to 2 h, and late reactions 3–6 days after infusions. The symptoms of both types of reactions are similar and comprise shivering, fever, urticarial exanthema, and cardiovascular signs such as tachycardia and hypotension. In a report on 25 patients with reactions to HSA, 9 developed early and 16 developed late reactions (Ring 1978a). Of the 9 patients exhibiting early reactions, 6 had been previously exposed to HSA. A history of allergy was found in 22 of the 25 patients, and an overrepresentation of autoimmune diseases could be noted. No significant differences between sexes and age groups were seen. Early reactions are mostly caused by 20% and late ones by 5% HSA solutions (Ring et al. 1974). In another study Ring et al. (1979) describe six patients, three reacting to HSA (severity grade II, III, and IV) and three to PPF (severity grade I, II, and III). All reactions occurred within 2–15 min after the onset of the infusion. All reactions were reversible by treatment with epinephrine, corticosteroid, or resuscitation. Without exception, a history of allergy was present in these cases, comprising asthma, hay fever, drug, plant, or food allergies. Three of the six patients had earlier received HSA infusions without showing adverse signs.

ALVING et al. (1978) reported 23 cases of hypotension of varying degree after PPF infusion. These were all connected with surgical interventions. In eight cases PPF was administered before cardiovascular bypass, in five during bypass, in five during general surgical procedures, and in the remaining five cases, shortly after operation. The average age of the patients undergoing bypass was 53 years (male: female ratio 11:1), and that of the other surgical patients was 49 years (male:female ratio 1:1). The rate of administration was usually 50 ml/min and hypotension occurred within 2 min after starting infusion. In patients who could be treated by discontinuation of the infusion, blood pressure rose to normal within about 5 min. Four of the patients required resuscitation.

The first case of an anaphylactoid reaction to the intravenous diagnostic administration of $^{99}Tc^m$-labeled human albumin microspheres was recently reported (LITTENBERG 1975). The symptoms comprised flush, severe bronchospasm, and rapid fall of blood pressure to unmeasurable levels. The patient recovered following treatment with epinephrine, benadryl, and hydrocortisone.

IV. Results of Diagnostic Tests

1. Skin Tests

Intracutaneous skin tests with 0.05 ml 0.5% HSA solution were performed on six patients with reactions to HSA (RING et al. 1974). Four of these gave a positive immediate skin response. In 20 volunteers similar intracutaneous tests were all negative. Skin tests seem to have a certain predictive value, especially in early HSA reactions.

The important role of aggregates as elicitors of skin reactions to HSA (RING 1978 a) is evident from results obtained in patients challenged intradermally with the following HSA preparations: monomeric HSA (2 in 12), albumin aggregates (9 in 12), and commercial HSA solution (5 in 12). The figures in parentheses indicate the frequency of positive immediate skin reactions.

2. Specific Antibodies

Using Ouchterlony gel double diffusion, no precipitating antibodies against monomeric HSA solution were found in sera of patients with anaphylactoid reactions to HSA (RING et al. 1979).

3. Lymphocyte Transformation Test

As evident from Fig. 1 in which the antigenic stimulatory action of various HSA preparations on lymphocytes of reactors to HSA is presented, HSA solution con-

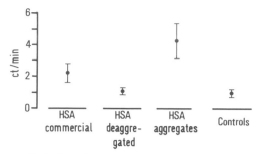

Fig. 1. ^3H-Thymidine uptake in lymphocyte cultures of patients with clinical human serum albumin (HSA) incompatibility after stimulation with different HSA fractions; final HSA concentration in the culture: 2.5 mg% ($n=7$). (Ring 1978 a)

taining a high amount of aggregates and commercial HSA both produced significant stimulation. Deaggregated HSA gave a negative lymphocyte transformation test (Ring 1978 a).

V. Potential Pathomechanisms

The presence of aggregates in protein solutions has to be considered as a potential risk factor for elicitation of anaphylactoid reactions. It has been shown, for example, that infusions of HSA solution containing aggregates into nonimmunized dogs produce anaphylactoid symptoms (Ring et al. 1977 b). These aggregates were produced by heat denaturation of monomeric HSA. Aggregates are also considered to be responsible for anaphylactoid reactions following intravenous infusion of gamma-globulin in humans (Barandun et al. 1962; Janeway et al. 1968; Ellis and Henney 1969). Ishizaka (1963) has extensively investigated the biologic effects of aggregated IgG. Such aggregates are known to activate plasma enzyme systems, e.g., the complement system (Müller-Eberhard 1976), and to release mediators from mast cells. Concerning early reactions to HSA and PPF solutions, aggregates are also regarded as elicitor agents (Ring et al. 1979; Ring and Richter 1980). Positive skin tests in reactors with aggregate-rich, but not with monomeric HSA, are in favor of such a view. IgA deficiency could be ruled out as pathogenic factor. It is known that anaphylactic reactions occur in IgA-deficient patients, infused with blood or plasma preparations (Leikola et al. 1973) and that they are due to the presence of anti-IgA antibodies (Wells et al. 1977).

Another potential triggering mechanism is sensitization of the patient to HSA modified by stabilizers such as caprylate (Ring et al. 1979). The immunogenicity of caprylate-modified HSA has been demonstrated to be much higher than that of monomeric HSA (Hossaini et al. 1977). Furthermore, caprylate-specific antibodies and autoagglutinins to HSA have been described in humans and animals (Golde et al. 1971, 1973). The anaphylactoid reactions in humans could thus be explained by the interaction of HSA with specific antibodies of IgE or other Ig classes, with subsequent mediator release. The frequent occurrence of a history of allergy in such patients may suggest participation of IgE. In addition, the genetic polymorphism of HSA has to be considered as a potential cause of immunogenicity and adverse reactions (WEITKAMP et al. 1973).

An important contribution to the elucidation of the triggering mechanism underlying hypotensive reactions to PPF has been made recently (ALVING et al. 1978). These workers were able to show a general correlation between levels of Hageman factor fragments (prekallikrein activator) and the incidence and severity of adverse reactions. A total of 13 batches of PPF from one manufacturer were implicated in 23 hypotensive incidents. All batches showed prekallikrein activator activity, probably generated by contact with foreign surfaces during some stages of the manufacturing procedure. The levels of bradykinin and kallikrein were low. Earlier, high levels of bradykinin had been shown to occur in some batches of PPF. This exogenous bradykinin would produce only a transitory vasodilator and hypotensive effect, because of rapid inactivation by kininases (VANE 1969). In contrast, the prekallikrein activator, present in certain batches of PPF, would be expected to induce a more persistent hypotensive response because of the establishment of a positive feedback mechanism (COLMAN et al. 1971). These results allow one to draw the conclusion that Hageman factor fragments may also have been of pathogenic importance in adverse reactions reported in an earlier study by BLAND et al. (1973). These workers investigated the effect on arterial blood pressure of HSA and PPF in 11 patients undergoing total cardiopulmonary bypass for correction of acquired heart disease. Whereas no significant change was seen after rapid infusion of 50 ml 5% HSA, decreases of varying extent were produced by three batches of PPF solution in the same patients. One batch gave significant decrease in all 11 patients and the other two in 3 and 4 respectively. The observed absence of hypotensive effect of HSA in this study is in accord with the observations of ALVING et al. (1978) and of HEINONEN et al. (1981), showing that prekallikrein activator activity rarely occurs in albumin. This is confirmed by LÜBEN et al. (1981), who further conclude that trace amounts of prekallikrein activator cannot be related to side reactions with HSA. In a recent editorial (COLMAN 1978) it is pointed out that albumin should be preferred to PPF as a plasma volume expander because of the lower incidence of hypotensive adverse reactions. This viewpoint is however still under discussion.

D. Dextran

I. Physicochemical and Pharmaceutical Aspects

The raw material for production of clinical dextran is native dextran, which was originally described as an undesirable viscous substance, occasionally clogging pipes in sugar factories. PASTEUR (1861) showed that the formation of such slimes was due to microbial action. The name dextran was coined by SCHEIBLER (1869), who demonstrated the strong dextrorotary properties of this polysaccharide, which is produced enzymatically from sucrose by the action of *Leuconostoc* (JEANES et al. 1954) and other bacteria. Native dextrans are water-soluble polysaccharides of $\bar{M}_w$ $10–100 \times 10^6$ daltons and are composed of glucose units linked together by α 1–6 bonds into thread-like macromolecules. They are branched to varying extent and the branches may be attached to the main chain by α 1–2, 1–3, or 1–4 linkages.

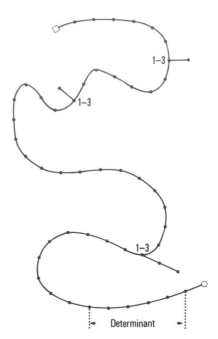

Fig. 2. Schematic picture of dextran B 512 molecule showing randomly coiled main chain composed of α 1–6 linked glucose units, and with reducing and non-reducing end groups. The distribution of α 1–3 linked side chains and the approximate size of an antigenic determinant are also indicated. *Circle* = reducing; *square* = non-reducing end group. (Hedin and Richter 1977)

To be clinically useful, dextrans have to be partially hydrolyzed to a molecular weight range comparable to that of plasma proteins. Furthermore, ethanol fractionation and extensive purification is required. The clinical dextrans used today are prepared from native dextran produced by the *Leuconostoc mesenteroides* NRRL B 512 strain (see Fig. 2). This dextran is only slightly branched, possessing 1 side chain for every 20 glucose units. Of the side chains, 85% comprise only 1–2 glucose units (Larm et al. 1971).

Dextran is an uncharged polymer. Sterilized solutions are stable and can be stored for many years over a wide temperature range. Only upon strong and repeated temperature changes may formation of flakes occur. The latter can be redissolved upon heating. The pH of dextran solutions is 4–5, but dextran infusion does not affect the pH of blood, because of the buffer capacity of the latter. Commercial dextran preparations are available as solutions in physiologic saline, other balanced electrolytes, or sugar solutions. The concentration of colloid varies between 3% and 10%. Such preparations represent dextran fractions of $\bar{M}_w$ 40,000, 60,000, 70,000, 75,000, and 110,000 daltons. They are designated as dextran 40, 60, etc. Examples of trade names are Rheomacrodex, Longasteril, Schiwadex, Macrodex, Lomodex, and Onkovertin. Recently, dextran 1 of $\bar{M}_w$ 1,000 (Promit 15%) has been introduced for prophylaxis of severe dextran reactions. It is given as 20 ml i.v.

injection 2 min before infusion of clinical dextran (RICHTER and HEDIN 1982; RENCK et al. 1983a).

II. Immunochemistry and Immunology

The dextran molecule represents a chain of repetitive antigenic determinants. The size of these determinants corresponds to short sequences of the dextran molecule, comprising 3–7 glucose units (KABAT 1957, 1966; KABAT and MAYER 1961). Evidence for this size was obtained from hapten inhibition tests, showing that precipitation between antidextrans and high molecular weight dextran was increasingly inhibited by isomaltose oligosaccharides of increasing size. In dextran produced by *L. mesenteroides* NRRL B 512, predominantly one type of determinant is present: α 1–6 linked glucose units (see Fig. 2). In branched dextrans, additional determinants are represented by the disaccharides at branch points, containing α 1–2, 1–3, and 1–4 linkages. To conclude, antigenic determinants of dextran can be located along the chain (RICHTER 1974) or terminally and at branch points (CISAR et al. 1975).

Dextran belongs to the thymus-independent antigens (BACH 1976) which induce formation of IgM antibodies in low concentrations. They easily induce tolerance in experimental animals (HOWARD et al. 1975). However, when coupled to protein, they become thymus dependent and induce formation of large amounts of IgG antibodies (RICHTER and KÅGEDAL 1972). The immunogenicity of dextran in animals (HOWARD et al. 1975) and humans (KABAT and BEZER 1958) is molecular weight dependent. Whereas native, high molecular weight dextran induces formation of small amounts of circulating antibodies in humans (ALLEN and KABAT 1957, 1958), single or repeated doses of clinical size dextran do not induce antibody formation (KABAT and BEZER 1958; GRÖNWALL 1959).

Naturally occurring dextran-reactive antibodies are frequently present in the sera of normal humans (KABAT and BERG 1952, 1953; MAURER 1953; GRABAR 1955; JACOBSSON and WIKSTRÖM 1958; JACOBSSON and ZSIGA 1958; FROM et al. 1961), and in various animal species (GRABAR 1955). With the sensitive method of passive hemagglutination we could demonstrate dextran reactive antibodies in 75% of normal human subjects, high titers of 256–2,048 comprising 11% (HEDIN and RICHTER 1982). Such antibodies may be induced either by high molecular weight dextran originating from dental plaque (GIBBONS and BANGHART 1967; FREEDMAN et al. 1978), food additives, or contaminants of commercial sucrose (NEILL et al. 1939) or by cross-reactive bacteria, e.g., pneumococci type II, XII, XX, and XXII, *Salmonella typhosa*, streptococci, and *Klebsiella* (ZOZAYA 1932; NEILL et al. 1939; SUGG and HEHRE 1942; HEHRE and NEILL 1946; NEILL and ABRAHAMS 1951; BRYAN and SCUDDER 1952; GOODMAN and KABAT 1964). Cross-reactivity between antisera to teichoic acids and dextrans has also been demonstrated (KNOX and WICKEN 1972).

III. Clinical Aspects

Adverse reactions to dextran, designated as anaphylactoid or anaphylactic, have been reported since the introduction of dextran into clinical use. During the early

1950s, mild reactions were frequently seen with the branched dextran used at that time (WILKINSON and STOREY 1953). Change to the nearly linear dextran B 512, however, markedly reduced the incidence of such reactions (WILKINSON 1956). The increasing use of clinical dextran B 512 during the last decade for plasma substitution, thromboprophylaxis, and improvement of blood flow has, however, shown that both mild and severe reactions do occur (BAILEY et al. 1967; BRISMAN et al. 1968; BAUER and ÖSTLING 1970; KOHEN et al. 1970; WEBSTER et al. 1973; MISGELD and MENDE 1974; AANDERUD and GRAN 1975; KRENZELOK and PARKER 1975; WALDHAUSEN et al. 1975; LAXÉNAIRE et al. 1976; VELTMANN and MUERTZ 1976; ADAR and SCHNEIDERMAN 1977; FURHOFF 1977; MENZANO et al. 1977; LJUNGSTRÖM et al. 1983a). All commercially available clinical dextrans of varying average molecular weight have the potential to elicit adverse reactions. A tendency for increased incidence with increasing $\bar{M}_w$ can, however, be noted (THORSÉN 1954; RING and MESSMER 1977). It should be mentioned that anaphylactoid reactions induced by iron dextran (BECKER et al. 1966; LEWINTER 1970) and dextran 70, used for hysterosalpingography (KNUDTSON and TAYLOR 1976) have also been reported.

The anaphylactoid symptoms vary from skin manifestations to cardiovascular shock, sometimes leading to cardiac arrest. Severe reactions usually start after infusion of a few milliliters, emphasizing the necessity of close supervision of the patient during the first 50 ml of the infusion (RING and MESSMER 1976). The frequency distribution of individual symptoms in 208 cases of anaphylactoid dextran reactions was as follows: tachycardia 57%, hypotension 48%, flush 45%, dyspnea 38%, nausea 29%, urticaria 21%, and fever 6%. Chronic inflammatory diseases were observed in 80% of the patients with severe reactions (RING 1978a). No preference of dextran reactions for association with certain categories of disease, classified according to the ICD system of WHO, was, however, apparent (HEDIN et al. 1976). No significant differences between sexes and age groups were found. FURHOFF (1977) reported that the severity of reactions increased with age. The median age of five lethal cases was found to be 79 years. Dextran reactions are observed both in conscious and anesthetized patients (SHEPHARD and VANDAM 1964; BAUER and ÖSTLING 1970; CARLSSON et al. 1972; HEDIN et al. 1976; GODENSCHWEGER et al. 1978, LJUNGSTRÖM et al. 1983a). A history of allergy was found in 40% of patients with grade I reactions, whereas the frequency of allergic disposition in grade II–IV reactions was comparable to that of a normal population (RING 1978a). A similar overrepresentation of atopic patients in grade I reactions was found in another series of reactors to dextran (HEDIN 1977).

IV. Results of Diagnostic Tests

1. Skin Tests

Intracutaneous skin tests with 0.05 ml Macrodex were performed in 37 patients, who had experienced anaphylactoid reactions to dextran (HEDIN et al. 1976). The incidence of positive wheal and flare responses was 11% at 0–7 days, and 32% at 1–12 months after the reaction. In normal human subjects, positive skin tests with clinical dextran have been reported in 6%–19% (BRYAN and SCUDDER 1952; MEISSNER 1961). From these findings it is concluded that skin tests are of limited value for prediction of anaphylactoid dextran reactions.

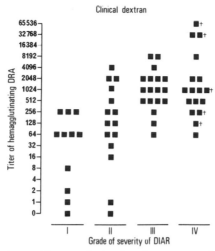

Fig. 3. Relation between titers of hemagglutinating dextran-reactive antibodies (DRA) in sera of dextran reactors ($n=61$) and severity of dextran-induced anaphylactoid reactions (DIAR). Titers were estimated on sera obtained prior to the reaction. (HEDIN et al. 1981 a)

2. Specific Antibodies

a) Reaginic Dextran-Reactive Antibodies

Serum samples from 100 dextran reactors collected from four different countries over a 5-year period were assayed by the radioallergosorbent technique (RAST). In 75% dextran-specific IgE levels were low and did not deviate from the normal range (HEDIN et al. 1976). Of the dextran reactors, 25% showed slightly increased specific IgE levels. Compared with specific IgE levels in atopic subjects, e.g., patients sensitive to Timothy grass pollen, the increase found in these dextran reactors is considered as liminal. These sera were also assayed by passive cutaneous anaphylaxis in monkeys (HEDIN et al. 1976). No immediate skin reactions were observed with any of the sera tested upon intravenous challenge with Macrodex at 3 and 24 h after sensitization. These findings indicate absence of dextran-reactive reaginic antibodies with both short and long latency, later confirmed by another method (KRAFT et al. 1982).

b) Hemagglutinating Dextran-Reactive Antibodies

Serum samples from 123 dextran reactors were assayed for dextran-reactive antibodies by passive hemagglutination (HEDIN et al. 1976). Human blood group O red cells were sensitized to dextran by incubation with stearoyldextran. A positive relationship was found between titers of hemagglutinating dextran reactive antibodies and increasing severity of the dextran reaction. High titers were found in all patients with severe reactions, in whom, by chance sera could be obtained prior to the reaction (HEDIN and RICHTER 1982; see Fig. 3). On the other hand, sera of dextran reactors taken shortly after the reaction had appreciably lower titers, indicating neutralization of antibodies by the infused clinical dextran. Since high titers of dextran-reactive antibodies also occur in about 11% of normal human subjects and the incidence of severe dextran reactions is much lower it is evident that use of passive hemagglutination delineates a risk group, but does not allow one to predict individual dextran reactions. Since passive hemagglutination detects the sum of IgG, IgA, and IgM class antibodies, differentiation of dextran reactive antibodies into classes and subgroups has been studied by the authors in collaboration with Dr. D. Kraft, using the red-cell-linked antigen antiglobulin reaction. Results show that high titers of dextran reactive antibodies of the IgG and sometimes IgA class are prevalent in dextran reactors (Hedin et al. 1979; Kraft et al. 1982). Within the IgG class the IgG_2 subgroup dominates.

3. Lymphocyte Transformation Test

In efforts to elucidate whether this test can be used as a diagnostic method for dextran allergy, lymphocytes of 19 dextran reactors and 30 normal subjects were studied. No mitogenic effect of dextran 60 (Macrodex) or dextran 40 (Rheomacrodex) at concentrations between 2×10^{-4} and $3 \times 10^{-9} M$ was, however, demonstrable (Ring 1978 b). Negative results in the lymphocyte transformation test were also obtained in three patients with dextran reactions, studied by Kohen et al. (1970).

V. Potential Pathomechanisms

It was suggested many years ago that the specific antibody-combining properties of dextrans represent a theoretical source of danger for individuals possessing high titers of circulating dextran-reactive antibodies at the time of clinical dextran infusion (Hehre and Sugg 1950). For clinical non-B 512 dextran, Kabat et al. (1957) reported a positive correlation between presence of preformed precipitating dextran-reactive antibodies and systemic allergic reactions. After introduction of the less branched, nearly linear B 512 dextran into clinical use, the incidence of allergic reactions was considerably reduced (Wilkinson 1956). From the fact that the great majority of individuals with high titers of precipitating dextran-reactive antibodies tolerated B 512 dextran infusion, Jacobsson (1959) concluded that the presence of such antibodies seems not to explain the occurrence of dextran reactions, except in some cases of allergic disorders. From our recent accumulated data on the sera of dextran reactors (Fig. 3) strong evidence is, however, obtained for participation of preformed hemagglutinating dextran-reactive antibodies in the elicitation of severe dextran-induced anaphylactoid reactions (Hedin and Richter 1982). In such cases a significant decrease of Clq levels was also found, suggesting complement activation via the classical pathway. The antibody and complement findings allow one to postulate that generation of specific immune complexes is the first step in a series of events, finally leading to mediator release which is responsible for the clinical signs. Histopathologic findings with total occlusion of the pulmonary circulation in fatal dextran reactions are in accord with such a hypothesis (Ziegler 1978; Revenäs et al., unpublished). Consequently, we consider that severe dextran reactions should be classified as aggregate anaphylaxis (Becker and Austen 1976). Interference with immune complex formation would therefore be a theoretical possibility to prevent or mitigate dextran reactions. This could be achieved by application of the hapten inhibition principle (RICHTER et al. 1980a, b). In a canine model of aggregate dextran anaphylaxis, hapten treatment markedly reduced both the incidence and severity of the anaphylactic reaction (MESSMER et al. 1980b; SEEMANN et al. 1978; SCHWARZ and RASCHAK 1978; SCHWARZ et al. 1981). Clinical multicenter trials comprising more than 100,000 patients have shown the efficacy of hapten administration in prevention of dextran anaphylaxis in humans (MESSMER et al. 1980a, b; HEDIN et al. 1981b; GRUBER et al. 1982; RICHTER and HEDIN 1982; LAUBENTHAL et al. 1982a, b, 1983; LJUNGSTRÖM et al. 1983b; RENCK et al. 1983a, b). The prophylactic effect was found to be dose dependent. The incidence of severe dextran reactions was reduced by at least 50% with a 10 ml preinjection of Dextran 1 (Promit = haptendextran $\bar{M}_w$ 1,000) and by 90%–97% with a 20 ml dose. The latter dose is now recommended for routine prophylaxis of severe dextran reactions. The applications of hapten inhibition represents a new basic approach to eliminate adverse drug reactions, which are antibody dependent.

It should be pointed out that available data clearly show that dextran reactions are not mediated by specific reagins. This is in contrast to certain other drug reactions in which IgE antibodies could be demonstrated, permitting one to classify such reactions as cytotropic anaphylaxis (PHILLS and PERELMUTTER 1974; KRAFT et al. 1976). Since it is known that native dextran can activate the alternative pathway of complement in vitro (PILLEMER et al. 1955), it was hypothesized that dextran reactions might be triggered in a similar way. However, we could show that clinical dextran does not activate the alternative pathway. We also established complement profiles in sera of dextran reactors to study this possibility (HEDIN 1977). In addition, anaphylatoxin inactivator levels were determined, since low levels might lead to high serum concentrations of anaphylatoxins with potential shock-producing activity. A significant decrease in the levels of Clq was found in grade II, III, and IV reactions but not in grade I reactions. No further significant differences in complement protein concentrations including factor B were demonstrable. Thus, evidence for activation of the classical pathway but not of the alternate pathway was obtained. Normal anaphylatoxin inactivator levels were found in 100 dextran reactors, suggesting that deficiency of the anaphylatoxin inactivator does not play any pathogenic role in dextran reactions (HEDIN 1977). In another study, activation of factor B and conversion of C3 were found in 5 of 12 dextran reactors (JOHNSON and LAURELL 1974). The latter data may suggest either direct activation by dextran of the alternate pathway, or activation of the classical pathway by immune complexes.

The question of the elicitory role of impurities in drug allergy has always to be considered (DE WECK 1969). In the case of dextran, we have used various immunologic methods to study this problem (RICHTER 1970; HEDIN et al. 1976; HEDIN 1977; HEDIN and RICHTER 1977; RING et al. 1977a). We conclude that in severe reactions, contaminants do not play a causal role, since: (1) the reactions start after infusion of a few drops only; (2) no batch dependence is observed; (3) no contamination with pyrogens is found; and (4) the immunologic findings incriminate the dextran molecule itself as elicitor agent. In mild reactions, however, in which the immunologic background is uncertain, the elicitory role of impurities cannot be completely dismissed. To guarantee a dextran of high purity, an immunochemical test based on reversed single radial immunodiffusion (RSRI) and using antisera to non-dextran components of *Leuconostoc mesenteroides* NRRL B 512, was recently described (Hedin and Richter 1977; Richter 1980).

VI. Miscellaneous

The clinical applications of dextran have been reviewed by Grönwall (1957), Gruber (1969), Ingelman et al. (1969), Lutz (1975), and Thorén (1978). For some pharmacologic and biologic effects of dextran, see the following literature: hemostasis and coagulation (Bygdeman and Eliasson 1967; Åberg et al. 1977; Alexander 1978), red cell aggregation (Thorsén and Hint 1950; Richter 1966), enzymatic degradation in tissues (Ammon 1963), intravascular persistence (Arturson and Wallenius 1964), and kidney function (Matheson 1966; Giromini et al. 1967). Anaphylactoid reactions to dextran occur regularly in rats (Vorhees et al. 1951) and are probably due to release of vasoactive mediators in this species, mediated via plasma enzyme systems (West 1977; Briseid et al. 1978).

E. Gelatin Derivatives

I. Physicochemical and Pharmaceutical Aspects

Gelatin is prepared from animal tissues rich in collagen, e.g., skin, cartilage, and bones. The collagen molecule is a rigid rod of molecular weight 300,000 daltons. It is a fibrous protein, composed of three peptide chains, arranged in a helical fashion (Lundsgaard-Hansen et al. 1969). Hydrolysis of collagen yields crude gelatin as a polymolecular solution of isolated peptide chains, which have a molecular weight of about 100,000. In contrast to other proteins, gelatin contains mainly proline, hydroxyproline, lysine, and alanine. Aromatic amino acids such as tyrosine and tryptophan are present in very small amounts, if at all (Schwick and Heide 1969). At room temperature, native gelatin forms a rigid gel. To be clinically useful, gelatin therefore has to be modified. Three types of preparations are commercially available as infusion solutions: (1) Plasmagel, Neoplasmagel, and Physiogel are modified fluid gelatin derivatives prepared by succinylation of gelatin; (2) Haemaccel is a gelatin derivative composed of peptide chains of $\bar{M}_w$ 12,000–15,000 daltons cross-linked with hexamethylene diisocyanate (urea bridges); (3) Gelifundol represents a third type of derivative, oxypolygelatin, which is gelatin cross-linked by glyoxal and subsequently degraded by oxidation and heating. The average molecular weight, $\bar{M}_w$, of all these preparations varies between 30,000 and 35,000 daltons. The concentration of colloid is 3.0%–5.5% with a pH of 7.0–7.25.

II. Immunochemistry and Immunology

Early studies indicated that gelatin was not immunogenic (Boyd 1956). Use of more sensitive methods, e.g., passive hemagglutination, showed, however, that gelatin may induce formation of specific antibodies in humans (Maurer 1960). The cause of the weak immunogenicity of gelatin was shown to be the absence or scarcity of aromatic amino acids, as demonstrated by Sela and Arnon (1960). These

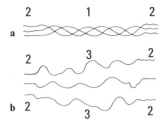

Fig. 4. Localization of three different types of antigenic determinants in native collagen (**a**) and denatured collagen, i.e., gelatin (**b**): (*1*) helical, conformation dependent; (*2*) terminal, non-helical, conformation independent, low cross-reactivity; (*3*) central, exposed upon denaturation, conformation independent, high cross-reactivity. (BEIL et al. 1973)

authors substituted gelatin with tyrosine and were able to show that introduction of only 2% of this amino acid increased the immunogenicity of gelatin considerably. The clinical gelatin preparations used today appear to be nonimmunogenic in humans (MAURER and LEBOVITZ 1956; PICCININO and DI STASIO 1963).

Recent extensive research on the immunogenicity of collagen has been conducted by TIMPL and collaborators (TIMPL et al. 1968; BEIL et al. 1973; HAHN et al. 1975; WICK et al. 1975; BECKER et al. 1976; WICK et al. 1976). It can be shown that the distinct structural features of helical native and non-helical denatured collagen, i.e., gelatin, are reflected by three different types of antigenic determinants. As shown in Fig. 4, the conformation-dependent determinant resides in the helical part of native collagen. The terminal regions of native collagen harbour non-helical, conformation-independent determinants. Upon denaturation of collagen, a new distinct determinant is revealed which is also conformation independent. Apparently, for degraded and cross-linked gelatin preparations, the central antigenic determinants are of greatest interest, especially in view of the fact that antibodies to central antigenic determinants exhibited strong interspecies cross-reactions (TIMPL et al. 1968; BEIL et al. 1973). The presence of central determinants in gelatin offers the theoretical possibility of interaction with preformed gelatin-reactive antibodies.

Naturally occurring gelatin-reactive antibodies have been found in sera of different animal species and in humans (MAURER 1954a, b, 1958, 1960). Horse, dog, pig, monkey, guinea pig, cat, and rat are species in which such antibodies could be demonstrated, whereas they were absent in sera of cattle, chicken, sheep, rabbit, crab, and shark. In humans, preformed gelatin-reactive antibodies occurred in individuals who had never been injected with gelatin derivatives and were especially abundant in patients with rheumatoid arthritis and degenerative joint diseases (MAURER 1960; see Table 4). In this connection, the demonstration of antibody-like cold insoluble globulin with gelatin-binding properties in humans must also be taken into consideration (DESSAU et al. 1978). Cold insoluble globulin has been shown to be identical with fibronectin, a glycoprotein normally found in plasma and on certain cell surfaces (FURIE et al. 1980).

Recently, interesting results have been obtained in a comparative study on the immunogenicity of gelatin and the three types of clinically used gelatin derivatives (SONNEBORN et al. 1978). In rabbits and guinea pigs, marked humoral immune re-

Table 4. Preformed precipitating gelatin-reactive antibodies in sera of normal human subjects and patients with rheumatoid arthritis and degenerative joint diseases. (MAURER 1960)

Group	Subjects	Subjects with antibody N in serum (%)			
		0–4.9 µg/ml	5.0–9.9 µg/ml	10.0–14.9 µg/ml	>15.0 µg/ml
Normal subjects	113	23.9	41.6	20.4	14.2
Rheumatoid arthritis	97	30.9	12.4	29.9	26.8
Degenerative joint diseases	29	6.9	6.9	34.5	51.7

sponses were obtained with diisocyanate cross-linked gelatin (Haemaccel) and modified fluid gelatin (Plasmagel) whereas gelatin and oxypolygelatin (Gelifundol) induced weak responses. Similar results were obtained in corresponding anaphylactic shock experiments. The antibodies induced by Haemaccel and Plasmagel were to a large extent specific for the immunizing antigen. This indicates that new antigenic determinants have been generated by introduction of the cross-linking substituents. The results of SONNEBORN et al. (1978) are in contrast to earlier work in which no antibody response was obtained in rabbits and guineapigs, following immunization with Haemaccel (SCHWICK and HEIDE 1969). The differences are probably explained by differences in the immunization schemes used.

III. Clinical Aspects

All three types of chemically modified gelatin derivatives have the potential to elicit anaphylactoid reactions (BORTOLUZZI et al. 1967; MEISEL and ZÖCKLER 1971; LÖDING and LAWIN 1972; MÜLLER and DIETZEL 1972; LUND 1973; LANGREHR et al. 1975; NEUMANN 1975, RING et al. 1975 b; SCHÖNING and KOCH 1975; WISBORG 1975; RING and MESSMER 1976; TSUJI et al. 1976; SCHÖNING et al. 1982). SCHÖNING and KOCH (1975) found no correlation of the frequency of side effects in orthopedic patients to age or general surgical risk. RING (1978 a) described seven cases of adverse reactions to gelatin derivatives and found no association with specified types of disease. Similar findings were reported by TSCHIRREN et al. (1973/1974), who registered 14 allergic episodes with Physiogel; 10 of these occurred during general anesthesia and 4 in non-anesthetized patients. In contrast, SCHMIDT and PFLÜGER (1971) and SCHMIDT and RIEBER (1980) observed preferential association of reactions with malignomas and arterial occlusive disease upon infusion of oxypolygelatin. Predominance of skin manifestations was a characteristic of these reactions. SCHÖNING and KOCH (1975) and SCHMIDT and RIEBER (1980) found that the preferred sites for skin eruptions were thorax, neck, head, and upper extremities. The efflorescences consisted of urticarial wheals and erythema, either in patches or as flush.

Anaphylactoid reactions to gelatin preparations usually occur in the initial phase of the infusion, but reactions starting after infusion of the second or third unit have also been reported (TSCHIRREN et al. 1973/1974; LUNDSGAARD-HANSEN and TSCHIRREN 1980).

It is generally accepted that gelatin derivatives are endowed with low immunogenicity, but occasional sensitization may occur. One such case has been described by BENBUNAN et al. (1976). A leukemic patient had inadvertently been given Plasmagel subcutaneously in minute amounts together with incomplete Freund's adjuvant. This resulted in formation of specific precipitating antibodies and subsequent intravenous infusion of Plasmagel led to a severe anaphylactic shock.

No atopic background is usually demonstrable in patients experiencing anaphylactoid reactions to gelatin derivatives. RING (1978a) found no history of allergy in six of seven patients with reactions of grade II to III.

IV. Results of Diagnostic Tests

1. Skin Tests

RING (1978a) demonstrated positive immediate skin reactions in three of seven reactors to gelatin derivatives upon intradermal injection of 1:10 or 1:100 dilutions of Haemaccel and Gelifundol. TSCHIRREN et al. (1973/1974) reported positive scratch and intracutaneous tests in 5 of 14 reactors to Physiogel. In a case of Haemaccel reaction, presenting with urticaria, respiratory distress, and edema of the face, a positive skin test was obtained with a 1:10,000 dilution of Haemaccel (LUND 1973). To summarize, positive skin reactions are reported in less than half of patients with anaphylactoid reactions to gelatin preparations.

2. Specific Antibodies

No specific IgE antibodies have been demonstrable in sera of reactors to gelatin preparations (RING 1978a) and total IgE levels were within the normal range. Hemagglutinating gelatin-reactive antibodies (IgG, IgA, and IgM classes) could be demonstrated both in reactors and non-reactors to gelatin derivatives (RICHTER et al. 1977). The highest titer, 1:320, was encountered in a patient with a grade III reaction to Haemaccel. Specific precipitating antibodies could be detected in a patient who had received Plasmagel inadvertently in minute amounts together with incomplete Freund's adjuvant subcutaneously (BENBUNAN et al. 1976). Subsequent intravenous infusion of Plasmagel led to a severe anaphylactic reaction.

3. Lymphocyte Transformation Test

This test was negative in patients who had experienced anaphylactoid reactions to gelatin derivatives, indicating absence of specific cell-mediated hypersensitivity (RING 1978a). Further, the T- and B-cell functions were considered normal as measured by stimulation of the lymphocytes with phytohemagglutinin and pokeweed mitogen.

V. Potential Pathomechanisms

LORENZ and co-workers (1972) have developed a sensitive and specific method for determination of plasma histamine levels and have provided evidence in extensive studies that gelatin preparations are capable of releasing histamine upon intravenous infusion in dogs and humans (MESSMER et al. 1970; LORENZ 1975; LORENZ et al. 1974, 1976, 1978). In patients with anaphylactoid reactions they could establish a positive correlation between severity of symptoms and plasma histamine levels. Whereas concentrations of 8 ng/ml were associated with anaphylactoid symptoms, no such symptoms were seen with concentrations below 2 ng/ml. Since the causal role of released histamine for elicitation of anaphylactoid symptoms to gelatin derivatives was considered highly probable, prophylaxis by use of H_1 and H_2 receptor blockers was proposed (LORENZ et al. 1977). A first application of this measure in a randomized controlled single-blind trial in 50 volunteers showed that anaphylactoid reactions following rapid infusion of Haemaccel could be prevented ($P < 0.05$). Furthermore, by reducing the amount of crosslinking reagent during manufacture, a preparation giving only minor adverse reactions was obtained (SCHÖNING and LORENZ 1981).

No evidence has been found for a causal role of IgE class antibodies in anaphylactoid reactions to gelatin derivatives (RING 1978a). Preformed gelatin-reactive antibodies of IgG, IGA, and IgM classes were, however, demonstrable in reactors as was a transient neutralization of antibodies following infusion of gelatin preparations. This implies that clinically used gelatin derivatives may have specific antigenic or haptenic properties. Consequently, it is feasible that formation of specific immune complexes may be induced in connection with infusion of modified gelatin preparations. One of the theoretically possible pathomechanisms is therefore elicitation of the anaphylactoid reaction via immune complexes with subsequent release of mediators–so-called aggregate anaphylaxis (BECKER and AUSTEN 1976). The occurrence of both a high incidence of gelatin-reactive antibodies in patients with degenerative joint diseases (MAURER 1960) and the high rate of anaphylactoid reactions to modified gelatin reported in orthopedic patients (SCHÖNING and KOCH 1975) is in accord with such a hypothesis. With regard to Haemaccel, no correlation was found between the collagen binding capacity of sera of reactors and occurrence of adverse reactions (ADELMANN-GRILL and SCHÖNING 1981). No indications for activation of the complement system were found in four reactors to gelatin derivatives (RING 1978a).

The role of impurities in elicitation of anaphylactoid reactions to modified fluid gelatin has been discussed by LUNDSGAARD-HANSEN and TSCHIRREN (1978, 1980). They point out that the accumulations of reactions, which they observed, could be due to variations in contaminant levels between batches. The fact that a number of the severe reactions were elicited only after infusion of the second or third unit is in favor of the view that the gelatin derivative itself is not the responsible agent.

In conclusion, different pathomechanisms can be envisaged. The observed histamine release may either be due to a direct action of some component of the gelatin preparation on mast cells and basophils, or be a consequence of formation of specific immune complexes.

VI. Miscellaneous

The clinical applications of gelatin derivatives have been reviewed by GRUBER (1969), LUNDSGAARD-HANSEN et al. (1969), LUTZ (1975), and LUNDSGAARD-HAN-

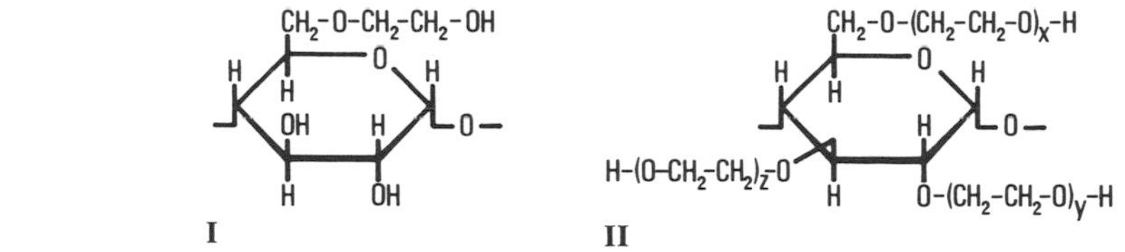

Fig. 5. Formula I shows the formerly widely accepted structure for a glucose residue in hydroxyethylstarch, substituted only at C-6. Formula II represents a revised structure for a glucose residue carrying additional substituents at C-2 and C-3. (Banks et al. 1973)

Sen and Tschirren (1978). For particular pharmacologic and biologic effects of gelatin derivatives, see the following literature: red cell aggregation (Thorsén and Hint 1950) and kidney function (Griem et al. 1964a, b, c; Cottier et al. 1966).

F. Hydroxyethylstarch

I. Physicochemical and Pharmaceutical Aspects

Hydroxyethylstarch (HES) is prepared from the amylopectin of waxy maize starch by hydrolysis and subsequent treatment with ethylene oxide. Amylopectin is a branched polyglucose composed of chains of α 1–4 linked glucose residues, to which a number of branches are attached by α 1–6 linkages (Aspinall 1970). When soluble amylopectin is intravenously injected into animals, it is rapidly degraded by α-amylase and is therefore unsuitable as a plasma substitute. For this reason Wiedersheim (1957) suggested substitution of amylopectin with hydroxyethyl groups to slow down the action of amylase and so extend its persistence in the circulation. He showed that such HES preparations had useful properties as plasma expanders and were relatively nontoxic. These results were subsequently confirmed and extended (Thompson et al. 1962, 1964, 1970).

The substitution pattern is more complex than suggested by the designation hydroxyethylstarch, since individual glucose units may carry one, two, or three substituents and since the length of an individual substituent may exceed that of a hydroxyethyl group (Banks et al. 1973; Fig. 5). It is possible to prepare HES of different average molecular weights by varying the time of hydrolysis and to control persistence time in the circulation by varying the degree of substitution. The latter indicates the number of substituents in relation to the number of glucose units; e.g., a degree of substitution of 0.7 means that seven out of ten glucose units carry hydroxyethyl groups.

Three kinds of HES preparations are at present used clinically. One resembles dextran 70 in duration and magnitude of volume replacement. $\bar{M}_w$ is 450,000 daltons and the degree of substitution is 0.75 (Plasmatonin, Plasmasteril, Volex). These preparations are available as 6% solutions in 0.9% saline. HES solutions have been reported to possess high stability and to remain free of visible precipitates after months of shaking and temperature cycling (Lee-Benner and Walton 1965). Recently two other HES preparations of $\bar{M}_w$ 40,000 daltons (Expafusin, 6%) and $\bar{M}_w$ 200,000 daltons (Haes-Steril, 10%) have been introduced. The degree of substitution is 0.50–0.55.

II. Immunochemistry and Immunology

HES represents a highly branched bush-like molecule composed of hydroxyethyl-ated glucose units linked together by α 1–4 bonds with side chains attached to the main chains by α 1–6 linkages. Experimental results have shown that HES is a poor immunogen. Precipitating antibodies could be demonstrated in humans neither after intravenous infusion of large doses (Brickmann et al. 1966) nor following immunization with milligram doses of clinically used HES preparations (Maurer and Berardinelli 1968). The latter workers also showed that no specific antibody formation could be induced in guinea pigs and rabbits following immunization with clinically used HES preparations or a high molecular weight HES fraction. When HES is covalently coupled to protein, however, specific antibodies to this polysaccharide could be induced in rabbits following immunization with such conjugates (Richter and de Belder 1976). In contrast, non-hydroxyethylated starch is nonimmunogenic (Allen and Kabat 1957; Sorg et al. 1970), even after conjugation to protein (Richter and de Belder 1976). This implies that introduction of hydroxyethyl groups has conferred immunogenicity to the starch molecule. The anti-HES antibodies gave specific precipitates with clinical HES (Volex) or with HES fractions of $\bar{M}_w$ 26,600–1,920,000 daltons in gel diffusion tests, whereas no precipitates were obtained with amylopectin and glycogen. Results of these experiments indicate that the antigenic determinants of HES most probably consist of short sequences of hydroxyethylated glucose units. From its physicochemical properties HES would be expected to belong to the group of thymus-independent antigens (Andersson and Blomgren 1971; Bach 1976).

Naturally occurring HES-reactive antibodies have been shown to occur in sera of normal human subjects (Richter et al. 1977). Using passive hemagglutination, preformed HES-reactive antibodies of low titer could be demonstrated in 26% of sera of 268 normal human subjects. Highest titers, comprising 1% of the sera tested, ranged from 1:4 to 1:8 (Ring and Richter 1980).

III. Clinical Aspects

The clinical symptoms of anaphylactoid reactions observed in connection with HES infusions comprise skin eruptions and cardiovascular changes (Metcalf et al. 1970; Schöning and Koch 1975; Ring et al. 1976; Matthiessen et al. 1977/1978; Ring 1978 a; Beez and Dietl 1979). In a report on eight cases the symptoms were restricted to the site of infusion and the skin in three patients, while five responded with hemodynamic changes (Ring et al. 1976). Tachycardia up to 150 beats/min and hypotension with decrease of systolic pressure by 20 mmHg down to unmeasurable values were observed in six and four patients respectively. One nonanesthetized patient developed anaphylactoid shock after infusion of 10 ml HES solution; the patient recovered after treatment with 500 mg intravenous prednisolone. It is of interest that in four patients immediate local pain with subsequent inflammatory swelling and redness of the infused vein was observed. This symptom is seen only rarely in reactions to other plasma substitutes. Six reactions occurred after infusion of only small amounts, 10–100 ml HES. No sex prevalence was noted. Six of the eight patients were under general anesthesia and two were premedicated, but conscious. A history of allergy was present in four cases.

In another study on 150 orthopedic patients, four anaphylactoid reactions to HES preceding anesthesia were described (SCHÖNING and KOCH 1975). In all cases, macular erythema was the only symptom observed, with localization on the neck, shoulders, and anterior thorax. In one case, large symmetric maculae were found over the parotid glands, persisting for more than 35 min. No parotid swelling was present. In the other cases, the erythema disappeared after 6–8 min. MATTHIESSEN et al. (1977/1978) reported on a severe anaphylactoid reaction to HES in a 74-year-old man with occlusive arterial disease. Extensive flush, tachycardia, and protracted hypotension, which could be reversed only after 40 min intensive therapy, was seen. No pulmonary symptoms were registered.

IV. Results of Diagnostic Tests

1. Skin Tests

Upon intradermal injection of 0.05 ml undiluted clinical HES solution, positive immediate skin reactions were observed in five of eight reactors to HES, tested between 10 days and 2 months after the reaction (RING et al. 1976). Three of these patients, who exhibited grade II–III reactions also showed positive skin tests with a 1 : 10 dilution and two with a 1 : 100 dilution of clinical HES solution. These results indicate that skin tests may be of a certain diagnostic value for severe HES reactions.

2. Specific Antibodies

In agar gel double diffusion tests, no precipitating antibodies against HES were detected in sera of eight patients with anaphylactoid reactions to HES (RING et al. 1976). No tests with more sensitive techniques have been performed.

3. Lymphocyte Transformation Test

Negative results were obtained in this test after specific antigenic stimulation of lymphocytes from reactors to HES (RING et al. 1976). Furthermore, the T- and B-cell functions were considered normal, as measured by stimulation of the lymphocytes with phytohemagglutinin and pokeweed mitogen.

V. Potential Pathomechanisms

The pathomechanism of HES-induced anaphylactoid reactions is unknown. Since HES has been in general clinical use for a comparatively short time, only a few data are available for critical evaluation of the triggering mechanisms of adverse reactions. From the physicochemical properties of HES a few possible mechanisms may, however, be visualized. Comparing the occurrence in humans of preformed antibodies reactive with plasma substitutes, it is evident that both titers and frequency are highest for gelatin, intermediate for dextran, and lowest for HES. In this connection, it is interesting to note that upon rapid infusion of HES into hu-

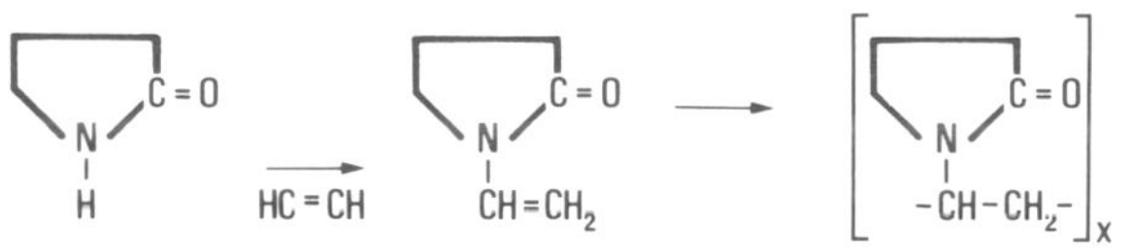

Fig. 6. Structure of pyrrolidone (I) and polymerization of vinylpyrrolidone (II) to polyvinyl-pyrrolidone (III)

man volunteers no histamine release was seen (Lorenz et al. 1975), whereas after rapid infusion of gelatin, increased plasma histamine levels were frequently observed (Lorenz et al. 1976). In comparable experiments dextran occupied an intermediate position. Considering the relative insignificance of HES-reactive antibodies and the absence of histamine release upon rapid infusion in humans, direct activation of the plasma enzyme systems (complement, kallikrein-kinin) by HES in a few predisposed individuals could be envisaged as possible pathogenetic factors. In contrast to clinical dextran, clinical HES preparations ($\bar{M}_w$ 450,000 daltons) can activate the alternative pathway of complement in vitro (Hedin unpublished). This fact, together with indications of corresponding in vivo activation in some HES reactors (Ring et al. 1976), is in favor of the view that complement activation via the alternate pathway may be the initiating step in triggering HES reactions. For review of potential pathomechanisms, see also Seidemann (1979).

VI. Miscellaneous

The clinical applications of HES have been reviewed by Lutz (1975) and Thompson (1978). For particular pharmacologic and biologic effects of HES see the following literature: hemostasis and coagulation (Alexander 1978), intravascular persistence in humans (Thompson et al. 1970; Boon et al. 1976), and storage in animals (Lindblad and Falk 1976).

G. Polyvinylpyrrolidone

Polyvinylpyrrolidone (PVP) was widely used during World War II and the Korean War as a plasma expander. Subsequently, PVP was extensively studied and it was found that this synthetic water-soluble polymer cannot be broken down in the body. Thus it is used today only to a limited extent. Since this substance illustrates the problems encountered in the use of completely synthetic colloids as plasma expanders, a short survey, mainly of historical interest, will be presented.

I. Physicochemical and Pharmaceutical Aspects

PVP is a completely synthetic macromolecule, produced by polymerization of vinylpyrrolidone (Fig. 6). It was introduced by Hecht and Weese (1943) as a plasma substitute. Its thread-like molecules are highly water soluble and form viscous solutions, which can be sterilized and are stable for many years. Preparations for-

Table 5. Physicochemical data of the most important polyvinylpyrrolidone preparations discussed in the literature. (GRUBER 1969)

Trade name	Concentration (%)	$\bar{M}_w$	Molecular weight distribution		Manufacturer
			10% Low molecular fraction	10% Top fraction	
Periston	4	25,000	4,100	189,000	Bayer, Leverkusen
Periston-N	6	~12,000			Bayer, Leverkusen
Neo Compensan					Heilmittelwerke, Vienna
Hämodyn,	4	50,000			Bayer, Leverkusen
Kollidan					BASF, Ludwigshafen
Plasgen	3.5	50,000	9,600	127,000	Kyorin, Tokyo
Plasgen-L	6	17,000			Kyorin, Tokyo
Isoplasma	4				Vifor, Geneva
Subtosan	3.5	50,000			Specia, Paris
Parenteral P	3.5	40,000			Serag-Wiessner, Naila, Munich
Compensan	4	30,000			Heilmittelwerke, Vienna
Kollosteril	3.5	30,000			Dr. Fresenius, Bad Homburg
Elo Compen	4	24,500			Leopold, Graz

merly used as expanders had $\bar{M}_w$ between 25,000 and 50,000 daltons, as shown in Table 5. The concentration of colloid in such solutions is 3.5%–4.0%. The colloid is dissolved in a balanced electrolyte solution. Trade names of PVP preparations are given in Table 5.

II. Immunochemistry and Immunology

The linear molecules of PVP resemble those of other repetitive polymers like dextrans, mannans, levans, etc. As antigens, many of such polymers are thymus-independent antigens. It was shown by GILL and KUNZ (1968) that PVP consistently elicited a moderate amount of antibody upon immunization of rabbits, using doses between 10 and 100 µg. In mice, PVP has been shown to produce a thymus-independent humoral antibody response (ANDERSSON 1969; ANDERSSON and BLOMGREN 1971). It is probable that the antigenic determinants comprise sequences on the molecular chain consisting of 3–6 vinylpyrrolidone residues.

III. Miscellaneous

RAVIN et al. (1952) used PVP labeled with ^{131}I and showed that molecules of $\bar{M}_w$ 40,000 daltons or less can be found in the tissues; studies by HECHT and SCHOLTAN (1959) with the newer PVP preparation of $\bar{M}_w$ 25,000 daltons indicate that about 20% is retained in the body. In animals and humans, the reticuloendothelial system and other tissues store PVP not eliminated by the kidney and may retain it for several years (Bargmann 1947; Ammon and Braunschmidt 1949; Hüsselmann 1952; Altemeier et al. 1954; Heckner and Gehlmann 1956; Upham et al. 1956; Towers 1957). Many authors regard the tissue deposition of PVP as irreversible. Some clinical findings are in accord with this view. A papular exanthema that remained unaltered for 4 years was observed by Dupont and Lachapelle (1964). It was caused by PVP, injected as plasma substitute. Lachapelle (1966) also reported a second case with skin storage of PVP. Similarly, a storage disease, with papular skin manifestations was observed following inadvertent repeated injections of small doses of high molecular weight PVP, used as a retarding medium (Reske-Nielsen et al. 1976). Storage of PVP in the kidneys has been reported by Grünfeld et al. (1968). Considerable interest was raised when animal experiments showed that Periston had oncogenic properties in animals (Hueper 1957; Lusky and Nelson 1957). Hueper (1961) could not, however, duplicate his experiments later. No evidence exists that PVP has ever caused a carcinoma in humans (Lindner 1960). Since PVP has no advantages over gelatin derivatives and dextran and because a considerable fraction is permanently stored, most clinicians no longer use PVP preparations.

H. Parenteral Nutrition

I. General Aspects

Sugars, amino acids, and fat emulsions are nowadays used clinically either separately or in suitable combinations for the purpose of intravenous feeding. When all nutrients absorbed from ordinary oral food are given by the intravenous route, this is designated "complete intravenous feeding". It can be given either via a peripheral or a central catheter, owing to the vein sparing effect of fat emulsions. According to Dudrick et al. (1968, 1969) the energy requirements may also be adequately provided by glucose and amino acids with a concomitant supply of all other nutrients, but no fat. Because of the hypertonic solutions required such intravenous feeding can be performed only via a central vein catheter.

Kausch (1911) first infused glucose for nutrition after surgical procedures, and Henriques and Andersen injected hydrolyzed protein into animals in 1913. Fat was infused experimentally in 1916 by Murlin and Riche and was used in humans following the results of Yamakawa's work in 1920. Early literature on parenteral nutrition has been documented by Geyer (1960) and more recent accounts have been given by Lee (1974), Zumtobel (1974), Ghadimi (1975), Fischer (1976), and Shenkin and Wretlind (1978).

Anaphylactoid reactions to sugars, amino acids, and fat emulsions are rare. With regard to sugars, the causal role of macromolecular contaminants in eliciting such reactions has been demonstrated in some cases. No anaphylactic shock due to amino acid mixtures has apparently been reported in the literature, but flush and urticaria may occur occasionally. For fat emulsions adverse reactions are dependent on their composition. Some emulsifiers may give rise to antibody formation and subsequently be responsible for development of allergic reactions.

II. Sugars

Infusion solutions containing sugars (monosaccharides) are generally well tolerated when they are administered at adequate concentrations and rates of infusion. In rare instances, anaphylactoid and anaphylactic reactions have been observed in connection with intravenous infusion of various sugars or sugar alcohols. The neutral, low molecular weight monosaccharides themselves have a low immunogenic potential. It is, however, known that antibodies specific for certain monosaccharides can be raised following immunization with protein–sugar conjugates (LANDSTEINER 1962). The raw material used for production of clinically employed monosaccharides often contains traces of macromolecular antigenic contaminants, which may not be completely eliminated during the manufacturing and purification process. Such contaminants are potential elicitors of anaphylactoid symptoms produced by sugar solutions in a few predisposed individuals.

1. Glucose

Adverse reactions associated with glucose injections have been reported in Bulgaria (PETKOV and NANKOW 1974). Analysis of the solutions revealed that 10 of 12 batches contained nitrogen. The authors conclude that the anaphylactoid reactions may be explained by the presence of protein contaminants.

PANDIT et al. (1976) have determined the incidence of adverse reactions to various intravenous fluids in a prospective study in India. The incidence of fever, rigors, and itching was 5.8% ($n = 138$) and 15.2% ($n = 59$) for glucose and glucose with saline in orthopedic patients. The corresponding incidence, expressed in terms of units infused, was 2.5% and 9%. Since fever and rigors were the predominant symptoms they were considered to be attributable to pyrogens or bacterial contamination.

2. Galactose

One case of anaphylactic shock has been reported in connection with intravenous infusion of galactose, given for examination of liver function (RUD 1968 a, b; CARPENTER 1968). Immediately after completed infusion of 67 ml 30% galactose solution infused over 3–4 min the patient developed a severe shock state. He complained of a burning sensation in his face and abdominal pains. Directly afterwards he became unconscious with impalpable pulse, apnea, and involuntary defecation and micturition. Intramuscular adrenaline and artificial respiration controlled the situation to some extent, but the patient developed acute lung edema. Only after aspiration of 1.5–2 l viscous bronchial secretion, as well as hyperbaric ventilation with oxygen, was his condition largely corrected. Upon examination, the galactose solution was found to be sterile and pyrogen free. Chromatography showed only one peak, corresponding to galactose. Plastic infusion sets of similar kind have repeatedly been used on the patient without reaction. Galactose from the same batch has been given to other patients without side effects. Some time after the incident, the patient received intradermal injections of 0.1 ml isotonic solutions of galactose from four different manufacturers. He reacted strongly positively to them all.

Table 6. Examples of α 1–6 glucan contaminant levels of sugars of varying provenience, estimated by reversed single radial immunodiffusion (RSRI). (RICHTER unpublished)

Type of sugar	α 1–6 Glucan	
	RSRI score	Parts/10^6
Sucrose, household, Denmark	0	0–6
Sucrose, United States	+	100
Sucrose, Roumania	0	0–6
Sucrose, Tate and Lyle, United Kingdom	+	75
Sucrose, Trinidad	+	400
Sucrose, Hopkins and Williams, United Kingdom	+	150
Granulated cane sugar, United States	+	400
Saccharose, purest, Merck, Germany	+	400
Dextrose, *USP*, United States	0	0–6
Dextrose, J.T. Baker, United Kingdom	0	0–6
D-Fructose, United States	+	400
Fructose, Kotka, Finland	0	0–6

Isotonic solutions of sodium chloride and glucose have no reaction. It seems that the patient exhibits a true hypersensitivity to galactose, but since galactose should be considered a monovalent hapten, some aberrant elicitation mechanism has to be called upon to explain this incident.

3. Invertose

A few cases of mild anaphylactoid reactions have been reported following infusion of invertose in Norway (LUNDE 1974). In Sweden, 13 incidents were reported during a 7-month period in 1973 (RICHTER et al. 1976). This corresponds to an incidence of 1 in 31,000 units infused. The symptoms comprised flushing, erythema, urticaria, dyspnea, fever, lumbar pain, and edema at the injection site. It is known that sucrose contains various polysaccharides as trace impurities. These comprise predominantly dextrans, but also levan, hemicellulose, and starch (NEILL et al. 1939; IMRIE and TILBURY 1972). Since impurities of this type were suspected as elicitors of the anaphylactoid reactions to invertose, the infusion solutions having caused reactions were tested for α 1–6 glucans by passive cutaneous anaphylaxis in guinea pigs and by a specially developed screen test based on reversed single radial immunodiffusion (RSRI). All sugar batches connected with reactions were found positive in these tests, which permits one to detect polysaccharides of the α 1–6 glucan type in concentrations exceeding 10 parts/10^6. Contaminant levels of various commercially available sucrose preparations are given in Table 6. The contaminants could be isolated from invert sugar solutions implicated in anaphylactoid reactions and structural analysis confirmed the presence of α 1–6 linked glucan, i.e., native dextran, with few branches and a molecular weight of $10–100 \times 10^6$ daltons (Fig. 7). This has been confirmed by BERGE et al. (1976).

Results strongly indicate a causal role for macromolecular contaminants as elicitors of anaphylactoid reactions to invertose solutions (RICHTER et al. 1976).

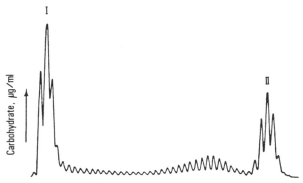

Fig. 7. Gel chromatographic detection of high molecular weight polysaccharides in invert sugar solutions implicated in anaphylactoid reactions in humans. Autoanalyzer tracing of the eluate from gel chromatography of ultrafiltrated residue from invert sugar solution. Eluted fractions were assayed for carbohydrate, using the anthrone reaction. The tracing demonstrates that the carbohydrate material in the sample consists of three main components. Peak I (56%) represents very high molecular weight material (MW > 10×10^6 daltons), since it is excluded from the gel matrix. Peak II (22%) corresponds to the sugars remaining in the sample. The broad band between these peaks very likely represents degraded material produced during inversion, i.e., acid hydrolysis (pH 1.5, 125 min, 71°–73 °C). (RICHTER et al. 1976)

Therefore a mandatory RSRI purity test for the sucrose raw material was introduced to prevent adverse reactions. This test procedure was incorporated into the PHARMACOPOEA NORDICA (1976). Among 1,636 samples of sucrose tested during one year, 272 gave positive results. The latter samples were found to contain α 1–6 glucans in concentrations of 12–400 µg/g sucrose and were rejected as raw material for invertose. Introduction of this control procedure reduced the frequency of reported reactions in Sweden about 20-fold to 1 in 575,000 units infused, as estimated during a 2-year period. It should be mentioned that symptoms began after infusion of 10–100 ml with RSRI positive invertose solutions. In the few mild reactions reported after introduction of the RSRI test symptoms appear only after infusion of more than 1 l solution. This indicates an inverse relationship between content of contaminants and time of onset of symptoms after the start of the infusion.

4. Mannitol

Rarely, anaphylactoid reactions following infusions of mannitol may also occur. This is illustrated by a case reported by SPAETH et al. (1967). A 65-year-old woman with glaucoma received a 20% solution of mannitol. About 3 min after starting the infusion the patient began to sneeze violently, her nose was running, and breathing became difficult; 3 min later, she became extremely anxious, dyspneic, cyanotic, and lost consciousness. Four large wheals developed on her chest. After discontinuation of the mannitol infusion, epinephrine was injected subcutaneously and the reaction slowly came under control. The patient had never to her knowledge received mannitol before. Skin tests with mannitol performed two months later were positive and suggested an immediate hypersensitivity. Since mannitol, like galactose, should be considered as a monovalent hapten, it seems unlikely that the reaction was mediated by specific antibodies. Some aberrant elicitation mechanism such as activation of plasma enzyme systems would thus be required to explain this incident.

III. Amino Acids

The use of L-amino acids constitutes part of the therapeutic measure of parenteral nutrition, which also includes fat emulsions and carbohydrates, i.e., sugars. Only with mixtures of amino acids is it possible to provide physiologic intravenous protein feeding. The modern use of intravenous amino acid nutrition was initiated by ELMAN (1937), following studies on casein hydrolyzates.

1. Physicochemical and Pharmaceutical Aspects

The two general types of amino acid preparations for intravenous feeding are protein hydrolyzates and mixtures of crystalline amino acids. Examples of raw material for preparation of protein hydrolyzates by enzymatic, acid, or other hydrolysis are casein and fibrin. One enzymatic casein hydrolyzate which has been widely used in Europe is Aminosol. This preparation is produced by a special method including dialysis, by which all the high molecular weight peptides and other substances, which might cause allergic reactions are removed. It contains about 67% free amino acids and 37% low molecular weight peptides (WRETLIND 1947).

Mixtures of crystalline amino acids offer the advantage of flexibility in composition. SHOHL and BLACKFAN (1940) first used a complete mixture of crystalline amino acids for parenteral nutrition. Since then, intravenous feeding with mixtures of crystalline amino acids has been extensively studied. Examples of commercially available amino acid mixtures are: Amigen, Aminosol, Trophysan, Neo-Aminosol, Freamine, Aminoplasmal. They contain 3.3%–10% amino acids. The pH of a 10% Aminosol solution is 5.0.

2. Adverse Reactions, Including Potential Pathomechanisms

Untoward reactions are considered to be of minor importance as evident from the following statement: "Adverse reactions to amino acid mixtures do not appear to constitute a problem when these materials are properly employed" (SCHINDEL 1977). In rare cases, nausea, flush or transient urticaria have been reported. In general, nausea is attributed to disturbances in electrolyte balance, infections, or too high infusion rate. With regard to mixtures of pure crystalline amino acids, there appears no theoretical reason why they should elicit allergic reactions, apart from the potential risk of traces of macromolecular contaminants. In practice the latter risk seems, however, negligible, since apparently no severe allergic reactions have been reported. In the case of amino acid mixtures prepared from protein hydrolyzates, traces of high molecular weight peptides would seem to present a somewhat greater potential risk. However, even with this type of preparations, no case of anaphylaxis has been reported during many years of clinical use (WRETLIND, personal communication). One factor explaining the absence of severe allergic reactions due to such preparations may be the dialysis step introduced as a safety measure in the manufacturing process.

Table 7. Composition of intravenous fat emulsions. (SHENKIN and WRETLIND 1978)

	Intralipid[a]	Lipiphysan[b]	Lipofundin[c]	Lipofundin S[c]
Soybean oil (g)	100 or 200			100 or 200
Cottonseed oil (g)		150	100	
Egg yolk phospholipids (g)	12			
Soybean lecithin (g)		20		
Soybean phospholipids (g)			7.5	7.5 or 15
Glycerol (g)	25			
Sorbitol (g)		50	50	
Xylitol (g)				50
DL-α-Tocopherol (g)		0.5	0.585	
Distilled water to a volume of (ml)	1,000	1,000	1,000	1,000

[a] Vitrum, Stockholm
[b] Egic, Loiret
[c] Braun, Melsungen; Lipofundin is no longer commercially available

IV. Fat Emulsions

1. Physicochemical and Pharmaceutical Aspects

Fat emulsions for intravenous nutrition (for review see HOLM et al. 1982; GRÜNERT 1982; SHENKIN and WRETLIND 1978; SAILER 1981) are prepared from vegetable oil, finely dispersed in water by an emulsifier, which also stabilizes the emulsion. To obtain isotonicity with the blood sorbitol, xylitol or glycerol is added in low concentrations. Examples of commercial fat emulsions are Intralipid-, Lipiphysan, and Lipofundin-S; for composition see Table 7. The emulsions contain soybean or cottonseed oil. As emulsifiers purified egg yolk, soybean phospholipids or lecithin are used. Recently an emulsion based on safflower oil with a very high content of unsaturated fatty acids and egg yolk emulsifier has been introduced under the trade name Liposyn (WONG and DEITEL 1981). Comparative electron microscopic studies on chylomicrons and Intralipid have been performed (SCHOEFL 1968; see SHENKIN and WRETLIND 1978). It was found that the particle size in Intralipid 10% was about the same as that of chylomicrons, whereas particles in Intralipid 20% were somewhat larger. Pronounced physical similarities exist between fat particles in the modern type of fat emulsions and natural chylomicrons, which have a diameter of 0.10–0.21 µm. In contrast, an earlier emulsion, Lipomul (now withdrawn from the market), from cottonseed oil had particles of a diameter exceeding 6 µm.

2. Immunochemistry and Immunology

In general, lipids are poor immunogens and antibodies against, for example, fatty acids and triglycerides are not known. This is partly due to their low molecular weight and to the difficulty of dispersing them so that potential antigenic determinants may become available. In contrast to proteins, large quantities of lipids are usually required for antibody production. For a recent review of immune reactions of lipids and lipid model membranes, see ALVING (1977). Early results of animal experiments on antibody production upon immunization with fats showed that protein impurities were the immunogenic components (UHLENHUTH and HAENDEL 1910; LANDSTEINER 1962). Occasionally, however, lipids may act as immunogens. Serologically active glycolipids occur in various microorganisms including mycoplasma (KENNY 1975), streptococci (BIRNBAUM-FEINMAN et al. 1973), and treponemas (DUPOUEY 1972). The lipid A component of lipopolysaccharides also belongs to the group of immunogenic lipids (see WESTPHAL 1975; GALANOS et al. 1977). Other examples are cardiolipin, the complex immunogenic phospholipid of tissue extracts which is used as antigen in the Wassermann reaction (PANGBORN 1942), and the antigenic phosphatide fraction or fractions prepared from human tubercle bacilli (ANDERSON et al. 1940). Further, it has been shown that immunogenicity could be conferred on certain lipids simply by mixing them with proteins in vitro. SACHS and KLOPSTOCK (1925) first obtained complement-fixing and flocculating immune sera in rabbits upon injecting cholesterol and lecithin together with serum of a foreign species (*Schleppereffekt*). It is interesting that LEVENE et al. (1927) could confirm immunogenicity of egg lecithin when using commercial preparations, whereas more purified preparations had no distinct immunizing effect. Another way to confer immunogenicity to some lipids is to couple them covalently to proteins (TAKETOMI and YAMAKAWA 1963; ARNON and TEITELBAUM 1974).

3. Clinical Aspects

When given in appropriate dosage and rate of infusion, modern fat emulsions are well tolerated. Reactions are generally rare, minor and easily managed. They can be differentiated into immediate and late (delayed) reactions (MEYLER 1964, 1968). Immediate reactions occur soon after infusion of a few milliliters. The following symptoms are observed: headache, lumbar pain, chest pain, dyspnea, cyanosis, tachycardia, hypotension, occasionally hypertension, chills, fever, oily taste, nausea, vomiting, flush, urticaria, and thrombophlebitis (HALLBERG et al. 1967; HARTMANN 1967; GÄRTNER et al. 1969).

The late reactions, sometimes designated the fat overloading syndrome, develop usually 5–25 days after the beginning of the infusions. In rare cases the interval may be as long as 10 weeks (ALEXANDER and ZIEVEL 1961). The fat overload syndrome was frequently seen with earlier fat emulsions but is no longer observed upon proper use of modern preparations. An exceptional case has been reported in a newborn child with multiple congenital defects (BELIN et al. 1976). Intralipid was tolerated for 4 months, but a severe overload syndrome suddenly developed, which was completely reversible, however. The following symptoms have been observed during the fat overload syndrome: fever, rigors, headache, sore throat, urticaria, excitability, tenderness of the neck, cyanosis, dyspnea, abdominal pain, nausea, vomiting, hyperlipemia, asthenia. In addition, hepatomegaly (WATKIN 1957) with or without impaired liver function, splenomegaly, progressive anemia (LE VEEN et al. 1961), angina pectoris, impaired blood clotting, and thrombocytopenia associated with bleeding preferentially from the gastrointestinal tract have been recorded (MEYLER 1968). Rarely, cholestatic jaundice develops (OLBING et al. 1969; ALLARDYCE 1982). In a few cases, a syndrome with severe, radiologically demonstrable pulmonary circulatory changes resembling disseminated intravascular coagulation has been described (HORISBERGER 1966). Reactions to fat emulsions are reversible following cessation of infusions. Side effects to emulsions prepared from cottonseed oil and soybean oil show a similar clinical picture (MEYLER 1968).

The clinical picture of six adverse reactions associated with the infusion of Lipiphysan prepared from cottonseed oil and soybean lecithin has been extensively described by NICOLAS et al. (1966). In two cases the reaction was observed in connection with the first and in one case after the third infusion. These patients had not received Lipiphysan earlier. Two of the patients had tolerated Lipiphysan earlier, but renewed infusion 10–15 days later provoked adverse reactions. In the sixth case a continuous series of 17 infusions was well tolerated but the unit 18 provoked a reaction. In this series of patients the symptoms corresponded to those described above: chills, flush, headache, episodes of hypo- and hypertension, tachycardia, vomiting, and body temperatures as high as 39.5 °C. All patients recovered from the intolerance reactions. GOULON et al. (1974) have reviewed the clinical data on nine cases of severe late reactions. Eight of these were caused by preparations stabilized with soybean lecithin and one with egg yolk lecithin.

Two severe acute reactions have recently been reported in connection with Intralipid therapy (JELLINEK 1976). A 22-year-old female developed an acute clinical illness resembling hypertensive encephalopathy. Symptoms comprised headache, focal and generalized convulsions, and persistent cortical blindness. Daily minor parietal attacks persisted for several years. In the second case, a 76-year-old male, quadriplegia developed suddenly during Intralipid infusion. After 1 month, the left side remained paralyzed but he had limited use of a spastic right arm and leg. It is concluded that Intralipid may have precipitated acute thromboembolic cerebral vascular disease in these two cases.

4. Incidence

An early cottonseed oil emulsion (Lipomul) caused adverse reactions in about 5% of cases (MEYLER 1960). The symptoms included nausea, vomiting, headache, fever, chills, and chest or back pain. The most frequent reactions consisted of slight rises in temperature. This preparation was withdrawn from use because of the high incidence of side effects. Intravenous infusion of soybean oil emulsion (Intralipid) in 400 cases was associated with mild reactions comprising subfebrile temperatures in 1% and sweating and an oily taste in the mouth in 3% (MEYLER 1966). In a later study of 2,800 infusions of Intralipid, the incidence of chills and febrile reactions were reported to be 1% and 1.7% respectively in postoperative and geriatric patients (SCHINDEL 1972). The incidence of immediate reactions to Lipofundin-S is less than 1% (GÄRTNER et al. 1969). Regarding long-term treatment modern fat emulsions are well tolerated.

5. Results of Diagnostic Tests

a) Skin Tests

NICOLAS et al. (1966) have performed intradermal skin tests in reactors and nonreactors to Lipiphysan and in apparently healthy volunteers. Positive delayed skin

Table 8. Antiglobulin consumption test performed on sera of reactors (group I) and non-reactors (group III) to Lipiphysan, and on subjects without previous exposure to Lipiphysan (group II). (Nicolas et al. 1966)

Subjects	Antiglobulin consumption in the presence of				Controls[a]
	Lipiphysan	Cottonseed oil	Soybean lecithin	α-Tocopherol	
Group I					
A	+ + + +	0	+ + +	0	0
B	+ + + +	0	+ + +	0	0
C	+ + + +	+	+ + +	+ + +	+ +
D	+ +	0	+ + +	0	0
Group II					
E	0	0	0	0	0
F	0	0	0	0	0
G	0	0	0	0	0
H	+	0	+ + +	0	0
J	0	0	0	0	0
K	0	0	0	0	0
Group III					
L	(+)	0	+	+ +	0
M	(+)	0	+	0	0
N	+	0	+ +	0	0
H	+ + +	0	+ + + +	0	0
J	+ + +	0	+ + +	0	0
K	0	0	0	0	0

[a] Controls = human red cells of group 0, Rh^+, incubated with serum of the individual studied

reactions appeared 24–36 h after intradermal injection into two reactors tested. Skin tests were negative in six non-reactors to Lipiphysan and in ten volunteers. The positive results in reactors indicate that Lipiphysan has the capacity to induce cell-mediated immunity.

b) Specific Antibodies

Titers of 1 : 100 –1 : 400 of anti-Lipiphysan antibodies could be demonstrated in sera of all five Lipiphysan reactors tested, using the antiglobulin consumption test (Nicolas et al. 1966). Sera of volunteers were similarly examined and in 27 of 28 individuals negative results were obtained. The test was slightly positive in one case. Six patients, who had tolerated eight to ten infusions of Lipiphysan, were also investigated 8–17 days after infusion for the presence of specific antibodies. High titers were demonstrable in three of the patients and low or zero titers in the remainder. The fact that patients with high titers of specific antibodies following repeated Lipiphysan infusion had low or zero titers before starting treatment shows that Lipiphysan is an immunogenic agent. Examples of tests for the presence of specific antibodies against the three components of Lipiphysan are given in Table 8. Results show that the soybean lecithin used as emulsifier is the responsible antigen. GOULON et al. (1974) were also able to demonstrate presence of anti-Lipi-physan antibodies in one reactor to Lipiphysan.

6. Potential Pathomechanisms

In dog toxicity tests over a four-week period with a dose of fat of $9 \text{ g kg}^{-1} \text{ day}^{-1}$, the following adverse signs were observed: marked anemia and leukocytosis, hypertriglyceridemia, vomiting, diarrhea, and blood in urine and faeces (JACOBSON and WRETLIND 1970). This clinical picture may be explained by extensive and disseminated fat embolism (OBEL 1970). These adverse reactions, which are reversible up to a certain grade of severity, would correspond to the late reactions or fat overloading syndrome observed in humans.

With regard to possible pathomechanisms for late reactions in humans, the following viewpoints are of interest. GOULON et al. (1974) suggest that decomposition of the fat emulsion caused by anti-emulsifier antibodies leads to liberation of fat with subsequent development of a syndrome resembling that of post-traumatic fat embolism or disseminated intravascular coagulation. The observed symptoms of anemia, thrombocytopenia, splenomegaly, and icterus resemble those seen in autoimmune diseases and could therefore indicate similar underlying immunopathologic changes. Some of the emulsifiers are antigenic lecithins and have the potential to become incorporated into the lipid domains of the red cell membrane. The circulating anti-Lipiphysan antibodies (anti-lecithin antibodies), which have been demonstrated in patients with adverse reactions to Lipiphysan (NICOLAS et al. 1966; GOULON et al. 1974) might then combine with specific antigen on the red cell or platelet surface. Such sensitized cells could then be agglutinated and lysed and thus give rise to the clinical symptoms of thrombocytopenia, anemia, and splenomegaly. Alternatively, damage to red cells could be caused by simple progressive incorporation of components of the fat emulsion following prolonged use.

The possible cause of the symptoms seen in immediate reactions may be direct release of vasoactive mediators by the emulsifier. Histamine liberation has been suggested by SCHUBERT and WRETLIND (1961). It is known that certain synthetic emulsifiers like Tweens are so-called macromolecular histamine releasers in dogs (HALPERN 1956). Similar action of other emulsifiers is therefore feasible in a few predisposed individuals. Among other potential mechanisms for elicitation of early reactions, liberation of ATP from blood cells (SCHUBERT and WRETLIND 1961) and formation of flocculates inducing ischemic changes (WADELL et al. 1957) have been proposed. Formation of circulating flocculates could also lead to activation of the plasma enzyme systems.

References

Aanderud L, Gran L (1975) Anafylactoide reaksioner etter dextran infusjon. Tidsskr Nor Laegeforen 95:1896–1897
Åberg M, Hedner U, Bergentz SE (1977) The effect of dextran on haemostasis and coagulation with special regard to factor VIII. Acta Univ Ups Symp 3:23–30
Adar R, Schneiderman W (1977) Severe anaphylaxis in cirrhotic patients receiving dextran 40. JAMA 237:119–120

Adelmann-Grill B, Schöning B (1981) Lack of evidence for immunological reactions to polygelatin. Dev Biol Stand 48:235–240

Alexander B (1978) Effects of plasma expanders on coagulation and hemostasis: dextran, hydroxyethylstarch, and other macromolecules revisited. In: Blood substitutes and plasma expanders. Liss, New York, pp 293–326

Alexander CS, Zievel L (1961) Fat infusion. Arch Intern Med 107:514–528

Allardyce DB (1982) Cholestasis caused by lipid emulsions. Surg Gynecol Obstet 154:641–647

Allen PZ, Kabat EA (1957) Studies on the capacity of some polysaccharides to elicit antibody formation in man. J Exp Med 105:383–394

Allen PZ, Kabat EA (1958) Persistence of circulating antibodies in human subjects immunized with dextran, levan and blood group substances. J Immunol 80:495–500

Altemeier WA, Schiff L, Gall EA, Gisueffi J, Hamilton D, Freiman D, Braunstein H (1954) Long term studies on the effect of polyvinylpyrrolidone retention in human patients. Surg Forum 4:724–730

Alving BM, Hojima Y, Pisano JJ, Mason BL, Buckingham RE, Mozen MM, Finlayson JS (1978) Hypotension associated with prekallikrein activator (Hageman-factor fragments) in plasma protein fraction. N Engl J Med 299:66–70

Alving CR (1977) Immune reactions of lipids and lipid model membranes. In: The antigens, vol 4. Academic Press, New York, pp 3–72

Ammon R (1963) Das Vorkommen von Dextranase im menschlichen Gewebe. Enzyme 25:245–251

Ammon R, Braunschmidt G (1949) Das Schicksal von Periston im Organismus. Biochem Z 319:370–377

Anderson RJ, Peck RL, Creighton MM (1940) The chemistry of the lipids of tubercle bacilli. LXI. The polysaccharide of the phosphatide obtained from cell residues in the preparation of tuberculin. J Biol Chem 136:211–227

Andersson B (1969) Induction of immunity and immunological paralysis in mice against polyvinylpyrrolidone. J Immunol 102:1309–1313

Andersson B, Blomgren H (1971) Evidence for thymus-independent humoral antibody production in mice against polyvinylpyrrolidone and E. coli lipopolysaccharide. Cell Immunol 2:411–424

Arnon R, Teitelbaum D (1974) Lipid-specific antibodies elicited with synthetic lipid conjugates. Chem Phys Lipids 13:352–366

Arturson G, Granath K (1972) Dextrans as test molecules in studies of the functional ultrastructure of biological membranes. Molecular weight distribution analysis by gel chromatography. Clin Chim Acta 37:309–322

Arturson G, Wallenius G (1964) The intravascular persistence of dextran fractions of different molecular size in normal humans. Scand J Clin Lab Invest 1:76–80

Aspinall GO (1970) Polysaccharides. Pergamon, Oxford

Bach J-F (1976) Immunologie. Flammarion, Paris

Bailey G, Strub RL, Klein RC, Salvaggio J (1967) Dextran-induced anaphylaxis. JAMA 200:889–891

Banks W, Greenwood CT, Muir DD (1973) The structure of hydroxyethylstarch. Br J Pharmacol 47:172–178

Barandun S, Kistler P, Jeunet F, Isliker H (1962) Intravenous administration of human gamma globulin. Vox Sang 7:157–174

Bargmann W (1947) Über Milzveränderungen nach Zufuhr des Blutflüssigkeitsersatzes Periston. Virchows Arch 314:162–166

Bauer Å, Östling G (1970) Dextran-induced anaphylactoid reactions in connection with surgery. Acta Anaesthesiol Scand [Suppl] 37:182–185

Bauer K (1974) A study on the determinant structure of human serum albumin. J Immunogenet 1:315–321

Bayliss WM (1916) Methods of raising a low arterial pressure. Proc R Soc London [Biol] 89:380–393

Becker CE, McGregor RR, Walker KS, Jandl JH (1966) Fatal anaphylaxis after intramuscular iron-dextran. Ann Intern Med 65:745–748

Becker EL, Austen KF (1976) Anaphylaxis. In: Miescher PA, Müller-Eberhard H-J (eds) Textbook of immunopathology, 2nd edn. Grune & Stratton, New York, pp 117–135

Becker U, Nowack H, Gay S, Timpl R (1976) Production and specificity of antibodies against the aminoterminal region in type III collagen. Immunology 31:57–65

Beez M, Dietl H (1979) Retrospektive Betrachtung der Häufigkeit anaphylaktoider Reaktionen nach Plasmasteril und Longasteril. Infusionsther Klin Ernaehr 6:23–26

Behrens PO, Spiekerman AM, Brown JR (1975) Structure of human serum albumin. Fed Proc 34:591

Beil W, Timpl R, Furthmayr H (1973) Conformation dependence of antigenic determinants on the collagen molecule. Immunology 24:13–24

Benbunan M, Pavie-Fischer J, Reviron J (1976) Réaction d'intolérance majeure liée à l'injection de gélatine fluide modifiée. Anesth Analg (Paris) 33:691–702

Berge A, Kristoffersen J, Backe-Hansen K, Wold JK (1976) Polysaccharide contaminants in ultra-pure grade sucrose with relation to anaphylactoid reactions in clinical use of invert sugar solutions. Acta Pharm Suec 13:459–468

Birnbaum-Feinman S, Prescott B, Cole RM (1973) Serological reactions of glycolipids from streptococcal L-forms. Infect Immun 8:752–756

Bland JHL, Laver MB, Lowenstein E (1972) Hypotension due to 5 per cent plasma protein fractions. N Engl J Med 286:109

Bland JHL, Laver MB, Lowenstein E (1973) Vasodilator effect of commercial 5 per cent plasma protein fraction solutions. JAMA 224:1721 1724

Böttiger LE, Furhoff AK, Holmberg L (1979) Fatal reactions to drugs. Acta Med Scand 205:451–456

Boon JC, Jesch F, Ring J, Messmer K (1976) Intravascular persistence of hydroxyethylstarch in man. Eur Surg Res 8:497–503

Bortoluzzi E, Carrera F, Finozzi CC, Galetti P, Longoni-Bortoluzzi S (1967) Nota su di un caso di schock anafilattico da polimero della gelatina (Emagel®). Studio clinico ed immunoematologico. Anesthesiol Rianim 8:73–75

Boyd WC (1956) Fundamentals of immunology. Interscience, New York

Brickman RD, Murray GF, Thompson WL, Ballinger WF (1966) The antigenicity of hydroxyethylstarch in humans. Studies in seven volunteers. JAMA 198:1277–1279

Briseid G, Briseid K, Toverud EL, Kristoffersen J (1978) Dextran-induced lowering of prekallikrein proactivator and prekallikrein in rat plasma. Acta Pharmacol Toxicol (Copenh) 42:93–102

Brisman R, Parks LC, Haller JA (1968) Anaphylactoid reactions associated with the clinical use of dextran 70. JAMA 204:824–825

Bryan GC, Scudder J (1952) Dextran and pneumococcus polysaccharide cross-reactivity in skin tests and serum precipitin tests. Ann NY Acad Sci 55:477–478

Bygdeman S, Eliasson R (1967) Effect of dextrans on platelet adhesiveness and aggregation. Scand J Clin Lab Invest 20:17–23

Carlsson C, Gustafson I, Nilsson E, Nordström L, Persson P-O, Söderberg M (1972) Anafylaktoid reaktion på dextran. Lakartidningen 69:3690–3692

Carpenter GG (1968) Anaphylactic shock after intravenous galactose. Lancet 2:972

Cisar J, Kabat EA, Dorner M, Liao J (1975) Binding properties of immunoglobulin combining sites specific for terminal or non-terminal antigenic determinants in dextran. J Exp Med 142:435–459

Colman RW (1978) Paradoxical hypotension after volume expansion with plasma protein fraction. N Engl J Med 299:97–98

Colman RW, Girey GJD, Zacest R, Talamo RC (1971) The human plasma kallikrein-kinin system. Prog Hematol 7:255–298

Cottier P, Basevi A, Schafroth HJ (1966) Die Wirkung eines Gelatine-Expanders, Physiogel, auf die Nierenfunktion. Helv Chir Acta 33:383–391

Dessau W, Jilek F, Adelmann BC, Hörmann H (1978) Similarity of anti-gelatin factor and cold insoluble globulin. Biochim. Biophys. Acta 533:227–237

de Weck AL (1969) Research in drug allergy: a search for impurities? Bayer Symp 1:302–308

Dudrick SJ, Wilmore DW, Vars HM, Rhoads JE (1968) Long-term total parenteral nutrition with growth, development, and positive nitrogen balance. Surgery 64:134–142

Dudrick SJ, Wilmore DW, Vars HM, Rhoads JE (1969) Can intravenous feeding as the sole means of nutrition support growth in the child and restore weight-loss in an adult? An affirmative answer. Ann Surg 169:974–984

Duma RJ (1976) Thomas Latta, what have we done? The hazards of intravenous therapy. N Engl J Med 294:1178–1180

Dupont A, Lachapelle J-M (1964) Dermite due to a drug deposit during diabetes insipidus therapy. Bull Soc Fr Dermatol Syphiligr 71:508–509

Dupouey P (1972) Structure antigènique des tréponèmes: mise en évidence d'un nouvel haptène lipidique dans Treponema reiteri. Ann. Inst Pasteur 122:283–295

Ellis EF, Henney CS (1969) Adverse reactions following administration of human gamma globulin. J Allergy 43:45–54

Elman R (1937) Urinary output of nitrogen as influenced by i.v. injection of a mixture of amino acids. Proc Soc Exp Biol Med 37:610–613

Fischer JE (1976) Total parenteral nutrition. Little Brown, Boston

Fisher MMcD (1975) Severe histamine mediated reactions to intravenous drugs used in anesthesia. Anesth Intensive Care 3:180–197

Freedman M, Birked D, Granath K (1978) Analyses of glucans from cariogenic and mutant streptococcus mutans. Infect Immun 21:17–27

Freeman MK (1979) Fatal reactions to haemaccel. Anaesthesia 34:341–343

From A, Grönwall A, Wallenius G, Zaar B (1961) On the antibody nature of a dextran-precipitable protein spontaneously occurring in normal human serum. Probl Gematol Pereliv Krovi 6:45–47

Furhoff A-K (1977) Anaphylactoid reactions to dextran. A report of 133 cases. Acta Anaesthesiol Scand 21:161–167

Furie MB, Frey AB, Rifkin DB (1980) Location of a gelatinbinding region of human plasma fibronectin. J Biol Chem 255:4391–4394

Gärtner C, Soballa G, Kösters B, Berg G (1969) Parenterale Ernährung im Rahmen einer Intensivpflegestation. Medizin und Ernährung 10:185–188

Galanos C, Lüderitz O, Rietschel ET, Westphal O (1977) Newer aspects of the chemistry and biology of bacterial polysaccharides, with special reference to their lipid A component. In: Goodwin TW (ed) Biochemistry of lipids II. International review of biochemistry 14:239–335

Geyer RP (1960) Parenteral nutrition. Physiol Rev 40:150–186

Ghadimi H (1975) Total parenteral nutrition – promises and premises. Wiley and Sons, New York Chichester

Gibbons R, Banghart S (1967) Synthesis of extracellular dextran by cariogenic bacteria and its presence in human dental plaque. Arch Oral Biol 12:11–24

Gill TJ, Kunz HW (1968) The immunogenicity of vinyl polymers. Proc Natl Acad Sci USA 61:490–496

Giromini M, Jungers P, Ducrot H (1967) Anurie provoquée par la perfusion de dextran de faible poids moléculaire. Nouv Press Med 75:2561–2562

Godenschweger I, Arlt E, Arlt B (1978) Unverträglichkeitsreaktionen nach Infusion kolloidaler Volumenersatzmittel während der Narkose. Fortschr Med 96:227–230

Golde DW, McGinniss MG, Holland PV (1971) Serum agglutinins to commercially prepared albumin. Am J Clin Pathol 55:655–658

Golde DW, Greipp PR, McGinniss MH (1973) Spectrum of albumin autoagglutinins. Transfusion 13:1

Goodman JW, Kabat EA (1964) Immunochemical studies on cross-reactions of antipneumococcal sera. IV. Cross-reactions of horse type 22 antipneumococcal serum with dextrans. J Immunol 93:213–219

Goulon M, Barrois A, Grosbuis S, Schortgen G (1974) Embolie graisseuse après perfusions répétées d'émulsions lipidiques. Nouv Presse Med 3:13–18

Grabar P (1955) Réactions de divers serums normaux avec des substances macromoléculaires naturelles ou synthétiques. Ann Inst Pasteur 88:11–23

Griem W, Czok G, Lang K (1964a) Histologische und physiologische Untersuchungen an Ratten nach Verabreichung des Plasmaexpanders Gelifundol. Anaesthesist 13:321–324

Griem W, Czok G, Lang K (1964b) Histologische und physiologische Untersuchungen an Ratten nach Haemaccel und Rattenserum-Injektionen. Anaesthesist 13:324–330

Griem W, Czok G, Lang K (1964c) Histologische und physiologische Untersuchungen an Ratten nach Verabreichung des Plasmaexpanders Plasmagel. Anaesthesist 13:330–333

Grönwall A (1957) Dextran and its use in colloidal infusion solutions. Almqvist & Wiksell, Stockholm

Grönwall A (1959) Antigenicity of Swedish clinical dextran (macrodex®) Acta Soc Med Ups 64:244–246

Grönwall A, Ingelman B (1944) Untersuchungen über Dextran und sein Verhalten bei parenteraler Zufuhr. I. Acta Physiol Scand 7:97–107

Gruber UF (1969) Blood replacement. Springer, Berlin Heidelberg New York

Gruber UF, Wettler H, Allemann U, Gerber H, Laubenthal H, Messmer K (1982) Prophylaxe allergischer Dextranreaktionen durch Vorinjektion von 20 ml Hapten bei 12000 Patienten in der Schweiz. Schweiz Rundschau Med (Praxis) 71:1092–1100

Gruber US, Saldeen T, Brokop T et al. (1980) Incidences of fatal postoperative pulmonary embolism after prophylaxis with dextran 70 and low dose heparin. An international multicenter study. Br Med J 10:69–72

Grünert A (1982) Die Applikation von Fettemulsionen in posttraumatischen und postoperativen Zuständen. In: Eckart J, Wolfram G (eds) Fett in der parenteralen Ernährung 2. Zuckschwerdt, München, pp 3–32

Grünfeld J-P, de Montera H, Berry J-P, Reveillaud R-J (1968) A propos d'une observation de thésaurismose par polyvinylpyrrolidone avec localisation rénale prédominante. J Urol Nephrol 74:656–665

Guynn JB, Poretz DM, Duma RJ (1973) Growth of various bacteria in a variety of intravenous fluids. Am J Hosp Pharm 30:321–325

Hahn E, Timpl R, Miller EJ (1975) Demonstration of a unique antigenic specificity for the collagen alpha 1(II) chain from cartilaginous tissue. Immunology 28:561–568

Hall CE, Hall O (1961) Experimental hypertension elicited by injections of methylcellulose. Experientia 17:544–545

Hall CE, Hall O (1965) Hypertensogenicity and aqueous solubility of polyvinyl alcohol polymers. Tex Rep Biol Med 23:423–434

Hallberg D, Holm J, Obel AL, Schuberth O, Wretlind A (1967) Fat emulsion for complete intravenous nutrition. Postgrad Med 4:307–316

Halpern BN (1956) Histamine release by long chain molecules. In: Histamine. Churchill Livingstone, Edinburgh London, pp 92–123

Harrison GA, Torda TA, Schiff P (1971) Hypotensive effects of stable plasma protein solutions (SPPS): a preliminary communication. Med J Aust 2:1308–1309

Hartmann G (1967) Fettemulsionen (Intralipid) in der inneren Medizin. Wien Med Wochenschr 177:51–55

Hecht G, Scholtan W (1959) Über die Ausscheidung von Polyvinylpyrrolidon durch die normale Niere. Z Exp Med 130:557–603

Hecht G, Weese H (1943) Periston, ein neuer Blutflüssigkeitsersatz. MMW 90:11–15

Heckner F, Gehlmann F (1956) Cytologische Beobachtungen zur Kollidonspeicherung. Z Gesamte Exp Med 127:213–226

Hedin H (1977) Dextran-induced anaphylactoid reactions in man. Immunological in vitro and in vivo studies. Acta Univ Ups Abstr Upps Diss Sci no. 432

Hedin H, Richter W (1977) Potential pathomechanisms of dextraninduced anaphylactoid reactions in man. Acta Univ Ups Symp 3:9–22

Hedin H, Richter W (1982) Pathomechanisms of dextran-induced anaphylactoid/anaphylactic reactions in man. Int Arch Allergy Appl Immun 68:122–126

Hedin H, Richter W, Ring J (1976) Dextran-induced anaphylactoid reactions in man. Role of dextran reactive antibodies. Int Arch Allergy Appl Immun 52:145–159

Hedin H, Kraft D, Richter W, Scheiner O, Devey M (1979) Dextranreactive antibodies in patients with anaphylactoid reactions to dextran. Immunobiology 156:289

Hedin H, Richter W, Kraft D (1981a) Pathomechanism of dextran-induced anaphylactoid reactions in man. Int Arch Allergy Appl Immunol (Suppl 1) 66:75–77

Hedin H, Richter W, Messmer K, Renck H, Ljungström KG, Laubenthal H (1981 b) Incidence, pathomechanism and prevention of dextran induced anaphylactoid/anaphylactic reactions in man. Dev Biol Stand 48:179–189

Hehre EJ, Neill JM (1946) Formation of serologically reactive dextrans by streptococci from subacute bacterial endocarditis. J Exp Med 83:147–162

Hehre EJ, Sugg JY (1950) Serological reactivity of dextran plasma substitute. Fed Proc 9:383

Heinonen J, Peltola K, Himberg J-J, Suomela H (1981) Hypotensive effect of prekallikrein activator (PKA) in plasma protein fractions (PPF). Dev Biol Stand 48:129–130

Henriques W, Andersen AC (1913) Über parenterale Ernährung durch intravenöse Injektion. Hoppe Seylers Z Physiol Chem 88:357–369

Hogan JJ (1915) The intravenous use of colloidal (gelatin) solutions in shock. JAMA 64:721–726

Holm E, Bässler KH, Staedt U, Leweling H, Striebel JP (1982) Parenterale Fettzufuhr bei der Leberzirrhose. In: Eckart J, Wolfram G (eds) Fett in der parenteralen Ernährung 2. Zuckschwerdt, München, pp 87–106

Horisberger B (1966) Severe pulmonary and cerebral circulation disorders after parenteral injection of a high dosage fat emulsion. A case of unusual therapeutic complication. Schweiz Med Wochenschr 96:1065–1069

Hossaini AA, Hazeghi K, Amiri P (1977) Experimental induction of caprylate dependent albumin antibodies. Transfusion 17:54–58

Howard JG, Vicari G, Courtenay B (1975) Influence of molecular structure on the tolerogenicity of bacterial dextrans. I. The α 1–6 linked epitope of dextran B 512. Immunology 29:585–597

Hueper WC (1942) Macromolecular substances as pathogenic agents. Arch Pathol 33:267–290

Hueper WC (1957) Experimental carcinogenic studies in macromolecular chemicals. Neoplastic reactions in rats and mice after parenteral introduction of polyvinylpyrrolidone. Cancer 10:8–18

Hueper WC (1961) Bioassay on polyvinylpyrrolidones with limited molecular weight range. J Nat Cancer Inst 26:229–237

Hüsselmann H (1952) Speicherungserscheinungen beim Menschen nach Periston. Klin Wochenschr 30:801–808

Hurwitz SH (1917) Intravenous injections of colloidal solutions of acacia in hemorrhage. JAMA 68:699–701

Imrie FKE, Tilbury RH (1972) Polysaccharides in sugar cane and its products. Sugar Technol Rev 1:291–386

Ingelman B, Grönwall A, Gelin L-E, Eliasson R (1969) Properties and applications of dextrans. Almqvist & Wiksell, Stockholm

Isbister JP, Biggs JC (1976) Reactions to rapid infusion of stable plasma protein solution during large volume plasma exchange. Anaesth Intensive Care 4:105–107

Ishizaka K (1963) Gammaglobulin and molecular mechanisms in hypersensitivity reactions. Prog Allergy 7:32–106

Jacobson S, Wretlind A (1970) The use of fat emulsion for complete intravenous nutrition. In: Body fluid replacement in the surgical patient. Grune & Stratton, New York, pp 334–347

Jacobsson L (1959) Studies on partially hydrolyzed dextran with special reference to its use for plasma volume determination in man. PhD dissertation, University of Uppsala

Jacobsson L, Wikström R (1958) The detection of dextran-reacting antibodies in human serum. Acta Soc Med Ups 63:180–187

Jacobsson L, Zsiga J (1958) Dextran-reacting antibodies in human serum. Acta Soc Med Ups 63:165–179

Janeway CA, Merler E, Rosen FS, Salmon S, Crain JD (1968) Intravenous gammaglobulin. N Engl J Med 278:919–923

Jeanes A, Haynes WC, Wilham CA et al. (1954) Characterization and classification of dextrans from ninety-six strains of bacteria. J Am Chem Soc 76:5041–5052

Jellinek EH (1976) Dangers of intravenous fat infusions. Lancet 2:967

Johnson U, Laurell AB (1974) Activation of complement in anaphylactoid reactions in connection with infusion of dextran. Scand J Immunol 3:673–676

Kaars-Sijpesteijn JA, Huizinga T (1975) Blood and blood products. In: Meyler's side effects of drugs, 8. Excerpta Medica, Amsterdam London New York, pp 721–737

Kabat EA (1957) Size and heterogeneity of the combining sites on an antibody molecule. J Cell Comp Physiol 50:79–102

Kabat EA (1966) The nature of an antigenic determinant. J Immunol 97:1–11

Kabat EA, Berg D (1952) Production of precipitins and cutaneous sensitivity in man by injection of small amounts of dextran. Ann NY Acad Sci 55:471–476

Kabat EA, Berg D (1953) Dextran – an antigen in man. J Immunol 70:514–532

Kabat EA, Bezer AE (1958) The effect of variation in molecular weight on the antigenicity of dextran in man. Arch Biochem Biophys 78:306–318

Kabat EA, Mayer M (1961) Experimental immunochemistry, 2nd edn. Thomas, Springfield

Kabat EA, Turino GM, Tarrow AB, Maurer PH (1957) Studies on the immunochemical basis of allergic reactions to dextran in man. J Clin Invest 36:1160–1170

Kausch W (1911) Über intravenöse und subkutane Ernährung mit Traubenzucker. Dtsch Med Wochenschr 37:8–9

Kenny GE (1975) Antigens of the Mycoplasmatales and Chlamydiae. In: The antigens, vol 3. Academic Press, New York, pp 449–478

Knox KW, Wicken AJ (1972) Reaction of dextrans with antisera to teichoic acids. Arch Oral Biol 17:1491–1494

Knudtson ML, Taylor PJ (1976) Überempfindlichkeitsreaktion auf Dextran 70 (Hyskon) während einer Hysteroskopie. Geburtshilfe Frauenheilkd 36:263–264

Kohen M, Mattikow M, Middleton E, Butsch DW, Wayne NJ (1970) A study of three untoward reactions to dextran. J Allergy 46:309–314

Kraft D, Wilson DW, Devey MI (1976) Penicillin allergy studies by a modified red cell linked antigen antiglobulin reaction. Int Arch Allergy Appl Immunol 52:248–256

Kraft D, Hedin H, Richter W, Scheiner O, Rumpold H, Devey MI (1982) Immunoglobulin class and subclass distribution of dextran reactive antibodies in human reactors and non reactors to clinical dextran. Allergy 37:481–489

Krenzelok EP, Parker WA (1975) Dextran 40 anaphylaxis. Minn Med 58:454–455

Lachapelle JM (1966) Thésaurismose cutanée par polyvinylpyrrolidone. Dermatologica 132:476–489

Landsteiner K (1962) The specificity of serological reactions, 2nd edn. Dover, New York

Langrehr D, Singbartl G, Neuhaus R (1975) Nebenwirkungen nach Dextran- und Gelatinepräparaten in der Infusionstherapie. Klinische Erfahrungen die der anaphylaktoiden Sofortreaktion. Klin Anaesthesiol Intensivther 9:73–87

Larm O, Lindberg B, Svensson S (1971) Studies on the length of side chains of the dextran elaborated by leuconostoc mesenteroides NRRL B 512. Carbohydr Res 20:39–48

Laubenthal H, Gerber H, Richter W, Kraft D, Peter K, Gruber UF, Messmer K (1982a) Effektivität der Haptenhemmung zur Prophylaxe der Dextrananaphylaxie. Ergebnisse der deutsch-schweizerischen multizentrischen Studie. Anaesthesist 31:503–504

Laubenthal H, Peter K, Messmer K (1982b) Prophylaxe der Dextrananaphylaxie. Münch Med Wochenschr 124:951–953

Laubenthal H, Peter K, Richter W, Kraft D, Selbmann HK, Messmer K (1983) Anaphylaktoide/anaphylaktische Reaktionen auf Dextran: Pathomechanismus und Prophylaxe. Diagnostik und Intensivtherapie 8:4–14

Laxénaire MC, Jacob F, Noël P (1976) Accidents anaphylactoides liés à l'emploi de dextran de poids moléculaire 40,000. Ann Anesthesiol Fr 17:101–104

Lee HA (1974) Parenteral nutrition in acute metabolic illness. Academic Press, New York

Lee-Benner L, Walton RP (1965) From the 3rd conference on artificial colloidal agents (1965), Washington, DC. National Academy of Science, National Research Council, Washington, DC pp 54–55

Leikola J, Koistinen J, Lehtinen M, Virolainen M (1973) IgA-induced anaphylactic transfusion reactions: a report of four cases. Blood 42:111–119

LeVeen HH, Harry H, Giordano P, Speltzer J (1961) The mechanism of removal of intravenously injected fat. Arch Surg 83:311–321

Levene PA, Landsteiner K, van der Scheer J (1927) Immunization experiments with lecithin. J Exp Med 46:197–204

Lewinter P (1970) Iron-dextran anaphylaxis. J Med Soc NJ 67:116–117

Lindblad G, Falk J (1976) Konzentrationsverlauf von Hydroxyäthylstärke und Dextran in Serum und Lebergewebe von Kaninchen und die histopathologischen Folgen der Speicherung von Hydroxyäthylstärke. Infusionstherapie 3:301–303

Lindner J (1960) Tierexperimentelle Untersuchungen zum Problem der sog. Polymerkrebse. Verh Dtsch Ges Pathol 44:272–280

Littenberg RL (1975) Anaphylactoid reaction to human albumin microspheres. J. Nucl Med 16:236–237

Ljungström KG, Renck H, Strandberg K, Hedin H, Richter W, Widelöf E (1983a) Adverse reactions to dextran in Sweden 1970–1979. Acta Chir Scand 149:253–262

Ljungström KG, Renck H, Hedin H, Richter W, Rosberg B (1983b) Prevention of dextran-induced anaphylactic reactions by hapten inhibition. I. Scandinavian multicenter study on the effects of 10 ml 15% Dextran 1 administered before Macrodex or Rheomacrodex. Acta Chir Scand 149:341–348

Löding HW, Lawin P (1972) Anaphylaktischer Schock in Narkose durch Oxypolygelatine. Z Prakt Anaesthesiol 7:283–287

Lorenz W (1975) Histamine release in man. Agents Actions 5/5:402–416

Lorenz W, Reimann H-J, Barth H, Kusche J, Meyer R, Doenicke A, Hutzel M (1972) A sensitive and specific method for the determination of histamine in human whole blood and plasma. Hoppe Seylers Z Physiol Chem 353:911–920

Lorenz W, Seidl W, Doenicke A et al. (1974) Elevated plasma histamine levels in surgery: causes and clinical significance. Klin Wochenschr 52:419–425

Lorenz W, Doenicke A, Freund M, Schmal A, Dormann P, Praetorius B, Schürk-Bulich M (1975) Plasmahistaminspiegel beim Menschen nach rascher Infusion von Hydroxyäthylstärke: Ein Beitrag zur Frage allergischer oder anaphylaktoider Reaktionen nach Gabe eines neuen Plasmasubstituts. Anaesthesist 24:228–230

Lorenz W, Doenicke A, Messmer K et al. (1976) Histamine release in human subjects by modified gelatin (haemaccel®) and dextran: an explanation for anaphylactoid reactions observed under clinical conditions? Br J Anaesth 48:151–165

Lorenz W, Doenicke A, Dittmann I, Hug P, Schwarz B (1977) Anaphylaktoide Reaktionen nach Applikation von Blutersatzmitteln beim Menschen. Verhinderung dieser Nebenwirkung durch Prämedikation mit H_1- und H_2-Rezeptorantagonisten. Anaesthesist 26:644–648

Lorenz W, Doenicke A, Reimann HJ, Schmal A, Schwarz B, Dorman P (1978) Anaphylactoid reactions and histamine release by plasma substitutes: a randomized controlled trial in human subjects and in dogs. Agents Actions 8:397–399

Lüben G, Quast U, Geiger H (1981) Prekallikrein activator levels and side effects with human albumin preparations. Dev Biol Stand 48:123–127

Lund N (1973) Anaphylactic reactions induced by infusion of haemaccel. Br J Anaesth 45:929

Lunde I (1974) Invertoseinfusioner/biverkninger. Tidsskr Nor Laegeforen 94:1926

Lundsgaard-Hansen P, Tschirren B (1978) Modified fluid gelatin as a plasma substitute. In: Blood substitutes and plasma expanders. Liss, New York, pp 227–257

Lundsgaard-Hansen P, Tschirren B (1980) Anaphylaktoide Reaktionen auf 102,787 Einheiten Gelatine. Allergologie 3:76–78

Lundgsgaard-Hansen P, Hässig A, Mitschmann H (eds) (1969) Modified gelatin as plasma substitutes. Karger, Basel

Lusky LM, Nelson AA (1957) Fibrosarcoma induced by multiple s.c. injections of carboxymethylcellulose, polyvinylpyrrolidone, and polyoxyethylene sorbitan monostearate. Fed Proc 16:318

Lutz H (1975) Plasmaersatzmittel. Thieme, Stuttgart

Matheson NA (1966) Renal effects of low molecular weight dextran. Monogr Surg Sci 3:303–364

Mathiessen H, Tempel G, Kolb E (1977/1978) Anaphylaktoide Reaktion nach Hydroxyäthylstärke. Anaesthesiol Intensivmed Prax 14:61–63

Maurer PH (1953) Dextran, an antigen in man. Proc Soc Exp Biol Med 83:879–884

Maurer PH (1954a) Antigenicity of gelatin in rabbits and other species. J Exp Med 100:515–523

Maurer PH (1954b) Antigenicity of oxypolygelatin and gelatin in man. J Exp Med 100:497–513

Maurer PH (1958) Antigenicity of gelatin. J Exp Med 107:125–131

Maurer PH (1960) Immunologische Untersuchungen mit Plasmaersatzmitteln. Klin Wochenschr 38:417–421

Maurer PH, Berardinelli B (1968) Immunologic studies with hydroxyethylstarch (HES), a proposed plasma expander. Transfusion 8:265–268

Maurer PH, Lebovitz H (1956) Studies on the antigenicity of modified fluid gelatin. J Immunol 76:335–341

McMillin RD, Hood TR, Griffen WO (1978) Systemic anaphylaxis secondary to the use of 5 per cent plasma protein fractions. Am J Surg 135:706–707

Meisel G, Zöckler H (1971) Anaphylaktische Reaktion nach der Gabe von Plasmaexpandern auf Gelatinebasis. Bibl Haematol 37:348–353

Meissner F (1961) Allergische Reaktionen nach Dextraninfusion. Allerg Asthmaforsch 4:33–38

Menzano A, Miletto A, Anselmetti G, Musto P, Zocche GP (1977) Considerazioni su due casi di reazione anafilattoide ai destrani. Minerva Anestesiol 43:667–672

Messmer K, Lorenz W, Sunder-Plassmann L, Klöverkorn WP, Hutzel M (1970) Histamine release as cause of acute hypotension following rapid colloid infusion. Naunyn Schmiedebergs Arch Pharmacol 267:433–445

Metcalf W, Papadopoulos A, Tuparo R, Barth A (1970) A clinicalphysiologic study of hydroxyaethylstarch. Surg Gynecol Obstet 131:255–267

Meyler L (1960) Miscellaneous agents. In: Meyler L (ed) Side effects of drugs. Excerpta Medica, Amsterdam London New York, pp 202–214

Meyler L (1964) Unclassified agents. In: Meyler L (ed) Side effects of drugs, 4th edn. Excerpta Medica, Amsterdam London New York, pp 332–344

Meyler L (1966) Unclassified drugs. In: Meyler L (ed) Side effects of drugs, vol V. Excerpta Medica, Amsterdam London New York, pp 527–534

Meyler L (1968) Unclassified drugs. In: Meyler L, Herxheimer A (eds) Side effects of drugs, vol VI. Excerpta Medica, Amsterdam London New York, pp 509–523

Misgeld V, Mende C (1974) Dextran-Unverträglichkeit. Med Klin 69:1452–1455

Messmer K, Ljungström KG, Gruber U, Richter W, Hedin H (1980a) Prevention of dextran induced anaphylactoid reactions by hapten inhibition. Lancet 1:975

Messmer K, Seemann C, Hedin H, Richter W, Peter K (1980b) Anaphylaktoide Reaktionen nach Dextran. II. Tierexperimentelle und klinische Ergebnisse der Prophylaxe durch Haptenhemmung. Allergologie 3:59–66

Mollison PL (1972) Blood transfusion in clinical medicine, 5th edn. Blackwell Oxford

Müller R, Dietzel W (1972) Bericht über einen allergischen Schock nach Infusion von Haemaccel. Anaesth Inform 8:335

Müller-Eberhard HJ (1976) The serum complement system. In: Miescher PA, Müller-Eberhard HJ (eds) Textbook of immunopathology, 2nd edn. Grune & Stratton, New York, pp 45–73

Murlin J, Riche JA (1916) The fat of the blood in relation to heat production, narcosis and muscular work. Am J Physiol 40:146

Neill JM, Abrahams I (1951) Reactions of dextrans with antiserums of rabbits immunized with S. typhi. Proc Soc Exp Biol Med 78:537–540

Neill JM, Hehre EJ, Sugg JY, Jaffe EM (1939) Serological studies on sugar. I. Reactions between solutions of reagent sucrose and type II antipneumococcus serum. J Exp Med 70:427–442

Neumann R (1975) Klinische Untersuchung über etwaige Nebenwirkungen einer Plasmaersatzlösung auf Gelatinebasis (bei Spinalanästhesie). Infusionstherapie 2:353–354

Nicolas F, Guimbretière J, Nicolas G, Guimbretière L (1966) Six réactions d'intolérance à une émulsion lipidique. Anesth Anal Reanim 23:647–661

Nilsson G, Nilsson K (1974) Molecular weight distribution determination of clinical dextran by gel permeation chromatography. J Chromatogr 101:137–153

Obel AL (1970) Morphological studies in longtime experiments with intravenous fat emulsions in dogs. In: Berg Advances in parenteral nutrition. Thieme, Stuttgart, pp 206–216

Olbing A, Engels AM, Doenges KG (1969) Hepato-zellulärer Ikterus nach wiederholter intravenöser Infusion von Fettemulsionen bei Kindern mit ausgedehnter Darmresektion. Dtsch Med Wochenschr 96:1825–1827

Pandit MD, Kamat LB, Thakkar DH (1976) Adverse reactions to transfusion fluids. A prospective survey. Antiseptic 73:181–184

Pangborn MC (1942) Isolation and purification of a serologically active phospholipid from beef heart. J Biol Chem 143:247–256

Pasteur L (1861) Sur la fermentation visqueuse et la fermentation butyrique. Bull Soc Chim Fr pp 30–31

Petkov P, Nankow K (1974) Investigation of side effects connected with locally (Bulgarian) produced glucose solution for injection. Farmatsiya (Sofiya) 24:9–12

Pharmacopoea Nordica Addendum (1976) Universitetsforlaget, Oslo, pp 30.10, 60.1

Phills JA, Perelmutter L (1974) IgE mediated and non-IgE mediated allergic type reactions to aspirin. Acta Allergol. 29:474–490

Piccinino F, Di Stasio G (1963) Assenza di movimento anticorpale (anticorpi devianti il complemento) in soggetti sottoposti a singole o ripetute somministrationi per via endovenosa di soluzioni colloidali di polimerizzati di gelatina scissa. Minerva Anestesiol 29:340–342

Pillemer L, Schoenberg MD, Blum L, Wurz L (1955) Properdin system and immunity. II. Interaction of the properdin system with polysaccharides. Science 122:545–549

Ravin HA, Seligman AM, Fine J (1952) Polyvinylpyrrolidone as a plasma expander. N Engl J Med 247:921–929

Renck H, Ljungström KG, Hedin H, Richter W (1983a) Prevention of dextran-induced anaphylactic reactions by hapten inhibition. III. A Scandinavian multicenter study on the effects of 20 ml Dextran 1, 15%, administered before dextran 70 or dextran 40. Acta Chir Scand 149:355–360

Renck H, Ljungström KG, Rosberg B, Dhuner KG, Dahl S (1983b) Prevention of dextran-induced anaphylactic reactions by hapten inhibition. II. A comparison of the effects of 20 ml dextran 1, 15%, administered either admixed to or before dextran 70 or dextran 40. Acta Chir Scand 149:349–353

Reske-Nielsen E, Bojsen-Möller M, Vetner M, Hansen JC (1976) Polyvinylpyrrolidone-storage disease. Acta Pathol Microbiol Scand [A] 84:397–405

Richter AW (1974) Cross-reactivity of synthetic linear dextran with anti-B 512 dextran. Int Arch Allergy Appl Immunol 46:438–447

Richter AW, De Belder AN (1976) Antibodies against hydroxyethylstarch produced in rabbits by immunization with a proteinhydroxyethylstarch conjugate. Int Arch Allergy Appl Immunol 52:307–314

Richter AW, Granath K, Östling G (1976) Anaphylactoid reactions in connection with infusion of invert sugar solutions are due to macromolecular contaminants. Int Arch Allergy Appl Immunol 50:606–612

Richter AW, Kågedal L (1972) Preparation of dextran protein conjugates and studies of their immunogenicity. Int Arch Allergy Appl Immunol 42:887–904

Richter W (1966) Normalizing effect of low molecular weight dextran fractions on the reduced suspension stability of human erythrocytes in vitro. Acta Chir Scand 131:1–8

Richter W (1970) Absence of immunogenic impurities in clinical dextran tested by passive cutaneous anaphylaxis. Int Arch Allergy Appl Immunol 39:469–478

Richter W (1980) A new immunochemical purity test for clinical dextran. Methodology and studies on clinical dextran preparations. Int Arch Allergy Appl Immunol 61:457–466

Richter W, Hedin HI (1982) Dextran hypersensitivity. (A review) Immunology Today 3:132–138

Richter W, Hedin H, Ring J (1977) Immunologische Befunde bei der Infusion kolloidaler Lösungen. Med Welt 28:1717–1719

Richter W, Hedin H, Ring J, Kraft D, Messmer K (1980a) Anaphylaktoide Reaktionen nach Dextran. I. Immunologische Grundlagen und klinische Befunde. Allergologie 3:51–58

Richter W, Seemann C, Hedin H, Ring J, Messmer K (1980b) Dextranunverträglichkeit. Immunologische, tierexperimentelle und klinische Studien. Med Welt 31:365–369

Ring J (1978a) Anaphylaktoide Reaktionen. In: Bergmann H (ed) Anaesthesiologie und Intensiv Medizin, vol 111. Springer, Berlin Heidelberg New York

Ring J (1978b) Lymphocyte transformation studies using B 512 dextran in dextran-allergic patients and normals. Clin Immunol Immunopathol 11:288–291

Ring J, Messmer K (1976) Anaphylaktoide Reaktionen nach Infusion kolloidaler Volumenersatzmittel. Intern Prax 16:579–588

Ring J, Messmer K (1977) Incidence and severity of anaphylactoid reactions to colloid volume substitutes. Lancet 1:466–469

Ring J, Richter W (1980) Wirkungsmechanismus unerwünschter Reaktionen nach Hydroxyäthylstärke (HÄS) und Humanalbumin. Intensivbehandlung. 5:85–92

Ring J, Seifert J, Lob G, Coulin K, Brendel W (1974) Humanalbuminunverträglichkeit. Klinische und immunologische Untersuchungen. Klin Wochenschr 52:595–598

Ring J, Seifert J, Lob G, Brendel W (1975a) Immunologische Untersuchungen bei Patienten mit klinischer Humanalbuminunverträglichkeit. Langenbecks Arch Chir [Suppl Chir Forum] 411–415

Ring J, Seifert J, Messmer K, Brendel W (1975b) Untersuchungen zur Frage der Nebenwirkungen bei Anwendung von Plasmaersatzmitteln. Klin Anaesthesiol Intensivther 9:58–72

Ring J, Seifert J, Messmer K, Brendel W (1976) Anaphylactoid reactions due to hydroxyethylstarch infusion. Eur Surg Res 8:389–399

Ring J, Hedin H, Richter W, Jesch F, Messmer K (1977a) Immunological properties of a high molecular weight component from yeast cell autolysate in dogs and evaluation of its potential role in human dextran reactions. Eur Surg Res 9:338–346

Ring J, Seifert J, Jesch F, Brendel W (1977b) Anaphylactoid reactions due to non-immune-complex serum protein aggregates. Monogr Allergy 12:27–35

Ring J, Stephan W, Brendel W (1979) Anaphylactoid reactions to infusions of plasma protein and human serum albumin. Role of aggregated proteins and of stabilizers added during production. Clin Allergy 9:89–97

Roelands JR, Moody MF, Cohen P (1974) Effects of repeated heating on human albumin. Vox Sang 26:415–424

Rud C (1968a) Anaphylactic shock after intravenous galactose. Lancet 2:515

Rud C (1968b) Anaphylactic shock after intravenous galactose. Lancet 2:1189

Sachs H, Klopstock A (1925) Die serologische Differenzierung von Lezithin und Cholesterin. Biochem Z 159:491–501

Sailer D (1981) Bedeutung von Fettemulsionen im Rahmen der parenteralen Ernährung. In: Hempel V, Clauberg G (eds) Fette in der parenteralen Ernährung, Symposium Tübingen 1979. Melsungen, Bibliomed Medizinische Verlagsges. pp 29–36

Scheibler C (1869) Untersuchungen über die Natur der gallertartigen Ausscheidung (sog. Froschlaich), welche bei der Saftgewinnung aus Rüben beobachtet wird. Verh Dtsch Zuckerind 24:309–315

Schindel L (1972) Intravenous infusion solutions and emulsions. In: Meyler L, Herxheimer A (eds) Side effects of drugs, VII. Excerpta Medica, Amsterdam London New York, pp 471–481

Schindel L (1977) Intravenous infusions – solutions and emulsions. In: Dukes MNG (ed) Side effects of drugs, annual 1. Excerpta Medica, Amsterdam Oxford, pp 252–261

Schmidt H, Pflüger H (1971) Nebenwirkungen bei Volumensubstitution mit Gelatinepräparaten. Med Welt 22:1073–1077

Schmidt H, Rieber W (1980) Häufigkeit und Schweregrad anaphylaktoider Reaktionen nach Gelatineinfusionen. Allergologie 3:71–75

Schoefl GI (1968) The ultrastructure of Chylomicra and of the particles in an artificial fat emulsion. Proc R Soc Lond [Biol] 169:147–152

Schöning B, Koch H (1975) Pathergiequote verschiedener Plasmasubstitute an Haut und
    Respirationstrakt orthopädischer Patienten. Anaesthesist 24:507–516
Schöning B, Lorenz W (1981) Prevention of allergoid (cutaneous anaphylactoid) reactions
    to polygeline (Haemaccel) in orthopaedic patients by premedication with H_1 and H_2 re-
    ceptor antagonists. Dev Biol Stand 48:241–249
Schöning B, Lorenz W, Doenicke A (1982) Prophylaxis of anaphylactoid reactions to a
    polypeptidal plasma substitute by H_1 plus H_2 receptor antagonists: synopsis of three
    randomized controlled trials. Klin Wochenschr 60:1048–1055
Schubert O, Wretlind A (1961) Intravenous infusions of fat emulsion phosphatides and
    emulsifying agents. Clinical and Experimental studies. Acta Chir Scand [Suppl] 278:1–
    21
Schwarz JA, Raschak M (1978) Vortrag; 14. Tagung der Deutschen Gesellschaft für Aller-
    gie- und Immunitätsforschung in Freiburg, Br., 1–4 Okt. 1978: Verhinderung Antikör-
    per-bedingter Dextran-Nebenwirkungen durch Hapten-Hemmung. – Eine experimen-
    telle Pilotstudie am wachen Hund (Abstr). Allergologie 1:184
Schwarz JA, Rother U, Koch W, Raschak M, Till G (1981) Verhinderung Antikörperbe-
    dingter Dextran-Nebenwirkungen durch Haptenhemmung mit Dextran 1 am Hund.
    Anaesthesist 30:297–303
Schwick HG, Heide K (1969) Immunochemistry and immunology of collagen and gelatin.
    Bibl. Haematol 33:111–125
Seemann C, Hedin H, Richter W, Ring J, Stippig S, Messmer K (1978) Vortrag; 14. Tagung
    der Deutschen Gesellschaft für Allergie- und Immunitätsforschung in Freiburg, Br., 1–4
    Okt. 1978: Haptenhemmung der Dextran-induzierten anaphylaktischen Reaktion beim
    Hund Abstr Allergologie 1:185
Seidemann J (1979) Hydroxyäthylstärke – ein neues interessantes kolloidales Volumener-
    satzmittel. Anaphylaktoide Reaktionen. Zentralbl Chir 104:1457–1464
Sela M, Arnon R (1960) The role of rigidity in the antigenicity of polypeptidyl gelatins. Bio-
    chem J 77:394–399
Shenkin A, Wretlind A (1978) Parenteral nutrition. World Rev Nutr Diet 28:1–111
Shepard DAE, Vandam LD (1964) Anaphylaxis associated with the use of dextran. Anes-
    thesiology 25:244–246
Shohl AT, Blackfan KD (1940) Intravenous administration of crystalline amino acids to in-
    fants. J Nutr 20:305–316
Silver H (1976) Autologous transfusion. JAMA 235:1611–1612
Sonneborn HH, de Weck AL, Toffler O (1978) Vergleichende Studie über die Immunoge-
    nität von Plasmaersatzlösungen auf Gelatinebasis im Tierexperiment. Infusionstherapie
    5:41–49
Sorg C, Rüde E, Westphal O (1970) Immunological properties of amylose, dextran and
    polyvinyl alcohol conjugate with polytyrosyl peptides. Eur J Biochem 17:85–90
Spaeth GL, Spaeth EB, Spaeth PG, Lucier AC (1967) Anaphylactic reaction to mannitol.
    Arch Ophthalmol 78:583–584
Sugg JY, Hehre EJ (1942) Reactions of dextran of leuconostoc mesenteroides with the
    antiserums of Leuconostoc and of types 2, 20 and 12 pneumococcus. J Immunol 43:119–
    128
Taketomi T, Yamakawa T (1963) Immunochemical studies of lipids. I. Preparation and im-
    munological properties of synthetic psychosine-protein antigens. J Biochem (Tokyo)
    54:444–451
Thompson WL (1960) Plasma substitutes. A review. J SC Med Assoc 56:456–472
Thompson WL (1978) Hydroxyethyl starch. In: Blood substitutes and plasma expanders.
    Liss, New York, pp 283–292
Thompson WL, Britton JJ, Walton RP (1962) Persistence of starch derivatives and dextran
    when infused after hemorrhage. J Pharmacol Exp Ther 127:39–45
Thompson WL, Wayt DH, Walton RP (1964) Bleeding volume indices of hydroxyethyl-
    starch, dextran, blood, and glucose. Proc Soc Exp Biol Med 115:474–477
Thompson WL, Fukushima T, Rutherford RB, Walton RP (1970) Intravascular persis-
    tence, tissue storage and excretion of hydroxyethylstarch. Surg, Gynecol Obstet
    131:965–972

Thorén L (1978) Dextran as a plasma volume substitute. In: Blood substitutes and plasma expanders. Liss, New York, pp 265–282

Thorsén G (1954) Dextran-position in therapy in Sweden 1953 and problems. Ann Chir Gynaecol Fenn [Suppl 5] 43:445–450

Thorsén G, Hint H (1950) Aggregation, sedimentation and intravascular sludging of erythrocytes. Acta Chir Scand [Suppl] 154

Timpl R, Wolff I, Wick G, Furthmayr H, Steffen C (1968) Immunogenicity and specificity of collagen. VII. Differences between various collagens demonstrated by cross-reactivity studies. J Immunol 101:725–729

Tomoda M, Inokuchi K (1959) Sodium alginate of lowered polymerization (alginon). J Int Coll Surg 32:621–635

Towers RP (1957) Lymph-node changes due to polyvinylpyrrolidone. J Clin Pathol 10:175–177

Tschirren B, Affolter U, Elsässer R, Freihofer UA, Grawehr R, Müller PH, Lundsgaard-Hansen P (1973/1974) Der klinische Plasmaersatz mit Gelatine. Zwölf Jahre Erfahrungen mit 39,320 Einheiten Physiogel. Infusionstherapie 1:651–662

Tsuji S, Shimizu H, Kuba T (1976) Anaphylactic shock due to haemaccel. Jpn J Anesthesiol 25:90

Tullis JL (1977) Albumin. I. Background and use. JAMA 237:355–362

Uhlenhuth P, Haendel D (1910) Untersuchungen über die praktische Verwertbarkeit der Anaphylaxie zur Erkennung und Unterscheidung verschiedener Eiweißarten. Z Immunforsch 4:761–816

Upham HC, Lovell FW, Detrick LE, Highby DH, Debley V, Haley TJ (1956) Tissue deposition of polyvinylpyrrolidone in normal and irradiated rabbits. Arch Int Pharmacodyn Ther 106:151–163

Vane JR (1969) The release and fate of vasoactive hormones in the circulation: the second Gaddum Memorial lecture. Br J Pharmacol 35:209–242

Veltmann G, Muertz R (1976) EKG-Veränderungen bei Dextran-Unverträglichkeit. Dtsch Med Wochenschr 101:1493–1495

Vorhees AB, Baker HJ, Pulaski EJ (1951) Reaction of albino rat to injections of dextran. Proc Soc Exp Biol Med 76:254–256

Waddell WR, Geyer RP, Olsen FR, Stare FJ (1957) Clinical observations on the use of non-phosphatide (pheronic) fat emulsions. Metabolism 6:815–821

Waldhausen E, Brinke G, Nagel A, Lohmann R (1975) Allergische Reaktionen nach Dextraninfusionen. Anesthesist 24:129–135

Watkin DM (1957) Clinical, chemical, hematologic and anatomic changes accompanying repeated intravenous administration of fat emulsions to man. Metabolism [Suppl] 6:785–806

Webster AL, Comfort PT, Fischer AJG (1973) Two cases (one fatal) of severe reactions to Rheomacrodex. S Afr Med J 47:2421–2422

Weitkamp LR, Arends T, Gallango ML, Neel JV, Schultz J, Shreffler DC (1972) The genetic structure of a tribal population, the Yanomama Indians. III. Seven serum protein systems. Ann Hum Genet 35:271–279

Weitkamp LR, Salzano FM, Neel JV, Porta F, Geerdinf RA, Tarnoky AL (1973) Human serum albumin: twenty-three genetic variants and population distribution. Ann Hum Genet 36:381–392

Wells JV, Buckley RH, Schanfield MS, Fudenberg HH (1977) Anaphylactic reactions to plasma infusions in patients with hypogammaglobulinemia and anti-IgA antibodies. Clin Immunol Immunopathol 8:265–271

West GB (1977) Anaphylactoid responses in rats. Int Arch Allergy Appl Immunol 55:542–545

Westphal O (1975) Bacterial endotoxins. Int Arch Allergy Appl Immunol 49:1–43

Wick G, Furthmayr H, Timpl R (1975) Purified antibodies to collagen: an immunofluorescence study of their reaction with tissue collagen. Int Arch Allergy Appl Immunol 48:664–679

Wick G, Nowack H, Hahn E, Timpl R, Miller EJ (1976) Visualization of type I and II collagens in tissue sections by immunohistologic techniques. J Immunol 117:298–303

Wiedersheim M (1957) An investigation of oxyethylstarch as a new plasma volume expander in animals. Arch Int Pharmacodyn Ther 111:353–361

Wilkinson AW (1956) Dextran without reactions. Lancet 2:604–606

Wilkinson AW, Storey ID (1953) Reactions to dextran. Lancet 2:956–958

Wisborg K (1975) Anaphylactic reaction induced by infusions of polygeline (haemaccel). Br J Anesth 47:1116–1117

Wretlind A (1947) Free amino acids in dialyzed casein digest. Acta Physiol Scand 13:45–54

Yamakawa S (1920) Nippon Naika Gakkai Zasshi 17:122–126

Ziegler HK (1978) Sektionsbefund bei Dextranzwischenfall. Med Klin 73:1089–1090

Zozaya J (1932) Immunological reactions between dextran polysaccharides and some bacterial antisera. J Exp Med 55:353–360

Zumtobel V (1974) Zur Verträglichkeit und Verwertung postoperativer parenteraler Fettgaben. In: Grundlagen und Praxis der parenteralen Ernährung. Thieme, Stuttgart

CHAPTER 21

Gastrointestinal Drugs

L. JUHLIN

A. Introduction

This review is based on information in the literature and on allergic reactions reported to the Swedish National Board of Health and Welfare from 1965 to 1979. All doctors in Sweden are supposed to report all severe side effects and side effects which are not well known, especially adverse reactions to new drugs. The effects are then judged as certain, probable, or possible. Only certain and probable allergic reactions will be considered here.

B. Antacids

Aluminium hydroxide, magnesium hydroxide, and magnesium carbonate are frequently dispensed in combinations and widely used as antacids. I have not seen any allergic reactions described toward these common drugs except one patient with fixed drug eruption after administration of both phenolphthalein and phenobarbital who also had a similar outbreak after magnesia magma administration (ABRAMOWITZ and RUSSO 1940). ARNDT and JICK (1976) found no cutaneous reactions in over 1,000 treated patients. In Sweden only two cases of exanthema were reported as possibly caused by an antacid. One patient developed angioedema after treatment with a preparation containing alginic acid (Gaviscon) and another developed urticaria after taking a combined tablet containing bismuth-based alkalis, liquorice, and cortex frangulae (Cavedess).

C. Gastric Antisecretory Drugs

The histamine H_2 receptor antagonist, cimetidine (Tagamet) is used to inhibit acid secretion. In 900 patients treated for gastric and duodenal ulcers a rash was seen in 2 patients and periorbitaledema and rash in 1 patient (SHARPE and HAWKINS 1977). DELAUNOIS (1978) reported a case of Quincke's edema and laryngospasm and AHMED et al. (1978) a case of Stevens–Johnson syndrome. In Sweden there are reports of one certain case of asthma, one of urticaria, and three cases of exanthema. In addition there has been a case of erythema nodosum, probably caused by cimetidine.

Leukopenia and agranulocytosis have recently been reported (KLOTZ and KAY 1978; POSNETT et al. 1979; AL-KAWAS et al. 1979). The neutropenia could involve a block of histamine-induced initiation of DNA synthesis in bone marrow stem cells (POSNETT et al. 1979) but other effects are possible (FRESTON 1979). Cases of thrombocytopenia have also been reported (MCDANIEL and STEIN 1979; IDVALL 1979) as well as acute pancreatitis (ARNOLD et al. 1978) and hepatitis (VILLENEUVE and WARNER 1979). PRIMACK (1978) described renal allograft rejection after administration of cimetidine which might have stimulated elements of the immune system. The febrile reactions observed might be due to blockade of histamine H_2 receptors in the thermoregulatory areas of the hypothalamus (NISTICÒ et al. 1978). Confusion after administration of cimetidine and brain stem dysfunction might suggest ischemia (CUMMING and FOSTER 1978).

Anticholinergic drugs used for the treatment of peptic ulcer include tertiary ammonium compounds such as atropine, belladonna, and scopolamine and quaternary ammonium compounds such as propantheline bromide, hyoscine-n-butyl bromide, and mepenzolate bromide. Scarlatiniform exanthema and urticaria have been mentioned in the literature (WISE and SULZBERGER 1933; ALEXANDER 1955; BRUINSMA 1977) but must be very rare. MATANIC (1956) described a patient with urticaria-like lesions and purpura who showed a positive intradermal reaction to atropine. Scopolamine given for analgesia during labor caused edema of the uvula and glottis in three patients (KIRSCHBAUM 1942; STEINBERG 1945; MAYER 1949).

Fixed drug eruptions have been described after atropine, belladonna, and scopolamine (CORNBLEET et al. 1955; WELSH 1961; KANDIL 1969; KAUPPINEN 1972). Single cases of dermatitis and purpura have also been seen (MATANIC 1956). The reactions reported in Sweden appear in Table 1.

D. Laxatives

Anthraquinones have cathartic properties and inhibit water and electrolyte absorption. The principal agents in this group are sagrada from *Rhamnus purshiana*, senna, and danthron. Dermatitis of the anal area has been described and found to be due to the formation of an irritant anthraquinone (DOEPFMER 1954; IPPEN 1959; BERGSTRÖM and HOLST 1972). Two cases of exanthema have been reported in Sweden.

Diphenylmethanes are another type of cathartic which include phenolphthalein, bisacodyl, and oxyphenisatin. The laxative properties of phenolphthalein were first described by VÁMOSSY (1902). It was, at that time, added in small amounts to wine in Hungary as a denaturant and to show that tax had been paid to the governement (WELSH 1961). That the drug can cause characteristic skin lesions was first observed by TRIMBLE (1909). Unaware of this report ABRAMOWITZ (1918) and FOX (1918) described a second case. In the following years several fixed cutaneous reactions to phenolphthalein were described (WELSH 1961). The lesions are one or several macular plaques varying in size from that of a pinhead to that of a palm. They appear any where on the skin and may involve the nails, but are most frequently seen in the mouth and on the genitals. Early lesions are red and sometimes itch. Later they become darker brownish or violaceous. In very pigmented patients the intensity of the blackness becomes deeper (BROWNE 1964). They persist for months after discontinuation of the drug and often leave residual pigmentation. When the patient takes the drug again the lesions recur in the same

Table 1. Allergic reactions to anticholinergic drugs reported to the Swedish National Board of Health 1967–1978

Drug	Type of reaction	Cases
Butylscopolamine	Anaphylactic shock	1
	Erythema multiforme	1
	Exanthema	1
Methylscopolamine	Exanthema	2
Hyocyamine sulfate	Exanthema	2
	Urticaria	1
Propantheline bromide	Exanthema	1
	Urticaria	1
Emepromium bromide	Agranulacytosis	1
	Thrombocytopenia	3
	Exanthema	1
Belladonna and phenobarbital	Stevens–Johnson syndrome	1
Isopromamideiodide and prochlorperazinemalente	Purpura	1
	Stevens–Johnson syndrome	1
	Exanthema	1
Clidinium bromide and chlordiazepozide	Exanthema	2
	Urticaria	1
Oxiphencyclimine and meprobamat	Agranulacytosis	1
	Stevens–Johnson syndrome	1

skin area. The fixed eruptions also appear as urticarial (CORSON and SIDLICK 1922; PHILLIPPS 1932), vesicular, postular, bullous, eczematous, and erythema multiforme-like lesions (WISE and SULZBERGER 1933; WELSH 1961). That the lesions can appear suddenly in an individual who has used phenolphthalein for years points to an allergic mechanism. Small amounts, which can be present in icing on cakes, candy, pink mouthwashes, toothpastes, and beverages can cause relapses (ABRAMOWITZ 1935).

Positive patch tests to phenolphthalein have been reported in some eczematous lesions (BERNSTEIN 1931; WISE and SULZBERGER 1933). False positive patch tests, reflecting epidermal hysteresis, have also been demonstrated after phenolphthalein administration (SHELLEY et al. 1972). WYATT et al. (1972) found that serum taken during exacerbations produced a local inflammation when injected intradermally. Possible cross-reaction with erythrosin which is used as a food and drug colorant has been reported (WILE 1936). Other rare allergic manifestations after phenolphthalein administration are urticaria, Stevens–Johnson syndrome, lupus erythematosus-like eruptions, and encephalitis (LINDEMAYR 1959; KENDALL 1954).

Bisacodyl can produce a generalized exanthema and six such cases have been reported in Sweden. Oxyphenisitin is no longer used since it can cause hepatitis (PEARSON et al. 1971; REYNOLDS et al. 1971).

Castor oil contains a triglyceride of ricinoleic acid which is hydrolyzed by intestinal lipases to glycerol and ricinoleic acid, which has cathartic effects. Allergic reactions such as angioedema, rhinitis, asthma, and scarlatiniform rashes have been described but seem to be rare reactions to this common laxative (BENNETT and SCHWARTZ 1934; BLANK 1945).

Surfactants such as dioctyl sodium sulfosuccinate are also used as laxatives. A case of anaphylactic shock has been reported in Sweden after administration of an enema. The preparation also contained sorbitol and benzoates as preservative.

Bulk-forming laxatives contain indigestible, unabsorbed polysaccharides. Among these drugs are carboxymethylcellulose, psyllium preparations, agar gums, and bran. Symptoms of asthma, rhinitis, ocularpruritus, and itching of hands and face have been observed after exposure to ispaghula powder, which consists of finely ground psyllium seeds (*Plantago ovata*). Psyllium is a member of the plantain weed familiy. The specificity of the reaction was proven by positive immediate skin tests and radioallergosorbent test (RAST) (BERNTON 1970; BUSSE and SCHOENWETTER 1975; MACHADO et al. 1979). The symptoms have been described in factory workers, nurses, and patients handling the laxatives. Examples of such psyllium preparations are Vi-Siblin, Metamucil, and Lunelax. Atopic subjects are more easily sensitized. It is advisable to use the granulated and less dusty forms of such bulk laxatives (MACHADO et al. 1979). Asthma, hay fever, and urticaria have also been seen after administration of laxatives containing gums like Indian (karaya) gum and tragacanth (BULLEN 1934; FEINBERG 1935; BOWEN 1939; FIGLEY 1940; GELFAND 1943; BROWN and CREPEA 1947).

E. Antidiarrheal Agents

Morphine and opiates decrease propulsive contractions and have long been used to arrest diarrhea. They are now often replaced by diphenoxylate and difenoxine, often in combination with atropine. Allergic side effects are unusual. Fixed drug eruption can occur from opium (WELSH 1961) but it is rare. In Sweden a few cases of urticaria, angioedema, exanthema, and purpura have been reported. A preparation containing diphenoxylate and atropine (Retardin) caused urticaria and angioedema in three patients and exanthema in one.

F. Anti-Inflammatory Drugs

Sulfasalazine (salicylazosulfapyridine, Salazopyrin) is a chemical combination of sulfapyridine and salicylate and is given orally in the treatment of inflammatory bowel disease. Sensitivity reactions are common and include exanthema, photosensitivity, urticaria, bronchospasm, pulmonary eosinophilia, hemolytic anemia, leukopenia, thrombocytopenia, and agranulocytosis. They have been reviewed by COLLINS (1968), DAS and DUBIN (1976), and MILLER (1977). Pulmonary eosinophila and hypersensitivity with symptoms of dyspnea and fever have been reported by several authors and summarized by TYDD (1976) and CONSTANTINIDIS (1976). Less frequent reactions are toxic epidermal necrolysis (STRÖM 1969; VÁRKONYI and TÖRÖK 1976), Stevens–Johnson syndrome (CARROL et al. 1966; STRÖM 1977), fibrosing alveolitis (DAVIES and MACFARLANE 1974), pulmonary vasculitis (ISENBERG et al. 1968), hepatitis (CHESTER et al. 1978; MIHAS et al. 1978; SOTOLONGO et al. 1978), pancreatitis (BLOCK et al. 1970), bloody diarrhea (WERLIN and GRAND 1978), neurotoxicity (WALLACE 1970), and lupus erythematosus (GRIFFITHS and KANE 1977; JAUP 1978). Recently male infertility due to sulfasalazine has also been

Table 2. Reactions to sulfasalazine reported in Sweden 1967–1978

Type of reaction	Cases
Skin	
Exanthema	44
Urticaria	5
Erythrodermia	4
Stevens-Johnson syndrome	4
Erythema multiforme	2
Lupus-like syndrome	3
Photosensitivity	1
Blood	
Agranulocytosis	17
Hemolytic anemia	10
Leukopenia	7
Thrombocytopenia	5
Aplastic anemia	1
Other	
Fever	25
Pulmonary reaction	5
Arthralgia	3
Nonspecificic allergies	6

reported in five patients (LEVI et al. 1979). The mechanism for the infertility was unknown. Erythema nodosum is reported as a complication of ulcerative colitis. It is possible that sulfasalazine could be responsible in some cases. The hypersensitivity reactions reported in Sweden are shown in Table 2.

Neomycin is used to alter the intestinal flora in preparation of the bowel for surgery and in hepatic coma. In patients with allergic contact dermatitis to neomycin it may cause a flare of the skin lesions (PIRILÄ and RANTANEN 1960; EKELUND and MÖLLER 1969). Nystatin is effective in eliminating moniliasis. Side effects are rare. A case of fixed drug eruption has been reported (KANDIL 1969).

Halogenated hydroxyquinolines act on microorganisms in the intestinal tract and have been used for "traveler's diarrhea." In Japan clioquinol (Vioform) has caused a subacute myelooptic neuropathy (SMON). The oral preparations have therefore been removed from the market in most countries. Clioquinol is still used topically and can cause contact dermatitis. A flare of contact dermatitis after oral intake has been reported (LEIFER and STEINER 1951; DOMAR and JUHLIN 1967; EKELUND and MÖLLER 1969).

G. Miscellaneous Drugs

Cholestyramin is a basic anion exchange resin which is used to ameliorate watery diarrhea in cases of ileal dysfunction, ileal resection, and vagotomy. It is also used to relieve pruritus due to elevated serum and skin levels of bile salts in patients with intrahepatic cholestasis and to lower cholesterol levels in familial hypercholesterolemia. One case of exanthema and one with Stevens–Johnson syndrome have been reported in Sweden.

Desferoxamine (Desferal) is a chelating agent used to remove excess iron from the body in conditions such as hemochromatosis and in acute iron poisoning. Erythema, probably mediated through histamine release and two cases of urticaria have been described after intramuscular injection (WESTLIN 1971). After oral treatment no allergic side effects are reported.

Penicillamine is a chelating agent which binds copper, mercury, zinc, and lead. It has been used to treat poisoning from these chemicals and also for disorders of copper metabolism such as Wilson's disease and primary biliary cirrhosis. Penicillamine has been tried in scleroderma and arthritis. Hypersensitivity reactions are common. About 20%–30% of the patients show hypersensitivity reactions suchs as morbilliform exanthema, urticaria, purpura, anorexia, lymphadenopathy, leukopenia, and thrombocytopenia (MEYBOOM 1975; BALME and HUSKISSON 1977). More severe skin symptoms associated with penicillamine therapy are Stevens–Johnson syndrome, pemphigus, myasthenia gravis, cholestatic jaundice (BARZILAI et al. 1978), nephropathy (LANGE 1978) and lupus-like syndrome (HARPEY et al. 1972).

Bronchial asthma has been described in a mother who had opened capsules of pancreatic extract, which had been prescribed for her children suffering from cystic fibrosis (SAKULA 1977). Piperazine is an anthelmintic drug. Single cases of angioedema, urticaria, exanthema, and erythema multiforme have been reported in Sweden. Suppositories and ointments used for the anal region can cause allergic contact dermatitis. Procaine, benzocaine, cinchocaine, and antimicrobial agents are the most common offenders. We have seen two cases of purpura and one case of urticaria caused by such suppositories.

Acknowledgements. This work was supported by grants from the Swedish Research Council.

References

Abramowitz EW (1918) Erythema multiforme associated with cutaneous pigmentation (melanin): clinical and pathologic report of five cases. J Cutan Dis 36:11–12

Abramowitz EW (1935) Reactions due to phenolphthalein. A study of their pathogenesis. Arch Dermatol Syphilol 31:777–795

Abramowitz EW, Russo JJ (1940) Fixed eruption from magnesium hydroxide. Polysensitivity. Arch Dermatol Syphilol 41:707–710

Ahmed AH, McLarty DG, Sharma SK, Masawe AEJ (1978) Stevens-Johnson syndrome treatment with cimetidine. Lancet 2:433

Alexander HL (1955) Reactions with drug therapy. Saunders, Philadelphia

Al-Kawas FH, Lenes BA, Sacher RA (1979) Cimetidine and agranulocytosis. Ann Intern Med 90:992–993

Arndt KA, Jick H (1976) Rates of cutaneous reactions to drugs. A report from the Boston collaborative drug surveillance program. JAMA 235:918–923

Arnold F, Doyle PJ, Bell G (1978) Acute pancreatitis in a patient treated with cimetidine. Lancet 1:382–383

Balme HW, Huskisson EC (1977) Side effects of penicillamine other than nephropathy and their management. In: Penicillamine research in rheumatoid disease. Fabritius, Oslo, pp 250–254

Barzilai D, Dickstein G, Enat R, Bassan H, Lichtig C, Gellei B (1978) Cholestatic jaundice caused by D-penicillamine. Ann Rheum Dis 37:98–100

Bennett RH, Schwartz E (1934) Castor bean dust sensitization. J Allergy 5:427–431

Bergström G, Holst R (1972) Perianala hudförändringar orsakade av antrakinon i avföringsmedel. Lakartidningen 69:28–29

Bernstein F (1931) Überempfindlichkeit gegen Phenolphthalein. Dermatol Z 62:368–369

Bernton HS (1970) The allergenicity of psyllium seed. Med Ann DC 39:313–317

Blank P (1945) Sensitization of the oral administration of castor oil. Ann Allergy 3:297

Block MB, Genant HK, Kirsner JB (1970) Pancreatitis as an adverse reaction to salicylazosulfapyridine. N Engl J Med 282:380–382

Bowen R (1939) Karaya gum as a cause of urticaria. Arch Dermatol Syphilol 39:506–509

Brown EB, Crepea SB (1947) Allergy (asthma) to ingested gum tragacanth. J Allergy 18:214–216

Browne SG (1964) Fixed eruption in deeply pigmented subjects: clinical observations on 350 patients. Br Med J 2:1041–1044

Bruinsma W (1977) A guide to drug eruptions. The file of adverse reactions to the skin. University of Amsterdam

Bullen SS (1934) Perennial hay fever from Indian gum (karaya gum). J Allergy 5:484–487

Busse W, Schoenwetter WF (1975) Asthma from psyllium in laxative manufacture. Ann Intern Med 83:361–362

Carroll OM, Bryan PA, Robinson RJ (1966) Stevens-Johnson syndrome associated with long-acting sulfonamides. JAMA 195:691–693

Chester AC, Diamond LH, Schreiner GE (1978) Hypersensitivity to salicylazosulfapyridine. Renal and hepatic toxic reactions. Arch Intern Med 138:1138–1139

Collins JR (1968) Adverse reactions to salicylazosulfapyridine (azulfide) in the treatment of ulcerative colitis. South Med J 61:354–358

Constantinides KA (1976) Eosinophilic pneumonia. An unusual side effect of therapy with salicylazosulfapyridine. Chest 70:315–316

Cornbleet T, Hoit L, Sickley JF (1955) Fixed eruption. Arch Dermatol 71:507–510

Corson EF, Sidlick DM (1922) Urticaria from habitual use of phenolphthalein. JAMA 78:882–883

Cumming WJK, Foster JB (1978) Cimetidine-induced brainsteam dysfunction. Lancet 1:1096

Das KM, Dubin R (1976) Clinical pharmacokinetics of sulphasalazine. Clin Pharmacokinet 1:406–425

Davies D, MacFarlane A (1974) Fibrosing alveolitis and treatment with sulphasalazine. Gut 15:185–188

Delaunois L (1978) Hypersensitivity to cimetidine. N Engl J Med 300:1216

Doepfmer R (1954) Zur Kenntnis des perianalen Istizin-Erythems. Hautarzt 5:278–279

Domar M, Juhlin L (1967) Allergic dermatitis produced by oral clioquinol. Lancet 1:1165–1166

Ekelund AG, Möller H (1969) Oral provocation in eczematous contact allergy to neomycin and hydroxy-quinolines. Acta Derm Venereol (Stockh) 49:422–426

Feinberg SM (1935) Karaya gum asthma. JAMA 105:505

Figley KD (1940) Karaya gum (Indian gum) hypersensitivity. JAMA 114:747–748

Fox H (1918) Erythema perstans following ingestion of phenolphthalein. J Cutan Dis 36:252–253

Freston JW (1979) Cimetidine and granulocytopenia. Ann Intern Med 90:264–265

Gelfand HH (1943) The allergenic properties of the vegetable gums. A case of asthma due to tragacanth. J Allergy 14:203–219

Griffiths JD, Kane SP (1977) Sulphasalazine-induced lupus syndrome in ulcerative colitis. Br Med J 2:1188–1189

Harpey JP, Caille B, Moulias R, Goust JM (1972) Drug allergy and lupus-like syndrome (with special reference to d-penicillamine). In: Dash CH, Jones HEH (eds) Mechanisms in drug allergy. Churchill Livingstone, Edinburgh London, pp 51–57

Idvall J (1979) Cimetidine-associated thrombocytopenia. Lancet 2:159

Ippen H (1959) Ätiologie und Pathogenese des sogenannten Istizin-Exanthemes. Dtsch Med Wochenschr 84:1062–1066

Isenberg JI, Goldstein H, Korn AR, Ozeran RS, Rosen V (1968) Pulmonary vasculitis – an uncommon complication of ulcerative colitis. N Engl J Med 279·1376–1377

Jaup H (1978) Salazosulfapyridin-induziertes Lupus-erythematodes-Syndrom bei Colitis ulcerosa. Dtsch Med Wochenschr 103:1211–1213

Kandil E (1969) Fixed drug eruptions. Dermatologica 139:37

Kauppinen K (1972) Cutaneous reactions to drugs. Acta Derm Venereol (Stockh) [Suppl] 52:68

Kendall AC (1954) Fatal case of encephalitis after phenolphthalein ingestion. Br Med J 2:1461–1462

Kirschbaum HM (1942) Scopolamine in obstetrics. Am J Obstet Gynecol 44:664–672

Klotz SA, Kay BF (1978) Cimetidine and agranulocytosis. Ann Intern Med 88:579

Lange K (1978) Nephropathy induced by D-penicillamine. Contrib Nephrol 10:63–74

Leifer W, Steiner K (1951) Studies in sensitization to halogenated hydroxy-quinolines and related compounds. J Invest Dermatol 17:233–240

Levi AJ, Fisher AM, Hughs L, Hendry WF (1979) Male infertility to sulphasalazine. Lancet 2:276–277

Lindemayr W (1959) Arzneiexantheme. Dermatol Venerol 3/1:327–383

Machado L, Zetterström O, Fagerberg E (1979) Occupational allergy in nurses to a bulk laxative. Allergy 34:51–55

Matanic V (1956) L'urticaire provoquée par l'atropine avec fin létale. Int Arch Allergy 8:262–270

Mayer EC (1949) Edema of the uvula, a manifestation of scopolamine sensitivity. Calif Med 71:146–147

McDaniel JL, Stein JJ (1979) Thrombocytopenia with cimetidine therapy. N Engl J Med 300:864

Meyboom RHB (1975) Heavy metal antagonists. In: Dukes MNG (ed) Meyler's side effects of drugs, 8. Excerpta Medica, Amsterdam London New York, pp 529–542

Mihas AA, Goldenberg DJ, Slaughter RL (1978) Sulfasalazine toxic reactions. Hepatitis, fever and skin rash with hypocomplementemia and immune complexes. JAMA 239:2590–2591

Miller B (1977) Wirkung und Nebenwirkungen der Therapie mit Salizylazosulfapyridin. In: Kremer K, Kivelitz H (eds) Colitis ulcerosa. Thieme, Stuttgart, pp 71–86

Nisticò G, Rotiroti D, de Sarro A, Naccari F (1978) Mechanism of cimetidine-induced fever. Lancet 2:265–266

Pearson AJG, Grainger JM, Scheuer PJ, McIntyre N (1971) Jaundice due to oxyphenisatin. Lancet 1:994–996

Phillipps FA (1932) Toxic effects of phenolphthalein. Lancet 1:803

Pirilä V, Rantanen A (1960) Root canal treatment with bacitracinneomycin as cause of flare-up of allergic eczema. Oral Surg 13:589–593

Posnett DN, Stein RS, Graber SE, Krantz SB (1979) Cimetidine-induced neutropenia. A possible dose related phenomenon. Arch Intern Med 139:584–586

Primack WA (1978) Cimetidine and renal-allograft rejection. Lancet 1:824–825

Reynolds TB, Peters RL, Yamade S (1971) Chronic active and lupoid hepatitis caused by a laxative, oxyphenisation. N Engl J Med 285:813–820

Sakula A (1977) Bronchial asthma due to allergy to pancreatic extract. Lancet 2:193

Sharpe PC, Hawkins BW (1977) Efficacy and safety of cimetidine. Long-term treatment with cimetidine. In: Burland WL, Simkins MA (eds) Cimetidine. Proc Second Int Symp on Histamine H_2-receptor Antagonists. Excerpta Medica, Amsterdam London New York, pp 358–366

Shelley WB, Schlappner OLA, Heiss HB (1972) Demonstration of intercellular immunofluorescence and epidermal hysteresis in bullous fixed drug eruption due to phenolphthalein. Br J Dermatol 86:118–125

Sotolongo RP, Neefe LI, Rudzki C, Ishak KG (1978) Hypersensitivity reaction to sulfasalazine with severe hepatotoxicity. Gastroenterology 75:95–99

Steinberg M (1945) Edema of the uvula and glottis; a reaction to demerol-scopolamine anesthesia. Am J Obstet Gynecol 50:542–545

Ström J (1969) Toxic epidermal necrolysis (Lyell's syndrome). A report on four cases with three deaths. Scand J Infext Dis 1:209–216

Ström J (1977) Aetiology of febrile mucocutaneous syndromes with special reference to the provocative role of infections and drugs. Acta Med Scand 201:131–136

Trimble WB (1909) Purpura. J Cutan Dis 27:306

Tydd TF (1976) Sulphasalazine lung. Med J Aust 1:570–573

Vámossy Z (1902) Über ein neues Abführmittel (Purgen). Ther Ggw 4:201–202

Várkonyi V, Török I (1976) Salazopyrin okozta Lyell-syndroma. Orv Hetil 117:971–973

Villeneuve JP, Warner HA (1979) Cimetidine hepatitis. Gastroenterology 77:143–144

Wallace IW (1970) Neurotoxicity associated with a reaction to sulphasalazine. Practitioner 204:850–851

Welsh AL (1961) The fixed eruption. A possible hazard of modern drug therapy. Thomas, Springfield

Werlin SL, Grand RJ (1978) Bloody diarrhea – a new complication of sulfasalazine. J Pediatr 92:450–451

Westlin WF (1971) Desferoxamine as a chelating agent. Clin Toxicol 4:597–602

Wile UJ (1936) Discussion case presentation. Arch Dermatol Syphilol 33:1089–1090

Wise F, Sulzberger MB (1933) Drug eruptions. I. Fixed phenolphthalein eruptions. Arch Dermatol Syphilol 27:549–567

Wyatt E, Greaves M, Søndergaard J (1972) Fixed drug eruption (phenolphthalein). Evidence for a blood born mediator. Arch Dermatol 106:671–673

CHAPTER 22

Intolerance to Food and Drug Additives

L. JUHLIN

A. Introduction

Fresh farm and dairy products are increasingly being replaced by manufactured and prepared convenience foods. With this change there has been an increased use of food additives. We have now more than 2,500 chemicals that can be added to enhance the quality and facilitate the preparation of food. The largest group consists of 1,200 flavoring agents. The main types of additives and their amounts are listed in Table 1. Their chemical structure, properties, occurrence, and regulatory status are described in two books edited by FURIA (1972) and FURIA and BELLANCA (1971). Hypersensitivity reactions to such products have been reported, especially for coloring agents, preservatives, and antioxidants. These chemicals can also be added to drugs in quantities which are high enough to produce symptoms (JUHLIN et al. 1972). The structures of some common offenders are given in Fig. 1.

B. Symptoms of Intolerance

I. Hyperkinetic Behavior Disturbance

This syndrome is mainly seen in children who show an increase of purposeless physical activity and reduced attention. The diagnosis is not easy to make, since

Table 1. Food additives used in the United States in 1967. (ANGELINE and LEONARDOS 1973)

Type	Amount $(kg \times 10^6)$
Thickeners and stabilizers	138
Nutrient supplements, protein additives, enzymes	109
Flavoring agents and enhancers	100
Surfactants	73
Leavening, bleaching, and maturing agents	51
Buffers, acids, alkalies	46
Coloring agents	36
Preservatives	17
Antioxidants	7
Miscellaneous (sorbitol, anticaking agents, dough conditioners)	31
Total	608

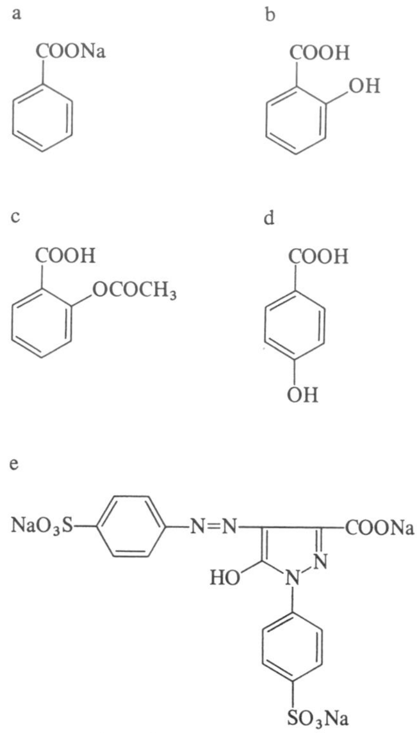

Fig. 1a–e. Chemical structures of (**a**) sodium benzoate, (**b**) salicylic acid, (**c**) acetylsalicylic acid, (**d**) 4-hydroxybenzoic acid, and (**e**) tartrazine

similar symptoms may be due to simple restlessness caused by such factors as hunger or lack of understanding by teachers or parents. Hyperactive children often have learning difficulties and some have complex behavior problems. Estimates of the prevalence of hyperactivity vary from 3% to 15% (SCHRAG and DIVOKY 1975). The syndrome is more common in males with a male: female ratio ranging from 4:1 to 9:1. The cause of the symptoms are probably multifactorial. It has been described in terms of brain injury caused by trauma, virus infections and social and dietary factors.

That dyes, preservatives and other additives as well as salicylates are responsible was first postulated by FEINGOLD at a meeting in 1973. It received widespread publicity and was published in the Congressional Report (BEAL 1973). FEINGOLD (1975) claimed a dramatic and rapid improvement in 25%–50% of hyperactive children after they were given a diet free from artificial food colors and flavors. The first two scientific studies designed to test Feingold's hypothesis came from Australia (COOK and WOODHILL 1976; SALZMAN 1976). They found a marked improvement of the children after adoption of the Feingold diet (as scored by their mothers). Both studies were critically analyzed in a guest editorial (WERRY 1976). In another study by CONNERS et al. (1976) there was a significant reduction in hyperactivity as judged by teacher ratings. A diminution of symptoms was also found by BRENNER (1977). To eliminate bias by parents and teachers two other studies were later published. WILLIAMS et al. (1978) showed some improvement of the test scores in 25% of the children. The most rigidly controlled and comprehensive study was reported by HARLEY et al. (1978). The teachers and special observers could detect no differences in the children's behavior when on the special diets, but the parents by contrast scored their children less active on the diet.

Thus the evidence to date indicates that there might be a scarcely significant relationship between diet and behavior, but the food additive controversy is not yet settled as pointed out in an editorial by BIERMAN and FURUKAWA (1978). The antioxidants butylhydroxyanisole (BHA) and butylhydroxytoluene (BHT) have been added to the list of agents which should be avoided, but there is no evidence that they can influence behavior. The amount of color tested is often 100 mg, which usually exceeds the daily intake, especially when taken repeatedly. One should also differentiate between azo dyes and other chemical types of dye. An excellent review of these problems has recently been published by LIPTON et al. (1979).

II. Contact Dermatitis

Contact dermatitis to additives in food and drugs has been described, but is rare (FISCHER 1973). It is more common to additives used in topical medications and cosmetics (WILKINSON 1972). Here we are dealing with a lymphocyte-mediated allergy where sensitization of the patients occurs after repeated local contact of the skin with the chemical.

1. Dyes

In patients sensitive to p-phenylenediamine, the intake of certain azo dyes caused a flare of their dermatitis (BAER and LEIDER 1949; SIDI and AROUETE 1959). The cross-reactivity between various allergenic dyes has been tested by WEIRICH (1961). Contact dermatitis to azo dyes employed in the textile and leather industries was described by SUURMOND et al. (1967). ROELEVELD and VAN KETEL (1976) reported a patient with a dermatitis caused by a yellow shirt. The patch test was positive to the azo dye, tartrazine. Interestingly the eruptions worsened after drinking orange juice which could have contained tartrazine. CALNAN (1976) found positive patch tests to quinazoline yellow which is used in foods, drugs, and cosmetics. GRATER (1976) reported 133 positive reactions to a set of such dyes.

2. Antioxidants

ROED-PETERSEN and HJORT (1976) and FISCHER (1976) have demonstrated contact dermatitis to antioxidants which are hidden sensitizers in topical medications and in foods. Antioxidants are usually phenols such as BHA, BHT, nordihydroguaiaretic acid (NGDA), and gallate esters. BURCKHARDT and FIERZ (1964) and BRUN (1964, 1970) described contact dermatitis from gallate esters in margarine. α-Tocopherol has been used extensively in food and topical applications but only a few cases of contact dermatitis have been reported (BRODKIN and BLEIBERG 1965; AELING et al. 1973; MINKIN et al. 1973; MARZULLI and MAIBACH 1974; ROED-PETERSEN and HJORT 1976).

3. Preservatives

Preservatives such as parabens, i.e., esters of *p*-hydroxybenzoic acid are used in the pharmaceutical and cosmetic industry as well as in foods. Allergic reactions to parabens have been reported with increasing frequency from the United States (Fischer 1973). Contact allergy to sorbic acid has also been reported but seems to be rare (Hjort and Trolle-Lassen 1962; Klaschka and Beiersdorff 1965; Fischer et al. 1971; Saihan and Harman 1978; Brown 1979). That the dermatitis should flare up or get worse after intravenous or oral ingestion of such preservatives has not been reported.

4. Flavors

Cinnamon and cinnamic aldehyde are used in cooking, bakeries, confectionery, soft drinks, vermouth, chewing gum, ice cream, mouthwashes, toothpicks, tooth-pastes, and cosmetics. Allergic contact dermatitis has been described by several authors. Leifer (1951) reviewed the literature and described a case where ingestion of cinnamon produced a flare of a dermatitis owing to previous topical sensitization. Further cases were reported by Hjort (1961), Schorr (1975), Magnusson and Wilkinson (1975), and Drake and Maibach (1976). Cinnamon cross-reacts with balsam of Peru (Hjort 1961). The ingestion of quinine which is used as a bitter flavor in "tonic water" may produce contact dermatitis in sensitized individuals (Fischer 1966). Cyclamates have been used as sweetening agents and documented cases of photodermatitis have been described (Kabori and Araki 1966; Lamberg 1967).

5. Stabilizers

Ethylenediamine hydrochloride is used in topical preparations and is a common sensitizer (Epstein and Maibach 1968). Sensitive patients can react with dermatitis when the ethylenediamine is taken systemically (Provost and Jillson 1967). It may cross-react with ethylenediamine tetraacetate (EDTA) which is used as a preservative in eyedrops and in the cosmetic industry (Raymond and Gross 1969). EDTA is also used as a sequestrant in food systems; it acts synergistically to several antioxidants and may be present in fats, oils, salad dressings, meat, seafood, vegetables, beverages, and dairy products (Furia 1972).

III. Recurrent Urticaria and Angioedema

Urticaria is a common symptom and 20% of people have had, have or will have it. Urticaria is usually easy to diagnose. The wheals are elevated, red, warm, and often itch when they develop. The symptoms are a sign of histamine release. In acute urticaria the cause of histamine release is often an allergic reaction to a drug or food. In recurrent or chronic urticaria, the mechanism is more complicated and rather uncertain. In many cases the complement system is involved (Laurell et al. 1977). The coagulation system is also involved in certain patients with the formation of fibrin microclots in vitro when the patient's blood is exposed to bacterial endotoxin (JUHLIN and SHELLEY 1977). Such asteroid fibrin bodies are not seen in healthy volunteers but are common in blood from patients with vasculitis. The center of the oriented fibrin star formation is usually a monocyte (SHELLEY and JUHLIN 1977).

Before the diagnosis of recurrent urticaria is made we have to exclude urticaria caused by heat, cold, pressure, urticaria pigmentosa, and hereditary angioedema. The remaining cases of urticaria that continue for more than 2–3 months are generally called recidivating if the periods without lesions are longer than those with the wheals, and chronic if the periods free of urticaria are shorter. Strict differentiation between these types of urticaria is often difficult, hence they are classified together as recurrent urticaria. Certain foods and drinks are mentioned by 40% of our patients as possible agents which might worsen or provoke their urticaria (JUHLIN 1980). However, real allergy to foods was seen in only 2% of the patients studied by CHAMPION et al. (1969). Exacerbation of the urticaria is common after administration of salicylates and also after ingestion of a number of food additives. At present the only way one can determine such a hypersensitivity is through provocation tests. Several such studies have now been published.

An urticarial reaction to an azo dye, tartrazine, was first reported by LOCKEY (1959). SAMTER and BEERS (1968) found that some of their aspirin-sensitive patients with urticaria also reacted to tartrazine. We found that seven of ten patients with aspirin intolerance reacted to tartrazine (JUHLIN et al. 1972). Some of the patients also reacted to benzoic acid and its derivatives. In a selected sample of 52 patients with chronic urticaria studied by MICHAËLSSON and JUHLIN (1973) half the patients reacted within 14–20 h with urticaria to different azo dyes and benzoic acid compounds. The doses used in the provocation test were easily exceeded in daily life by the consumption of foods and drugs. For one azo dye, tartrazine, a positive reaction with urticaria was obtained in 36% of the patients tested. Lower figures for tartrazine (13%–21%) were reported by THUNE and GRANHOLT (1975) and WARIN and SMITH (1976). A possible reason for our higher figures is that many of the patients were referred to us for investigation because they had a history of angioedema or hypersensitivity to aspirin or azo dyes.

Since our first publication in 1973 we have investigated 330 patients treated for chronic urticaria in the clinic from 1974 to 1979 (JUHLIN 1981). The various food additives were given in coded, white, opaque capsules with lactose as placebo. A reaction was judged positive if the patient developed urticaria within 24 h. The reactions were judged by various doctors as positive, questionable, and negative. The results appear in Table 2. Retesting of patients with questionable reactions was not done in most cases, which might explain the high number of reactions judged as uncertain. This sample is also selected. Aspirin-, benzoate-, and azo dye-reacting patients had often been taken care of by the referring hospital. Several patients were now referred because they had a negative history of aspirin or azo dye hypersensitivity, which might explain the decrease in the percentage of patients reacting to aspirin and azo dyes.

From 1974 to 1978 one or more clearly positive provocation tests were found in 31% of the patients tested and 36% of the patients did not react to any of the provocations. The same figure was recently reported by AUGUST (1979). DOEGLAS

Table 2. Provocation tests in patients with recurrent urticaria: test period 1974–1978

Substance	Result (%)			Patients
	Positive	Uncertain	Negative	
Lactose	5	16	79	191
Azo dyes	18	14	68	179
Benzoates	11	18	71	172
Aspirin	22	14	64	149
Annatto, β-carotene	10	14	76	112
BHT, BHA	15	12	73	156
Sodium glutamate	7	12	81	72
Sodium nitrite, nitrate	6	12	82	60
Sorbic acid	9	14	77	115
Quinoline yellow	13	15	72	91
Yeast	16	14	70	57

(1975a, b) performed provocation tests in 131 patients with chronic urticaria or physical urticaria. He found reactions to aspirin in patients with chronic urticaria, pressure urticaria, and cholinergic urticaria. A total of 23 patients were also tested with tartrazine and benzoates. A positive reaction was found in 30% to benzoates and also to tartrazine. MIKKELSEN et al. (1978) challenged 61 consecutive patients who had chronic urticaria or angioedema to various food colors. They described reactions to annatto extract in 26% of the patients. The dose of dye was the same as used in 25 g butter. Positive reactions were also found in the following percentages: to tartrazine 11%; Sunset Yellow 17%; Food Red 17%, 16%; amaranth 9%; Ponceau 4R 15%; erythrosine 12%; and Brilliant Blue 14%.

The results of provocation tests with food additives in chronic urticaria has also been reported by other Danish authors. BRODTHAGEN et al. (1974) found positive reactions in 30% of his patients and KAABER (1978) found one or more precipitating factors in 35% of 65 patients. When the reactions to various dyes were analyzed in 23 positive patients, 3 reacted to tartrazine and 3 to other azo dyes; 5 reacted to annatto, 3 to erythrosine, and 2 to sodium benzoate. From France, MEYNADIER et al. (1979) recently reported one or more positive reactions in 17 of 24 cases with chronic urticaria. An urticarial reaction was seen after ingestion of aspirin in 10, food colors in 11, and preservatives in 6 patients.

In a questionaire to French dermatologists, on the subject of reactions to food colors, 64 positive responses and 33 negative responses were obtained but many cases were not proven (GOUNELLE DE PONTANEL et al. 1977). CASTELAIN (1977) reported 84 positive tests to various dyes in 66 patients. SETTIPANE et al. (1976) exposed 13 patients who had improved on a diet without artificial colors to as little as 0.15 mg of tartrazine in an oral double-blind study. Three of them had an exacerbation of urticaria within 3 h. Further cases of hypersensitivity to food colors have been reported by other authors (CALAS and CASTELAIN 1958; FISCHERMAN and COHEN 1973; GIRARD 1974; HUBBARD 1975; SETTIPANE and PUDUPAKKAM 1975; GRATER 1976; DRY and PRADALIER 1977; FERNANDES et al. 1977; LOCKEY 1977; BERNSTEIN et al. 1978; WELIKY et al. 1978; MONCRET-VAUTRIN and AUBERT 1978;

PELLEGRIN 1979). Urticaria to antioxidants like BHT and BHA was reported in 10%–12% of cases by THUNE and GRANHOLT (1973) and JUHLIN (1977). FISCHER-MAN and COHEN (1977) tested urticaria patients with a bleeding time test. They found that patients which were intolerant to BHT and BHA often cross-reacted to various additives such as Tween-80, sodium propionate, triglycerides, oleic acid, stearic acid, and olive oil.

Patients with chronic urticaria have been shown to improve on a diet free from azo dyes and preservatives (THUNE and GRANHOLT 1975; ROS et al. 1976; WARIN and SMITH 1976; DOEGLAS 1977; FREEDMAN 1977a; RUDZKI 1977; AUGUST 1979). The prognosis of chronic urticaria was studied by CHAMPION et al. (1969). They found that it depended on the duration of the disease. If the urticaria had lasted for 4 months, it was expected that about 25% of patients should be free from symptoms after 12 months. The finding of an abrupt change to complete freedom from symptoms within a few days in 12% of patients and that 50% got much better points to the importance of the diet (THUNE and GRANHOLT 1975). WARIN and SMITH (1976) found that 35 of 45 patients recovered or improved considerably on the diet. Similar results were also reported by GERMAN (1978). In a follow-up study on patients with chronic urticaria by ROS et al. (1976), the effect of the diet was most impressive in the 57% of patients who were much better, which meant that they only had reactions when they ingested something containing azo dyes or benzoates by mistake.

IV. Asthma, Rhinorrhea, and Nasal Polyps

Aspirin is known to cause serious reactions in certain patients with asthma (COOKE 1919). The patients can also have rhinorrhea and nasal polyps that may precede the bronchoconstrictor type of intolerance to aspirin for months or years. This triad of symptoms is common in middle-aged women. The aspirin-sensitive patients often show intolerance to other analgesics (SMITH 1971). SPEER (1958) reported that color additives can precipitate asthma. Aspirin-sensitive patients with asthma also cross-react to tartrazine in 8%–15% of the cases (CHAFFEE and SETTI-PANE 1967; SAMTER and BEERS 1967; HOSEN 1972; SETTIPANE and PUDUPAKKAM 1975; DELANEY 1976) and to various benzoates (JUHLIN et al. 1972; ROSENHALL and ZETTERSTRÖM 1973). Hypersensitivity to food colorants, preservatives, and analgesics was studied in 504 patients with asthma and rhinitis by ROSENHALL (1977). Hypersensitivity to at least one of the substances was found in 106 patients. In 33 patients sensitive to tartrazine 42% were intolerant to aspirin and 39% to sodium benzoate. Rosenhall also tested his patients with other azo dyes such as Sunset Yellow and New Coccine as well as the non-azo dyes carmine and patent blue. The method of examination and reproducibility of the results were studied in detail. Dietary treatment was found to be effective in some patients in preventing exacerbations of the disease but on the whole had no influence on the course of the disease or the need for medication.

STENIUS and LEMOLA (1976) tested 140 asthmatics for sensitivity to aspirin and tartrazine. Most of the patients sensitive to tartrazine also reacted to aspirin. In one-third of the tartrazine-sensitive patients a history of reaction to colored additives in food and drinks was obtained. They recommended that tests for sensitivity to analgesics and certain food additives should be done routinely in asthmatics, in order to give advice on medication and suitable diet to these patients.

FREEDMAN (1977b) found that among 272 patients with asthma 11% had attacks of asthma shortly after ingestion of orange soft drinks. Since they did not react to oranges or pure orange juice it seemed likely that the symptoms were caused by food additives. A total of 14 of the patients agreed to undergo challenge tests. Positive provocation tests were obtained to sulfur dioxide in eight, sodium benzoate in four, and tartrazine in one patient. This is the first report to describe asthma after ingestion of beverages containing sulfur dioxide. The reaction to sulfur dioxide was immediate and suggests inhalation or sublingual absorption.

Reactions to tartrazine have also been described in children (SPEER 1958). VEDANTHAN et al. (1977) found no adverse response after tartrazine provocation in 56 asthmatic children. SYVÄNEN and BACKMAN (1978) reported 32 children with asthma where intolerance to aspirin was seen in 33%, to sodium benzoate in 18%, and to tartrazine in 20%. ØSTERBALLE et al. (1979) in a primary screening found that 11 of 46 children with asthma had positive reactions to aspirin benzoates or dyes. In a double-blind retesting with placebo, however, only 3 of 46 children reacted. Similar results were reported by WEBER et al. (1979) in 45 patients with moderately severe asthma.

Gum acacia and tragacanth are used in tablets, suppositories, vaginal jellies, and diabetic foods as excipients. A few cases of asthma have been reported to such vegetable gums (GELFAND 1943). BROWN and CREPEA (1947) reported a patient who was sensitive to tablets containing 0.005 mg tragacanth.

V. Purpura

CRIEP (1971) reported a case of recurrent allergic purpura after tartrazine ingestion. Seven patients with allergic purpura after ingestion of azo dyes and benzoates were reported by MICHAËLSSON et al. (1974). This type of purpura is also known as Schönlein–Henoch purpura or allergic vasculitis. The mild purpuric reactions were more easily revealed in skin pretreated with a nicotinic acid ester (JUHLIN and MICHAËLSSON 1971). The patients improved on a diet free from the additives. A case of anaphylactoid purpura provoked by tartrazine and benzoates has been reported by KUBBA and CHAMPION (1975). Purpura has also been described for quinine in tonic water (BELKIN 1967). Exclusion of food and drug additives has been found by us to be of importance in clearing several patients of purpura and vasculitis.

VI. Other Symptoms of Intolerance

Anaphylactic shock reactions claimed to be caused by tartrazine and Sunset Yellow were reported in a patient receiving an enema of liquid castile soap (TRAUTLEIN and MANN 1978). Tests with components of the soap showed marked wheal and flare reactions to the dyes. It should be pointed out that positive skin test reactions to azo dyes are not found in patients with urticaria and asthma.

HAGERMAN (1970) reported exacerbation of acne after a few days of exposure to azo dyes. Itching, skin rash, and fever were reported in three patients with immediate hypersensitivity to plant substances (acacia and tragacanth) used as fillers and adhesives in prednisone tablets (RUBINGER et al. 1978).

Erythema multiforme-like symptoms were demonstrated to F. D. and C. Green No. 5 (Fast Green) which is a non-azo dye, approved for use in food, drugs and cosmetics in the United States (GRATER 1976). Quinine present in bitter drinks may induce fixed reactions, toxic epidermal necrolysis, or a scarlatiniform rash (DERBES 1964; CALNAN and CARON 1961; CALLAWAY and TATE 1974).

After provocation tests in patients with urticaria, various other symptoms such as sneezing, hoarseness, nasal congestion, sweating, irritability, and sensations of swelling, drowsiness, or heaviness in the head may be noted (MICHAËLSSON and JUHLIN 1973). Such symptoms are, however, difficult to evaluate. Diffuse symptoms after administration of 50 mg tartrazine have also been reported by NEUMAN et al. (1978). Dextrose was used as placebo but details of its clinical effect were not described. Further studies in this area seem warranted.

In 1960 there were epidemics in Germany and Holland called the margarine disease. The disease had a clinical picture similar to erythema multiforme and was attributed to an emulsifier used in the preparation of a certain brand of margarine. The Dutch epidemic was reviewed by MALI and MALTEN (1966). They emphasized that opinions were divided as to the etiological significance of margarine.

Fixed drug eruptions, i.e., skin lesions which recur in the same area when a chemical is taken, have been described in a patient taking capsules colored by amaranth and tartrazine (KLEVANSKY and KINGSLEY 1964).

C. Mechanisms

The exact mechanism for intolerance to azo dyes and benzoates is still unknown. Since cross-reactions to various analgesics and anti-inflammatory drugs such as aspirin, indomethacin, dextropropoxyphene, phenylbutazone, menfenamate, ibuprofen, and sodium salicylate also occur, a nonallergic mechanism seems probable for most patients. A chemical resemblance can clearly be seen only between benzoates and salicylates (Fig. 1). When azo dyes are taken orally there will be an azoreductive cleavage in the intestinal tract into sulfanilic acid and a pyrazolone derivative which can be further hydrolyzed to sulfophenylhydrazine (RYAN et al. 1969). Some azo dyes can form aniline compounds, which could explain their cross-reactions with preservatives (WALKER 1970).

Most patients with chronic urticaria show a heightened delayed reaction to the intradermally injected kinin releaser, kallikrein (JUHLIN and MICHAËLSSON 1969). This suggests that a temporary decrease of a circulating kallikrein inhibitor might be involved. Thus, an erratic metabolic interference with the inhibitors in serum could be a hypothetical explanation for the intolerance to aspirin and additives. In patients with chronic urticaria, low levels of the antitrypsin and antichymotrypsin levels have been described (DOEGLAS and BLEUMINK 1975). This, however, did not correlate with the increased sensitivity to intracutaneously injected kallikrein. The intimate relationship of the kallikrein–kinin system to the prostaglandin system has recently been reviewed (NASJLETTI and MALIK 1979). Prostaglandins might act as modulators and mediators of the actions of kinins. In asthmatic intolerance, an abnormal blocking of prostaglandin E_2 (which is a bronchodilator) has been proposed as a possible explanation (SETTIPANE et al. 1974). Such a mechanism in asthma seems logical since antiphlogistic drugs which, like aspirin, induce urticaria and asthma are also good inhibitors of microsomal prostaglandin synthetase, but weaker inhibitors of this enzyme (like acetaminophen and salicylamide) often fail to produce allergic symptoms (SZCZEKLIK et al. 1975, 1977). Nevertheless, it is difficult to understand why some people react adversely to aspirin-like drugs while others improve. An inborn error of reactivity or deficiency of a certain receptor must then be postulated in sensitive patients. The adverse reactions to tartrazine seem not to be mediated through an inhibition of the prostaglandin pathway (GERBER et al. 1979). These authors believe that the tartrazine sensitivity coexists with that of aspirin and might have an allergic basis.

Several investigations have been concerned with the question wether specific immunoglobulins are involved in these adverse reactions. Antibodies of the immunoglobulin E class do not seem to be involved in the reaction (WELTMAN et al. 1978; BERNSTEIN et al. 1978).

WELIKY et al. (1978, 1979) applied paper disk radioimmunoassay methods to measure tartrazine-specific IgD and IgE antibodies. Both sensitive patients and healthy control subjects had such antibodies but interestingly, after absorption with a tartrazine–protein conjugate, the levels of serum IgD-specific antibody in sensitive patients were clearly distinguishable from those in controls. This seems to be the first report associating hypersensitivity to a low molecular weight chemical with IgD.

D. Diagnosis of Intolerance

Symptoms of asthma and rhinorrhea usually occur within the first hours after taking the additives and then disappear. In patients with urticaria and angioedema, however, the symptoms are often delayed and are most evident the following night or morning. The may then sometimes continue for several days. It is important to take a careful history, but only half the patients with intolerance to aspirin and 21% of those sensitive to azo dyes and benzoates were aware of it (ROS et al. 1976). That so many patients did not know of their sensitivity is probably because the additives were hidden in so many drugs, foods, and drinks. The recent introduction of labeling all products intended for consumption has been found to be of great help for the patient.

If in doubt from the history of the patient, the only way to determine hypersensitivity is through provocation tests. A challenge test battery with several controls is used (Table 3). We prefer to have patients in the hospital for their own safety and so that they can be followed closely during the 2-week test period. The time in the hospital may prove less than the loss of working days from the urticaria itself.

At least a week before admission the patient should be on a diet free from dyes and preservatives. The patient should avoid antihistamines for 3 days before admission. The test should be done when the patient has minimal or no abnormal skin findings. Table 3 shows the substances used in the present challenge test series.

Table 3. Test battery for patients with recurrent urticaria

Day	Substance	Amount (mg)
1	Control (lactose)	100, 100
2	Azo dyes: Tartrazine	0.1[a], 1, 10
	New Coccine	0.1[a], 1, 10
	Sunset Yellow	0.1[a], 1, 10
3	Control (lactose)	100, 100
4	Benzoates: Sodium benzoate	50, 500
	4-Hydrobenzoic acid	50, 200
5	Carotene, canthaxanthin	100, 100
6	Annatto	5, 10
7	BHT–BHA	1, 10, 50, 50
8	Yeast extract	600
9	Control (lactose)	100, 100
10	Aspirin	0.1[a], 1, 10, 100, 250[b], 500[b]

[a] 0.1 mg only in patients with a history of asthma
[b] Not given to patients with a history of asthma and severe aspirin reactions

The substances are given in gelatin capsules whitened with titanium dioxide; lactose or starch can be added to complete the capsule filling. In this way the patient – and, ideally, the observing physician – cannot recognize the compound.

We usually start with lactose. Additional or increased doses are given at 1-h intervals. Provocation tests are judged positive when the patients develop signs of asthma, urticaria, or angioedema. Other allergic signs may be noted. These include hoarseness, wheezing, rhinitis, sneezing, nasal congestion, increased tear secretion, and reddening of the eyes. Subjective symptoms such as irritability and tiredness are also noted but difficult to evaluate. Judging whether a reaction is positive or negative is not always easy, and repeated provocations with placebo and additives may be necessary.

E. Food and Drug Labeling

Information on the occurrence of additives in food and drugs is of the utmost importance for sensitive patients. They improve if they can be on a diet free from the chemicals to which they react. Such additives should at least not be allowed in drugs used for treatment of urticaria, asthma, and rhinitis. The amount of dye earlier found in some antihistamines used for urticaria or β-stimulators used for asthma is enough to provoke the patient's symptoms and prevent their disappearance. In Sweden, colorants and preservatives are listed in Colors and Preservatives in Drugs, an annual publication which has been of great help for both doctors and patients. Here, the problem with azo dyes in drugs has tended to disappear since 1978, when such additives were, to a large degree, forbidden. In foods, azo dyes are only permitted in caviar, preserved cocktail cherries, so-called fruit cocktails, and alcoholic drinks. The regulations about food colors in Sweden and the labeling on the European market have been published with summaries and tables in English

(AHLBORG et al. 1974, 1975; AHLBORG and DICH 1978). The comprehensive handbooks edited by FURIA (1972) and FURIA and BELLANCA (1971) give almost 2,000 pages of detailed and valuable information. A one-page summary of importance for the allergist is given by MITCHELL (1971). Recent reviews on the occurrence of food additives and contaminants in the United States have been published by CAMPBELL et al. (1977), MILLER (1978), and CHOPRA (1979). It should be added that labeling of tartrazine in drugs has been required by the FDA from June 1980.

Consumers' organizations have asked whether all additives are necessary. It is evident that preservatives and antioxidants serve an important function. They account, however, for only 6% of the total value of additives used (GROSE 1977). The use of several other types of additive like colors, stabilizers, emulsifiers, thickeners, anticaking agents, and antifoaming agents have been debated. The Joint FAO/WHO Expert Committee on Food Additives has helped in explaining the reasoning of the experts and is offering solutions to the problem. Each of the additives permitted by the EEC is now given a number (E-number). Manufacturers with an export trade must therefore label their products. The list of ingredients is not impossibly long, so that anyone can check the specific additives. The shops, at least in Sweden, supply a list identifying the E-numbers. Our experience after 3 years with such a system has proved to be most beneficial for the group of consumers who show adverse reactions to certain chemicals. Allergic patients still suffer from problems with natural ingredients like egg, milk, soy, corn, and fish which are often hidden in various foods. Who would expect that fish meal can be used to "enrich" your morning toast? Here labeling could be further improved to help the allergic patient.

Acknowledgement. This work was supported by grants from the Swedish Research Council.

References

Aeling JL, Panagotacos PJ, Andreozzi RJ (1973) Contact dermatitis to vitamin E aerosol deodorant. Arch Dermatol 108:578–580

Ahlborg UG, Dich J (1978) The use of food additives in Sweden. Arch Toxicol [Suppl] 1:305–308

Ahlborg UG, Byfors I, Dich J, Eriksson H-B (1974) Use of food colours in Sweden. Var Foda 26:194–217

Ahlborg UG, Albanus L, Slorach S (1975) New regulations concerning food colours. Var Foda 27:2–31

Angelini JF, Leonardos GP (1973) Food additives – some economic considerations. Food Technol 24:40–50

August PJ (1979) Successful treatment of urticaria due to food additive with sodium cromoglycate and an exclusion diet. In: Pepys J, Edwards AM (eds) The mast cell, its role in health and disease. Pitman Medical, Tunbridge Wells

Baer R, Leider M (1949) The effects of feeding artificial food azodyes in paraphenylendiamine-hypersensitive subjects. Br J Dermatol 13:223–232

Beal JG (1973) Food additives and hyperactivity in children. Congressional Rec S 1973 6 (Oct 30)

Belkin GA (1967) Cocktail purpura. An unusual case of quinine sensitivity. Ann Intern Med 66:583–586

Bernstein IL, Johnson CL, Gallagher JS, Archer D, Johnson H (1978) Are tartrazine reactions mediated by IgE? J Allergy Clin Immunol 61:191

Bierman CW, Furukawa CT (1978) Food additives and hyperkinesis: are there nuts among the berries. Pediatrics 61:932–934

Brenner A (1977) A study of the efficacy of the Feingold diet on hyperkinetic children. Clin Pediatr 16:652–656

Brodkin RH, Bleiberg J (1965) Sensitivity to topically applied vitamin E. Arch Dermatol 92:76–77

Brodthagen H, Thormann J, Veien NK (1974) Urticaria. Farvestoffer og antihistaminica. Ugeskr Laeger 136:1307

Brown EB, Crepea SB (1947) Allergy (asthma) to ingested gum tragacanth. J Allergy 18:214–216

Brown R (1979) Another case of sorbic acid sensitivity. Contact Dermatitis 5:268

Brun R (1964) Kontaktekzem auf Laurylgallat und p-Hydroxy-Benzoe-Säure-Ester. Berufs-dermatosen 12:281–284

Brun R (1970) Eczéma de contact à un antioxydant de la margarine (gallate) et changement de métier. Dermatologica 140:390–394

Burchhardt W von, Fierz U (1964) Antioxydanten in der Margarine als Ursache von Ge-werbsekzemen. Dermatologica 129:431–432

Calas E, Castelain PY (1958) Intolérance à des colorants pharmaceutiques utilisés pour l'en-robage des comprimés. Bull Soc Fr Dermatol Syphiligr 65:69–71

Callaway JL, Tate WE (1974) Toxic epidermal necrolysis caused by "gin and tonic". Arch Dermatol 109:909

Calnan CD, Caron GA (1961) Quinine sensitivity. Br Med J 2:1750–1751

Calnan CD (1976) Quinazoline yellow SS in cosmetics. Contact Dermatitis 2:160–166

Campbell AD, Horwitz W, Burke JA, Jelinek, CF, Rodricks JV, Shibko SJ (1977) Food ad-ditives and contaminants. In: Hall VF (ed) Handbooks of physiology, sect. 9. Reactions to environmental agents, Williams & Wilkins, Baltimore, pp 167–179

Castelain PY (1977) L'allergie aux colorants alimentaires. Med Nutr 13:112–113

Chafee FH, Settipane GA (1967) Asthma caused by FD & C approved dyes. J Allergy 40:65–72

Champion RH, Roberts SOB, Carpenter RG, Roger JH (1969) Urticaria and angi-edema; a review of 554 patients. Br J Dermatol 81:588–597

Chopra JG (1979) The role on food and drug administration in food allergy. Ann Allergy 42:1–4

Colors and Preservatives in Drugs (1978) Läkemedelsinformation AB Stockholm

Conners CK, Goyette CH, Southwick DA, Lees JM, Andrulonis PE (1976) Food additives and hyperkinesis: a controlled doubleblind experiment. Pediatrics 58:154–166

Cook PS, Woodhill JM (1976) The Feingold dietary treatment of the hyperkinetic syn-drome. Med J Aust 2:85–90

Cooke RA (1919) Allergy in drug idiosyncrasy. JAMA 73:759–760

Criep LH (1971) Allergic vascular purpura. J Allergy Clin Immunol 48:7–12

Delaney JC (1976) Response on patients with asthma and aspirin idiosyncrasy to tartrazine (a dye commonly used in food and drug industries). Practitioner 217:285–287

Derbes VJ (1964) The fixed eruption. JAMA 190:765–766

Doeglas HMG (1975a) Chronic urticaria, clinical and pathogenetic studies in 141 patients. Thesis, University of Groningen

Doeglas HMG (1975b) Reactions to aspirin and food additives in patients with chronic ur-ticaria, including the physical urticarias. Br J Dermatol 93:135–144

Doeglas HMG (1977) Dietary treatment of patients with chronic urticaria and intolerance to aspirin and food additives. Dermatologica 154:308–310

Doeglas HMG, Bleumink E (1975) Protease inhibitors in plasma of patients with chronic urticaria. Arch Dermatol 111:979–985

Drake T, Maibach HJ (1976) Allergic contact dermatitis and stomatitis caused by a cinna-mic aldehyde flavoured toothpaste. Arch Dermatol 112:202–203

Dry J, Pradalier A (1977) A propos des additifs alimentaires et de leur rôle allergénique. Rev Fr Allergol 17:123–125

Epstein E, Maibach HI (1968) Etylendiamine-allergic contact dermatitis. Arch Dermatol 98:476–478

Feingold B (1975) Why your child is hyperactive. Random House, New York

Fernandes B, Figueiredo E, Girard JP (1977) Etude de quelques additifs alimentaires en tant que facteurs étiologiques de l'urticaire chronique et de l'oèdeme angioneurotique. Rev Fr Allergol 17:127–131

Fischer AA (1966) Systemic eczematous "contact-type" dermatitis medicamentosa. Ann Allergy 24:406–420

Fischer AA (1973) Contact dermatitis. Lea & Febiger, Philadelphia

Fischer AA (1976) Reactions to antioxidants in cosmetics and foods. Cutis 17:21–28

Fischer AA, Pascher F, Kanof NB (1971) Allergic contact dermatitis due to ingredients of vehicles. Arch Dermatol 104:286–290

Fischerman EW, Cohen GN (1973) Aspirin and other cross-reaction small chemicals in known aspirin-intolerant patients. Ann Allergy 31:476–484

Fischerman EW, Cohen GN (1977) Chronic and recurrent urticaria: new concepts of drug-group sensitivity. Ann Allergy 39:404–414

Freedman BJ (1977a) A dietary free from additives in the management of allergic disease. Clin Allergy 7:417–421

Freedman BJ (1977b) Asthma induced by sulphur dioxide, benzoate and tartrazine contained in orange drinks. Clin Allergy 7:407–415

Furia TE (1972) Handbook of food additives, 2nd edn. CRC Press, Cleveland

Furia TE, Bellanca N (1971) Fenaroli's handbook of flavor ingredients. CRC Press, Cleveland

Gelfand HH (1943) The allergenic properties of the vegetable gums. A case of asthma due to tragacanth. J Allergy 14:203–206

Gerber JG, Payne NA, Oelz O, Nies AS, Oates JA (1979) Tartrazine and the prostaglandin system. J Allergy Clin Immunol 63:289–294

German DF (1978) Practical diagnosis and management of chronic urticaria. Ann Allergy 40:299

Girard JP (1974) Réactions allergiques aux additifs alimentaires. Med Hyg 32:1953–1957

Gounelle de Pontanel H, Vigne J, Letourmy P (1977) Une enquête auprès des dermatologues francais sur les allergies, notamment par colorants alimentaires. Med Nutr 13:107–110

Grater W (1976) Hypersensitive skin reactions to FD & C dyes. Cutis 17:1163–1165

Grose D (1977) Our polluted food-fact or fancy? Food additives – is there a spectre at the feast? R Soc Health J 97:193–196

Hagerman G (1970) Reaktionen auf Farben und Geschmacksmitteln in Arzneimitteln. Arch Klin Exp Dermatol 237:170–172

Harley JP, Ray RS, Tomasi L et al. (1978) Hyperkinesis and food additives: testing the Feingold hypothesis. Pediatrics 61:818–828

Hjort N (1961) Eczematous allergy to balsam, allied perfumes and flavoring agents. Acta Derm Venerol (Stockh) [Suppl] 41:102–105

Hjort N, Trolle-Lassen C (1962) Skin reactions to preservatives with special regard to paraben esters and sorbic acid. Arch Pharm Chem 69:9–16

Hosen H (1972) The relationship of FD & C dyes and respiration allergy. J Asthma Res 10:131–134

Hubbard RD (1975) Urticaria due to food dyes. Cutis 14:748–749

Juhlin L (1977) Clinical studies on the diagnosis and treatment of urticaria. Ann Allergy 39:356–361

Juhlin L (1981) Recurrent urticaria: clinical investigation of 330 patients. Br J Dermatol 104:369–381

Juhlin L, Michaëlsson G (1969) Cutaneous reactions to kallikrein, bradykinin and histamine in healthy subjects and in patients with urticaria. Acta Derm Venereol (Stockh) 49:26–36

Juhlin L, Michaëlsson G (1971) Abnormal cutaneous reactions to a nicotinic acid ester. Acta Derm Venereol (Stockh) 31:448–452

Juhlin L, Shelley WB (1977) Oriented fibrin crystallization: a phenomenon of hypersensitivity to bacteria in psoriasis, vasculitis and other dermatoses. Br J Dermatol 96:577–586

Juhlin L, Michaëlsson G, Zetterström O (1972) Urticaria and asthma induced by food- and drug-additives in patients with aspirin hypersensitivity. J Allerg Clin Immunol 50:92–98

Kaaber K (1978) Farvestoffer og konserveringsmidler ved kronisk urticaria. Vaerdien af provokationsforsog og eliminationsdiet. Ugeskr Laeger 140:1473–1476

Kahori T, Araki H (1966) Photoallergy in dermatology. J Asthma Res 3:213–216

Klaschka F, Beiersdorff HU (1965) Allergic eczema reaction through sorbic acid used as preservative of external medicaments. MMW 107:185–188

Klevansky H, Kingsley HJ (1964) Fixed drug eruptions caused by dyes. S Afr Med J 38:216

Kubba R, Champion RH (1975) Anaphylactoid purpura caused by tartrazine and benzoates. Br J Dermatol [Suppl 11] 93:61–62

Lamberg SI (1967) A new photosensitizer. The artificial sweetener cyclamate. JAMA 201:747–750

Laurell AB, Mårtensson U, Sjöholm AG (1977) Studies of C 1 subcomponents in chronic urticaria and angioedema. Int Arch Allergy Appl Immunol 54:434–442

Leifer W (1951) Contact dermatitis due to cinnamon. Recurrence of dermatitis following oral administration of cinnamon oil. Arch Dermatol 64:52–55

Lipton MA, Nemeroff CB, Mailman RB (1979) Hyperkinesis and food additives. In: Wurtman RJ, Wurtman JJ (eds) Nutrition and the brain, vol 4, Raven, New York, pp 1–27

Lockey SD (1959) Allergic reactions due to FD & C yellow No. 5 dye, tartrazine, an aniline dye used as a coloring and identifying agent in various steroids. Ann Allergy 17:719–721

Lockey SD (1977) Hypersensitivity to tartrazine (FD & C yellow No. 5) and other dyes and additives present in foods and pharmaceutical products. Ann Allergy 38:206–210

Magnusson B, Wilkinson DS (1975) Cinnamic aldehyde in toothpaste. 1. Clinical aspects and patch tests. Contact Dermatitis 1:70–76

Mali JWH, Malten KE (1966) The epidemic of polymorph toxic erythema in the Netherlands in 1960. Acta Derm Venereol (Stockh) 46:123–135

Marzulli FN, Maibach HI (1974) Status of topical parabens: skin hypersensitivity. Int J Dermatol 13:397–399

Meynadier J, Guilhou J, Meynadier J, Lavanture N (1979) L'urticaire chronique. Ann Dermatol Venereol 106:153–158

Michaëlsson G, Juhlin L (1973) Urticaria induced by preservatives and dye additives in food and drugs. Br J Dermatol 88:525–532

Michaëlsson G, Pettersson L, Juhlin L (1974) Purpura caused by food and drug additives. Arch Dermatol 109:49–52

Mikkelsen H, Larsen JC, Tarding F (1978) Hypersensitivity reactions to food colours with special reference to the natural colour annatto extract (butter colour). Arch Toxicol [Suppl] 1:141–143

Miller JB (1978) Hidden food ingredients, chemical food additives and incomplete food labels. Ann Allergy 41:93–98

Minkin W, Cohen HJ, Frank SB (1973) Contact dermatitis from deodorants. Arch Dermatol 107:774–775

Mitchell JC (1971) The skin and chemical additives to foods. Arch Dermatol 104:329–330

Moncret-Vautrin DA, Aubert B (1978) Le risque de sensibilisation aux colorants alimentaires et pharmaceutiques. Masson, Paris

Nasjletti A, Malik KU (1979) Relationships between the kallikrein-kinin and prostaglandin systems. Life Sci 25:99–110

Neuman I, Elian R, Nahum H, Shaked P, Creter D (1978) The danger of "yellow dyes" (tartrazine) to allergic subjects. Clin Allergy 8:65–68

Østerballe O, Taudorf E, Haahr J (1979) Asthma bronchiale af konserveringsmidler, farvestoffer og acetylsalicylsyre hos børn. Ugeskr Laeger 141:1908–1910

Pellegrin A (1979) Deux observations nouvelles d'allergie à la tartrazine. Ann Med Intern 130:211–214

Provost TT, Jillson OF (1967) Ethylendiamine contact dermatitis. Arch Dermatol 96:231–234

Raymond JZ, Gross PR (1969) EDTA: preservative dermatitis. Arch Dermatol 100:436–440

Roed-Petersen J, Hjort N (1976) Contact dermatitis from antioxidants. Hidden sensitizers in topical medications and foods. Br J Dermatol 94:233–241

Roeleveld CG, van Ketel WG (1976) Positive patch test to the azodye tartrazine. Contact Dermatitis 2:180

Ros AM, Juhlin L, Michaëlsson G (1976) A follow-up study of patients with recurrent urticaria and hypersensitivity to aspirin, benzoates and azo dyes. Br J Dermatol 95:19–24

Rosenhall L (1977) Hypersensitivity to analgetics, preservatives and food colorants in patients with asthma or rhinitis. Acta Univ Ups 269:1–117

Rosenhall L, Zetterström O (1973) Astma utläst av analgetika, livsmedelsfärg och konserveringsmedel. Lakartidningen 70:1417–1419

Rubinger D, Friedlander M, Superstine E (1978) Hypersensitivity to tablet additives in transplant recipients on prednisone. Lancet 2:689

Rudzki E (1977) Przewlekla pokrzywka wywolana przez aspiryne i dodatki pokarmowe. Przegl Dermatol 64:163–166

Ryan AJ, Welling PG, Wright SE (1969) Further studies on the metabolism of tartrazine and related compounds in the intact rat. Food Cosmet Toxicol 7:287

Saihan EM, Harman RRM (1978) Contact sensitivity to sorbic acid in "Unguentum Merck". Br J Dermatol 99:583–584

Salzman LK (1976) Allergy testing, psychological assessment and dietary treatment of the hyperactive child syndrome. Med J Aust 2:248–251

Samter M, Beers RF Jr (1967) Concerning the nature of intolerance to aspirin. J Allergy 40:281–293

Samter M, Beers RF Jr (1968) Intolerance to aspirin. Ann Intern Med 68:975–983

Schorr WF (1975) Cinnamic aldehyde allergy. Contact Dermatitis 1:108–111

Schrag P, Divoky D (1975) The myth of the hyperactive child. Partheon, New York, p 35

Settipane GA, Pudupakkam RK (1975) Aspirin intolerance. III. Subtypes, familial occurrence and cross-reactivity with tartrazine. J Allergy Clin Immunol 56:215–221

Settipane GA, Chafee FC, Klein DE (1974) Aspirin intolerance. II. A prospective study in atopic and normal population. J Allergy Clin Immunol 53:200–204

Settipane GA, Chafee FH, Postman IM et al. (1976) Significance of tartrazine sensitivity in chronic urticaria of unknown etiology. J Allergy Clin Immunol 57:541–546

Shelley WB, Juhlin L (1977) Induction of fibrin thrombi by monocytes. Nature 270:343–344

Sidi E, Arouete J (1959) Sensibilisation aux colorants azoïques et au groupe de la para. Nouv Presse Med 67:2067–2069

Smith AP (1971) Response of aspirin-allergic patients to challenge by some analgesics in common use. Br Med J 2:494–496

Speer F (1958) The management of childhood asthma. Thomas, Springfield

Stenius BSM, Lemola M (1976) Hypersensitivity to acetylsalicylic acid (ASA) and tartrazine in patients with asthma. Clin Allergy 6:119–129

Suurmond D, Verspijk Mijnssen GAW (1967) Allergic dermatitis due to shoes and a leather prothese. Dermatologica 134:371–378

Syvänen P, Backman A (1978) Abstract. Nordic congress of allergology, Copenhagen, p 58

Szczeklik A, Gryglewski RJ, Czerniawska-Mysik G (1975) Relationship of inhibitor of prostaglandin biosynthesis by analgesics to asthma attacks in aspirin-sensitive patients. Br Med J 1:67

Szczeklik A, Gryglewski RJ, Czerniawska-Mysik G (1977) Clinical patterns of hypersensitivity to nonsteroidal anti-inflammatory drugs and their pathogenesis. J Allergy Clin Immunol 60:276–284

Thune P, Granholt A (1975) Provocation tests with antiphlogistic and food additives in recurrent urticaria. Dermatologica 151:360–367

Trautlein JJ, Mann WJ (1978) Anaphylactic shock caused by yellow dye (FD & C No. 5 and FD & C No. 6) in an enema (case report). Ann Allergy 41:28–29

Vedanthan PK, Menon MM, Bell TD, Bergin D (1977) Aspirin and tartrazine oral challenge: incidence of adverse response in chronic childhood asthma. J Allergy Clin Immunol 60:8–13

Walker R (1970) The metabolism of azo-compounds: a review of the literature. Food Cosmet Toxicol 8:659–676

Warin RP, Smith RI (1976) Challenge test battery in chronic urticaria. Br J Dermatol 94:401–406

Weber RW, Hoffman M, Raine DA Jr, Nelson HS (1979) Incidence of bronchoconstriction due to aspirin, azo dyes, non-azo dyes and preservatives in a population of perennial asthmatics. J Allergy Clin Immunol 64:32–37

Weirich EG (1961) Untersuchungen zum Allergencharakter der Pyrazolfarbstoffe. Arch Klin Exp Dermatol 213:445–454

Weliky N, Heiner DC, Tamura H, Anderson S (1978) Tartrazinespecific IgD and IgE antibodies. J Allergy Clin Immunol 61:190–191

Weliky N, Heiner DC, Tamura H et al. (1979) Correlation of tartrazine hypersensitivity with specific serum IgD levels. Immunol Commun 8:65–71

Weltman JK, Szaro RP, Settipane GA (1978) An analysis of the role of IgE in intolerance to aspirin and tartrazine. Allergy 34:273–281

Werry JS (1976) Food additives and hyperactivity. Med J Austr 2:281–282

Wilkinson DS (1972) Sensitivity to pharmaceutical additives. In: Dash CH, Jones HEH (eds) Mechanisms in drug allergy. Churchill Livingstone, Edinburgh London

Williams JI, Cram DM, Tausig FT, Webster E (1978) Relative effects of drugs and diet on hyperactive behaviours: an experimental study. Pediatrics 61:811–817

CHAPTER 23

Vitamins

W. Schalch and L. Dostálová

A. Introduction

In a book devoted to a discussion of drugs and drug effects it may, at first glance, be surprising to find a group of physiologic substances like the vitamins. Originally vitamins were regarded as nutritive elements rather than as drugs or drug-equivalent compounds. We feel, therefore, that it is very important to reevaluate the position of the vitamins within the class of biologically active substances. The vitamins comprise a group of widely different chemical compounds and because of this variety, are somewhat difficult to define comprehensively. So far, the most generally accepted definition of vitamins is that given by Folkers (1969): "A vitamin is an organic substance of nutritional nature, which is present in low concentration as a natural component of enzyme systems and catalyzes required reactions, and may be derived externally to the tissue or by intrinsic biosynthesis." To this definition it should be explicitly added that the intake of vitamins is essential for the maintenance of life and the well-being of the individual. In a book dealing with drug allergy in general and in a chapter presenting a discussion of allergic reactions to vitamins in particular, it is important to appreciate the dichotomy of the vitamins primarily as essential nutritive factors and only secondarily as drug-equivalent compounds. This feature clearly separates the vitamins from all of the other compounds discussed in this volume, which have no relation at all to nutrition in the sense the vitamins have.

We would like to preface the description of allergic reactions to the various vitamins with a brief general consideration of the drug nature of vitamins and of the theoretical and conceptual problems posed by the induction of allergic responses to vitamins. According to a widely accepted definition, a drug is any substance or mixture of substances administered to humans for the diagnosis, treatment, investigation, or prevention of disease, or for the modification of physiologic functions (Graham 1979). In the sense of this definition vitamins can be regarded as drugs owing to their ability to abrogate specific deficiency symptoms. Thus, it was already common practice before the beginning of this century to use lime juice or lemon juice as a very effective means of preventing and curing scurvy (Lind 1953) and to prescribe cod liver oil for the treatment of rickets (Trousseau 1861), to cite only two early examples. More will be found in a paper by Chick (1975), dealing with the discovery of vitamins.

The capability of vitamins to cure nutrition-induced deficiency diseases does not reside, however, in some pharmacodynamic action independent of their nutritional effect. It is, therefore, generally agreed that vitamins are not to be regarded as drugs when ingested in amounts designed to treat vitamin deficiency diseases or to match daily requirements under normal conditions. In this respect, full emphasis is given to their nutritional value rather than to their pharmacologic action. But it also has to be taken into account that borderline cases may exist where it is difficult to assign to the vitamins an unambiguous status as either drug-equivalent compounds or as nutrients. Although governmental regulations differ from country to country, a basic general guideline for making this distinction are the "Recommended Dietary Allowances (RDA)" published in the United States by the National Academy of Sciences (1980). With these recommendations in mind, an intake of vitamins exploiting their pharmacodynamic effects, i.e., an intake in dosages significantly exceeding the RDA, might be regarded as a drug-equivalent use of vitamins.

I. The Drug-Equivalent Use of Vitamins

Soon after the chemical structures of the first vitamins were identified, one application of vitamins emerged that went beyond their classical nutritional use in the treatment of specific deficiency diseases. This was the use of vitamins in treating diseases unrelated to nutrition (non-nutritional pharmacologic use). Early crystallizations of those ideas are reviewed by Gordon (1947) and a more recent review of the pharmacologic use of vitamins appeared in 1976 (Körner and Völlm). The use of vitamins in dermatology has been treated by Fishman and Goldstein (1968). The most prevalent drug-equivalent uses of individual vitamins are referred to in Table 1, where the RDA of each individual vitamin can also be seen. In this chapter only a general survey of the drug-equivalent use of vitamins is given.

The non-nutritional use of vitamins covers the treatment of pathophysiologic states (such as are induced by inborn errors of metabolism) and the deficiencies due to impaired absorption, transfer, and/or utilization as well as increased excretion of one or more vitamins. The therapy of these disease states is basically a form of replacement and substitution therapy. A more specific drug-equivalent use of vitamins, aimed at the alleviation of specific non-nutritional and non-deficiency diseases, tries to exploit specific pharmacodynamic effects totally different from the vitamins' nutritional action. However, the nature and presence of these effects has not been unequivocally demonstrated, so far, for each individual vitamin and is, therefore, widely disputed. The most spectacular example of a suggested vitamin use which is clearly of a drug-equivalent nature is the megadose treatment proposal. Pauling started the discussions on the pharmacologic and toxicologic effects of vitamins with his publications about orthomolecular therapy in psychiatric medicine (Pauling 1968) and the common cold (Pauling 1974). As defined by Pauling (1968) orthomolecular psychiatric therapy comprises: "A treatment of mental disease by provision of optimum molecular environment for the mind." It is not the purpose of this chapter to review the appropriate scientific papers that provide evidence for and against the question as to whether or not there is a demonstrable abnormality in vitamin content or function in certain diseases such as mental illness. However, because of the very high doses used or proposed in this kind of therapy, it clearly constitutes drug-equivalent use of the vitamins concerned. A further example of a drug-equivalent use of vitamins is the treatment of

Table 1. Drug-equivalent use of individual vitamins

Vitamin	Indication for treatment	Active form	Pharmaceutical forms	Pharmacologic daily doses	Recommended daily dietary allowances (NATIONAL ACADEMY OF SCIENCES 1980)	
					Infants and children	Adults
A	Supplement: vitamin A deficiency states (malnutrition), impairment of absorption or transport Therapy: nyctalopia, difficulties of adaptation to darkness, xerophthalmia, severe skin or mucosa damages, follicular hyperkeratosis, acne, inner ear deafness, tinnitus	Retinyl palmitate, retinyl acetate	Tablets, capsules, drops, emulsion, suspension, ointment, ampules	7,500–100,000 IU	420–700 µg	800–1,000 µg
B_1	Supplement: vitamin B_1 deficiency states, impaired absorption or increased requirements (pregnancy, lactation, alcoholism) Therapy: beriberi, Wernicke's encephalopathy, neuritis, polyneuritis (alcoholic and toxic), neuralgia, myalgia, myocardia, disorders of the intermediate metabolism	Thiamine chloride and hydrochloride, thiamine mononitrate, cocarboxylase, thiamine pyrophosphate	Tablets, sugar-coated pills, dragées, ampules	50–300 mg	0.3–1.2 mg	1.0–1.4 mg
B_2	Supplement: vitamin B_2 deficiency states, impaired absorption, increased requirements	Riboflavin 5′-phosphate sodium, riboflavin	Tablets, ampules	10–30 mg	0.4–1.4 mg	1.2–1.6 mg

Table 1 (continued)

Vitamin	Indication for treatment	Active form	Pharmaceutical forms	Pharmacologic daily doses	Recommended daily dietary allowances (NATIONAL ACADEMY OF SCIENCES 1980)	
					Infants and children	Adults
	Therapy: paralgesia, cramps in the lower extremities, keratitis, glossitis, cheilitis, seborrhea, hemeralopia, conjunctivitis					
B_6	Supplement: vitamin B_6 deficiency states, impaired absorption, therapy with vitamin B_6 antagonists, increased requirements (pregnancy, lactation), increased stimulation with exogenic estrogens, X-ray therapy Therapy: vitamin B_6-dependent hypochrome anemia and convulsions in infants, seborrheic dermatitis, glossitis, neuritis peripherica, decreased formation of antibodies, cerebral convulsions with EEG changes	Pyridoxine hydrochloride	Tablets, ampules, sugar-coated pills, suppositories	20–600 mg	0.3–1.6 mg	2.0–2.2 mg
B_{12}	Supplement: vitamin B_{12} deficiency states, increased requirements (pregnancy)	Hydroxocobalamin, cyanocobalamin hydroxocobalamin	Tablets, drops, ampules, capsules	10–1,000 µg[a]	0.5–3.0 µg	3.0 µg

	Therapy: malabsorption of vitamin B_{12}, i.e., in pernicious or other macrocytic anemias, sprue, gastrointestinal pathology or surgery, enteropathy concomitant with folic acid deficiency, stimulation of hematopoiesis	acetate				
C	Supplement: vitamin C deficiency states, impaired absorption increased requirements (pregnancy lactation, premature babies, surgical shock, heavy physical work, infection, convalescence) Therapy: scurvy, prescurvy, paradontosis, gingivitis, hemorrhagic diathesis	Ascorbic acid, sodium ascorbate, calcium ascorbate	Tablets, ampules, capsules, effervescent tablets	100–1,000 mg[a]	35–45 mg	60 mg
Biotin	Supplement: biotin deficiency states, increased requirement (alcohol abuse, treatment with biotin antagonists) Therapy: impairment of absorption of biotin in gastrointestinal pathology or surgery, seborrheic dermatitis, anorexia, intoxication	Biotin	Tablets	2.5 mg	35–120 µg	100–200 µg[b]
Folic acid	Supplement: folic acid deficiency states, impaired absorption, increased requirements (pregnancy, increased stimulation with exogenic estrogens) treatment with folic acid antagonists	Folic acid, sodium folate, tetrahydrofolic acid, folinic acid	Tablets, ampules	5–15 mg	30–300 µg	400 µg

Table 1 (continued)

Vitamin	Indication for treatment	Active form	Pharmaceutical forms	Pharmacologic daily doses	Recommended daily dietary allowances (National Academy of Sciences 1980)	
					Infants and children	Adults
	Therapy: gastrointestinal surgery, enteropathies, folic acid-dependent anemia					
Nicotinic acid	Supplement: nicotinamide deficiency, impaired absorption, increased requirements. Therapy: pellagra, vasomotoric headache, migraine, schizophrenia	Nicotinamide	Tablets	200–1,000 mg	6–16 mg	13–18 mg
Panthothenic acid	Supplement: panthothenic acid deficiency states. Therapy: postoperative intestinal dystonia, paralytic ileus, for promoting the formation of granulation tissue and epithelization	D-Panthenol	Tablets, ointment, ampules	200, 500, 1,000 mg	2–7 mg	4–7 mg[b]
D	Supplement: vitamin D deficiency states, impaired absorption, increased requirements. Therapy: rickets, hypoparathyroidism, osteomalacia	Cholecalciferol, 25-hydroxycholecalciferol, 1,25-dihydroxycholecalciferol, ergocalciferol	Ampules, capsules, tablets, drops	500–500,000 IU	400 IU	200 IU

E	DL-α-tocopheryl acetate	Dragées, chewable dragées, ampules, drops	10–1,000 mg[a]	3–7 mg	8–10 mg
	Supplement: vitamin E deficiency states in impaired resorption or transport Therapy: during a diet with a high proportion of polyunsaturated fats, in A-β-lipoproteinemia, in premature babies and neonates with high hemolysis rate, in claudicatio intermittens, vascular disease, cardiopathies, collagenoses, morbus Dupuytren, fertility disturbances				
K	Phytomenadione (vitamin K_1)	Chewable dragées, ampules, drops	10–40 mg[a]	10–100 µg	100–200 µg
	Supplement: vitamin K deficiency states, impaired absorption, increased requirements Therapy: vitamin K_1-dependent disorders of clotting, neonatal bleeding, hepatopathies				

[a] In particular cases, pharmacologic daily doses in excess of the stated upper limits may be administered

[b] A recommended daily allowance has not been established; the numbers given will meet the needs of almost all healthy people

drug-induced vitamin deficiencies. This interesting interaction of vitamins and drugs has been comprehensively treated by Roe (1976). Examples of these deficiencies are the vitamin B_6 depletion observed in women using oral contraceptive agents, the folic acid deficiency encountered most frequently in alcoholics as reported by Bonjour (1980) and the folic acid deficiencies observed during methotrexate treatment (Groff and Blakley 1978; Rosenblatt 1978).

II. Allergic Reactions to Vitamins

Vitamins were identified originally as natural products nontoxic in physiologic amounts; they are still believed to be for the most part harmless. But recent publications reflect the emergence of a new consciousness that is increasingly alert to the possible existence of harmful effects of vitamins, though not only of vitamins. Regarding "adverse" effects of vitamins, we shall in the present work be concerned exclusively with allergic and allergoid reactions to these substances.

Vitamins, in the first instance, are essentially food constituents. From this nutritional point of view an obvious possible cause of allergic reactions to vitamins could be the presence of a food allergy. In our extensive survey of the literature, however, not a single case of a food allergy was found that could be interpreted as implicating one or more vitamins as the causative agent.

Nor have vitamins been implicated in the pathogenesis of food allergy in the most recent review concerned with immunology of the gastrointestinal tract (Bleumink 1979). In recent work, the application of biochemical testing as well as immunologic investigations have indicated that food allergy per se is a relatively rarely observed phenomenon (Bleumink 1979). In the second place, vitamins have drug-equivalent uses and the question arises whether allergic reactions occur in these circumstances.

A feature vitamins have in common with drugs is their low molecular weights, ranging from 205 daltons for vitamin B_6 to 1,360 daltons for vitamin B_{12}. Intimately linked to this property is their poor or absent immunogenicity. It has long been known (Landsteiner 1945) that small molecules acquire an immunogenic potential only when covalently bound to some macromolecular carrier, be it a protein, a polysaccharide, or a biologic particle (including fractions thereof) such as a blood cell or a bacterium, to cite only two examples.

As outlined by de Weck (1971) in one of his basic contributions to our understanding of drug reactions, the ability of a simple chemical to induce an immune response, and consequently allergic reactions, rests on its ability to form those macromolecular conjugates in vivo or on the presence in the final pharmaceutical preparation of substances with chemical reactivity towards body constituents. For this to occur, it is either necessary that the vitamins possess some intrinsic chemical reactivity, contain some reactive decomposition product or byproduct, or that a reactive species is metabolically created in vivo (the reactive metabolite).

When dealing with the individual vitamins we will review briefly what is known about such potentially reactive vitamin metabolites formed in vivo and the most likely reactive decomposition products, aggregation products, or byproducts formed in vitro. We will then also refer to possible intrinsic chemical reactivities of the individual vitamins themselves.

A second important condition to be fulfilled for a macromolecular substance to be immunogenic is that it has to be recognized by the immune system of the host as foreign, because there is normally no immune response against constituents of the host except in autoimmune disease. This principle of self and non-self discrimination was recognized by BURNET (1959) and formulated as the clonal selection theory. Put shortly, this theory states that the distinction between self and non-self is made by the body's immune system during embryonic and neonatal life. All lymphocytes which by means of their specific surface receptors encounter antigens during this period become, by some not yet fully understood mechanisms, paralyzed and are eliminated. In this way the body loses immunocompetence for all substances encountered during embryonal development. In recent years, it has become evident that self-reactive B-lymphocyte clones are not eliminated, but are merely unreactive under normal circumstances. Accordingly, activation of these B-cell clones in a variety of ways (helper T-cells, B-cell antigens, polyclonal activation, etc.) could easily lead to the formation of auto-antibodies against self-constituents, including vitamins. However, when lymphocytes come into contact with antigens *after* this period when the immune system is matured, an immune response and consequently immunologic memory necessary for the induction of allergic responses is established.

The vitamins – although not synthesized by the body – are present throughout embryonic development. Consequently an immune response to them should not occur, even when they are presented as a possible immunogenic conjugate with a macromolecular body-derived carrier. A response could be established only if, after the maturation of the immune system, new metabolites and new macromolecular conjugates were to emerge. To the best of our knowledge, however, no reports exist of vitamin metabolism changing with adolescence and thus creating metabolites unknown to the immune system.

The above examples clearly demonstrate the uniqueness of vitamins as being essentially self-components in the immunologic sense. This feature evidently separates them from the common drugs, which, unlike the vitamins, are not present during the whole lifetime of the organism. Rather are drugs present for limited periods only; they constitute a group of substances foreign to the body and may consequently become immunogenic when in conjugation with a protein, cell, or polysaccharide (macromolecular conjugate). From these theoretical considerations we can conclude that an allergy to vitamins ought to be a highly improbable phenomenon, as becomes particularly clear when the vitamins are regarded as essentially constituents of the body itself. Thus, every immune response arising against them could be called an autoimmune disease. Conceptually, an allergy to vitamins, therefore, can arise from the creation of new metabolites or decomposition products formed in vitro, or by the emergence of forbidden anti-vitamin lymphocyte clones which produce the corresponding antibodies.

Vitamin allergy – when it occurs – is by definition an immunologic phenomenon. Here we wish to recall the guidelines DE WECK (1971) has given for the classification of drug reactions. According to DE WECK, a factor of the utmost importance in reaching an objective diagnosis of allergic reactions to drugs is the conclusive demonstration of the presence of specific immunologic agents, that is, antibodies or sensitized cells. In the past, sensitive methods have been developed for

the assay of specific antibodies in allergic diseases. We refer to the original literature for discussion of these techniques (Soloshenko et al. 1971; Semenovich et al.
1976; Ring 1978; Rand et al. 1979; Schroeder et al. 1979; Kleinhans 1979 a;
Prish and Hughes 1979). For the clinical diagnosis of allergic diseases we refer to
a treatise by Fuchs (1979). But it has to be kept in mind that it is not easy, in most
cases, to isolate clearly one particular vitamin as the causative agent of an allergic
reaction to a pharmaceutical preparation incorporating a mixture not only of several vitamins but also of vitamins plus various additives.

A problem which will not be given close attention in this discussion of allergic
reactions to vitamins is the relation of the atopic individual to this kind of drug
reaction. Recent evidence indicates that atopy has a distinctly genetic basis (reviewed by Oprée 1979) and the incidence of drug allergies in general and of vitamin
allergies in particular could be higher in this genetically related population. While
elevated IgE antibody levels dominate discussions of vitamin allergies in the atopic
patient, it is also important to emphasize the purely pharmacologic effects of vitamins. By this we mean a vitamin-induced, nonspecific histamine liberation which
mimics an allergic mechanism without being dependent on the presence of specific
antibodies or cells. Nutrition as one of those nonimmunologic factors in allergy has
been discussed by Currier (1970), who gives a short review of what is known
about the effects of individual vitamin deficiencies in generating immune responses
to a variety of antigens.

In the sections which follow, we will critically discuss typical examples of suggested vitamin allergy and assess the observed phenomena as to a definite allergic
genesis. In this discussion we will apply the rigid criteria proposed by de Weck
(1971) for classifying observed reactions as allergic reactions against vitamins. In
the past, a considerable number of review articles have been published covering the
literature on adverse effects of vitamins, including allergic reactions (Meyler 1952,
1957, 1958, 1960, 1963, 1966; Alexander 1955; Pedersen 1966; Dalderup 1968,
1972; Randazzo et al. 1972; Nater 1975, 1977, 1978; Hellriegel and Reuter
1975, 1978; Reuter and Hellriegel 1977, 1979). The present work will deal with
13 vitamins in particular: A, D, E, and K of the fat-soluble vitamins, and B_1, B_2,
B_6, B_{12}, C, biotin, folic acid, nicotinic acid, and pantothenic acid of the water-soluble vitamins. Not all untoward reactions to drugs, however, are due to allergy and
such terms as "idiosyncrasy", "intolerance", and "toxicity" are not necessarily synonymous with allergy and will not be considered in this chapter.

B. Vitamin A

I. Physicochemical and Pharmacologic Aspects

Vitamin A (retinol) is a fat-soluble, long chain alcohol (molecular weight 286.4 daltons) which exists in a number of isomeric forms. The most active and the form

most frequently found in mammalian tissues is the all-*trans*-retinol. Retinol forms pale yellow crystals and is soluble in fat and organic solvents but insoluble in water. It is often found in an esterified form and esters such as the acetate and palmitate are sometimes preferred for nutritional and medical use. Retinol is sensitive to oxygen, acids, and ultraviolet light. One of the main sources of vitamin A is liver. Vitamin A is absorbed in its free form. Absorption is accelerated in the presence of emulsifying agents, e.g., bile. After absorption the vitamin is deposited in the parenchymal cells of the liver as an ester of long chain fatty acids, mainly retinyl palmitate. It is subsequently carried in the blood bound to retinol-binding protein (RBP). A detailed treatise on the metabolism of vitamin A was published by OLSON (1967). The role vitamin A plays in the vision process is undisputed as is its involvement in the maintenance of epithelial tissues. The mechanistic role vitamin A plays in other biologic systems, however, is not yet fully understood.

Deficiency of vitamin A leads to degenerative lesions in the epithelium, xerophthalmia being the classical vitamin A deficiency disease. The drug-equivalent uses of vitamin A can be seen in Table 1.

II. Allergic Reactions to Vitamin A

Early reports of allergoid reactions to vitamin A are vague. COPE (1942) reports a contact dermatitis due to cod liver oil, which had been applied for the treatment of an ulcer on the leg. In patch tests the patient was negative to petrolatum, hydrous wool fat, and cholesterolized petrolatum. In view of the high content of vitamin A in cod liver oil (85,000 IU/100 g) vitamin A was tentatively suspected as the causative agent: conclusive evidence, however, has not been presented. Recently, sensitivity to vitamin A has been reported by GREENBAUM (1979) in a 9-month-old boy who showed a rash typical of a topic dermatitis. Interestingly, the problem resolved on a diet free of foods containing vitamin A. Prick tests showed equivocal reactions to house dust and dust mites and were negative for more than 40 foods tested. When the child returned to a normal diet and was challenged with commercial preparations of vitamin A drops, the symptoms recurred. Again, in this report, no conclusive evidence for an immunologically allergic nature of the observed reactions could be presented. There are some reports of allergic reactions during vitamin A acid therapy (LINDGREN et al. 1976; KAIDBEY et al. 1975; JORDAN et al. 1975; KRUEGER et al. 1972). A recent review covering the adverse reactions to vitamin A acid was published by HEEL et al. (1977).

In conclusion, the presence of true allergic reactions to vitamin A has, so far, not been unequivocally proven by the demonstration of specific antibodies or cells sensitized to vitamin A. On the other hand, however, vitamin A has been the only vitamin against which antibodies have been induced in rabbits (CONRAD and WIRTZ 1973) by injection of vitamin A acid covalently coupled to human serum albumin. One reason for the low or absent sensitization capability of retinol may be the fact that in the body vitamin A is being transported in close non-covalent association with RBP; for reviews see GOODMAN (1974) and DeLUCA et al. (1979). The influence of this close association with serum proteins, however, on the induction of immunologic responses against vitamins has not been investigated. Vitamin A appears to be an adjuvant (DRESSER 1968; SPITZNAGEL and ALLISON 1970) and this has been explained by the lysosome-labilizing action of retinol. This effect, however, seems to be without influence on the allergenic properties of vitamin A.

C. Vitamin B$_1$

I. Physicochemical and Pharmacologic Aspects

Vitamin B$_1$ (thiamine, aneurine) has the molecular structure of a pyrimidine and a thiazole ring bridged by a methylene group; the molecular weight is 337.3 daltons. It contains a quarternary nitrogen atom. The water-soluble, white, crystalline solid is stable in acidic solution but less stable in neutral or alkaline solution. Thiamine is present in high concentrations in yeast, in the pericarp, and germ of cereals. Whole rice and wheat flour are the main sources for this vitamin, but it is present in practically all plant and animal tissues.

Thiamine is mainly absorbed by an active transport mechanism from the small intestine. Only when high doses are present is transport effected passively by diffusion. The body is incapable of storing the free vitamin, and excretes excess quantities of it readily in the urine. Within the body, thiamine is transformed by phosphorylation into the active coenzyme thiamine pyrophosphate (TPP, cocarboxylase). Small amounts of this phosphorylated form occur in all animal cells. Thiamine pyrophosphate plays a key role in the oxidative decarboxylation of α-ketoacids to aldehydes and, therefore, is essential for carbohydrate metabolism. In 1 day about 1 mg thiamine – independent of the amount ingested – is metabolized. Of the over 20 different metabolites the following have been identified (Neal and Sauberlich 1973): 2-methyl-4-amino-5-pyrimidine carboxylic acid, 4-methylthiazole-5-acetic acid, 2-methyl-4-amino-5-hydroxymethylpyrimidine, 5-(2-hydroxyethyl)-4-methylthiazole, 3(2′-methyl-4′-amino-5′-pyrimidylmethyl)-4-methylthiazole-5-acetic acid (thiamine acetic acid), and 2-methyl-4-amino-5-formylaminomethylpyrimidine. To our knowledge, it has not been investigated whether these metabolites under physiologic conditions can form immunogenic covalent conjugates with plasma proteins or blood cells. This seems fairly unlikely in view of the chemical structure of these substances. The same applies to free thiamine, for which a definite intrinsic chemical reactivity has not been reported.

When dealing with allergic reactions to vitamin B$_1$ an obvious first question is where and when the body has been exposed to this vitamin. As vitamin B$_1$ is an essential food constituent, exposure occurs during the whole lifetime at relatively low dosages. Food allergy caused by thiamine, however, has not been reported so far. An exposure to higher concentrations of thiamine is encountered in the drug-equivalent use of this vitamin. The classical use is the thiamine treatment of beriberi, a disease which can be endemic, especially among populations whose staple cereal in the diet is rice. This disease is the classical B$_1$ avitaminosis, its prevalent feature being a polyneuritis. From this symptom the name aneurin, synonymous with thiamine, is derived, reflecting the relation of vitamin B$_1$ to the nervous system.

At present, the important clinical indication areas for therapy with thiamine are the beriberi of alcoholics and Wernicke's encephalopathy (KÖRNER and VÖLLM 1976). In both cases, therapy is started with daily doses of at least 50–100 mg (in severe cases up to 200 mg) thiamine administered parenterally. Therapy is then continued with oral doses of 100–300 mg daily. Neuritis accompanying pregnancy responds particularly well to vitamin B$_1$ therapy. In some severe disorders of the intermediate metabolism (e.g., diabetic acidosis, severe hepatic malfunction), the necessary phosphorylation of thiamine in the organism is no longer ensured. Thiamine has, therefore, to be administered directly in its active form, thiamine pyrophosphate (TPP, cocarboxylase). Instances of toxicity of thiamine have been reported, primarily showing effects on the cardiovascular and nervous systems (UNNA 1972; DiPALMA and RITCHIE 1977).

II. Allergic Reactions to Vitamin B$_1$

Thiamine is the vitamin which has most frequently given rise to reactions, which have been classified as allergic on the basis of a variety of criteria. Those reactions range from quite mild symptoms to fatal cases. LAWS (1941) reported a case in which a patient who had not previously suffered allergic symptoms received a series of daily *subcutaneous* injections of 25 mg doses of thiamine hydrochloride over a period of 10 days, followed by weekly injections for a period of 10 weeks. Then thiamine medication was terminated. When injections were resumed 10 months later there were no marked local reactions, but occasionally the site of injection would itch for several hours. During this course of treatment the patient noticed that soon after leaving the doctors's office she sneezed violently several times, this occurring after each injection of thiamine. Thirty minutes after the last of these injections she developed several nasal symptoms, generalized urticaria, facial edema, dyspnea, and cyanosis, culminating in collapse. Epinephrine was given within a few minutes, and at the end of 5–6 h the entire reaction had subsided. In intradermal tests a large urticarial wheal resulted. Passive transfer (Prausnitz–Küstner test) was made to a nonallergic individual, and at the end of 48 h the sensitized sites reacted strongly when the same preparation of thiamine was introduced.

SCHIFF (1941) refers to a similar case in which a patient received a series of *intramuscular* injections of 25 mg dosages within a period of 7 months using three different commercial preparations. After the last injection, nausea, vomiting, profuse sweating, and collapse occurred showing the signs of severe shock. On closer interrogation, it was found that the patient had had several brief episodes of nasal symptoms and nausea after the previous injections. An intradermal test with an aqueous solution of thiamine hydrochloride was also positive in this case. In view of the rapidity with which the reaction occurred, the author assumed that some of the thiamine hydrochloride solution must have been administered intravenously at the last injection.

In the following case (TEMIME and CASTELAIN 1960), a 67-year-old patient developed nausea and generalized pruritus after *oral* ingestion of one vitamin B$_1$ tablet. On the next day the patient, nevertheless, received an *intramuscular* injection

of vitamin B_1 which resulted in anaphylactic shock with loss of conciousness for
4 h followed by Quincke's edema. Mills (1941) reported the first death after the
intramuscular injection of thiamine. Acharya et al. (1969) reports a fatal anaphylactic reaction which occurred after ingestion of a 100 mg tablet of vitamin B_1. The
case history revealed that the patient had taken one tablet containing 100 mg thiamine daily for 15 days, 2 months previously. On the day of admission she had taken
one tablet in the morning. Post-mortem examinations showed evidence of a recent
thrombus in one of the arteries. This report is the first and, so far, only report of
a severe reaction after the *oral* ingestion of thiamine preparations. *Oral* vitamin B_1
might cause allergic reactions in the same way as does oral penicillin. But in view
of the total amount of thiamine which is ingested around the world, we can safely
consider this to be an extremely rare occurrence.

Most of the cases of anaphylactic or anaphylactoid reactions to vitamin B_1 described in the literature took place after a series of injections, although a few occurred after only one injection. As a rule, the undesirable reactions started a few
minutes after the injection, but some may occur after up to 1 h, which is extremely
dangerous because in such cases the patient is no longer under the doctor's observation. Previous allergic conditions do not seem to be of appreciable importance
with regard to the likelihood of allergic reactions following the administration of
vitamins. Several authors have tried conducting intradermal tests with vitamin B_1
solutions in order to determine the presence of allergy. A number of such tests have
been discussed; Kalz (1942) maintains that thiamine always tends to give false
positive reactions, while Stiles (1941) stresses that false positive reactions can be
avoided by using solutions containing less than 5 mg thiamine per ml.

An interesting experiment was carried out by Seusing (1951) in a patient who
developed severe urticaria after the first *intravenous* injection of thiamine. An intradermal test with vitamin B_1 at a dilution of 1:400,000 in 0.9% sodium chloride
was negative, whereas vitamin B_1 dissolved in the patient's own serum gave a
strong positive reaction; the serum alone gave a negative reaction. Jolliffe (1941)
obtained a positive skin test with the solvent, chlorbutanol, used in the relevant vitamin preparation, whereas vitamin B_1 yielded a negative reaction. These cases illustrate the complexity of allergic reactions to vitamin B_1. The problem centers on
the significance of positive skin reactions, since their appearance in most cases was
the criterion by which sensitivity was judged. In view of the experiments reported
by Seusing (1951), it is conceivable that a combination of thiamine with protein
might have been generated which is antigenic to the host. The evidence, however,
is not conclusive and the anaphylactogenic properties of thiamine require further
investigation. If thiamine is an obligate wheal-producing agent (Kalz 1942), positive intradermal tests as well as positive passive transfer tests, as reported by a number of authors (Laws 1941; Mitrani 1944; Shapero and Gwinner 1947; Engelhardt and Baird 1949; Tetreault and Beck 1956; Hoigné and Naegeli 1957),
may not be valid proof of individual sensitivity.

How far the acetylcholine-like activity of thiamine, postulated by Kalz (1942),
can be used to explain the observed anaphylactoid phenomena has not been discussed in the literature. The same applies to its curare-like effects, as reported by
Barazzone and Lambelet (1954), as well as to its effects on nervous tissue (Cooper and Pincus 1979). Neither does the literature consider the role thiaminases

might play in the generation of allergenic thiamine derivatives. That thiaminases exist in humans was demonstrated by the isolation from human feces of certain bacteria which elaborated enzymes capable of destroying thiamine (EVANS 1975).

On the basis of thin layer chromatographic analysis, the anaphylactoid properties of thiamine preparations were ascribed by BLUM et al. (1974) to an impurity migrating in the neighborhood of pure thiamine. This impurity was postulated to act in the sense of a systemic anaphylactoid substance. Later this product was identified as 2′-demethylthiamine. Further investigations of this compound, however, could not confirm its anaphylactogenic properties in a reproducible manner.

In conclusion we can say that the pathogenetic mechanism of the anaphylactoid phenomena connected with the use of vitamin B_1 is not yet clear. To our knowledge, antibodies against vitamin B_1 have not been demonstrated unequivocally. Nevertheless, the occurrence of anaphylactoid reactions after vitamin B_1 administration are a real, although so far, unresolved problem. POLLITT (1968) reported that the risk of such reactions is negligible when thiamine is given intravenously *together* with other members of the vitamin B complex. Interestingly, reports of adverse reactions against vitamin B_1 become increasingly rare after 1970. The decreased use of thiamine, especially parenterally, for various functional disorders, may have resulted in a reduction of the incidence of anaphylactoid as well as toxic reactions (DiPALMA and RITCHIE 1977) to vitamin B_1.

D. Vitamin B_2

I. Physicochemical and Pharmacologic Aspects

Vitamin B_2, riboflavin, is an isoalloxazine derivative with a ribitol side chain; the molecular weight is 376.4 daltons. The orange–yellow crystals melt with decomposition at about 280 °C. At ordinary temperatures, it is thermally stable and unaffected by atmospheric oxygen. It is very slightly soluble in water, the solution exhibiting a strong yellow–green fluorescence. It is insoluble in organic solvents, stable in strongly acid solution, unstable in the presence of alkali or when exposed to light or ultraviolet radiation. Riboflavin is widely distributed in all leafy vegetables, in the flesh of warm-blooded animals and in fish.

Riboflavin can be synthesized by bacteria within the intestinal tract of many species. In humans, however, enterosynthesis is not sufficient to meet the whole body requirement which is about 1.4 mg/day. Free vitamin B_2 is phosphorylated in the intestinal mucosa during absorption. It is stored in small quantities in the liver, spleen, kidney, and cardiac muscle. Riboflavin is eliminated in the urine. The active coenzyme forms of riboflavin are riboflavin 5′-phosphate, also called flavin mononucleotide (FMN) and flavinadenin dinucleotide (FAD) which form the prosthetic group of several different enzyme systems (flavoproteins) all concerned with hydrogen transport. In both animals and humans, riboflavin is essential to growth and life. The drug-equivalent use of riboflavin can be seen in Table 1.

II. Allergic Reactions to Vitamin B$_2$

As early as 1942, studies by UNNA and GRESLIN have shown that riboflavin is an exceptionally nontoxic compound. Rats and dogs tolerated single oral doses of 10 g/kg and 2 g/kg, respectively. Giving 34 mg/kg to mice intraperitoneally, which is the equivalent of 20 g/day for humans, had no apparent adverse effects. HORWITT (1972) ascribed the relative innocuousness of riboflavin to its low solubility in polar as well as in nonpolar solvents. This low solubility may also be the reason why allergic reactions to riboflavin have so far not been reported. This is interesting because chemically reactive riboflavin derivatives can be created by light, which might produce immunogenic protein conjugates with distinct immunochemical determinants cross-reacting with riboflavin.

E. Vitamin B$_6$

I. Physicochemical and Pharmacologic Aspects

Vitamin B$_6$ comprises a group of three slightly different compounds: pyridoxine (molecular weight 205.6 daltons), pyridoxal, and pyridoxamine. These substances are colorless crystals, soluble in water and alcohol, both as free bases and as the commonly available hydrochlorides. They are resistant to normal heat but are decomposed by alkalis and ultraviolet light. Pyridoxine hydrochloride decomposes at its melting point (204°–205 °C). The three forms are widely distributed in low concentrations in all animal and plant tissues. The vitamin is rapidly absorbed but little is known about the factors influencing its absorption. About 70% of the vitamin is excreted in the urine as the inactive metabolite 4-pyridoxic acid. Within the body, vitamin B$_6$ is rapidly converted into the coenzymes pyridoxal 5′-phosphate and pyridoxamine 5′-phosphate. In the form of these coenzymes vitamin B$_6$ is directly involved in important metabolic conversions such as transaminations, decarboxylations, and deaminations. In humans, it has proved difficult to induce deficiency symptoms, whereas some more or less specific lesions can be induced by the administration of the pyridoxine antagonist, deoxypyridoxine. The drug-equivalent uses of the vitamin B$_6$ group can be seen in Table 1.

II. Allergic Reactions to Vitamin B$_6$

In connection with the use of the vitamin B$_6$ group, only one report describing an anaphylactoid reaction has been published (DANILOV 1973); its allergic nature has, however, not been confirmed by further tests. KADLEC and HANSLIAN (1965) reported an allergy observed in a vitamin B$_6$ factory. The causative agent, however, was not one of the B$_6$ group vitamins itself but an intermediate product.

F. Vitamin B$_{12}$

I. Physicochemical and Pharmacologic Aspects

The compounds active as vitamin B$_{12}$ are of a complicated chemical structure, the best known and most important being cyanocobalamin (molecular weight 1355.4 daltons), the others differing only slightly from it. Cyanocobalamin is a red, crystalline, hygroscopic substance, freely soluble in water and alcohol but insoluble in acetone, chloroform, or ether. It is labile in strong acid, alkali, and light. The structure of cyanocobalamin bears a relationship to the porphyrins, but with a central cobalt atom. In its natural form, vitamin B$_{12}$ is probably bound to peptides or proteins.

Vitamin B$_{12}$ is synthesized in large quantities by the intestinal flora, particularly in ruminants. The exact amount of vitamin B$_{12}$ required by the normal human is not known. The absorption of vitamin B$_{12}$ from the gastrointestinal tract is dependent on the presence of a gastric mucoprotein called "intrinsic factor." Calcium ions seem to be necessary for the interaction of vitamin B$_{12}$ with this intrinsic factor. Vitamin B$_{12}$, which is absorbed only in the ileum, is stored in the liver. There are two transport proteins for vitamin B$_{12}$: transcobalamin I and II, the latter being physiologically more important. Vitamin B$_{12}$ plays an important role in the metabolism of functional groups with one carbon atom such as the methyl group and, therefore, is related to folic acid. The exact mechanism of action, however, is still only poorly understood.

II. Allergic Reactions to Vitamin B$_{12}$

The first report of sensitivity to vitamin B$_{12}$ was published by YOUNG et al. (1950). He described a patient who was extremely sensitive to liver extract and vitamin B$_{12}$ concentrate from streptomycin broth but not to crystalline vitamin B$_{12}$. Skin tests were positive with liver extract as well as *Streptomyces* vitamin B$_{12}$ concentrate, whereas crystalline vitamin B$_{12}$ and streptomycin induced no reactions. Allergic reactions to vitamin B$_{12}$ were reported by BRODULIN (1961), who described a case where anaphylactic shock developed 3 min after injection of 200 µg vitamin B$_{12}$ in a 29-year-old patient. After skin testing, anaphylactic symptoms recurred, associated with local redness and swelling. Another case of severe anaphylaxis after vitamin B$_{12}$ administration (intramuscularly) is reported by HOVDING (1968). The patient, a 67-year-old man with pernicious anemia, was treated with intramuscular injections of liver extract and 0.2 mg cyanocobalamin at intervals of 2–8 weeks over a period of 1 year, when the treatment was changed to hydroxocobalamin. Until the third and last injection of hydroxocobalamin 6 months later, he had never shown any adverse reaction either to the liver extract or to the different preparations of vitamin B$_{12}$. Within a few minutes of receiving the last injection of hydroxocobalamin, however, he developed symptoms of severe anaphylactic shock. After the administration of 0.75 ml adrenaline he slowly recovered. The author discusses his findings critically, particularly emphasizing the role impurities might play. Vitamin B$_{12}$ is produced by biosynthesis and BEDFORD (1952) suggested that carryover impurities are responsible for the antigenic properties of vitamin B$_{12}$.

Another possible explanation of the observed reactions are the additives in pharmaceutical preparations. Thus LAGERHOLM et al. (1958) reported a case of hypersensitivity to benzyl alcohol added as a preservative to vitamin B$_{12}$ preparations, resulting in urticaria after injection. HOVDING (1968), however, was not able to demonstrate a positive skin reaction either with benzyl alcohol or with cobalt chloride. However, skin tests with commercial brands of cyanocobalamin and hydroxocobalamin as well as with purified cyanocabalamin and hydroxocobalamin were positive. MALTEN (1975) reports a flare reaction in a woman due to the third injection of 250 µg vitamin B$_{12}$. Prick and patch tests, however, remained negative. A recent short review of reactions after administration of vitamin B$_{12}$ preparations was published by MEUWISSEN (1978). An extensive review covering the literature up to 1975 was presented by FAIVRE et al. (1975). The authors conclude that, despite the widespread use of vitamin B$_{12}$ preparations, cases of accidents after vitamin B$_{12}$ administration are very rare, but nevertheless are a potential risk. Therefore, skin and immunologic tests should be made prior to administration and especially parenteral application of the vitamin. The authors do not make an explicit statement as to a definite allergic mechanism of the observed phenomena.

NAVA (1971) suggested a definitive allergy to the vitamin B$_{12}$ molecule or to a vitamin B$_{12}$ protein complex. In his report, the hypersensitivity to vitamin B$_{12}$ of 110 people was induced by occupational exposure to cyanocobalamin in 50 cases and by drug-equivalent exposure in 60 cases. He could exclude the possibility of an allergy to additives and impurities of fungal (*Streptomyces*) origin. An interesting case was noted by JAMES and WARIN (1971) where a woman responded with anaphylaxis and chronic severe urticaria to *parenteral* as well as *oral* administration of vitamin B_{12}. Intradermal prick tests with cyanocobalamin and hydroxocobalamin were negative in this case. Interestingly, GILLHESPY (1955) had reported the oral route of administration as being well tolerated by patients sensitive to the injection. Skin tests also were negative in a case of anaphylactic shock reported by AUZÉPY et al. (1974), as in the cases reported by SAIF et al. (1975) and DALLY and GAULTIER (1976). PEVNY et al. (1977) report on a case of delayed hypersensitivity to vitamin B_{12} under a long-term and high dosage treatment.

In conclusion, we want to emphasize that there are only a few reports on adverse allergic effects of vitamin B_{12} preparations, when taking into account the widespread use of this vitamin. Moreover, a distinct immunologic mechanism has not been proven, even in cases where highly purified cobalamines have been used. Thus, in only one report (UNGLEY 1955) is a Prausnitz–Küstner test mentioned, this being positive. Most of the cases of reactions against vitamin B_{12}, in our view, are, therefore, reflections of idiosyncratic or intolerance phenomena.

G. Vitamin C

I. Physicochemical and Pharmacologic Aspects

Ascorbic acid (molecular weight 176.1 daltons) is the enolic form of 3-keto-1-gulo-furanolactone. Only the L-isomer has vitamin C activity. The endiol groups at the second and third carbon atoms are sensitive to oxidation and can easily be converted into a diketo group. The resultant dehydro-L-ascorbic acid is just as effective against scurvy as the reduced substrate. Ascorbic acid is a white, odorless, crystalline substance, which is reasonably stable in air, but which rapidly deteriorates in aqueous solution in the presence of air. It is heat labile. Ascorbic acid is insoluble in benzene, chloroform, ether, petroleum ether, or fat. Vitamin C is widely distributed in high concentrations, particularly in citrus fruits and green vegetables. Unlike most animals, humans are unable to synthesize ascorbic acid. Ascorbic acid is readily absorbed from the intestinal tract by an active transport mechanism. In persons whose tissue is saturated with it after either oral or parenteral administration, ascorbic acid is excreted rapidly in the urine. It appears that limited stores of ascorbic acid are held in the body. To a limited degree ascorbic acid is also excreted in sweat and feces. The definite biochemical function of ascorbic acid is still unknown, but it is believed that it plays a role in hydroxylation reactions. For the current drug-equivalent uses of ascorbic acid, Table 1 may be consulted.

II. Allergic Reactions to Vitamin C

Cases of allergic reactions to ascorbic acid are very rare. Early observations reported rubelliform, morbilliform, and scarlatiniform exanthemas, urticaria, and edema
after vitamin C use (WIDENBAUER 1936 a, b). Positive skin reactions were reported
by RUST (1954) in seven cases and by PANZANI (1961) in one case. In this latter case,
the skin test was a passive transfer test (Prausnitz–Küstner) but the data presented
are too scarce to demonstrate a definite immunological etiology of the observed
reactions. The same holds for three cases of respiratory and cutaneous allergy reported recently by VASSAL (1975).

Although allergic reactions to vitamin C have been reported only in very few
cases in humans there are numerous publications (albeit controversial) about possible effects of ascorbic acid on the metabolism of histamine, the well-known mediator of allergic disease, and on prostaglandins. These studies have been carried
out predominantly in the guinea pig. VUKUSIC et al. (1970) observed a suppressive
effect of vitamin C on sensitization and on the intensity of anaphylactic reactions
of guinea pigs to ovalbumin. Ascorbic acid was also found to prevent bronchoconstriction induced by 5-hydroxy-tryptamine, bradykinin, and histamine by DAWSON
and WEST (1965) and by ZUSKIN et al. (1973). This inhibitory action was ascribed
by SHARMA and WILSON (1977) and SHARMA et al. (1976) to an inhibition of prostaglandin formation. HITCHCOCK (1975), however, found a stimulation of immunologic histamine release and production of prostaglandin F by ascorbic acid. In
a study on humans, no protective effect of vitamin C (500 mg) against ragweed
antigen-induced bronchospasm could be observed by KORDANSKY et al. (1979)
whereas BIANCO et al. (1977) showed prevention of a prostaglandin F-induced
bronchoconstriction by ascorbic acid in asthmatic patients. The pharmacodynamic role of ascorbic acid in direct and indirect mediator metabolism clearly
requires further investigation. Interestingly, as has been pointed out by CHATTER-
JEE (1973), those animals which have lost the capacity to synthezise ascorbic acid
are just those in which histamine exerts a strong vasoactive effect as the primary
mediator of the anaphylactic reaction.

In conclusion, allergic reactions to ascorbic acid with a proven immunologic
pathogenesis have, so far, not been reported. An indirect involvement of ascorbic
acid in the production of the allergic response has, however been suggested by WIL-
SON (1976a) and reviewed by THOMAS and HOLT (1978). In this context, it is worth
mentioning that ascorbic acid is being used for the determination of reaginic antibodies of the IgE class in diagnostic tests of atopic allergy. This test, called the leukocyte ascorbic acid uptake direct antigen challenge test (LAADACT), was established by WILSON (1974) and WILSON et al. (1975). It measures the inhibition of the
uptake of ascorbic acid by leukocytes from atopic subjects, when incubated in
ascorbic acid in the presence of specific antigen. A LAADACT is considered positive when the ascorbic acid uptake by leukocytes is reduced by 20% or more in the
presence of antigen. In non-atopic subjects, the test is negative in the presence of
the same antigen. When results from the LAADACT are compared with results
from skin tests (WILSON 1976a) and, more importantly, with results from radioallergosorbent tests (RAST) (WILSON 1976b, c), high IgE concentrations were significantly correlated with positive LAADACT reactions in all cases. While this test

might be useful in the diagnosis of atopic allergy, its underlying mechanism has not yet been definitely elucidated.

H. Biotin

Biotin is a cyclic derivative of urea with an attached thiophen ring; the molecular weight is 244.3 daltons. There are eight different isomers of which only one, the so-called (+)-biotin, is found naturally and has vitamin activity. The fine, colorless needles are slightly soluble in water, more soluble in alcohol, but practically insoluble in organic solvents. It is stable to heat and not decomposed by acid or alkali. The vitamin is widely distributed in small concentrations in all animal and plant tissues, one of its main sources being eggs. Biotin is readily absorbed from the small intestine. The vitamin plays a key role in intermediary metabolism and is particularly involved in carboxylation and transcarboxylation reactions (MURTHY and MISTRY 1977).

Allergic reactions to biotin have not been reported so far. BONNET and FLORENS (1969) explicitly emphasized that biotin did not induce allergy in their studies on the effect of biotin in the treatment of acne and eczema. Biotin is tolerated by humans and by various laboratory animals without any side effects, even at high doses (GYÖRGY and LANGER 1968; WRIGHT 1956).

J. Folic Acid

I. Physicochemical and Pharmacologic Aspects

Folic acid is pteroyl monoglutamic acid, molecular weight 441.4 daltons. It is a yellow–orange, crystalline powder, tasteless and odorless, insoluble in alcohol, ether, and other organic solvents. It is slightly soluble in hot water. Pteroylglutamic acid is a combination of the pteridine nucleus, p-aminobenzoic acid, and glutamic acid. If the glutamic acid is replaced, the vitamin effect is lost; on the other hand pteroic acid, both in combination with three molecules of glutamic acid (pteroyltriglutamic acid) and with seven glutamic acid molecules (pteroylheptaglutamic acid) are biologically active. Folic acid is stable to heat in neutral and alkaline solution, but unstable in acid solution. The vitamin is present in green vegetables, liver, and kidney. No direct studies have been made of the absorption of folic acid. The vitamin does not seem to be stored in the liver. The function of folic acid is to act as a carrier of "reactive" fragments containing single carbon atoms for methylation reactions.

II. Allergic Reactions to Folic Acid

Mitchell et al. (1949) reported one case presumed to be a hypersensitivity to folic acid. The patient had hyperthyroidism and had developed granulocytopenia from thiouracil. For this, 5 mg folic acid was given orally three times a day. Thiouracil was given concomitantly for 2 weeks when a pruritic maculopapular eruption appeared, which faded 36 h after folic acid was stopped. When the drug was resumed 1 and 2 weeks later, the first dose of 50 mg synthetic folic acid given *intravenously* caused flushing and dizziness. The following day, immediately after the second dose, dyspnea, substernal oppression, and marked tachycardia occurred. Later, an intradermal skin test with folic acid gave a large reaction. No precipitins, however, were found in the blood and passive transfer was not successful. One other case where the passive transfer (Prausnitz–Küstner test) was also negative is reported by Rausch (1956). In this case, the clinical picture was a severe life-threatening anaphylactic shock after the *intravenous* injection of folic acid. The author ascribed the symptoms to an allergic mechanism only on the basis of an intracutaneous test.

Intracutaneous testing was also the method with which Chanarin et al. (1957) observed a sensitivity to orally ingested folic acid in a healthy male. Free antibody, specific for folic acid could not be detected with a precipitation nor with a hemagglutination technique. The authors, therefore, are cautious in ascribing the symptoms to an allergic reaction and speak only of a sensitivity to folic acid. A further report about sensitivity to folic acid was published by Mathur (1966). He describes a 9-month-old child who had a generalized urticarial rash which disappeared after 4 days. After 1 week, a 5 mg folic acid tablet was given, which again produced urticaria. Later on, sensitivity to folic acid was confirmed by an intradermal test. This author as well as Chanarin et al. (1957) emphasize that the purest form of folic acid then available contained about 3% impurities. It is, therefore, not proven whether folic acid itself was the causative agent in both cases. In a report by Levander-Lindgren (1957), the role folic acid plays in the observed "hypersensitivity to folic acid" is also obscure, mainly because in this case even the applied skin tests were negative. Woodliff and Davis (1966) investigated three patients with a history suggesting allergy to folic acid. However, they admit that there might have been some other cause.

In conclusion, in spite of the extensive use of folic acid since its synthesis in 1945, only six vague reports about a possible allergy to folic acid have been published. Conclusive evidence for a real allergic pathogenesis of the observed reactions, however, has not been presented.

K. Nicotinic Acid and Nicotinamide

R = −OH (acid)

R = −NH₂ (amide)

I. Physicochemical and Pharmacologic Aspects

Nicotinic acid is pyridine-β-carboxylic acid (molecular weight 123.1 daltons) and nicotinamide is the corresponding amide (molecular weight 122.1 daltons). Both are white, crystalline solids soluble in water. They are very stable: not heat labile, nor sensitive to light, air, or alkali. Intestinal production of the vitamin by intestinal bacteria is of only minor importance in the human. Intestinal absorption of nicotinic acid is normally very efficient. The vitamin is converted in the body into the coenzymes nicotinamide adenine dinucleotide (NAD) and nicotinamide adenine dinucleotide phosphate (NADP); though these are widely distributed, no true storage occurs. A small amount of nicotinic acid or amide is excreted, the largest portion as N-methylnicotinamide. As an indispensable component of the NAD- or NADP-dependent dehydrogenases, nicotinamide plays an important central role in oxidative and reductive metabolism.

II. Allergic Reactions to Nicotinic Acid and Nicotinamide

There are only a few reported instances of hypersensitivity to nicotinic acid. RACH-MILEWITZ and GLUECK (1938) describe the occurrence of urticarial dermatitis, with flushing and severe pruritus, in a patient with pellagra who had taken nicotinic acid 100 mg/day for some time. WATROUS (1939) described a few cases of exanthema with itching in industrial workers who had been exposed to nicotinic acid, while no reaction was observed in their colleagues who had been exposed to nicotinic acid under the same conditions. PELNER (1947) reports on two patients who developed shock after *intravenous* injection of nicotinic acid in doses of 5–25 mg. Both patients had previously taken nicotinic acid by mouth with mild side effects, one with swelling of the lower lip, and the other with coughing and vertigo. The first patient developed shock only 2 min after the first injection of nicotinic acid, so that it can be assumed that this person had been sensitized through taking nicotinic acid by mouth. In the other patient, shock developed after the fourth injection. POWERS (1948) also reported a case of shock after *intravenous* nicotinic acid. FEINBERG (1948) reports on a patient who received 150 mg three times a day. In this case, shock occurred after the sixth dose, while 6 weeks later an intradermal skin test gave a marked reaction.

A distinct allergic–immunologic pathogenesis of all these reported cases is not established because skin tests were the only evidence, antibodies not having been investigated. Interestingly, there exist three reports on anti-allergic effect of nicotinic acid (KODA et al. 1972; PARROT et al. 1974; BEKIER and MASLINSKI 1974). The mechanism of the antihistaminic action of nicotinamide is, however, not known. There seems to be a relation between the inhibitory effect of nicotinamide on rat liver phosphodiesterase and cyclic adenosine monophosphate, a known mediator of smooth-muscle relaxation.

L. Pantothenic Acid

$$HOH_2C - \underset{\underset{CH_3}{|}}{\overset{\overset{CH_3}{|}}{C}} - CHOH - CO - NH - CH_2 - CH_2 - CO_2H$$

From the two optically active isomers of pantothenic acid (molecular weight 219.2 daltons) only the dextrorotatory form is effective as a vitamin. The free acid is a pale yellow, viscous oil, soluble in water and alcohol, insoluble in benzene and chloroform, and unstable to acids, bases, and heat. Pantothenic acid occurs in all animal and plant tissues and is, as the name implies, ubiquitous. Pantothenic acid, its salts, and the corresponding alcohol (panthenol) are absorbed from the intestinal tract, probably by diffusion. Within the tissues the vitamin is converted to coenzyme A (CoA). Pantothenic acid is the essential component of CoA, important in intermediary metabolism. Pantothenic acid is tolerated without any reactions, even at very high doses and is, therefore, considered nontoxic (GREENGARD 1970). Allergic or allergoid reactions have not been reported so far.

M. Vitamin D

This vitamin is present in nature in several forms. All are sterols and occur only in the animal organism. The active synthetic compounds for therapy in the human are vitamin D_2 (ergocalciferol, molecular weight 396.7 daltons) and vitamin D_3 (cholecalciferol, molecular weight 384.6 daltons). They occur as colorless crystals, insoluble in water, but readily soluble in alcohol and other organic solvents. Normal adults obtain adequate amounts of vitamin D by exposure to sunlight. The normal human requirement is not yet clearly established and a daily requirement of 10 µg cholecalciferol has been suggested. Vitamin D is absorbed from the intestinum, fats being necessary for this to occur. The vitamin is intimately involved in the metabolism of calcium and phosphorus. Reports of allergic reactions against the D vitamins have, so far, not been published.

N. Vitamin E

I. Physicochemical and Pharmacologic Aspects

Naturally occurring vitamin E comprises a series of compounds called tocopherols. Among the richest sources are cereal germs and most oilseeds. α-Tocopherol (molecular weight 430.7 daltons), which possesses the highest vitamin E activity, is a yellow oil, insoluble in water, but soluble in organic solvents. It is readily oxidized and, therefore, is also used as an antioxidant. A vitamin E deficiency disease has not been reported in humans although it may be readily induced in experimental animals by feeding them an appropriate diet. The absorption of tocopherol, similar to that of other fat-soluble vitamins, is probably linked to fat absorption and facilitated by the presence of bile salts. The mechanism of action of vitamin E is still far from clear. Undisputed, however, is the function it fulfills because of its redox properties.

II. Allergic Reactions to Vitamin E

The first report of a suggested adverse reaction to vitamin E was published by BRODKIN and BLEIBERG (1965) who describe a case of contact allergy to synthetically produced α-tocopherol as follows.

The patient, an 18-year-old white female stenographer, reported that she has first experienced swelling and itching of the left ear lobe five months previously, which had subsided with a salve, allergy pills, and a spray prescribed by her general physician. This eruption had recurred approximately three days before she consulted us. For several years, the patient had applied a variety of topical medications for "lumps" which she occasionally felt in her ear lobes. Significant physical findings were limited to the left ear lobe and helix and consisted of erythema, edema, vesiculation, and crusting. The diagnosis of acute allergic eczematous contact dermatitis was made. She was patch tested to standard testing dilutions of lanolin, phenol, and menthol, and to Tashan Cream, undiluted, by standard closed patch test methods. All patch tests were negative except for the one to Tashan Cream which showed erythema, edema, and vesiculation. The manufacturers of Tashan Cream were contacted and supplied the ingredients of their formulation which consists of 17 chemicals. The materials were applied as closed patch test and the only significant reaction was to α-tocopherol. This consisted of intense erythema and edema. The eruption responded to avoidance of Tashan Cream and symptomatic topical and systemic therapy.

A contact dermatitis occurring after the use of a deodorant was reported by MINKIN et al. (1973), but without suggesting an underlying allergic mechanism for the observed symptoms. All three cases reported were severe enough to require systemic administration of corticosteroids. A further instance of allergic contact dermatitis to vitamin E in an aerosol deodorant has been reported by AELING et al. (1973). The three patients in this instance were also patch tested to DL-α-tocopherol and showed marked positive reactions. Interestingly, one patient developed dermatitis after the first exposure to the aerosol and it is not known how he became sensitized to the molecule. No symptoms were observed after oral ingestion of vitamin E. Sensitization, however, can also be induced by patch testing itself, as reported by ROED-PETERSEN and HJORTH (1975). An interesting case is reported by JAMES (1978). Malignant hyperthermia under general anaesthesia occurred in a 69-year-old patient who had been taking 400 mg α-tocopheryl acetate daily. He showed an increased vitamin E serum level. The high dose had been well tolerated without allergic symptoms and it is difficult to assess whether the vitamin E could have been the cause of the malignant hyperthermia, which might also have been induced by general anesthetics and muscle relaxants used in surgery. Subsequent investigation by muscle biopsy of the three children of the patient demonstrated in two of them a susceptibility to malignant hyperthermia. It, therefore, seems likely that the hyperthermia was due to a genetically determined susceptibility and not to vitamin E (JAMES 1979).

A group of 21 infants weighing less than 1,500 g received 75–150 mg/kg vitamin E and the only related side effect was mild erythema at the injection site (GRAEBER et al. 1977). Vitamin E allergy in creams (SCHORR 1975) and in soaps (FISHER 1975) has been reported but without thorough immunologic analysis. BRIGGS and BRIGGS (1974) point out that little is known of the toxicity of tocopherol oxidation products, which may be present in old vitamin E preparations. These substances can also have a distinct sensitization capacity. A genetically interesting case was reported by KASSEN and MITCHELL (1974) who observed contact urticaria from a vitamin E preparation in two siblings. Patch tests to vitamin E and vehicle, however, have not been carried out in this case. The mother never noticed adverse reactions after application of vitamin E preparations. All authors insist that adverse reactions, including allergic phenomena to tocopherol are extremely rare. Moreover, in no case has a definite involvement of reaginic antibody or cells specific for vitamin E been demonstrated.

O. Vitamin K

I. Physicochemical and Pharmacologic Aspects

The general term vitamin K is now used to describe not a single chemical entity, but a group of quinone compounds which have characteristic antihemorrhagic effects. These compounds are all related to 2-methyl-1,4-naphthoquinone. The most important form of vitamin K which occurs naturally is vitamin K_1 (molecular weight 450.7 daltons). It is soluble only in organic solvents. Many related active substances have been synthesized, some of them being water soluble. Vitamin K_1 is distributed fairly widely in nature, one of the main sources being pig liver. Vitamin K_2 is synthesized by many bacteria including some of the normal intestinal flora. Like all oil-soluble vitamins, vitamin K is absorbed only in association with the dietary fats and requires the presence of bile salts for adequate uptake from the intestinal tract. The vitamin is utilized in the liver but, as only very little is stored, depletion occurs rapidly when absorption is reduced. The involvement of vitamin K in blood homeostasis was already recognized by DAM (1929) and its most important physiologic function is in the production of certain coagulation factors in the blood (BOUVIER and MAURICE 1964). Therefore, the most prevalent drug-equivalent uses of this vitamin are connected with anticoagulation therapy and/or with the treatment of coagulopathies.

II. Allergic Reactions to Vitamin K

Side effects of vitamin K are reported to be rare (HELLRIEGEL and REUTER 1975; REUTER and HELLRIEGEL 1979), examples being cases of Kernicterus in the newborn due to a high dose of vitamin K (20 mg *intramuscularly*) and skin reactions.

These have been described by TEXIER et al. (1974), MAEDA (1969), HEYDENREICH (1977), and BULLEN et al. (1978). Interestingly, an allergic mechanism has not been implicated in those reactions. This probably reflects the more critical assessment of intradermal and patch tests as to the allergic origin of the observed symptoms. BULLEN et al. (1978) emphasize that, especially with substances insoluble in water, the role of the additives has to be considered seriously. Some non-aqueous solvents, including vegetable oils, are known to cause allergic reactions and local tissue reactions (SPIEGEL and NOSEWORTHY 1963). In cases where adverse reactions to vitamin K are reported, intradermal tests are not described very precisely, a common feature being itching, erythema, and induration. In conclusion, according to BULLEN et al. (1978), the pathogenesis of the reactions after vitamin K treatment remains uncertain and it is suggested that large doses are implicated and the reactions are probably not immunologically determined.

Two of the early cases, where an immunologic mechanism has been explicitly suggested, are that of an occupational exposure to vitamin K, as reported by JIRASEK and SCHWANK (1965), and that of allergy after treatment with vitamin K_1 and liver extract by CARTON (1965). In the latter case, a definite participation of vitamin K_1 is difficult to establish because of the use of a multicompound mixture. In the case of the occupational exposure, the authors reported a group sensitization to menadiol (vitamin K_4) and menadion (vitamin K_3), but not to phylloquinone (vitamin K_1). The authors claim that the skin tests were suggestive of toxic–allergic reactions rather than of a pure allergic reaction.

Two cases of allergy to vitamin K_1 were reported by SCHÖPF (1977). They used skin tests for the evaluation of the reactions in their patients who did not have a history of atopy. The authors also tested the response of lymphocyte cultures to vitamin K_1, without being able to demonstrate a stimulation subsequent to phylloquinone addition. They conclude that it is not possible to characterize the underlying immune reaction unequivocally. They were not able to show the presence of specific antibody by immunodiffusion according to the method of Ouchterlony. But this technique is probably too insensitive when searching for specific immunoglobulins in allergy. BARNES and SARKANY (1976), however, were able in one case to demonstrate a vitamin K_1-specific lymphoblastic transformation in culture, whereas this test was negative in the remaining three patients who were positive in intradermal tests with vitamin K_1 preparations.

P. Conclusions

In the present chapter, we have reviewed the literature on allergic and allergoid reactions to vitamins. The majority of reports of such reactions deal with thiamine, whereas no similar reports have been published for vitamin B_2, vitamin B_6, biotin, the vitamin D group, and pantothenic acid. Reactions to the remaining vitamins have been described but, as has been shown, most have to be considered as allergoid manifestations rather than as true allergic reactions. One reason for this apparent low incidence of allergic reactions to vitamins, in addition to the immunologic reasons given in the introduction, might be the type of diagnostic procedures used. We do not wish to recapitulate all the diagnostic procedures applied in the evaluation of drug allergy as this topic has been treated elsewhere in this volume. We shall only comment briefly on the diagnostic value of skin tests (for a comprehensive treatment, see Pepys 1975).

In the investigation of allergic and allergoid reactions to vitamins, classical skin tests (such as the prick, scratch and patch tests) have been by far the most commonly used test techniques. Passive transfer tests (Prausnitz–Küstner test) and radioallergosorbent tests (RAST), however, have only been carried out in a few cases. Only these latter test methods demonstrate the presence of reaginic antibodies unequivocally. Clear-cut evidence for the presence of vitamin-specific antibodies, however, has not been forthcoming in a single instance. This means that, according to the rigid criteria for the classification of allergic reactions to drugs (De Weck 1971), definite proof of an allergic pathogenic mechanism of reactions observed after vitamin use does not exist so far.

Skin tests, together with the case history, remain the only investigational procedures on which the diagnosis of vitamin allergies has normally been based in practice. In this context, the point made by Kleinhans (1979b) has to be emphasized, namely that exanthema caused by a drug is not necessarily due to an allergic reaction, even if it is clinically manifested as an itching urticarial wheal. The same applies to the anaphylactoid reactions. Mast cell degranulation, with its concomitant release of allergic mediators is responsible for urticarial skin eruptions as well as anaphylactic reactions. Degranulation, however, can also be induced by other means than an antigen–antibody reaction. In a way similar to mast cell degranulation, mediators can also be liberated from blood basophils.

The complement system can also be activated without a preceding immune reaction, and activated complement components (C3a, C5a) can induce histamine liberation and allergoid reactions. Accordingly, the clinical pictures described as allergic reactions to vitamins, and especially the anaphylactoid reactions after administration of vitamin B_1, should be attributed to an allergoid reaction until the presence of vitamin-specific antibodies has been unequivocally demonstrated. There have been no detailed investigations, so far, of the direct mast cell degranulating ability of vitamins. Therefore, it is not yet possible to come to any definite conclusion on this point. Reactions can also be caused by the vehicles used as well as by possible decomposition products.

We wish to stress the difficulty of reaching an objective allergic diagnosis for immediate hypersensitivity based exclusively on skin tests. In cases of contact dermatitis, however, patch tests performed with proper controls in a normal population, in order to avoid toxic concentrations, are usually considered reliable. Considering the widespread use of vitamins in nutrition as well as in therapy, reports of allergic of allergoid reactions are comparatively rare. We conclude that, from the viewpoint of allergic reactions, the vitamins are safe nutrients as well as safe drug-equivalent compounds.

References

Acharya V, Store SD, Golwalla AF (1969) Anaphylaxis following ingestion of aneurine hydrochloride. J Indian Med Assoc 52:84–85

Aeling JL, Panagotacos PJ, Andreozzi RJ (1973) Allergic contact dermatitis to vitamin E aerosol deodorant. Arch Dermatol 108:579–580

Alexander HL (1955) Reactions with drug therapy. Saunders, Philadelphia London

Auzepy P, Veissieres J-F, Deparis M (1974) Choc anaphylactique dû à l'hydroxocobalamine. Nouv Presse Med 3:152

Barazzone V, Lambelet F (1954) Accidents mortels après injection de thiamine. Nouv Presse Med 62:1867–1868

Barnes HM, Sarkany I (1976) Adverse skin reaction from vitamin K_1. Br J Dermatol 95:653–656

Bedford PD (1952) Side effects of a preparation of vitamin B_{12}. Br Med J 1:690–692

Bekier E, Maslinski C (1974) Antihistaminic action of nicotinamide. Agents Actions 4/3:196

Bianco S, Robuschi M, Grugni A, Allegra L (1977) Prevention of prostaglandin F 2 α induced broncho constriction by ascorbic-acid in asthmatic patients. Int Res Commun Syst 5:33

Bleumink E (1979) Food allergy and the gastrointestinal tract. In: Immunology of the gastrointestinal tract. Asquith & Gell, Edinburgh London New York

Blum KU, Kasemir H, Scharfe W (1974) Untersuchungen zur Pathogenese der anaphylaktischen Reaktionen nach Thiamin-Applikation. Verh Dtsch Ges Inn Med 80:1569

Bonjour JP (1980) Vitamins and alcoholism, II. Folate and vitamin B_{12}. Int J Vitam Nutr Res 50:96–121

Bonnet J, Florens A (1969) Le bépanthêne et la biotine dans quelques indications de la pratique dermatologique courante. Gaz Med Fr 76:1201–1203

Bouvier CA, Maurice PA (1964) Liver and blood coagulation. In: The liver, vol II. Academic Press, New York London

Briggs M, Briggs M (1974) Are vitamine E supplements beneficial? Med J Aust 1:434–437

Brodkin RH, Bleiberg H (1965) Sensitivity to topically applied vitamin E. Arch Dermatol 92:76–77

Brodulin YD (1961) Anaphylactic shock as a complication of vitamin B_{12}. Klin Med 8:139–141

Bullen AW, Miller JP, Cunliffe WJ, Losowsky MS (1978) Skin reactions caused by vitamin K in patients with liver disease. Br J Dermatol 98:561–565

Burnet FM (1959) The clonal selection theory of acquired immunity. Cambridge University Press, Cambridge

Carton MFX (1965) Réaction allergique au cours d'un traitement: vitamine K_1 + extrait de foi. Bull Soc Fr Dermatol Syphilol 72:228

Chanarin I, Fenton JCB, Mollin DL (1957) Sensitivity to folic acid. Br Med J 1:1162–1163

Chatterjee IB (1973) Evolution and the biosynthesis of ascorbic acid. Science 182:1271–1272

Chick H (1975) The discovery of vitamins. Prog Food Nutr Sci 1:1–20

Conrad DH, Wirtz GH (1973) Characterization of antibodies to vitamin A. Immunochemistry 10:273–275

Cooper JR, Pincus JH (1979) The role of thiamine in nervous tissue. Neurochem Res 4:223–239

Cope EP (1942) Contact dermatitis due to cod liver oil. Arch Dermatol Syphilol 42:140–141

Currier WD (1970) Nonimmunologic factors in allergy. Part 2. Nutrition. Trans Am Soc Ophthalmol Otolaryngol Allergy 11:78–89

Dalderup CBM (1968) Vitamins. In: Side effects of drugs, 6. Excerpta Medica, Amsterdam London New York, pp 573–582

Dalderup CBM (1972) Vitamins. In: Side effects of drugs, 7. Excerpta Medica, Amsterdam London New York, pp 507–515

Dally S, Gaultier M (1976) Choc anaphylactique dû à l'hydroxocobalamine. Nouv Presse Med 5:1917

Dam H (1929) Cholesterinstoffwechsel im Hühnerei und Hühnchen. Biochem Z 215:475–492

Danilov LN (1973) Anaphylactic shock during vitamin B_6 treatment. Klin Med 51:139

Dawson W, West GB (1965) The importance of bradykinin in anaphylactic shock. J Pharm Pharmacol 17:246–277

De Luca LM, Glover J, Heller J, Olson JA, Underwood B (1979) Recent advances in the metabolism and function of vitamin A and their relationship to applied nutrition. In: A report of the international vitamin A consultative group (IVACg) Nutrition Found Inc, New York

de Weck AL (1971) Drug reactions. In: Immunological diseases. Little Brown, Boston

Di Palma JR, Ritchie DM (1977) Vitamin toxicity. Annu Rev Pharmacol Toxicol 17:133–148

Dresser DW (1968) Adjuvanticity of vitamin A. Nature 217:527–529

Engelhardt HT, Baird VC (1949) Sensitivity to thiamine hydrochloride. Ann Allergy 4:291–292

Evans WC (1975) Thiaminases and their effects on animals. Vitam Horm 33:467–504

Faivre M, Saif N, Barral C (1975) Accidents de la vitamine B_{12}. Lyon Med 233:897–993

Feinberg SM (1948) Anaphylactic shock due to nicotinic acid. NY State J Med 48:635

Fisher AA (1975) Contact dermatitis in surgeons. J Dermatol Surg 1:63–67

Fishman L, Goldstein M (1968) Vitamins in dermatology. J Med Assoc Ga 57:342–346

Folkers K (1969) Survey on the vitamin aspects of coenzyme Q. Int J Vitam Nutr Res 39:334–352

Fuchs E (1979) Klinische Diagnostik der Allergosen. Prax Pneumol 33:268–276

Gillhespy RO (1955) Reaction to vitamin B_{12}. Lancet 1:1076

Goodman DeW S (1974) Vitamin A transport and retinol-binding-protein metabolism. Vitam Horm 32:167–180

Gordon ES (1947) Nutrition and vitamin therapy in general practice. Year Book Publishers, Chicago

Graeber JE, Williams ML, Oski FA (1977) The use of intramuscular vitamin E in the premature infant. J Pediatr 90:282–283

Graham JDP (1979) An introduction to human pharmacology. Oxford University Press, Oxford New York Toronto

Greenbaum J (1979) Vitamin A sensitivity. Ann Allergy 43:93–99

Greengard P (1970) Water soluble vitamins. I. The vitamin B complex. In: The pharmacological basis of therapeutics, 4th edn. Collier Macmillan, London Toronto

Groff JP, Blakley RL (1978) Rescue of human lymphoid cells from the effects of methotrexate in vitro. Cancer Res 38:3847–3853

Gyoergy P, Langer BW (1968) Biotin. XII. Pharmacology. In: The vitamins, 2nd edn., Academic Press, New York London

Heel RC, Brodgen RN, Speight TM, Avery GS (1977) Vitamin A acid: a review of its pharmacological properties and therapeutic use in the topical treatment of acne vulgaris. Drugs 14:401–419

Hellriegel KP, Reuter H (1975) Side effects of vitamins. In: Meyler's side effects of drugs, 8. Excerpta Medica, Amsterdam London New York, pp 799–811

Hellriegel KP, Reuter H (1978) Vitamins. In: Side effects of drugs, annual 2. Excerpta Medica, Amsterdam London New York, pp 305–309

Heydenreich G (1977) A further case of adverse skin reaction from vitamin K_1. Br J Dermatol 97:697

Hitchcock M (1975) Stimulation of immunologic histamine (H) release and production of prostaglandin $F_2 \alpha$ ($PGF_2 \alpha$) by ascorbic acid. Fed Proc 34:798

Hoigné R, Naegeli H (1957) Schockzustände bei Sensibilisierung auf Arzneimittel. Helv Med Acta 24:27–38

Horwitt MK (1972) Vitamin B_2: pharmacology and toxicology. Vitamins 5:85–87

Hovding G (1968) Anaphylactic reaction after injection of vitamin B_{12}. Br Med J 610:102

James J, Warin RP (1971) Sensitivity to cyanocobalamin and hydroxocobalamin. Br Med J 5756:262

James P (1978) Vitamin E and malignant hyperthemia. Br Med J 1:1345

James P (1979) Vitamin E and malignant hyperthermia. Br Med J 1:200

Jirasek L, Schwank R (1965) Berufskontaktekzem durch Vitamin K. Hautarzt 18:353–355

Jordan WP, Higgins M, Dvorak J (1975) Allergic contact dermatitis to all-trans-retinoic acid; epicutaneous and leukocyte migration inhibition testing. Contact Dermatitis 1:306–310

Kadlec K, Hanslian L (1965) Gruppenallergie gegen Pyridinderivate. Hautkrankheiten 13:283–288

Kaidbey KH, Kligman AM, Yoshida H (1975) Effects of intensive application of retinoic acid on human skin. Br J Dermatol 92:693–701

Kalz F (1942) Thiamine hydrochloride – an obligate wheal producing agent. J Invest Dermatol 5:135–137

Kassen B, Mitchell JC (1974) Contact urticaria from a vitamin E preparation in two siblings. Contact Dermatitis Newslett 16:482

Kleinhans D (1979a) Die Bedeutung des Radio-Allergo-Sorbens-Tests (RAST) in der Allergiediagnostik. Therapiewoche 29:3608–3622

Kleinhans D (1979b) Anaphylactoide Arzneimittelreaktionen. Therapiewoche 29:5492–5494

Koda A, Shimazawa T, Watanabe S, Yanagihara A (1972) Anti-allergic effect of nicotinic acid derivatives and related compounds of Mephenesin. Jpn J Pharmacol 22:111

Körner WF, Völlm J (1976) In: Klinische Pharmakologie und Pharmakotherapie. Urban & Schwarzenberg, Munich Berlin Vienna

Kordansky DW, Rosenthal RR, Norman PS (1979) The effect of vitamin C on antigen-induced bronchospasm. J Allergy Clin Immunol 63:61–64

Krueger GG, Molk L, Kahn G (1972) Exacerbation of atopic dermatitis. Arch Dermatol 105:405–406

Lagerholm B, Lodin A, Gentele H (1958) Hypersensitivity to phenylcarbinol preservative in vitamin B_{12} for injection. Acta Allergol 12:295–296

Landsteiner K (1945) In: The specificity of serological reactions. Harvard University Press, Cambridge

Laws CL (1941) Sensitization to thiamine hydrochloride. JAMA 117:176

Levander-Lindgren M (1957) Hypersensitivity to folic acid in a case of erythroblastomatosis. Acta Med Scand 157:233–234

Lind J (1953) In: A treatise of the scurvy. Millow, London

Lindgren S, Groth O, Molin L (1976) Allergic contact response to vitamin A acid. Contact Dermatitis 2:212–217

Maeda M (1969) Vitamin K_1-eruption followed by eczematous dissemination. Jpn J Dermatol 79:313

Malten KE (1975) Flare reaction due to vitamin B_{12} in a patient with psoriasis and contact eczema. Contact Dermatitis 1(5):325–326

Mathur BP (1966) Sensitivity of folic acid: a case report. Indian J Med Sci 20(2):133–134

Meuwissen JHJM (1978) Allergische reacties veroorzaakt door vitamine B_{12}. Ned Tijdschr Geneeskd 122:685

Meyler L (1952) Side effects of drugs. Elsevier, Amsterdam Houston London New York

Meyler L (1957) Side effects of drugs, 1. Excerpta Medica, Amsterdam London New York, pp 102–106

Meyler L (1958) Side effects of drugs, 2. Excerpta Medica, Amsterdam London New York, pp 151–154

Meyler L (1960) Side effects of drugs, 3. Excerpta Medica, Amsterdam London New York, pp 189–193

Meyler L (1963) Side effects of drugs, 4. Excerpta Medica, Amsterdam London New York, pp 299–305

Meyler L (1966) Side effects of drugs, 5. Excerpta Medica, Amsterdam London New York, pp 393–397

Mills CA (1941) Discussion on vitamin therapy. JAMA 117:1500–1502

Minkin W, Cohen HJ, Frank SB (1973) Contact dermatitis from deodorants. Arch Dermatol 107:774–775

Mitchell DC, Vilter RW, Vilter CF (1949) Hypersensitivity to folic acid. Ann Intern Med 31:1102–1105

Mitrani MM (1944) Vitamin B_1 hypersensitivity with desensitization. J Allergy 15:150–153

Murthy PNA, Mistry SP (1977) Biotin. Prog Fed Nutr Sci 2:405–455

Nater JP (1975) Drugs used on the skin. In: Meyler's side effects of drugs, 8. Excerpta Medica, Amsterdam London New York, pp 331–405

Nater JP (1977) Drugs used on the skin. In: Side effects of drugs, annual 1. Excerpta Medica, Amsterdam London New York, pp 124–139

Nater JP (1978) Drugs used on the skin. In: Side effects of drugs, annual 2. Excerpta Medica, Amsterdam London New York, pp 130–143

National Academy of Sciences (1980) Recommended dietary allowances, ninth revised edition. National Academy of Sciences, Washington, DC

Nava C (1971) Allergic reaction to vitamin B_{12}. Med Lav 62:285–291

Neal RA, Sauberlich HE (1973) Thiamin. In: Modern nutrition in health and disease, 5th edn, Lea & Febiger, Philadelphia

Olson JA (1967) The metabolism of vitamin A. Pharmacol Rev 19:559–596

Opree W (1979) Pathogenese atopischer Erkrankungen aus immunologischer Sicht. Verlag Chemie, Weinheim New York

Panzani MR (1961) Un cas d'asthma par sensibilisation à l'acide L-ascorbique. Nouv Presse Med 69:1928

Parrot J-L, Wyczolkowska A, Santais MC, Ruff F (1974) The action of nicotinamide on the release of histamine. Agents Actions 4:202

Pauling L (1968) Orthomolecular somatic and psychiatric medicine. J Vital Subst Dis Civiliz 14:1

Pauling L (1974) Early evidence about vitamin C and the common cold. J Orthomol Psychiatry 3:139

Pedersen JT (1966) Allergiske reaktioner efter vitamindgift (en oversigt og et tilfaelde). Ugeskr Laeger 128:708–709

Pelner L (1947) Anaphylaxis to the injection of nicotinic acid (niacin), successful treatment with epinephrine. Ann Intern Med 26:290–304

Pepys J (1975) Skin tests in diagnosis. In: Clinical aspects of immunology, 3rd edn. Blackwell, Oxford

Pevny I, Hartmann A, Metz I (1977) Vitamin B_{12} (Cyanocobalamin) Allergie. Hautarzt 28:600–603

Pollitt NT (1968) Large intravenous dosage of thiamine. JAMA 203:175

Powers BR (1948) Circulatory collapse following intravenous administration of nicotinic acid. Ann Intern Med 29:558–560

Prish WE, Hughes EG (1979) Specific IgE antibodies to platinum salts in sensitized workers. Clin Allergy 9:109–117

Rachmilewitz M, Glueck HI (1938) Treatment of pellagra with nicotinic acid. Br Med J 2:346–348

Rand S, Collin WS, Fireman P (1979) IgE and IgG antibodies in allergic children immunized with alum or fluid diphtheria and tetanus toxoid. J Allergy Clin Immunol 63:147

Randazzo SD, Giardina A, Cavallaro A (1972) Dermatosi iatrogene da vitamine. G Ital Dermatol 47:350–354

Rausch F (1956) Anaphylaktischer Schock nach Folsäure. Ther Ggw 95:53–55

Reuter H, Hellriegel KP (1977) Vitamins. In: Side effects of drugs, annual 1. Excerpta Medica, Amsterdam London New York, pp 274–280

Reuter HD, Hellriegel KP (1979) Vitamins. In: Side effects of drugs, annual 3. Excerpta Medica, Amsterdam London New York, pp 298–309

Ring J (1978) RIST, PRIST, RAST und so weiter. Dtsch Med Wochenschr 103:365–368

Roe DA (1976) Drug-induced nutritional deficiencies. AVI, Westport, Conn

Roed-Petersen J, Hjorth N (1975) Patch test sensitization from D,L-alpha-tocopherol (vitamin E). Contact Dermatitis 1:391–393

Rosenblatt DS (1978) Folinic acid inhibits the accumulation of methotrexate polyglutamates by cultured human cells. Clin Res 26:875A

Rust S (1954) Über allergische Reaktionen bei Vitamintherapie. Z Hautkr 17:317–319

Saif N, Faivre M, Barral C, Lery N (1975) Chocs après la vitamine B_{12}. Bull Med Leg Toxicol Med 18:65–67

Schiff L (1941) Collapse following parenteral administration of solution of thiamine hydrochloride. JAMA 117:609

Schoepf H (1977) Allergie gegen Vitamin K_1. Z Hautkr 52:703–705

Schorr WF (1975) Allergic skin disease caused by cosmetics. Am Fam Physician 12:90–95

Schroeder H, Belin L, Lanner A (1979) Comparison between skin prick test, RAST-based methods, and rocket electrophonesis for assay of allergen extract potency. J Allergy Clin Immunol 63:194

Semenovich NI, Samoilova LN, Kakoeva LD (1976) Blastic lymphocyte transformation test for drug allergy. Ter Arkh 48:103–108

Seusing J (1951) Allergisches Verhalten gegen Vitamin B$_1$ (Aneurin, Thiamin). Klin Wochenschr 29:394

Shapero W, Gwinner MW (1947) Sensitivity to thiamine hydrochloride. Ann Allergy 5:349–352

Sharma SC, Wilson CWM (1977) The relationship of L-ascorbic acid to the antigen-antibody reaction. Ir J Med Sci 146:310

Sharma SC, Garg SK, Wilson CWM (1976) The effect of L-ascorbic-acid on the in-vitro production of prostaglandin E and prostaglandin F by the guinea-pig lung. Int Res Commun Syst 4:573

Soloshenko EN, Brailovskii AY, Bazarnova MA (1971) Tests of lympho blastic transformation in drug allergy. Klin Med 49:131–135

Spiegel AJ, Noseworthy MM (1963) Use of non-aqueous solvents in parenteral products. J Pharm Sci 52:917–927

Spitznagel JD, Allison AC (1970) Mode of action of adjuvants: Retinol and other lysosomelabilizing agents as adjuvants. J Immunol 1:128 139

Stiles MH (1941) Hypersensitivity to thiamine chloride with a note on sensitivity to pyridoxine. J Allergy 12:507–509

Temime P, Castelain PY (1960) Accident anaphylactique après la vitamine B$_1$ avec oedème de Quincke. Nouv Presse Med 68:2058

Tetreault AF, Beck IA (1956) Anaphylactic shock following intramuscular thiamine chloride. Ann Intern Med 45:134–138

Texier L, Gauthier Y, Gauthier O (1974) Sclérodermies lombofessières consécutives à des injections intramusculaires de la vitamine K$_1$. Bordeaux Med 7:1571–1583

Thomas WR, Holt PG (1978) Vitamin C and immunity: an assessment of the evidence. Clin Exp Immunol 32:370–379

Trousseau A (1861) Clin Med Hôtel-Dieu Paris. Baillière, Paris

Ungley CC (1955) The chemotherapeutic action of vitamin B$_{12}$. Vitam Horm 13:137–211

Unna KR (1972) Thiamine, pharmacology and toxicology. The vitamins, chemistry, physiology, phathology, methods 5, 2nd edn. academic Press, New York London, pp 150–155

Unna K, Greslin JG (1942) Studies on the toxicity and pharmacology of riboflavin. J Pharmacol Exp Ther 76:75–80

Vassal P (1975) A propos de trois allergies respiratoires et cutanées à l'acide ascorbique. Rev Fr Allergol 16:103

Vukusic Z, Pavlovic S, Stojanovic D, Draskovic S (1970) The effect of vitamin C on the course of sensitization and on the intensity of anaphylactic reaction. Jugosl Physiol Pharmacol Acta 6:431–436

Watrous RM (1939) Dermatitis from industrial contact with nicotinic acid (B$_3$). JAMA 112:2132

Widenbauer F (1936a) Ascorbinsäurestudien an Säuglingen. Klin Wochenschr 15:815–817

Widenbauer F (1936b) Toxische Nebenwirkungen von Ascorbinsäure. C-Hypervitaminose? Klin Wochenschr 15:1158–1159

Wilson CWM (1974) The relationship between allergic symptoms and vitamin C. Clin Allergy 4:221–223

Wilson CWM (1976a) The role of ascorbic acid in allergic reaction. Proc Nutr Soc 35:121 A

Wilson CWM (1976b) The relationship of the leucocyte ascorbic acid direct antigen challenge test (LAADACT) to the clinical manifestations of allergic sensitivity. Clin Allergy 6:414–415

Wilson CWM (1976c) The role of ascorbic acid in drug sensitivity. Br J Clin Pharmacol 3:963P

Wilson CWM, Loh HS, Watters K (1975) Vitamin C metabolism and atopic allergy. Clin Allergy 5:317–324

Woodliff HJ, Davis RE (1966) Allergy to folic acid. Med J Aust 1:351–352

Wright LD (1956) The metabolism of biotin. Symposium on vitamin metabolism. National Vitamin Foundation, New York, Nutrition Symposium Series

Young WC, Ulrich CW, Fouts PJ (1950) Sensitivity to vitamin B_{12} concentrate. JAMA 143:893–894

Zheltakov MM, Skripkin IK, Somov BA, Butov IS (1969) Allergic reactions due to group B vitamins. Vestn Dermatol Venerol 43:62–65

Zuskin E, Lewis AJ, Bouhuys A (1973) Inhibition of histamine-induced airway constriction by ascorbic acid. J Allergy Clin Immunol 51:218–226

CHAPTER 24

Corticotrophins and Corticosteroids

J. CHARPIN, A. ARNAUD, and J. AUBERT

A. Frequency of Accidents due to Corticotrophins

ACTH (adrenocorticotrophic hormone, corticotrophin) was introduced in the treatment of allergic conditions in 1949. From 1949 to 1961, the use of natural, unpurified ACTH caused many allergic accidents; the frequency was estimated differently:

 4 Cases of sensitization in 19 patients (TRAEGER 1950)
 6 Cases in 113 (STEVENSON 1951)
 7 Cases in 208 (BROWN and HOLLANDER 1951)
 1 Case in 38 (ARBESMANN et al. 1952)
 3 Cases in 35 (BRODEWALL 1954)
10 Cases in 106 (ARNOLDSON 1955)

This frequency was higher when the patients were atopic and still higher when they had received long-term steroid therapy. In one of our groups of patients (CHARPIN et al. 1961, 1964; CHARPIN and AUBERT 1971), of 113 patients undergoing long-term steroid therapy, and receiving one intramuscular injection of impure depot ACTH monthly, we observed 43 allergic accidents (38%). WOLFROMM and HERMAN (1967) observed 7 accidents in a group of 19 asthmatics treated with steroids for more than 6 months and then deprived of the drug.

The incidents or accidents ranged from an itching eruption, localized at the needle puncture, to severe shocks with general malaise, dyspnea, and abdominal pains. Lethal accidents were reported by HILL and SWINBURN (1954), VAN UFFORD (1952), WILSON (1951), HALPERN et al. (1961). Escalation often occurred in these accidents, for instance, one injection gave a generalized pruritus or an urticaria, the second injection, performed without taking this alarm signal into account, produced a severe accident.

The mechanism of these accidents was studied by us (CHARPIN et al. 1964) and by many others. The solvents used and the animal species from which the extract comes, play no role. The impurities not entirely eliminated during the extraction, constituting up to 95% of the drug (DUCHAINE et al. 1962), played a dominant role. RAJKA (1961) separated by electrophoresis, two fractions, one fairly pure, the other rich in impurities. The latter regularly elicited positive reactions in patients allergic to ACTH. We will see, further on, that the results obtained with highly purified ACTH extracts confirmed these results.

Actually, all of this work is part of the history of the problem. In the last ten years a new series of facts have appeared:

1. Preparation of a corticotrophin, highly purified and less allergenic

2. Synthesis in 1961 by SCHWYZER and KAPPELER (SCHWYZER 1964) of a chain
   formed by the first 24 amino acids. BELL, as early as 1956, showed that it was
   common to all animal species
3. Synthesis in 1963 by SCHWYZER and SIEBER of the complete chain of 39 amino
   acids with molecular weight 4,567 daltons
4. Synthesis of a chain of 25 amino acids, slightly modified: the pentacosapeptide,
   which was never made available commercially.

With highly purified forms of natural ACTH accidents were less frequent than
with the older extracts.

In a group of 38 patients presenting definite accidents of sensitization to the
older extracts, and still reacting positively to tests (it is necessary in fact, to remember the instability of some ACTH allergies) 14 tests were negative; 24 tests were
positive with a dilution of 1:100 of this naturally extracted hormone. In a series
of 168 asthmatics where 1,267 injections of purified ACTH were given, only 6 presented definite allergic reactions (2 of these 6 patients formerly were allergic to impure ACTH). PANZANI (1966) reported comparable results. However, since then,
we have observed a lethal allergic reaction in a 71-year-old man, provoked by perfusion of purified natural ACTH. However, these accidents now belong to the history of allergy to corticotrophin, as these purified extracts have been replaced by
synthetic molecules.

The study of synthetic chains and of the frequency of the accidents they may
produce can be approached in different ways: by considering subjects known to be
allergic to natural ACTH, by controlling that they are still reacting positively to
natural ACTH, and by giving them intradermal tests with synthetic materials
(CHARPIN and AUBERT 1969, 1971; CHARPIN et al. 1967, 1973). Of 58 patients
known to be allergic to ACTH (of which 38 still react positively to this extracted
hormone) 48 showed totally negative tests, 9 had one positive test to a 1:10, and
1 patient a positive test to a 1:100 dilution of synthetic ACTH.

Known allergic subjects can also be treated with these synthetic molecules. Of
our 58 allergic patients, 44 were treated carefully with ordinary tetracosapeptide
(0.125 mg the first day, 0.125 mg the second and third days, then 1 mg a day, intramuscularly or by perfusion). The total dose received was variable, 0.125–45 mg.
The tolerance was excellent, 39-fold. The treatment was stopped four times because
of incidents.

Finally in our initial trial of Synacthen, 107 asthmatics nonallergic to ACTH,
received β-1,24-corticotrophin, for 21 patients in its ordinary form, and for 86 in
depot form. A total of 10 incidents were observed, 7 difficult to interpret, while 3
were likely to be allergic accidents. The new synthetic β-1,24-corticotrophin causes
a very low number of allergic incidents. However, we have to keep in mind the
possibility of these incidents and one should ask every patient "have you had any
incident before, from Synacthen", especially if intravenous infusion of β-1,24-cor-
ticotrophin is planned.

B. Clinical Aspects of Allergic Reactions to ACTH

In this section, we shall no longer consider accidents due to the old form of ACTH,
but deal only with accidents due to the new, synthetic forms. We shall give three
clinical examples of allergic accidents certainly due to synthetic corticotrophin.

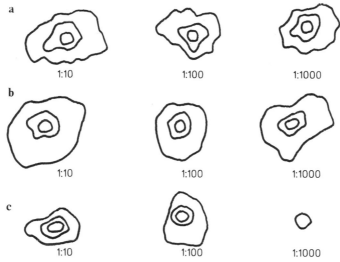

Fig. 1. Skin reactions to (**a**) purified natural ACTH, (**b**) tetracosapeptide, and (**c**) pentacosapeptide in an allergic patient. The numbers below the diagrams indicate the dilutions

Case 1. A 56-year-old woman, suffering from asthma with permanent dyspnea and undergoing long-term steroid therapy received a monthly injection of 1 mg depot tetracosapeptide. On 8 November 1968, she had her ninth injection without incident. On 8 December 1968, 15 min after the tenth injection, cutaneous pruritus, generalized eruption, and dyspnea developed. The patient did not inform us of the incident and on 8 January 1969, she had the eleventh injection, resulting in eruption and immediate acute dyspnea. In 48 h, she improved and was cured within 12 days. On 13 March 1969, skin tests were positive (Fig. 1) with 1 : 100 and 1 : 1,000 dilutions of tetracosapeptide. She was hospitalized again on 10 December 1969 for an acute attack of asthma. For 14 days she received DW 75 pentacosapeptide, first at very small doses (25 IU) then for the last six injections 200 IU daily, without any incident.

Case 2. A 53-year-old woman undergoing long-term steroid therapy for asthma with permanent dyspnea, received, from 15 September 1967 until January 1969, 16 monthly 1 mg tetracosapeptide injections. Then she had an injection every two weeks. The 21st injection on 10 March 1969, was followed by lumbar pains and vomiting but no eruption. On 24 March 1969, 0.25 mg depot tetracosapeptide was injected; the same phenomena followed the next day with Quincke's edema and generalized urticaria. Tests were positive to 1 : 100 dilution of tetracosapeptide.

Case 3. A 58-year-old woman undergoing long-term steroid therapy for severe asthma with permanent dyspnea had never received ACTH before hospitalization because of an asthma attack on 24 June 1970. On 3 July 1970, at the very beginning of the perfusion, she had heat sensations then general pruritus, finally eruption on the superior members with very marked oppression. Perfusion was stopped. On 4 July 1970, she was still taking steroids; skin test reactions were negative to DW 75, positive to 1 : 10 dilution of tetracosapeptide, and negative at 1 : 100. She received 25, then 100 IU pentacosapeptide without any incident.

We see in these three cases some of the usual characteristics of these accidents. The most frequent incidents appear on the skin:
1. Pruritus around the site of intramuscular injection
2. Generalized pruritus with or without erythema
3. Typical urticaria with or without angioedema.

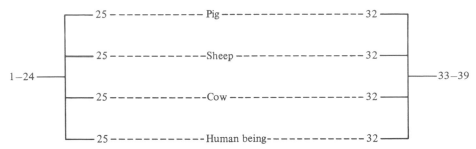

Fig. 2. Schematic structure of ACTH showing the constant portions of the sequence (1–24 and 33–39) and the variation of the central portion (25–32) from species to species

Ser	Tyr	Ser	Met	Glu	His	Phe	Arg
1	2	3	4	5	6	7	8

Try	Gly	Lys	Pro	Val	Gly	Lys	Lys
9	10	11	12	13	14	15	16

Arg	Arg	Pro	Val	Lys	Val	Tyr	Pro
17	18	19	20	21	22	23	24

Fig. 3. The 1–24 sequence in ACTH

Typical asthma is frequently observed. It appeared twice in our three cases, twice in two patients of GRILLIAT et al. (1973), seven times out of the eleven cases reported by BENOS et al. (1973). Sometimes, a real shock occurs, mainly after intravenous infusion and the patient may die (UZZAN, personal communication; MOHR 1975; PORTER and JICK 1977; DURIGON et al. 1978). But usually, this is not the first accident observed, it comes after a pruritus or an urticaria which the patient has neglected to mention.

C. Etiology and Physiopathology of Accidents

As we have shown, the incidents with natural ACTH were mainly due to impurities, and highly purified natural extracts are less dangerous. As for synthetic ACTH, let us first recall the structure of the ACTH chain (Fig. 2). Chain 1–24 is common to the different species (Fig. 3); chain 25–32 (Fig. 4) is variable; chain 33–39 (Fig. 5) is common to the different species. As for the pentacosapeptide (Fig. 6) we see that the amino acids 1 and 4 have been changed and that in position 25 a valinamide has been added, but, as already indicated, this excellent synthetic ACTH was never made available commercially.

What is the possible antigenicity of this ACTH molecule and its different portions? We need to, on one hand, recall the work of researchers who have used dif-

Pig	Asp	Gly	Ala	Glu	Asp	Gluta	Leu	Ala
Sheep	Ala	Gly	Gly	Asp	Asp	Glu	Ala	Ser
Cow	Asp	Gly	Glu	Ala	Glu	Asp	Ser	Ala
Human being	Ala	Ala	Gly	Glu	Asp	Gluta	Ser	Ala
	25	26	27	28	29	30	31	32

Fig. 4. The 25–32 sequences in porcine, ovine, bovine, and human ACTH

Glu	Ala	Phe	Pro	Leu	Glu	Phe
33	34	35	36	37	38	39

Fig. 5. The 33–39 sequence in ACTH

D–Ser			Nor						
~~L–Ser~~	Tyr	Ser	~~Met~~	Glu	His	Phe	Arg	Try	Gly
1	2	3	4	5	6	7	8	9	10
Lys	Pro	Val	Gly	Lys	Lys	Arg	Arg	Pro	Val
11	12	13	14	15	16	17	18	19	20
				Val					
Lys	Val	Tyr	Pro	~~Asp~~					
21	22	23	24	25					

Fig. 6. The sequence in pentacosapeptide showing how this differs from the 1–25 sequence in ACTH

ferent segments of the ACTH chain as antigens, and on the other hand, recall what we may learn of the pathogenic aspects from the clinical observations. We must keep in mind that these two ways of approaching the problem are not necessarily compatible. The fact that one or another fragment of the ACTH chain is experimentally antigenic and gives rise to anti-ACTH antibodies does not necessarily imply that in humans this fragment gives rise to an immediate reaginic allergy.

FELBER et al. (1966) showed that β-1,39-corticotrophin is as antigenic as the purified ACTH extract. The β-1,24 fragment is hardly antigenic but can compete

Table 1. Biologic activity concentrated in the first part, 1–24, of the ACTH molecule, the last part, 22–39 having immunogenic properties and no hormonal activity. (Imura et al. 1965, 1967)

	Biologic activity	Immunologic activity
Natural ACTH		
Ovine	+ +	+ +
Human	+ +	+ +
Porcine	+ +	+ +
Fraction 22–39	0	+ +
Synthetic ACTH[a]		
Fractions 1–17	0	0
1–19	+ +	0
1–24	+ +	+
1–26	+ +	+
1–39	+ +	+ +

[a] Porcine type

with the entire molecule in fixing anti-ACTH antibodies; this is something which the isolated sequences 1–10 and 11–24 cannot do.

Imura et al. (1965, 1967) studied the biologic action and the immunologic activity of three natural corticotrophins (ovine, human, and porcine) and of six synthetic chains with 17, 19, 24, 26 (human type) and 39 (porcine type) amino acids, and of a sequence 23–39 (ovine type) as shown in Table 1. The biologic activity of the ACTH extract is equivalent to the synthetic chains with 24, 26, and 39 amino acids. It is decreased by half for the chain with 19. There is no activity for the chain with 17 and for the sequence 22–39 (ovine). As for the immunologic activity, it is identical for the synthetic chain with 39 amino acids and the ACTH extracts, weak for the chains with 26 and 24 amino acids, absent for the chains with 19 and 17 amino acids, but strong for the fragment 22–39.

Gelzer (1968) observed, in one rabbit of four, the formation of complement-fixing antibodies by injecting with an adjuvant β-1,24-corticotrophin linked to rabbit albumin serum. If this linkage with rabbit albumin serum is not achieved, there is no appearance of antibodies. It is the terminal part of the section 17–24 which appears to be antigenic. Finally, Salvin and Liauw (1967) showed that delayed sensitivity can be induced by the molecule with 39 as well as the molecule with 24 amino acids. When fragmenting the latter, it appears that only the segment 11–24 is antigenic, particularly its extremity 17–24. From these experimental studies, principally concerned with anti-ACTH antibodies, we can remember that the antigenicity of the ACTH molecule is due to the 17 terminal amino acids 22–39.

In the clinical field, we have seen:

1. that patients allergic to old, natural ACTH rarely had significant reactions to skin tests performed with a 1:100 dilution of β-1,24-corticotrophin. This happened once in a series of 58 patients allergic to old ACTH

2. that a great majority (40 of 44 in one study) of patients allergic to natural ACTH tolerate synthetic ACTH perfectly well
3. that asthmatic patients treated with synthetic ACTH sometimes, experience incidents which may evoke an allergic phenomenon. The nature of the incidents has to be interpreted carefully.

Synthetic β-1,24-corticotrophin is well known as a histamine liberator for mast cells. As early as 1969, JAQUES and BRUGGER had thoroughly studied the malaise often accompanied by a kind of flush, which can appear in humans after an injection of some polypeptide chains, particularly corticotrophin, and which may be due to histamine release. However, in some clinical cases, the fact that several injections are well tolerated and that the severity of incidents increases gradually is a good argument for an allergic mechanism. The findings of GIRARD et al. (1973) were about the same as ours (CHARPIN et al. 1974). We tried to appreciate the nature and the significance of antibodies present in the sera of 44 patients who had received a long course of treatment with synthetic β-1,24-corticotrophin. The level of plasma antibodies directed against this molecule was measured by radioimmunoassay. Such antibodies were present in 10 patients. There does not seem to be any correlation between the antibodies which belong to the IgG class and allergic sensitization to synthetic β-1,24-corticotrophin. These antibodies do not neutralize the corticotropic effect of synthetic β-1,24-corticotrophin and our results are identical on this point to those of LANDON et al. (1965). Among these 44 patients there were 10 who were allergic to β-1,24-corticotrophin. We could not study in this group the eventual presence of antibodies belonging to IgE class.

As for the synthetic β-1,39-corticotrophin, we injected this synthetic hormone into ten patients allergic to natural ACTH and found no positive skin test. We treated one of these patients with the entire synthetic molecule without any incident. This fits well with the idea that the numerous accidents formerly obtained with extracted ACTH were due to impurities and not to the hormone itself. The synthesis of the complete chain of 39 amino acids by SCHWYZER and SIEBER (1963) was a superb achievement in biochemistry but had no therapeutic interest. As we have mentioned, AUBERT and FELBER (1969) and FELBER et al. (1966) clearly demonstrated that β-1,39-corticotrophin, which would, on the other hand, be very expensive, is as antigenic as the extracted hormone but not for the same reasons.

D. Diagnosis of Allergy to ACTH

The diagnosis is not difficult. The one problem is not to forget to ask the patient "have you experienced any incident after your previous injections of Synacthen?" It is often more difficult, as we have just stated, to appreciate the nature of the accident: direct histamine release or type I allergy? Skin tests, if properly used, give very interesting information. If they are positive with 1:100 or 1:1,000 dilutions, they confirm that the patient is sensitive to β-1,24-corticotrophin (Fig. 3) but this can be due either to allergy or to histamine release by the mast cells of the skin.

To know if there is really an antigen–antibody reaction it is necessary to use other methods. A Prausnitz–Küstner reaction was used with success in one of the cases related by PATRIARCA et al. (1974). In our cases, we have never succeeded in obtaining a positive radioallergosorbent test (RAST), but it was obtained in one case observed by Sonneville et al. (1976).

E. Therapy

There is no special treatment. Antihistamines and corticosteroids are very efficent and epinephrine is advisable in the rare cases of acute shock with or without edema of the larynx. After the accident, it is usually possible to treat the patient without the help of corticotrophin. However, in some cases, this treatment may appear necessary and in these cases desensitization has been attempted [with success in two cases of multiple sclerosis observed by Patriarca et al. (1974)].

F. Allergy to Corticosteroids

Allergy to corticosteroids is extremely rare. Clinically, several types of symptoms supposedly of an allergic nature, have been related to the administration of corticosteroids.

I. Neurologic Symptoms

Neurosensitive troubles, which occur during the intravenous injection of sodium succinate hydrocortisone include: sharp loin pains, psychomotor agitation, weakness followed by loss of consciousness, and tremor. This form was notably described by Kounis (1976), who was able to reproduce the symptoms twice in the same patient by intravenous administration of hydrocortisone, even though the drug, when injected intramuscularly, was well tolerated. These symptoms, comparable to those described by Batchelor et al. (1951) could probably be related to intravenous administration of substances having a crystalline structure. They have no bearing on allergy.

II. Contact Dermatitis

Eczematous skin lesions are characterized by their chronic evolution and their frequent spread, despite the topical administration of corticosteroids. They are caused, as was shown by Hjorth and Trolle-Lassen (1963), by parabens contained in corticosteroid ointments. Patch tests done with different types of parabens yielded positive responses. Local application of pure corticosteroids, without preservatives, brought about rapid healing. This type of allergy, falsely related to corticosteroids, was particularly studied by Shorr (1968); 1% of his patients treated for chronic dermatitis suffered from this allergy.

III. Anaphylactoid Reactions

This type of reaction consists of the isolated or associated occurrence of urticaria, angioedema, cardiovascular collapse and severe bronchospasm. These reactions were first reported by HOLLANDER (1953) and by KING (1960). They seemed to occur either rarely upon oral administration or, more frequently, during intra-articular injections of hydrocortisone. The responsibility of the administered corticosteroids is sometimes doubted since some patients are simultaneously receiving several drugs (hyaluronidase, local anesthetics). In the case reported by O'GARRA (1962), the diluent of the corticosteroid appeared to be responsible. The well-documented observation of MENDELSON et al. (1974) concerns an asthmatic patient who presented with urticaria, angioneuroedema, and severe bronchospasm a few minutes after intravenous administration of Solu-Medrol. This drug contains methylprednisolone sodium succinate, associated with preservatives amongst which are found methyl- and propylparaben. This intolerance was confirmed twice, once upon intravenous administration and once upon oral administration of 40 mg Solu-Medrol. Intravenous challenges with the diluent of the drug, as well as those of diverse corticosteroids with different chemical structures, gave negative results. Cutaneous tests done with powder or with tablets of methylprednisolone and hydrocortisone gave an immediate positive response; skin tests performed with the same medications in solution were negative. Passive cutaneous transfer of the positive skin reactions gave negative results in three recipients. These conflicting results are not uncommon, as is well known in studies of drug allergy. More recently, PARTRIDGE and GIBSON (1978) reported two cases of severe asthma induced by intravenous administration of hydrocortisone sodium phosphate in patients sensitive to aspirin. Such reactions were previously related by NAGEL (1977) to paraben allergy.

In summary, it seems that immunologic mechanisms can explain some accidents induced by topical or systemic administration of corticosteroids. These reactions are exceptionally due to the corticosteroids themselves but generally seem to be related to the preservatives.

References

Arbesman CE, Schneider AM, Greene DG, Osgood H (1952) Intraveinous ACTH and oral cortisone in the treatment of bronchial asthma. J Allergy 23:293

Arnoldsson H (1955) Allergische Reaktionen auf ACTH. Acta Allergol 8:369

Aubert L, Felber JP (1969) Studies on ACTH binding antibodies. Characterization of immunological specificities. Acta Endocrinol (Copenh) 62:521

Batchelor RCH, Horne GO, Rogerson HG (1951) An unusual reaction to procaine penicillin in aqueous suspension. Lancet 2:195

Benos S, Koutsoukos A, Kelaidis E (1973) Reactions allergiques observées cours de l'administration intermittente à longue échéance du Tetracosactide-retard. Rev Fr Allergol 13:107

Brodewall EK (1954) Allergic reactions due to corticotrophin. North Am Med 51:303

Brown EM, Hollander JL (1951) Allergy to ACTH and the use of beef ACTH. In: Proceedings, II clinical ACTH conference. Blakiston Division, McGraw-Hill, New York Philadelphia, p 391

Charpin J, Aubert J (1969) Allergie au tetracosapeptide. Marseille Med 106:881

Charpin J, Aubert J (1971) Allergy to ACTH and its prevention. In: New concepts in allergy and clinical immunology. Proceedings of the VII International Congress of Allergology, Florence, 12–17 October 1970. Excerpta Medica, Amsterdam London New York, p 224

Charpin J, Zafiropoulo A, Blanc M (1961) Accidents allergiques dûs à l'ACTH. In: Charpy J (ed) Thérapeutique dermatologique et allergologique, vol 1. Masson, Paris, p 153

Charpin J, Zafiropoulo A, Aubert J, Ohresser P, Boutin C (1964) Données actuelles concernant l'allergie à l'ACTH. Nouv Presse Med 72:3025

Charpin J, Aubert J, Boutin C (1967) The allergenic properties of the newer adrenocortico-
    trophic hormones. Acta Allergol 22:289
Charpin J, Aubert J, Boyer J, Vague P (1973) Synthetic A.C.T.H. preparations in respira-
    tory diseases. In: Schuppli R (ed) ACTH a practical review of progress to date. Huber,
    Berne
Charpin J, Vague P, Aubert J, Vervloet D, Anfosso-Capra F, di Campo C (1974) Anticorps
    anti-beta 1–24 corticotrophine de synthèse. Biomedecine 21:349
Duchaine J, Spapen R, Jacques M (1962) L'allergie à l'A.C.T.H. Etude expérimentale. Rev
    Fr Allergol 2:15
Durigon M, Dumont G, Barres D (1978) Un cas de mort subite après injection de tetraco-
    sactide. Bull Med Leg Toxicol Med 21:333
Felber JP, Ashcroft SHJ, Villaneuva A, Vannotti A (1966) Antibodies to synthetic cortico-
    trophin. Nature 211:654
Gelzer J (1968) Immunochemical study of beta-corticotropin (1–24) tetracosapeptide. Im-
    munochemistry 5:23
Girard J, Lipchitz L, Nars PW (1973) Propriétés allergeniques de l'ACTH. In: Schuppli R
    (ed) ACTH a practical review of progress to date. Huber, Berne
Grilliat JP, Moneret-Vautrin DA, Pupil P, Viniaker H, Delrous JL (1973) Allergie au Sy-
    nacthène. Ann Med Nancy 12:1419
Halpern BN, Jacob M, Binaghi B, Marquet V (1961) Etude clinique et expérimentale de l'al-
    lergie provoquée par la corticostimuline hypophysaire A.C.T.H. Rev Fr Allergol 1:188
Hill BHR, Swinburn PD (1954) Death from corticotrophin. Lancet 1:1218
Hjorth N, Trolle-Lassen C (1963) Skin reactions to ointment bases. Trans St John's Hosp
    Dermatol Soc 49:127
Hollander JL (1953) Proceedings of the eighth international congress of rheumatic diseases.
    Med Hyg
Imura H, Sparks LL, Grodsky GM, Forsham PH (1965) Immunologic studies of
    adrenocorticotropic hormone (ACTH) of biologic and immunologic activities. J Clin
    Endocrinol 25:1361
Imura H, Sparks LL, Tosaka M, Hane S, Grodsky GM, Forsham PH (1967) Immunologic
    studies of adrenocorticotropic hormone (ACTH): effect of carboxypeptidase digestion
    on biologic and immunologic activities. J Clin Endocrinol 27:15
Jaques R, Brugger M (1969) Synthetic polypeptides related to corticotrophin acting as his-
    tamine liberators. Pharmacology 2:361
King RA (1960) A severe anaphylactoid reaction to hydrocortisone. Lancet 2:1093
Kounis NG (1976) Untoward reactions to corticosteroids: intolerance to hydrocortisone.
    Ann Allergy 36:203
Landon J, Wynn V, Wood JB (1965) Adrenal response to infused corticotropin in subjects
    receiving glucocorticoids. J Clin Endocrinol 25:602
Mendelson LM, Meltzer EO, Hamburger RN (1974) Anaphylaxis like reactions to cortico-
    steroid therapy. J Allergy Clin Immunol 54:125
Mohr PD (1975) Allergic reactions to tetracosactrin. Br Med J 4:162
Nagel JF, Fuscaldo JT, Fireman P (1977) Paraben allergy. JAMA 237:1594
O'Garra JA (1962) Anaphylactic reactions to hydrocortisone injections. Br Med J 1:615
Panzani R (1966) Une nouvelle A.C.T.H. purifiée dans le traitement de la maladie asthma-
    tique. Etude clinique. Rev Fr Allergol 6:93
Partridge MR, Gibson GJ (1978) Adverse bronchial reactions to intravenous hydrocor-
    tisone in two aspirine-sensitive asthmatic patients. Br Med J 1:1521
Patriarca G, Venuti A, Schiavino D (1974) Desensitizing treatment in allergy to synthetic
    corticotrophin: study of three cases. Acta Allergol 29:469
Porter J, Jick H (1977) Drug-related deaths among medical in patients. JAMA 237:879
Rajka G (1961) On the prophylaxy in ACTH allergy. Acta Allergol 16:159
Salvin SB, Liauw HL (1967) Hypersensitivity to peptide fragments. Int Arch Allergy Appl
    Immunol 31:366
Schorr WF (1968) Paraben allergy. A cause of intratacle dermatitis. JAMA 204:859
Schwyzer R (1964) Synthetic peptides with ACTH activity. Am Rev Biochem 33:274

Schwyzer R, Sieber P (1963) Total synthesis of adrenocorticotrophic hormone. Nature 199:172

Sonneville A, Garrigue MA, Lamisse F, Baudouin J, Muh JP, Gutman N, Ginies G (1976) Etat de mal asthmatique par hypersensibilité réaginique au synacthene. Diagnostic assuré par le RAST. Rev Med Tours 10:1086

Stevenson CR (1951) Discussion in: Proceedings of the second clin. ACTH conference. Blakiston, Philadelphia, p 395

Traeger C (1950) Proceeding of the first clin. ACTH conference. Blakiston, Philadelphia, pp 356–358

Van Ufford QWJ (1952) Sudden death during prolonged treatment with ACTH. Int Arch Allergy Appl Immunol 3:229

Wilson LA (1951) Protein shock from intravenous ACTH. Lancet 261:478

Wolfromm R, Herman D (1967) L'allergie médicamenteuse à l'ACTH, ses manifestations cliniques, ses moyens de prévention. Sem Hop Paris 43:1252

CHAPTER 25

Hypersensitivity Reactions to Hormones

M. C. Conroy and A. L. de Weck

The hormones, naturally occurring products of endocrine glands, are secreted into the blood and exert their effects on specific target tissue. Since hormones are an integral part of the organism, antibodies to endogenous hormones rarely occur. When present, these antibodies usually contribute to the pathologic processes associated with autoimmune diseases such as Hashimoto's thyroiditis, Graves' disease, and some types of Addison's disease or diabetes mellitus, rather than to those associated with allergic disease (VOLPE 1977).

Exogenous hormones on the other hand, administered for replacement therapy, diagnostic purposes, or to achieve a specific pharmacological effect, occasionally induce immediate-type reactions. Allergic-like reactions following administration of hormone extracts, the prostaglandins, steroids, and oral contraceptive drugs are discussed here, with special emphasis on immunochemical, pharmacological, clinical, and diagnostic aspects. Because of the chronic use of insulin and adrenocorticotropic hormone and the special problems accompanying their use, these two hormones are discussed separately (Chaps. 24 and 26).

A. Protein and Polypeptide Hormones

I. Immunochemical and Pharmacological Aspects

Structural and pharmacological similarities between hormones from various species allow the use of animal extracts for treating certain hormonal imbalances and insufficiencies in man. Improved extraction and protein purification techniques, the development of synthetic peptides, and increased awareness of the potential risk of allergic reactions have decreased the number of adverse reactions to hormonal therapy. The current literature cites relatively few instances in which protein hormones, e.g., calcitonin, parathyroid hormone, and antidiuretic hormone, have elicited allergic reactions. Those peptide hormones administered only once for diagnostic purposes are rarely accociated with allergic reactions (DE LANGE and DOORENBOS 1968, 1975; VON EICKSTEDT 1980). In addition, the failure to develop allergic reactions to certain hormones, such as gonadotropins, may be a form of immune tolerance resulting from exposure to high concentrations of the hormone in early fetal life (DEVLIN 1975).

Most protein and polypeptide hormones exert their pharmacological effects by binding to specific hormone receptors on the plasma membrane (see CATT et al. 1979 for review). In the appropriate tissues in vitro, calcitonin, parathyroid hormone, and antidiuretic hormone stimulate cAMP formation. Calcitonin, a 32

amino acid polypeptide synthesized by the parafollicular cells of the thyroid, inhibits bone resorption and increases urinary calcium and phosphorus output.
Bovine and porcine calcitonin differ from the human hormone in almost 60% of
the amino acid residues. Salmon calcitonin, although having only 50% homologous structure, is the most active of the animal calcitonins and has the longest half-
life in man (QUEENER and BELL 1975; DEFTLOS 1978). This latter form of calcitonin
is used in the treatment of Paget's disease.

Parathyroid hormone, a single chain polypeptide hormone with 84 amino acid
residues, regulates the calcium ion concentration in the extracellular fluid by
promoting mobilization of calcium from bone. The biological activity resides in the
first 34 residues, and hormones from bovine, porcine, and human sources cross-
react with the same antibody.

In humans and most mammals, antidiuretic hormone activity resides in the
nonapeptide, 8-arginine vasopressin, although the analog, 8-lysine vasopressin (lypressin) is also active. The major site of action of this hormone following its release
from the posterior pituitary during conditions of water deprivation is the renal collecting duct. Antidiuretic hormone increases cAMP concentrations and ultimately
increases the permeability of the tubular epithelial cell membrane to water (see
STREWLER and ORLOFF 1977, for review). Various forms of this hormone have been
used in the treatment of diabetes insipidus. Originally, powdered extracts of bovine
posterior pituitary, which also contained contaminating proteins, were administered as "snuff." Oxytocin-free bovine pituitary extracts in aqueous solution (pitressin) or in a water insoluble form suspended in oil (pitressin tannate) are now
administered by injection; synthetic lypressin is given as a nasal spray. Allergic
reactions to all these forms of antidiuretic hormone have been observed.

II. Clinical Aspects

Antibodies developing during treatment with calcitonin are occasionally associated with resistance to this drug (SINGER and BLOCH 1972). Despite the immunogenicity of the hormone, actual reports of allergic reactions to calcitonin therapy
are rare. STURTRIDGE et al. (1977) observed no allergic reactions in 28 patients who
were followed for 9–42 months while taking calcitonin for Paget's disease. Of the
16 patients with various malignancies treated with calcitonin daily for 21–70 days,
PENDE et al. (1976) reported that two developed allergic reactions and had to be
taken off treatment.

Since parathyroid hormone is not used in routine therapy, but in the diagnosis
of hyperparathyroidism, its potential for immunogenicity is limited. Nevertheless,
O'ROURKE et al. (1973) reported that intravenous injection of parathyroid hormone elicited an anaphylactic-type reaction in a patient. The patient had never received this hormone and had no history of atopy, but had received multiple blood
transfusions in the past. Diagnostic tests (Sect. A.III) confirmed the presence of
IgE antibodies, which were presumed responsible for the reaction.

Allergic reactions to pituitary extracts have also been reported. OSVATH et al.
(1970) observed severe anaphylactic shock in a child treated with posterior pitu-

itary for the first time. The child's only previous exposure had been to one unit of Glanduitrin (extract of bovine pituitary) during the diagnosis of diabetes insipidus. The authors noted the novelty of this child's response since it was directed against the active component of the pituitary snuff and not against contaminating proteins. LAWRENCE et al. (1972) described a patient who, after nearly a year of treatment, developed urticaria with pruritis, wheezing, and shortness of breath following an injection of pitressin tannate. This patient, as well as the patients treated by LIPPMANN et al. (1973) and MIMICA et al. (1968), tolerated lypressin spray, which successfully controlled the diabetes.

In the past, insufflation of pituitary snuff occasionally resulted in asthma and other types of respiratory involvement. More serious complications associated with nasal insufflation of pituitary snuff include miliary shadowing in the lungs, bronchospasm, and eosinophilia (PEPYS et al. 1966; MAHON et al. 1967; BUETIKOFER et al. 1970; GERMOUTY et al. 1972). Impaired respiratory function was often accompanied by positive skin tests and precipitating antibody to the pituitary extracts. Although alternative therapy such as lypressin spray could usually be substituted, discontinuation of the pituitary snuff did not guarantee return of normal lung function.

Allergic reactions to thyroid hormones per se have not been reported, although ROMANSKI and WALCZYNSKI (1966) suggested that these hormones may influence the susceptibility of children to urticarial lesions. In a group of 103 children treated with thyroid preparations, 43 developed urticaria, but none had bronchial symptoms. The authors noted that this incidence of urticaria was much higher than might be expected in a nontreated population of children and that the complete absence of bronchial symptoms was remarkable. They postulated that excess thyroid hormones might create a favorable environment for the development of urticaria. Further studies would be required to substantiate this hypothesis.

III. Results of Diagnostic Tests

Routine diagnostic tests can identify not only the sensitizing antigens in various hormone preparations, but potentially allergic patients. Using partially purified fractions of parathyroid hormone and a solid phase immunosorbent test, O'ROURKE et al. (1973) showed the presence of reaginic antibodies in serum from their patient. Negative skin tests to extracts of other beef tissues such as bovine serum albumin, beef muscle, and insulin supported the diagnosis of allergy to the specific parathyroid hormone structure. PURNELL et al. (1968) successfully used skin testing to identify patients at risk for immediate-type reactions. All 56 patients with negative skin tests to parathyroid hormone were treated without ill effects. Treatment was withheld from the two patients with positive skin tests.

Strongly positive skin tests and histamine release from basophils confirmed a sensitivity to pitressin in a patient who had anaphylactic shock following administration of this hormone (LAWRENCE et al. 1972). The presence of reaginic-like antibodies to pituitary protein and to lysine vasopressin has also been confirmed by PK tests (OSVATH et al. 1970).

B. Prostaglandins

I. Immunochemical and Pharmacological Aspects

The naturally occurring prostaglandins, all derived from prostanoic acid, can be divided into four series, A, B, E, and F, depending on the arrangement of groups around the cyclopentane ring. Prostaglandins are not stored intracellularly, but are synthesized by a variety of tissues from essential fatty acid precursors immediately before release. The pharmacological effect of the prostaglandin depends not only on its structure but also on the nature of the target tissue itself. Thus PgE_2 is most frequently a bronchodilator in the lung, $PgF_{2\alpha}$, a bronchoconstrictor. Both of these prostaglandins, however, have been used for therapeutic abortion and the induction of labor because of their constrictive effect on uterine smooth muscle in vivo.

Because of their size and presence in nearly every tissue, it is unlikely that prostaglandins are immunogenic in man. True allergic reactions, involving reaginic antibodies, have not been reported, though bronchoconstriction and urticaria remain toublesome side effects.

The prostaglandins produced following cell activation mediate not only immediate-type reactions, but inflammatory reactions as well. Greaves and Kingston (1975) suggested that prostaglandins may also make tissues more sensitive to the action of other mediators. However, whether prostaglandin infusion actually lowers the threshold of bronchial tissue to the effects of other mediators has not yet been established.

II. Clinical Aspects

The bronchoconstrictive side effect of $PgF_{2\alpha}$ may preclude its use in certain patients, especially those with bronchial asthma. Severe bronchospasm was noted in otherwise healthy individuals who received $PgF_{2\alpha}$ for therapeutic abortion (Fishburne et al. 1972; Bouillon and Van Assche 1980). These reactions were successfully controlled with hydrocortisone and antihistamines. Gillespie et al. (1971) described the use of an "unnatural" prostaglandin, ω-homo PgE_1, for therapeutic abortion. Significant skin flushing occurred at the effective infusion dose of 5 µg/min. One of the three patients in this study developed urticarial skin reactions which responded to an antihistamine injection.

III. Results of Diagnostic Tests

The instances of anaphylactic-like reactions just cited represent direct, albeit unintentional, "challenges" resulting in changes of respiratory function or urticaria. Deliberate provocation with $PgF_{2\alpha}$ produces similar bronchial effects. Nine of 11 volunteers infused with $PgF_{2\alpha}$ developed bronchoconstriction in proportion to the amount of drug administered (Smith 1972). Mathe et al. (1973) reported a controlled study designed to investigate the influence of inhaled aerosols of $PgF_{2\alpha}$, E_2, and histamine on airway coductance in ten asthmatics and in ten controls. There was a marked increase in sensitivity to $PgF_{2\alpha}$ among the asthmatics. Although inhalation of the aerosols produced bronchoconstriction in both groups, the asthmatics responded to concentrations of $PgF_{2\alpha}$ 8,000 times lower than the concentrations which decreased the airway conductance in healthy controls. These reports emphasize not only the bronchoconstrictive effect of prostaglandins on nonatopic individuals, but also the apparent increased sensitivity in certain groups of patients.

C. Adrenocorticosteroids

I. Immunochemical and Pharmacological Aspects

The adrenal cortex produces many steroids, but only a few have significant hormonal activity. Aldosterone, which regulates sodium and potassium balance, and the glucocorticoids, which increase the amounts of circulating glucose, fatty acids, and amino acids, are among the most important. Synthetic analogs of the glucocorticoids are not only more specific, but have greater activity than the natural hormones. Prednisone, prednisolone, and dexamethasone, for example, have greater anti-inflammatory activity but less salt-retaining capacity and a three- to ninefold longer half-life than cortisol and cortisone.

The corticosteroids exert their pharmacological effect by modifying RNA and protein synthesis in target tissue. After binding to the specific cytoplasmic protein receptors, the steroid-receptor complex is transported to the nucleus, where it binds to the nuclear chromatin, thereby altering the transcription of RNA. Since the steroids are not stored, the steroid concentration in the plasma is maintained by regulation of steroid biosynthesis.

Steroids are administered therapeutically in chronic and acute adrenal insufficiency. In addition, glucocorticoids are often administered for their anti-inflammatory effect to treat rheumatoid and osteoarthritis, bronchial asthma, and certain skin diseases or malignancies.

Although the glucocorticoids are too small to be immunogenic themselves, BUNDGAARD (1980) has recently shown that degradation products of corticosteroids, viz. 21-dehydro-corticosteroids or steroid-glyoxals, present as impurities or formed by spontaneous oxidation, can react irreversibly with the arginine residues in proteins. The steroid-glyoxal which forms stable conjugates with human serum albumin under physiological conditions of pH and temperature may thus function as a hapten in the induction of antibody (and allergic) responses.

II. Clinical Aspects

The severity and type of symptoms in corticosteroid sensitivity are related to the dose of drug and the method of administration. Topical application of steroid creams occasionally produces local contact allergy (COSKEY 1978; BRANDAO and CAMARASA 1979), while systemic administration results in more severe generalized reactions.

Urticaria, increased asthmatic symptoms, tremor, and loss of consciousness following an intravenous dose of hydrocortisone have been described (MENDELSON et al. 1974; KUONIS 1976). PARTRIDGE and GIBSON (1978) observed a patient who developed severe airflow obstruction and another in whom urticaria followed hydrocortisone injection for treatment of asthma. HAYHURST et al. (1978) noted that hydrocortisone aggravated bronchospasm in two aspirin-sensitive patients.

ALANI and ALANI (1972) reported that 0.3% of 1,835 patients with contact dermatitis had positive patch tests to topical steroids. Since these drugs are frequently used to treat various allergic reactions, it is difficult to identify allergic reactions to the drugs themselves. In those instances in which a patient's condition becomes worse following steroid administration, a hypersensitivity to the drug should be suspected (KUONIS 1976; HAYHURST et al. 1978; PARTRIDGE and GIBSON 1978).

III. Results of Diagnostic Tests

1. Cutaneous Tests

Patch tests are often useful in the diagnosis of drug allergies. Both BRANDAO and CAMARASA (1969) and COSKEY (1978) were able to distinguish sensitivity to the drug from sensitivity to the vehicle or solvent with this method. The results of intradermal skin tests, however, are occasionally ambiguous. Patients with systemic reactions to hydrocortisone can have negative skin tests to the drug (KUONIS 1976; HAYHURST et al. 1978), or react to some but not other formulations (MENDELSON et al. 1974).

2. Direct Challenge

These tests were either performed deliberately under carefully monitored conditions or unintentionally and then analyzed retrospectively. When the history of sensitivity was uncertain, direct challenge was often warranted. MENDELSON and HAYHURST used this method to establish that their patients were sensitive to the steroids in question (MENDELSON et al. 1974; HAYHURST et al. 1978). In direct challenge tests, the route of administration is important. Patients who react to intravenous challenge are often able to tolerate oral challenge with the same or related drugs (MENDELSON et al. 1974; PARTRIDGE and GIBSON 1978).

D. Sex Steroids and Oral Contraceptive Drugs

I. Immunochemical and Pharmacological Aspects

Because they are close structural derivatives of the natural hormones, synthetic estrogens and progestins are probably poorly immunogenic. Nonetheless, there is no literature on the role of oral contraceptive drugs (OCDs) as either antigens or haptens (PELIKAN 1970) despite their use by over 50 million women worldwide (MURAD and HAYNES 1980).

The mechanism of action of OCDs is similar to that of the other steroids: the molecules bind tightly to specific cytoplasmic receptors, and translocation of this complex into the nucleus produces the specific biochemical events in the target cell. Administration of estrogens and progestins inhibits secretion of follicle-stimulating hormone and leutenizing hormone from the pituitary and thus prevents ovulation, the basis for using estrogens and progestins as contraceptive drugs.

The ability of sex hormones to precipitate an allergic reaction or to influence the immune response is not clear. There are, however, reports suggesting that OCDs, in addition to eliciting allergic reactions, may either adversely affect or improve already existing allergic rhinitis. Some of these reports are included below.

II. Clinical Aspects

Allergic reactions to synthetic estrogens and progesterones include severe angioedema and anaphylactic shock. In one patient, parenteral administration of the long-acting progestin medroxyprogesterone resulted in numbness and tingling of extremities followed rapidly by urticaria and facial edema (BROOKS 1974). Within several months the patient also developed arthralgia suggestive of a "serum sickness-like" reaction. Since the patient had not previously received exogenous progesterone or a structurally related drug, BROOKS noted that a true anaphylactic reaction due to prior sensitization was unlikely. Similarly, there was sufficient data to support the diagnosis of serum sickness in this patient. It is likely that this patient, like the two described by FARAH and SHBAKLU (1971), suffered from an autoimmune disorder.

Hemodynamic and metabolic observations of a woman in whom anaphylactic shock followed injection of estradiol benzoate were reported by HANASHIRO and WEIL (1967). Their patient had received hormonal therapy for the past 7 years without incident. One week prior to the injection which caused collapse, the patient experienced mild allergic symptoms after treatment.

Several groups have noted a relationship between the use of OCDs and changes in allergic symptoms. ABRAMSON and SCHULTZ (1971) also suggested that synthetic steroids or their by-products may aggravate side effects of OCDs, especially in atopic women. They reported that of a group of 15 women taking OCDs, the 7 with side effects (e.g., vision problems, headache, leg pain) were also atopic. FALLIERS (1974), noting the effect of pregnancy on allergy, studied the allergic histories of women taking OCDs. Three women with severe chronic asthma since childhood improved on OCDs, whereas 11 with no prior history of allergy developed either rhinitis (nine) or eczema/urticaria (two). Ten of these 11 had positive skin tests. Only two of the five women who discontinued OCDs experienced a decrease in their allergic symptoms.

Although many side effects are associated with OCDs, the incidence of actual allergic reactions to the hormones themselves appears to be low. CHILLA and HAUBRICH (1975) questioned 460 women in a survey and determined that the symptoms of the 67 women who were allergic were not the result of hormonal therapy. In 1977 FROUCHTMAN et al. published the results of a study to assess the incidence of allergies to medication in allergic patients. Of 500 selected case histories, they reported only one patient with "crisis of vasomotor rhinitis due to birth control pills."

III. Results of Diagnostic Tests

Many physicians confirm allergy to a specific medication by direct provocation tests. WOLF (1967) established Ovulen as a cause of angioedema in a patient to whom he reintroduced the drug during a symptom-free period. TROMOVITCH and HEGGLI (1967) reproduced an urticarial reaction in a patient with an injection of progesterone. FARAH and SHBAKLU (1971) elicited urticarial lesions with progesterone given intramuscularly to their patient, who they suspected was sensitive to the hormone.

PELIKAN (1978) studied the effect of OCDs in nasal provocation tests in women who observed a worsening of nasal symptoms while taking OCDs. Of the group of 15 women, 13 had positive nasal provocation tests, compared with only three positive challenge tests among 34 atopic women without increased rhinitis after OCDs. All other controls had negative provocation tests.

As in other types of drug hypersensitivity, skin testing often yields variable results. FARAH and SHBAKLU (1971) reported positive skin tests on intradermal injections of progesterone and confirmed the sensitivity of both their patients by passive cutaneous transfer tests. FALLIERS (1974) noted that 10 out of 11 women with either allergic rhinitis/asthma or urticaria had strong positive wheal and erythema reactions. In contrast, the patients treated by PELIKAN (1978) did not show a good correlation between the results of nasal provocation and either scratch or patch tests.

Other tests more commonly associated with delayed hypersensitivity have also been used in the diagnosis of OCD hypersentivity. SAVAL et al. (1970) found that the lymphocytes of two patients thought to be sensitive to OCDs had increased ^{3}H-thymidine incorporation in vitro. Lymphocytes from controls, including three men, six women not taking OCDs, and six women taking OCDs (two had "other side effects"), had no stimulation with OCDs. The authors pointed out that this test was useful in distinguishing to which component in the medication the patient might be sensitive, but that it offered no insight into the degree of sensitivity or the type of symptoms.

ABRAMSON and SCHULZ (1971) found precipitating antibodies to OCDs in sera from women with the most severe side effects due to these drugs. These sera were negative when tested in immunodiffusion using nonrelevant steroids. FARAH and SHBAKLU (1971) detected antibodies to progesterone in serum from two patients with autoimmune progesterone urticaria.

E. Conclusion

Allergic or immediate-type reactions to hormones are as varied as the hormone preparations themselves. In many cases the presence of reaginic antibody or positive skin tests confirm the diagnosis of allergy to the hormone. Occasionally, immediate reactions occur very early in treatment or may represent an intolerance to pharmacological doses of the hormone. Thus although immediate-type reactions to hormone administrations are quite rare, the literature cited here emphasizes potential problems which may occur during their routine use.

References

Abramson FD, Schultz JS (1971) Oral contraceptive side-effects and allergy: an immune aetiology? Lancet 2:1374–1375

Alani MD, Alani SD (1972) Allergic contact dermatitis to corticosteroids. Ann Allergy 30:181–185

Bouillon R, Van Assche FA (1980) Miscellaneous hormones. In: Dukes MNG (ed) Side effects of drugs annual 4. Excerpta Medica, Amsterdam London New York, pp 311–315

Brandao FM, Camarasa FM (1979) Contact allergy to hydrocortisone 17-butyrate. Contact Dermatitis 5:354–356

Brooks GG (1974) Anaphylactoid shock with medroxyprogesterone acetate: a case report. J La State Med Soc 126:397–399

Buetikofer E, de Weck AL, Scherrer M (1970) "Pituitary snuff taker's lung". Schweiz Med Wochenschr 100:97–101

Bundgaard H (1980) The possible implication of steroid-glyoxal degradation products in allergic reactions to corticosteroids. Arch Pharm Chem Sci Ed 8:83–90

Catt KJ, Harwood JP, Aguilera G, Dufau ML (1979) Hormonal regulation of peptide receptors and target cell responses. Nature 280:109–116

Chilla R, Haubrich J (1975) Vasomotorische Rhinitis. Eine Nebenwirkung hormonaler Kontrazeption? HNO 23:202–206

Coskey RJ (1978) Contact dermatitis due to multiple corticosteroid creams. Arch Dermatol 114:115–117

Deftlos LJ (1978) Calcitonin in clinical medicine. Adv Intern Med 23:159–193

De Lange WE, Doorenbos H (1968) Hormones and synthetic substitutes. In: Meyler L, Herxheimer A (eds) Side effects of drugs. Excerpta Medica, Amsterdam London New York, pp 383–421

De Lange WE, Doorenbos H (1975) Miscellaneous hormones. In: Dukes MNG (ed) Meyler's side effects of drugs. Excerpta Medica, Amsterdam London New York, pp 928–933

Devlin JG (1975) Hormone resistance and hypersensitivity. In: Gell PGH, Coombs RRA, Lachmann PJ (eds) Clinical aspects of immunology. Blackwell Scientific, Oxford, pp 963–986

Falliers CJ (1974) Oral contraceptives and allergy. Lancet 2:515

Farah FS, Shbaklu Z (1971) Autoimmune progesterone urticaria. J Allergy Clin Immunol 48:257–261

Fishburne JI, Brenner WE, Braaksma JT, Hendricks CH (1972) Bronchospasm complicating intravenous prostaglandin $F_{2\alpha}$ for therapeutic abortion. Obstet Gynecol 39:892–896

Frouchtman R, Olive A, Mones L (1977) Alergia a medicamentos. Aportación a su estudio en 500 enfermos con diversas alergosis. Allergol Immunopathol (Madr) 5:1–14

Germouty J, Demonet B, Tuffery-Boussinesq M (1972) Sur une fibrose pulmonaire secondaire a l'inhalation de poudre de post-hypophyse. Rev Tuberc Pneumol 36:867–880

Gillespie A, Beazley JM, Van Dorp DA (1971) The use of an "unnatural" prostaglandin in the termination of pregnancy. J Obstet Gynaecol 78:301–304

Greaves MW, Kingston WP (1975) Prostaglandins as mediators of sustained inflammation in the skin. Int J Dermatol 14:338–340

Hanashiro PK, Weil MH (1967) Anaphylactic shock in man: report of two cases with detailed hemodynamic and metabolic studies. Arch Intern Med 119:129–140

Hayhurst M, Braude A, Benatar SR (1978) Anaphylactic-like reaction to hydrocortisone. S Afr Med J 18:259–260

Kuonis NG (1976) Untoward reactions to corticosteroids: intolerance to hydrocortisone. Ann Allergy 36:203–206

Lawrence GD, Hsu T-H, Lichtenstein LM (1972) Diabetes insipidus with hypersensitivity to pitressin: an immunological study. Johns Hopkins Med J 131:172–177

Lippmann M, Morgan WKC, Murphy DM (1973) Drug-induced pulmonary disease. Ann Intern Med 78:616

Mahon WE, Scott DJ, Ansell E, Manson GL, Fraser R (1967) Hypersensitivity to pituitary snuff with miliary shadowing in the lungs. Thorax 22:13–20

Mathe AA, Hedquist P, Holmgren A, Svanborg N (1973) Bronchial hyperreactivity to prostaglandin $F_{2\alpha}$ and histamine in patients with asthma. Br Med J 1:193–196

Mendelson LM, Meltzer EO, Hamburger RN (1974) Anaphylaxislike reactions to corticosteroid therapy. J Allergy Clin Immunol 54:125–131

Mimica N, Wegienka LC, Forsham PH (1968) Lypressin nasal spray: usefulness in patients who manifest allergies to other antidiuretic hormone preparations. JAMA 203:286–287

Murad F, Haynes RC Jr (1980) Estrogens and progestins. In: Gilman AG, Goodman LS, Gilman A (eds) The pharmacological basis of therapeutics. Macmillan, New York, pp 1420–1447

O'Rourke JN, Booth BH, Patterson R (1973) An anaphylactic reaction to parathyroid hormone. J Allergy Clin Immunol 52:55–59

Osvath P, Kovacs K, Lerhner J, Godo B (1970) Development of atopic allergy to synthetic lysine vasopressin in a child suffering from Hand-Schüller-Christian disease. Allerg Asthma 16:97–101

Partridge MR, Gibson GJ (1978) Adverse bronchial reactions to intravenous hydrocortisone in two aspirin-sensitive asthmatic patients. Br Med J 10:1521–1522

Pelikan Z (1978) Possible immediate hypersensitivity reaction of the nasal mucosa to oral contraceptives. Ann Allergy 40:211–219

Pende G, Barreca T, Di Benedetto G (1976) Effects of calcitonin on bone metastases from malignant tumors. Erba, Milan, pp 117–126

Pepys J, Jenkins PA, Lachmann PJ, Mahon WE (1966) An iatrogenic autoantibody: immunological responses to "pituitary snuff" in patients with diabetes insipidus. Clin Exp Immunol 1:377–389

Purnell DC, Jones JD, Becker KL (1968) Response to parathyroid hormone infusion in primary hyperparathyroidism. J Clin Endocrinol 28:567–574

Queener SF, Bell NH (1975) Calcitonin: a general survey. Metabolism 24:555–567

Romanski B, Walczinski Z (1966) Allergy in children with struma juvenile treated with thyroid hormones. Bull Pol Med Sci Hist 9:92–94

Savel H, Madison JF, Meeker CI (1970) Cutaneous eruptions and in vitro lymphocyte hypersensitivity associated with oral contraceptives and mestranol. Arch Dermatol 101:187–190

Singer FR, Bloch KJ (1972) Antibodies and clinical resistance to salmon calcitonin (SCT). Clin Res 20:220

Smith AP (1972) Side-effects of prostaglandins. Lancet 2:655

Strewler GJ, Orloff J (1977) Role of cyclic nucleotides in the transport of water and electrolytes. Adv Cyclic Nucleotide Res 8:311–361

Sturtridge WC, Harrison JE, Wilson DR (1977) Long-term treatment of Paget's disease of bone with salmon calcitonin. Can Med Assoc J 117:1031–1034

Tromovitch TA, Heggli WF (1967) Autoimmune progesterone urticaria. Calif Med 106:211–212

Volpe R (1977) The role of autoimmunity in hypoendocrine and hyperendocrine function. Ann Intern Med 87:86–99

Von Eickstedt K-W (1980) Miscellaneous hormones. In: Dukes MNG (ed) Meyler's side effects of drugs. Excerpta Medica, Amsterdam London New York, pp 719–726

Wolf RL (1967) Angioneurotic edema from an oral contraceptive. JAMA 201:162

CHAPTER 26

Allergy to Insulin

J. Aubert and J. Charpin

A. Epidemiology and Frequency of Allergic Reactions

The frequency of allergic reactions after insulin injection appears to have decreased constantly since the drug was first used (Joslin et al. 1922).

The appearance of purified (repeatedly recrystallized) insulins and more recently of monocomponent insulins has brought about a diminution in the rates of local reactions, formerly observed at the site of injection in 40%–56% of cases (Paley and Tunbridge 1952), and generalized reactions such as urticaria or anaphylactic shock (Feinglos and Jegasothy 1979; Jorpes 1949; Kreines 1952; Ljung 1952; Mirouze et al. 1973; Sherman 1954; Wolfromm and Nataf 1965; Liebermann et al. 1971; de Shazo 1978).

B. Clinical Aspects

From a clinical point of view, two main types of reaction can be observed:

1. A local reaction at the injection site, often painful but usually diminishing with continued treatment. This kind of reaction, formerly very frequent, still occurs today. It may be of the immediate type (Goldstein 1971) or the delayed type (Frei et al. 1965).

2. A generalized reaction, manifested by a generalized urticaria or Quincke's edema, or sometimes taking the form of anaphylactic shock with digestive and respiratory symptoms (Aubert et al. 1968; Capbell et al. 1930; Hanaver and Baston 1961; Rose and Barron 1955). Although these manifestations are rare (estimated at 1 or 2 per 1,000 in 1965) they are still observed, even with monocomponent insulins.

C. Immunological, Pharmaceutical, and Pharmacological Aspects

The majority of reactions observed, particularly the local ones, have been attributed to the impurities present in the injected products. However, we now know that insulin itself can be responsible for sensitization (Minars et al. 1974; Diem and Teuscher 1979). Insulin is composed of 51 amino acids divided into two chains: chain A is composed of 21 amino acids and chain B of 30. It appears that the antigenic properties of insulin and the formation of anti-insulin antibodies are linked to chain A (Halpern and Bourdon 1966) but an epitope on Chain B is probably involved in cell-mediated reactions (Faulk et al. 1975; MacCuish et al. 1975).

This intrinsic insulin antigenicity seems to be confirmed by the fact that the use of monocomponent insulin can be followed by a local reaction with eosinophilic

Table 1. The A8–A10 sequences of different insulins

Insulin	A8	A9	A10
Bovine	Alanine	Serine	Valine
Ovine	Alanine	Glycine	Valine
Porcine	Threonine	Serine	Isoleucine
Human	Threonine	Serine	Isoleucine

infiltration which from an immunological view point appears not be an Arthus phenomenon but to depend upon the presence of anti-insulin IgE (Kumar 1977; Patterson et al. 1973).

It equally appears that sensitization is usually specific for insulin from a given species, and that there may be no coexisting sensitivity to insulins from other species, including man. However, this is not always the case, and patients sensitive to porcine and/or bovine insulin may also react to human insulin (Diem and Teuscher 1979).

Variations amongst the species exist on the A-chain sequence (Table 1).

Exceptionally, zinc has been considered as a cause of allergic reactions to insulins (Feinglos and Jegasothy 1979), but the interpretation is difficult since zinc appears also to be an obligate mitogen (Diem et al. 1982).

D. Results of Diagnostic Tests

Clinical observation is generally sufficient in orienting the diagnosis. It can be confirmed by cutaneous tests, the lymphocyte stimulation test (Federlin 1971; Halpern et al. 1971; Diem et al. 1982), or the inhibition of leukocytic migration and also by the determination of insulin-specific IgE using the RAST technique (Kumar 1977; Patterson et al. 1973).

Indeed, the presence of insulin-specific IgE has been reported in the great majority of insulin-treated patients, with and without insulin allergy (Kumar 1977), so that their diagnostic value only appears when their titer and the titer of concomitant "blocking" anti-insulin IgG is known.

Various investigators (Halpern et al. 1967; Federlin et al. 1969; Federlin 1971; Feinglos and Jegasothy 1969; Faulk et al. 1975; MacCuish et al. 1975; Diem and Teuscher 1979; Diem et al. 1982) have shown that insulin of porcine or bovine origin can induce lymphocyte transformation in lymphocytes from diabetic patients with both immediate- or delayed-type hypersensitivity to commercial insulin. Such cell-mediated reactions to insulin in vitro have also been reported in untreated diabetics; they are rather common in insulin-treated diabetics even without any evidence of allergy in vivo (MacCuish et al. 1975).

E. Special Considerations

Insulin allergy cannot be disassociated from resistance to insulin due to other anti-insulin antibodies.

An allergic reaction to insulin can be followed by resistance to insulin, with, as was shown by DOLOVITCH et al. (1970), the presence of IgG, IgA, IgM, and IgE antibodies directed against the insulin itself and not against its impurities (DE SHAZO 1978).

It seems that significant proportion (40%) of patients treated with insulin develop positive cutaneous tests to it, and are carriers of IgE anti-insulin antibodies without, however, developing generalized allergic reactions (LAMKIN et al. 1976). This "tolerance" can be explained by the coexistence of IgG-type blocking antibodies (KUMAR 1977; PATTERSON et al. 1973; MATTSON et al. 1975).

References

Aubert J, Codaccioni JL, Charpin J (1968) Allergie à l'Insuline Soc Franç Allergie, meeting of 16.11.1968

Capbell WR, Gardiner WJ, Scott DA (1930) Reactions after administration of crystalline insulin. J Clin Invest 9:28

De Shazo RD (1978) Insulin therapy and insulin resistance. Two immunologic reactions. Postgrad Med 63:85

Diem P, Teuscher A (1979) Immunologische Untersuchungen mit vollsynthetischem humanem Insulin bei Patienten mit Diabetes mellitus. Schweiz Med Wochenschr 109:1814

Diem P, Spengler H, de Weck AL (1982) Lymphocyte transformation by insulin and insulin zinc suspensions. Clin Exp Immunol 50:155

Dolovitch J, Schnatz JD, Reisman RE, Uags Y, Arbesman C (1970) Insulin allergy and insulin resistance. J Allergy Clin Immunol 46:127

Faulk WP, Girard JP, Welscher HD (1975) Cell-mediated immunity to insulin and its polypeptide chains in insulin-treated diabetics. Int Arch Allergy Appl Immunol 48:364

Federlin K (1971) Immunopathology of insulin. In: Gross F, Labhart A, Mann T, Samuels LT, Zander J (eds) Monographs on endocrinology vol 6. Springer, Berlin Heidelberg New York

Federlin K, Kriegbaum D, Flad HD (1969) Lymphozytentransformation in vitro bei verschiedenen Formen der Insulinallergie. Therapiewoche 45:2042

Feinglos MN, Jegasothy BV (1979) Insulin allergy due to zinc. Lancet 1:122

Frei PC, Cruchaud S, Vannotti A (1965) Allergie à l'insuline de type cellulaire. Rev Fr Etud Clin Biol 10:1083

Goldstein HH (1971) Allergy and diabetes. In: Marble A, White P, Bradley RF, Krall LP (eds) Joslini's diabetes mellitus. Lea and Febiger, Philadelphia

Halpern BN, Bourdon M (1965) L'antigénicité de l'insuline. XVIèmes Journées de Diabétologie de l'Hôtel-Dieu

Halpern B, Ky NT, Amache N (1967) Diagnosis of drug allergy in vitro with the lymphocyte transformation test. J Allergy 40:168

Hanaver L, Baston JM (1961) Anaphylactic shock following insulin injection. Diabetes 10:105

Joslin EP, Gray H, Root HF (1922) Insulin in hospital and home. J Metab Res 1:651

Jorpes JE (1949) Recrystallized insulin for diabetic patients for insulin allergy. Arch Intern Med 83:363

Kreines K (1952) The use of various insulins in insulin allergy. Arch Med Scand 48:260

Kumar D (1977) Anti-insulin IgE in diabetics. J Clin Endocrinol Metab 45:1159

Lamkin N, Lieberman P, Hashimoto K, Marohashi M, Sullivan P (1976) Allergic reaction to insulin. J Allergy Clin Immunol 58:213

Lieberman P, Patterson R, Metz R, Lucena G (1971) Allergic reactions to insulin. JAMA 215:1106

Ljung O (1952) Recrystallized insulin in insulin allergy. Acta Med Scand 48:260

MacCuish AC, Jordan J, Campbell CJ, Duncan LJP, Irvine WJ (1975) Cell-mediated immunity in diabetes mellitus. Lymphocyte transformation by insulin and insulin fragments in insulin-treated and newly-diagnosed diabetics. Diabetes 24:36

Mattson JR, Patterson R, Roberts M (1975) Insulin therapy in patients with systemic aller-
    gy. Arch Intern Med 135:818
Minars S, Shifu Y, Escobar MR (1974) Biphasic local reaction to a new insulin (U.100). J
    Allergy Clin Immunol 56:411
Mirouze J, Orsetti A, Schmouker Y, Cartrye-Almes N (1973) Diabète sucré, son traitement
    par les insulines purifiées monocomposées. Nouvelle Presse Méd 2:1981
Paley RG, Tunbridge RE (1952) Dermal reactions to insulin therapy. Diabetes 1:22
Patterson RC, Mellies CJ, Roberts M (1973) Immunologic reactions against insulin: II. IgE
    anti-insulin, insulin allergy and combined IgE and IgG immunologic insulin resistance.
    J Immunol 110:1135
Rose C, Barron J (1955) Anaphylactic shock as a complication of insulin comatherapy. Br
    Med J 1:583
Sherman WB (1954) A case of coexisting insulin allergy and insulin resistance. J Allergy
    22:49
Wolfromm R, Nataf P (1965) Allergie à l'insuline. VIèmes Journées de Diabétologie de
    l'Hôtel-Dieu

CHAPTER 27

Radiologic Contrast Media

J.-P. Girard and L. Gamba

A. Introduction

The radiographic contrast media currently used in diagnostic medicine are almost all derivatives of triiodobenzoic acid; they have frequently been found to cause unpredictable adverse reactions following intravascular application. As early as 1931, Horsters described a lethal anaphylactic reaction following intravenous injection of such a chemical. A large series of untoward reactions to contrast media was reported by Hultborn (1939), suggesting an allergic mechanism. Such a pathogenic hypothesis was later also proposed by several authors (Dolan 1940; Braunbehrens 1940; Pässler 1952). Up to now, however specific antibodies against contrast media have seldom been found (Bauer and Deutsch 1975; Kleinknecht et al. 1974) and delayed hypersensitivity mechanisms have never been demonstrated.

It has been reported that contrast media bind to serum proteins (Lasser and Lang 1966; Lasser and Lang 1970), activate or inhibit various enzymes (Lasser 1968; Lasser and Lang 1966), induce histamine release (Ansell 1970; Lasser 1968) and perhaps increase vascular permeability (Lasser 1968). Most investigators consider that contrast media act as nonspecific histamine-releasing agents, possibly through the activation of complement factors (Till et al. 1978). Adverse reactions to contrast media are frequent. According to most clinical surveys, mild reactions such as flushing, nausea, or headache occur in approximately 3%–10% of all patients. The incidence of more severe reactions, such as hypotensive shock, asthma, cardiac arrest, or convulsions is 1 in 2–15,000 and the incidence of deaths is 1 in 10–40,000 (Witten 1975; Ansell 1970).

Considering the increasing use of contrast media in diagnostic medicine, there is a need for better information not only for radiologists but also for practioners. In this short review, the various pathogenic mechanisms and the means of prevention will be reviewed.

B. Chemical Structures of Contrast Media

All the products available for intravascular injection are water soluble, whereas the chemicals given by oral route are lipid soluble. Their basic structure is made up of a benzene nucleus with three iodine atoms in positions 2, 4, and 6 (these provide the necessary radiologic contrast). Position 1 is an acidic site which seems to play a role in solubilizing the product. Different chains may occupy positions 3 and 5 and their nature seems to influence the general tolerance of the specific chemicals. There are numerous variations on the basic structure, most of these being salts of sodium or methylglucamine. It appears that the sodium compounds provote fewer untoward effects that the methylglucamine salts (LASSER et al. 1971; ANSELL 1970).

C. Clinical Manifestations

There is a large variety of clinical manifestations related to the side effects of contrast media (ANSELL 1970; EPSTEIN 1977; TILL et al. 1978; WITTEN 1975). The incidence and the clinical type vary considerably with different types of chemicals and also with the route of administration. For instance, EPSTEIN (1977) reported an overall incidence of 5% of adverse reactions on analysis of 32,000 intravenous urographies. However, the incidence increases to 13% for patients known to have previously developed adverse reactions to iodine and 20% in the case of previous side effects of contrast media. The extreme limits of adverse effects in large, unselected groups of patients is reported to be 3%–8.5% (ANSELL 1970; WITTEN 1966; WITTEN 1975).

Clinical symptoms are usually classified in three differents categories:
1. Minor symptoms: nausea and vomitting; simple malaise; urticaria; non-urticarial skin rash; pain at the site of injection; hot flushes.
2. Intermediate symptoms: severe vomiting; angioedema; bronchospasm; urticaria and fever; loss of consciousness, headache, thoracic and abdominal pain.
3. Severe symptoms: convulsions; vascular shock; cardiac arrest; pulmonary edema; arrhythmia.

According to ANSELL (1970), the incidence of severe symptoms is 0.04% (10,000 cases) and 1.7% in the report of EPSTEIN (1977) (32,000 cases). Lethality also varies greatly between different reports. WOLFROMM et al. (1960) reported 15 fatalities on a total of 912,000 intravenous urographies whereas ANSELL observed a higher incidence with 8 fatalitiess for 318,000 intravenous urugraphies. It is noteworthy that the fatalities are observed mainly with elderly patients and in most of those cases, death occurs within a few minutes after the injection has been performed. According to ANSELL (1970) the death rate failed to decrease with the introduction of some newer contrast media, this in spite of the improvement in techniques of emergency care.

D. Pathogenic Mechanisms

I. Hypersensitivity Mechanisms

Most of the adverse reactions to contrast media mimic allergic manifestations. Therefore, this type of mechanism has been considered by several authors. According to LANG et al. (1974) and TILL et al. (1978), contrast media are of low molecular weight and can function as haptens. Considering their binding properties to proteins (LASSER and LANG 1970), they may develop full antigenicity. Iodine, whose antigenicity is well known, was considered as the major antigenic determinant of the molecule (ZWEIMANN et al. 1975). This hypothesis was reinforced by the observation that adverse reactions to contrast media are considerably more frequent

Table 1. Skin tests and lymphocyte transformation test (LTT) in 120 cases of adverse reactions to contrast media

Type of reaction	Patients	Number of positive results[a]	
		Skin tests	LTT
Allergic:	54		
Urticaria			
Anaphylactic shock		21	40
Asthma			
Nonallergic:	66		
Vagal reactions			
Nausea, vomiting			
Headache		13	9

[a] Tests were counted positive when stimulation index > 1.5

among patients who have previously developed allergic reactions to other drugs, especially penicillin (ANSELL 1970).

In fact, IgG and IgE antibodies specific for contrast media have been demonstrated by several authors (TILL et al. 1978; FISCHER and DOUST 1972; BAUER and DEUTSCH 1975; KLEINKNECHT et al. 1974), but these results could not be confirmed by others (LASSER et al. 1971; LASSER 1968). Lasser (1968) reported positive lymphocyte transformation in vitro in the presence of methylglucamine and diodone, a result which was confirmed in our laboratory.

For several years, the lymphocyte transformation test has been done routinely in cases of adverse reactions to contrast media, together with cutaneous scratch tests using soluble media at a dilution of 1:5,000. In this study, 120 patients were examined for the presence of an allergic factor in the pathogenesis of their clinical manifestation. Four different media were tested (Biligrafin, Telepaque, Urografin, Angiografin) and the patients divided into two groups according to the type of clinical reaction ("allergic" or "nonallergic", Table 1).

The results demonstrate a rather high incidence of positive lymphocyte transformation tests among patients from the supposed allergic group whereas it was negligible among the nonallergic group. The incidence of positive skin tests was low in both groups, which demonstrates that skin-sensitizing antibodies might be part of the pathogenesis (WAKKERS-GARRITSEN et al. 1976) only in some infrequent situations. The interpretation of the positive lymphocyte transformation test is difficult. However, when extrapolating the observations on allergic reactions to other drugs (GIRARD et al. 1976), one can expect that at least in some cases, true hypersensitivity may be present. Finally, the inidence of positive tests was very similar with all the four media tested.

Besides the low incidence of positive immunologic tests, one major argument against the allergic hypothesis is that in most cases of adverse reactions to contrast media, the symptoms occur following the first administration of the chemical (SANDSTRÖM 1955; LAWRENCE 1959; SAMTER and BEERS 1968). Furthermore, according to SANDSTRÖM (1955), in an analysis of 1,557 patients who had undergone several L.V.U. intravenous urographies and developed an adverse reaction on one occasion, the recurrence of such a reaction seems to be rather unusual. One can answer these different arguments by pointing out that iodine in various forms is widely represented in food and drugs; this could lead to sensitization to that antigenic determinant. On the other hand, physicians familiar with the problem of hypersensitivity to drugs know that a renewed allergic reaction in a patient who has developed a previous reaction to a specific drug is unpredictable and may occur in no more than 30%–35% of cases (Cuevas and Girard 1978). However, hypersensitivity is by no means the only way to develop an adverse reaction to contrast media, which exhibit a variety of biologic properties, now to be described.

II. Direct Histamine Release

The histamine-releasing property of contrast media was first demonstrated experimentally by Mann (1961). He was able to show that contrast media and histamine-releasing agents induced identical symptoms when injected intravenously and that the intensity of the symptoms was dose dependent with both types of drug. Another good argument was advanced by Lang (1965), who demonstrated that the lung is an important reservoir of histamine. He also observed that bronchospasm induced by contrast media often follows intravenous injection of the chemical, whereas this rarely occurs after intra-arterial administration. However, this hypothesis was criticized by several authors (Peters et al. 1966; Bentley 1968; Lang and Walters 1970), who were unable to demonstrate an elevated blood histamine level, following intravenous administration of contrast media. It is possible, however, that histamine is rapidly destroyed (Rockoff et al. 1970a) and the only possibility would be its determination in situ. Furthermore, besides histamine, other vascular mediators could be responsible for the bronchospasm (Rockoff et al. 1970b).

In animal experiments, Rockoff et al. (1971a) were able to demonstrate that methylglucamine contrast media, when injected in to the pulmonary artery, released a significant amount of histamine as determined in the aorta. Curiously, this experiment could not be duplicated when using the sodium salt, in spite of the fact that these compounds induced histamine release from mast cells in vitro (Rockoff et al. 1970a; Rockoff et al. 1971b). Rockoff et al. (1971a) were also able to demonstrate that the histamine-releasing property was independent of the osmolarity and pH of the injected substance. In most of the reports dealing with histamine release by contrast media, it is concluded that this unique property cannot explain the pathogenesis of the whole variety of adverse reactions (Lasser et al. 1971; Rockoff et al. 1970a; Rockoff et al. 1971a, b) to contrast media.

III. Activation of Complement Factors

In a recent paper, Till et al. (1978) were able to demonstrate that iodinated contrast media such as methylglucamine diatrizoate and sodium ioglycamate activate serum complement in vitro. This was shown by a dose-dependent decrease of total hemolytic complement activity in normal serum, conversion of C4 and C6 activity, conversion of C3 to C3b and generation of C5-derived chemotactic and smooth-muscle contracting activity. Complement activation took place even in sera depleted in immunoglobulins and properdin. These results suggest a mechanism of activation differing from the classical and alternate pathways. These authors also demonstrated the clinical relevance of the in vitro findings. Five patients who had developed an adverse reaction to contrast media were tested for complement activity. All these patients were shown to have a 20%–40% drop in total serum complement (CH 50) levels 20 min following injection and exhibited substantial amounts of complement-derived chemotactic activity in their serum, whereas control sera failed to do so.

This finding raises an important question. Evidently, this mechanism is taking place in only a fraction of individuals receiving contrast media. Therefore, this seems to exclude the hypothesis of a general property of these chemicals. There seem to be additional factors present in those subjects which allow the activation of complement sequences, i.e., a genetically determined enzymatic defect or eventually an immunologically induced helper factor. Whether these complement-activating properties of contrast media, as shown to be present in some individuals (release of anaphylatoxin), are related to the experimentally demonstrated histamine release, is not yet known.

IV. Inhibition of Acetylcholine Esterase

A few years ago, LASSER and LANG (1966) demonstrated that cholinesterase activity was strongly inhibited by contrast media, thus potentiating the parasympathetic activity. In testing contrast chemicals, these authors were able to divide the substances into two groups, one with a strong inhibitory activity (Telepaque, Orabilix, Cholographin, Diodrast, Methylglucamin) and the second with a much weaker inhibitory activity (Hypaque, Angiografin, Angiocontrast). Interestingly, they were able to demonstrate a clear-cut relationship between the inhibitory activity and the corresponding rat LD_{50} values. They concluded that all the pathologic changes resulting from adverse reactions to contrast media, such as peripheral vasodilation, increased flow, hypotension, rhinorrhea and lacrimation, bronchoconstriction, convulsive activity, and urticaria could be explained on the basis of potentiation of cholinergic activity.

However, the problem seems to be more complicated, since it was shown later on that contrast media depress the specific activity of several other enzymes such as β-glucuronidase, glucose-G-phosphate dehydrogenase, and lysozyme. In each instance, the greatest inhibition occurred with the medium that showed the strongest binding to serum albumin and the lowest LD_{50} (LASSER and LANG 1966; LASSER 1968).

The variety of biologic properties of contrast media suggests that the pathogenesis of the known adverse reactions is multifactorial, involving several enzymatic systems. This could partially explain the fibrinolysis, hemorrhagic accidents, and hemolysis which are sometimes observed (LASSER 1968; STUHL et al. 1965; BERNSTEIN and GANS 1966; COHEN et al. 1969). In any case, these reported properties become manifest only in a small proportion of individuals receiving contrast media. This observation suggests a peculiar genetic background among these individuals, explaining their unique susceptibility to these chemicals. In this context, analysis of familial susceptibility to contrast media together with studies on HLA typing or genetic pharmacology are urgently needed.

E. Diagnostic Tests

I. Skin Tests

Skin tests have been performed by a large number of investigators, including us. According to most reports, they are of low value and sometimes may even be dangerous (WITTEN 1975; BRASCH and CALDWELL 1976; DAVIES et al. 1975). When performed at higher concentrations (1:100–1:500), they cause, in almost all recipients, a local inflammatory response which probably reflects their histamine-releasing properties. On the other hand, when performed at a 1:5,000 concentration, they sometimes, although rarely, induce a typical wheal and flare reaction which may be due to the presence of specific IgE antibodies. On some occasions, delayed reactions (tuberculin type) can also be observed, which suggests the occurrence of cell-mediated hypersensitivity reactions.

For several years, we have been interested in the problem of allergic reactions to food additives. Among the coloring agents, erythrosin is the most frequently responsible for allergic reactions (especially chronic urticaria). Erythrosin is a tetraiodofluorescein and because of the iodine content of the molecule, we became interested in testing contrast media in erythrosin allergic patients and in testing erythrosin in patients suspected of hypersensitivity to contrast media. We discovered that in approximately 80% of patients, skin tests were positive to both classes of reagents, suggesting a cross-antigenicity between the two classes of chemicals (GIRARD, unpublished).

II. Lymphocyte Transformation Test

In spite of difficulties in interpreting the results, the lymphocyte transformation test should be performed in every situation where the clinical picture suggests an immunologic mechanism. Although a positive result does not exclude the involvement of other pathogenic mechanisms, it may represent an alarm signal in case of further radiologic investigations with contrast media. We are now adapting the procedure of macrophage migration inhibition factor production for the determination of hypersensitivity to contrast media. This procedure offers several advantages over the lymphocyte transformation test: the excellent reproducibility, the rapidity of execution (24 h), and the low cost of the test.

III. Provocation Tests

In several reports, the use of provocation tests was suggested, especially in the case of positive skin tests. Conjunctival provocation tests or intravenous injection of a small dose of the product have been proposed. There is general agreement that this procedure is not very reliable and sometimes dangerous (KELLY et al. 1978;

FISCHER and DOUST 1972). A careful clinical history is of major importance if one is to appreciate the nature of a previous reaction and to prescribe special care in case of further radiologic examinations with contrast media (EPSTEIN 1977).

F. Prevention

I. Risk Factors

It has been assumed that patients with some preexisting clinical allergic states are at extremely high risk of reaction when given injections of an iodinated contrast medium. This assumption was based on the presumed allergic pathogenesis of reactions to media and on the belief that hypersensibility to iodine, iodine salts, iodine-containing drugs, and seafood could be expected to predict a comparable reaction to contrast media. This view was challenged and could not be confirmed by SANDSTRÖM (1955). However, in a recent prospective study of 10,000 patients, WITTEN (1975) demonstrated that reactions are approximately twice as frequent in patients with known clinical hypersensitivity states than in those without, a result which has been confirmed by others. Considering the incidence of reactions in patients with selected types of allergies, such as asthma, hay fever, food allergies, or iodine hypersensitivity, an even higher incidence of reactions could be demonstrated (WITTEN 1975). In the same report, patients who had experienced an adverse reaction and who received a second administration of contrast media were examined. It appears that only approximately one-third of these patients developed a second reaction, a result which corresponds to that observed in allergic reactions to other drugs. On the other hand, the second reaction was never more severe than was the first.

Therefore, it is apparent that previous reactions to contrast media are not an absolute contraindication to further radiologic examination with media. However, reexamination should be done only when an absolute medical indication exists and after having clearly informed the patient about the potential hazards of the test.

II. Premedication

Attempts to prevent reactions by premedication with various drug mixtures have been advocated. On the basis of available studies, the value of premedication appears limited and seems to be rarely systematically applied.

There is a definite controversy about the use of antihistaminic agents. Although they are capable of minimizing some minor side effects, they are by no means capable of preventing vascular shock. Furthermore, they may represent a potential risk owing to their sensitizing properties (ANSELL 1970). For these reasons, the use of antihistaminic agents is highly recommended by some authors (EPSTEIN 1977; SANDSTRÖM 1955; SCHATZ et al. 1975) and definitely rejected by others (ANSELL 1970; DAVIES et al. 1975; WITTEN 1975).

The preventive effect of corticosteroids, on the other hand, is widely accepted by radiologists. This premedication is recommended in a highly selected group of patients considered to be at high risk, especially in those who have experienced a severe reaction after a previous examination with contrast media. According to

LASSER (1977), the beneficial effect of corticosteroids is explained by their stabilizing properties on cell membranes and lysosomes. A possible inhibitory effect on complement activation was also considered (JENNINGS 1966). According to several reports (LASSER et al. 1977), two procedures can be applied. The first implies the use of large doses of corticosteroids (30 mg/kg or more) and the second more usual doses (1 mg/kg). Paradoxically, high doses seem to potentiate the effect of contrast media on complement activation. Therefore, it is recommended that a few hours before the reexamination the patient is given one or two normal doses of corticosteroids (1 mg/kg); a 3-day premedication with low (or in some cases high) doses may be even better.

Finally, especially with patients at high risk, it is recommended to have available an anesthesiologist and all the facilities of an intensive care unit.

References

Ansell G (1970) Adverse reactions to contrast agents; scope of problem. Invest Radiol 5:78–84

Bauer K, Deutsch E (1975) Antikörper-ähnliche Aktivität von monoklonalem IgM-Paraprotein gegen Röntgenkontrastmittel, die 3-Amino-2,4,6-trijodbenzoesäure-Gruppen enthalten. Verh Dtsch Ges Inn Med 81:1224–1226

Bentley P (1968) Liberation of histamine as a mechanism of the toxic action of radiopaque diagnostic agents. PhD thesis, Ann Arbor University Microfilms

Bernstein EF, Gans H (1966) Anticoagulant activity of angiographic contrast media. Invest Radiol 1:162–168

Brasch RC, Caldwell JL (1976) The allergic theory of radiocontrast agent toxicity; demonstration of antibody activity in several patients suffering major radiocontrast agent reactions. Memorial Award Lecture, Association of University Radiologists, Boston

Braunbehrens H (1940) Allergische Zwischenfälle bei intravenöser Pyelographie. MMW 3:1203

Cohen LS, Kokko JP, Williams WH (1969) Hemolytic and hemoglobinuria following angiography. Radiology 92:329–332

Cuevas M, Girard JP (1978) Diagnostic et prévention des allergies médicamenteuses aux pénicillines. Actua 10:6

Davies P, Roberts MB, Roylance J (1975) Acute reactions to urographic contrast media. Br Med J 2:434–437

Dolan LP (1940) Allergy death due to intravenous use of diodrast; suggestions for possible prevention. JAMA 114:138

Epstein N (1977) Acute reactions to urographie contrast media. Ann Allergy 39

Fischer HW, Doust VL (1972) An evaluation of pre-testing in the problem of serious and fatal reactions to excretory urography. Radiology 13:497

Girard JP, Cattin S, Cuevas M (1976) Immunological mechanisms and diagnostic tests in allergie drug reaction. Ann Clin Res 8:74

Horsters H (1931) Anaphylaktisches Zustandbild nach Injektion von monojodmethansulfosaurem Natrium (Abrodil). Med Klin 27:203

Hultborn KA (1939) Allergische Reaktionen bei Kontrastinjektionen für die Urographie. Acta Radiol 20:263

Jennings JF (1966) The effect of hydrocortisone on immune lysis of cells induced by cytotoxic antibody and complement in vitro. J Immunol 96:409–414

Kelly JF, Patterson R, Liebermann P, Mathison DA, Stevenson DD (1978) Radiographic contrast media studies in high risk patients. J Allergy Clin Immunol 62:181

Kleinknecht D, Deloux J, Hoberg JC (1974) Acute renal failure after intravenous urography: detection of antibodies against contrast media. Clin Nephrol 2:116–119

Lang EK (1965) Clinical evaluation of side-effects of radiopaque contrast media administered via intravenous and intra-arterial routes in the same patients. A preliminary report. Radiology 85:666–668

Lang J, Lasser EC, Talner LB (1974) Inorganic iodide in contrast media. Invest Radiol 9:51

Lang J, Walters AJ (1970) Are contrast media histamine releasers? Invest Radiol 5:277

Lasser EC (1968) Basic mechanisms of contrast media reactions. Theoretical and experimental considerations. Radiology 91:63–65

Lasser EC, Lang J (1966) Inhibition of acetylcholinesterase by some organic contrast media. A preliminary communication. Invest Radiol 1:57–69

Lasser EC, Lang J (1970) Physiological significance of contrastprotein interactions. I. Study in vitro of some enzyme effects. Invest Radiol 5:514–518

Lasser EC, Walters A, Reuter SR, Lang J (1971) Histamine release by contrast media. Radiology 100:683–686

Lasser EC, Lang J, Sovak M, Kolb W, Lyon S, Hamlin AE (1977) Steroids: theoretical and experimental basis for utilization in prevention of contrast media reaction. Radiology 125:1–9

Lawrence HS (1959) Delayed hypersensitivity and the behaviour of the cellular transfer system in animal and man. In: Shaffer JH, Lo Grippo GA, Chase MW (eds) Mechanisms of hypersensitivity. Henry Ford Hospital International Symposium. Churchill, Livingstone Edinburgh London, p 453

Mann MR (1961) The pharmacology of contrast media. Proc R Soc Med 54:473

Pässler HW (1952) Die Angiographie zur Erkennung. Behandlung und Begutachtung periferer Durchblutungsstörungen. Fortsch Roentgenstr 67

Peters GA, Hodgson JR, Donovon RJ (1966) The effect of premedication with chlorpheniramine on reactions to methylglumine iodipamide. J Allergy 38:74

Rockoff SD, Brasch R, Kuhn C, Chraplyvy M (1970a) Contrast media as histamine liberators. I. Mast-cell histamine release in vitro by sodium salts of contrast media. Invest Radiol 5:503–509

Rockoff SD, Brasch R, Kuhn C, Chraplyvy M (1970b) Contrast media as histamine liberators. II. Histamine release into venous plasma during intravenous urography in man. Invest Radiol 5:510–513

Rockoff SD, Brasch R, Kuhn C, Chraplyvy M (1971a) Contrast media as histamine liberators. III. Histamine release and some associated hemodynamic effects during pulmonary angiography in the dog. Invest Radiol 6:110–114

Rockoff SD, Brasch R, Kuhn C, Chraplyvy M (1971b) Contrast media as histamine liberators. IV. In vitro mast cell histamine release by methylglucamine salts. Invest Radiol 6:186–191

Samter M, Beers RS Jr (1968) Intolerance to aspirin – clinical studies and consideration of its pathogenesis. Ann Intern Med 68:975

Sandström C (1955) Secondary reactions from contrast media and the allergy concept. Acta Radiol 44:233–241

Schatz M, Patterson R, O'Rourke J, Nickelsen J, Northup C (1975) The administration of radiographic contrast media to patients with a history of a previous reaction. J Allergy Clin Immunol 55/5:358–366

Stuhl L, Gillot C, Sotty M (1965) Mise en évidence d'un processus fibrinolytique au cours des intolérances aux produits iodés de contraste et des états allergiques. Nouv Presse Méd 73:2297–2300

Till G, Rother V, Gemsa D (1978) Activation of complement by radiographic contrast media generation of chemotactic and anaphylatoxis activities. Int Arch Allergy Appl Immunol 56:543–550

Wakkers-Garritsen BC, Houwerzidi J, Nater JP, Wakkers PJM (1976) IgE-Mediated adverse reactivity to a radiographic contrast medium. Ann Allergy 36:122–126

Witten DM (1966) Micro-autoradiographic study of the distribution of tritiated sodium diatrizoate in the canine kidney. Invest Radiol 1:271

Witten DM (1975) Reactions to urographic contrast media. JAMA 231

Wolfromm R, Dehouve A, Degaud F, Wattez E, Lang R, Crehalet A (1960) Les accidents graves par injection intraveineuse de substances iodées pour urographie. J Radiol Electrol 47:346

Zweiman B, Miskin MM, Hildreth EA (1975) An approach to the performance of contrast studies in contrast material reactive persons. Arch Intern Med 83:159

Subject Index

Handbook of Experimental Pharmacology

Continuation of "Handbuch der experimentellen Pharmakologie"

Editorial Board
G.V.R.Born, A.Farah,
H.Herken, A.D.Welch

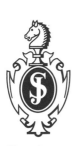

Springer-Verlag
Berlin
Heidelberg
New York

Handbook of Experimental Pharmacology

Continuation of "Handbuch der experimentellen Pharmakologie"

Editorial Board
G.V.R.Born, A.Farah,
H.Herken, A.D.Welch

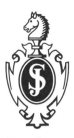

Springer-Verlag
Berlin
Heidelberg
NewYork

ce Library